**Second Edition**

# Anatomy
## Simplified

- Covers extensively theory and practical aspects
- Contents designed as per the latest CBME Guidelines | Competency Based Undergraduate Curriculum for the Indian Medical Graduate

**Second Edition**

# Anatomy

# Simplified

- Covers extensively theory and practical aspects
- Contents designed as per the latest CBME Guidelines | Competency Based Undergraduate Curriculum for the Indian Medical Graduate

**Lalitha A Kulkarni**

MBBS MS (Anatomy) DNB (Anatomy) MS (ENT) DNB (ENT)

Ex-Senior Resident
Department of Anatomy
JIPMER, Puducherry

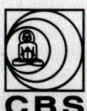

**CBS Publishers & Distributors** Pvt Ltd

New Delhi • Bengaluru • Chennai • Kochi • Kolkata • Mumbai
Hyderabad • Jharkhand • Nagpur • Patna • Pune • Uttarakhand

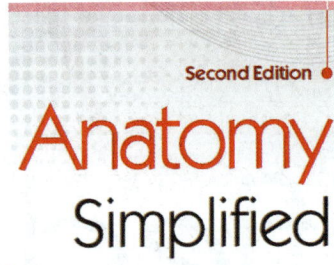

# Anatomy
## Simplified

**Second Edition**

**ISBN:** 978-81-948986-0-3

Copyright © Author and Publisher

**Second Edition: 2021**
First Edition: 2015

Published by Satish Kumar Jain and produced by Varun Jain for

**CBS Publishers & Distributors Pvt Ltd**

4819/XI Prahlad Street, 24 Ansari Road, Daryaganj, New Delhi 110 002, India.
Ph: 011-23289259, 23266861, 23266867
Fax: 011-23243014

Website: www.cbspd.com
e-mail: delhi@cbspd.com; cbspubs@airtelmail.in.

*Corporate Office:* 204 FIE, Industrial Area, Patparganj, Delhi 110 092
Ph: 011-4934 4934    Fax: 011-4934 4935

e-mail: publishing@cbspd.com; publicity@cbspd.com

*Branches*

- **Bengaluru:** Seema House 2975, 17th Cross, K.R. Road, Banasankari 2nd Stage, Bengaluru 560 070, Karnataka
  Ph: +91-80-26771678/79        Fax: +91-80-26771680        e-mail: bangalore@cbspd.com
- **Chennai:** 7, Subbaraya Street, Shenoy Nagar, Chennai 600 030, Tamil Nadu
  Ph: +91-44-26680620, 26681266      Fax: +91-44-42032115        e-mail: chennai@cbspd.com
- **Kochi:** 42/1325, 1326, Power House Road, Opp KSEB, Ernakulum, Kochi 682 018, Kerala, India
  Ph: +91-484-4059061-65,67        Fax: +91-484-4059065        e-mail: kochi@cbspd.com
- **Kolkata:** 6/B, Ground Floor, Rameswar Shaw Road, Kolkata-700014 (West Bengal), India
  Ph: +91-33-2289-1126, 2289-1127, 2289-1128        e-mail: kolkata@cbspd.com
- **Mumbai:** PWD Shed, Gala no 25/26, Ramchandra Bhatt Marg, Next to JJ Hospital Gate no. 2, Opp. Union Bank of India, Noorbaug Mumbai-400009, Maharashtra
  Ph: +91-22-24902340/41/42        Fax: +91-22-24902342        e-mail: mumbai@cbspd.com

*Representatives*

| | | | | | |
|---|---|---|---|---|---|
| • Hyderabad | 0-9885175004 | • Jharkhand | 0-9811541605 | • Nagpur | 0-9421945513 |
| • Patna | 0-9334159340 | • Pune | 0-9623451994 | • Uttarakhand | 0-9716462459 |

*Printed at* HT Media Ltd, Greater Noida, UP, India

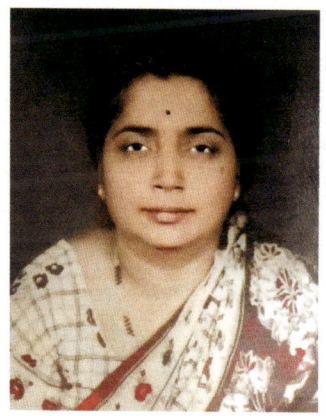

to

*my mother late Mrs Usha A Kulkarni*
*who strongly felt education is the real ornament of daughter.*
*My mother was my first teacher who introduced me to true values of life.*
*Being poised in every situation of life is the real success of life.*
*She always said one's hobbies and books are the true companions in life.*

## MOTHER'S SYMBOL

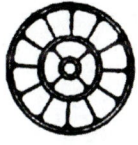

The central circle represents the Divine Consciousness.

The four petals represent the four powers of the Mother.

The twelve petals represent the twelve powers of the Mother manifested for Her work.

Aurobindo Ashram, Puducherry

# Preface to the Second Edition

The first edition of this book was well accepted by the first year students of all disciplines of medicine; however students felt the need of practicals of anatomy to be dealt with in a similar fashion so that the whole subject of anatomy was made easy and reproducible in exams. Therefore, this second edition not only covers the theory portions but also the practical portions of anatomy. That is the whole of anatomy under one roof!

The subject of anatomy is presented in an organised and a student-friendly manner. As you sail through the book, the whole subject becomes easy.

To begin with, key to anatomy unravels the logic behind the anatomy jargon so that students can easily remember anatomy more by understanding than by rote. Any subject if remembered with understanding is difficult to forget; and anatomy is such a subject which you need to apply all throughout your medical career.

The regions of the body are dealt with under separate sections; for example, upper limb, lower limb, abdomen and pelvis, thorax, head and neck, neuroanatomy, embryology, and histology. Each section splits the regional information by and large in the following format—key osteology questions, key short notes, key long questions, key diagrams with MCQ tips, MCQs, dissection of that particular region, osteology in detail again and the section ends with surface anatomy. The chapter on dissection deserves a special mention; after reading this chapter an apparent comparison can be drawn with live surgeries. In the chapter on dissection, incision markings are given in the form of schematic diagrams and then notes are provided regarding the crucial structures encountered in that particular region. A special term vivisection introduced under this chapter will assist the student to understand that dissection on cadavers and operations carried on patients are similar. Many a time postgraduate students pay through their nose for workshops to learn surgeries, and miss this opportunity in dissection hall to practise dissection on cadavers. Master in dissection and you will be master in surgery. Another section which needs a special mention and is dealt with differently is surface anatomy, I have not only provided the points to be marked on the body of a living subject theoretically but also shown the same on the living subject by means of clinical photography. This section gives you an edge over layman in the first year of your medical profession itself. It makes the anatomy subject lively and interesting. There are times in *viva voce* when you are asked to demonstrate muscle actions of extremities. In reply, clinical photographs are provided depicting particular muscle action.

To meet the need of the hour, i.e. to fair well in competitive exams, the region wise MCQs and key diagrams with MCQ tips are also provided. This chapter revision just before any exam (class test, university exam, PG entrance, or DNB exam) will make students confident to face the exams.

Another challenge in anatomy is embryology, this book covers the same mostly in a Socratic method. Practicals of embryology are given in the form of pictures for embryology models. One part of embryology model is unlabelled and the other is labelled. Students will get a feel of exam when they see the unlabelled model and they can practise answering the model.

Anatomy is a vast subject to remember and reproduce in exams. Apart from making the language of anatomy easy I have provided mnemonics here and there to remember topics in sequence.

Special emphasis on illustrations which form the cornerstone of anatomy memory is given for each topic. Anatomy can be best remembered by drawing diagrams.

The book ends with literal meanings of Greek and Latin words used in anatomy.

Overall personally I want every student to breeze through medical career and enjoy anatomy subject. This is my modest intention behind writing the book *Anatomy Simplified*.

Please remember dear students "What man has done man can do."

**Lalitha A Kulkarni**
e-mail: lalita.joshi@hotmail.com

# Preface to the First Edition

Anatomy Simplified is a book meant for students of 1st year MBBS, dental, ayurvedic, homeopathic and students preparing for entrance examinations. Since the book also deals with surgical anatomy, it will be useful for students doing postgraduation in surgical discipline.

The book covers examination-oriented topics in Socratic method, in the form of 'questions and answers'. The book prepares the students even for 'viva voce' and makes students feel confident to appear for the examinations.

Certain topics like, neurobiotaxis, humeral torsion, surgical anatomy, and hearsay topics dealt in dissection hall are also covered up in the book. Key diagrams, which form the basis of the book, will make it simple to remember 'anatomy'.

Most of the sections are arranged into five chapters namely Key Questions, Short Notes, Long Questions, Key Diagrams with MCQ Tips and MCQs, which will enable the students to prepare for all types of examinations including *viva voce* and to acquire knowledge in a simple and systematic way. Separate Glossary for Neuroanatomy section is given considering its importance. Sections VII and VIII deal with Embryology and Histology. Section IX deals with the meanings of few Greek and Latin words used in anatomy.

Always a subject studied in own language is easy, similarly an attempt is made to make 'anatomy language' easy. It is difficult to make the subject easy, but if the student adopts right method of learning, it becomes *Anatomy Simplified*.

Lalitha A Kulkarni

# Preface to the First Edition

# Acknowledgements

At the outset, I express my deep gratitude to my father, Shri Arvind Gajanan Kulkarni, who has been a constant source of inspiration all throughout my educational journey. He told me stories of my grandfather who was a schoolteacher in a small village of Satara (Maharashtra) and who walked miles to take home tuitions. My father feels women education is the only ladder to uplift the status of women in society. He always tells me, be positive in every situation of life. Positive attitude is in his blood (his blood group is also B+); he also has a subtle sense of humour and these are his secrets of successful life. It is only because of my father what I am today!

The next person who was directly involved in my book project is my husband, Shri Hemant Joshi, a Chartered Accountant, LLB by profession; who spared time even at odd hours to help me. He always encouraged me to devote time on priority to my book. Without his support this project would not have seen light of the day.

I thank my all teachers throughout my medical career who not only critically acclaimed my educational achievements but also blessed me in my every venture.

I shall remain indebted to all the staff of CBS Publishers and Distributors for their painstaking efforts to make my dream into reality.

Last but not the least I am indebted to all my students who have been the real reason behind the genesis of this book. It is only because of the love of students and my desire to fulfil their requirements of the subject I could pen down this book *Anatomy Simplified*.

**Lalitha A Kulkarni**

# Contents

Preface to the Second Edition                                    vii

Preface to the First Edition                                      ix

## Section I: Key to Anatomy                                       1

## Section II: General Anatomy                                     5
Introduction                                                      7

## Section III: Upper Limb                                        37
  1. Key Osteology Questions                           39
  2. Key Short Notes                                    44
  3. Key Long Questions                                 77
  4. Key Diagrams with MCQ Tips                         87
  5. MCQs                                               92
  6. Dissection                                         98
  7. Osteology                                         121
  8. Surface Anatomy                                   134

## Section IV: Lower Limb                                        141
  9. Key Osteology Questions                          143
 10. Key Short Notes                                        150
 11. Key Long Questions                                     180
 12. Key Diagrams with MCQ Tips                             195
 13. MCQs                                                   203
 14. Dissection                                             212
 15. Osteology                                              233
 16. Surface Anatomy                                        248

## Section V: Abdomen and Pelvis                                 255
 17. Key Osteology Questions                                257
 18. Key Short Notes                                        260
 19. Key Long Questions                                     300
 20. Key Diagrams with MCQ Tips                             339
 21. MCQs                                                   347
 22. Dissection                                             352
 23. Osteology                                              382
 24. Surface Anatomy                                        384

## Section VI: Thorax                                            391
 25. Key Osteology Questions                                393

26. Key Short Notes                                                398
27. Key Long Questions                                             415
28. Key Diagrams with MCQ Tips                                     430
29. MCQs                                                            435
30. Dissection                                                      439
31. Osteology                                                       448
32. Surface Anatomy                                                 452

## Section VII: Head and Neck                                      457
33. Key Osteology Questions                                        459
34. Key Short Notes                                                 481
35. Key Long Questions                                             534
36. Key Diagrams with MCQ Tips                                     581
37. MCQs                                                            593
38. Dissection                                                      608
39. Osteology                                                       638
40. Surface Anatomy                                                 653

## Section VIII: Neuroanatomy                                      659
41. Key Questions                                                  661
42. Key Short Notes                                                 667
43. Key Long Questions                                             695
44. MCQs                                                            707
45. Glossary                                                        711
46. Neuroanatomy Specimens                                         713

## Section IX: Embryology                                          719
47. General Embryology Key Questions                               721
48. Systemic Embryology                                            749
49. MCQs                                                            792
50. Embryology Models                                              802

## Section X: Histology                                            853
51. Histology Slides                                               855

## Section XI: Great Vessels of the Body                           875
52. Pulmonary Trunk, Aorta and Vena Cavae                          877

## Section XII: Radiological Anatomy                               887
53. Basics of Radiological Anatomy                                 889

*Literal Meanings of Anatomical Words*                             893

*Index*                                                            901

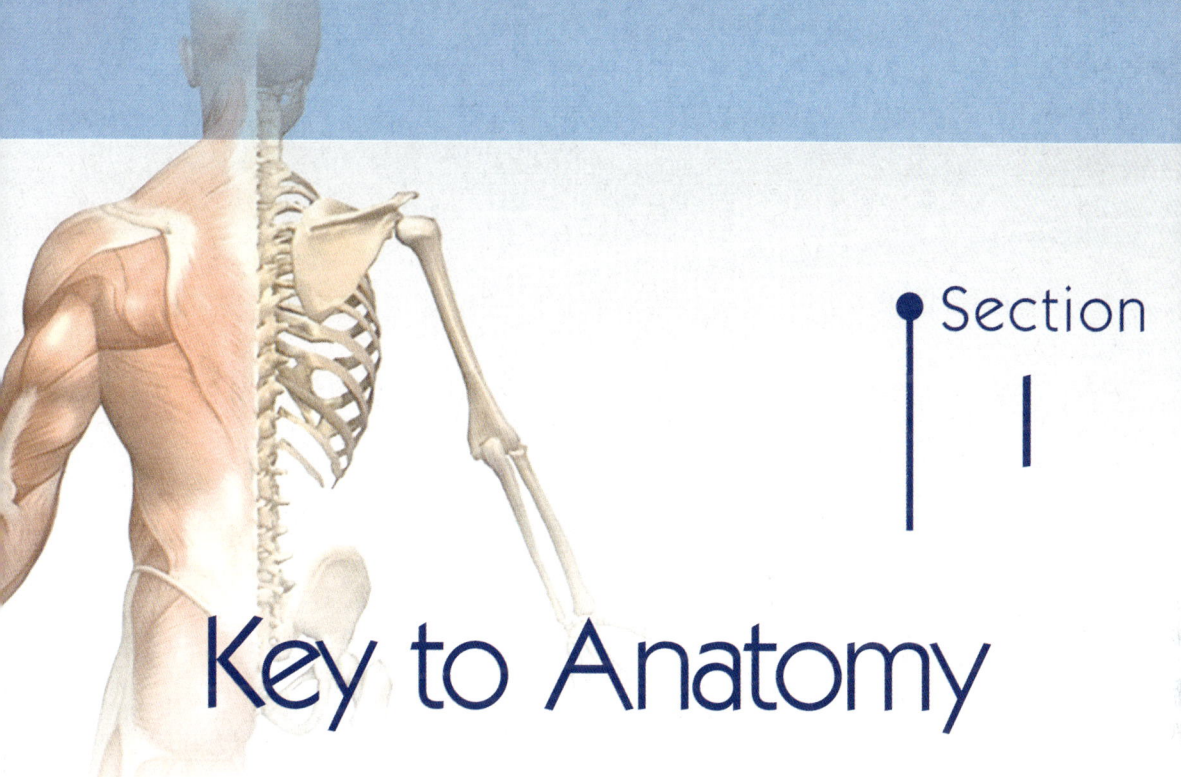

Section

I

# Key to Anatomy

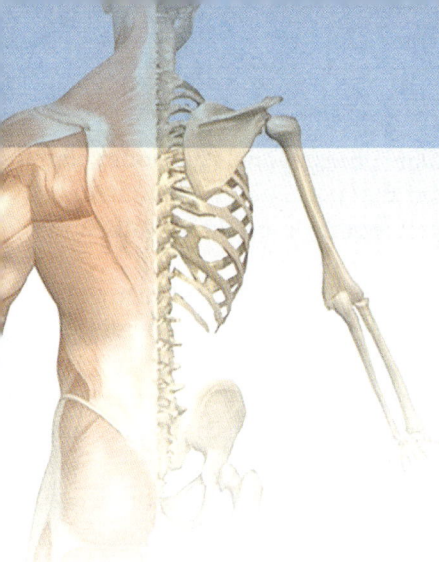

# Key to Anatomy

## ARCHITECTURE OF BODY

A building has iron beams, bricks, cement, etc. and this is gross anatomy of building. Similarly, a human body is made-up of bones, muscles, arteries, veins, nerves and lymphatics.

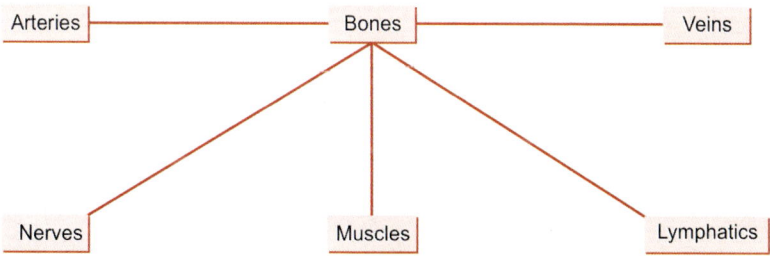

There is an architectural plan to any house; similarly body design is planned:
1. Skin is followed by subcutaneous tissue (superficial fascia), deep fascia, muscles, bone.
2. Artery is always in a deeper plane to be well-protected, since it provides nutrition to the various parts of body.
3. An artery is always accompanied by vein.
4. Veins are accompanied by lymphatics.
5. If you are discussing artery automatically, other relations are the remaining structures of body, i.e. vein, nerve, lymph; if lymph is discussed, other structures form the relations.
6. Names of the arteries are given by and large by the organs it supplies. For example, artery going to uterus-uterine artery, artery going to thyroid-thyroid artery, etc.
7. Ligament connecting radius to ulna is named as radioulnar ligament; ligament connecting tibia to fibula is named as tibiofibular ligament.
8. Name given to any neurovascular bundle is according to the region it is present, e.g. femoral region-femoral artery, femoral vein, femoral nerve; axillary region-axillary artery, axillary vein, axillary nerve.

9. Regions are described in the form of triangles, quadrangular spaces, tunnels depending on its appearance to make it easy for studying the anatomy of that particular region.

10. Any region is described under the following subtitles (like a room)—roof, floor, walls, and contents.

11. Triangle has three sides, mostly formed by muscles, roof is formed by skin and subcutaneous nerves and vessels, floor is bone with its attachments, and contents will always be arteries, veins, nerves, and lymph nodes.

12. Bones always give attachments to two structures—muscles and ligaments.

13. Any muscle is described under the following headings—attachments, nerve supply, and action. Sometimes relations form an important description of the muscle.

14. An artery or a nerve have the following subtitles—origin, course, relations, and branches like a river.

15. Any organ in the body should be dealt in the following manner—location, gross features, relations, blood supply, lymphatic drainage, and applied anatomy.

16. Above all, the best way to learn anatomy is by teaching anatomy and drawing diagrams repeatedly.

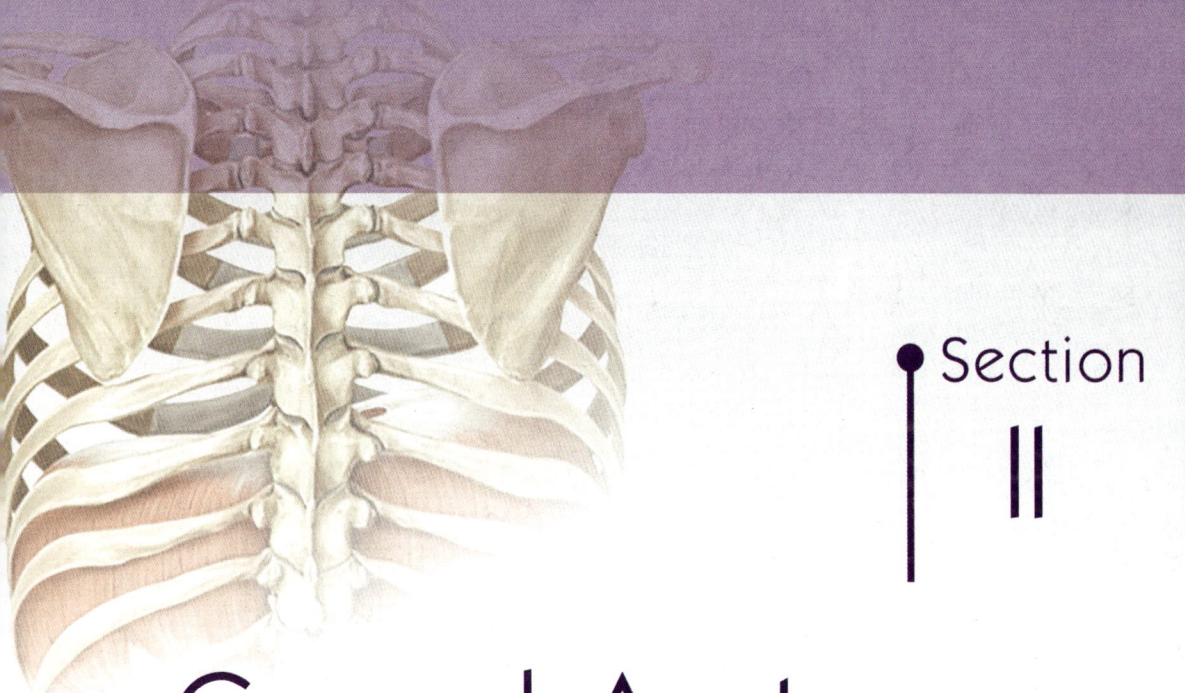

# General Anatomy

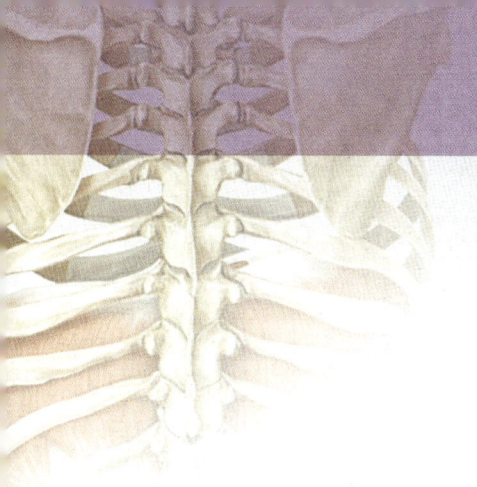

# Introduction

## KEY GENERAL ANATOMY TOPICS

### Anatomy Definition

Anatomy is a Greek word. The literal meaning of the word is:
- ANA—through
- TOMY—cutting.

It means by cutting through the cadaver, i.e. by doing dissections one can acquire the knowledge of anatomy.

### Anatomy Classification

Anatomy can be studied under following subdivisions:
1. Gross anatomy—as seen by naked eyes (grossly, as in dissection hall).
2. Microscopic anatomy (histology)—as seen under microscope.
3. Developmental anatomy (embryology)—study of growing embryo.
4. Surface anatomy—marking deep structures on skin.

### 1. ANATOMICAL POSITION

- Student should remember that even if dissections are done with the body lying on the table, the anatomical terms are in reference to anatomical position.
- Anatomical position is described as follows:
  - Body upright
  - Upper limbs hanging on sides
  - Forearm supinated
  - Palms facing forwards
  - Eyes staring straight forwards
  - Feet close to each other.

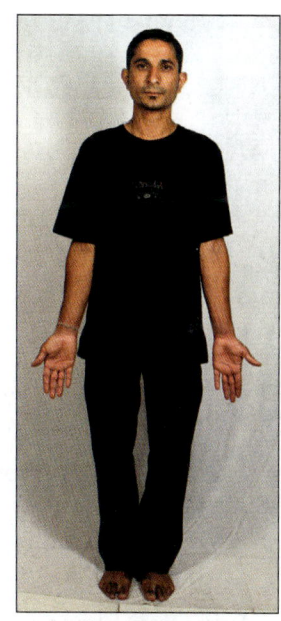

Anatomical position

Student should be able to demonstrate the position when asked in *viva voce*

7

## 2. ANATOMICAL TERMS

- **Superior/cephalic**—towards the head
- **Inferior/caudal**—towards the feet
- **Anterior/ventral**—towards the front
- **Posterior/dorsal**—towards the back
- **Median**—midline
- **Medial**—towards the midline
- **Lateral**—away from midline
- **Proximal**—towards the root of structure
- **Distal**—away from root of structure
- **Sagittal plane**—vertical plane parallel to median plane
- **Coronal plane**—vertical plane perpendicular to median plane

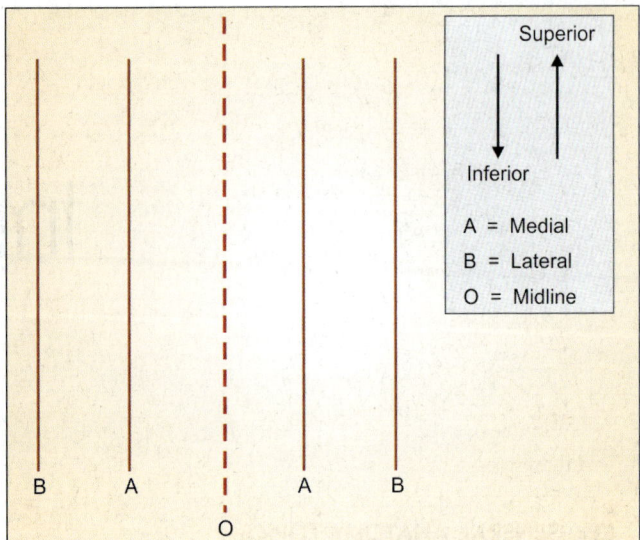

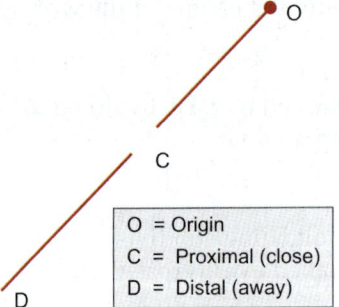

## 3. TERMS RELATED TO MOVEMENTS

- **Flexion**—bending forwards
- **Extension**—bending backwards
- **Abduction**—movement away from mid-plane
- **Adduction**—movement towards the mid-plane
- **Pronation**—hand moves backwards so that palm faces posteriorly
- **Supination**—hand moves in front, to lie in anatomical position.

## BODY STRUCTURE

- The bones, i.e. skeleton forms the backbone of the whole body, on which the body is supported. Apart from the bones, other body structures include—muscles (motor of body, bringing about action), nerves (which carry the sensations), arteries (provide nutrition to body parts), veins and lymphatics ( constitutes the drainage system of body).

- Irrespective of the region we deal, body structures remain the same and the names given to the various structures are according to the region, e.g. axillary region, an artery, vein, lymph nodes, or a nerve in that region is named accordingly, i.e. axillary artery, axillary vein, axillary lymph nodes, axillary nerve.
- Muscle is by and large named by its attachments, e.g. coracobrachialis the name itself will tell you the attachment, i.e. it is attached between coracoid process to the brachium bone, i.e. humerus. The same holds true for the ligaments, e.g. Tibiofibular the name itself implies its attachments, i.e. the ligament lies between tibia and fibula.
- Certain Greek and Latin words are used to describe plane of location of structures, i.e. profunda means deep so a muscle or artery in a deeper plane in the brachium is named as profunda brachii.

## 4. BONES

### a. Functions

- Gives shape to the body
- Provides surface for attachment of muscles and their action
- Protect vital organs like brain, spinal cord
- Certain bones have the marrow cells which produce red blood cells
- Bones are the major storage site of calcium and phosphorous.

### b. Classification

*Based on the Shape of Bone*

- Long bones, e.g. humerus, femur
- Short bones, e.g. tarsal, carpal bones
- Flat bones, e.g. skull vault, ribs, sternum
- Irregular bones—hip bone
- Long short bones, e.g. metacarpals, metatarsals.

*Peculiar Bone Types*

- Pneumatic bones—these bones contain air spaces within, e.g. maxilla, sphenoid
- Sesamoid bones (like sesame seeds)—these bones develop within the tendon of muscles, e.g. Patella in quadriceps muscle.

*Based upon the Location*

- Axial skeleton—comprises of skull, vertebral column, thoracic cage
- Appendicular skeleton—comprises the limb bones.

*Based upon the Ossification Type*

- Membranous bones—develop within the membranous framework, e.g. facial bones, vault
- Cartilaginous bones—cartilaginous framework transforms into bone, e.g. all limb bones, vertebrae, ribs
- Membranocartilaginous—bone partly develops from cartilage and partly from membrane, e.g. clavicle, mandible.

*Based upon the Macroscopic Structure* (when vertical section of long bone is taken)

- Compact bone—it appears dense but porous largely appreciated in the outer cortex of long bone
- Spongy (= Cancellous) bone comprises of meshwork of trabeculae containing marrow spaces.

### c. Parts of Developing Bone (diagram below)

### d. Parts of Adult bone (diagram below)

### e. Blood Supply of Long Bone

Bone has rich blood supply with arteries named according to the portion of bone it supplies. Metaphyseal arteries have hair pin bends and nutrient artery pecuralities are:

- Enters the shaft at an angle
- Nutrient artery foramen is directed away from the growing end of long bone (to the elbow i go, while flee away from the knee), e.g. growing end of humerus is upper end.

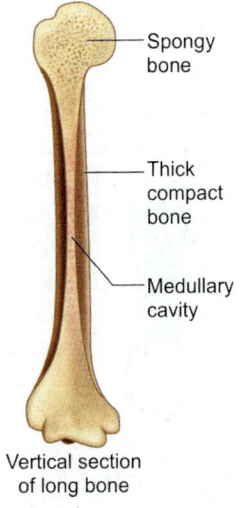

Vertical section of long bone

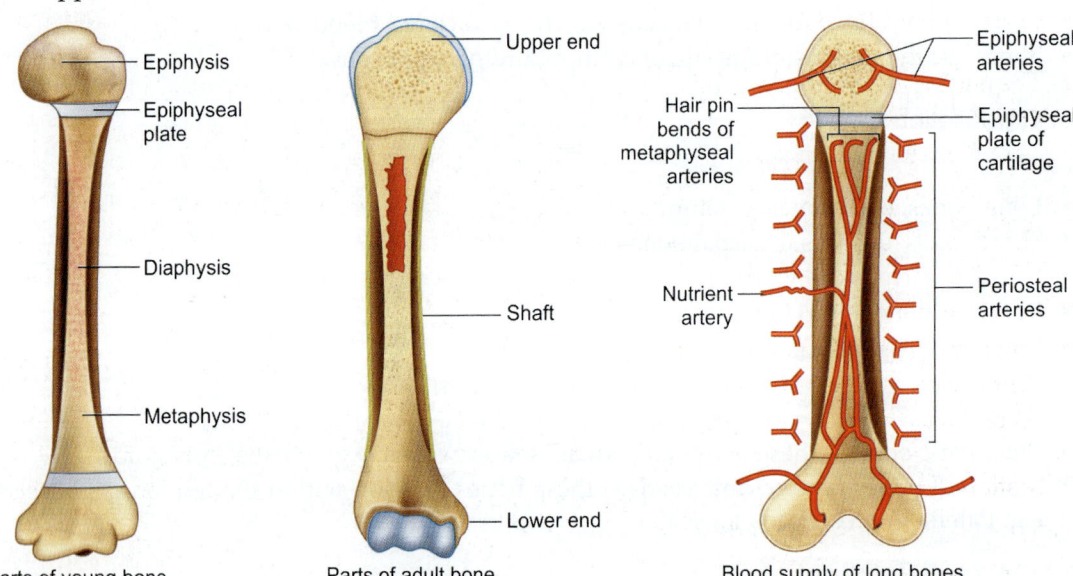

Parts of young bone   Parts of adult bone   Blood supply of long bones

### f. Ossification

- Bones, to begin with, appear in the form of mesodermal condensations, which further metamorphose into bone. This conversion of mesoderm model to directly into bone, without passing into an intermediate stage of cartilage are known as membrane bones.
- Most of the bones first undergo a cartilaginous transformation from the mesodermal model, (around 2nd month of intrauterine life). This further develops into a bone. This is known as intracartilaginous or endochondral ossification.
- Ossification begins around a certain point where blood vessels are present and where the osteoblasts lay bony lamellae. This site is known as the centre for ossification. When present

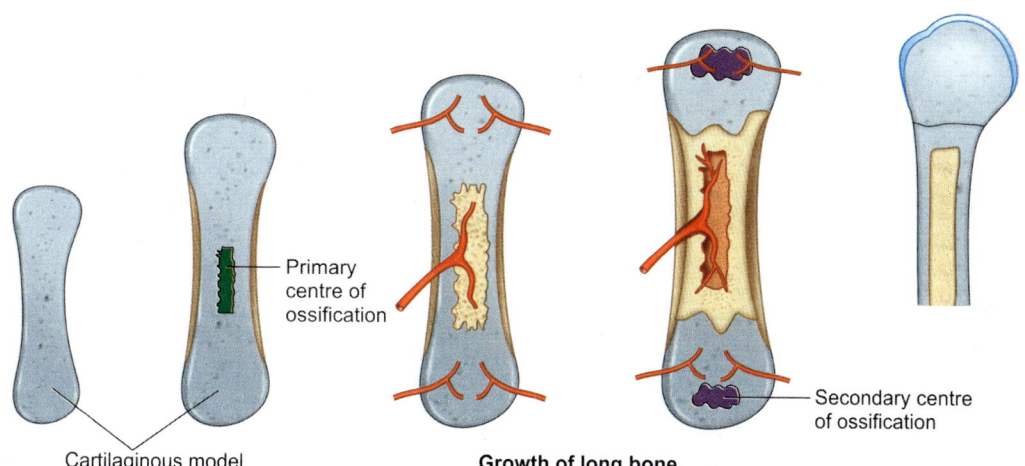

Primary centre of ossification

Secondary centre of ossification

Cartilaginous model

**Growth of long bone**

before birth it is known as primary centre, while when it appears after birth it is known as secondary centre. By and large primary centre of ossification appears around 8th week of intrauterine life, while secondary centre appears around puberty

- Primary centre forms the shaft of the long bone while the secondary centre forms the ends of the long bone.
- The ends of the bone fuse with the shaft by the age of 25 years after which the bone does not grow.
- The secondary centres which appear earlier are last to fuse is the basic law of ossification.
- The end of the bone where the epiphysis does not fuse with the shaft, i.e. the epiphysis remains unfused with the diaphysis is the growing end of the bone.

## LAWS OF OSSIFICATION

- The law states that the centre of ossification which appears first is last to unite.
- Primary centre is the centre that appears before birth.
- Secondary centre appears after birth.

### Exception for the Rule

Fibula bone violates the law of ossification as follows: Centre of ossification for distal end appears first and also unites early.

### Composition of Bone Marrow

It is a soft pulpy tissue found in the marrow cavities of long bone and spaces in the trabeculae of all bones. It is of 2 types—red and yellow.

### Features

In fetal life and at birth the whole skeletal system is made-up of red bone marrow; by 25 years of age it is replaced by yellow bone marrow except in certain bones ribs, sternum, vertebra, cranium, scapula, pelvis, cranial bones and proximal ends of long bones.

Fibula violates the laws of ossification

*Differences*

| Red bone marrow | Yellow bone marrow |
|---|---|
| • Loosely woven connective tissue | It is thick connective tissue |
| • Haemopoietic cells and sinusoids | Contains supporting blood vessels |
| • No fat cells | Lot of fat cells in adults |
| • Found in all bones in fetal life | |

## Peculiarity

No lymph vessels are seen in bone marrow (also in cartilage and nervous system).

## 5. CARTILAGE

a. It is connective tissue made-up of cells known as chondrocytes and gel-like matrix made-up of mucopolysaccharide. Matrix has fibres within, the fibres could be collagenous or elastic fibres. Cartilage is firm (not hard like bone).

b. *Pecularities:* Cartilage has no blood vessels and no lymphatics and no nerves, thus a cartilage cannot regenerate, is insensitive and gets its nutrition by diffusion through the matrix.

c. *Types:*
   • Hyaline cartilage, e.g. articular surfaces of joints, trachea
   • Fibrocartilage, e.g. pubic symphysis, temporomandibular joints
   • Elastic cartilage, e.g. pinna, external auditory meatus.

## 6. EPIPHYSIS

a. Ends of long bone which develop from secondary centres are known as epiphyses

b. *Types:*
   • **Pressure epiphysis** is articular and takes part in weight transmission, e.g. head and neck of femur
   • **Traction epiphysis** is non-articular, not involved in weight transmission, develop at the site of muscle attachment due to the pull of muscle, e.g. trochanters of femur, tubercles of humerus
   • **Atavistic epiphysis** is a separate bone which fuses with other bone, e.g. coracoid process of scapula, lateral tubercle of talus
   • **Aberrant epiphysis** occasionally present, e.g. head of first metacarpal.

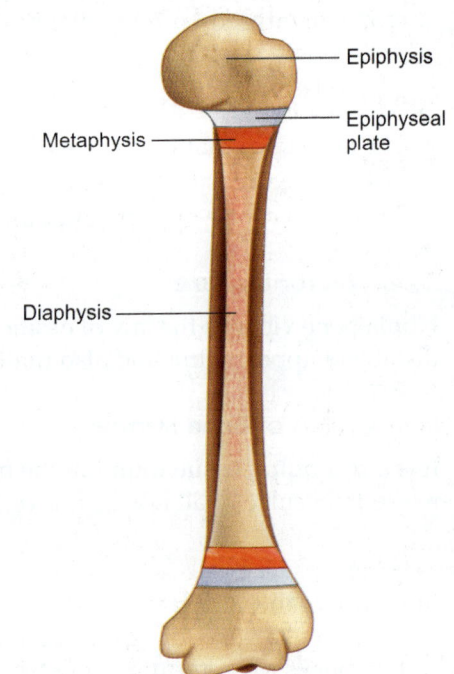

Parts of young bone

## 7. JOINTS

a. *Definition:* Joint is a junction of 2 or more bones
b. *Classification:* Based upon the structure

### Synovial Joints

*Structure:* Articular surfaces are held together by capsule and are lined from within by synovial membrane which secretes synovial fluid. Articular surfaces are covered by hyaline cartilage (synovial membrane does not cover the cartilage surface).

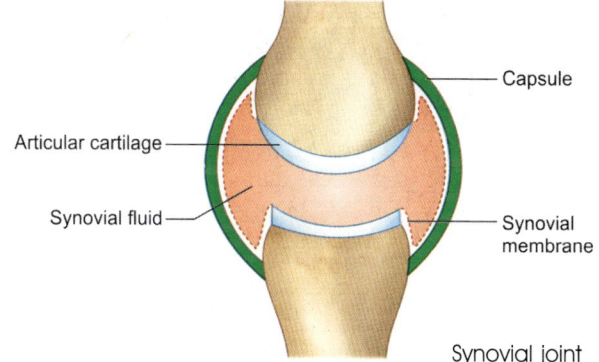

Synovial joint

- **Synovial joint subtypes:** Ball and socket type, e.g. Shoulder joint, hip joint.

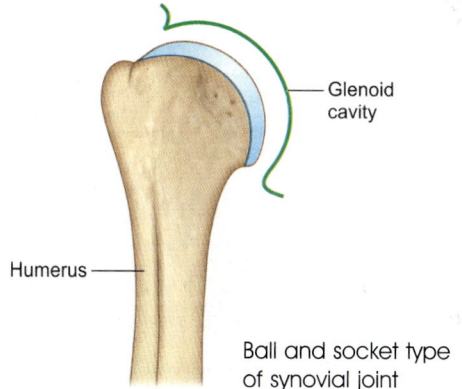

Ball and socket type of synovial joint

- **Saddle-shaped joint**, e.g. first carpometacarpal joint, sternoclavicular joint.

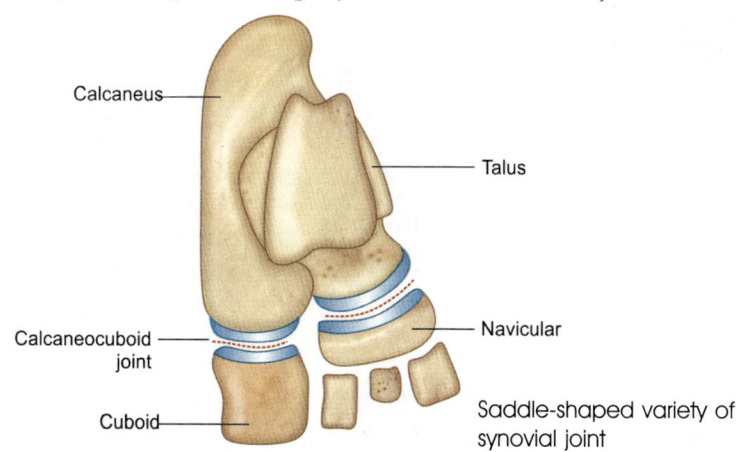

Saddle-shaped variety of synovial joint

- **Condylar variety**—have reciprocally curved articular surfaces, e.g. knee joint, temporomandibular joint.

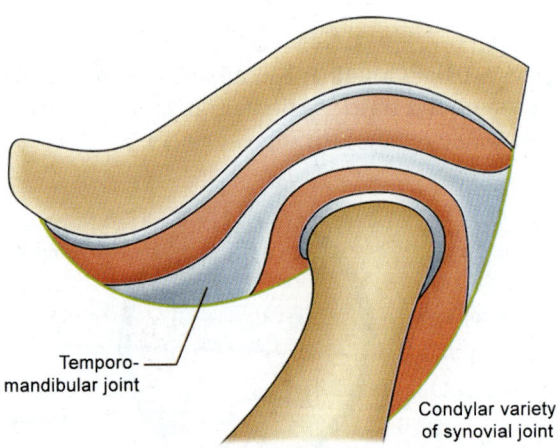

Condylar variety of synovial joint

- **Ellipsoid joint variety**—articular surfaces are oval, convex fitting into elliptical concave surface hence the name, e.g. wrist joint, atlanto-occipital joint.

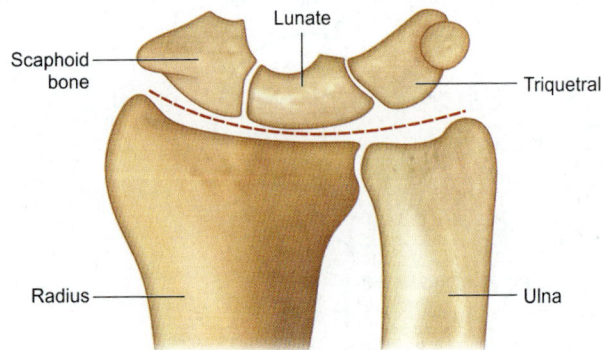

Ellipsoid variety of synovial joint

- **Hinge joint**—articular surfaces are pulley-shaped and these joints permit movements in one direction only (like a door) along transverse axis, e.g. elbow joint, ankle joint, interphalangeal joints.

Hinge variety of synovial joint

- **Pivot joint**—articular surfaces are around central bony pivot surrounded by annular ligaments, e.g. superior and inferior radioulnar ligament, atlantoaxial ligament.

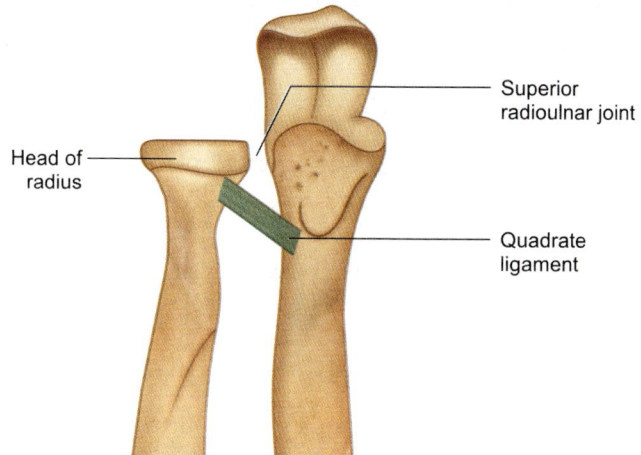

Pivot variety of synovial joint

- **Plane synovial joints**—articular surfaces are flat reciprocally, e.g. intertarsal, intercarpal joints.

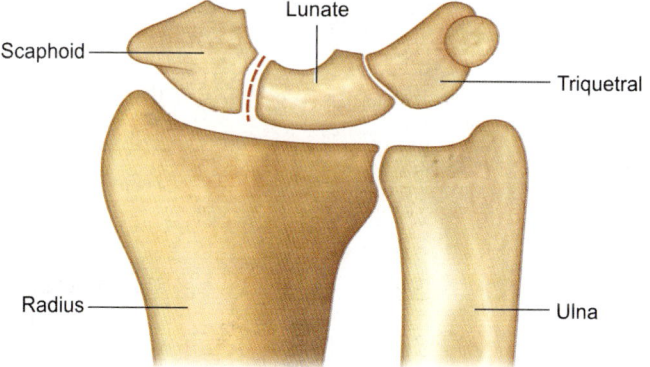

Plane variety of synovial joint

## Cartilaginous Joints

*Subtypes:*

- **Primary cartilaginous type**—bones are joined by cartilage (as though there is cartilage glue on the articular surfaces). These joints are immovable and may be temporary in nature, e.g. epiphyseal plate between the epiphysis and diaphysis.
- **Secondary cartilaginous joint**—in this variety articular surfaces are covered with hyaline cartilage and united by a disc of fibrocartilage.

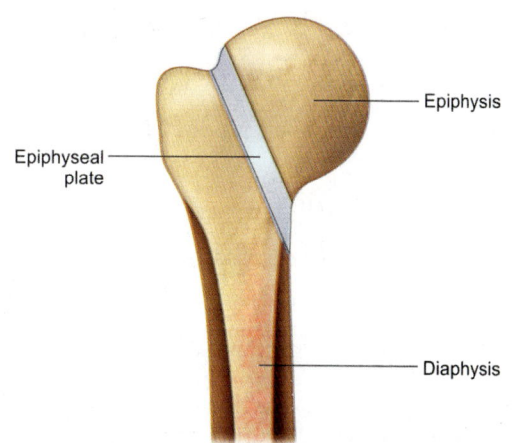

Primary cartilaginous joint

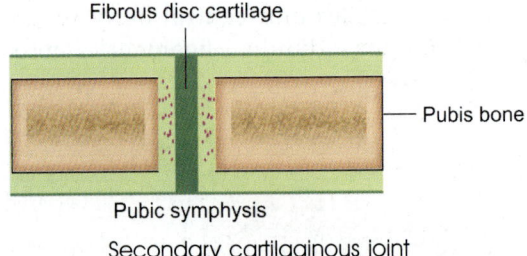

Fibrous disc cartilage

Pubis bone

Pubic symphysis

Secondary cartilaginous joint

Typically, these joints lie in median plane and are permanent in nature, e.g. symphysis pubis manubriosternal joint, joints within the vertebrae.

## Fibrous Joints

### Subtypes of Fibrous Joints

- **Sutures**—bony surfaces are united by fibrous tissue. Sutures could be plane, serrated.

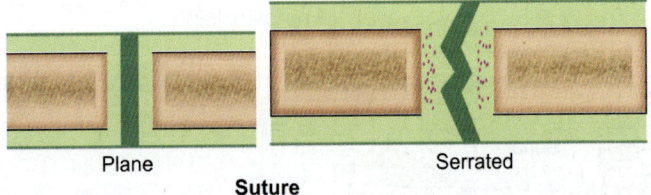

Plane                    Serrated

**Suture**

- **Syndesmosis**—bones are bound by interosseous membranes, e.g. inferior tibiofibular joint.

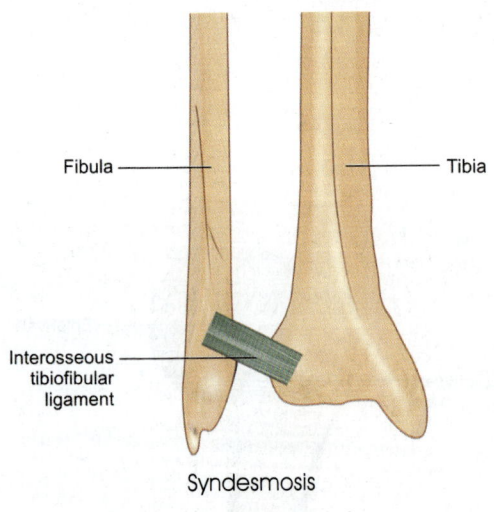

Fibula

Tibia

Interosseous tibiofibular ligament

Syndesmosis

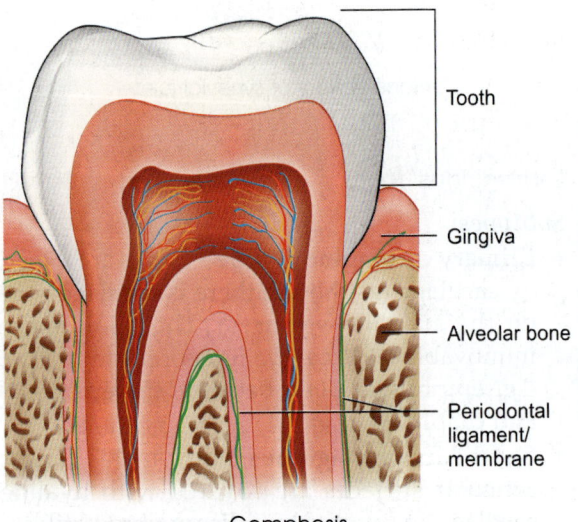

Tooth

Gingiva

Alveolar bone

Periodontal ligament/ membrane

Gomphosis

- **Gomphosis**—peg and socket joint, e.g. tooth and alveolar process.

*Based on the Number of Bones Articulating*

- **Simple joint**—only two bones articulate, e.g. intercarpal, interphalangeal joints
- **Compound joint**—more than two bones articulate, e.g. knee joint, elbow joint, wrist joint
- **Complex joint**—joint cavity is divided by intra-articular disc, e.g. temporomandibular joint, sternoclavicular joint.

*Based upon the Location*

- **Axial skeleton**—intervertebral joints, skull and vertebral joints, e.g. atlantoaxial
- **Appendicular skeleton**—the joints of upper and lower limbs.

*Based upon the Mobility*

- **Synarthrosis**—these are immovable joints, e.g. sutures of skull
- **Amphiarthrosis**—partially movable and partially immovable (like amphibian animals living in water and also on land), e.g. cartilaginous joints, pubic symphysis
- **Diarthrosis**—freely movable synovial joints, e.g. shoulder joint, hip joint.

*Based upon the Range of Movements*

- **Uniaxial joint**—movement of the joint is possible only along one axis like a hinge, e.g. interphalangeal joint
- **Biaxial joint**—movement is possible along 2 axes, e.g. wrist joint
- **Multiaxial joint**—movements possible along 3 axes (anteroposterior, transverse, vertical axes), e.g. shoulder joint.

## HILTON'S LAW

Law deviced by John Hilton, states that the nerve supplying the muscles which cross a particular joint also supplies the joint and the skin in proximity to the joint, e.g. elbow joint, biceps brachii muscle crosses the joint and is supplied by musculocutaneous nerve (muscles which cross the joint also bring about movement at that joint).

## VERTEBRAL COLUMN

Vertebral column comprises of 7 cervical vertebrae, 12 thoracic vertebrae, 5 lumbar vertebrae, sacrum and coccyx.

### Vertebral Column Curvatures

- Thoracic and pelvic curves are primary curves and concave ventrally.
- Cervical and lumbar curves are secondary curves
- Cervical curve is well-developed after the child starts holding his head, while lumbar curve is well-developed when the child starts walking by 1 to 2 years
- Cervical curve extends from C1 to T2, thoracic curve extends from T2 to T12. Lumbar curve extends from T12 to lumbosacral angle, and the pelvic curve extends from lumbosacral joint to coccygeal apex.

## 8. MUSCLES

### Definition

Muscles are the contractile components of the body which bring about all the movements (voluntary and nonvoluntary) in the body, e.g. writing with hands, picking up glass of water, all gastrointestinal movements are considered involuntary (not in one's control), etc.

### Classification

#### *Voluntary and Involuntary Muscles*

- Muscles which bring about movements under one's free will, i.e. any action like taking a book, picking glass of water are voluntary activities brought about by voluntary muscles
- Actions not under own control like breathing—diaphragm contracts, heart beats non-stop by virtue of cardiac muscle.

#### *Structural Classification*

- Striated variety has 2 subtypes—skeletal muscle and cardiac muscle
- Nonstriated is equivalent to smooth muscle.

#### *Skeletal Muscle*

Under microscope, skeletal muscles can be appreciated as bundle of multinucleated muscle fibres, with nuclei located peripherally

#### *Cardiac Muscle*

Under microscope cardiac muscle is seen as: Made-up of short, branched muscle fibres, and characterised by single nuclei, and intercalated disc.

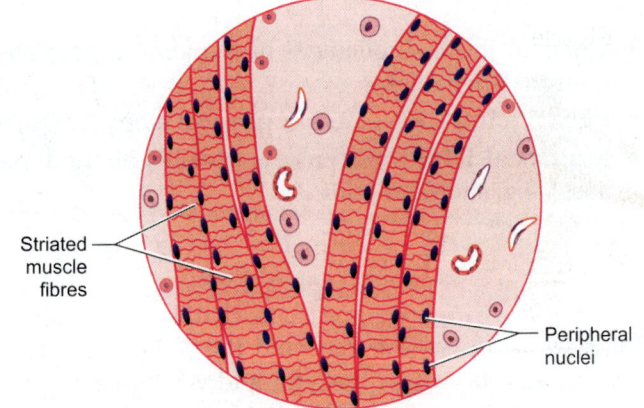

Striated muscle fibres

Peripheral nuclei

Skeletal muscle as seen under microscope

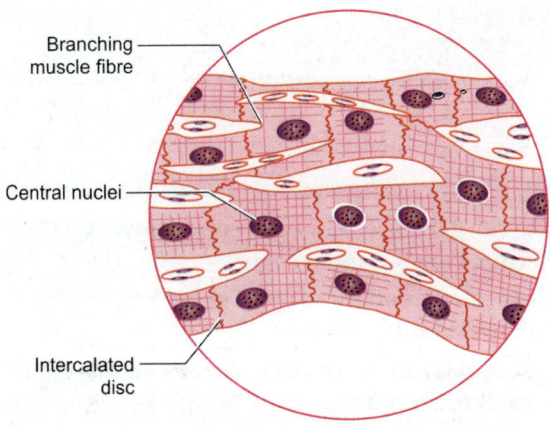

Branching muscle fibre

Central nuclei

Intercalated disc

Cardiac muscle as seen under the microscope

*Smooth Muscle*

These are spindle-shaped muscle fibres with centrally placed oblong nuclei.

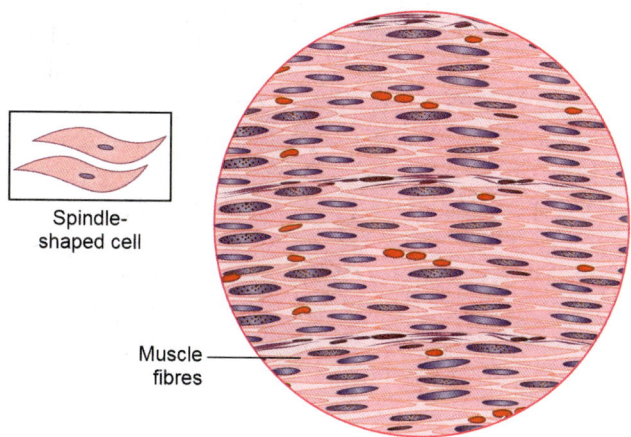

Smooth muscle as seen under the microscope

*Depending on Arrangement of Muscle Fibre Bundles (= fasciculi)*

- Muscle fibres may run parallel to the pull of muscle fibres, e.g. strap muscles of neck-thyrohyoid.

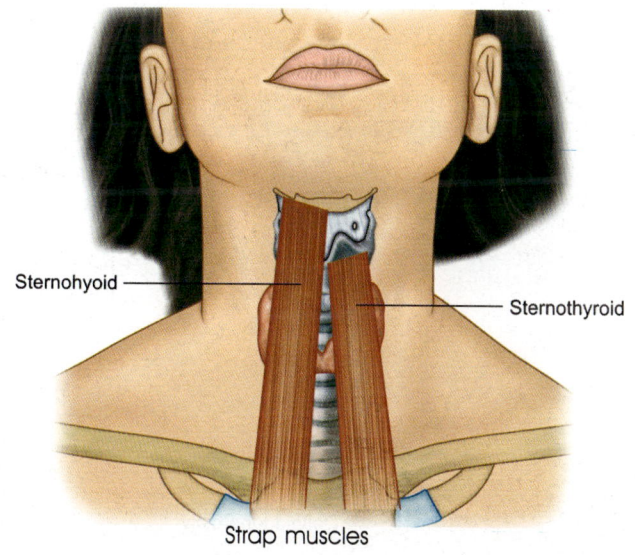

Strap muscles

- Muscle fibres may run oblique to the line of pull of muscle fibres. Subtypes of this pattern are as follows:
  - Unipennate, e.g. palmar interossei, flexor pollicis longus, extensor digitorum longus.

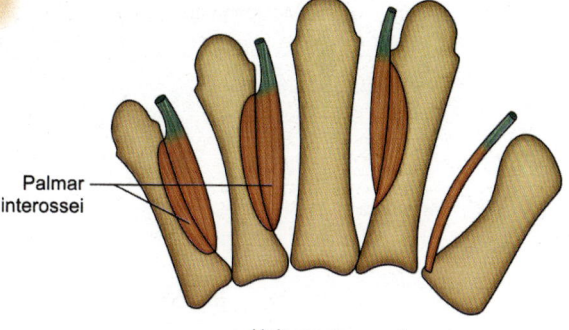

Unipennate muscle

– Bipennate, e.g. biceps brachii.

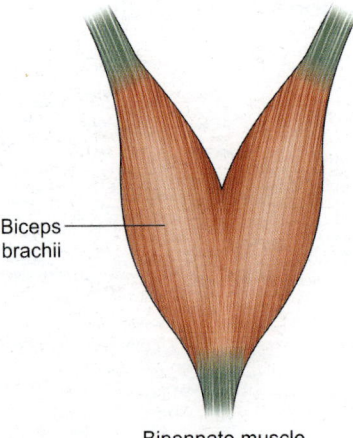

Biceps brachii

Bipennate muscle

– Multipennate, e.g. deltoid.

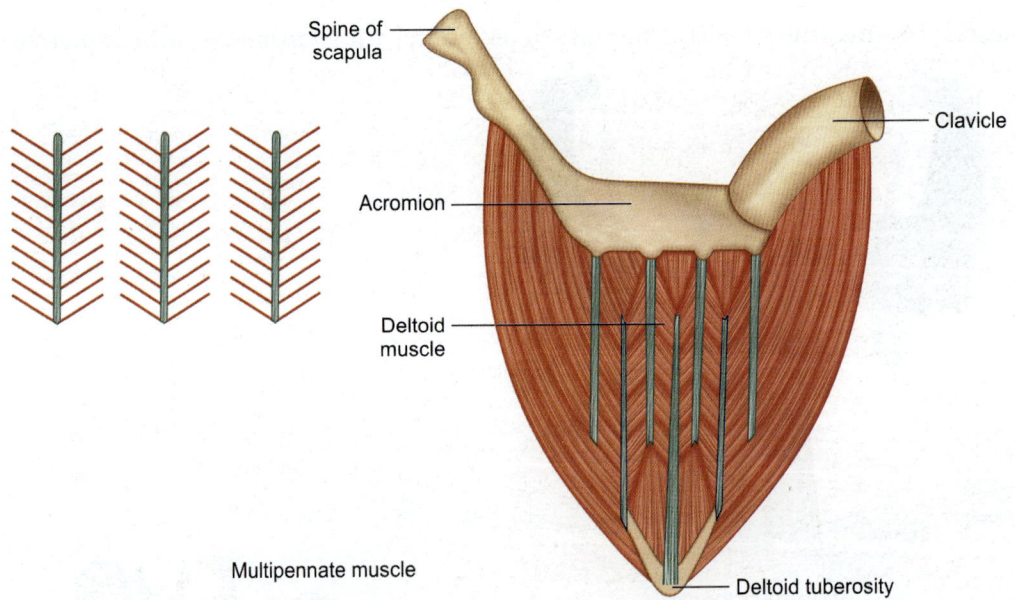

Spine of scapula

Clavicle

Acromion

Deltoid muscle

Multipennate muscle

Deltoid tuberosity

– Circumpennate, e.g. tibialis anterior.

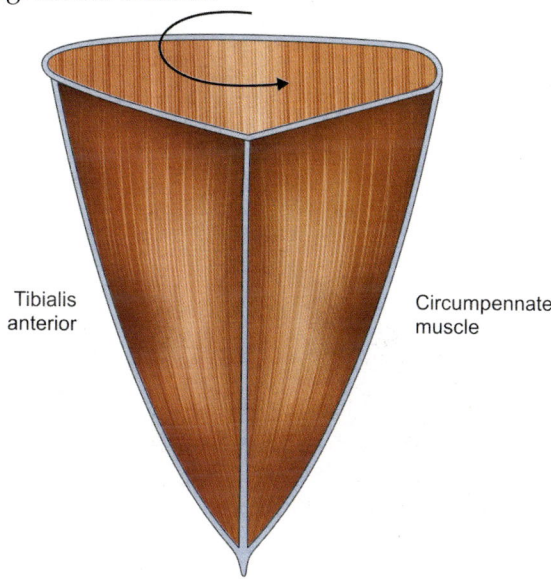

Tibialis
anterior

Circumpennate
muscle

– Fusiform, e.g. digastric muscle.

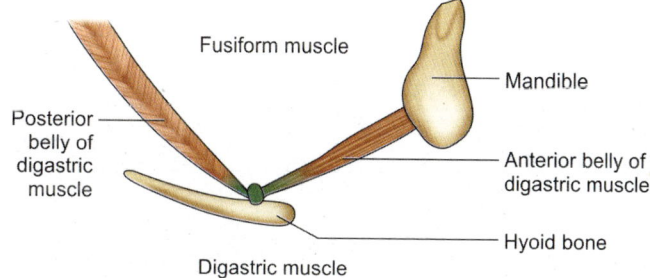

Fusiform muscle

Mandible

Posterior
belly of
digastric
muscle

Anterior belly of
digastric muscle

Hyoid bone

Digastric muscle

– Circular arrangement, e.g. orbicularis oculi.

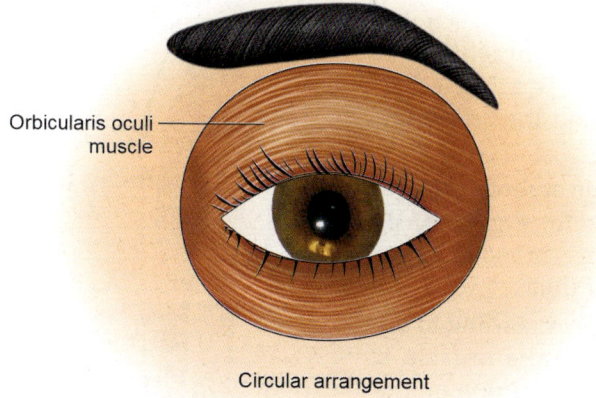

Orbicularis oculi
muscle

Circular arrangement

– Twisted pattern of fasciculi, e.g. lattisimus dorsi.

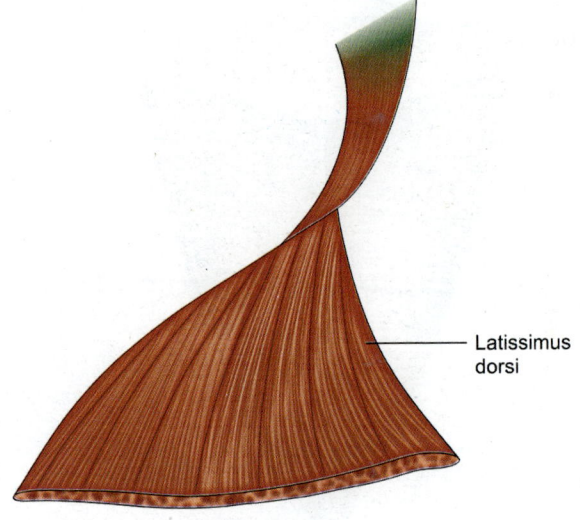

Latissimus
dorsi

Spiral fasciculi

**Depending upon the action it exerts on the joint it crosses**, the muscles are classified as SHUNT and SPURT muscles. It is mechanical classification depending on laws of physics.

| Shunt muscle | Spurt muscle |
|---|---|
| • Proximal attachment close to the joint it crosses | Proximal attachment is away from the joint it crosses |
| • Distal attachment is away from the joint it crosses | Distal attachment is close to the joint it crosses |
| • Stabilises joint | Movement occurs along line of pull of muscle |
| • For example, brachioradialis | For example, biceps brachii |

• **Remember:**
– Names of the muscle can be given according to the bones to which it is attached, e.g. coracobrachialis it means the muscle is attached to coracoid process and the brachium, (arm, humerus).
– Names can be given according to the location of muscle, e.g. tibialis anterior it means muscle is on anterior surface of tibia.
– Names can be given according to the region, e.g. temporalis muscle it occupies the temporal region on the scalp.

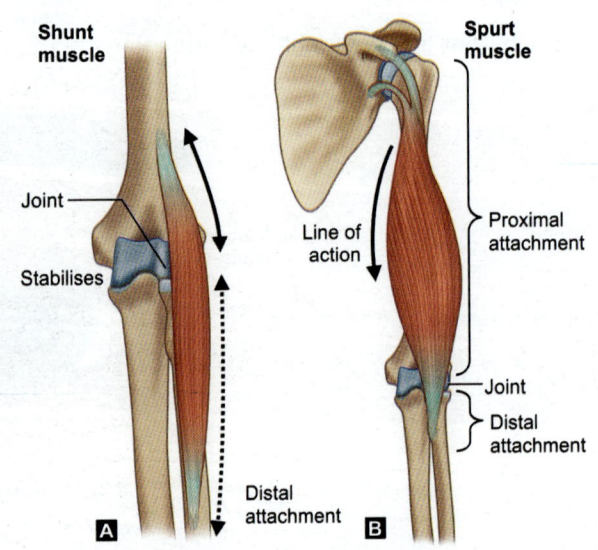

- Names can be given depending upon the compartment the muscle occupies and action it performs, e.g. extensor digitorum it means muscle is in the extensor compartment bringing about extension of digits.

## Difference between Tendons and Muscles

| Tendons | Aponeurosis |
|---|---|
| • Integral part of muscle | Direct or indirect connection with the muscle |
| • Cord like | Sheet like |

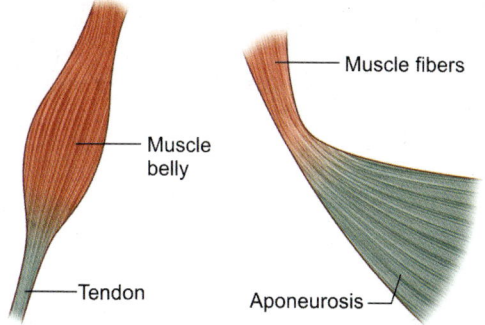

Tendon and aponeurosis

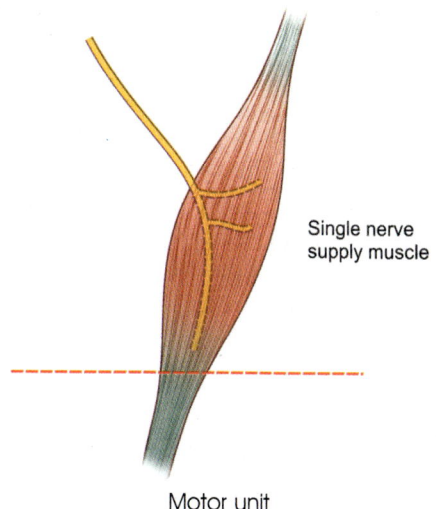

Motor unit

*Motor unit, single nerve injury:* Division of muscle with single nerve supply causes paralysis of the distal portion of muscle.

*Segmental innervation of muscle:* Division of muscle with segmental nerve supply causes no muscle paralysis.

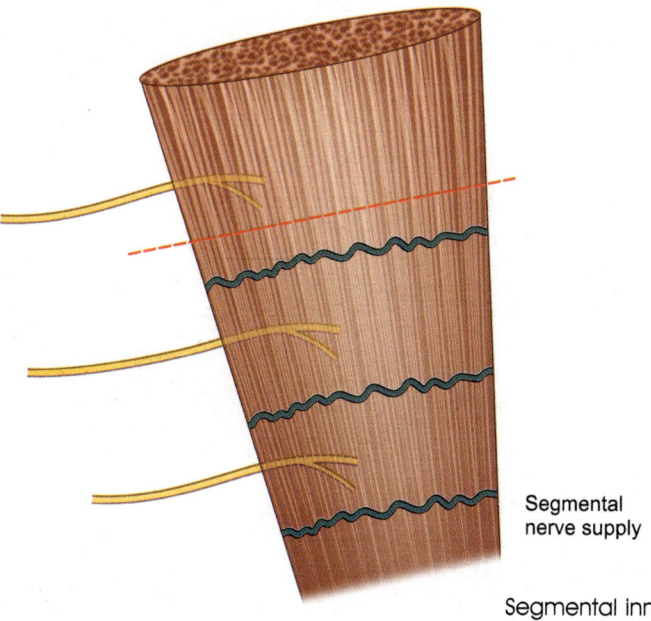

Segmental innervation of muscle

## 9. ARTERIES

### Definition

Arteries carry the oxygenated blood away from the heart, to provide nutrition to all parts of the body.

### Features

- Arteries have abundance of elastic tissue
- Arteries repeatedly branch to end in minute vessels known as arterioles, rich in smooth muscle
- Arteries are thick walled, lumen is smaller than the vein and have no valves
- All arteries have 3 layers when seen under microscope—tunica adventitia, tunica media and tunica intima
- Arteries get nutrition by small arteries named as vasa vasorum
- Non-myelinated sympathetic nerve fibres supply the arteries these are named as vasa nervorum.

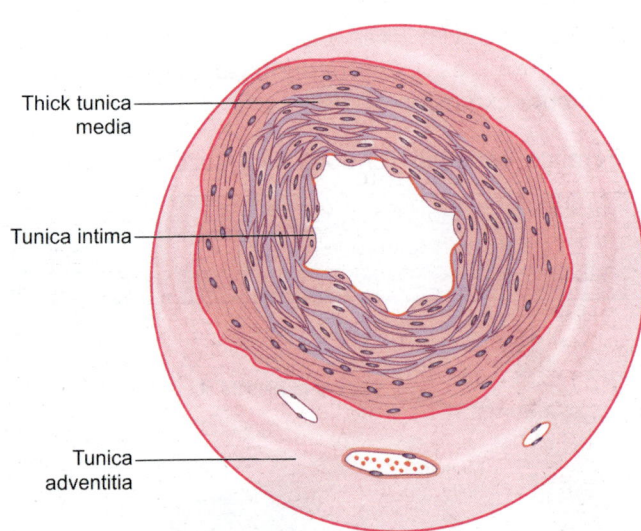

Artery as seen under microscope

## 10. VEINS

### Definition

Veins carry deoxygenated blood from different parts of the body to the heart.

### Features

- Veins are thin walled and have larger lumen within.
- Veins have valves allowing unidirectional flow of blood.
- Venous pressure is low (7 mm Hg).
- Muscular and elastic content of the vein is much less compared to the artery, smallest veins are known as venules.
- Veins normally have dead space around for dilatation during the venous return.
- Veins are also made-up of tunica adventitia, tunica media and tunica intima. However, the layers cannot be clearly demarcated and tunica adventitia is thicker.

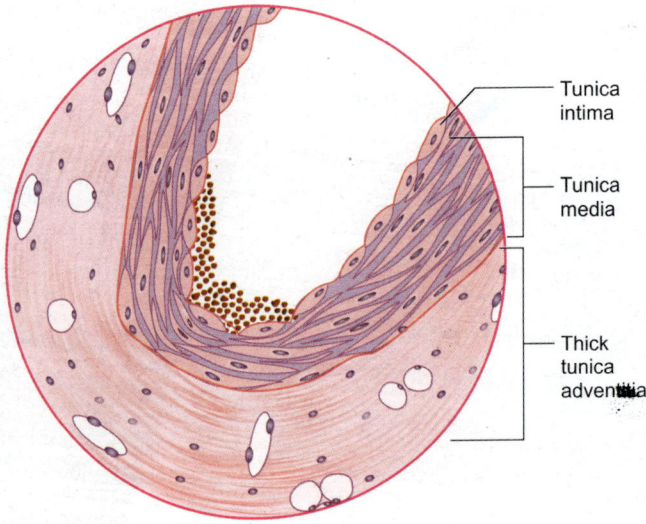

Vein as seen under microscope

## 11. CAPILLARIES

### Definition

These are communicating channels between the arterioles and the venules, at tissue level where the actual transport of oxygen or metabolites takes place.

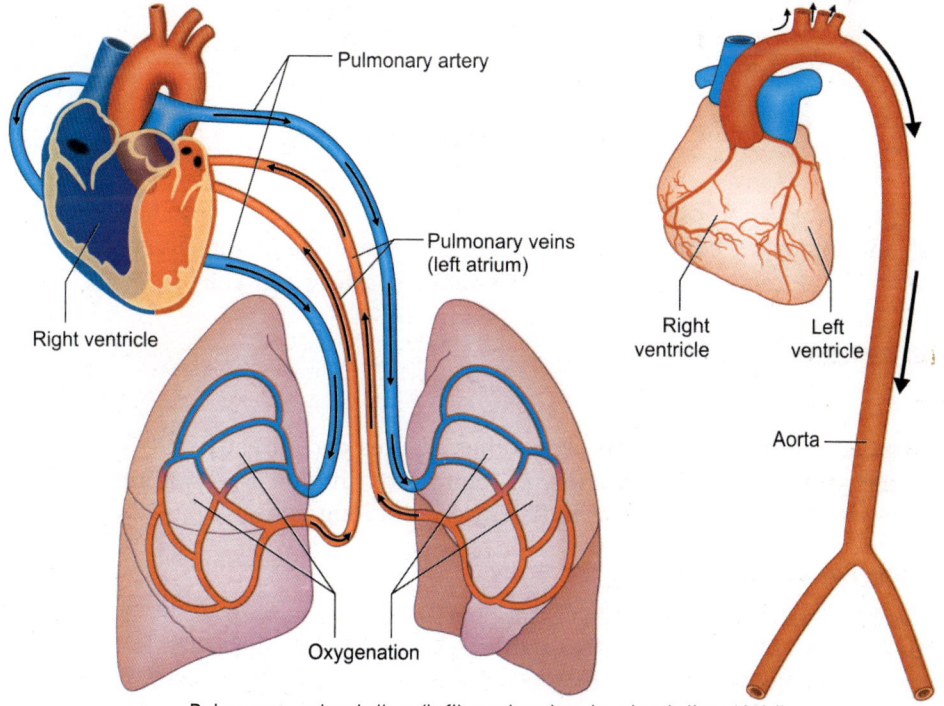

- **Meta-arterioles:** It is a small vessel in microcirculation which links arterioles and capillaries.
- **Precapillary sphincter:** The point where capillary begins there is a smooth muscle band which is known as precapillary sphincter. It regulates the flow of blood in capillaries.

### Types of Circulation

- Systemic—the blood gets distributed to the whole body from the heart, i.e. pure blood is distributed from left ventricle through aorta to all parts of the body and impure blood returns back through superior and inferior vena cava to the right atrium.
- Pulmonary—the blood from right ventricle goes to the lungs via pulmonary artery gets purified in lungs and returns to the left atrium via pulmonary veins.
- Portal circulation—it ends and begins as capillaries and is a part of systemic circulation.

### Types of Circulation

Pulmonary circulation (left) and systemic circulation (right)

| | Vascular system | Lymphatic system |
|---|---|---|
| Formed by function | Heart and blood vessels supplies oxygenated blood to all organs and collects deoxygenated blood from them | Lymph nodes and lymph vessels drains tissue fluid |
| | Pulmonary system | Systemic system |
| | Carry deoxygenated blood from right ventricle to lungs for purification then to left atrium the oxygenated blood | Carries oxygenated blood from left ventricle to all parts of body |

## 12. TYPES OF ANASTOMOSIS

### Definition

Communication between the vessels in the body is known as anastomosis. Presence of such communications help distribute blood via other route distal to the block.

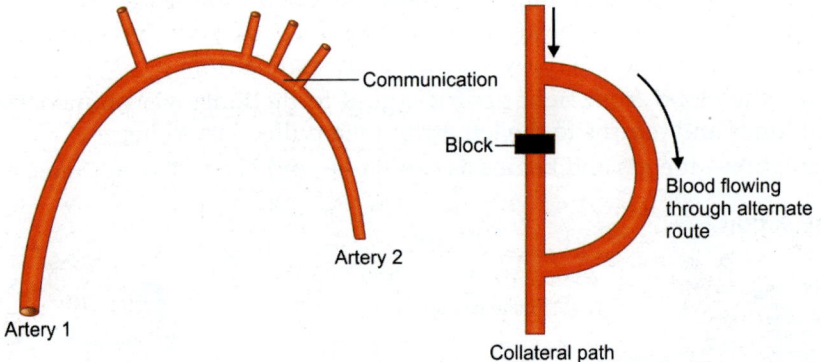

Types of anastomosis

### Types

- Arterial anstomosis is communication between the arteries, e.g. palmar arch
- Venous anastomosis is communication between the veins, e.g. dorsal venous arch
- Arteriovenous shunts are communications between artery and vein.

## 13. END-ARTERIES

### Definition

Arteries which do not communicate with other arteries and directly end on the organs are known as end arteries, e.g. central artery of retina, labyrinthine artery of internal ear, striate arteries going to the cerebrum, metaphyseal arteries of long bones.

### Clinical Terms Related to Vessels in the Body

- Thrombosis—formation of clots in vessels
- Infarction—death of an organ or tissue due to lack of blood supply
- Aneurysm—dilated blood vessel due to weakness in blood vessel wall
- Lymphedema—swelling caused in a body part due to obstruction of lymph.

## 14. LYMPHATICS

### Definition

Lymphatic system of the body is the drainage system of the body in close association with the veins (drains the toxins within the body). The fluid is the lymph which is clear and colourless (however intestinal lymph is milky and known as chyle) the cells are the lymphocytes T and B.

### Components

It comprises of lymph nodes (arranged in groups and named accordingly, e.g. in axilla, axillary nodes, in inguinal region, inguinal lymph nodes, etc.), lymphatic vessels (lymphatic duct, thoracic duct) and lymphatic organs like thymus, spleen, bone marrow.

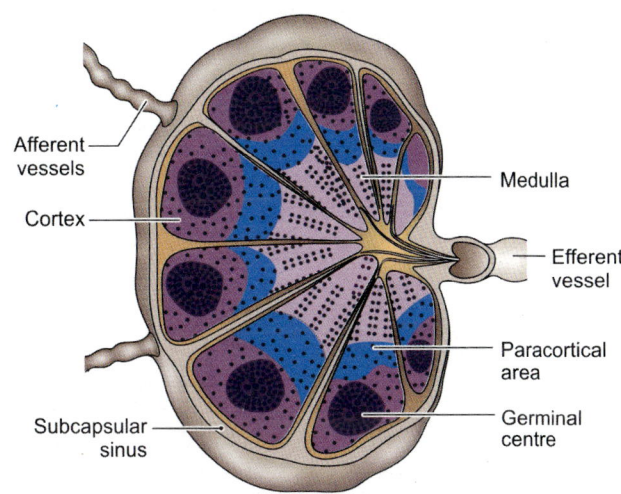

### Structure of Lymph Nodes

- Cut section of reniform lymph node shows cortex and medulla with afferent and efferent channels.
- Lymph node is covered by capsule and distinctly has subcapsular space = sinus except in the hilum.

Structure of lymph node

### Drainage Area of Lymphatic Ducts Broadly

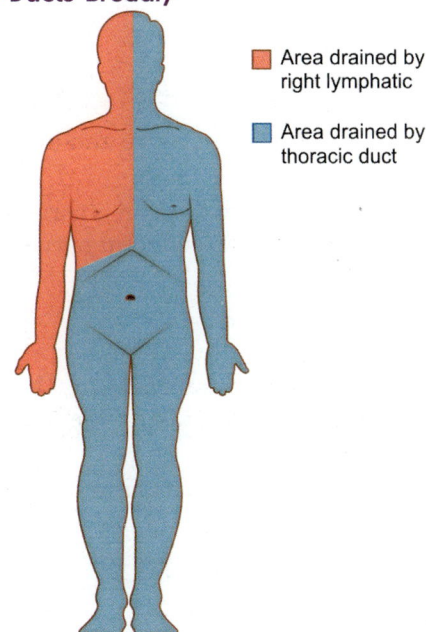

■ Area drained by right lymphatic

■ Area drained by thoracic duct

Pattern of whole body

## 15. NERVOUS SYSTEM

This system deals with the sensitivity, conductivity and responsiveness in the body (like electrical wires in the house).

### Classification

- Central nervous system (CNS)—comprises of brain and spinal cord.
- Peripheral nervous system (PNS)—comprises of 12 pairs of cranial nerves, 31 pairs of spinal nerves, and autonomic system which has sympathetic (thoracosacral outflow) and para-sympathetic (craniosacral outflow) components.

### Reflex Arc

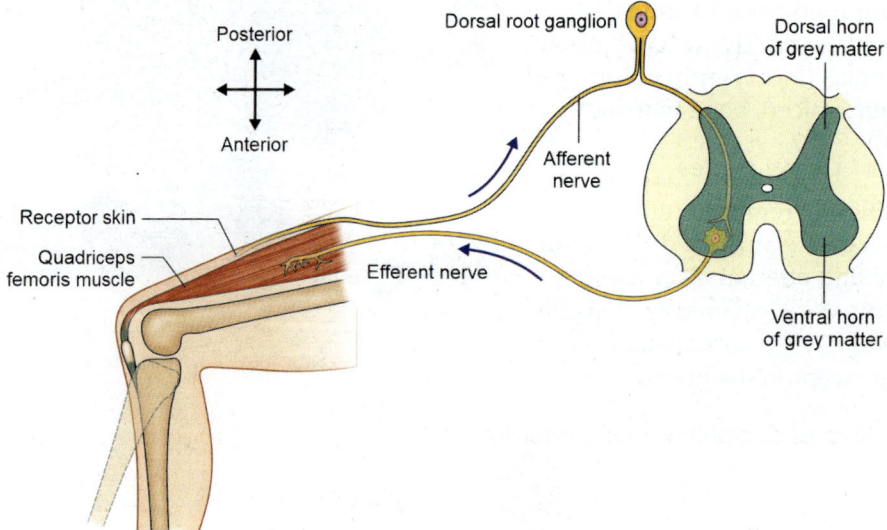

- Nerve carrying the impulse to CNS is afferent nerve and impulse going away from CNS is efferent nerve.
- The diagram depicts how the sensation from the skin is carried towards the central nervous system, integrated there and then reaction via efferent nerve like movement of certain part is brought about.

### Spinal Nerve

- Student should know how the spinal nerve branches out. The branches are known as rami, if the branch is anterior it is known as ventral rami if the branch is posterior it is known as dorsal rami.
- In any plexus, e.g. brachial it would be mentioned ventral rami of spinal nerve C5, so student should understand that it is the anterior branch of that particular nerve.

### Neuron

- Cells of the nervous system are known as neuron. They form the structural and functional components of nervous system.

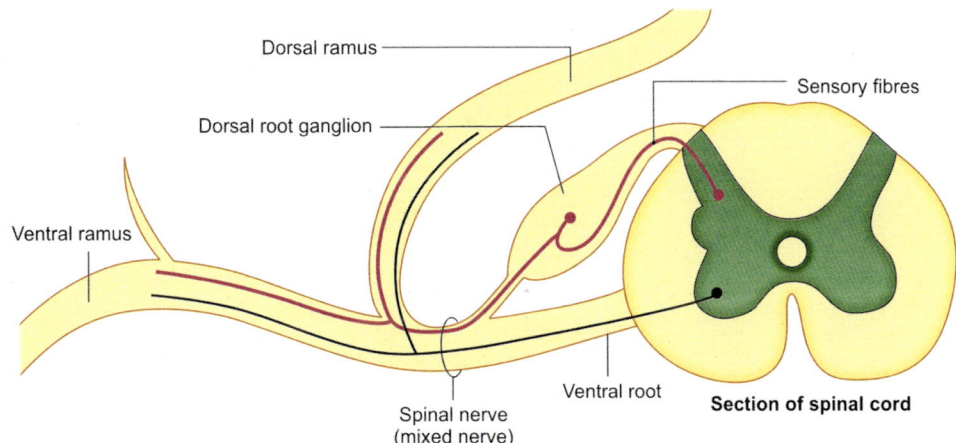

Section of spinal cord

- Neuron has a cell body and processes coming out of the body, dendrite and axon (axon carries impulse away from the cell body, dendrite carries impulse towards cell body).

## Nuclei

Collection of cell bodies of neuron within CNS is known as nuclei.

## Ganglia

Collection of cell bodies of neuron within the PNS is known as ganglia.

## Neuroglial Cells

Neuroglial cells are the supporting cells of nervous system, e.g. Schwann cells, microglia, macroglia, astrocytes, oligodendrocytes.

## Types of Neuron

- *Unipolar*—these neuron type have only single process, e.g. mesencehalic nucleus

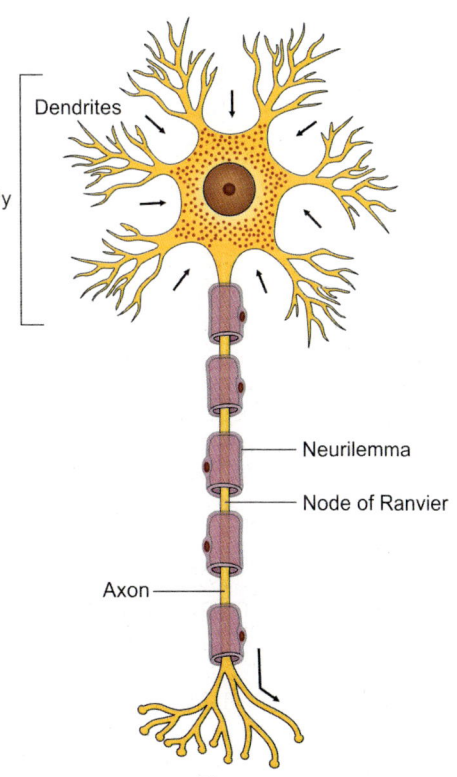

Neuron

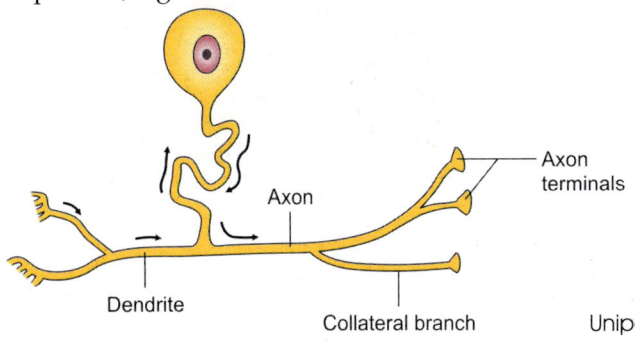

Unipolar neuron

- *Pseudounipolar* have process at one end of cell but it bifurcates, e.g. spinal ganglia

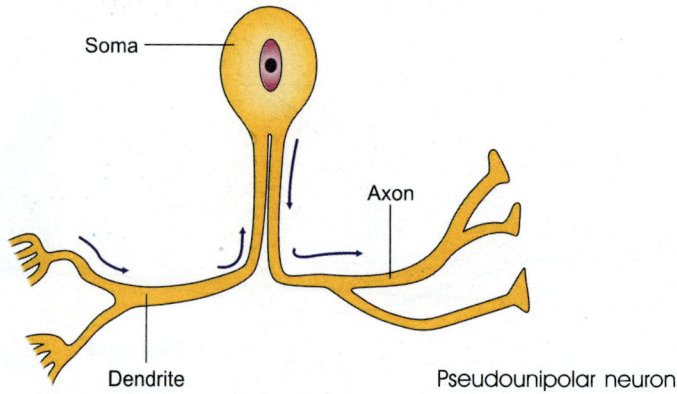

Pseudounipolar neuron

- *Bipolar* having processes at both the ends, e.g. spiral ganglia, vestibular ganglia

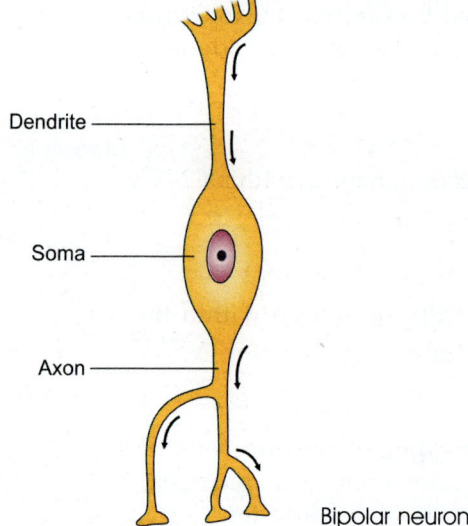

Bipolar neuron

- *Multipolar* having processes from several sites of the cell, e.g. neurons of cerebrum, cerebellum

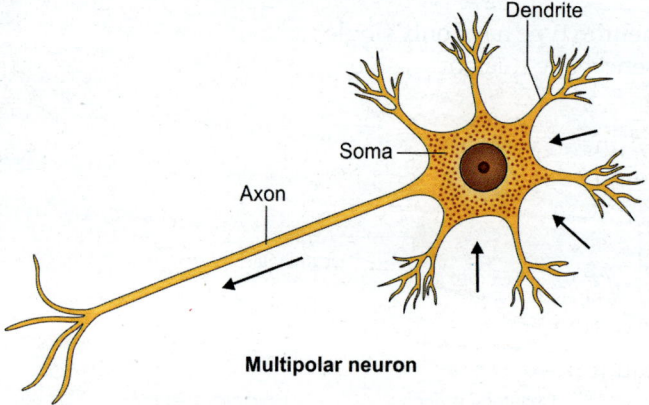

Multipolar neuron

- **Remember:** When we say nerve, e.g. facial nerve we are referring to the axon of the nerve while the cell body if in CNS is known as the nuclei of the nerve.

## Nerve Types

- Thick nerve fibres are covered by myelin sheath hence this nerve is termed myelinated nerve
- Thin nerve fibres have no myelin sheath thus termed nonmyelinated
- Nerves with long axon are termed Golgi type I nerves
- Nerves with short axon are termed Golgi type II nerves.

## Types of Synapse

Synapse is a junction between 2 neurons. Broadly 2 types are recognised: Axodendritic and axosomatic.

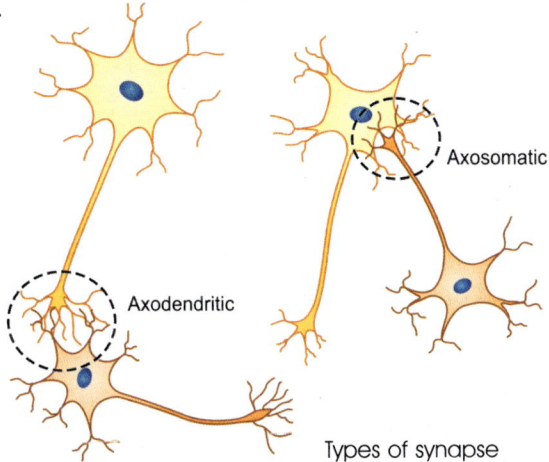

Types of synapse

| Spinal ganglion | Sympathetic ganglion |
|---|---|
| • Unipolar | Multipolar |
| • Found on dorsal root at intervertebral foramen | Found on sympathetic chain |
| • Sensory | Relay stations |
| • No synapse | Synapse ++ |

## Referred Sites with the Nerves Responsible for the Phenomenon of Referred Pain

### Referred Pain in Body

It is topic of special interest by virtue of its presentation. A pain originating in part of body is felt elsewhere. Anatomical basis for this phenomenon is the common nerve pathway both the sites share, i.e. they share same root value.

### Common Referred Pain Sites in the Body

a. Ear
b. Left upper arm and forearm
c. Left shoulder tip

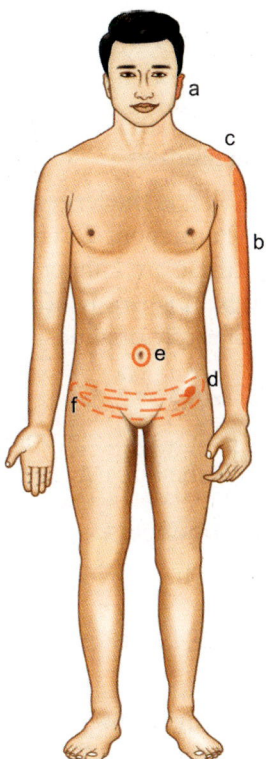

d. Hip joint
e. Periumbilical
f. Groin.

### Common Areas of Referred Pain in the Body

Pain is referred from following areas to above-mentioned sites, i.e. referees:

a. **To the ear** from tooth, temporomandibular joint, larynx auriculotemporal nerve(V) and vagus(X) are nerves involve.

b. **To the left arm and forearm,** cardiac pain is radiated to this region by virtue of C3, C4 C5 roots which are common to phrenic nerve and the dermatomes of upper limb.

c. Left shoulder tip pain due to splenic rupture is by virtue of the phrenic nerve C3, C4, C5.

d. **Periumbilical region** receives pain from appendix, kidney colon common root values sharing this pain are T10, T11, L1.

e. **Pain to the groin from loin** is radiated from ureter, kidney by virtue of common root value T10, T11, L1.

f. Pain can be referred to hip joint from knee joint by the common obturator L2, L3, L4 nerve sending branches to both the joints.

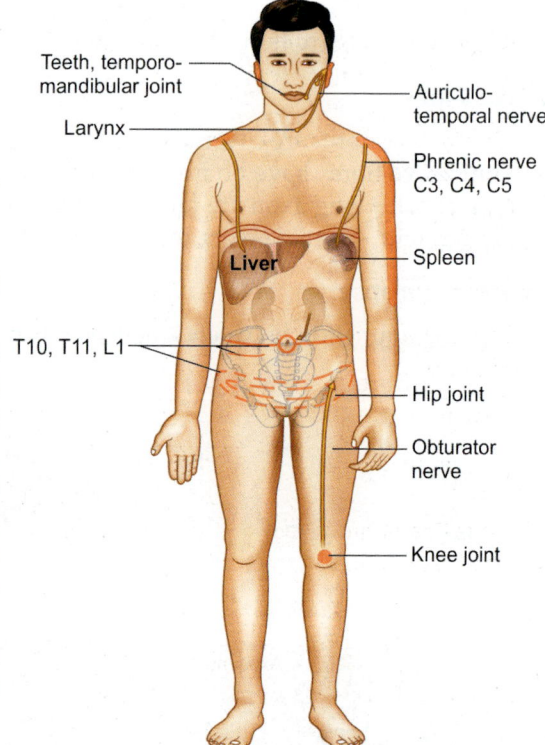

Teeth, temporo-mandibular joint
Larynx
Auriculo-temporal nerve
Phrenic nerve C3, C4, C5
Liver
Spleen
T10, T11, L1
Hip joint
Obturator nerve
Knee joint

## 16. SKIN

### Peculiarities

- Skin is the largest organ of the body
- Permanent skin folds can be recognised all over the body these are Langer's skin
- Skin is firmly attached to the underlying deep fascia at the site of joint.

### b. Types

- Thick skin, e.g. sole, nape of neck
- Thin skin, e.g. eyelids.

### c. Appendages of Skin

Nails, hair, sweat glands.

### PRINCIPLES OF SKIN INCISIONS

There are tensions lines or cleavage lines or Langer's lines on skin of the body. They coincide with the direction of collagen fibres in the dermis.

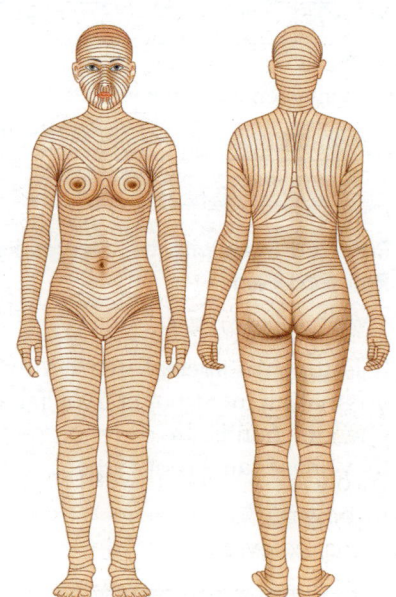

Cleavage lines on skin

Skin incisions during surgery should be along these lines to avoid postoperative scarring and better wound healing.

## 17. FASCIA

### Superficial Fascia

It is the connective tissue below the skin containing fat (like when you peel orange fruit outer covering the white fibres within the fruit and binding the individual pieces of orange are same like fascia in the body).

### Deep Fascia

It a tough fibrous tissue investing the deeper structures of body like muscle, or binding neurovascular bundle.

### MODIFICATIONS OF DEEP FASCIA

Deep fascia is modified in different regions of the body in different forms, e.g. intermuscular septae, retinaculi, fibroareolar sheath like carotid sheath.

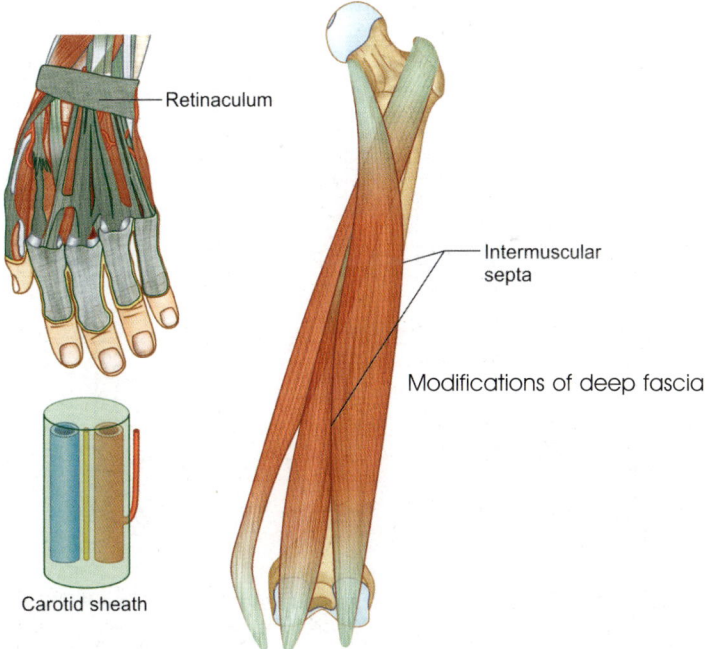

Retinaculum

Intermuscular septa

Modifications of deep fascia

Carotid sheath

### BASICS OF DISSECTIOIN

As one cannot learn driving by reading a book on driving similarly one cannot grasp anatomy by only reading. By doing dissections one can actually see the structures, appreciate the relations by naked eyes. Thus, it becomes very easy to remember anatomy.

To make dissections easy, stepwise approach to every region will be discussed.

*Latin:* **Dissecare to cut to pieces.**

## Cadaver Selection

- Unclaimed bodies
- Dead bodies with no history of death due to communicable diseases
- Not decomposed bodies.

## Embalming

It is a technique to preserve dead body.

## Embalming Fluid

- Formaldehyde
- Methanol
- Ethanol
- Dyes
- Odorants.

## Anatomy Act

It provides the supply of unclaimed bodies to medical and teaching institution for the purpose of anatomical examination and dissection.

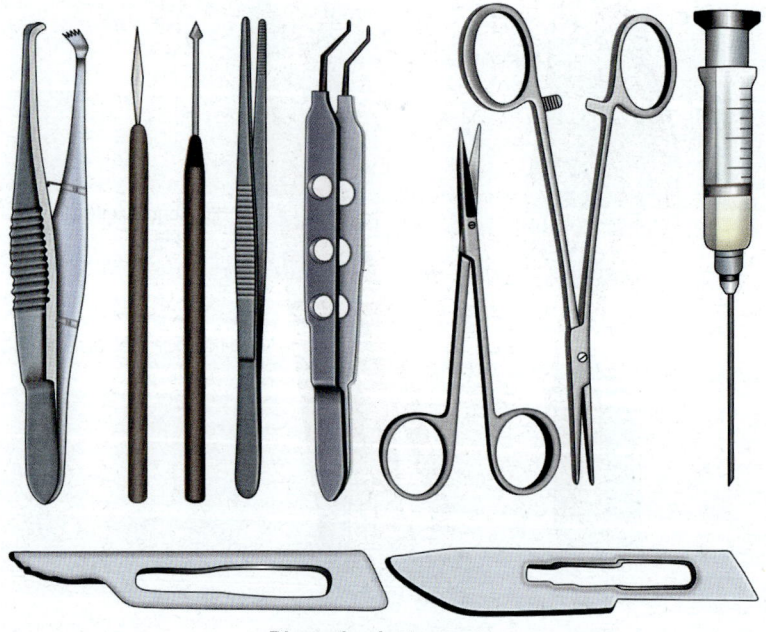

**Dissection instruments**

## Dissection Tools

- Scalpel
- Blade No. 21, 20, 12, 15
- Forceps (toothed, plain)
- Scissors (small iris, styli)
- Bone cutter, probe, syringe needle.

## Structures Encountered after Incising the Skin

- Superficial fascia
- Deep fascia
- Muscles
- Bone.

  Superficial fascia resembles the white fibres of orange, after peeling it; the way one separates the orange pieces similarly one has to separate the fascia between the neurovascular bundle to study individual structure.

## Principles of Dissection

- While incising the skin, hold scalpel like a pen and with a firm, controlled movement cut the skin
- Below the skin is superficial fascia
- Then comes deep fascia
- Incisions on fascia should be sharp with the knife
- Blunt (finger) dissection can be adopted to separate structures bound in sheath
- Nerve feels like a thick cord, (solid) when held in fingers
- Vessels feel like empty lumen, collapsed pipe when held in fingers
- Muscle is the fleshy structure, with cord like glistening tendon
- Membranes look shiny white
- *Anatomy knowledge will make you good physician*
- *Dissections will help you to be good surgeon. Surgery means dissection in living, i.e. vivisection.*

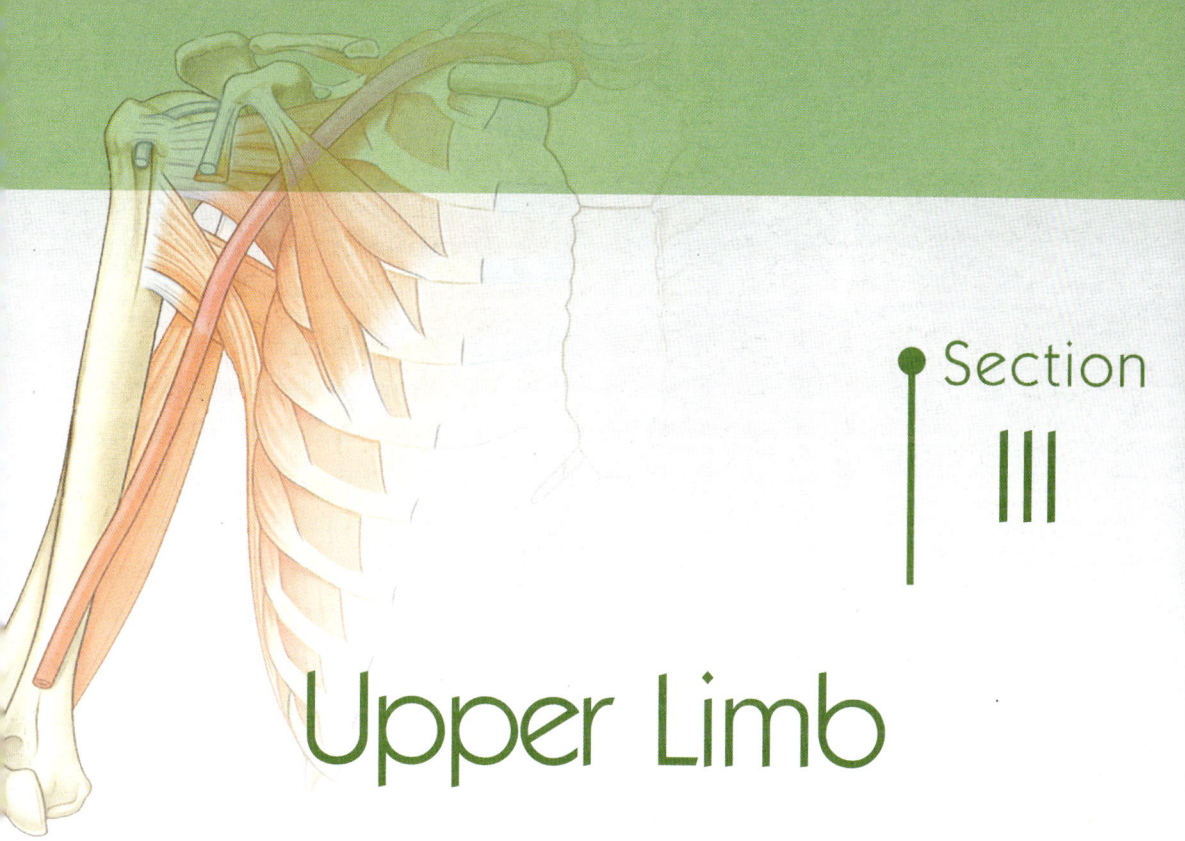

# Upper Limb

# Key Osteology Questions

## Q. Surfaces of clavicle

Ans.

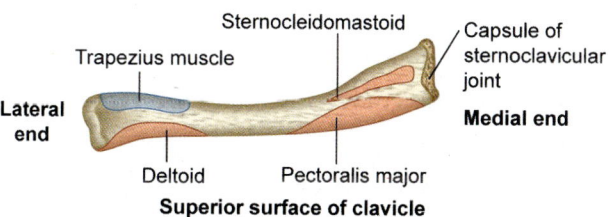

**Superior surface of clavicle**

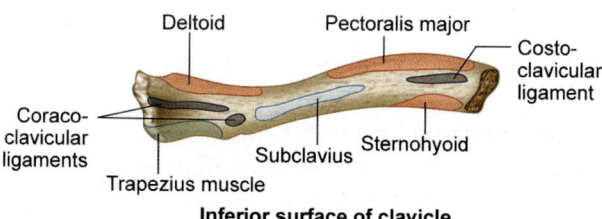

**Inferior surface of clavicle**

## Q. Which long bone in the body is placed horizontally?

**Ans.** Clavicle is the long bone placed horizontally.

## Q. What is the literal meaning of clavicle?

**Ans.** Clavicle means 'key'.

**Q. What are the peculiarities of clavicle?**

**Ans.**
- Clavicle is the only long bone that lies horizontally
- It is subcutaneous
- It is the first bone to ossify
- Most of it ossifies in the membrane
- It has two primary centres of ossification
- It usually has no medullary cavity
- It is the only bone pierced by a nerve (supraclavicular nerve).

**Q. How does the clavicle differ in females?**

**Ans.** The female clavicle is shorter, thinner, less curved and smoother, and its acromial end is lower than the sternal end.

**Q. How does one determine the sex of clavicle?**

**Ans.** Midshaft circumference is the most reliable single indicator of determining the sex of clavicle.

**Q. How does the clavicle differ in labourers?**

**Ans.** The clavicle is thicker and more curved in labourers.

**Q. What is the meaning of coracoid process?**

**Ans.** Coracoid process means 'beak like'.

**Q. What are the attachments on coracoid process?**

**Ans.** Following structures are attached on coracoid process:
- Coracobrachialis
- Pectoralis minor and short head of biceps brachii
- Coracohumeral, coracoclavicular, coracoacromial ligaments.

**Q. Paralysis of which muscle causes 'winging of scapula'?**

**Ans.** Paralysis of serratus anterior muscle causes 'winging of scapula'.

**Q. What is the literal meaning of scapula?**

**Ans.** Scapula means 'to dig'.

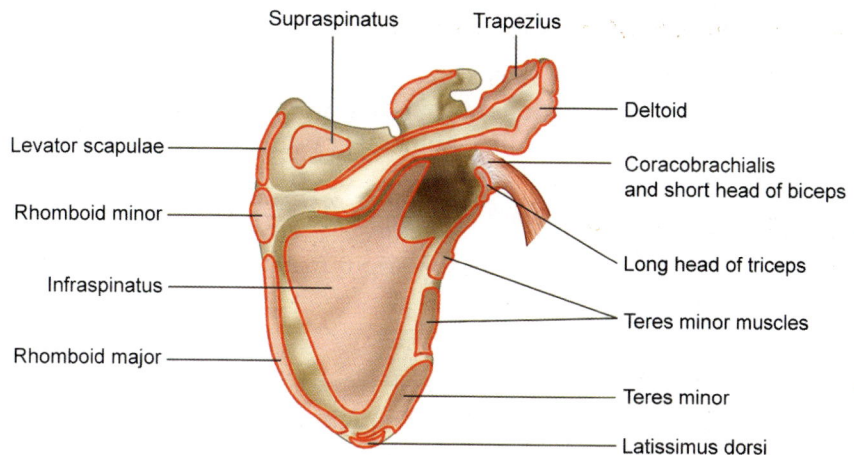

Supraspinatus  Trapezius

Levator scapulae

Rhomboid minor

Infraspinatus

Rhomboid major

Deltoid

Coracobrachialis
and short head of biceps

Long head of triceps

Teres minor muscles

Teres minor

Latissimus dorsi

**Dorsal surface of scapula**

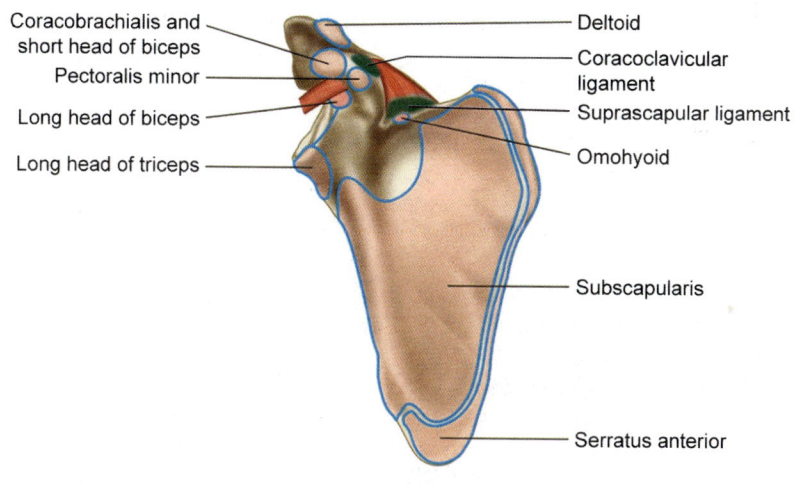

Coracobrachialis and
short head of biceps

Pectoralis minor

Long head of biceps

Long head of triceps

Deltoid

Coracoclavicular
ligament

Suprascapular ligament

Omohyoid

Subscapularis

Serratus anterior

**Costal surface of scapula**

## Q. Which group of muscles constitute the 'rotator cuff'?

**Ans.** Supraspinatus, infraspinatus, teres minor, subscapularis constitute the 'rotator cuff'.

## Q. Which nerves are directly related to humerus?

**Ans.**
- At the surgical neck—axillary nerve
- At the radial groove—radial nerve
- At the medial epicondyle—ulnar nerve.

**Q. What are the contents of intertubercular sulcus?**

**Ans.** The contents of intertubercular sulcus are:
- Tendon of long head of biceps with its synovial sheath.
- Ascending branch of anterior circumflex humeral artery.

**Q. Which is the common flexor origin?**

**Ans.** Medial epicondyle is the common flexor origin from where superficial flexors of the forearm arise.

**Q. Which is the common extensor origin?**

**Ans.** Lateral epicondyle is the common extensor origin from where superficial extensors of the forearm arise.

**Q. What is attached to the radial tuberosity?**

**Ans.** The biceps brachii is inserted onto the rough posterior part of radial tuberosity, while the anterior part is covered by a bursa.

**Q. Name the carpal bones.**

**Ans.** *Mnemonics*      *Structure*

| *Mnemonics* | *Structure* |
|---|---|
| "She | Scaphoid |
| Looks | Lunate |
| Too | Triquetral |
| Pretty | Pisiform |
| Try | Trapezium |
| To | Trapezoid |
| Catch | Capitate |
| Her" | Hamate |

**Q. Which of the carpal bone is a sesamoid bone?**

**Ans.** Pisiform bone is a sesamoid carpal bone, which develops in the tendon of flexor carpi ulnaris.

**Q. When does the pisiform bone ossify?**

**Ans.** Pisiform bone ossifies at the age of 12 years.

**Q. Which is the key carpal bone?**

**Ans.** Capitate is the key carpal bone.

**Q. What is attached to the hook of hamate?**

**Ans.** Flexor retinaculum is attached to the hook of hamate.

**Q. What is wrist complex?**

**Ans.** Wrist complex comprises of radiocarpal joint and midcarpal joint.

**Q. What is angle of humeral torsion?**

**Ans.** In lower mammals, the longest axes of proximal and distal humeral articular surfaces make an angle of approximately 90°. But in human beings, the head end has rotated laterally for about 164°. This is humeral torsion.

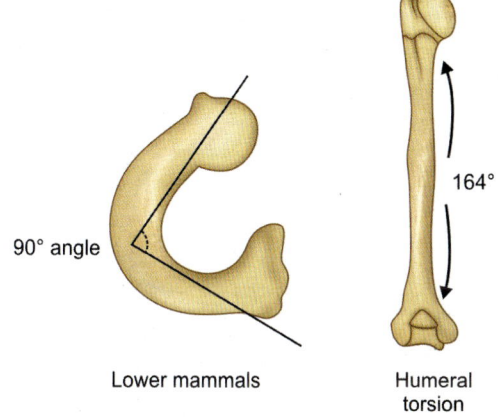

90° angle

164°

Lower mammals

Humeral torsion

Angle of humeral torsion

**Q. Which carpal bone gets fractured commonly on an outstretched hand?**

**Ans.** Scaphoid bone gets fractured commonly on an outstretched hand.

**Q. Where do you look for tenderness in cases of scaphoid bone fracture?**

Ans. One looks for tenderness in anatomical snuffbox for scaphoid bone fracture.

## MUSCLES

### Q. Pectoralis major muscle

**Ans.** Pectoralis major muscle is the chief muscle in front of the chest.

#### Attachments

*From*

- Anterior surface of medial half of clavicle
- Half side of the anterior surface of sternum
- Second to sixth costal cartilage
- A few fibres from aponeurosis of external oblique muscle.

*To*

Lateral lip of bicipital groove.

#### Nerve Supply

Medial and lateral pectoral nerves.

#### Action

Mainly adduction, medial rotation and flexion of arm.

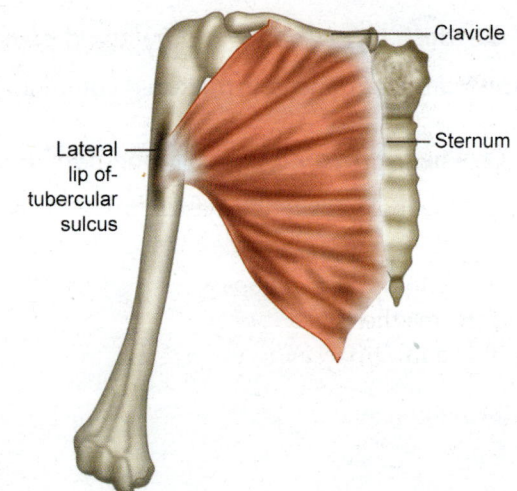

Clavicle

Lateral lip of- tubercular sulcus

Sternum

Pectoralis major attachment

### Q. Serratus anterior

**Ans.** Serratus anterior is a large muscular sheet extending from ribs to scapula.

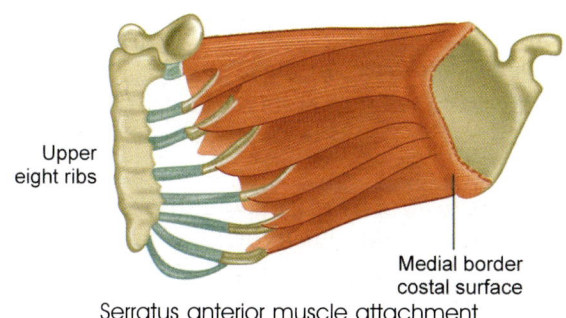

Serratus anterior muscle attachment

## Attachments

*From*

Upper eight ribs and intervening intercostal fascia.

*To*

Costal surface of scapula along its medial border.

## Nerve Supply

Long thoracic nerve (of Bell).

## Action

- Serratus anterior helps in pushing and punching movements
- It stabilises scapula during weight lifting
- It helps during forced inspiration.

## Applied Anatomy

When the muscle gets paralysed, the medial margin of scapula becomes prominent. This is known as 'winging of scapula'.

### Q. Deltoid

**Ans.** Deltoid means shaped like a delta (triangular):
- It forms the contour of the shoulder joint
- It is a multipennate muscle.

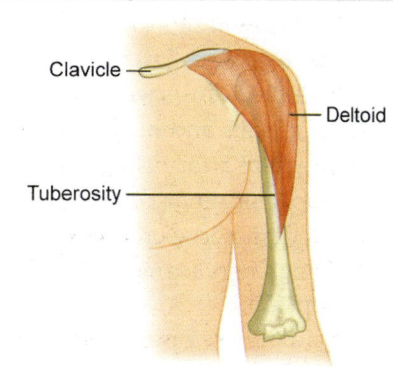

Deltoid attachments

## Attachments

*From*
- Anterior border of lateral one-third of clavicle
- Lateral border of acromion
- Crest of spine of scapula.

*To*

Deltoid tuberosity on humerus.

## Nerve Supply

Axillary nerve.

## Action

- Acromial fibres are powerful abductors of the arm
- Anterior fibres are flexors and medial rotators of the arm.

## Applied Anatomy

- Injury to axillary nerve leads to atrophy of deltoid muscle giving rise to bony prominences in shoulder region resembling shoulder dislocation
- Intramuscular injections are given in the lower half of muscle to avoid injury to the axillary nerve.

### Q. Coracobrachialis

**Ans.** Coracobrachialis is the key muscle of anterior compartment of arm.

## Attachments

*From*
Tip of coracoid process.

*To*
Middle third of humerus medially.

## Nerve Supply

Musculocutaneous nerve.

## Action

Flexes the arm.

## Peculiarities of Coracobrachialis

1. Coracobrachialis is pierced by musculocutaneous nerve.
2. Morphologically, it represents the medial compartment of arm.
3. *At the level of its insertion:*
   a. Deltoid is inserted.
   b. Brachialis and medial head of triceps begins.
   c. Brachial artery changes its course.
   d. Superior ulnar collateral artery originates.
   e. Median nerve crosses the brachial artery.
   f. Ulnar nerve pierces the medial intermuscular septum.
   g. Radial nerve pierces the lateral intermuscular septum.
   h. Nutrient artery enters.

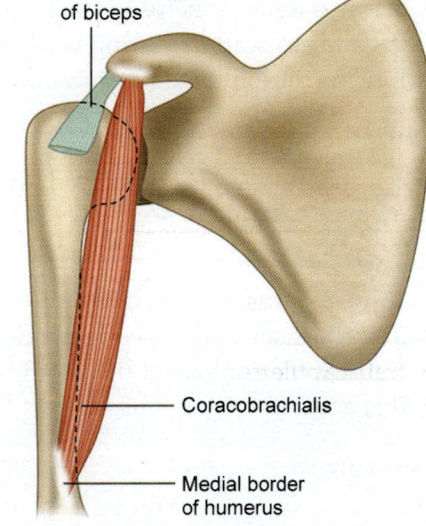

Coracobrachialis attachments

### Q. Biceps brachii

**Ans.** Biceps brachii is the muscle of anterior compartment of arm.

## Attachments

*From*

Biceps brachii has two heads of origin:
1. Short-head arises from tip of coracoid process
2. Long-head arises from supraglenoid tubercle of scapula and glenoid labrum.

*To*

Radial tuberosity (it gives off bicipital aponeurosis at this point).

## Nerve Supply

Musculocutaneous nerve.

## Action

- Stronger supinator when the forearm is flexed
- It is also flexor of the elbow.

## Applied Anatomy

When the arm gets fixed in abduction due to biceps tendon dislocation, it can be replaced by flexing the forearm and rotating the limb.

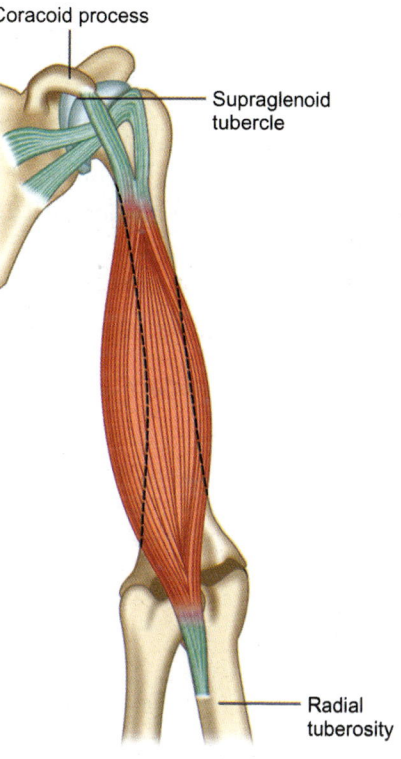

Attachments of biceps brachii

### Q. Rotator cuff

**Ans.** Rotator cuff is a fibrous sheath formed by four flattened tendons, which merge with the capsule of shoulder joint and strengthen it.
The muscles, which form the cuff, are:
- Supraspinatus
- Infraspinatus
- Teres minor
- Subscapularis.

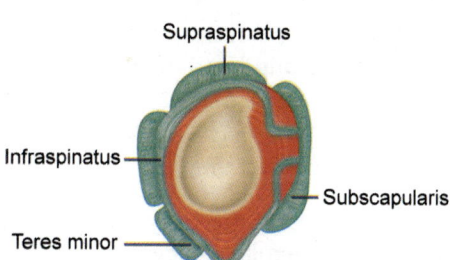

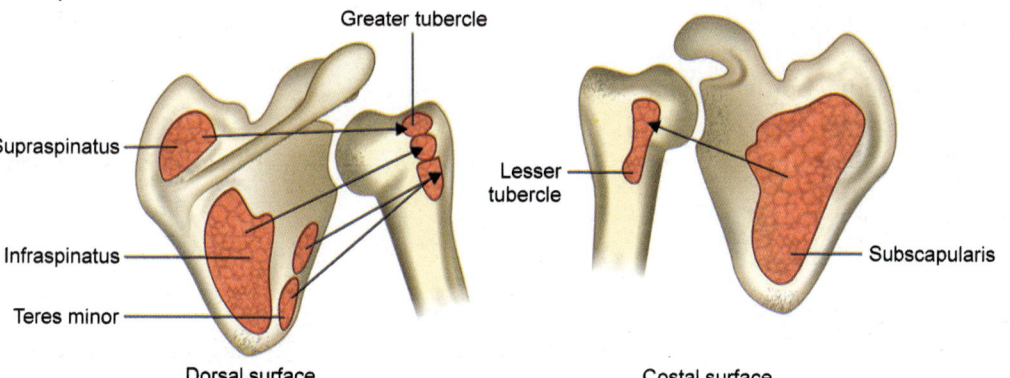

Rotator cuff muscle attachments

The muscles forming the cuff arise from scapula and get inserted onto the greater and lesser tubercles of humerus. The cuff strengthens the shoulder joint all around except inferiorly.

### Applied Anatomy

Inferior dislocations of shoulder joint are common, since:
- Capsule is lax (loose) inferiorly
- Cuff strengthens the joint all around except inferiorly.

### Q. Intermuscular spaces

**Ans.** There are three intermuscular spaces in the scapular region. They are given below.

### 1. Quadrangular Space

*Boundaries*

- *Superiorly:* Teres minor
- *Inferiorly:* Teres major
- *Medially:* Long-head of triceps
- *Laterally:* Surgical neck of humerus.

*Contents*

- Axillary nerve
- Posterior circumflex humeral vessels.

### 2. Upper Triangular Space

*Boundaries*

- *Medially:* Teres minor
- *Laterally:* Long-head of triceps
- *Inferiorly:* Teres major.

*Contents*

Circumflex scapular vessels.

### 3. Lower Triangular Space

*Boundaries*

- *Medially:* Long-head of triceps
- *Laterally:* Medial border of humerus
- *Superiorly:* Teres major.

*Contents*

- Radial nerve
- Profunda brachii vessels.

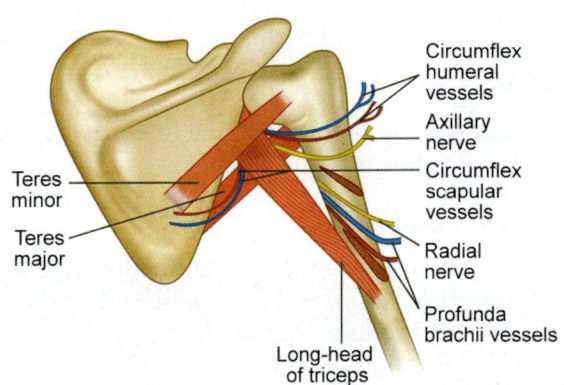

Intermuscular spaces in scapular region

### Q. Palmar interossei

**Ans.** There are four muscles placed between the shafts of metacarpal bones. They are numbered from lateral to medial side.

## Attachments

*From*

- I medial side of base of first metacarpal bone
- II medial half of the palmar aspect of the shaft of second metacarpal bone
- III lateral part of the palmar aspect of fourth metacarpal
- IV lateral part of the palmar aspect of the shaft of the fifth metacarpal.

*To*

- I medial side of the thumb
- II medial side of index finger
- III lateral side of fourth digit
- IV lateral side of fifth digit
- Middle finger has no insertion of any palmar interossei
- Each muscle is also inserted into dorsal digital expansion.

## Nerve Supply

All palmar interossei are supplied by deep branch of ulnar nerve.

## Action

All palmar interossei adduct the digits to the midline (**Mnemonic:** PAD).

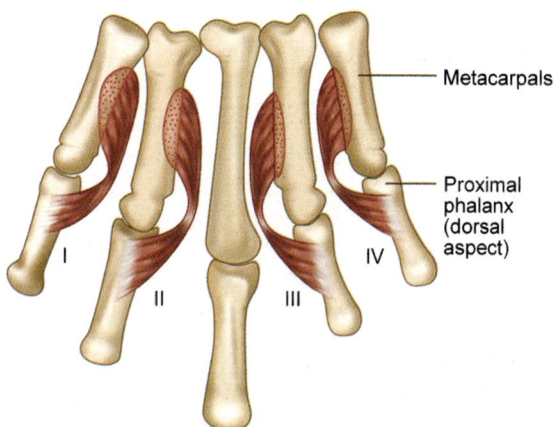

Palmar interossei attachments

## Q. Dorsal interossei

**Ans.** Dorsal interossei are four small muscles placed between the metacarpal bones.

## Attachments

*From*

- I shafts of first and second metacarpal
- II shafts of second and third metacarpal
- III shafts of third and fourth metacarpal
- IV shafts of fourth and fifth metacarpal.
- Each muscle is inserted into dorsal digital expansion and the base of proximal phalanx.

*To*

- I lateral side of index finger
- II lateral side of middle finger
- II medial side of middle finger
- IV medial side of fourth digit.

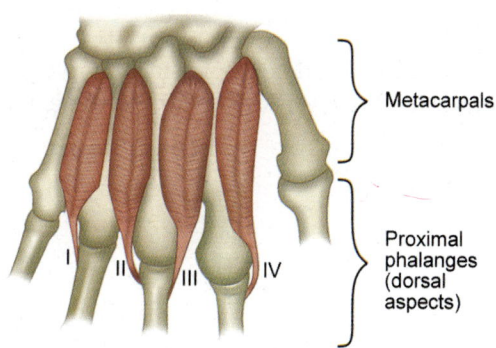

Dorsal interossei attachments

## Nerve Supply

All dorsal interossei are supplied by deep branch of ulnar nerve.

## Action

All dorsal interossei abduct the digits mnemonic (DAB).

## Applied Anatomy

- Paralysis of intrinsic muscles of the hand causes 'claw hand', in which there is hyperextension of metacarpophalangeal joints and flexion at interphalangeal joints
- Dorsal interossei are tested by asking the patient to spread out the fingers against resistance
- Palmar interossei are tested by placing a piece of paper in between the fingers (paper test).

### Q. Lumbricals

**Ans.** Lumbricals are four small muscles, which take origin from the tendons of flexor digitorum profundus.

## Attachments

*From*

- I lateral side of tendon of index finger
- II lateral side of tendon of middle finger
- III and IV adjacent sides of tendon of ring and little finger.

*To*

The tendons pass backwards on the lateral side of II, III, IV and V metacarpophalangeal joint to get inserted on the dorsal digital expansion.

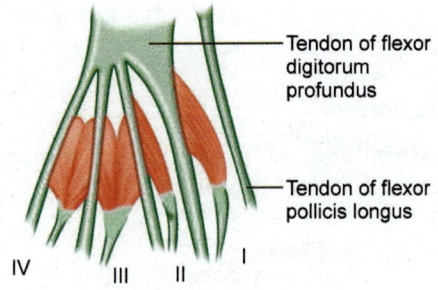

Tendon of flexor digitorum profundus

Tendon of flexor pollicis longus

IV　III　II　I

Lumbrical attachments

## Nerve Supply

- First and second supplied by median nerve
- Third and fourth supplied by deep branch of ulnar nerve.

## Action

The lumbricals flex the metacarpophalangeal joint and extend the interphalangeal joint (lumbricals connect the flexors to the extensors).

# NERVES

## Q. Axillary nerve

**Ans.** Axillary nerve is also known as circumflex humeral nerve.

### Origin

Axillary nerve is a branch of posterior cord of brachial plexus.

### Root Value

C5 and C6

### Course

Axillary nerve begins in the axilla and winds around the surgical neck of humerus. Thus, the nerve has a short course and ends by giving muscular, vascular, cutaneous and articular branches.

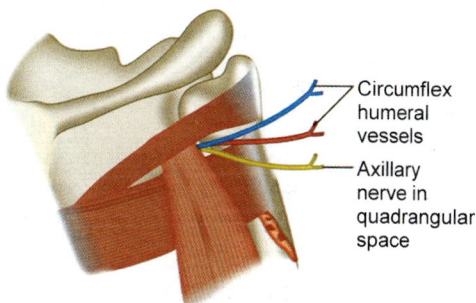

Axillary nerve in quadrangular scapular space

### Relations

In the axilla and upper arm, it is lateral to the radial nerve, posterior to the axillary artery and anterior to the subscapularis.

As it winds around the surgical neck of humerus, it passes through the quadrangular space. Quadrangular space is bounded by:
- *Superiorly:* Teres minor
- *Medially:* Long-head of triceps
- *Inferiorly:* Teres major.

### Branches

- Muscular branches to deltoid and teres minor
- Upper lateral cutaneous branch to the arm
- Articular branch to the shoulder joint
- Vascular branch to the posterior circumflex humeral artery.

### Applied Anatomy

Axillary nerve may get injured by dislocation of the shoulder joint or by fracture of the surgical neck of the humerus. Axillary nerve injury causes following disability:
- Loss of abduction at the shoulder joint
- Loss of contour of the shoulder
- Sensory loss over upper part of the arm.

## Q. Musculocutaneous nerve

**Ans.** Musculocutaneous nerve is the key nerve of the front of the arm.

## Origin

Musculocutaneous nerve is a branch of lateral cord of brachial plexus.

## Root Value

C5, C6, C7.

## Course

From the lower part of axilla, it courses downwards and laterally up to the middle third of arm, where it gives off muscular and cutaneous branches.

## Relations

Musculocutaneous nerve accompanies axillary artery in the axilla and pierces coracobrachialis before entering the arm. Following are the relations in axilla:

- *Anteriorly:* Pectoralis major
- *Posteriorly:* Subscapularis
- *Medially:* Axillary artery; lateral root of median nerve
- *Laterally:* Coracobrachialis.

In the arm, it runs downwards and laterally between biceps and brachialis and then gets lateral to the tendon of biceps.

It terminates by piercing the deep fascia 2 cm above the bend of forearm by becoming lateral cutaneous nerve of forearm.

Musculocutaneous nerve course and origin

## Branches

- Muscular branches to coracobrachialis, biceps and brachialis
- Cutaneous as the lateral cutaneous branch of the forearm
- Articular branch to the elbow joint
- A branch to the humerus, which enters along with the nutrient artery.

## Q. Ulnar nerve

**Ans.** Ulnar nerve is also described as 'musician nerve'.

## Origin

Ulnar nerve originates from the medial cord of brachial plexus.

## Root Value

C8, T1.

## Course

Overall the nerve lies on the medial side of arm and forearm.

From its origin in the axilla, it lies on the medial side of arm then runs downwards to lie behind the medial epicondyle and again on the medial side of the forearm and hand.

## Relations

In the axilla, the nerve lies medial to axillary artery and then medial to the brachial artery up to midarm, where the nerve pierces the medial intermuscular septum and runs distally to lie behind the medial epicondyle.

It enters the forearm between the two heads of flexor carpi ulnaris and descends on the medial side of the forearm on the flexor digitorum profundus; and 5 cm above the wrist, it gives off the dorsal cutaneous branch of hand.

It enters the hand by running superficial to flexor retinaculum and lateral to pisiform bone and terminates into superficial and deep branches.

## Branches

- Muscular branches to flexor carpi ulnaris and medial half of flexor digitorum profundus
- Palmar cutaneous branch supplies the skin over the hypothenar eminence and medial 1½ finger
- Dorsal branch supplies ulnar 2½ fingers and adjoining area of dorsum of hand
- Articular branch to the elbow joint and wrist
- Superficial terminal branch supplies palmaris brevis and medial palmar skin
- Deep terminal branch, which supplies adductor pollicis, all interossei, third and fourth lumbricals muscle of the hand.

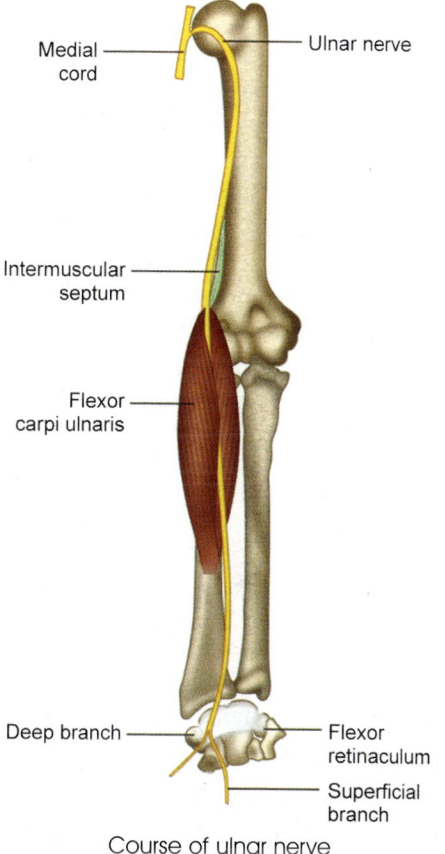

Course of ulnar nerve

## Applied Anatomy

Injury to ulnar nerve causes 'claw hand' involving mainly little and ring finger.

## Q. Median nerve

**Ans.** Median nerve is also described as 'labourer's nerve'.

## Origin

Median nerve has two roots of origin—one from lateral cord and another from medial cord.

## Root Value

C5, C6, C7, C8, T1.

## Course

Overall the nerve lies in the middle portion of arm and forearm in close relation to brachial artery and then enters the hand by-passing deep to the flexor retinaculum.

## Relations

The two roots unite either anterior or lateral to third part of axillary artery:

1. In the arm it lies initially lateral to brachial artery then it crosses the artery and becomes medial to the artery.
2. It enters the forearm between the two heads of pronator teres and lies lateral to the ulnar artery and descends between flexor digitorum superficialis and flexor digitorum profundus.
3. About 5 cm proximal to flexor retinaculum, it becomes superficial projecting laterally from behind the tendon of palmaris longus. It runs deep to flexor retinaculum to enter the palm and immediately terminates into medial and lateral branches.

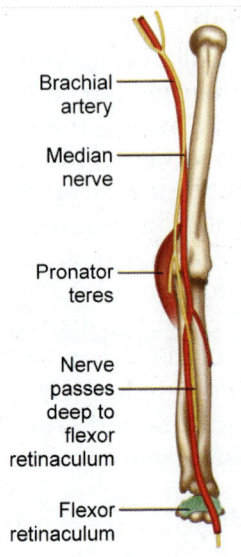

Median nerve origin and course

## Branches

- Muscular branches to superficial flexors of the forearm (except flexor carpi ulnaris) and lateral half of flexor digitorum profundus
- Muscular branches to thenar muscles in the hand
- Anterior interosseous nerve
- Palmar cutaneous branch
- Articular branch supplying elbow joint and proximal radioulnar joint.

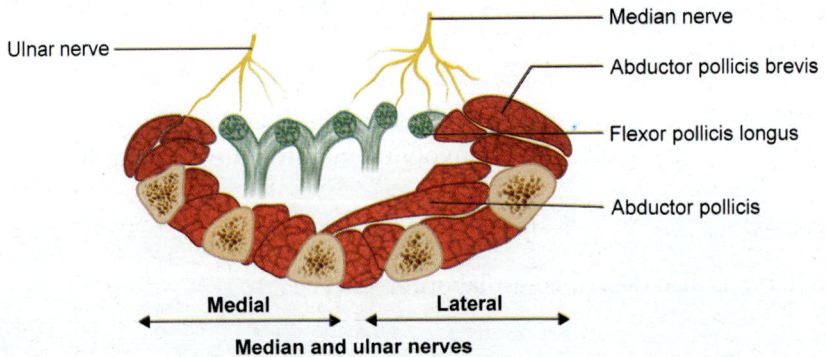

Median and ulnar nerves

## Applied Anatomy

1. *Ape thumb deformity:* In this deformity, the thumb lies in line with the other metacarpals due to paralysis of opponens pollicis.
2. *Pen test:* In this test, the patient keeps the palm on the table. If the patient cannot touch the pen kept above the palm it implies that abductor pollicis brevis is paralysed.
3. It is mainly responsible for coarse movements of the hand and hence, it is known as 'labourer's nerve'.

## Q. Cutaneous innervation of palm

**Ans.**

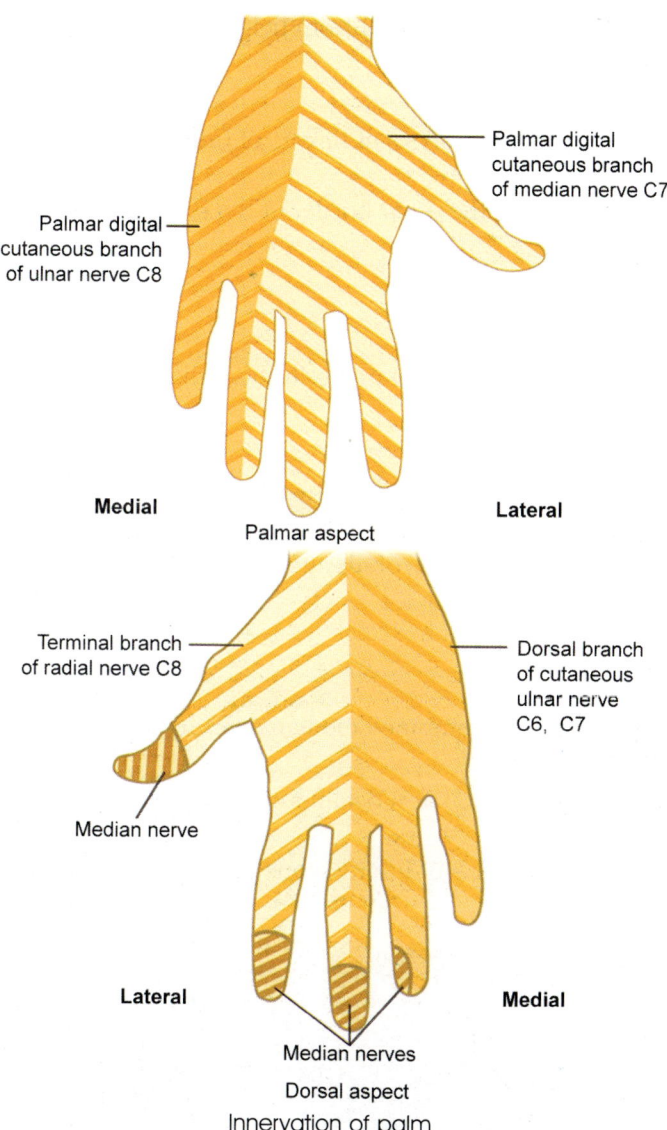

Palmar digital cutaneous branch of median nerve C7

Palmar digital cutaneous branch of ulnar nerve C8

**Medial**

**Lateral**

Palmar aspect

Terminal branch of radial nerve C8

Dorsal branch of cutaneous ulnar nerve C6, C7

Median nerve

**Lateral**

**Medial**

Median nerves

Dorsal aspect

Innervation of palm

## Q. Erb's paralysis

**Ans.** Erb's paralysis is an upper trunk brachial plexus injury:
- *Cause:* It is due to traction on arm at birth or fall on the shoulder
- *Roots:* Involved are C5, C6
- *Deformity:* Leads to typical 'porter tip' or 'policeman tip' deformity wherein arms hang by the side in adducted and medially rotated position (deltoid and lateral rotators are paralysed):
  – Extension of elbow (flexor paralysed)
  – Pronated forearm (supinator paralysed).

### Q. Klumpke's Paralysis

**Ans.** Klumpke's paralysis is due to lower trunk brachial plexus injury:
- *Cause:* Due to hyperabduction of arm (fall from height or birth injury)
- *Roots:* Involved are C8, T1
- *Deformity:*
  - Clawing of the hand due to paralysis of flexors of fingers, wrist and intrinsic muscles of the hand
  - Cutaneous anesthesia along the ulnar border of the forearm and hand
  - Horner's syndrome.

### Q. Wrist drop

**Ans.** Wrist drop is due to injury to radial nerve in the radial groove of humerus.
- *Cause:* It is due to midfracture of humerus
- *Roots:* Involved are C5, C6, C7, C8, T1
- *Deformity:* Hand is flexed at the wrist and is flaccid due to paralysis of extensors of elbow, wrist and interphalangeal joints along with supinator and brachioradialis.

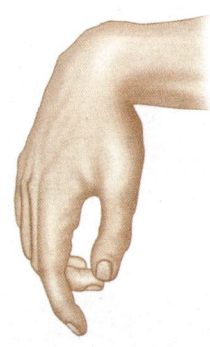

Wrist drop

### Q. Claw hand

**Ans.** Claw hand is a post effect of combined median and ulnar nerve lesion at elbow or lesion of medial cord of brachial plexus.

*Deformity:* There is hyperextension at wrist and metacarpophalangeal joints, and flexion at interphalangeal joint.

This deformity is due to paralysis of interosseous and lumbricals.

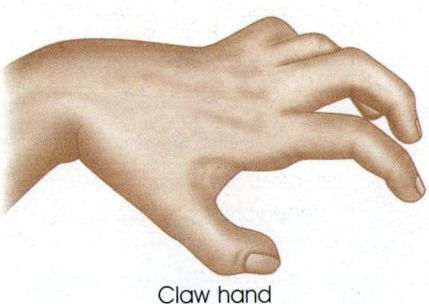

Claw hand

### Q. Carpal tunnel syndrome

**Ans.** Carpal tunnel syndrome is produced due to compression of median nerve in carpal tunnel.

Patient complains of painful paresthesia and numbness affecting the lateral 3½ fingers, which characteristically wakes up the patient at night because of tissue fluid accumulation. Patient also complains of inability to perform fine movements.

On examination, there is wasting of thenar eminence and hypoesthesia over radial 3½ fingers.

Skin over thenar eminence is not affected, since it is supplied by palmar cutaneous branch of median nerve, which takes origin proximal to carpal tunnel. Nerve conduction studies help to diagnose carpal tunnel syndrome.

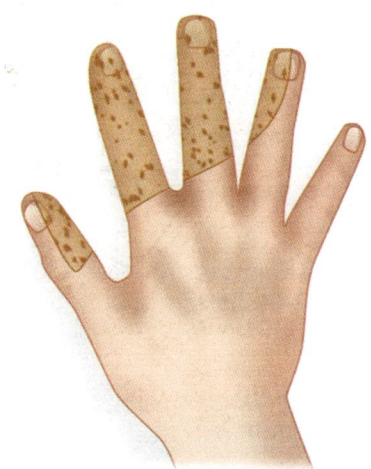

Area of sensory loss following division of median nerve

## ARTERIES

### Q. Scapular anastomosis

**Ans.** Scapular anastomosis occurs between first part of subclavian artery and third part of axillary artery.

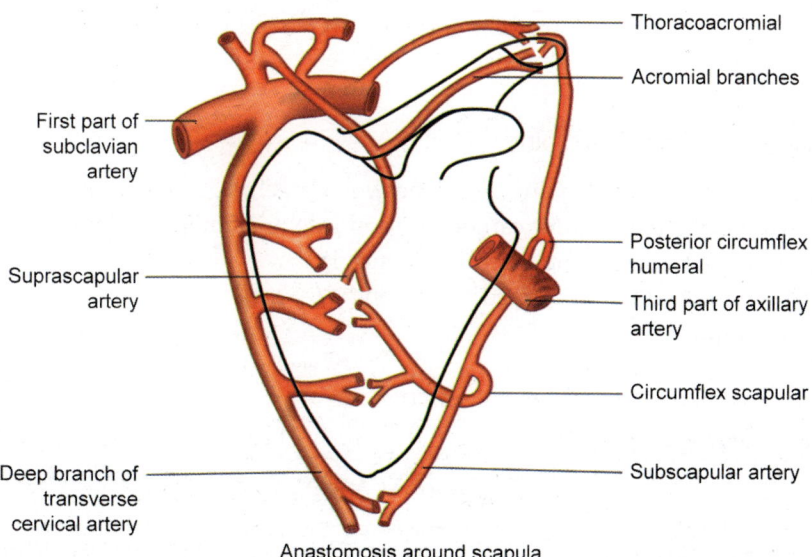

Anastomosis around scapula

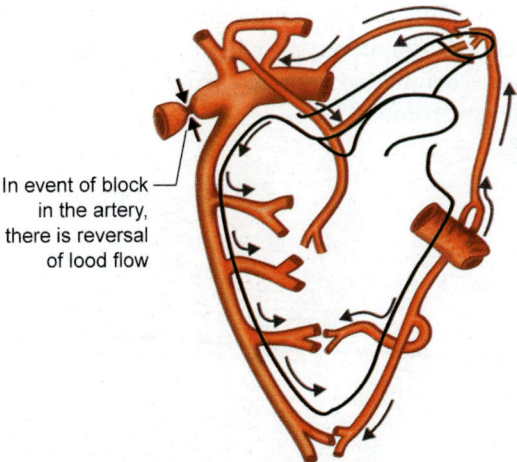

In event of block in the artery, there is reversal of lood flow

Functional anastomosis in event of block

Anastomosis over the scapula can be divided into anastomosis in two areas:
- Anastomosis around the body of scapula
- Anastomosis around the acromion process.

1. **Anastomosis around body of scapula occurs between following branches:**
   a. **First part of subclavian artery**            **Third part of axillary artery**
      - Suprascapular                                Posterior circumflex humeral
      - Deep branch of transverse cervical           Subscapular

2. **Anastomosis around acromion process:**
   a. Suprascapular                                  Posterior circumflex humeral
   b. Thoracoacromial.

### Surgical Importance

In event of blockage of any of the artery mentioned above in figure, blood can still flow to the upper limb through scapular anastomosis.

### Q. Anastomosis around elbow joint

**Ans.** Anastomosis around elbow joint occurs between brachial, radial and ulnar arteries. Anastomosis around the elbow joint can be divided into anastomosis in three areas:
1. Anastomosis in front and behind lateral epicondyle
2. Anastomosis in front and behind medial epicondyle
3. Above the olecranon process.

### Anastomosis in Front and Behind Lateral Epicondyle

| Front of lateral epicondyle | Behind lateral epicondyle |
|---|---|
| From above—anterior descending branch of profunda brachii | From posterior—descending branch of profunda brachii |
| From below—radial recurrent | From below—interosseous recurrent |

## Anastomosis in Front and Behind Medial Epicondyle

| Front of medial epicondyle | Behind medial epicondyle |
|---|---|
| From above—inferior ulnar collateral | From above—superior ulnar collateral |
| From below—anterior ulnar recurrent | From below—posterior ulnar recurrent |

## Above the Olecranon Process

A descending branch of profunda brachii anastomoses with a branch from inferior ulnar collateral artery.

## Surgical Importance

Due to rich collateral system around the elbow occlusion of brachial artery does not cause gangrene of the distal portion of the limb. However, laborers may experience forearm claudication (pain) during strenuous work.

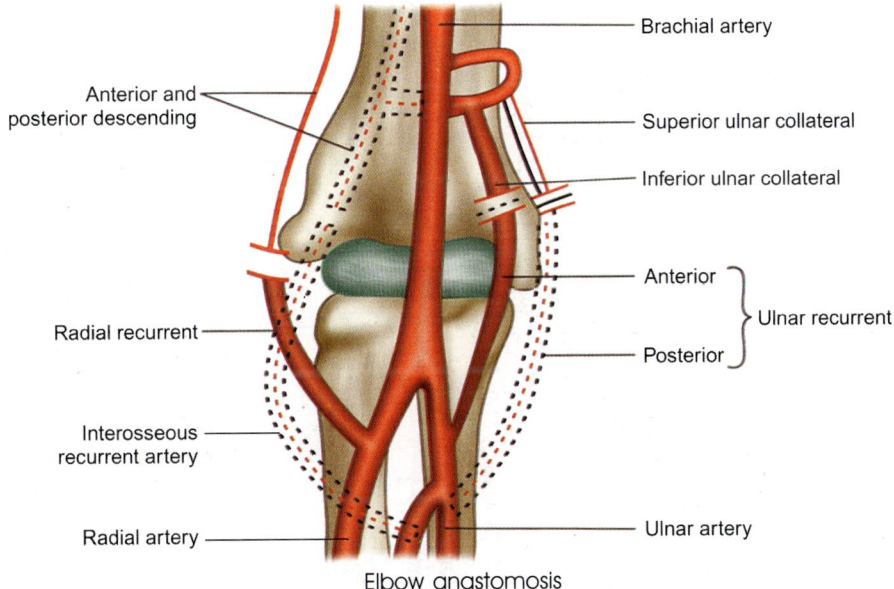

Elbow anastomosis

## Q. Superficial and deep palmar arch

**Ans.** Superficial and deep palmar arch represents anastomosis between radial and ulnar arteries.

## Superficial Palmar Arch

### Formation

Superficial palmar arch is a direct continuation of ulnar artery beyond flexor retinaculum. On the lateral side, it is completed by one of the following branches of radial artery:
- Superficial palmar branch
- Radialis indicis
- Princeps pollicis.

*Relations*

Arch lies between palmaris brevis, palmar aponeurosis in front and flexor tendons behind.

*Branches*

Digital branches supply medial 3½ fingers.

## Deep Palmar Arch

*Formation*

Deep palmar arch is a continuation of radial artery beyond the gap between the two heads of adductor pollicis. It is completed by deep branch of ulnar artery.

*Relations*

The arch lies at the level of proximal border of extended thumb. The deep branch of ulnar nerve lies within its concavity.

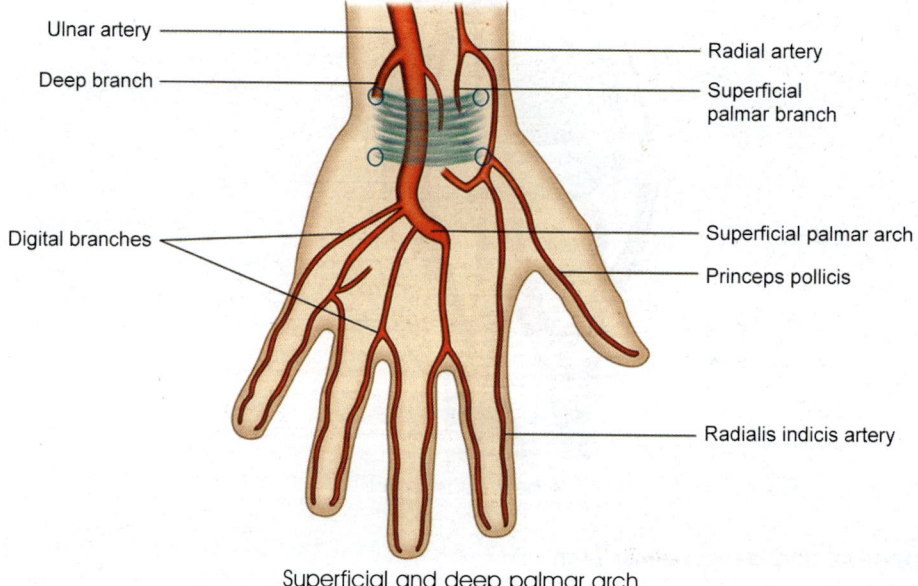

Superficial and deep palmar arch

*Branches*

- Three palmar metacarpal arteries
- Three perforating branches
- Recurrent branches.

*Surgical Importance*

In direct wounds of palmar arches, ligation of one of the forearm artery may be ineffective due to anastomosis between radial and ulnar arteries.

# VEINS

### Q. Cephalic vein

**Ans.** Cephalic vein is preaxial vein of the upper limb and is superficial.

## Course

Cephalic vein begins from lateral end of dorsal venous arch and courses laterally upwards to end in axillary vein.

## Relations

1. Cephalic vein runs upwards through the roof of anatomical snuffbox, winds around the lateral border of distal forearm to appear in front of elbow and lateral to biceps brachii.
2. After piercing the deep fascia at the lower border of pectoralis major, it lies in the deltopectoral groove.
3. It reaches the infraclavicular fossa, where it pierces clavipectoral fascia.
4. At the elbow, most of the venous blood is directed into the basilic vein via median cubital vein.
5. Lateral cutaneous nerve of forearm accompanies cephalic vein.

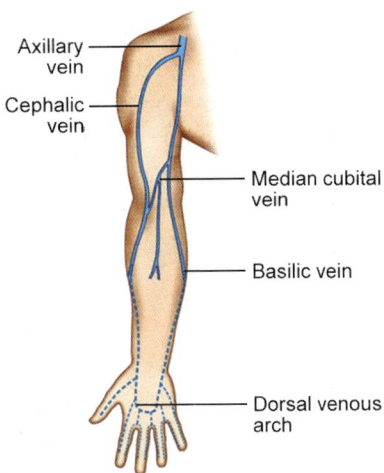

Veins of upper limb

## Applied Anatomy

Cephalic vein many times communicates with the external jugular vein by means of a small vein in front of clavicle. In radical surgeries, when axillary vein is sacrificed, this communicating vein enlarges and drains the complete upper limb.

### Q. Basilic vein

**Ans.** Basilic vein is the postaxial vein of upper limb and is superficial.

## Course

Basilic vein begins from the medial end of dorsal venous arch and runs along back of medial border of forearm to wind the elbow to continue in front till middle of the arm where it pierces the deep fascia to drain into axillary vein.

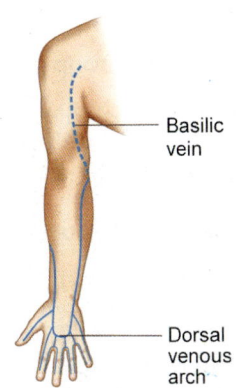

Basilic vein of upper limb

## Relations

1. Basilic vein lies along the medial side of brachial artery up to the lower border of teres major.
2. A few centimetres above the elbow it is joined by the median cubital vein.
3. It is accompanied by posterior branch of medial cutaneous nerve of the forearm.

## Applied Anatomy

1. Veins of the upper limb provide good access for intravenous supplementation.
2. Venous graft (reverse side) can be used in surgeries like stapedectomy for closing oval window.

# LYMPH NODES

### Q. Axillary lymph nodes

**Ans.** Axillary lymph nodes are divided into five groups:
1. Anterior group (pectoral)
2. Posterior group (scapular)
3. Lateral group
4. Central group
5. Apical group (infraclavicular).

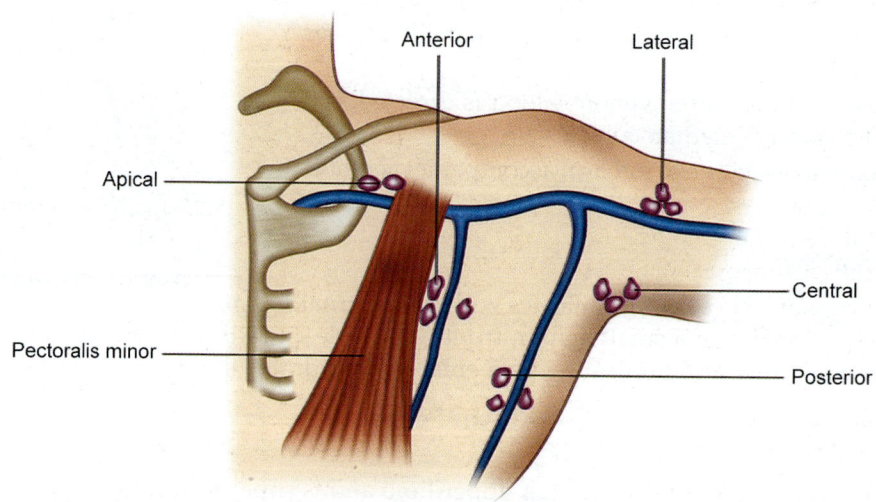

Axillary lymph nodes

## Anterior Group

Anterior group lymph node lies along lateral thoracic vein and are in direct contact with the axillary tail of the breast. They drain upper half of the anterior wall of the trunk and major part of the breast.

## Posterior Group

Posterior group lies along the subscapular vein and can be palpated along posterior fold of axilla. They drain upper half of the posterior wall of the trunk and axillary tail of breast.

## Lateral Group

Lateral group lies along the axillary vein in the upper part of the arm. It receives lymph from the upper limb.

## Central Group

Central group lies in the fat of axilla and is closely related to intercostobrachial nerve. They receive lymph from above-mentioned nodes.

## Apical Group

Apical group lies along the axillary vein and receives lymph from central group, upper part of breast and thumb.

## Applied Anatomy

- Axillary abscess may arise due to suppuration of lymph nodes
- Malignancy involving drainage areas of axillary lymph nodes can give rise to enlargement of lymph nodes.

### Q. Lymphatic drainage of breast

**Ans.** Breast cancer is staged depending upon the number, size and fixity of axillary lymph nodes. Treatment of breast cancer is planned according to the stage of the disease. Lymph from the breast drains into following group of lymph nodes:

- 70% drains into axillary lymph nodes
- 20% drains into internal mammary lymph nodes
- 5% drains into posterior intercostal lymph nodes
- The axillary lymph nodes and the internal mammary lymph nodes are involved comparatively early; only later the supraclavicular lymph nodes, the opposite breast and the mediastinum are involved
- Some lymph reaches subdiaphragmatic and subperitoneal lymph plexus.

## Lymphatic Vessels of the Breast

Superficial lymphatics drain the skin over the breast except the nipple and areola. Deep lymphatics drain the parenchyma of the breast, areola and nipple.

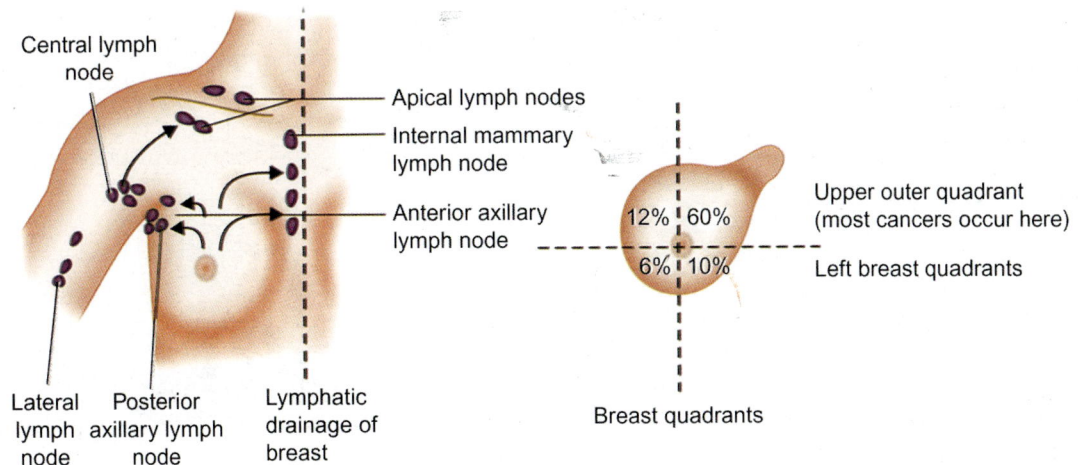

Central lymph node

Apical lymph nodes

Internal mammary lymph node

Anterior axillary lymph node

Upper outer quadrant (most cancers occur here)

12% | 60%

6% | 10%

Left breast quadrants

Lateral lymph node    Posterior axillary lymph node    Lymphatic drainage of breast

Breast quadrants

## Virchow's Node

Virchow's node is an enlarged left supraclavicular node infiltrated with metastatic cancer from gastrointestinal tract (GIT) predominantly. Metastases to supraclavicular nodes also occurs from lungs, breast or genital cancers.

## JOINT

### Q. Radioulnar joints

**Ans. Superior Radioulnar Joint**

*Type*

Pivot type of synovial joint.

*Articular Surfaces*

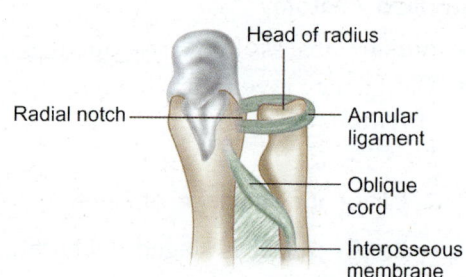

Superior radioulnar joint

They are:
- Head of radius
- Radial notch on ulna and annular ligament.

*Ligaments*

Ligaments joining the articular surfaces are annular ligament and quadrate ligament.
- Annular ligament: It encircles the head of radius and is attached to radial notch of ulna and capsule of elbow joint
- Quadrate ligament: Extends from neck of radius to radial notch.

*Nerve Supply*

- Musculocutaneous nerve
- Median nerve
- Ulnar nerve.

*Blood Supply*

Elbow anastomosis.

*Action*

The actions include:
- Pronation
- Supination.

### Inferior Radioulnar Joint

*Type*

Pivot type of synovial joint.

*Articular Surfaces*

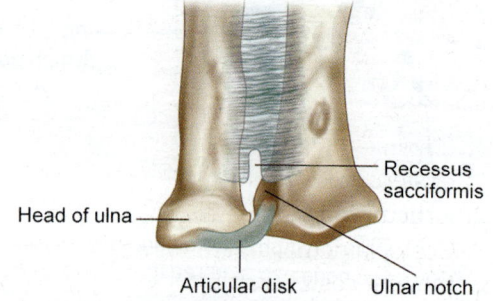

They are:
- Head of ulna
- Ulnar notch on radius.

*Ligaments*

Ligaments joining the articular surfaces are given below:
- Capsular ligament: Surrounds the joint
- Articular disk: Extends from base of styloid process to ulnar notch.

*Blood Supply*

Interosseous vessels.

*Nerve Supply*

Interosseous nerve.

*Actions*

- Pronation
- Supination.

## Q. Sternoclavicular joint

**Ans.**

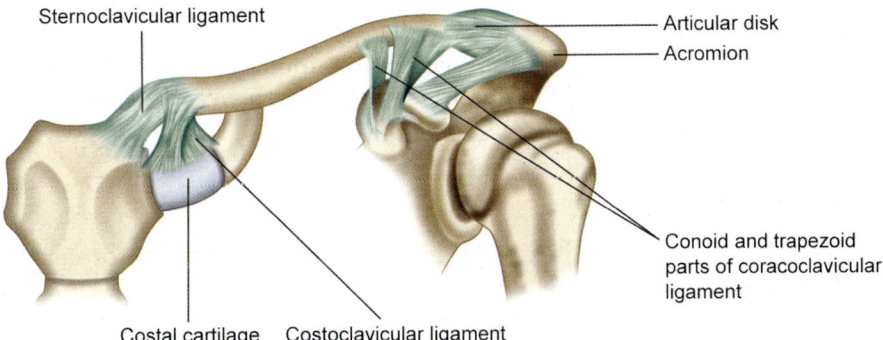

## Type
- Synovial joint
- Compound joint
- Complex joint.

## Articulating Bones
- Medial end of clavicle
- Clavicular notch of manubrium sterni
- Upper surface of first costal cartilage.

## Ligaments
1. Capsule is attached laterally to the margins of medial end of clavicle. Medially to the margins of sternum and on first costal cartilage.
2. Articular disk is the key bond between articular surfaces.
3. Costoclavicular ligament is attached above to the medial end of clavicle and inferiorly to the first costal cartilage.

## Nerve Supply

Medial supraclavicular nerve.

## Blood Supply

Internal thoracic and suprascapular vessels.

## Movements

1. Movements do not occur singularly at sternoclavicular joint, but collectively at the shoulder girdle.
2. Shrugging off shoulders, i.e. elevation of scapula is brought about by trapezius and levator scapula.
3. Depression of scapula is brought about by lower fibres of serratus anterior and pectoralis minor.
4. Pushing and punching movements are brought about by serratus anterior and pectoralis minor.
5. Retraction of scapula is brought about by rhomboids and trapezius.

## Applied Anatomy

- Clavicle by and large gets dislocated at its medial end
- The weight of the upper limb is transmitted from scapula to clavicle through coracoclavicular ligament and from clavicle to the first rib by costoclavicular ligament
- The clavicle fracture is often between these two ligaments.

### Q. Abduction at shoulder joint

**Ans.** Abduction at shoulder joint is a complex movement which can for convenience be separated into two coordinated movements.

$$[Total—120°(90° + 30°)]$$

## Movement at Glenohumeral Joint

Allows about 120° of abduction being limited by impingement of the greater tubercle of the humerus on the acromion process.

Abduction at glenohumeral joint is a coordinated movement involving deltoid muscle and the rotator cuff:

1. Rotator cuff holds the head in the socket.
2. Deltoid with supraspinatus brings about abduction.
3. Deltoid plus supraspinatus allows only 90° of abduction. Further movement is restricted due to the impingement of greater tubercle of humerus on the acromion.

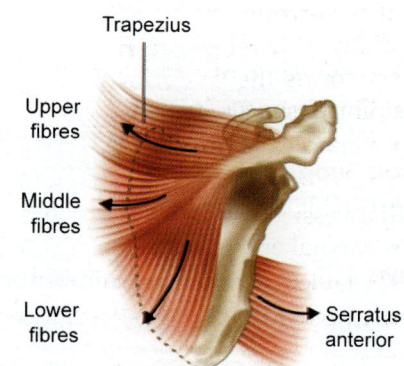

Muscles bringing about scapular rotation

4. Further 30° abduction takes place only when the humerus rotates externally so that greater tubercle lies posterior acromion.
5. Infraspinatus and teres minor also act as short external rotators. While subscapularis as internal rotator.

## Movement at Scapulothoracic Linkage

1. Upward rotation of scapula is accomplished by synchronous action of two muscles—trapezius and serratus anterior.
2. Basic action of trapezius is to rotate the scapula resulting in the glenoid fossa pointing upwards.
3. This upward rotation of scapula brings about further abduction.

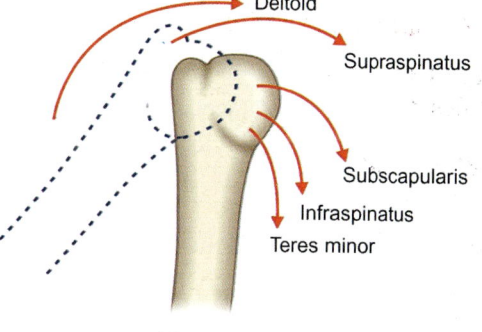

Muscle couple

### Q. First carpometacarpal joint

**Ans. Type**

Synovial joint—saddle variety.

## Articulating Surfaces

- Distal surface of trapezium
- Proximal surface of the base of first metacarpal bone.

## Peculiarity

First carpometacarpal joint has a separate joint cavity.

## Ligaments

*Capsular ligament:* It surrounds the joint and binds the articulating surfaces. It is thick, but loose.

Lateral, anterior and posterior ligament: All these ligaments strengthen the joint capsule.

## Relation

Joint is surrounded by muscles going to the thumb. Medially, it is related to first dorsal interossei. Radial artery forms the posterior relation of the joint in the anatomical snuffbox.

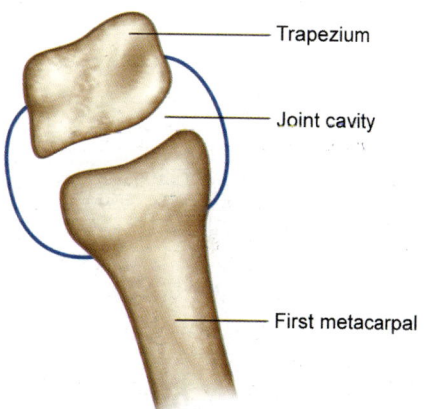

First carpometacarpal joint cavity

## Blood Supply

Radial vessels.

## Nerve Supply

Median nerve.

## Movement

1. Flexion and extension is brought about by the flexor pollicis tendons and extensor pollicis tendons respectively.
2. Adduction and abduction brought about by muscles supplying the pollex.
3. Opposition is brought about by mainly opponens muscle.
4. Circumduction is combination of above movements.

# MISCELLANEOUS

## Q. Clavipectoral fascia

**Ans.** Clavipectoral fascia is a bilaminar fibrous sheath extending from clavicle to axillary fascia. It lies deep to the clavicular portion of pectoralis major muscle.

### Attachments

- Medially, it is attached to the first rib and costoclavicular ligament
- Laterally, it is attached to the coracoid process and coracoclavicular ligament
- Above it splits to enclose subclavius muscle
- Below it splits to enclose pectoralis minor muscle
- Behind it merges with investing layer of deep cervical fascia.

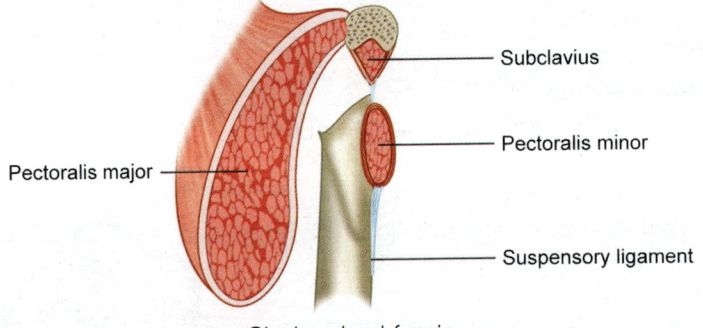

Clavipectoral fascia

### Structures Piercing Clavipectoral Fascia

- Lateral pectoral nerve
- Cephalic vein
- Thoracoacromial vessels
- Lymphatics passing from the breast and pectoral region to the apical group of axillary lymph nodes.

## Q. Coracoid process

**Ans.** Literal meaning of coracoid is 'bird's beak-like'. It is an atavistic type of epiphysis. It is a projection on costal surface of scapula.

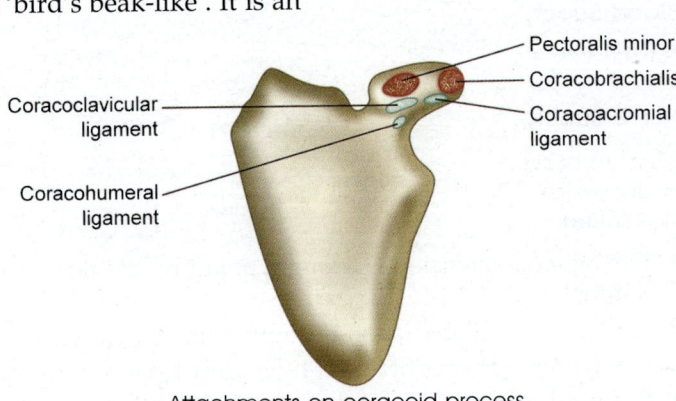

Attachments on coracoid process

### Attachments

1. *Muscles:*
   - Pectoralis minor
   - Coracobrachialis.
2. *Ligaments:*
   - Coracoclavicular
   - Coracoacromial
   - Coracohumeral.

### Q. Cubital fossa

**Ans.** Cubital fossa is a triangular hollow in front of the elbow.

### Boundaries

- *Base:* An imaginary line joining the two epicondyles
- *Laterally:* Medial border of the brachioradialis
- *Medially:* Lateral border of pronator teres
- *Apex:* Intersection of medial and lateral border.

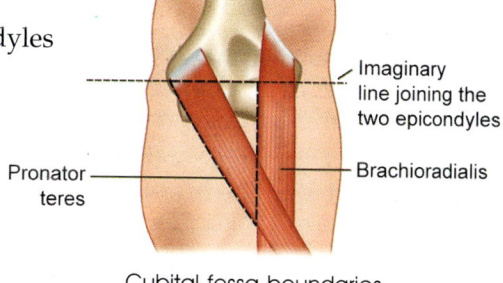

Cubital fossa boundaries

### Roof

- Basilic vein
- Cephalic vein
- Median cubital vein
- Medial and lateral cutaneous nerve of forearm.

### Floor

- Brachialis muscle
- Supinator muscle.

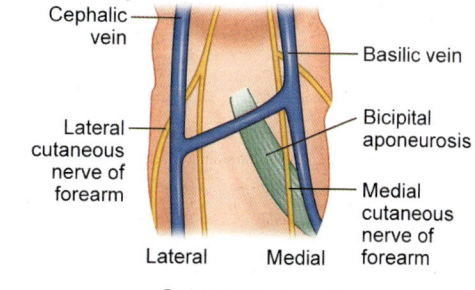

Cubital fossa roof

### Contents

- Termination of brachial artery
- Origin of radial and ulnar arteries
- Tendon of biceps brachii muscle
- Radial nerve
- Median nerve.

### Applied Anatomy

- Median cubital vein is an easily accessible vein for injecting intravenous fluids
- Blood pressure is recorded by auscultating brachial artery.

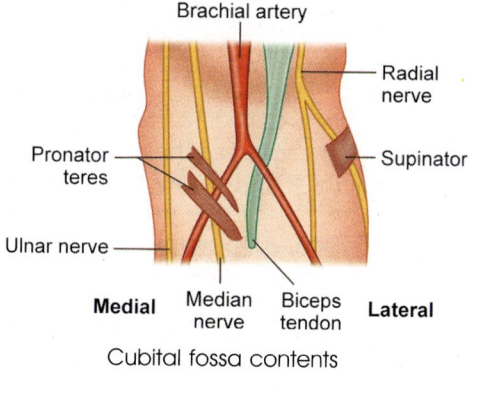

Cubital fossa contents

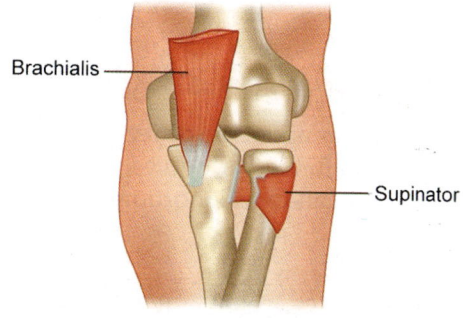

Cubital fossa floor

## Q. Flexor retinaculum

**Ans.** Flexor retinaculum is fibrous sheath, which connects the corner carpal bones and converts the anterior concavity into a tunnel (when one holds a ball in the hand the depression in between the thenar and hypothenar eminence marks the flexor retinaculum).

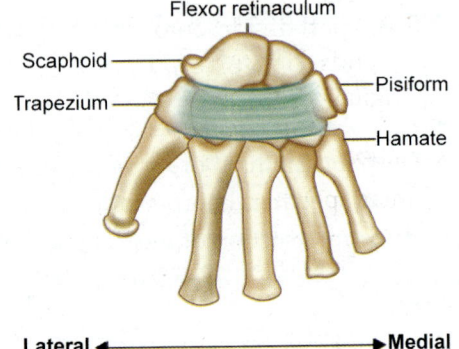

### Attachments

- *Medially:* Pisiform bone and hook of hamate
- *Laterally:* Tubercle of scaphoid and crest of trapezium.

### Relations

Structures passing superficial and deep to flexor retinaculum are:

| Superficial | Deep |
|---|---|
| Tendon of palmaris longus | Median nerve |
| Palmar cutaneous branch of median and ulnar nerve | Tendon of flexor digitorum superficialis and profundus |
| Ulnar vessels | Tendon of flexor pollicis longus |
|  | Radial and ulnar bursa |

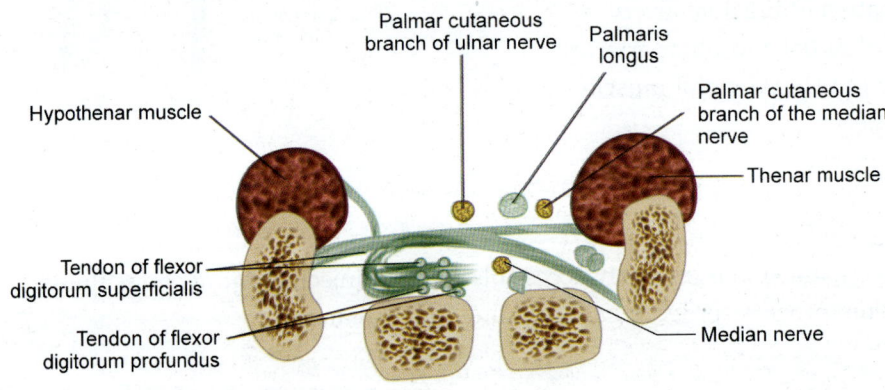

Relation of flexor retinaculum

## Q. Palmar aponeurosis

**Ans.** Palmar aponeurosis represents the deep fascia like in any other part of the body and is superficial to vessels, nerves, muscles and tendons. It has central thick and strong portion and lateral thin and weak portion.

### Peculiarities

1. It is derived from palmaris longus tendon.
2. Proximally, it is attached to flexor retinaculum.

3. Distally, it divides opposite to the heads of metacarpals into four slips. Each slip has a superficial and deep part. The superficial part is attached to the skin of palm and fingers, and deep part divides into two processes, which are continuous with the fibrous flexor sheaths.
4. It sends slips to deep transverse metacarpal ligament.
5. Digital vessels, nerves and tendons of lumbricals pass through the interval between the slips.

## Function

Palmar aponeurosis improves the grip of the hand.

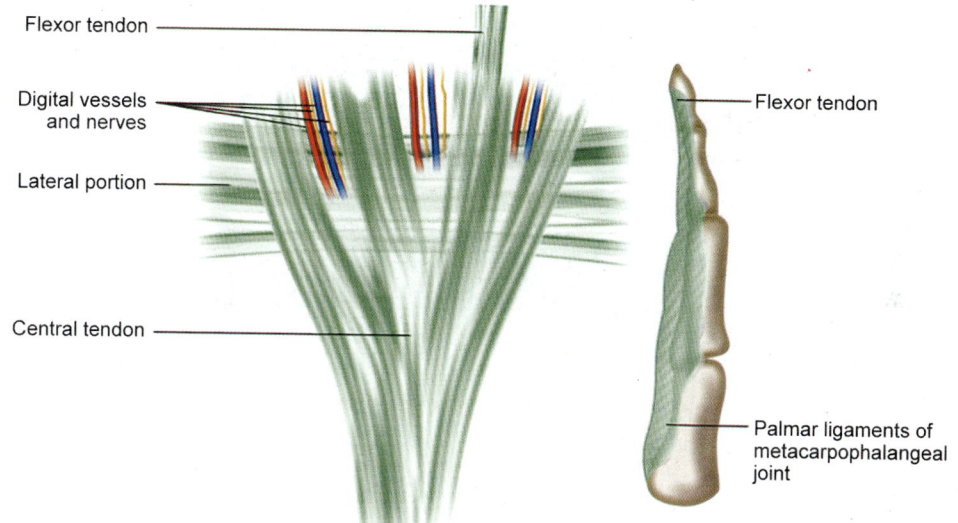

Palmar aponeurosis (parts and attachments)

## Applied Anatomy

Attachments of palmar aponeurosis are of surgical importance, in pathological contracture of palmar fascia (Dupuytren's contracture). In this condition, the proximal and intermediate phalanges of the fingers are acutely flexed because palmar fascia is attached to them. The distal phalanx remains extended as the fascia has no attachment to it.

## Q. Interosseous membrane

**Ans.** The interosseous membrane connects the shafts of the radius and ulna (appears very shiny in the cadaver).

- It is attached to the interosseous borders of radius and ulna
- The fibres run downwards, forward and medially (like hands in the pocket).

## Functions

- It connects the radius to the ulna
- It provides base for attachments of muscles
- It transmits the force applied to the radius.

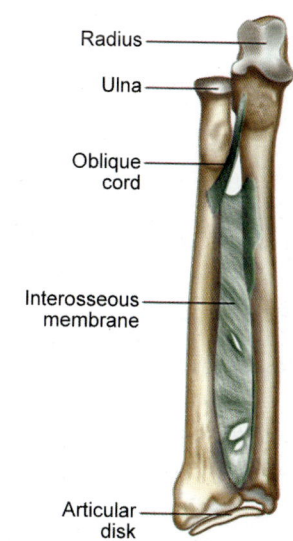

Interosseous membrane

## Q. Anatomical snuffbox

**Ans.** Anatomical snuffbox can be appreciated in fully extended thumb. In earlier days, during dissections, anatomists would keep the snuff in this depression. Hence, it is known as anatomical snuffbox.

### Roof

Cephalic vein, skin, superficial fascia, cutaneous branches of radial nerve.

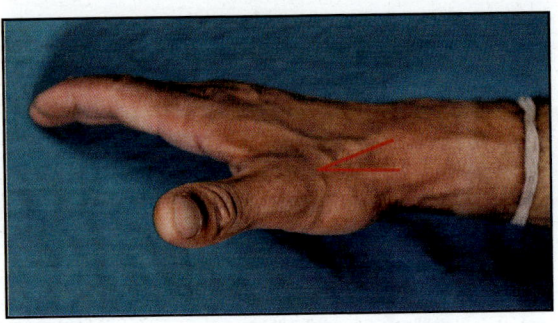

### Boundaries

- *Anteriorly:* Extensor pollicis brevis tendon and abductor pollicis longus tendon
- *Posteriorly:* Extensor pollicis longus tendon.

### Floor

*Scaphoid bone:* Tubercle, radial styloid, trapezium, base of thumb metacarpal.

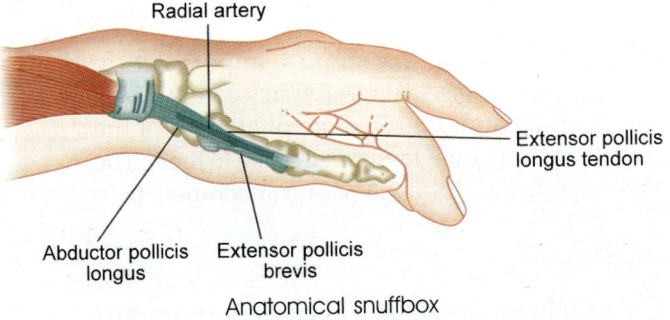

Anatomical snuffbox

### Contents

Radial artery.

### Surgical Importance

- Tenderness can be elicited in this area in cases of scaphoid bone fracture due to out stretched hand injury
- One needs to retract the tendons in this area and incise the radial collateral ligament to approach wrist joint from lateral side.

## Q. Carrying angle

**Ans.** Carrying angle is a peculiar feature of the elbow region. It is produced due to:

1. Projection of medial trochlear edge about 6 mm beyond its lateral edge.

2. Obliquity of coronoid's superior articular surface.

When forearm is fully extended and supinated it diverges laterally forming the so called the 'carrying angle' with the arm.

Tilt of humeral and ulnar surface is almost the same thus, the angle disappears in full flexion.

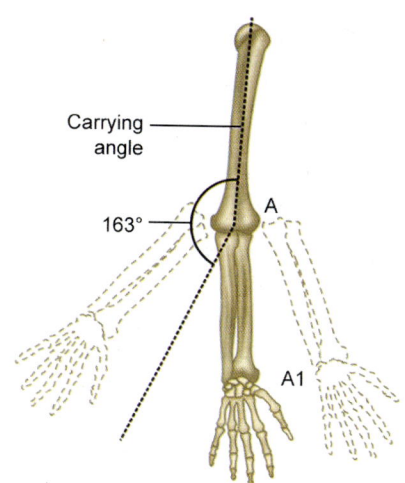

Formation of 'carrying angle'

### Applied Anatomy

- Carrying angle may vary in cases of fractures involving supracondylar area of humerus
- If the angle is increased it is known as cubitus valgus deformity
- Reversal of angle is known as cubitus varus deformity.

## Q. Extensor retinaculum

**Ans.** Extensor retinaculum is an oblique fibrous band on the back of wrist, which is nothing, but the modification of the deep fascia (like a friendship band). It holds the extensor tendons in position.

### Attachments

- Laterally, it is attached to lower 2–5 cm of the anterior border of radius
- Medially, it is attached to the triquetrum and pisiform.
- It is not attached to the lower end of ulna and thus it permits free movements of radius around ulna during pronation and supination.

### Peculiarities

1. The retinacula send down septa, which are attached to the longitudinal ridges on the radius. Thus, the back of the wrist is divided into six osteofascial compartments.
2. Each compartment is lined by synovial sheath.

## Q. Fibrous flexor sheath

**Ans.** Fibrous flexor sheath is the deep fascia of the digits. Proximally, it is continuous with the palmar aponeurosis.

### Peculiarities

- The sheath is thin against the interphalangeal joints
- It is arranged transversely across the phalanges and cruciate against the joint.

### Applied Anatomy

Tenosynovitis is an inflammatory condition of fibrous flexor sheath due to bacterial infection.

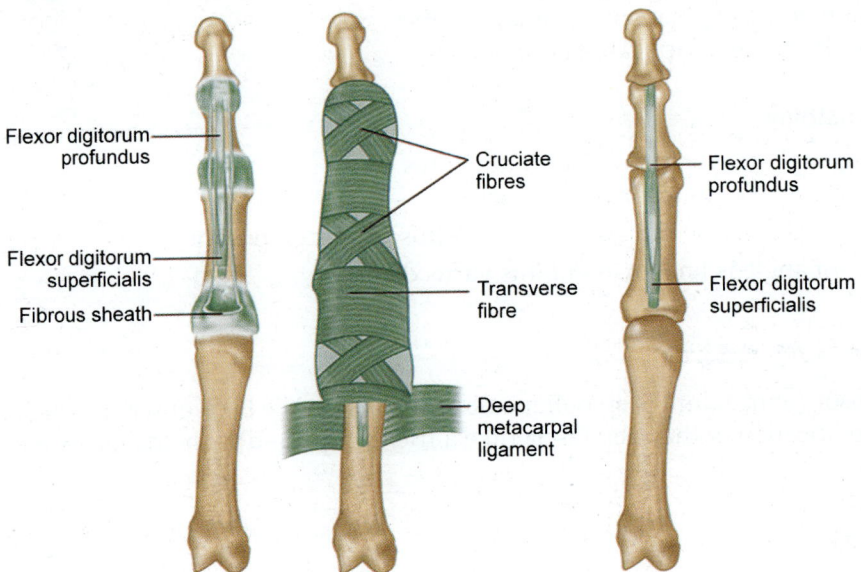

Arrangement of fibrous flexor sheath

## Q. Digital synovial sheath

**Ans.** Synovial sheaths line the flexor tendons of the digits.

### Arrangement

- Synovial sheaths of second, third and fourth digits are independent and terminate proximally at the level of head of the metacarpals
- Synovial sheath of little finger is continuous with the ulnar bursa
- Synovial sheath of thumb is continuous with the radial bursa.

### Applied Anatomy

- Infections of little finger and thumb can spread to the palm and distal forearm
- Incision to drain digital synovial sheath is taken on the distal interphalangeal crease

- To drain the ulnar bursa, an incision is taken along the lateral margin of hypothenar eminence
- To drain the radial bursa, an incision is taken along the medial margin of thenar eminence.

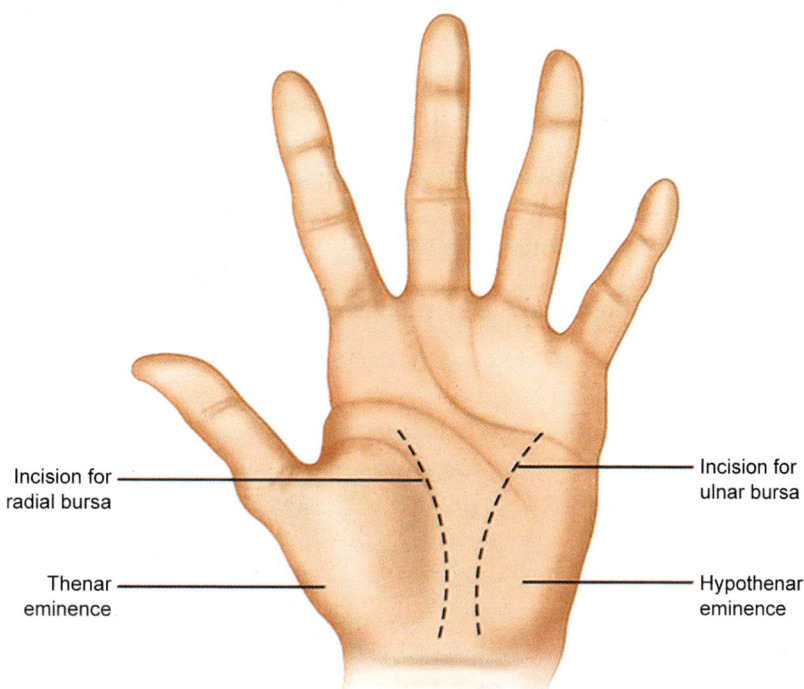

## Q. Dorsal digital expansion

**Ans.** Dorsal digital expansion is a hood-like fibrous expansion on the extensor aspect of the hand against the metacarpophalangeal joint. It receives insertion of dorsal interossei and lumbrical.

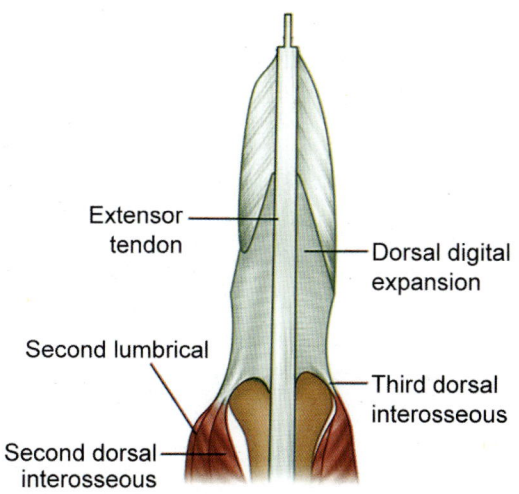

### Q. Space of whitlow

**Ans.** Space of whitlow is a space over the tip of the fingers and the thumb on its palmar aspect.

The fat in this region is divided into compartments by virtue of septae (fibrous strands) going from the skin to the periosteum of terminal phalanx. Terminal branch of digital artery passes through this space.

### Applied Anatomy

- Infection of this space gives rise to severe throbbing pain due to the typical arrangement of the septa
- The artery reaching the space is an end artery thus infection of this space can lead to tissue necrosis, if left untreated
- To drain the infection in this area, the incision is given laterally.

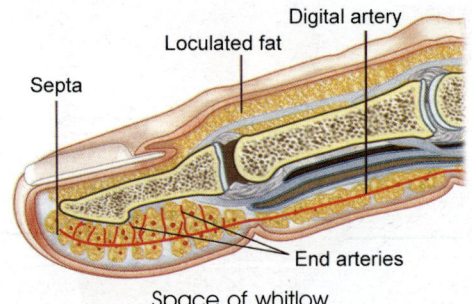

Space of whitlow

# Key Long Questions

**Q. Describe the formation and branches of brachial plexus. Add a note on its applied aspect.**

**Ans.** Brachial plexus is a network of nerves in the upper arm very close to the axillary artery. The parts of the brachial plexus can be simulated to parts of the tree (namely—roots, trunk and branches).

## Roots

Anterior primary rami of spinal nerves C5, C6, C7, C8, T1, contribute to the formation of brachial plexus (C4 and T2 may sometimes contribute in its formation).

## Trunks

- C5, C6 join to form upper trunk
- C7 forms middle trunk
- C8, T1 join to form lower trunk.

## Divisions

Each trunk bifurcates into anterior and posterior divisions.

## Cords

- Lateral cord is formed by the union of anterior division of upper and middle trunk
- Medial cord is continuation of anterior division of lower trunk
- Posterior divisions of all trunks form the posterior cord.

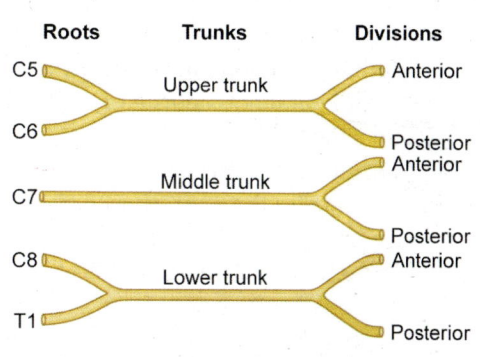

Framework of brachial plexus

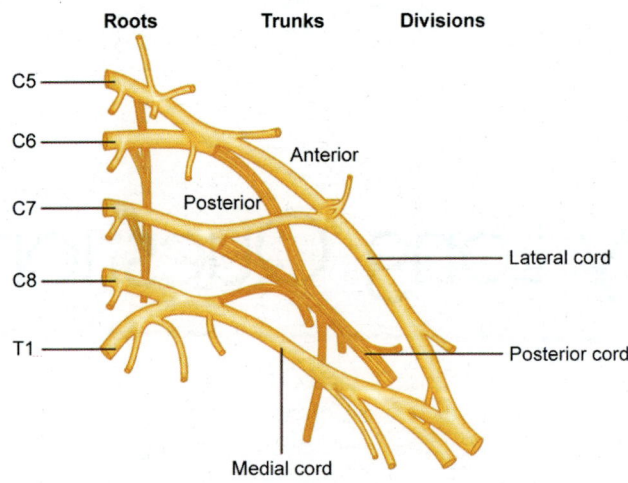

Brachial plexus showing trunk and cord formation

## Branches

Branches arise from the roots, trunk and cords of brachial plexus.

- Branches from the roots are:
  - Nerve to serratus anterior
  - Nerve to rhomboids.
- Branches from the trunk are:
  - Suprascapular nerve
  - Nerve to subclavius.
- Branches from the lateral cord are:
  - Lateral pectoral nerve
  - Musculocutaneous nerve
  - Lateral root of median nerve.

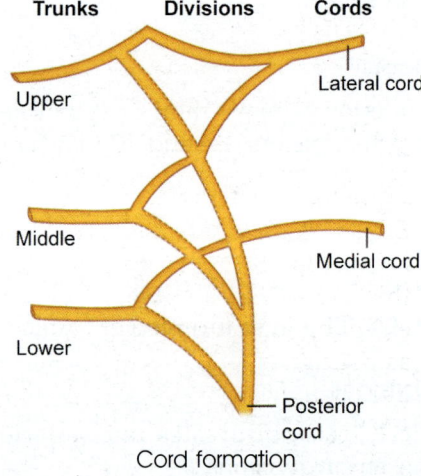

Cord formation

| Mnemonic |
| --- |
| Love me Lucy |
| L—Lateral pectoral nerve |
| M—Musculocutaneous nerve |
| L—Lateral root of median nerve |

- Branches from the medial cord are:
  - Medial pectoral nerve
  - Medial cutaneous nerve of arm
  - Medial cutaneous nerve of forearm
  - Ulnar nerve
  - Medial root of median nerve.
- Branches from the posterior cord are:
  - Upper subscapular
  - Nerve to latissimus dorsi
  - Lower subscapular
  - Axillary nerve
  - Radial nerve.

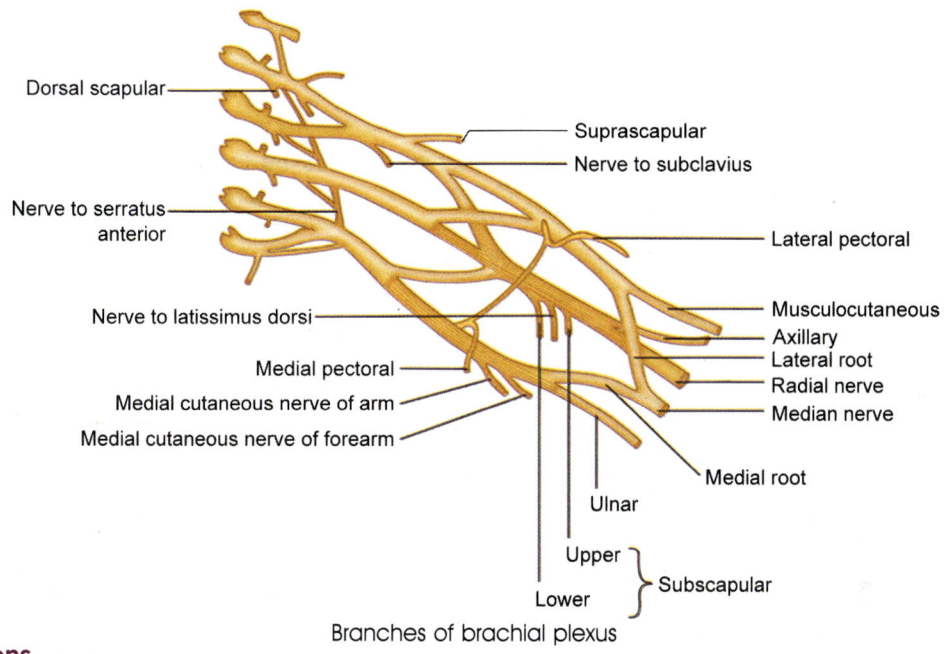

Branches of brachial plexus

## Relations

Axillary vessels lie entangled within the cords and branches of brachial plexus.

### Brachial Plexus Injuries

1. *Horner's syndrome:* Injury at the root of brachial plexus leads to Horner's syndrome. It is characterised by miosis (contraction of pupil), ptosis (drooping of eyelid), enophthalmos (sunken eyeball) and anhidrosis (lack of sweating).
2. *Erb's paralysis:* It is due to injury of upper trunk at Erb's point (compare in neck Erbs' point, p-614). Erb's point is a conglomeration of six nerves. It is here that the upper trunk usually stretches. In this deformity, the upper limb is adducted, extended and pronated. It is popularly known as policeman's tip or porter tip deformity (it is like trying to take tips secretly).
3. *Klumpke's paralysis:* It is due to injury of lower trunk of brachial plexus. Deformity produced due to lower trunk injury is claw hand, anesthesia over the ulnar border of forearm and hand.
4. *Injury to nerve supplying serratus anterior muscle:* It leads to 'winging of scapula'. In this deformity, the medial border of scapula becomes prominent. The patient cannot perform pushing and punching movements and cannot abduct the arm.
5. Cords can get injured due to dislocation of humerus. Injury to lateral cord will amount to loss of flexion of forearm. Injury to medial cord will amount to claw hand mainly.

> ### Q. Describe axillary artery in detail (origin, parts, relations and branches).

**Ans.** Axillary artery is the principal artery of the upper limb.

## Origin

Axillary artery is a continuation of subclavian artery.

## Extent

Axillary artery extends from outer border of first rib to lower border of teres major.

## Parts

For the sake of simplification, axillary artery is divided into three parts by 'pectoralis minor muscle'.

## Relations

Axillary artery is closely related to cords and branches of brachial plexus (roots and trunks of brachial plexus are not related to the axillary artery). In fact, the cords and branches entangle the axillary artery.

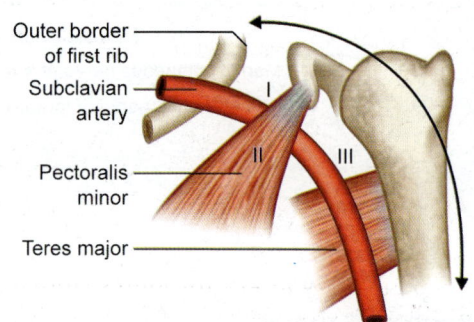

Parts of axillary artery

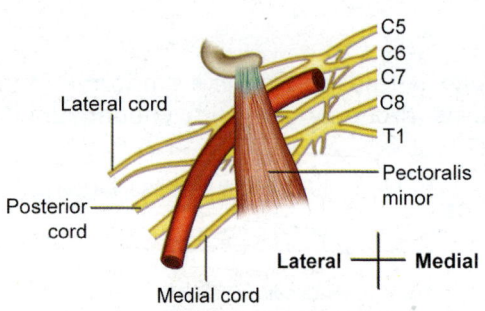

Relation of axillary artery to brachial plexus

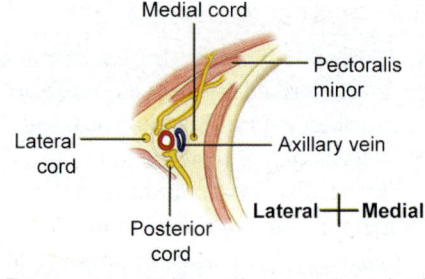

Transverse section of second part of axillary artery

**All throughout, medial cord with its branches is related medially to the artery. While lateral cord with its branches is related laterally and posterior cord with its branches is related posteriorly.**

## Branches

- *First part has one branch:* Superior thoracic artery.
- *Second part has two branches:*
  a. Acromiothoracic artery
  b. Lateral thoracic artery.
- *Third part has three branches:*
  a. Subscapular artery
  b. Anterior circumflex humeral artery
  c. Posterior circumflex humeral artery.

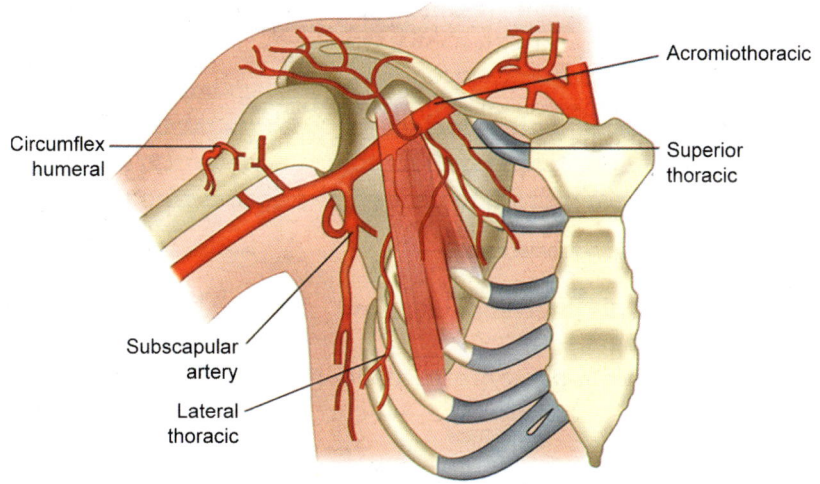

Branches of axillary artery

## Applied Anatomy

1. When axillary artery gets blocked, a collateral circulation develops between subclavian and axillary artery through scapular anastomosis.
2. Hilton's method of drainage should be adopted in cases of axillary abscess (i.e. blunt dissection).

> **Q. Explain radial nerve in detail (course, relations, branches). Add a note on its applied anatomy.**

**Ans.** Radial nerve is the main nerve of the extensor compartment of the arm.

## Origin

Posterior cord of brachial plexus.

## Root Value

C5, C6, C7, C8, T1.

## Course and Relations

1. In the axilla, it lies behind the third part of axillary artery and in front of subscapularis, latissimus dorsi and teres major.
2. In the upper arm, it lies behind the brachial artery and passes posterolaterally through the lower triangular space and then traverses the spiral groove.
3. At the level of insertion of coracobrachialis, the nerve pierces the lateral intermuscular septum and becomes anterior.

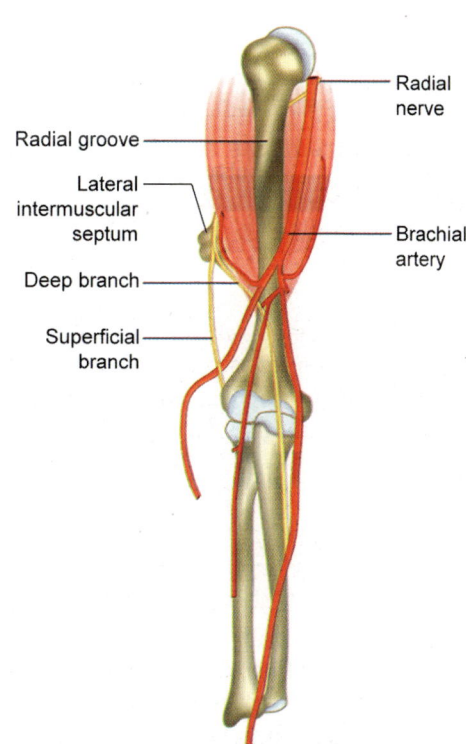

Radial nerve (course)

4. In the cubital fossa, the nerve lies between brachialis, brachioradialis and extensor carpi radialis longus. At the level of lateral epicondyle it gives off the posterior interosseous nerve, which leaves the fossa by piercing the supinator.
5. It terminates by dividing into posterior interosseous nerve (deep branch) and superficial cutaneous branch.

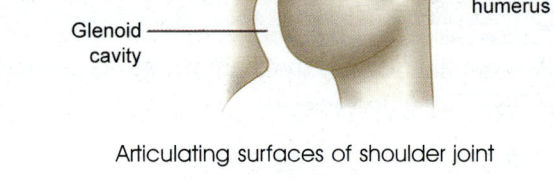

Radial nerve in cubital fossa

### Branches

- *Muscular:* Triceps brachialis, brachioradialis and extensor carpi radialis longus
- *Cutaneous:* Posterior cutaneous nerve of arm and forearm, and lower lateral cutaneous nerve of arm
- *Articular:* Elbow joint.

### Applied Anatomy

Radial nerve is commonly damaged in the radial groove due to intramuscular injections in the arm and sleeping in the armchair in a drunken state, i.e. crutch paralysis or saturday night palsy. This leads to wrist drop and sensory loss on the back of forearm.

### Q. Describe in detail shoulder joint.

**Ans.**

### Type

Synovial joint of ball and socket variety.

### Articulating Surfaces

- Glenoid cavity of scapula
- Head of humerus.

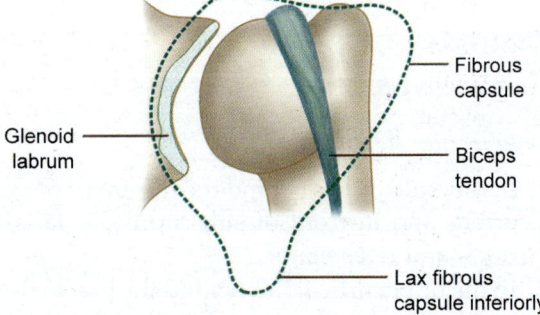

Articulating surfaces of shoulder joint

### Nature

Shoulder joint is structurally a weak joint. The head of the humerus is four times the size of glenoid cavity. However, due to the disparity in size, the mobility of the joint is enhanced.

### Ligaments

1. *Fibrous capsule:* It is attached along the margins of glenoid cavity of scapula. The supraglenoid tubercle is within the capsule:
   a. On the humerus it is attached to the anatomical neck. Attachment is deficient superiorly for the passage of tendon of biceps. While the capsule loosely hangs inferiorly up to the surgical neck of humerus.
   b. Anteriorly, the capsule is supplemented by glenohumeral ligament.

Fibrous capsule of shoulder joint

2. *Coracohumeral ligament:* It extends from root of the coracoid process to the neck of humerus, opposite the greater tubercle.
3. *Transverse humeral ligament:* It bridges the upper part of bicipital groove.
4. *Glenoid labrum:* It lines the glenoid cavity and deepens it.

## Relations

Rotator cuff muscles, i.e. supraspinatus, infraspinatus, teres minor and subscapularis surround the shoulder joint. Rotator cuff muscles are covered by bulky deltoid muscle. Axillary neurovascular bundle gets related inferiorly.

Several bursae are related to the joint. Important bursae are subacromial, subscapularis and infraspinatus. The last two may communicate with the joint.

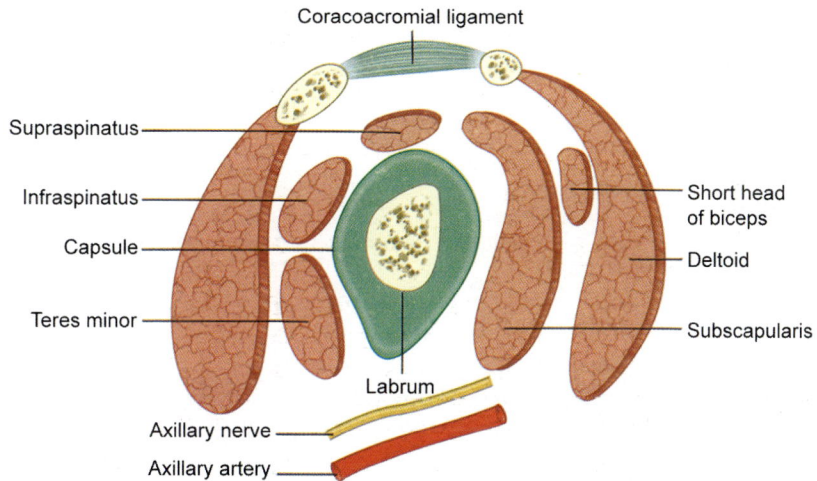

## Blood Supply

- Circumflex humeral vessels
- Supra and subscapular vessels.

## Nerve Supply

- Axillary nerve
- Musculocutaneous nerve
- Suprascapular nerve.

## Action

The key muscles and action are mentioned below:
- Flexion—pectoralis major, deltoid
- Extension—deltoid, latissimus dorsi
- Adduction—pectoralis major, latissimus dorsi
- Abduction—deltoid, supraspinatus, serratus anterior, trapezius
- Medial rotation—pectoralis major, latissimus dorsi, deltoid, teres major
- Lateral rotation—deltoid, infraspinatus, teres minor.

## Applied Anatomy

1. Inferior and recurrent dislocations are common due to the laxity of capsule.
2. *Chronic tendonitis (painful arc syndrome):* This syndrome is characterised by chronic thickening of the tendon of supraspinatus resulting in a typical impingement syndrome. The inflamed area is located by palpation of tender spot on the shoulder joint.
3. *Frozen shoulder:* Chronic inflammation of shoulder joint leads to adhesions between the rotator cuff muscles and humeral head.
4. Aspiration of shoulder joint is done by inserting a needle 1 cm inferior and lateral to the coracoid process.
5. Shoulder joint can be approached from front or behind, i.e. anterior exposure, posterior exposure, transacromial exposure.
6. Shoulder tip pain could be referred from the diaphragm, since the phrenic nerve and supraclavicular nerve have the same root value (C3, C4).

### Q. Describe in detail elbow joint.

**Ans.**

### Type

Synovial joint of hinge variety.

### Articulating Surfaces

- Capitulum and trochlea of humerus
- Head of the radius and trochlear notch of ulna.

### Nature

Elbow joint is in connection with the superior radioulnar joint. Humeroradial, humeroulnar and superior radioulnar joints are together known as cubital articulation.

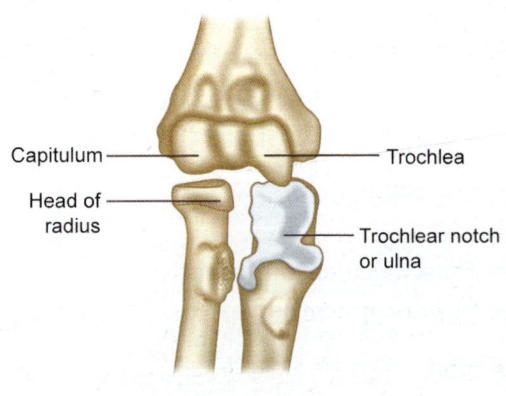

Articulating surfaces

### Ligaments

1. **Fibrous capsule:** Superiorly, it is attached to the lower end of humerus and includes radial fossa, coronoid fossa and olecranon fossa within it:
   a. Inferomedially, it is attached to the rim of trochlear notch.
   b. Inferolaterally, it is attached to the annular ligament of the superior radioulnar joint.
   c. Capsule is reinforced anteriorly and posteriorly by ligaments carrying the same name (anterior ligament, posterior ligament).
2. **Ulnar collateral ligament:** It is a triangular ligament. Above, it is attached to the medial epicondyle and below it splits into anterior, posterior and oblique bands.
3. **Radial collateral ligament:** It extends from lateral epicondyle to the annular ligament.

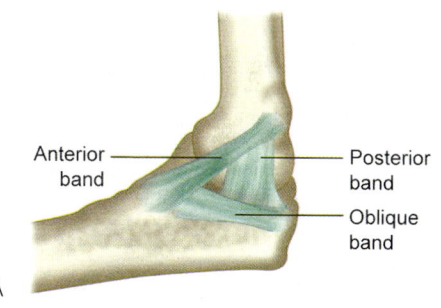

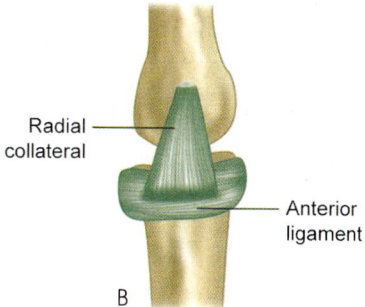

Ligaments of elbow joint

## Relations

- Anteriorly—cubital fossa with its contents
- Medially—ulnar nerve and common flexor origin
- Laterally—supinator and common extensor origin.

## Blood Supply

Anastomosis around the elbow joint between brachial, ulnar and radial.

## Nerve Supply

Ulnar, radial and median nerve.

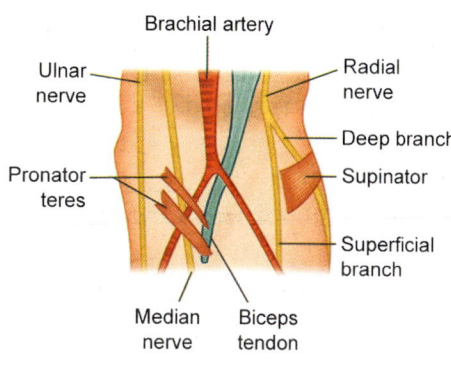

Cubital fossa with its contents

## Action

- Flexion—brachialis, biceps, brachioradialis
- Extension—triceps, anconeus.

## Applied Anatomy

- Posterior dislocation of elbow joint is common and is accompanied by fracture of coronoid process
- Subluxation is common in children
- Tennis elbow—abrupt pronation may lead to pain and tenderness over the lateral epicondyle.

## Q. Describe in detail wrist joint (radiocarpal joint).

**Ans.**

## Type

Synovial joint of ellipsoid variety.

## Articulating Surfaces

- Inferior surface of lower end of radius and articular disk of radioulnar joint
- Scaphoid, lunate, triquetral bones.

## Ligaments

- *Fibrous capsule:* It surrounds the articular surfaces
- *Palmar radiocarpal ligament:* It is a fibrous band extending from radius to lunate bone
- *Dorsal radiocarpal ligament:* It is the mirror image of palmar ligament on dorsal side
- *Radial collateral ligament:* It is attached above to the styloid process of radius and below to the lateral side of scaphoid bone
- *Ulnar collateral ligament:* It is attached above to the styloid process of ulna and below to the triquetral and pisiform bone.

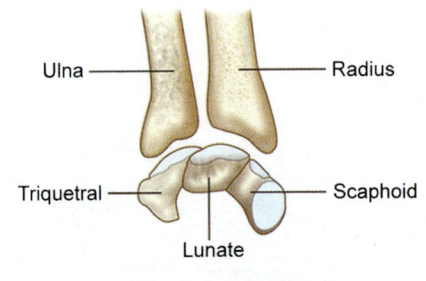

Articulating bones

## Relations

Anteriorly, it is related to the flexor tendons and posteriorly, it is related to the extensor tendons.

## Blood Supply

Anterior and posterior carpal arch.

## Nerve Supply

Anterior and posterior interosseous nerve.

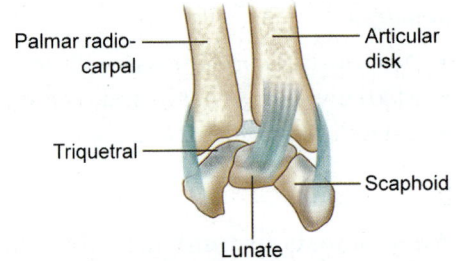

Ligaments of wrist joint

## Action

- Flexion and extension by the flexor and extensor tendons of the hand respectively.
- *Abduction:*
  - Flexor carpi radialis
  - Extensor carpi radialis longus
  - Abductor pollicis longus
  - Extensor pollicis brevis.
- *Adduction:*
  - Flexor carpi ulnaris
  - Extensor carpi ulnaris.

  Flexion is combined with adduction and extension with abduction.

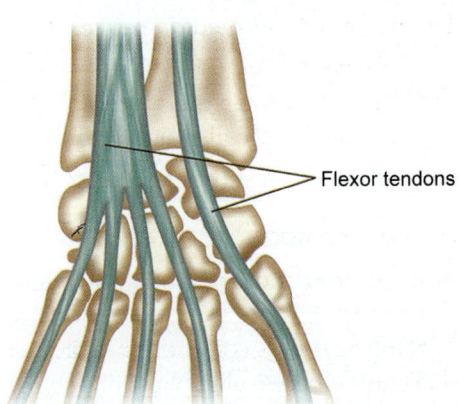

Anterior relations of wrist joint

## Applied Anatomy

- *Ganglion:* It is a commonest cystic swelling on the back of the wrist.
- *Madelung's deformity:* It is a congenital subluxation or dislocation of lower end of ulna.
- *Rheumatoid arthritis:* It commonly affects the wrist joint.

**Wrist complex comprises of 2 joints—radiocarpal joint and midcarpal joint.**

# Key Diagrams with MCQ Tips

**Ans.**

- Inserted on costal surface of scapula along its medial border
- Long thoracic nerve of Bell (C5, C6, C7) supplies the muscle
- Injury to above nerve leads to 'winging of scapula'.

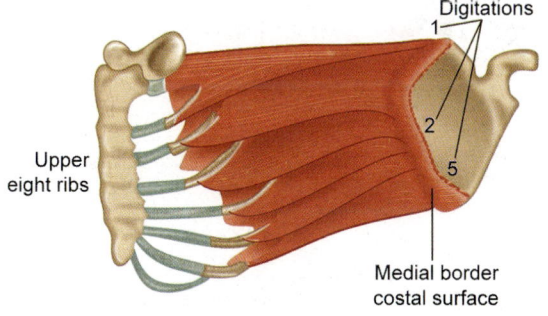

Digitations
1
2
5
Upper
eight ribs
Medial border
costal surface

**Q. Trapezius**

**Ans.**

- Also known as shawl muscle
- Supplied by spinal part of accessory nerve
- Elevates and retracts the scapula.

**Q. Dorsal interossei**

**Ans.**

- Bipennate muscles taking origin from adjacent sides of metacarpal bones

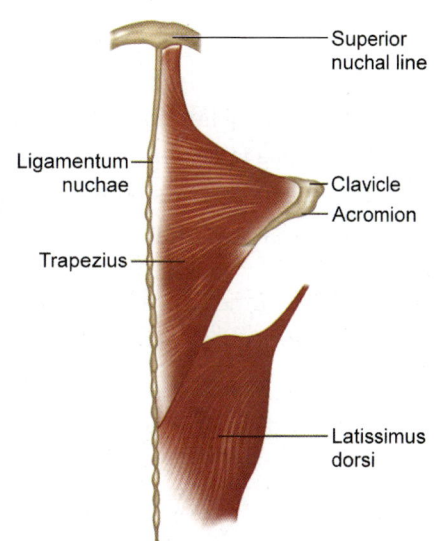

Superior
nuchal line

Ligamentum
nuchae

Clavicle
Acromion

Trapezius

Latissimus
dorsi

- Deep branch of ulnar nerve supplies all the interossei
- Abducts digits away from midline [i.e. dorsal interossei abduct (DAB)].

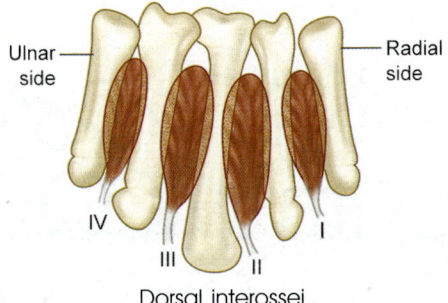

Dorsal interossei

## Q. Palmar interossei

**Ans.**
- Unipennate muscles between the shafts of metacarpal
- Deep branch of ulnar nerve supplies all the interossei
- Adduct digits toward midline [i.e. palmar interossei adduct (PAD)].

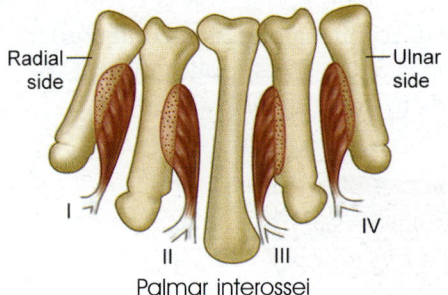

Palmar interossei

## Q. Cubital fossa

**Ans.**
- Brachial artery lies medial to biceps tendon
- Ulnar nerve is posterior to medial epicondyle
- Median nerve passes between two heads of pronator teres
- Radial nerves divides into superficial and deep branches
- The deep branch goes below the upper border of supinator.

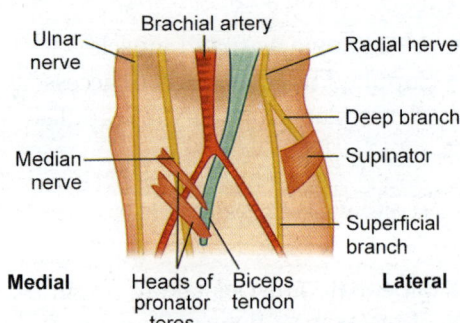

## Q. Insertion of flexor digitorum superficialis

**Ans.**

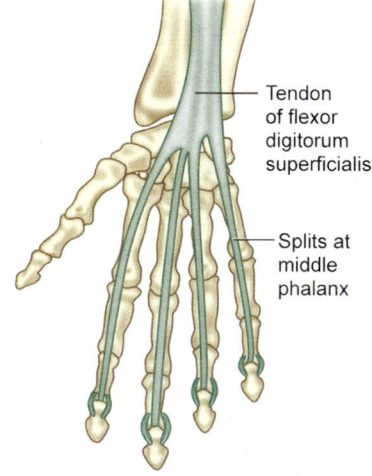

Tendon
of flexor
digitorum
superficialis

Splits at
middle
phalanx

Flexor digitorum superficialis

## Q. Flexor digitorum profundus

**Ans.**

- Flexor digitorum profundus is a hybrid muscle
- Medial half supplied by ulnar nerve
- Lateral half supplied by median nerve
- The tendon goes below the split end of flexor digitorum superficialis.

## Q. Lymphatic drainage of breast

**Ans.**

- To axillary lymph nodes 75%
- To internal thoracic (mammary) nodes 20%
- To posterior intercostal nodes 5%
- Subareolar plexus of Sappey is present

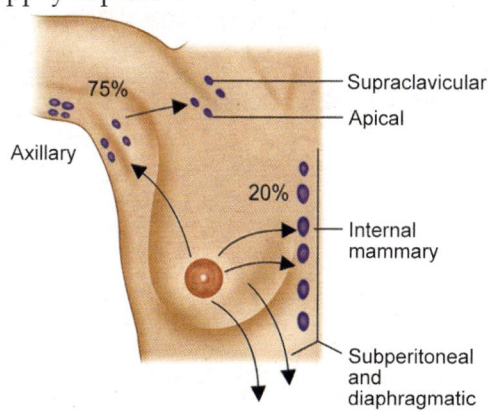

Supraclavicular

Apical

75%

Axillary

20%

Internal
mammary

Subperitoneal
and
diaphragmatic

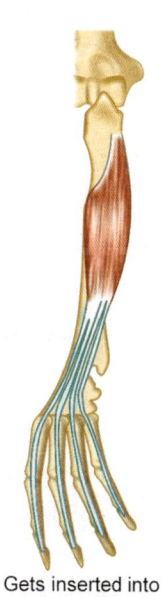

Gets inserted into
terminal phalanx

Flexor digitorum
profundus

- Radial incisions are taken to avoid cutting of lactiferous ducts
- Lymphatics from lower and inner quadrants of breast may communicate with subdiaphragmatic and subperitoneal plexus
- Staging of breast cancer depends on nodal status (size, number, fixity).

### Q. Shoulder girdle

**Ans.**
- Connects upper limb with axial skeleton
- Two joints:
  a. Sternoclavicular (synovial, compound, complex, type main bond of union is articular disk)
  b. Acromioclavicular (plane synovial type).

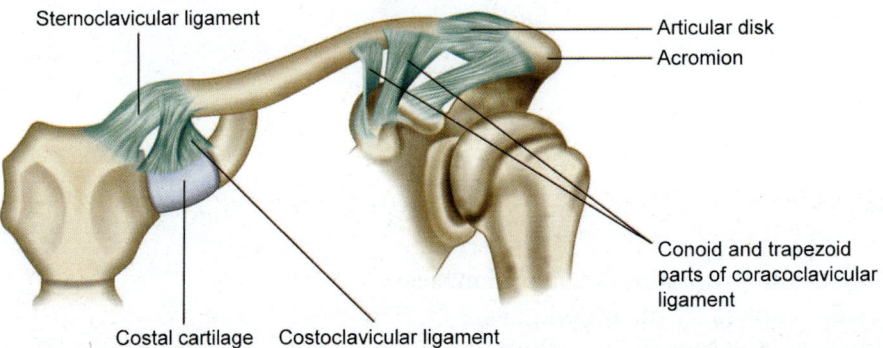

### Q. Medial epicondyle-common flexor origin.

### Q. Lateral epicondyle-common extensor origin.

### Q. Capitate key carpal bone, first to ossify.

### Q. Pisiform-sesamoid bone in tendon of flexor carpi ulnaris, last to ossify.

### Q. Palmaris brevis-subcutaneous muscle of upper limb.

## Q. Epiphyseal lines and capsular attachments

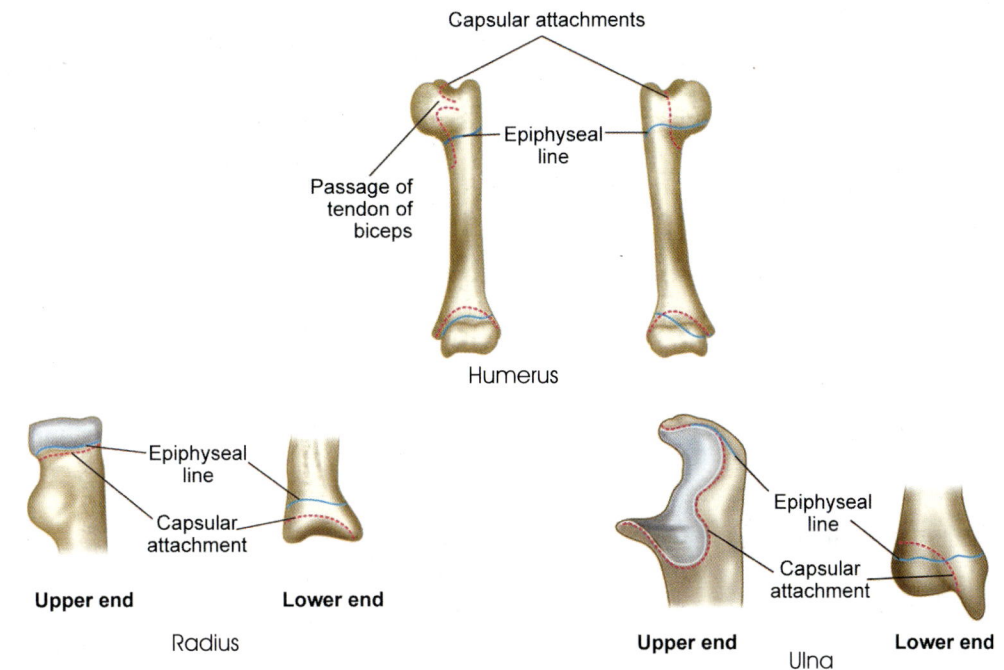

Capsular attachments

Epiphyseal line

Passage of tendon of biceps

Humerus

Epiphyseal line

Capsular attachment

Upper end          Lower end

Radius

Epiphyseal line

Capsular attachment

Upper end          Lower end

Ulna

## Q. Dermatomes of upper limb

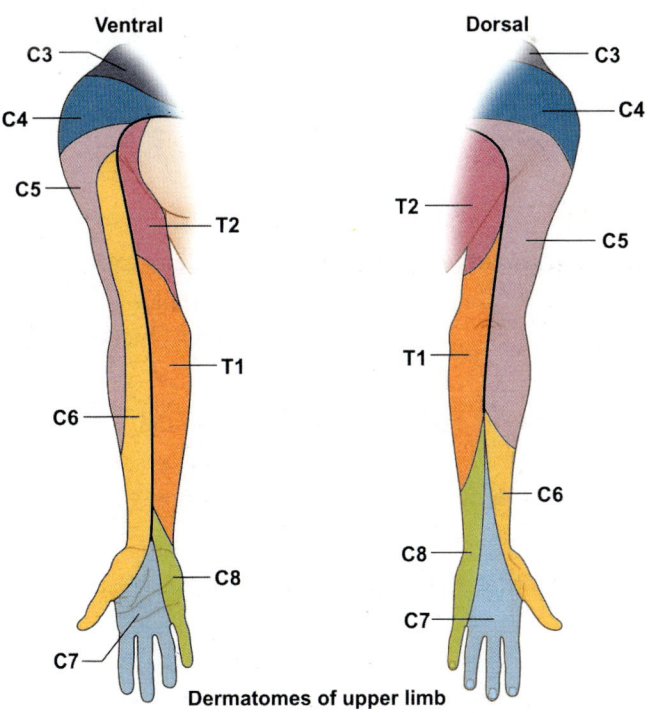

Ventral

C3
C4
C5
T2
T1
C6
C8
C7

Dorsal

C3
C4
C5
T2
T1
C6
C8
C7

Dermatomes of upper limb

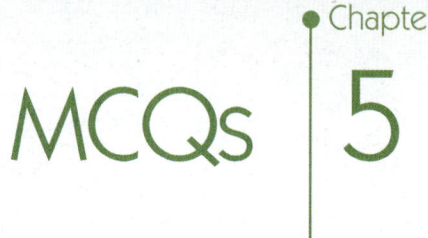

1. **The literal meaning of the word clavicle is ....................**
   - a. Lock
   - b. Key
   - c. Shield
   - d. Pyramid

   **Answer: b**

2. **The most reliable single indicator to determine sex of the clavicle is ....................**
   - a. Length of the bone
   - b. Thickness of the bone
   - c. Midshaft circumference of the bone
   - d. Curvature of the bone

   **Answer: c**

3. **Literal meaning of scapula is ....................**
   - a. To dig
   - b. To throw
   - c. To screw
   - d. To poke

   **Answer: a**

4. **Following are the attachments on the coracoid process except ....................**
   - a. Coracobrachialis
   - b. Pectoralis minor
   - c. Pectoralis major
   - d. Short head of biceps

   **Answer: c**

5. **Injury to .................... nerve causes 'winging' of scapula.**
   - a. Ulnar nerve
   - b. Long thoracic nerve of Bell
   - c. Phrenic nerve
   - d. Median nerve

   **Answer: b**

6. **Following muscles constitute the 'rotator cuff' except ....................**
   - a. Supraspinatus
   - b. Subscapularis
   - c. Suprascapularis
   - d. Infraspinatus

   **Answer: c**

7. **The nerve related to the surgical neck of humerus is** .....................

    a. Axillary nerve          c. Ulnar nerve

    b. Radial nerve           d. Median nerve

**Answer: a**

8. **Following nerve is related to the posterior aspect of medial epicondyle** ....................

    a. Median             c. Radial

    b. Ulnar              d. Medial cutaneous nerve of arm

**Answer: b**

9. **Pisiform bone is a sesamoid bone, which develops in the tendon of** ....................

    a. Flexor carpi radialis        c. Flexor digitorum profundus

    b. Flexor digitorum superficialis      d. Flexor carpi ulnaris

**Answer: d**

10. **Key carpal bone is** ....................

    a. Pisiform            c. Hamate

    b. Capitate           d. Trapezium

**Answer: b**

11. **Coracobrachialis muscle is pierced by following nerve** ....................

    a. Radial             c. Musculocutaneous

    b. Ulnar              d. Lateral cutaneous nerve of arm

**Answer: c**

12. **Middle finger receives insertion of which palmar interossei** ....................

    a. I                c. III

    b. II               d. None

**Answer: d**

13. **All palmar interossei** .................... **the digits.**

    a. Abduct            c. Flex

    b. Adduct            d. Extend

**Answer: b**

14. **All dorsal interossei** .................... **the digits.**

    a. Abduct            c. Flex

    b. Adduct            d. Extend

**Answer: a**

15. **All interossei are supplied by** .................... **nerve.**

    a. Median            c. Ulnar

    b. Radial             d. Musculocutaneous

**Answer: c**

16. **Paper test is used to test the action of** .....................
    a. Adductor pollicis
    c. Dorsal interossei
    b. Palmar interossei
    d. Opponens pollicis

    **Answer: b**

17. **The lumbricals have the following action** .....................
    a. Extend MP joint and flex IP joint
    c. Extend MP joint and extend IP joint
    b. Flex MP joint and extend IP joint
    d. Flex MP joint and also flex IP joint

    **Answer: b**

    MP, metacarpophalangeal; IP, interphalangeal.

18. **Musculocutaneous nerve descends in the arm between two muscles namely** ....................
    a. Coracobrachialis and brachialis
    c. Brachialis and biceps
    b. Pectoralis major and subscapularis
    d. Biceps and coracobrachialis

    **Answer: c**

19. **The key nerve of the front of arm is** .....................
    a. Musculocutaneous
    c. Median
    b. Ulnar
    d. Radial

    **Answer: a**

20. **The musculocutaneous nerve pierces** ..................... **muscle.**
    a. Biceps
    c. Coracobrachialis
    b. Pectoralis
    d. Brachialis

    **Answer: c**

21. **Musculocutaneous nerve is the branch of** ..................... **cord of brachial plexus.**
    a. Medial
    c. Posterior
    b. Lateral
    d. Anterior

    **Answer: b**

22. **Musician's nerve is** .....................
    a. Musculocutaneous nerve
    c. Radial nerve
    b. Ulnar nerve
    d. Median nerve

    **Answer: b**

23. **Ulnar nerve enters the forearm between the two heads of** .....................
    a. Flexor digitorum superficialis
    c. Flexor carpi ulnaris
    b. Flexor carpi radialis
    d. Flexor digitorum profundus

    **Answer: c**

24. **Median nerve lies between the two heads of** .....................
    a. Flexor carpi ulnaris
    c. Pronator teres
    b. Flexor carpi radialis
    d. Supinator

    **Answer: c**

**25. Median nerve originates from two cords ......................**

a. Medial cord and posterior cord
b. Medial cord and lateral cord
c. Lateral cord and posterior cord
d. Medial, lateral and posterior cord

Answer: b

**26. Roots involved in Erb's paralysis are ......................**

a. C5, C6
b. C6, C7
c. C8, C9
d. C4, C5

Answer: a

**27. Central group of axillary lymph node is related to following nerve ......................**

a. Axillary nerve
b. Radial nerve
c. Musculocutaneous nerve
d. Intercostobrachial nerve

Answer: d

**28. Clavipectoral fascia encloses ...................... muscles.**

a. Subclavius and pectoralis major
b. Pectoralis minor and subclavius
c. Pectoralis major
d. Coracobrachialis

Answer: b

**29. Coracoid process is ...................... type of epiphysis.**

a. Atavistic
b. Pressure
c. Traction
d. Aberrant

Answer: a

**30. First carpometacarpal joint...................... type of joint.**

a. Ball and socket
b. Condyloid
c. Saddle
d. None of the above

Answer: c

**31. The upper trunk of brachial plexus is formed by union of ......................**

a. C4, C5
b. C5, C6
c. C6, C7
d. C8, T1

Answer: b

**32. Extent of the axillary artery is between ......................**

a. Outer border of first rib to lower border of teres major
b. First costal cartilage to upper border of teres major
c. Outer border of first rib to upper border of teres major
d. Inner border of first rib to lower border of teres major

Answer. a

**33. Axillary artery is divided into three parts by ...................... muscle.**

a. Pectoralis major
b. Pectoralis minor
c. Teres major
d. Teres minor

Answer. b

34. **Shawl muscle is ...................**

    a. Deltoid
    b. Pectoralis major
    c. Subscapularis
    d. Trapezius

    **Answer: d**

35. **Brachial artery is ..................... to biceps tendon.**

    a. Lateral
    b. Anterior
    c. Medial
    d. Posterior

    **Answer: c**

36. **The last carpal bone to ossify is .....................**

    a. Capitate
    b. Pisiform
    c. Hamate
    d. Scaphoid

    **Answer: b**

37. **An alcoholic, who under the influence, slept with his arm on the chair and woke up in the morning with inability to move the arm. It is due to pressure on .....................**

    a. Ulnar nerve
    b. Median nerve
    c. Radial nerve
    d. Interosseous nerve

    **Answer: c**

38. **A porter carrying heavy weights on shoulder was unable to do pushing movements. The nerve likely to be injured is .....................**

    a. Nerve to latissimus dorsi
    b. Nerve to serratus anterior
    c. Nerve to subscapularis
    d. Nerve to subclavius

    **Answer: b**

39. **Forceps were applied, while delivering a child. Later child develops 'claw hand'. This is due to injury to ..................... trunk of brachial plexus.**

    a. Upper
    b. Middle
    c. Lower
    d. All

    **Answer: c**

40. **Undue pressure was applied on head, while delivering the baby. Following which, a deformity, wherein abduction, flexion of arm was not possible (policeman's tip). This is due to injury to .....................**

    a. C4, C5
    b. C5, C6
    c. C7, C8
    d. C8, T1

    **Answer: b**

41. **A middle-aged woman wakes up in sleep with pain and tingling in hand. This is due to entrapment of ..................... nerve in hand.**

    a. Median
    b. Ulnar
    c. Radial
    d. Musculocutaneous

    **Answer: a**

42. In a patient of leprosy, a thick cord-like structure was palpated behind medial epicondyle the nerve affected is .....................

a. Ulnar
b. Radial
c. Musculocutaneous
d. Median

**Answer: a**

43. A 60-year-old female complains of swelling in breast. The area to be examined after breast examination is .....................

a. Abdomen
b. Pelvis
c. Axilla
d. Neck

**Answer: c**

44. Axillary abscess should be drained by blunt dissection (Hilton's method) due to presence of .....................

a. Axillary lymph nodes
b. Axillary artery and vein
c. Axillary nerve
d. Axillary lymphatic vessels

**Answer: b**

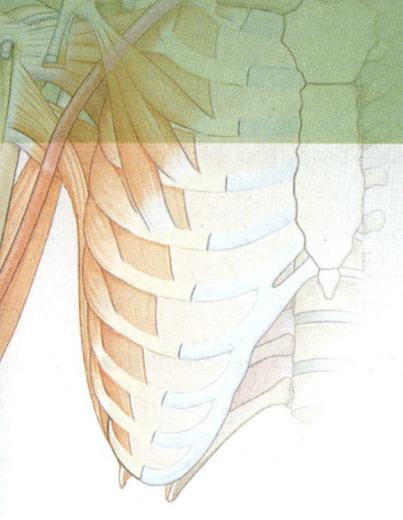

## 1. PECTORAL REGION

### a. Incision Markings

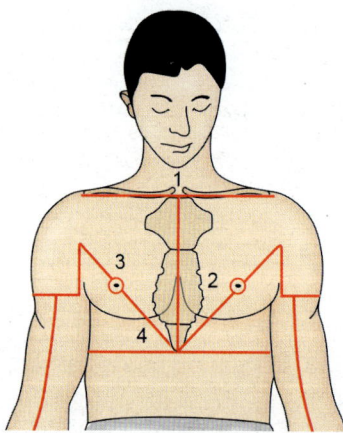

| | |
|---|---|
| 1 | = Along clavicle |
| 2 | = Midsternum |
| 3 | = Around nipple |
| 4 | = Along xiphoid process |

Incision markings for pectoral region

### b. Structures to be Identified

- **Supraclavicular nerves** in superficial fascia of upper flap
- Lateral cutaneous branches, of intercostal nerves in lower flap
- Breast in the form of fat it extends from margin of sternum to midaxillary line against 3rd to 5th ribs
- Clear the breast fat and you will see the **pectoralis major muscle:** It covers most of front of chest. Appreciate the attachments
- Lift the pectoralis major muscle by blunt dissection and you will appreciate a nerve, **medial pectoral nerve,** which appears there after piercing the pectoralis minor

- Deep fascia covering the pectoralis major muscle is continuous with the periosteum of clavicle and sternum
- Divide deep fascia to identify the cephalic vein
- Lymph nodes can be identified as tiny, inconspicuous, rounded bodies scattered in the body.

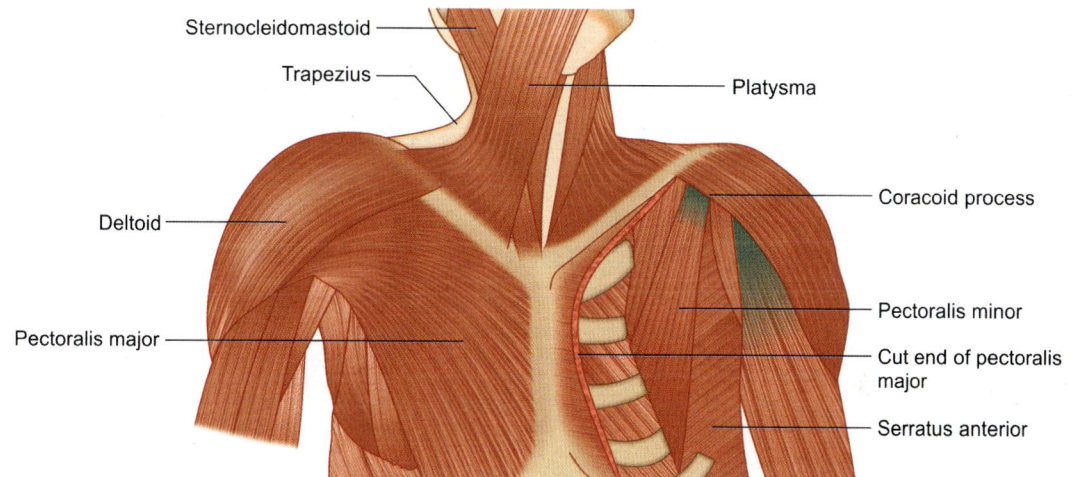

Superficial dissection of pectoral region

## c. Vivisection

*Radical mastectomy*: It is a surgery done in patients of breast cancer; it involves the same above dissection. Following structures are removed—whole breast, large portion of skin including nipple, all fat, fascia and lymph nodes.

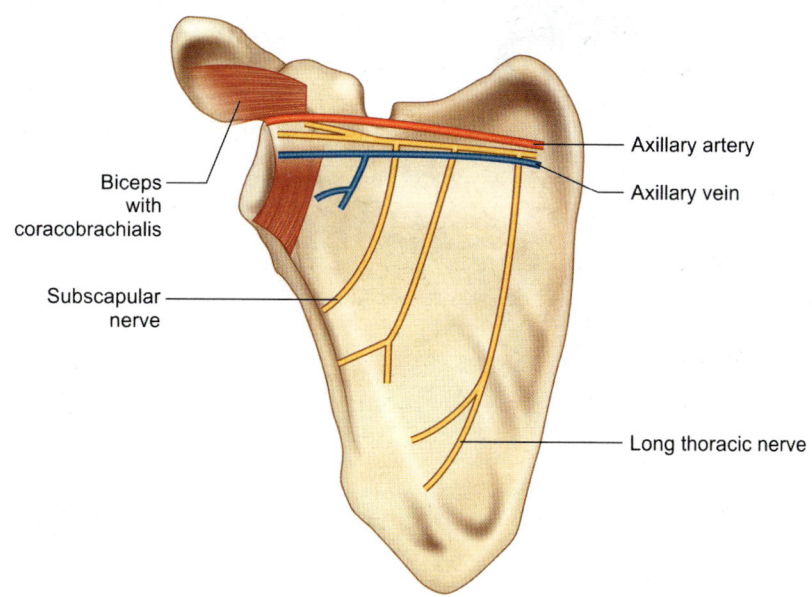

Deep structures of pectoral region

## d. Viva Questions

### Pectoralis Major Muscle

- It is a fan-shaped muscle in front of chest, extends from medial half of front of clavicle, anterior surface of sternum and upper six costal cartilages and aponeurosis of external oblique muscle to crest of greater tubercle of humerus
- Medial and lateral pectoral nerves
- Adductor and medial rotator of humerus.

### Pectoralis Minor Muscle

- Triangular muscle passes superolaterally from third to fifth rib, to coracoid process
- Medial pectoral nerve
- Pulls scapula downwards and forwards
- *Divides:* Axillary artery into 3 parts
- Clavipectoral fascia encloses the muscle.

### Lymph Nodes Draining the Breast

- Axillary nodes
- Posterior intercostal nodes
- Internal mammary nodes.

### Radial Incisions are Taken on Breast to avoid Cutting of Lactiferous Duct

## 2. AXILLARY REGION

### a. Incision Markings

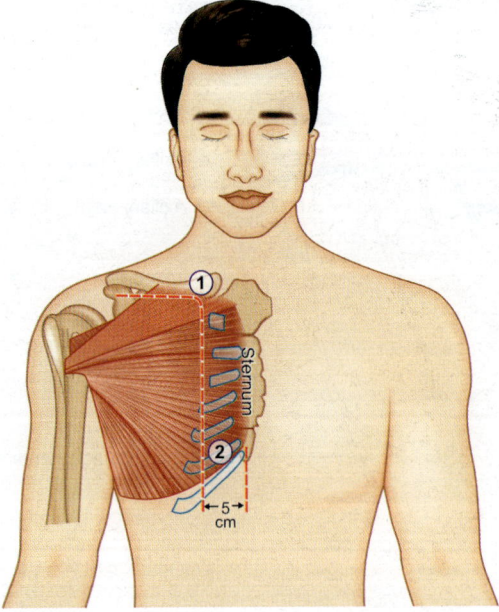

| 1. | Cut clavicular head of pectoralis major below clavicle |
|----|--------------------------------------------------------|
| 2. | Another cut 5 cm from sternum |

Incisions on pectoralis muscle to expose axillary region

## b. Structures to be Identified

- **Medial pectoral nerve** pierces pectoralis minor to enter pectoralis major from its under-surface, below upwards
- Identify **clavipectoral fascia** and trace **pectoralis minor** to its attachments
- Follow **cephalic vein to axillary vein, locate thoracoacromial artery, lateral pectoral artery**

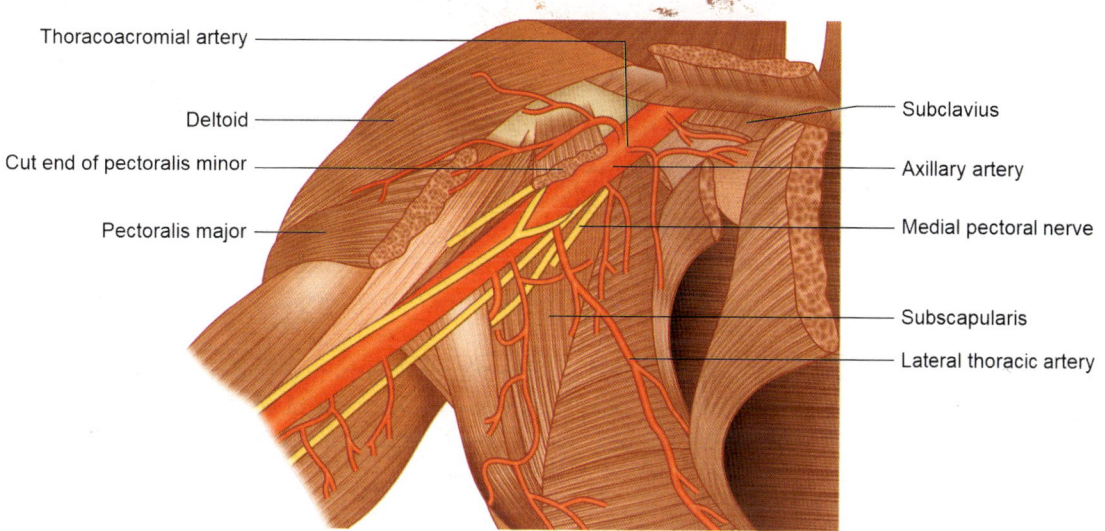

Structures under the cover of pectoralis major muscle

- Cut **clavipectoral fascia** just below clavicle to expose **subclavius muscle**
- Push a finger inferior to subclavius along the axillary vessels—you will reach the root of neck.

### Deep Dissection of Axilla

- Further you will be in **supra-clavicular triangle** by pushing finger medially between axillary artery and vein
- Remove the fat, lymph nodes from axilla to expose its contents
- Expose **coracobrachialis, short head of biceps** from tip of coracoid process
- Nerve piercing coracobrachialis is musculocutaneous nerve, axillary artery and median nerve is medial to above muscles
- Medial to axillary artery is axillary vein and medial cutaneous nerve of forearm lies between axillary artery and vein
- Medial cutaneous nerve of arm is medial to axillary vein. Follow the nerve which joins a branch of **intercostobrachial nerve** (= lateral cutaneous branch of 2nd intercostal nerve)
- Identify **lateral thoracic artery** and **nerve to serratus anterior (long thoracic nerve of Bell)** descending on lateral surface of serratus anterior muscle.

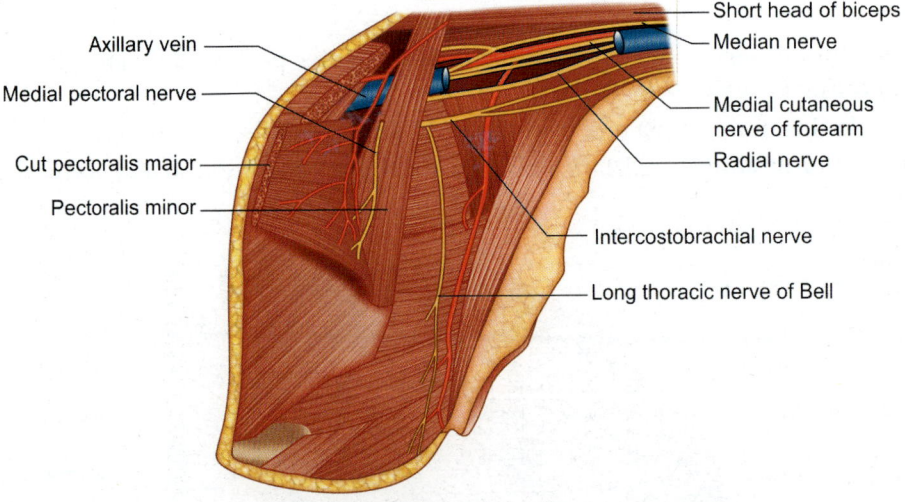

Deep dissection of axilla

### c. Vivisection

- Axillary abscess (Abscess = Pus in closed cavity) should be opened and drained by Hiltons method of drainage, i.e. do a blunt, finger dissection to open the abscess and drain the pus completely. No sharp instrument should be used in this region since there are major axillary vessels and branches of brachial plexus in this region.

- *Sentinel node biopsy:* Since the primary area of lymphatic drainage of breast is axilla, in cancer breast, axilla is primarily screened. The first node where the cancer spreads is known as sentinel node. (excision of the node or any swelling for study is known as biopsy.)

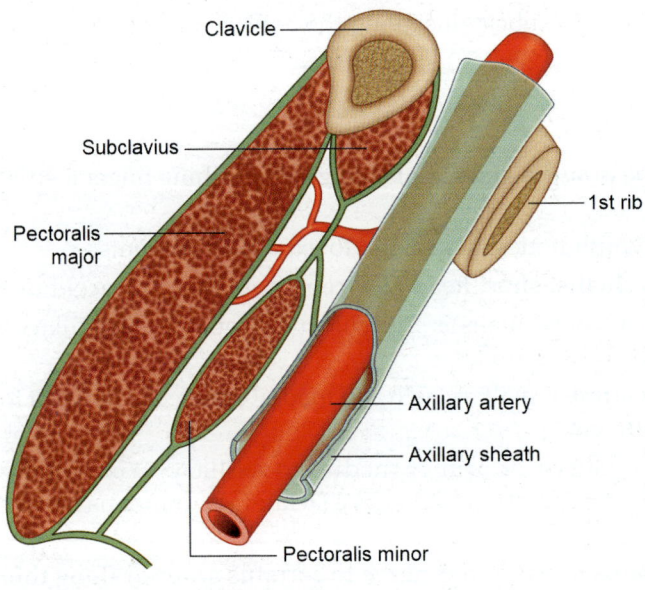

Clavipectoral fascia

## d. Viva Questions

- Axillary lymph nodes classification—anterior, posterior, central, apical, lateral
- Brachial plexus formation—ventral rami of C5, C6, C7, C8 and T1
- Brachial plexus branches—from each cord
  - Lateral cord—lateral pectoral nerve, lateral root of median nerve, musculocutaneous nerve (*Mnemonic:* Love me Lucy)
  - Medial cord—medial pectoral nerve, medial root of median nerve, ulnar nerve, medial cutaneous nerve of arm and forearm
  - Posterior cord—radial nerve, upper and lower subscapular nerve, nerve to latissimus dorsi, axillary nerve

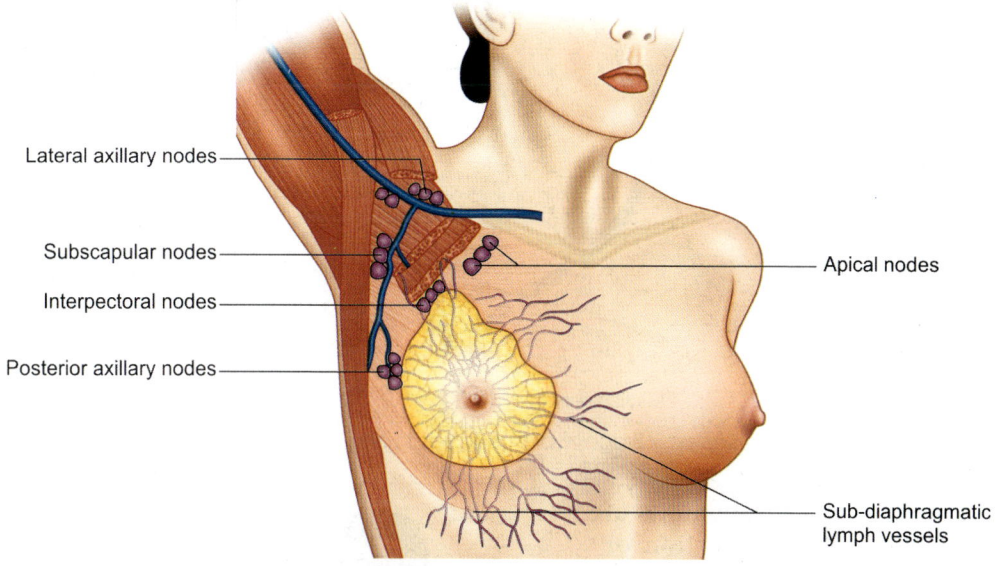

Axillary lymph nodes

- Coracoid process attachments—pectoralis minor, coracobrachialis, short head of biceps
- Intercostobrachial nerve is in close proximity to axillary tail of Spence
- Musculocutaneous nerve pierces the coracobrachialis muscle.

## 3. FRONT OF ARM

### a. Incision Markings

*Structures to be Identified*

- Cut the fascia on the anterior surface of the bulk muscle of arm, that muscle is **biceps brachii**, and fascia on the muscle is deep fascia.
- Lift the muscle forwards and you will see a prominent nerve, i.e. musculocutaneous nerve
- The muscle closely pasted to the humerus is **brachialis.**
- Follow the musculocutaneous nerve along with biceps and **coracobrachialis**, proximally and distally.
- The muscle which is pierced by the thick nerve is coracobrachialis.

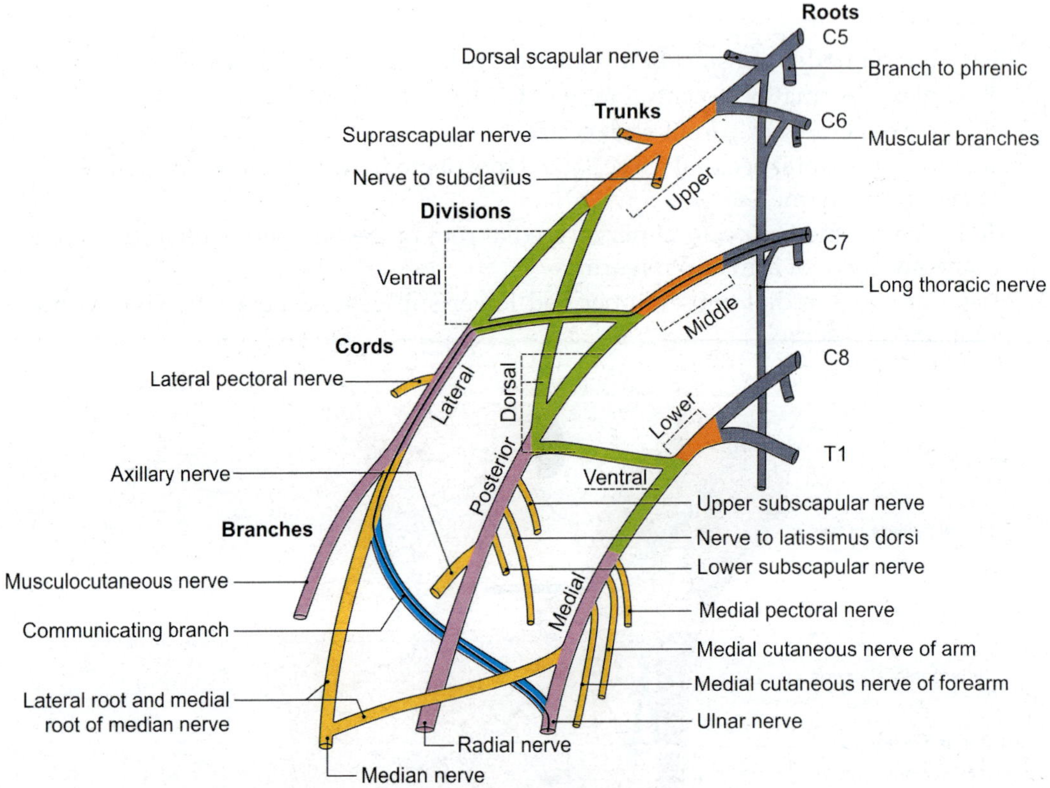

**Roots**
C5

Dorsal scapular nerve

Branch to phrenic

**Trunks**
C6

Suprascapular nerve

Muscular branches

Nerve to subclavius

Upper

**Divisions**

C7

Ventral

Long thoracic nerve

Middle

**Cords**
C8

Lateral pectoral nerve

Lateral

Posterior  Dorsal

Lower

T1

Axillary nerve

Ventral

Upper subscapular nerve

**Branches**

Nerve to latissimus dorsi

Lower subscapular nerve

Musculocutaneous nerve

Medial

Medial pectoral nerve

Communicating branch

Medial cutaneous nerve of arm

Medial cutaneous nerve of forearm

Lateral root and medial root of median nerve

Ulnar nerve

Radial nerve

Median nerve

Brachial plexus, cords trunks

- One cannot trace the tendons of biceps towards its insertion or origin, at this stage.
- Remove the fascia from the brachialis and then define brachioradialis, and extensor carpi radialis longus towards the lower part of arm. These muscles are present laterally and closely pasted to brachialis. One can do finger dissection to separate these muscles since there is **radial nerve** in this region and terminal branch of **profunda brachii** artery.
- Follow the radial nerve proximally and you will see it goes posterior to humerus.
- You will find the main neuro-vascular bundle deep to deep fascia, medial to biceps. Trace the contents above to axilla and below to cubital fossa.

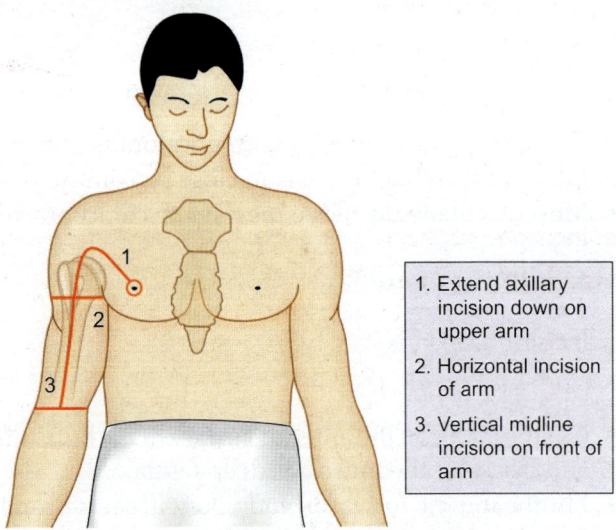

1. Extend axillary incision down on upper arm

2. Horizontal incision of arm

3. Vertical midline incision on front of arm

Incision markings on front of arm

## b. Vivisection

Fractures are common in this region, in cases of pathological fracture of humerus for open reduction one should know the muscles and the neurovascular bundle mentioned in the above dissection.

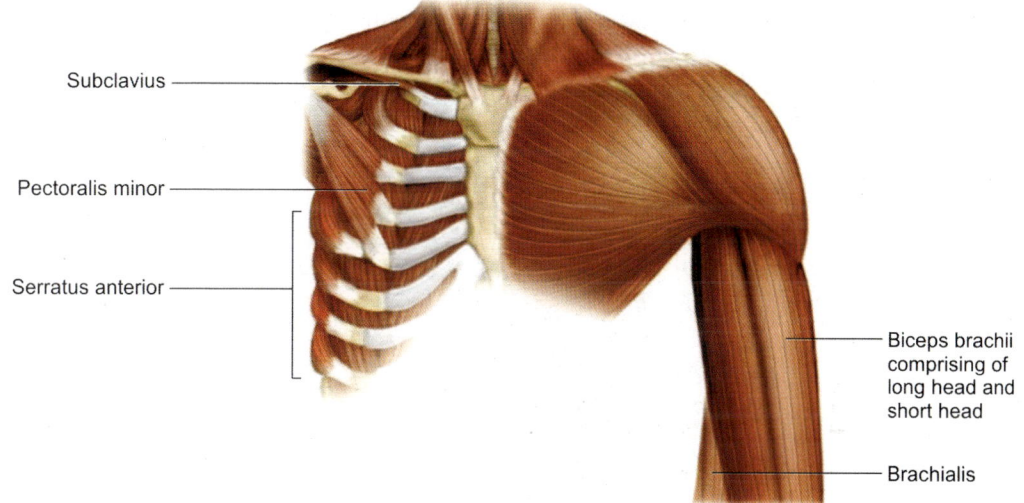

Muscles on front of the arm

## c. Viva Questions

- Coracobrachialis muscle attachments—the name itself will help you to remember the attachment, i.e. coracoid process to midbrachium
- Biceps form the bulk muscle of front of arm. It is the strong supinator and flexor of arm
- Biceps has two heads of origin, short head from coracoid process and long head from supra-glenoid tubercle and gets inserted to radial tuberosity. It crosses the shoulder and elbow joint and thus brings about movement over both the joints.

## 4. CUBITAL FOSSA

### a. Incision Markings

Incisions to be taken on cubital area.

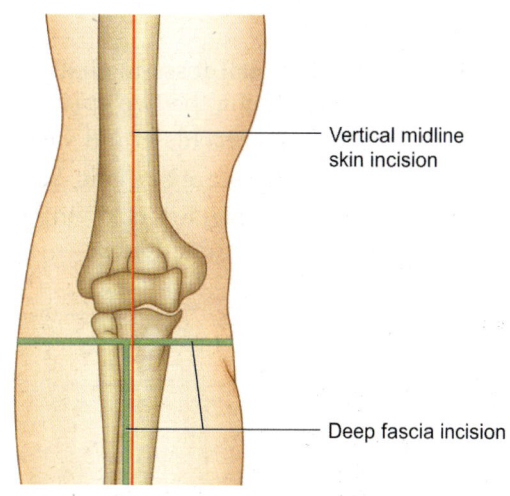

Cubital area

### b. Structures to be Identified

- Cut deep fascia vertically and transversely in front of elbow
- Separate the structures by finger dissection
- Identify the boundaries, **pronator teres** medially and **brachioradialis** laterally
- Appreciate the glistening white biceps tendon and aponeurosis
- **Brachial artery** is medial to **biceps tendon**
- Thick **median nerve** is medial to brachial artery.

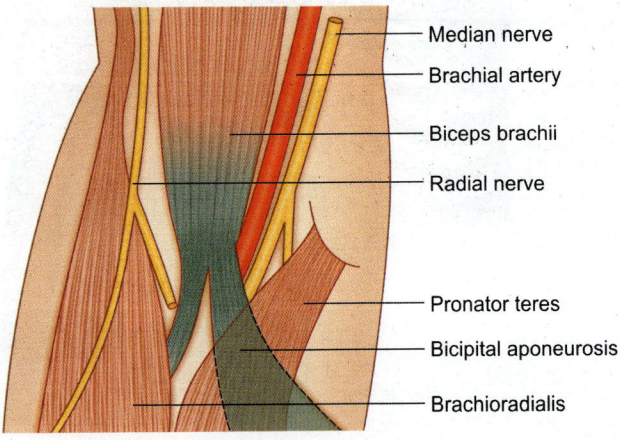

Median nerve
Brachial artery
Biceps brachii
Radial nerve
Pronator teres
Bicipital aponeurosis
Brachioradialis

Cubital fossa dissection

### c. Vivisection

- Superficial dissection is done in a procedure known as venesection, wherein a vein needs to be located for intravenous saline infusions in dehydrated patients
- Blood pressure is recorded by auscultating the brachial artery which is medial to the biceps brachii tendon.

### d. Viva Questions

- Boundaries of cubital fossa-medially pronator teres, laterally brachioradialis, base by an imaginary line joining the two epicondyles
- Floor is formed by brachialis and supinator muscles
- Superficial structures are cephalic, basilic vein and median cubital vein
- Median nerve, brachial artery dividing into ulnar and radial artery, and tendon of biceps are the contents of cubital fossa.

# 5. FRONT OF FOREARM

## a. Incision Markings

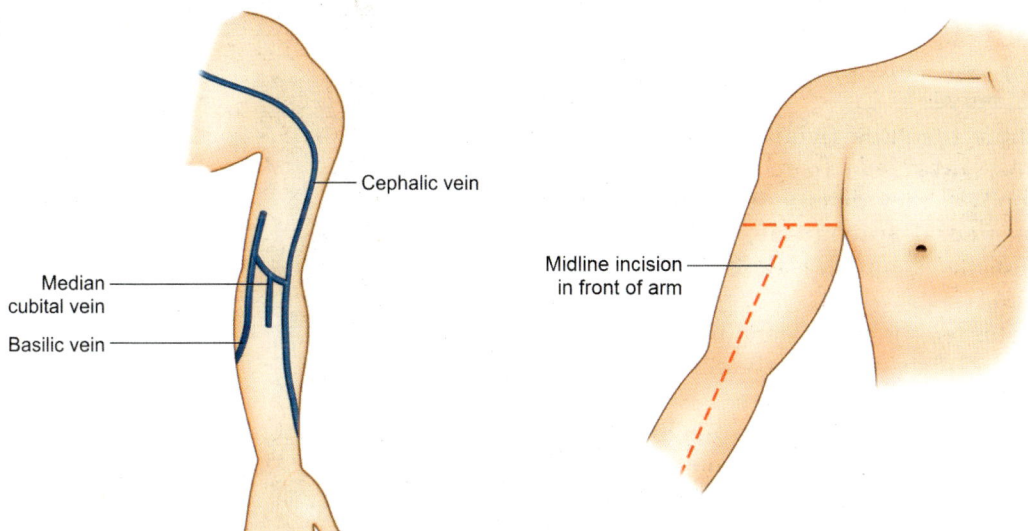

Superficial veins of arm and forearm

## b. Structures to be identified

### Superficial Plane

- Take a sharp cut on the deep fascia of the forearm from cubital fossa up to the proximal margin of **flexor retinaculum.**
- Make a horizontal cut proximal to the retinaculum.
- Reflect the flaps of fascia.
- The muscles you see medially are flexor group, and laterally are extensor group.
- First separate the most lateral and superficial muscle, **brachioradialis** and trace its attachments.
- At the site of lower attachment of brachioradialis separate the **abductor pollicis longus**, and **extensor pollicis brevis.**

Be careful about superficial **branch of radial nerve** at this point.

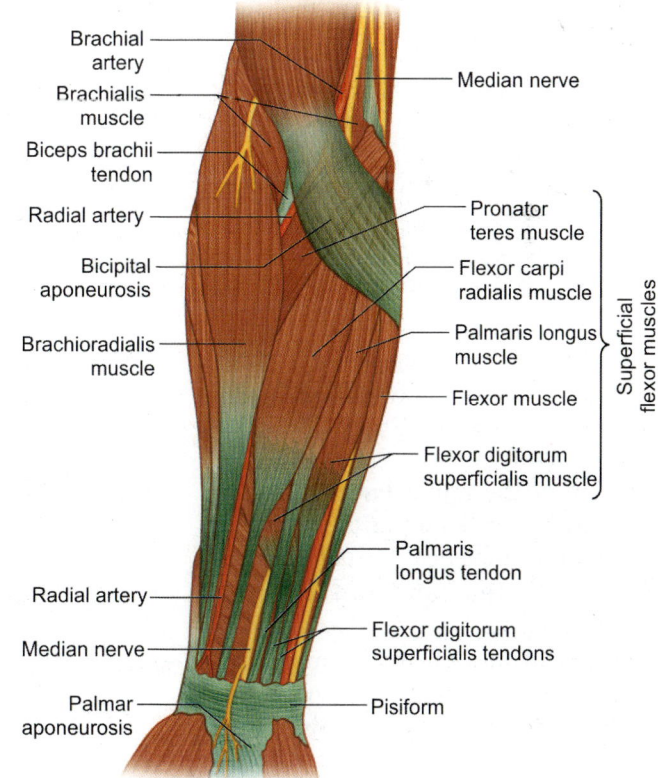

Superficial dissection front of forearm

- If you pull the brachioradialis away laterally, the extensor and flexor groups are identified separately. In the groove between the flexor and radial group one can identify **radial artery** and superficial branch of radial nerve.
- Separate the **superficial group of flexor muscles** from medial epicondyle, they diverge like a fan from **medial epicondyle**, with a vertical medial muscle is **flexor** carpi ulnaris.
- **Pronator teres** is most lateral half of forearm, placed obliquely across proximal convexity of radius.
- Medial to pronator teres is **flexor carpi radialis**, then, **palmaris longus,** followed by **flexor carpi** ulnaris.
- Locate **ulnar artery** and **ulnar nerve** which becomes superficial, between flexor carpi ulnaris tendon near the wrist and **flexor digitorum superficialis tendon**, just proximal to flexor retinaculum.

## Deep Plane

- Now cut transversely distal part of flexor digitorum superficialis, reflect the muscle laterally to expose the deep muscles of forearm.
- Separate the **median nerve** from the deep surface of flexor digitorum superficialis and trace the nerve proximally.
- Identify the **muscular branches of median nerve** and **anterior interosseous branch** near the cubital fossa.
- Follow **ulnar** and **radial artery** proximally.
- You will find glistening membrane in between bones ulna and radius this is **interosseous membrane** the nerve and artery on the membrane is **anterior interosseous nerve and artery.**

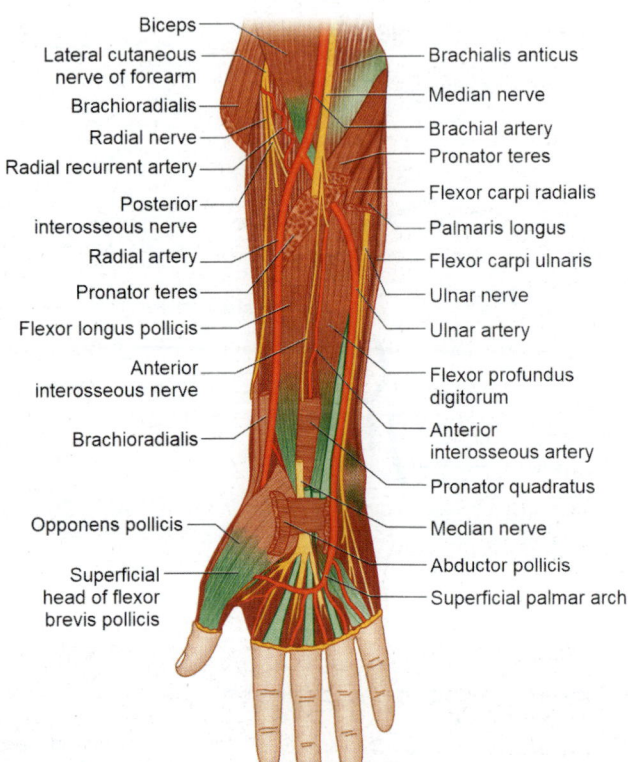

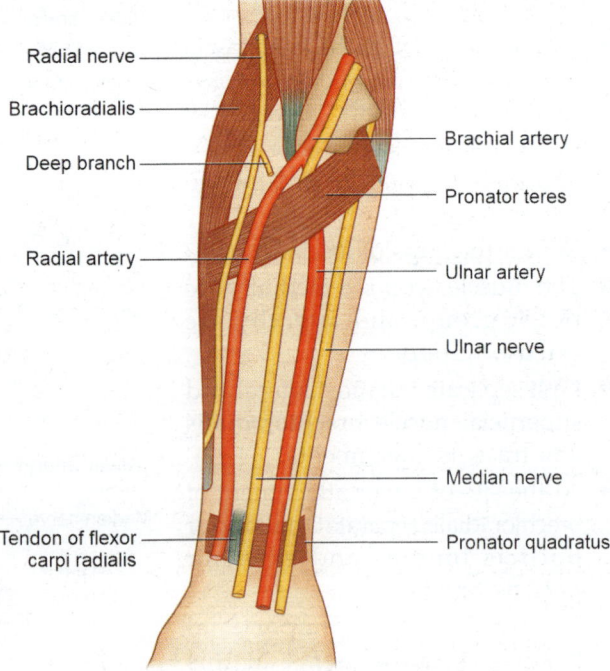

Deep dissection front of forearm

These vessels lie between flexor digitorum profundus medially and flexor pollicis longus laterally. **Pronator quadratus** is a rectangular muscle, in lower part of radius and ulna.

### c. Vivisection

- On incising the skin in front of forearm, for any kind of pathology like swelling, tumor removal, or fracture open reduction; surgeon should be aware of the structures in superficial plane and deep plane.
- Superficial group of muscles are, i.e. pronator teres, flexor carpi radialis, palmaris longus, flexor digitorum superficialis.
- Deep muscles are flexor digitorum profundus, flexor pollicis longus and pronator quadratus.
- Surgeon has to be vigilant about the neurovascular bundle in any region he is operating. In this region, he has to be careful about ulnar artery, radial artery and median nerve lying in deeper plane.

### d. Viva Questions

- Medial epicondyle is the common flexor origin for the superficial muscles of the front of forearm.
- Interosseous membrane is identified as a silvery white glistening membrane over the deep surface of forearm between radius and ulna bones. Fibres are directed downwards, forwards and medially (Like hands in pocket).
- The nerve and artery lying on the interosseous membrane is anterior interosseous nerve and artery.
- Supination and pronation movements occur at radioulnar joints.
- Hybrid muscle (= composite muscle) is muscle supplied by two nerves. Flexor digitorum profundus is a hybrid muscle supplied by median nerve (anterior interosseous branch) laterally and ulnar nerve medially. **Pectineus muscle in lower limb is another example of hybrid muscle it is supplied by femoral nerve and obturator nerve.**

### 6. FRONT OF HAND (PALM)

### a. Incision Markings

### b. Structures to be Identified

*Superficial Plane*

- Superficial fascia is in the form of dense fibrous bands binding the skin to the deep fascia. The skin is thick and hard, so you need to apply firm, uniform force using blade No. 21 to incise the skin on palm and reflect the skin.
- Identify the cutaneous muscle, **palmaris brevis.**

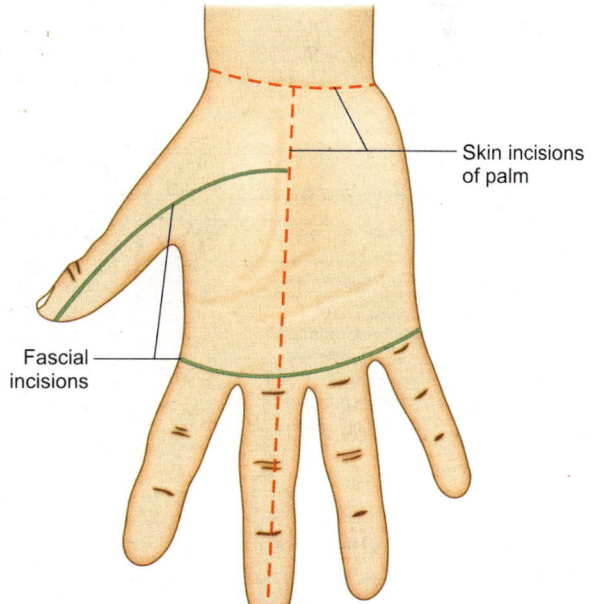

Skin incisions of palm

Fascial incisions

Skin and fascial incisions on front of palm

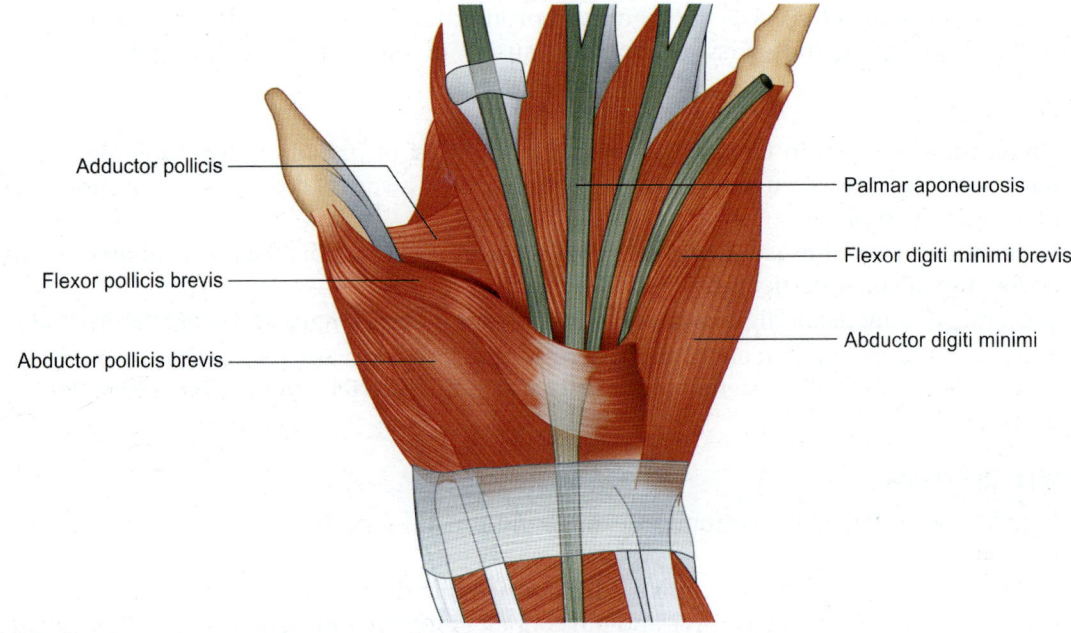

Adductor pollicis

Flexor pollicis brevis

Abductor pollicis brevis

Palmar aponeurosis

Flexor digiti minimi brevis

Abductor digiti minimi

Superficial plane front of palm

- Superficial metacarpal ligament stretches across base of digits; should be appreciated in superficial dissection.

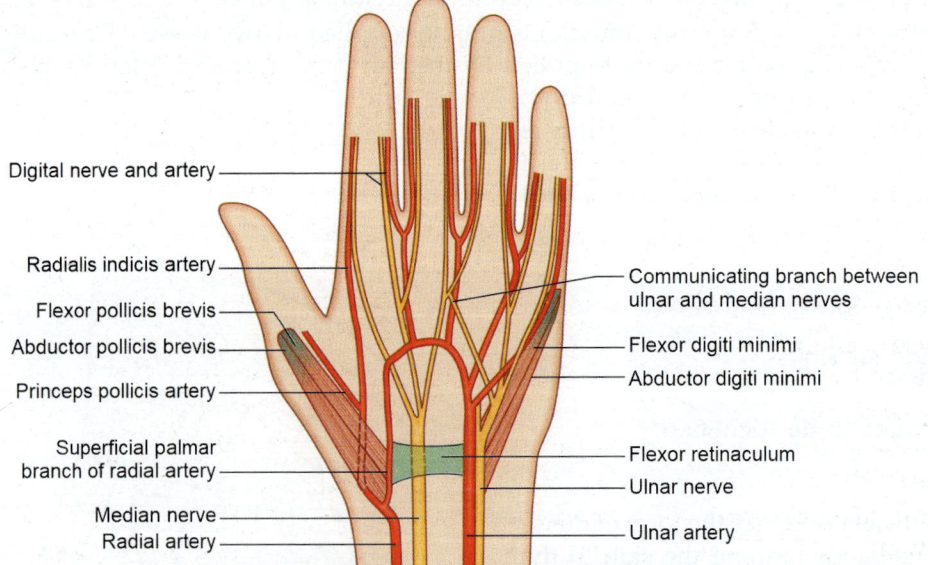

Digital nerve and artery

Radialis indicis artery

Flexor pollicis brevis

Abductor pollicis brevis

Princeps pollicis artery

Superficial palmar branch of radial artery

Median nerve

Radial artery

Communicating branch between ulnar and median nerves

Flexor digiti minimi

Abductor digiti minimi

Flexor retinaculum

Ulnar nerve

Ulnar artery

Intermediate level of dissection (2nd layer) front of palm

- Digital nerves and vessels can be seen.
- Appreciate the web-like triangular **palmar aponeurosis**. Apex blends with **flexor retinaculum** and **palmaris longus,** while the base divides into four slips against the head of metacarpals. Each slip divides into two slips and becomes continuous with fibrous flexor

sheaths of fingers. Digital nerves and vessels emerge from the slips. Identify the lumbrical muscles between the spaces of the slip.

## Deep Plane

- Reflect the palmar aponeurosis and you will see the **superficial palmar arch** as the continuation of ulnar artery.

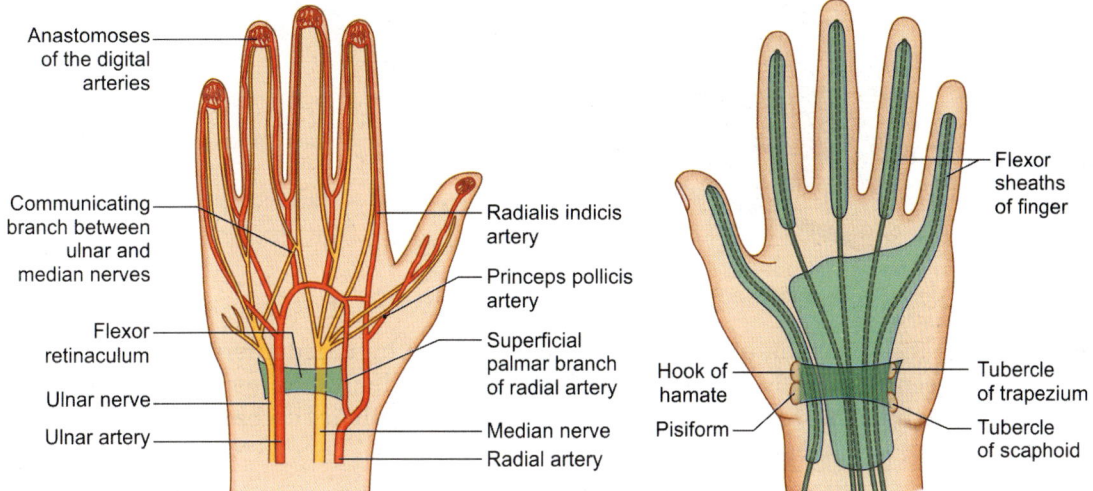

Structures seen after reflecting the palmar aponeurosis

- Flexor retinaculum, is a thick fibrous band connecting the corner carpal bones and converting the carpal arch into a tunnel. The flexor tendons of the digits pass through the tunnel. Ulnar nerve and artery are superficial to retinaculum medially. Divide the retinaculum vertically, between the thenar and hypothenar muscles. Beware of the median nerve it is deep to the retinaculum. Do not cut the nerve. Follow the tendon of **flexor digitorum profundus** to its insertion in distal phalanx. The tendon of **flexor digitorum superficialis** splits into two parts against the proximal phalanx and get inserted into middle phalanx.
- Separate the bundle of muscles of thenar eminence by finger dissection. The most anterior muscle is **abductor pollicis brevis**. The muscles below it are **opponens pollicis** and **flexor pollicis brevis.**
- Cut **flexor pollicis brevis** and reflect it to expose **flexor pollicis longus** and behind it is **adductor pollicis**.
- Separate the **abductor digiti minimi** from **flexor digiti minimi** of hypothenar eminence.
- Identify the **deep palmar branch of ulnar artery** and ulnar nerve between the **abductor digiti minimi** and **flexor digiti minimi**. Cut through the middle of abductor digiti minimi to expose opponens digiti minimi. Follow all the muscles to its attachments.
- Deepest muscle layer are the muscles in between the bones, these are known as **interossei (= palmar interossei)** appreciate the attachments.
- Synovial sheaths of fingers are best demonstrated by injecting air or water through hypodermis needle. While cutting the **fibrous flexor sheaths** please note that the sheath is thin against the joint while thick against the body of phalanges.

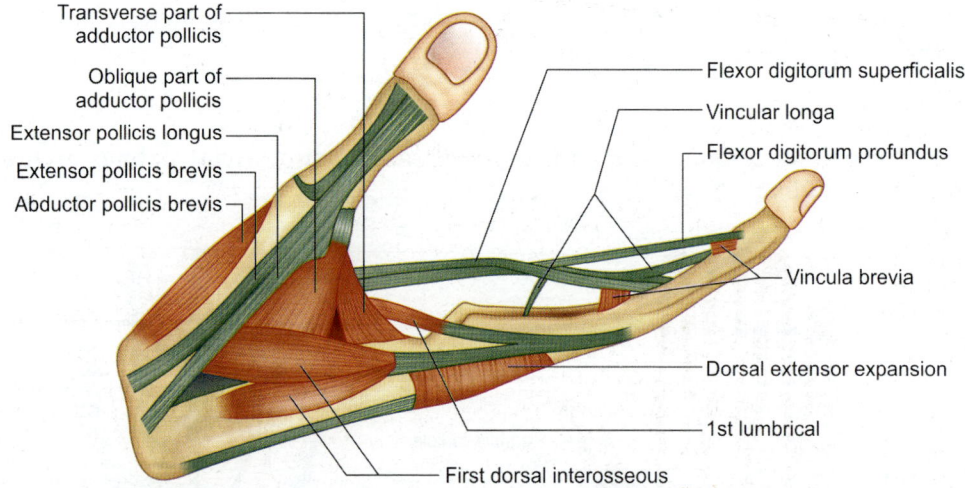

Transverse part of adductor pollicis

Oblique part of adductor pollicis

Extensor pollicis longus

Extensor pollicis brevis

Abductor pollicis brevis

Flexor digitorum superficialis

Vincular longa

Flexor digitorum profundus

Vincula brevia

Dorsal extensor expansion

1st lumbrical

First dorsal interosseous

Dissected side of hand—1st intermetacarpal space

- Appreciate the formation of **deep palmar arch**, formed by radial artery which enters the palm between two heads of first dorsal interossei muscle in first intermetacarpal space. Identify the branches, **princeps pollicis** and **indicis pollicis,** it completes the arch by anastomosing with the deep palmar branch of ulnar artery.

## c. Vivisection

- Ulnar bursa is drained by incising lateral margin of hypothenar eminence. Infection of this bursa is secondary to infection of little finger.

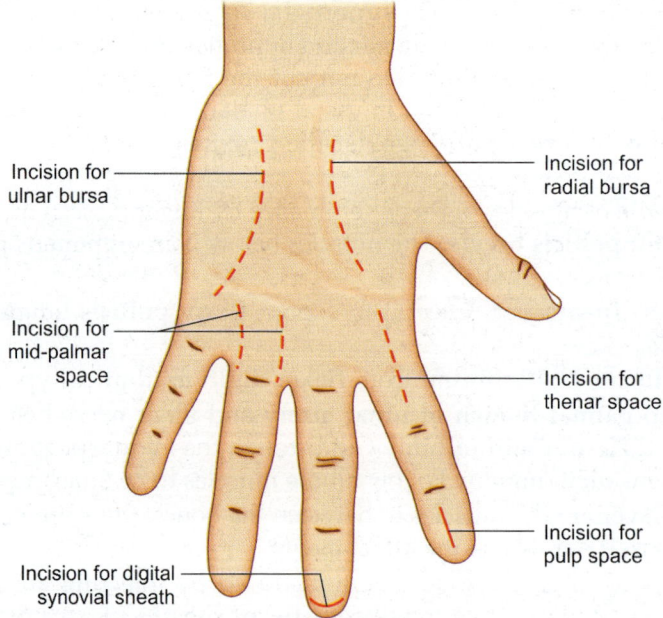

Incision for ulnar bursa

Incision for radial bursa

Incision for mid-palmar space

Incision for thenar space

Incision for pulp space

Incision for digital synovial sheath

Incisions for digital synovial sheath. Incisions for pulp space

- Radial bursa is drained by incising the medial margin of thenar eminence.
- Injuries of hand are common. Especially tendon divisions by cuts due to sharp objects is common. Repair of tendons is done by directly suturing the tendons.
- If only flexor superficialis tendon is cut no active intervention is needed.

### d. Viva Questions

- The patient is asked to touch a pen held in front of palm. This is the pen test to check the action of abductor pollicis brevis.
- Paper test—A thin paper is kept between fingers, to check the strength of palmar interossei. Patient is asked to hold paper in between the fingers.
- Inability to count fingers with the thumb is due paralysis of opponens pollicis.
- Median nerve is labourer's nerve since it controls coarse movements of hand.
- Ulnar nerve is musician's nerve it controls the fine movement.
- Median nerve lies deep to flexor retinaculum.
- Carpal tunnel syndrome is a median nerve entrapment syndrome.
- Dupuytren's contracture is due to contracture of palmar aponeurosis.
  It causes flexion of fingers since the aponeurosis is attached to proximal phalange through transverse metacarpal ligament. The contracture affects little and ring fingers. Surgical division of aponeurosis is done to straighten the fingers.

## 7. SCAPULAR REGION

### a. Incision Markings

*Structures to be identified:*

- Reflect the skin flaps laterally by doing blunt dissection which will involve more strength.
- Remove the deep fascia from the surface of trapezius, below the seventh cervical spine.
- Uncover **latissimus dorsi** now. Define its attachments.
- Reflect the **trapezius** by incising halfway between clavicle and spine of scapula horizontally and 5 cm from midline vertically.
- Identify the **superficial branch of transverse cervical** and **accessory nerve** on deep surface of trapezius muscle.
- Appreciate the muscles under the cover of trapezius namely—**levator scapulae, rhomboidus minor and rhomboidus major**, above downwards. Close to the lower end of

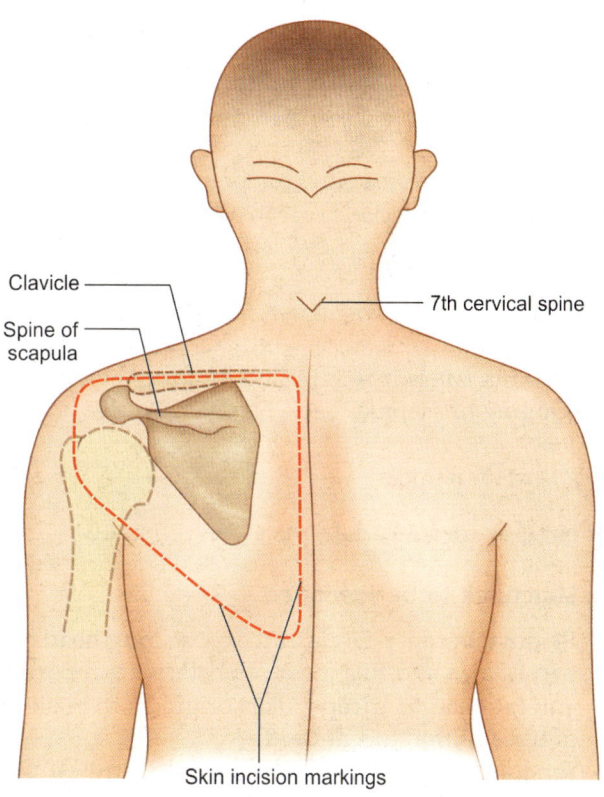

Skin incision markings

Skin incisions to be taken for scapular region

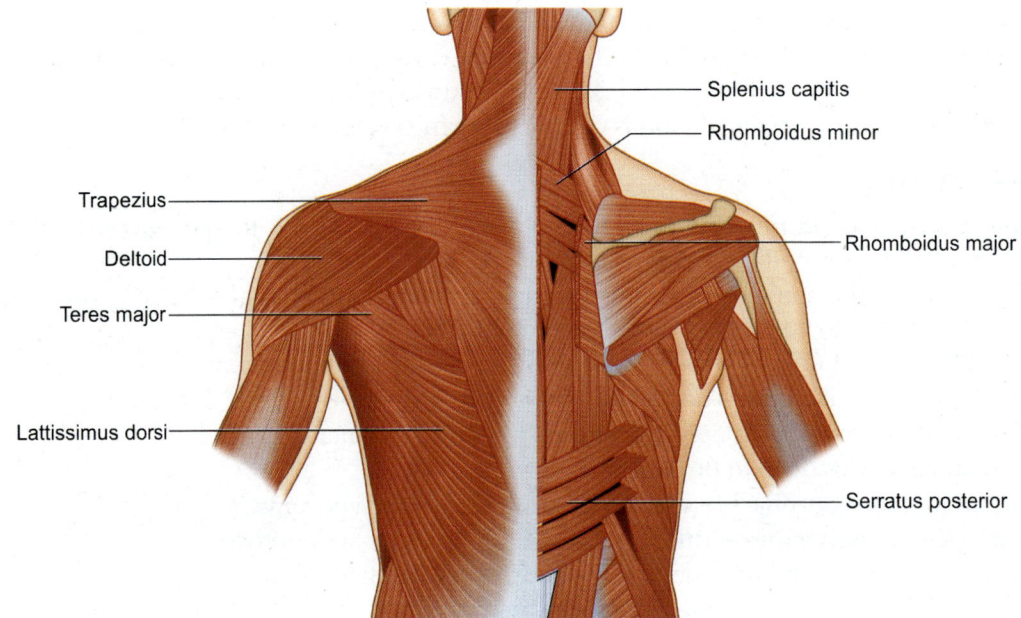

Superficial and deep muscles of the scapular region

levator scapulae muscle, locate the **dorsal scapular nerve** and identify the **deep branch of transverse cervical artery**. Easily one can lift the medial border of scapula and serratus anterior muscle. Study the attachments.

## b. Vivisection

While operating for any purpose in this region the surgeon needs to be aware of the neurovascular bundle, i.e. transverse cervical vessels, and dorsal scapular nerve.

## c. Viva Questions

- Trapezius is known as shawl muscle, supplied by spinal accessory nerve. Along with rhomboids and levator scapulae, it helps in shrugging of shoulders.
- Serratus anterior is supplied by long thoracic nerve (of Bell). Injury to this nerve leads to winging of scapula.

## 8. BACK OF ARM

### a. Incision Markings (refer Figure on next page)

### b. Structures to be Identified

- Remove the deep fascia and expose **long head of triceps**, which is medially placed in upper part of arm and fills most of posterior compartment.
- **Lateral head of triceps** takes origin from posterior surface of humerus between insertions of **teres minor** and **deltoid.**
- Separate the muscles on back of the arm by blunt dissection. Divide and reflect parts of lateral head of triceps to locate the groove containing **radial nerve** and **profunda brachii** artery. The medial head of triceps lies below the groove.

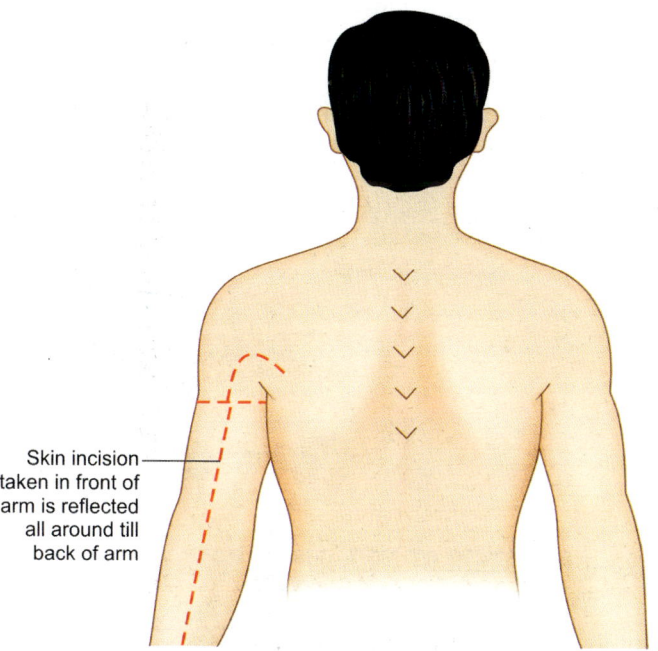

Back of arm—dissection

- Follow the radial nerve and appreciate the muscular branches.
- Locate the division of radial nerve into superficial and deep branches at the level of elbow joint.

## c. Vivisection

While operating on the back of arm the surgeon should be aware of the profunda brachii muscles and the radial nerve.

## d. Viva Questions

- Boundaries and contents of intermuscular spaces:
  - Upper triangular space—medially-teres minor, laterally long head of triceps, inferiorly teres major, circumflex scapular vessels.
  - Lower triangular space—medially-long head of triceps, laterally medial border of humerus, superiorly-teres major, radial nerve and profunda brachii vessels.

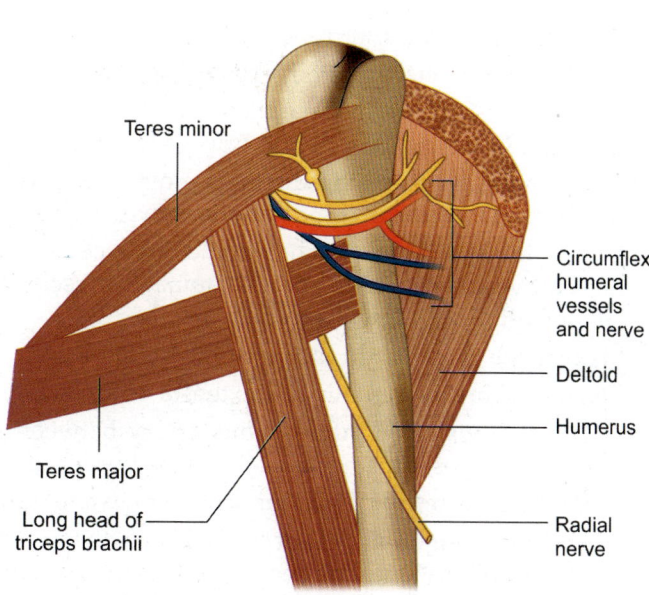

Intermuscular spaces on back of the arm

- Quandrangular space—superiorly teres minor, inferiorly-teres major, medially long head of triceps, laterally surgical neck of humerus, axillary nerve, posterior circumflex humeral vessels.
- Axillary nerve may get injured due to fractures of surgical neck of humerus.
- Radial groove structures are radial nerve, profunda brachii vessels.

## 9. BACK OF FOREARM

### a. Incision Markings

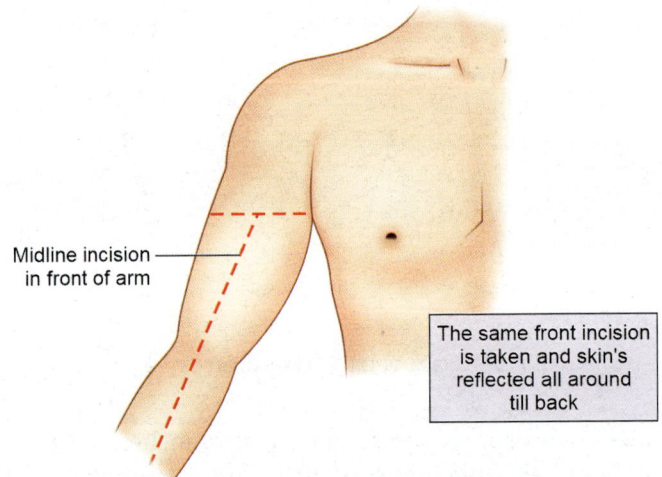

Midline incision in front of arm

The same front incision is taken and skin's reflected all around till back

Back of forearm-dissection

### b. Structures to be Identified

- Remove the deep fascia from back of the arm without dividing the extensor retinaculum.
- Define the proximal border of **extensor retinaculum** and demonstrate the **synovial sheaths.**
- Do finger dissections to separate the tendons near the wrist this will help you separate the superficial extensor muscles on back of forearm.
- Completely, separate the three anterolateral muscles—**brachioradialis, extensor carpi radialis, and extensor carpi radialis brevis** from extensor digitorum.
- Expose the **supinator** which lies under the cover of the extensor muscles. You will see a thick nerve at the distal border of supinator muscle, this is the **deep branch of radial nerve, i.e. posterior interosseous nerve.**
- Identify the muscular branches of the radial nerve.
- Retract the brachioradialis and extensor tendons laterally to locate the radial nerve.
- Locate the **posterior interosseous artery** between the radius and ulna, along with the posterior interosseous nerve at the distal border of supinator.
- Separate the **extensor digiti minimi** from **extensor digitorum tendon.**
- Just below the supinator the deep muscles of the back of forearm can be appreciated, namely-**abductor pollicis longus, extensor pollicis brevis, extensor pollicis longus, extensor indicis.** Trace the tendons of these muscles up to the extensor retinaculum.

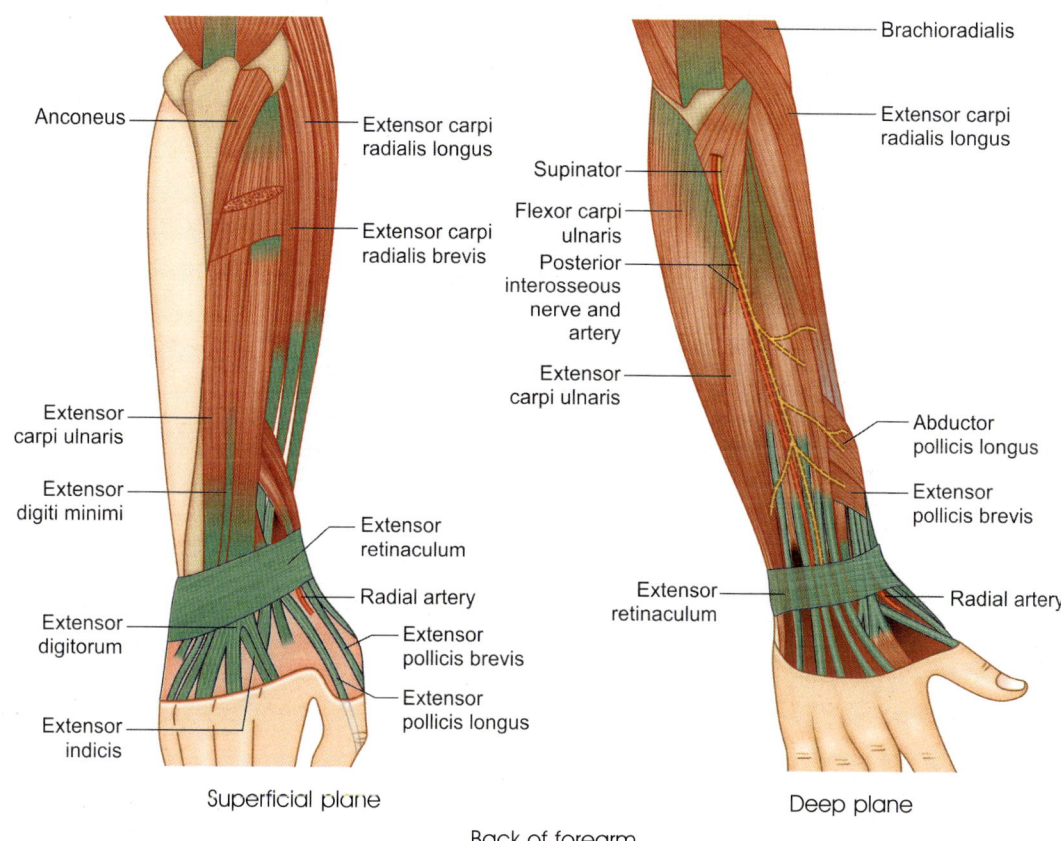

Anconeus

Extensor carpi radialis longus

Extensor carpi radialis brevis

Extensor carpi ulnaris

Extensor digiti minimi

Extensor digitorum

Extensor indicis

Extensor retinaculum

Radial artery

Extensor pollicis brevis

Extensor pollicis longus

Superficial plane

Brachioradialis

Extensor carpi radialis longus

Supinator

Flexor carpi ulnaris

Posterior interosseous nerve and artery

Extensor carpi ulnaris

Abductor pollicis longus

Extensor pollicis brevis

Extensor retinaculum

Radial artery

Deep plane

Back of forearm

## b. Vivisection

Ganglion is a very common swelling on the back of the wrist, it is excised for cosmetic reasons. While operating one has to be aware of the structures below the skin and be careful of the neurovascular bundle.

## c. Viva Questions

- You should be able to identify the supinator muscle on back of forearm near the elbow and the at the distal border is the deep branch of radial nerve, posterior interosseus nerve.

- Strong supinator of elbow is biceps brachii.

- Just above the extensor retinaculum are two tendons crossing—(namely extensor pollicis brevis and abductor pollicis longus) the extensor tendons going to the carpal bones. You should be able to identify the crossing tendons.

- Injury to radial nerve in axilla or arm leads to paralysis of the extensor muscles of the back of forearm producing wrist drop. This injury is above the origin of posterior interosseous nerve.

## 10. BACK OF HAND (DORSUM)

### a. Incision Markings

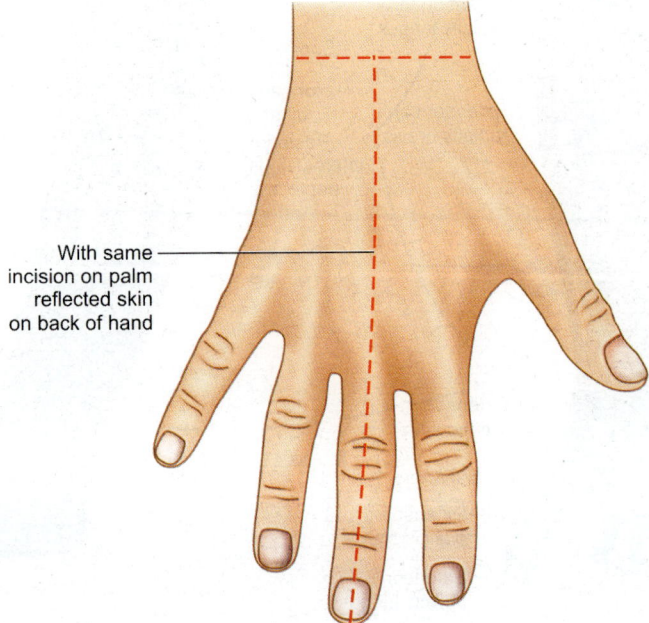

With same
incision on palm
reflected skin
on back of hand

Back of hand-dissection

### b. Structures to be Identified

- You can easily identify the extensor tendons on your own wrist and hand, i.e. index finger, little finger extensor tendons and 2 extensor tendons for the thumb.

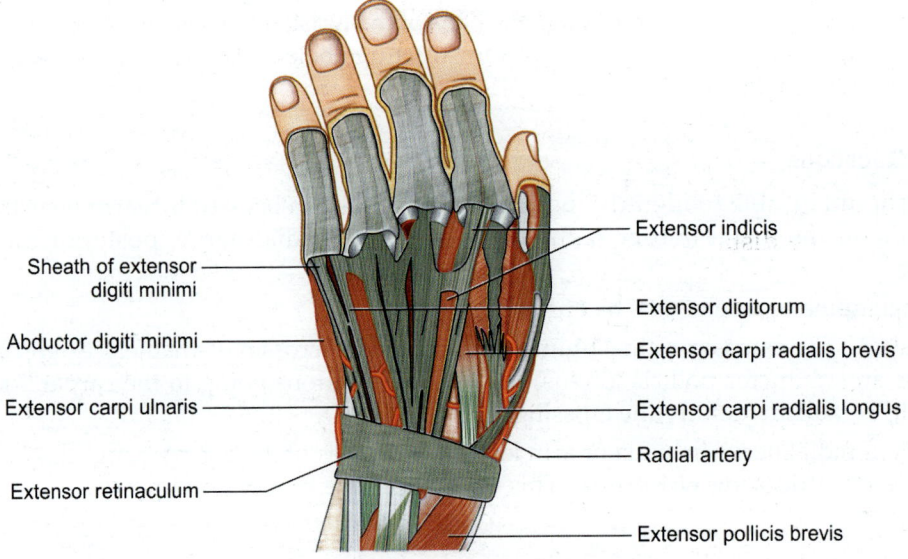

Sheath of extensor digiti minimi

Abductor digiti minimi

Extensor carpi ulnaris

Extensor retinaculum

Extensor indicis

Extensor digitorum

Extensor carpi radialis brevis

Extensor carpi radialis longus

Radial artery

Extensor pollicis brevis

Extensor tendons on back of hand

- Trace the **radial artery** from anterior surface of lower part of radius where it winds back, traverses the **anatomical snuffbox** deep to the tendons forming the boundaries of anatomical snuffbox. Identify carpal and digital branches.
- Follow the extensor tendons into the fingers and thumb. Appreciate that the extensor tendon expands against the metacarpophalangeal joints, like a hood. This expansion narrows against the proximal interphalangeal joint.

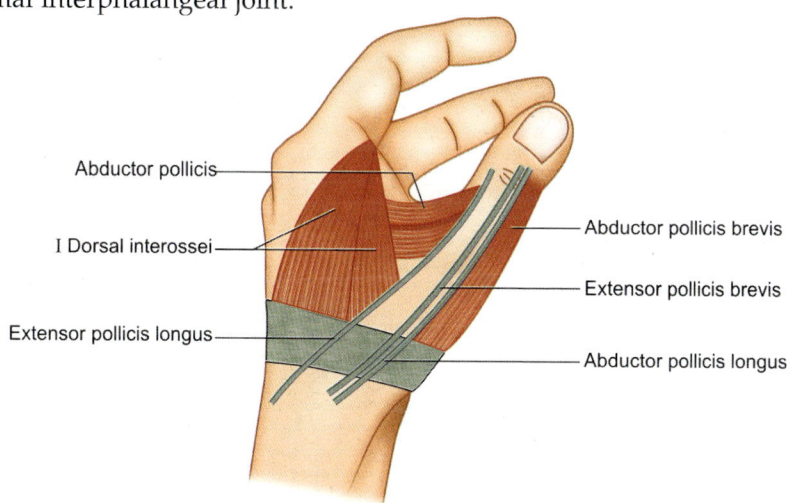

Dissected side of hand. Dorsal digital expansion

- Identify the tendon of lumbricals anteriorly, to the palmar surface of deep metacarpal ligament.
- Remove the fat and fascia from the intermetacarpal space and you will see the dorsal interossei muscle. Separate the muscle from adjacent metacarpal bones, turn it distally and this will expose the palmar interossei. Trace the palmar interossei tendon to extensor expansion.

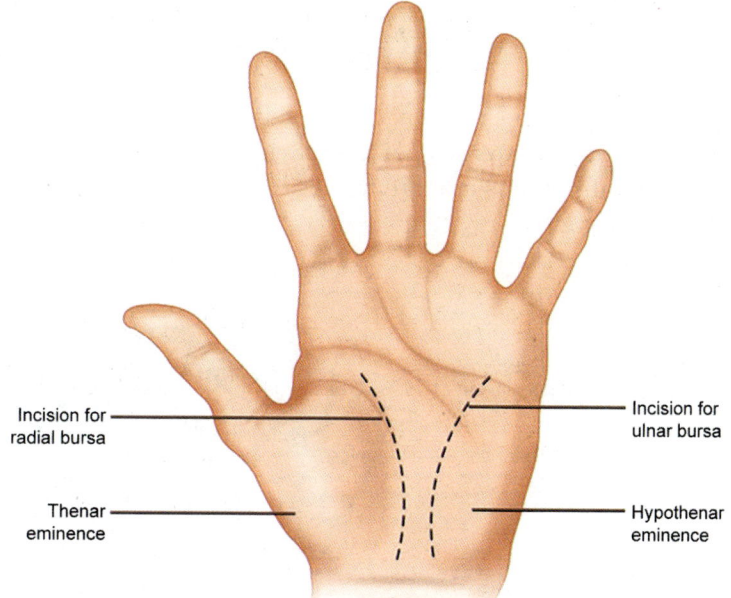

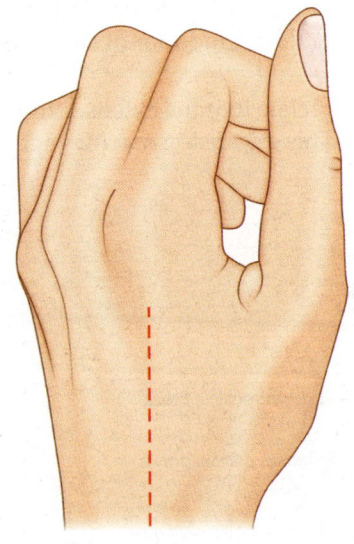

Incision for medial approach of wrist joint

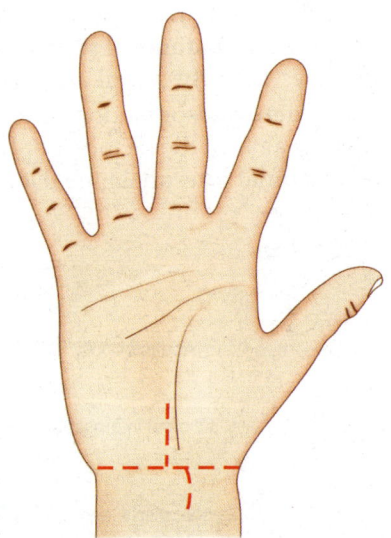

Incision for volar approach of wrist joint

## c. Vivisection

- While operating in lower part of forearm radially, surgeon needs to be careful about the radial artery in anatomical snuffbox.
- In case of tendon injuries, the skin is closed first then the tendon repair is done as a part of secondary intervention.

## d. Viva Questions

- Anatomical snuffbox-boundaries—anteriorly-abductor pollicis longus, extensor pollicis brevis and posteriorly-extensor pollicis longus, floor by extensor carpi radialis longus and brevis, contents radial artery, radial nerve. One looks for scaphoid fracture tenderness in this box.
- Extensor fascial compartments—from lateral to medial side
   i. Abductor pollicis longus, extensor pollicis brevis
   ii. Extensor carpi radialis longus and brevis
   iii. Extensor pollicis longus
   iv. Extensor digitorum, extensor indicis, poste rior interosseous nerve, anterior interosseous artery
   v. Extensor digiti minimi, extensor carpi ulnaris.

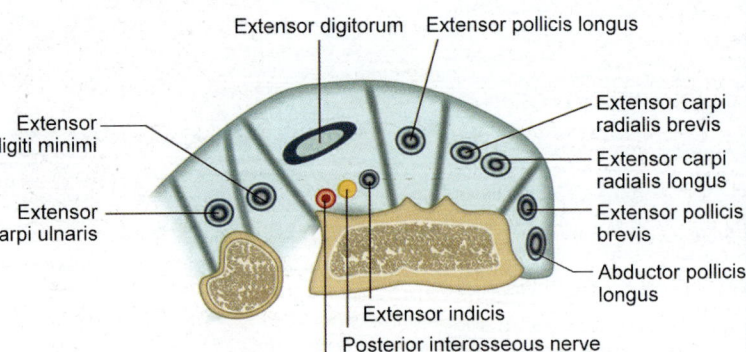

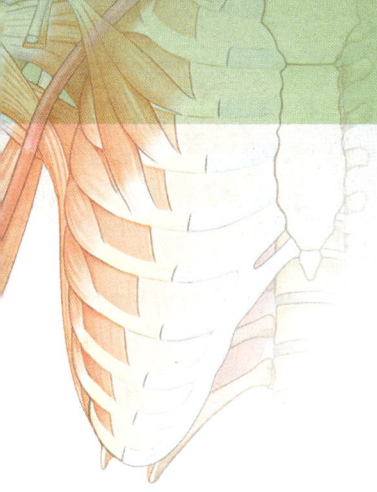

# Osteology |

### General Understanding

- Regarding any bone one should know—the side whether it belongs to right or left side, attachments (most crucial), ossification and any peculiarities.
- If the bone belongs to right side, hold it in the right hand, and if left side hold in left hand.
- Several points need to be clubbed together for side determination.
- Practically not possible to remember all the ossifications and only few important are repeatedly asked in the exams only these are dealt in this section.
- Clinical importance of certain bones one should know.
- Most commonly asked viva questions related to osteology are dealt in this section.
- Study the diagrams carefully and spend more time in understanding the diagrams. Diagram speaks 1000 words!
- Primary centre appears before birth generally, it is single, around 8th week of intrauterine life (IUL), secondary centre appears after birth. The centre which appears first fuses last, and by and large around puberty. In males, secondary centres merge with the shaft later than females, e.g. 14–15 years in females while 17–18 years in males.
- Most of the bones in the body develop from cartilaginous model, this is known as cartilaginous ossification. Few bones develop directly from connective tissue foundation these are the bones said to be developed from membranous ossification.

### Upper Limb

### 1. Clavicle (means—key)

It is a long bone.

*Side Determination*

- Medial end is large and stout, while lateral end is flat above downwards
- Shaft is convex forwards in its medial 2/3rd while concave forwards in its lateral 1/3rd
- Inferior surface, is grooved in its middle 1/3rd this is the, subclavian groove.

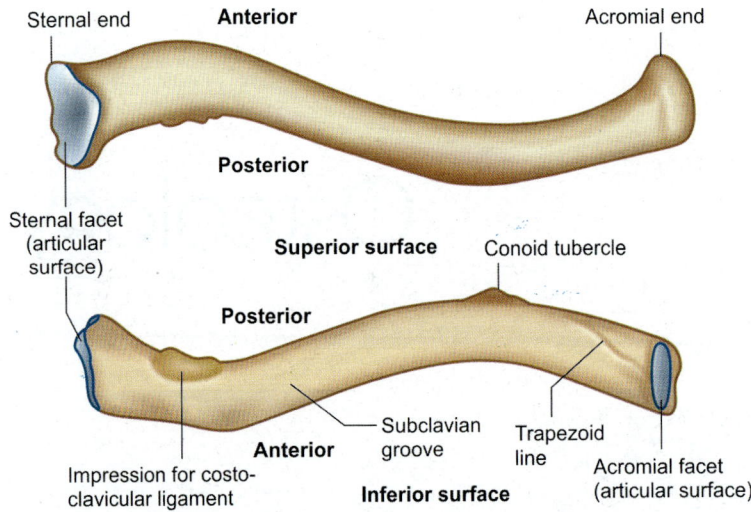

Clavicle—superior surface and inferior surface

## Attachments

- Muscle in the subclavian groove is subclavius.
- Attachments of pectoralis major, deltoid and trapezius are commonly asked in exams and if you study the diagram carefully one should be able to tell the attachments. Remember pectoralis muscle is the muscle of front of the chest, so obviously it will take origin from the front side of the bone, deltoid muscle forms the contour of the shoulder in and around the shoulder joint, so the attachments of this muscle are on all the bones in the shoulder region.

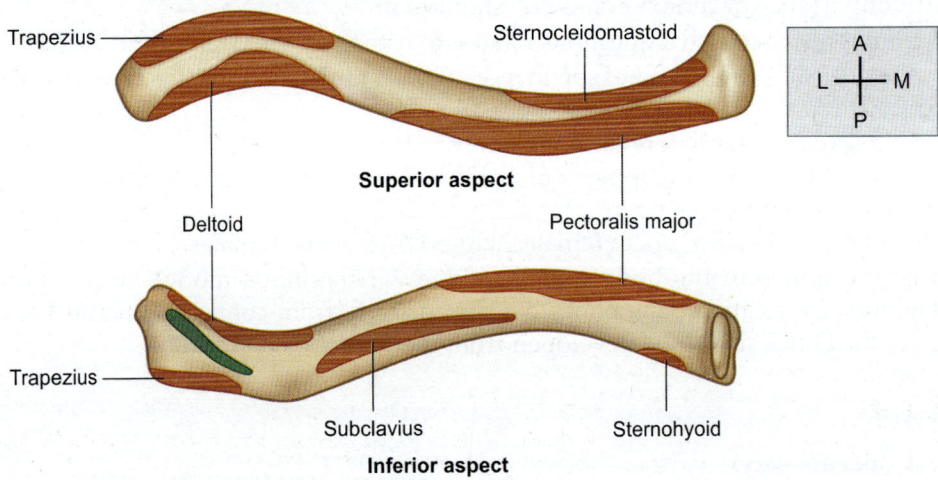

Clavicle-superior and inferior surface with muscle attachments

## Ossification

- Ossifies from 2 primary centres and 1 secondary centre
- The 2 primary centres appear for the shaft between 5th and 6th weeks of IUL and fuse by 1 and a half month
- Secondary centre for medial end appears around teen age and fuses by 21 to 22 years.

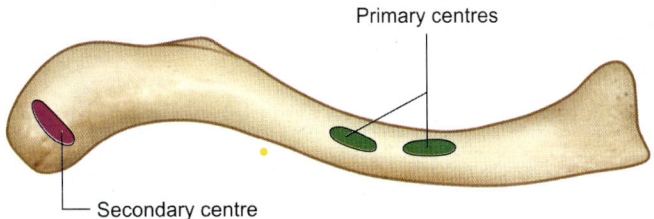

Clavicle showing primary and secondary centres

## *Peculiarities of Clavicle*

- Only long bone placed horizontally and sinuously curved
- The whole length of the bone is easily palpable, i.e. subcutaneous. (feel it on yourself)
- It is the first bone to ossify
- It is the only long bone having membranous ossification
- It is the only long bone which has 2 primary centres of ossification
- It has no medullary cavity
- It is the only bone pierced by nerve, i.e. supraclavicular nerves
- The weak point on the bone is at the junction of lateral and intermediate 1/3rd, thus a fall on outstretched hand will lead to break in the continuity of bone (= fracture) at this point
- Clavicle in females is shorter, thinner, less curved and smoother with its acromial end lower than the sternal end.

## 2. Scapula (means to dig)

It is a flat, triangular bone, on the posterior aspect of thoracic cage, lying against 2nd to 7th ribs.

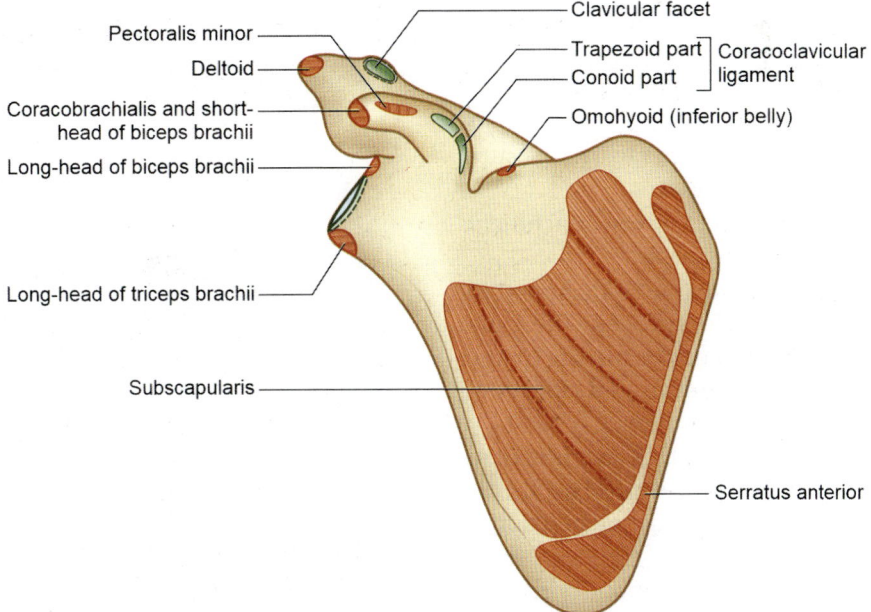

Scapula bone—anterior (costal) surface with muscle attachments

## Side Determination

- Spine of the scapula is on its dorsal aspect
- Glenoid cavity faces laterally, since it has to articulate with the humerus.

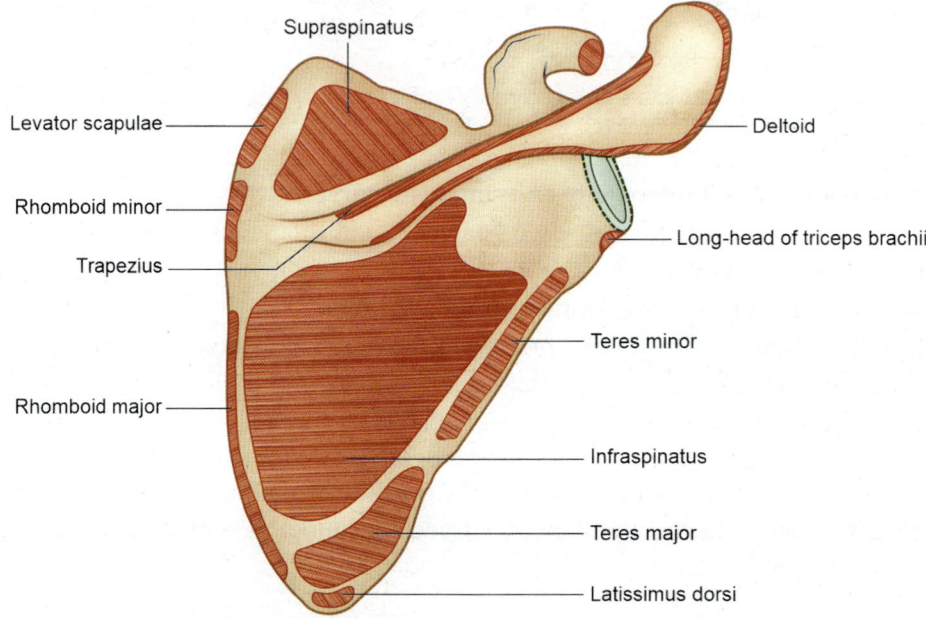

Scapula—dorsal surface with muscle attachments

## Attachments

- Coracoid process (beak like projection) provides attachment to coracobrachialis, short-head of biceps, pectoralis minor and coracoclavicular ligament.
- Subscapularis arises from most of the subcostal surface of scapula.
- Medial border in front gives attachment to serratus anterior muscle.
- Area above the spine gives attachment to supraspinatus muscle and below the spine is the area for infraspinatus muscle (name of the muscle is according to its location, above and below the spine).
- Supraglenoid tubercle gives attachment to long-head of biceps, while the infraglenoid tubercle gives attachment to long-head of triceps.
- Trapezius is attached to upper border of scapula, while lower border of scapula gives attachment to deltoid.
- Against the root of spine is the attachment of rhomboidus minor.

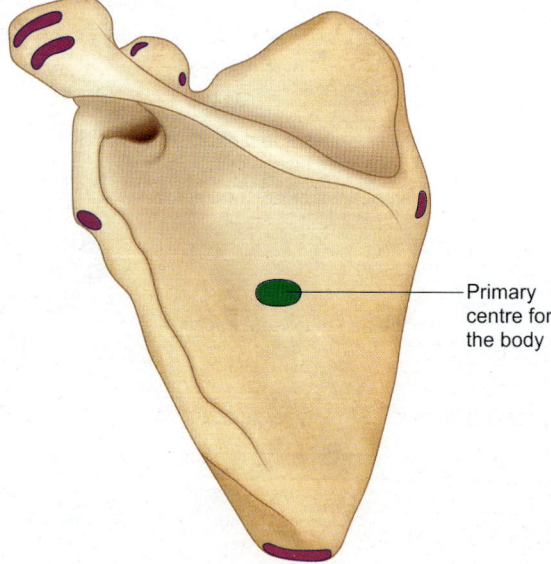

Scapula-dorsal surface showing primary and secondary centres of ossification

*Peculiarities*

- Supraglenoid notch is converted into supraglenoid foramen by a ligament which fills the gap. Suprascapular nerve lies within the foramen while the suprascapular artery and vein lie above the ligament
- Anatomical neck of scapula is the constriction around the rim of the glenoid cavity
- Capsular attachment around the glenoid cavity is lax inferiorly which permits good range of movements at the joint. (one should be able to mark it on the bone as shown in the figure)

*If your sleeves are tight in the underarm, your limb movement is restricted.*

*Ossification*

- This bone ossifies from 1 primary centre and 8 or more secondary centres
- Primary centre for the body appears in the body as usual during 8th week of IUL
- Secondary centres appear in coracoid process (2), acromion (2), lower part of glenoid rim, inferior angle and the adjacent medial border
- Secondary centre of coracoid process appears at 1st year and fuses by 15 years of age
- The other secondary centres appear around puberty and fuse by 25 years of age.

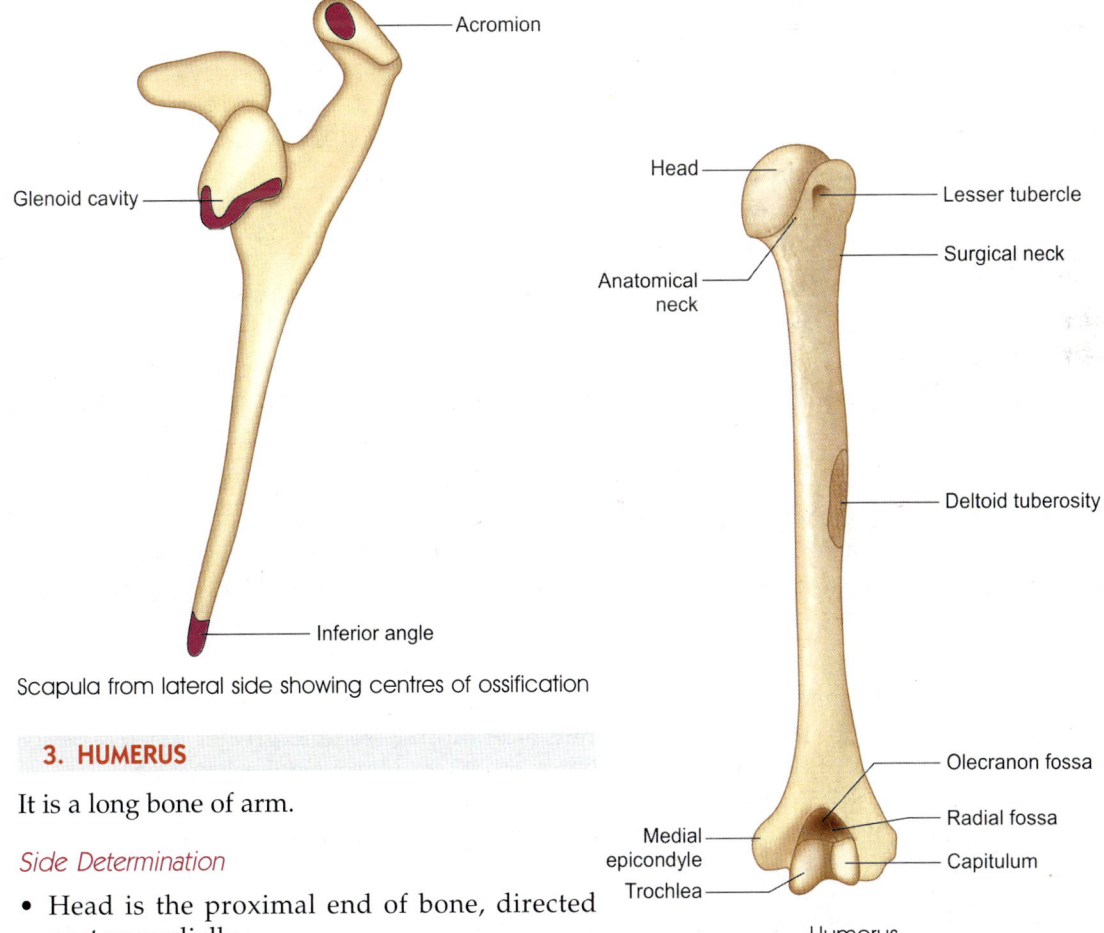

Scapula from lateral side showing centres of ossification

### 3. HUMERUS

It is a long bone of arm.

*Side Determination*

- Head is the proximal end of bone, directed posteromedially

Humerus

- Lower end is transversely expanded, with prominent medial epicondyle, 2 fossae facing forwards while 1 olecranon fossa posteriorly.

## Attachments

- Lesser tubercle—subscapularis.
- Greater tubercle—supraspinatus, infraspinatus, teres minor.
- Deltoid tuberosity—deltoid muscle.
- Anatomical neck—capsule of shoulder joint.
- In between the tubercles is the sulcus, hence named intertubercular sulcus. Lateral lip of sulcus gives attachment to pectoralis major medial lip to teres major and floor gives attachment to latissimus dorsi. (*Mnemonic:* **lady between 2 majors**)
- Medial epicondyle gives attachment to common flexor origin while lateral epicondyle to common extensor group muscles.
- Medial supracondylar ridge gives attachment to pronator teres.

Subscapularis
Supraspinatus
Pectoralis major
Lattisimus dorsi
Teres major
Deltoid
Brachialis
Pronator teres
Common flexor originator
Common extensor origin

Humerus with muscle attachments

## Peculiarities

- Angle of humeral torsion means, in lower animals the upper and lower ends of bone are at right angles to each other, however in human beings the proximal end of the bone appears to have rotated laterally to 164 degrees. This is angle of humeral torsion.
- Surgical neck is related to axillary nerve and posterior circumflex humeral vessels.

## Ossification

- Primary centre for shaft at 8th week of IUL.
- Secondary centres for head, within 6 months after birth, lesser and greater tubercle ossify by 2nd to 5th years of life. By 6th year, all fuse together to form single epiphysis.
- In the 1st year a centre appears for capitulum, and by 9–10 years for medial edge of trochlea, all fuse with each other by puberty to form single epiphysis and then fuse with rest of the shaft by 14 years in females and 16 years in males.
- Separate epiphysis appears for medial epicondyle which fuses with the shaft by 20 years.
- Distal epiphysis is the first to fuse with the shaft.

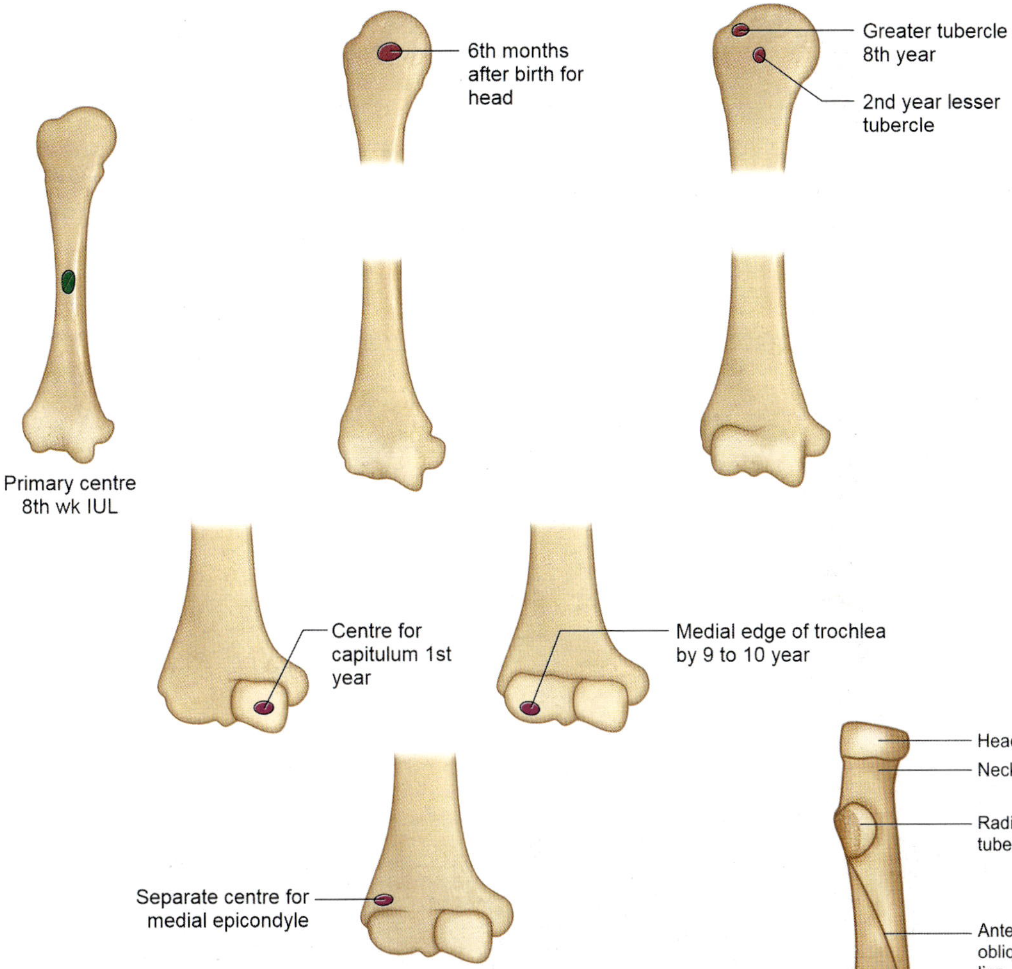

6th months
after birth for
head

Greater tubercle
8th year

2nd year lesser
tubercle

Primary centre
8th wk IUL

Centre for
capitulum 1st
year

Medial edge of trochlea
by 9 to 10 year

Separate centre for
medial epicondyle

Ossification of humerus-showing primary and secondary centres

## 4. RADIUS

It is one of the long bone of forearm, placed laterally.

### Side Determination

- Turban like appearance of head of radius forms the proximal end of radius while the distal end is expanded and has a pointed projection laterally styloid process
- Bulge, radial tuberosity is directed medially.

### Attachments

- Posterior, rough area of radial tuberosity gives attachment to biceps brachii muscle, anterior smooth portion related to bursa
- Area just behind the tuberosity provides attachment to supinator muscle.

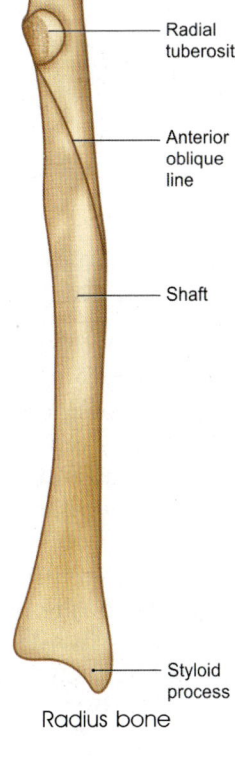

Head

Neck

Radial
tuberosity

Anterior
oblique
line

Shaft

Styloid
process

Radius bone

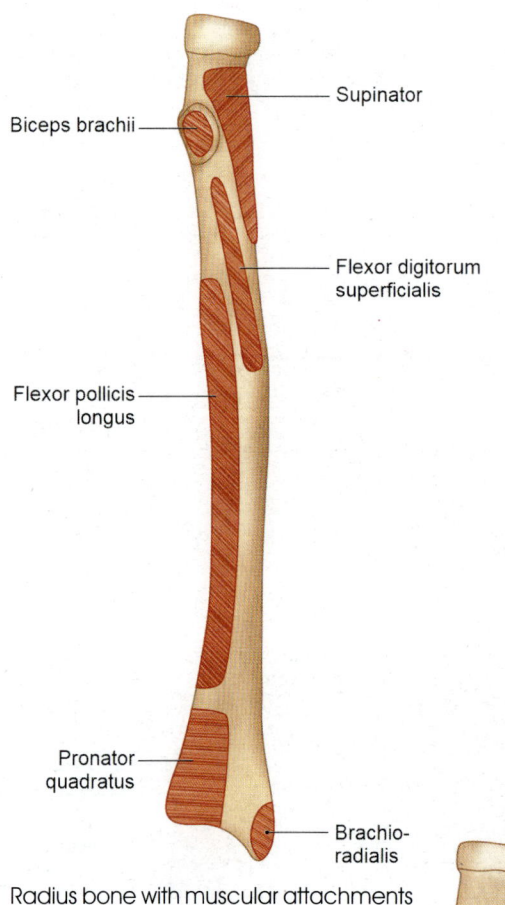

Biceps brachii

Supinator

Flexor digitorum superficialis

Flexor pollicis longus

Pronator quadratus

Brachio-radialis

Radius bone with muscular attachments

## Ossification

- 1 primary centre for the shaft appears in 8th week of IUL
- At the end of 1st year a secondary centre appears on the distal end of the bone while during the 4th year in proximal end
- Proximal centre fuses with the rest of the bone by 14–17 years, while the distal centre fuses with the rest of the bone by 17–19 years.

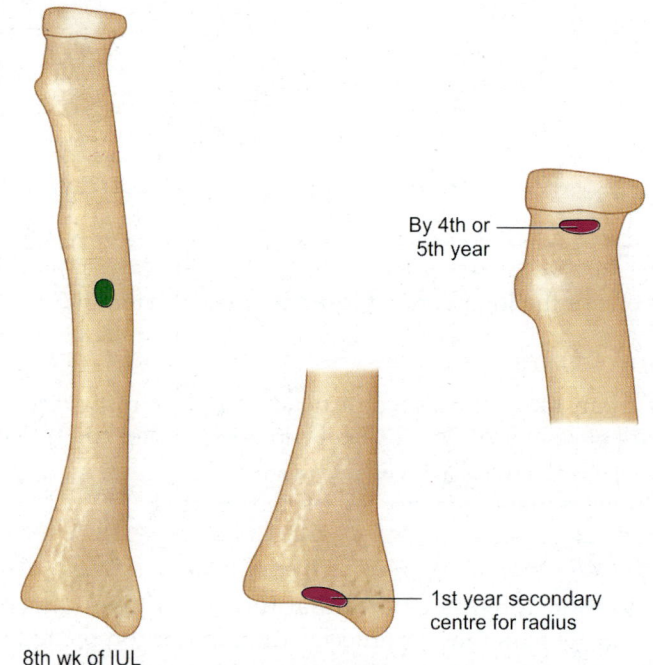

By 4th or 5th year

1st year secondary centre for radius

8th wk of IUL

Radius bone-showing primary and secondary centres of ossification

## 5. ULNA

It is the medially placed long bone of forearm.

### Side Determination

- Proximal part of the bone is hood-like having a prominent trochlear notch, and notch on the radial side for the radial bone
- Lateral border of the shaft is sharp, it is the interosseous border
- Distal part of the bone is small and rounded. With a small projection medially the styloid process.

### Attachments

- To the posterior 2/3rd of olecranon process triceps is attached, anconeus is just proximal to oblique line and lateral to olecranon
- Coronoid process and ulnar tuberosity have the attachment of brachialis muscle.

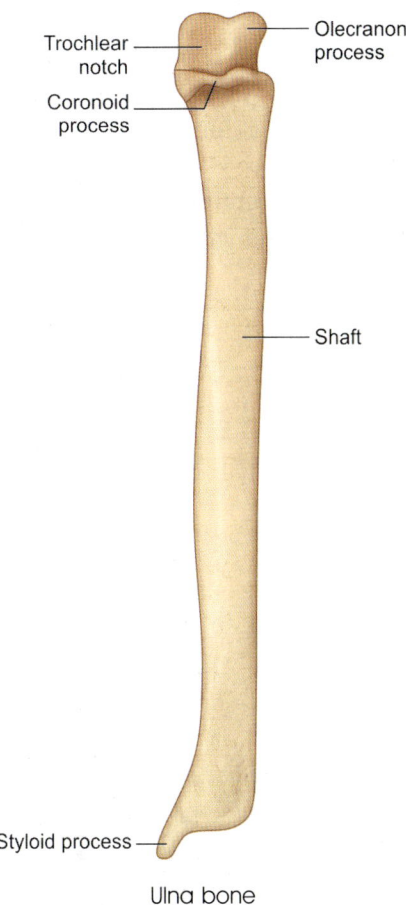

Ulna bone

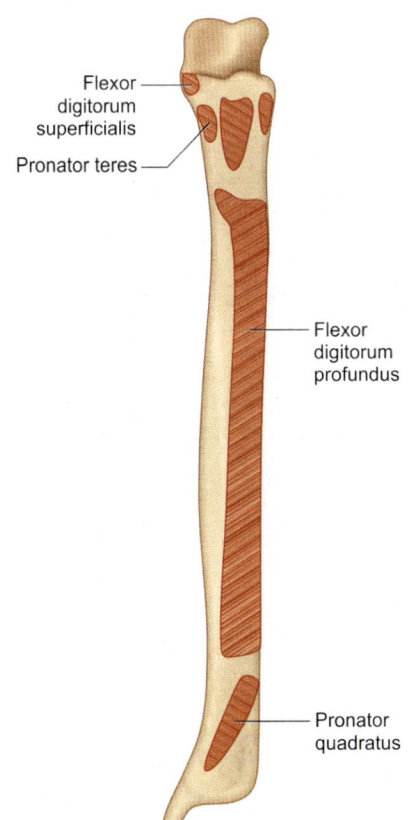

Ulna bone with muscular attachments

*Ossification*

- One primary centre for the shaft at 8th week of IUL
- One secondary centre around 5 to 6 years for distal end including styloid process
- Two centres for trochlear surface and one more centre on summit of olecranon, around 9 to 11 years
- Proximal centres merge with the shaft by 14–16 years
- Distal epiphysis unites with the shaft by 17–18 years.

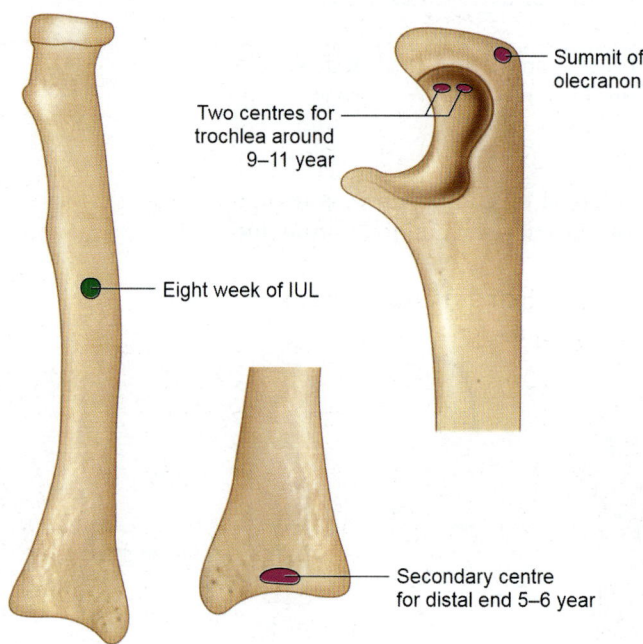

Two centres for trochlea around 9–11 year

Summit of olecranon

Eight week of IUL

Secondary centre for distal end 5–6 year

Ulna showing primary and secondary centres of ossification

## 6. CARPAL BONES

These are small irregular bones, forming proximal skeleton of hand.

### Number of Bones

| Mnemonic | Bones |
|----------|-------|
| She | Scaphoid |
| Looks | Lunate |
| Too | Triquetral |
| Pretty | Pisiform |
| Try | Trapezium |
| To | Trapezoid |
| Catch | Capitate |
| Her | Hamate |

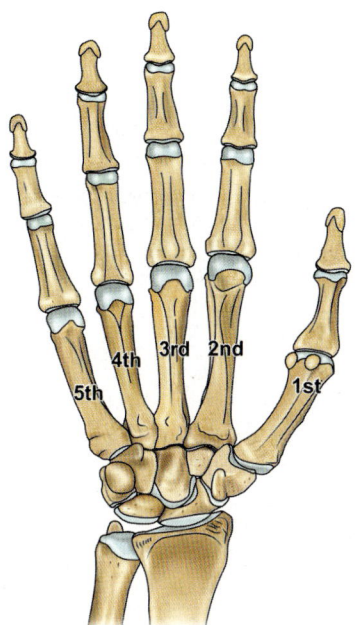

Skeleton of hand

## Identification Points of Carpal Bone

Only the exam-oriented points of important carpal bones are discussed in the following section.

### Scaphoid

*Literal meaning—boat-like*
- Largest carpal bone in proximal row
- Lateral surface is nonarticular
- Radial surface convex
- Medial surface is flat, semilunar
- Surface for capitate in front, is large, concave
- Surface for trapezium, trapezoid is convex
- Commonly fractured on an outstretched hand.

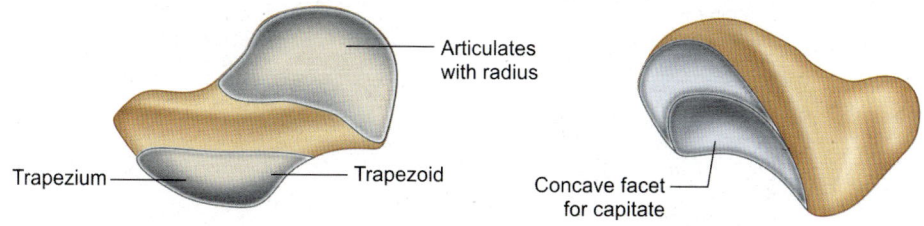

Scaphoid bone palmar and dorsal surfaces

## Lunate

*Literal meaning—half moon-shaped*
- Palmar surface is rough, larger, wider and triangular than dorsal surface
- Proximal surface is smooth and convex to articulate with the radius and articular disc
- Lateral surface has a small, semilunar facet for scaphoid
- Medial surface flat, square
- Distal surface is deeply concave for the head of capitate.

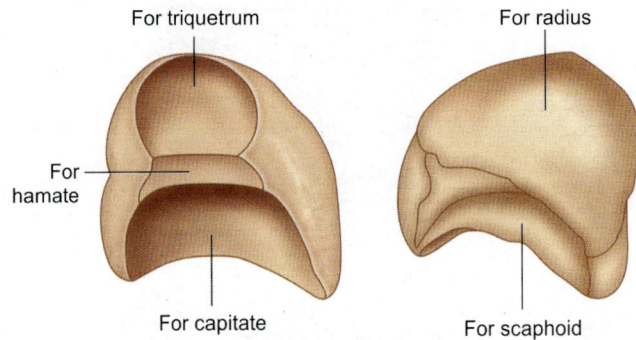

Lunate bone—proximal surface and distal surface

## Pisiform

*Literal meaning—pea-like*
- It is classified as sesamoid bone, developing in the tendon of flexor carpi ulnaris
- It ossifies at the age of 12 years
- One can assess the age of the patient from X-ray film, if the shadow of pisiform bone is visible: Age is 12 years.

## Capitate

It is the largest of all the carpal bones, hence considered as the key carpal bone.

## Hamate

This carpal bone can be easily identified by presence of prominent unciform hamulus, the uncinate process on the rough palmar surface of the bone.

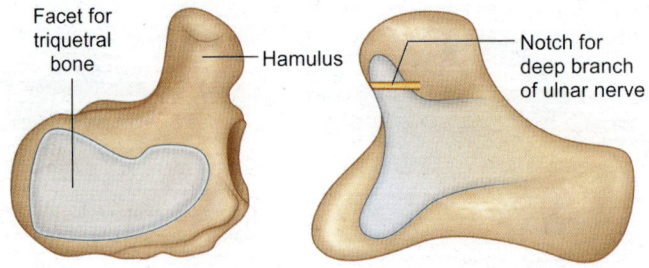

Hamate bone medial and radial surfaces

*Metacarpus*

These are short, long bones having the same parts as the long bone-upper end, (head) shaft and lower end (base).

*Ossification*

- Capitate is the first bone to ossify, while the pisiform is the last bone to ossify
- Each metacarpal has a primary centre for the shaft and secondary centre for the other metacarpals in the head except secondary centre for the first metacarpal is in the base.

# Surface Anatomy

## 8

Surface anatomy also referred as living anatomy is a very interesting way to learn anatomy on living. Student would get a feel of being a doctor and would have an upper edge over the lay man by able to tell what lies underneath the skin. Medicine is not Mathematics, wherein only approximate locations can be predicted not accurate. Knowledge of surface anatomy will prove very useful in clinics to come to the diagnosis of particular health condition.

*Only important exam-oriented topics and markings are discussed also remember markings are two-dimensional but organs underlying are three dimensional.*

## UPPER LIMB

### 1. Axillary Artery

*Position to be told to the subject:* Arms abducted with palms facing upwards

*Points to be marked on the body:* Photo showing points to be marked for
- Mid-point of clavicle
- Feel for the pulsations of the artery at the upper part of humerus, approximately pulsations can be felt at the junction of anterior 1/3 rd and posterior 2/3 rd of lateral wall of axilla.

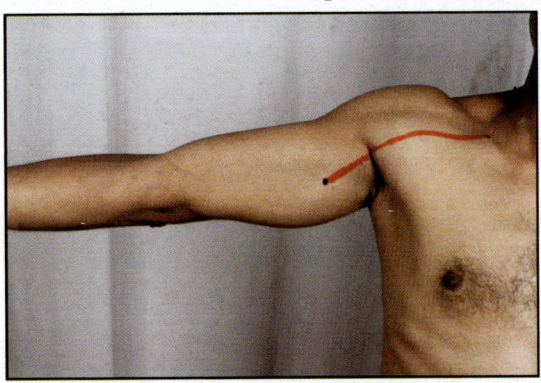

Photo showing points to be marked for axillary artery

## 2. Brachial Artery

*Position of the limb on the subject:* Since the artery is the continuation of axillary artery, end of axillary artery is the beginning of brachial artery, let the arm be abducted and ask the subject to flex the elbow tight so the biceps brachii tendon is seen prominently.

*Points to be marked*
- Upper part of upper limb at the junction of anterior 1/3rd and posterior 2/3rd of lateral wall of axilla
- Another marking just medial to the biceps brachii tendon.

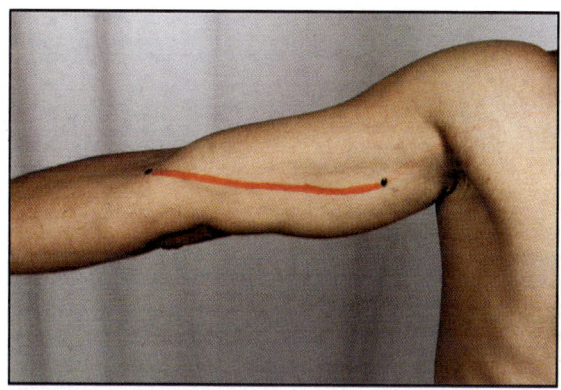

Photo showing points to be marked for brachial artery

## 3. Radial Artery

*Position to be taken by the subject:* Ask the subject to keep the forearm on the table with palm facing upwards and ask the subject to make a tight fist.

*Points to be marked*
- Brachial artery bifurcates to give rise to radial and ulnar artery. Thus, the end of brachial artery is the beginning of radial artery. So, the first marking is medial to the biceps brachii tendon.
- Another point lies at the wrist between lateral border of radius bone and tendon which can be easily seen on clenching the fist. This tendon is of the muscle flexor carpi radialis. One can feel for the radial artery pulsations.

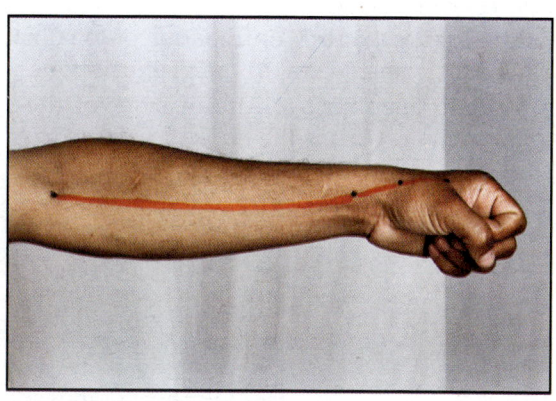

Photo showing points to be marked for radial artery

- Third marking can be done by turning the hand on oneside and a point marked at the styloid process.
- The artery enters the palm there onwards. Its end on dorsum of the hand is at the proximal end of the first intermetacarpal space.
  *(Very commonly asked in viva)*

### 4. Ulnar Artery

*Position of the subject:* Forearm extended and rested on the table with the palm facing upwards and ask the subject to flex the elbow so that the biceps tendon also becomes prominent.

*Points to be marked*

- Since the artery begins at the bifurcation of brachial artery the end of brachial artery is the beginning of the artery. The first point is medial to the biceps tendon.
- Second point is at the junction of upper 1/3rd and lower 2/3rd of the medial border of forearm.
- Third point is just lateral to the prominence of pisiform bone on the hand.

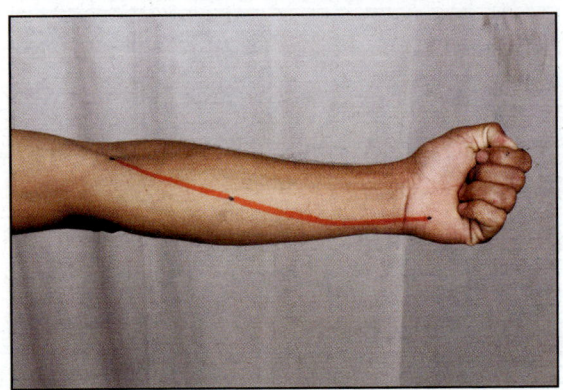

Photo showing points to be marked for ulnar artery

### 5. Superficial Palmar Arch

*Position of the limb:* Ask the subject to place his hand supported on table with palm facing upwards.

*Points to be marked*

- This arch is a direct continuation of the ulnar artery. Thus, the first point is the end of ulnar artery, i.e. just lateral to the pisiform bone
- Palpate deep, just a little in front of the earlier point and you can appreciate a bony prominence, this is the hook of hamate

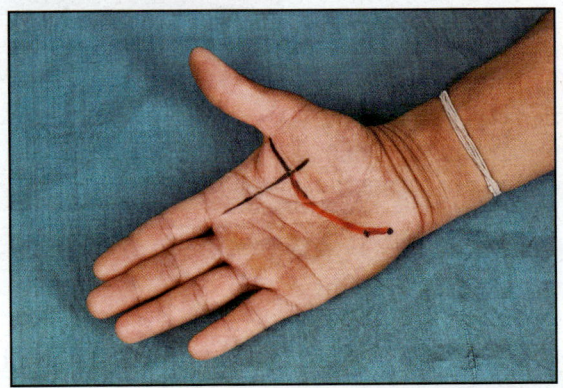

Photo showing points to be marked for superficial palmar arch

- Third point along the outer border of thenar eminence approximately the centre of the border at the point of intersection of the vertical line drawn from the index finger and horizontal line from the thumb
- Join the points with a convexity towards the digits.

## 6. Deep Palmar Arch

*Position to be taken by the subject:* Rest the hand on table with the palm facing upwards.

*Points to be marked*
- This arch is a continuation of the radial artery. The arch lies proximal to the superficial arch
- First point lies just distal to the hook of hamate this line can be extended horizontally for 4 cm and this marks the deep palmar arch.

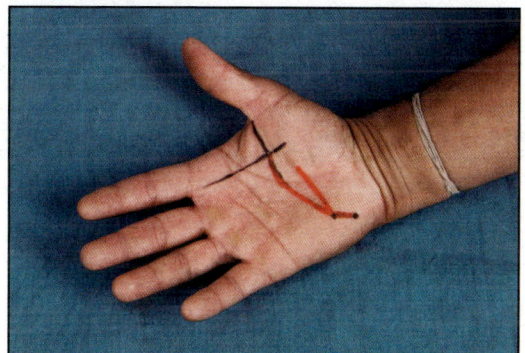

Photo showing points to be marked for deep palmar arch
*(Veins closely follow the arteries so the surface markings will by and large be the same)*

## 7. Anatomical Snuffbox

*Position of the hand:* Student should be able to demonstrate on himself the snuffbox (in olden times the dissectors would keep the snuff in this hollow to inhale, during long hours of dissection). Extend the thumb and you will appreciate the extensor tendons especially on thin individuals.

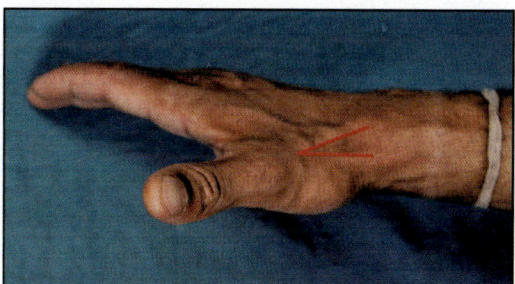

Photo showing anatomical snuffbox

*Viva questions:* Boundaries anteriorly extensor pollicis brevis, and abductor pollicis longus, posteriorly extensor pollicis longus, radial artery and a superficial branch of radial nerve are the contents of the box. On deep palpation in this area, the scaphoid bone is felt, and one can feel the pulsations of radial artery.

## 8. Flexor Retinaculum

*Position of the patient*
- Place the hand on the table with the palm facing upwards
- Ask the subject to make the pose of the hand as though he is holding a ball. The hollow between the thenar and hypothenar eminence is the area of flag like flexor retinaculum.

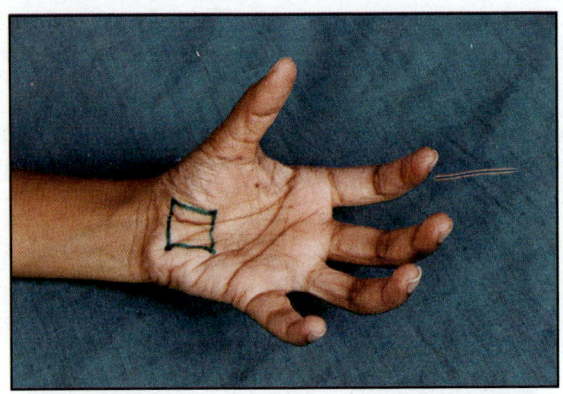

Photo showing markings of flexor retinaculum

*Points to be marked:*
- Pisiform bone
- Tubercle of scaphoid bone
- Hook of hamate
- Trapezium.

## 9. Extensor Retinaculum

*Position of the hand:* Ask the subject to place the hand on table with the palm downwards.

*Points to be marked:*
- On the back of the wrist the retinaculum extends in the form of band which lies between the radial and ulnar styloid process, and the band is 2 cm broad (it is like the way students wear the friendship band).

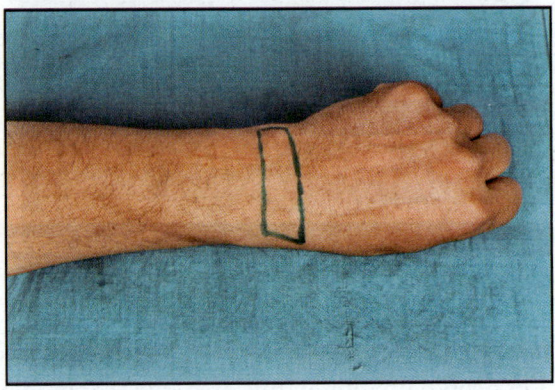

Photo showing markings of extensor retinaculum

## TESTING OF MUSCLES

- Trapezius—raise upper limb above the shoulders, i.e. above head, abduction, shrugging of shoulders
- Pectoralis major—bring arm on the chest

4 photos showing muscle action

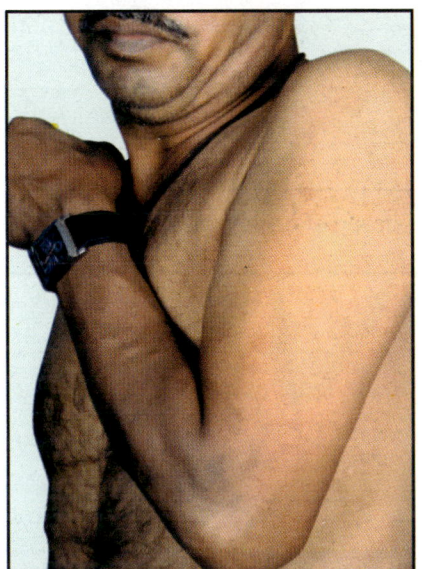

Photo 1—action of pectoralis major muscle

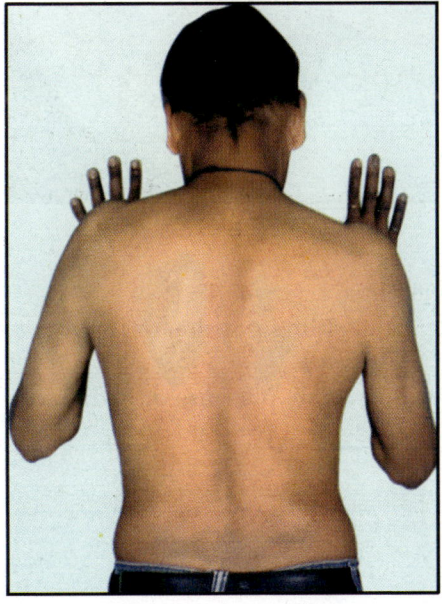

Photo 2—action of serratus anterior muscle

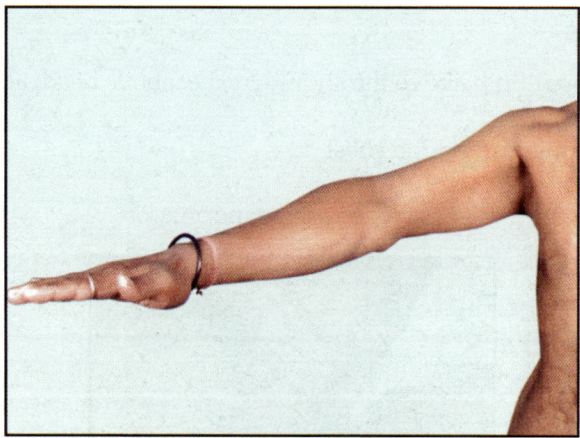

Photo 3—action of deltoid, abduction up to 90 degrees

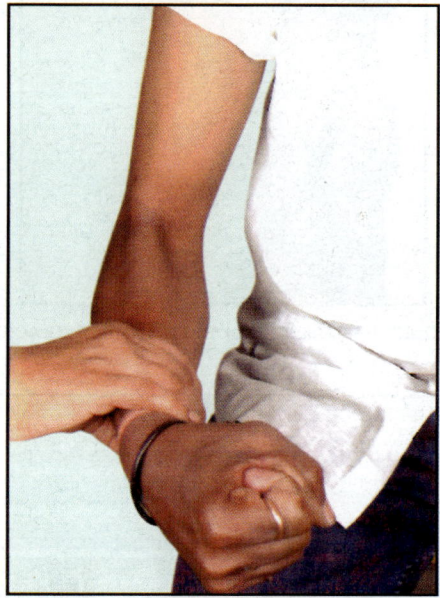

Photo 4—action of biceps brachii

- Serratus anterior—wall push-ups
- Latissimus dorsi—push-up from sitting position or holding a rope while climbing wall
- Deltoid—abduction up to 90 degrees
- Brachioradialis—flex elbow and apply pressure on radial side of forearm
- Biceps brachii—flex the elbow, against resistance.

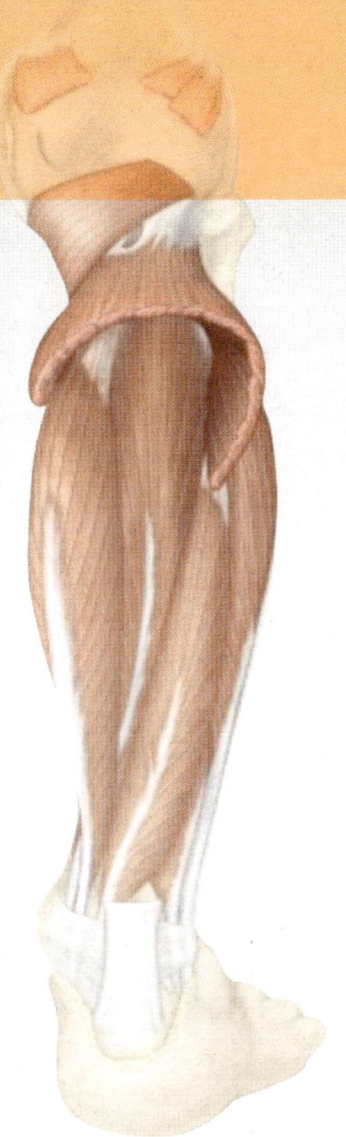

# Lower Limb

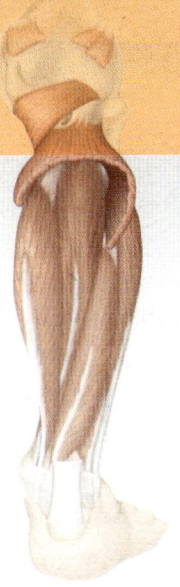

# Key Osteology Questions

## 9

**Q. What type of bone is hip bone?**

**Ans.** Hip bone is a large irregular bone.

**Q. Depict attachments on the iliac crest.**

**Ans.**

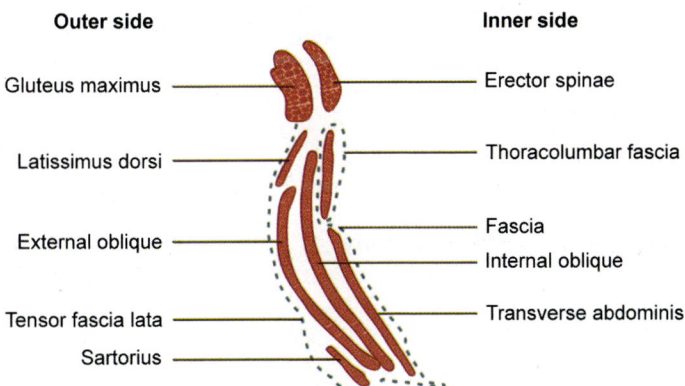

| Outer side | | Inner side |
|---|---|---|
| Gluteus maximus | | Erector spinae |
| Latissimus dorsi | | Thoracolumbar fascia |
| External oblique | | Fascia / Internal oblique |
| Tensor fascia lata | | Transverse abdominis |
| Sartorius | | |

**Q. Where is the tubercle of iliac crest located?**

**Ans.** The tubercle of iliac crest is located on the outerlip, 5 cm dorsosuperior to anterior superior iliac spine.

**Q. Is the summit of the iliac crest equivalent to the midpoint of the iliac crest?**

**Ans.** No, the summit of the iliac crest is little behind the midpoint of the iliac crest and is between L3 and L4.

**Q. Where is the auricular surface located? Why is it named so?**

**Ans.** Auricular surface is immediately anteroinferior to the iliac tuberosity. It is shaped like an ear (wide above and narrow below).

**Q. Where is the preauricular sulcus located?**

**Ans.** As the name indicates it is located before auricular surface, i.e. between auricular surface and upper border of greater sciatic notch. It is prominent in females and is one of the feature for sex determination of the pelvis.

**Q. What is attached to the preauricular sulcus?**

**Ans.** Ventral sacroiliac ligament and few fibres of piriformis are attached to the preauricular sulcus.

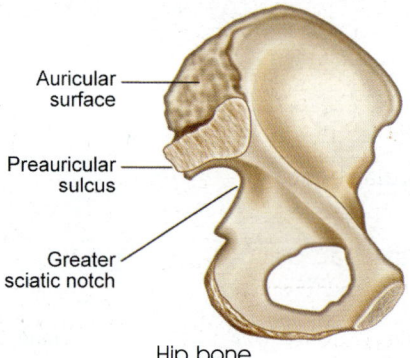

Hip bone

**Q. What type of joint is pubic symphysis?**

**Ans.** It is a fibrocartilaginous joint.

**Q. Depict the divisions of ischial tuberosity.**

**Ans.**

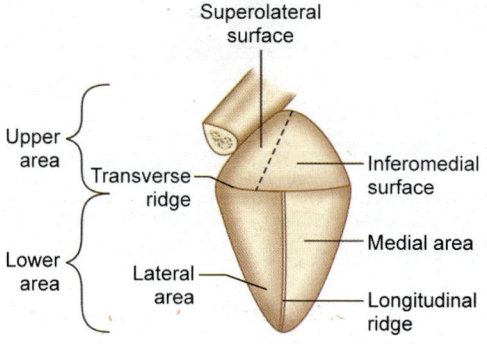

## Q. Depict the attachments on the ischial tuberosity.

**Ans.**

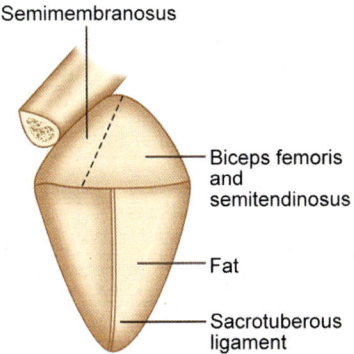

Semimembranosus

Biceps femoris and semitendinosus

Fat

Sacrotuberous ligament

## Q. What is attached to ischial spine?

**Ans.** Sacrospinous ligament is attached to the ischial spine.

## Q. What are the relations of ischial spine?

**Ans.** Internal pudendal vessels and nerve to obturator internus are related posteriorly. Coccygeus muscle and posterior fibres of levator ani are related anteriorly.

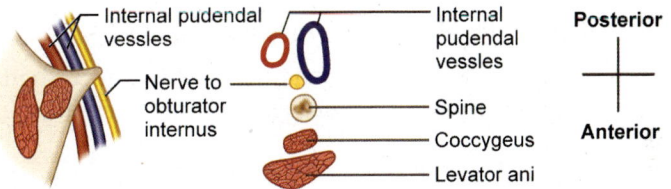

Internal pudendal vessles

Nerve to obturator internus

Internal pudendal vessles

Spine

Coccygeus

Levator ani

Posterior

Anterior

## Q. What is pelvic brim index?

**Ans.** Pelvic brim index = $\dfrac{\text{Anteroposterior diameter} \times 100}{\text{Transverse diameter}}$

## Q. How are the pelvis classified depending on pelvic brim index?

**Ans.** The pelvis are classified as follows:
- Platypellic—transversely long
- Mesatipellic—intermediate size
- Dolichopellic—anteroposteriorly long.

**Q. What are the differences between male and female pelvis?**

**Ans.**

| Criteria | Male | Female |
|---|---|---|
| Greater sciatic notch | Narrow | Wider |
| Acetabulum | Larger | Smaller |
| Iliac crest | More prominent | Less prominent |
| Iliac fossa | Shallow | Deeper |
| Pubic crest | Shorter | Longer |
| Ischiopubic rami | Everted | Not everted |
| Preauricular sulcus | Less prominent | More prominent |
| Ischial spine | Inturned | Straight, pointed |
| Obturator foramen | Large, oval | Small, triangular |

**Q. What is attached to the fovea of femoral head?**

**Ans.** The ligament of the head of femur is attached to the fovea of the femoral head.

**Q. Is the femoral head intracapsular?**

**Ans.** Femoral head is intracapsular.

**Q. What is the neck shaft angle and mention its significance?**

**Ans.** The femoral neck is at an angle with the shaft, this is the neck shaft angle. It is 125°. It facilitates the movement of hip joint thus helping the limb to swing freely away from the pelvis.

**Q. Depict the attachments on the greater trochanter.**

**Ans.**

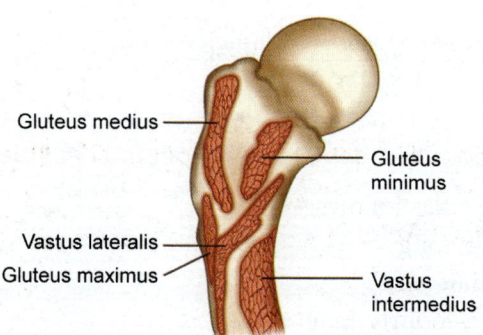

**Q. What is attached to trochanteric fossa?**

**Ans.** The tendon of obturator externus is attached to trochanteric fossa.

**Q. Mention the attachments on lesser trochanter.**

**Ans.** The anteromedial surface gives attachment to psoas major and iliacus, while the posterior surface gives attachment to adductor magnus.

**Q. What is angle of femoral torsion?**

**Ans.** The transverse axis of the head of femur makes an angle with the transverse condylar axis. This is the angle of femoral torsion.

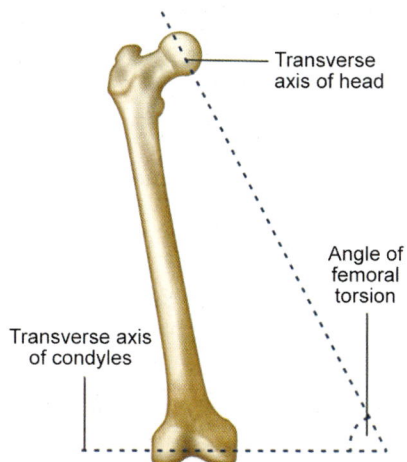

Transverse axis of head

Angle of femoral torsion

Transverse axis of condyles

**Q. What is attached to quadrate tubercle?**

**Ans.** Quadratus femoris is attached to the quadrate tubercle.

**Q. What is third trochanter?**

**Ans.** Gluteal tuberosity when prominent is known as third trochanter.

**Q. What is attached to adductor tubercle?**

**Ans.** Adductor magnus is attached to adductor tubercle.

**Q. What is the surgical importance of adductor tubercle?**

**Ans.** The knee joint line passes through the adductor tubercle.

**Q. What is the medicolegal importance of the lower end of femur?**

**Ans.** In a dead fetus, if the ossification centre is present on the lower end of femur it indicates that the child was alive at birth and one should suspect that it is an unnatural death. This is because ossification centre for lower end of femur appears just before birth.

## Q. Depict the attachments on linea aspera.

**Ans.**

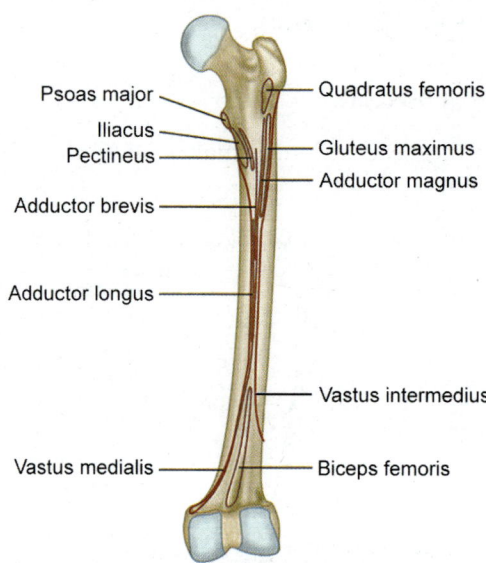

Psoas major — Quadratus femoris
Iliacus — Gluteus maximus
Pectineus — Adductor magnus
Adductor brevis
Adductor longus
Vastus intermedius
Vastus medialis — Biceps femoris

## Q. Which part of femur transmits more weight to tibia?

**Ans.** The lateral condyle of femur, which is large and in line with the shaft of femur transmits more weight to tibia.

## Q. What type of bone is patella?

**Ans.** Patella is a sesamoid bone, which develops in the tendon of quadriceps femoris.

## Q. Depict the proximal articular surface of tibia.

**Ans.**

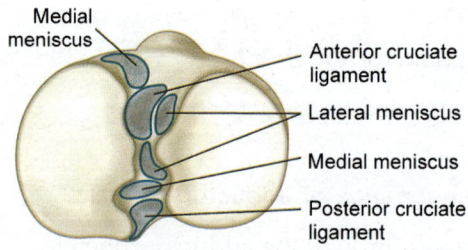

Medial meniscus
Anterior cruciate ligament
Lateral meniscus
Medial meniscus
Posterior cruciate ligament

*Mnemonic*

| | |
|---|---|
| "Medical | Medial meniscus anterior horn |
| College | Anterior Cruciate ligament |
| Lucknow | Anterior horn Lateral meniscus |
| Lucknow | Posterior horn Lateral meniscus |
| Medical | Posterior horn Medial meniscus |
| College" | Posterior Cruciate ligament. |

**Q. What is attached to the tibial tuberosity?**

**Ans.** Proximally ligamentum patellae are attached to the smooth part and the distal rough part is related to the infrapatellar bursa.

**Q. Which nerve is related to the head of fibula?**

**Ans.** Common peroneal nerve winds around the head of fibula.

**Q. What muscles are attached to talus bone?**

**Ans.** No muscles are attached to the talus bone.

**Q. Which tendon is related to sustentaculum tali?**

**Ans.** The tendon of flexor hallucis longus is related to sustentaculum tali.

**Q. What are the ligaments attached to sustentaculum tali?**

**Ans.** Inferiorly the margins of the groove give attachment to the deep part of flexor retinaculum and to its medial margin plantar calcaneonavicular ligament, superficial fibres of deltoid ligament and talocalcaneal ligament are attached.

**Q. What is attached to the navicular tuberosity?**

**Ans.** The tibialis posterior muscle is attached to the navicular tuberosity.

**Q. Compare carpal and tarsal bones.**

**Ans.** Following are the differences between carpal and tarsal bones:

| Criteria | Carpal | Tarsal |
| --- | --- | --- |
| Size | Small | Large, bulky |
| Arrangement | Retained primitive pattern | Primitive pattern not maintained |
| Weight transmission | Function not present | Involved in weight transmission primarily |
| Rows | Proximal, distal | No defined rows, Talus lies above calcaneum behind |

**Q. What is fabella?**

**Ans.** Fabella is a sesamoid bone developed in the lateral part of gastrocnemius tendon.

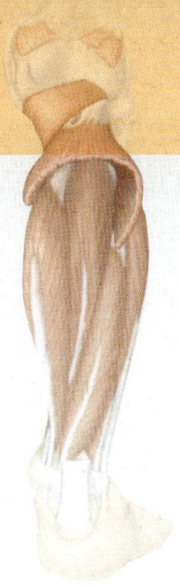

# Key Short Notes

## 10

## MUSCLES

### Q. Psoas Major

**Ans.** Psoas major is a long fusiform muscle extending from lumbar region to the upper thigh.

### Attachments

#### *Above*

Anterior surfaces and lower border of all transverse process of lumbar vertebra and their adjacent bodies and intervertebral disks.

The muscle descends along the pelvic brim, behind the midpoint of inguinal ligament and in front of hip joint capsule.

#### *Below*

Along with iliacus gets attached to the lesser trochanter.

### Relations in Lumbar Region

#### *Above*

Posterior to diaphragm, may be in contact with pleural sac.

#### *Anteriorly*

Kidney, psoas minor, renal vessels, ureter, gonadal vessels, genitofemoral nerve (right psoas related to inferior vena cava, left psoas to aorta).

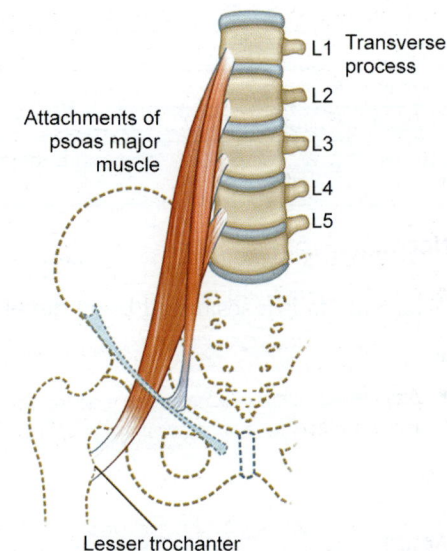

Relations of psoas major muscle

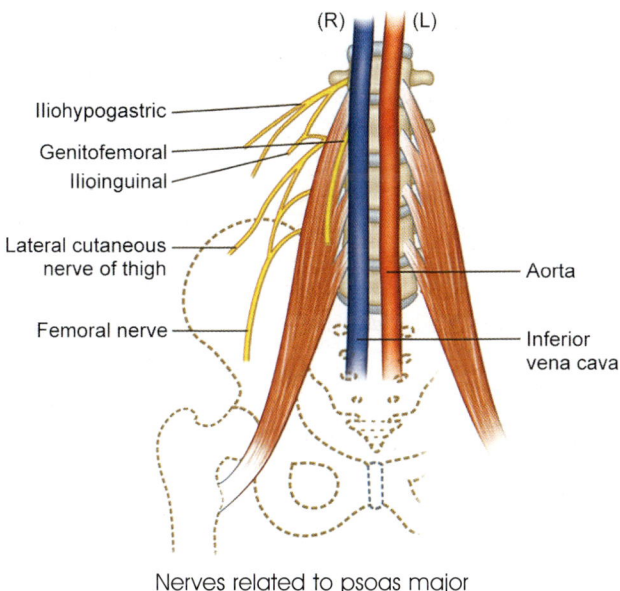

(R)          (L)

Iliohypogastric

Genitofemoral

Ilioinguinal

Lateral cutaneous
nerve of thigh

Aorta

Femoral nerve

Inferior
vena cava

Nerves related to psoas major

## Posteriorly

Transverse process of lumbar vertebra and quadratus lumborum.

The roots of lumbar plexus are within the muscle and branches emerge from its borders and surfaces.

## Medial

Lumbar vertebral bodies, sympathetic chain.

### Relations in hip region:
- *Anteriorly:* Fascia lata, femoral artery
- *Posteriorly:* Hip joint
- *Medially:* Pectineus, medial circumflex femoral vessels, femoral vein
- *Laterally:* Iliacus.

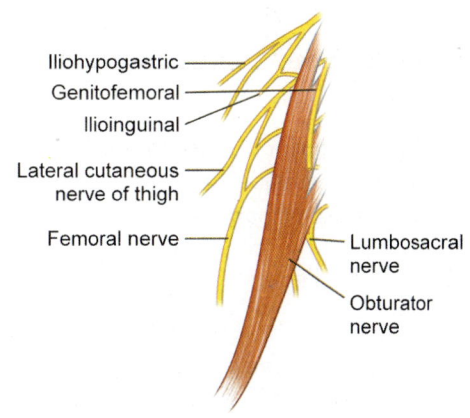

Iliohypogastric

Genitofemoral

Ilioinguinal

Lateral cutaneous
nerve of thigh

Femoral nerve

Lumbosacral
nerve

Obturator
nerve

Nerves related to psoas major

## Nerves Related to Psoas Major

- *Lateral border:* Iliohypogastric, ilioinguinal, lateral cutaneous nerve of thigh, femoral
- *Anterolateral:* Genitofemoral nerve surface
- *Medial border:* Obturator, accessory obturator, upper root of lumbosacral trunk.

**Nerve supply:** Ventral rami of L1, L2, L3.

## Action

Along with psoas it flexes the thigh on pelvis, helps in raising the trunk from lying position.

## Applied Anatomy

- In fracture neck of femur the limb is externally rotated and shortened, this is due to the action of psoas major, which acts as a lateral rotator.
- Psoas abscess—Abscess is collection of pus in closed cavity. The pus tracks down along the lower attachment of muscle; thus, there will be observable swelling on the medial side of the thigh.

## Q. Sartorius

**Ans.** The muscle is also known as Tailor's muscle. It extends in front of thigh diagonally.

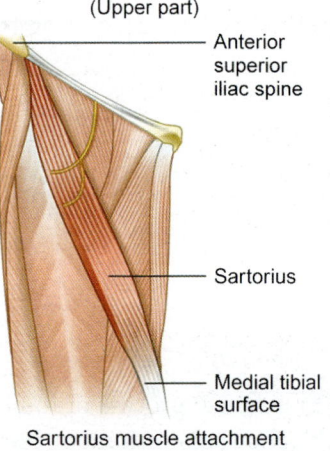

(Upper part)

Anterior superior iliac spine

Sartorius

Medial tibial surface

Sartorius muscle attachment

### Attachments

- *Above:* Anterior superior iliac spine
- *Below:* Medial tibial surface.

### Nerve Supply

Femoral nerve L2, L3.

### Action

Flexing the leg at knee, flexing the thigh on pelvis (like sitting on the floor cross-legged).

## Q. Quadriceps Femoris

**Ans.** As the name suggests it has four parts: rectus femoris, vastus medialis, vastus intermedius, vastus lateralis.

### Rectus Femoris

*Attachments*

- *Above:* Anterior inferior iliac spine and a few fibres from groove over acetabulum and fibrous capsule of hip joint.
- *Below:* Base of patella.

### Vastus Medialis

*Attachments*

- *Above:* Distal part of intertrochanteric line, spiral line, medial lip of linea aspera, medial supracondylar line, medial intermuscular septum
- *Below:* Medial border of patella.

### Vastus Intermedius

*Attachments*

- *Above:* Most of the anterior and lateral of femoral shaft, lateral intermuscular septum
- *Below:* Lateral border of patella.

## Vastus Lateralis

### Attachments

- *Above:* Intertrochanteric line, greater trochanter, lateral lip of gluteal tuberosity, lateral lip of linea aspera
- *Below:* Base of patella, lateral border.
  All the above muscles form a strong tendon and get attached to the patellar base.

### Nerve Supply

Femoral nerve, L2, L3, L4.

### Action

### Quadriceps Femoris

Extension of the knee.

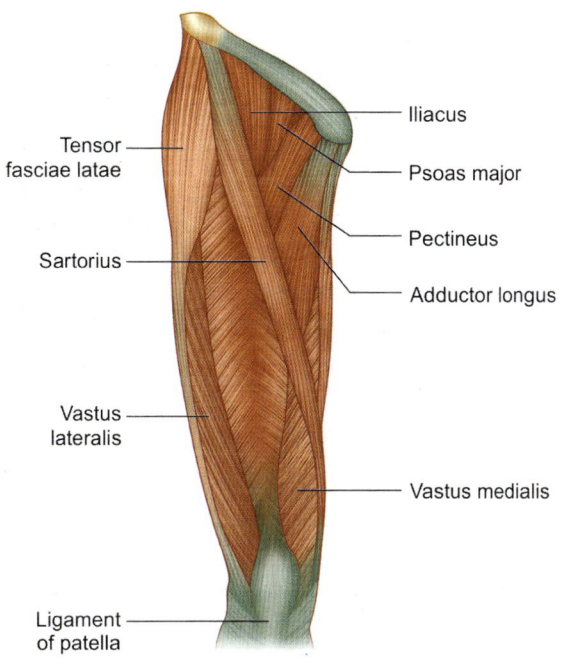

Tensor fasciae latae

Sartorius

Vastus lateralis

Ligament of patella

Iliacus

Psoas major

Pectineus

Adductor longus

Vastus medialis

Quadriceps femoris

## Q. Pectineus

**Ans.** Pectineus is a hybrid muscle.

### Attachments

- *Above:* Pecten pubis
- *Below:* Between lesser trochanter and linea aspera.

### Nerve Supply

Femoral nerve, obturator nerve.

### Action

Adduction of thigh also assists in flexion of pelvis.

## Q. Gluteus Maximus

**Ans.** The bulk of buttock is formed by gluteus maximus.

### Attachments

- *Above:* Posterior gluteal line and the area above it, a few fibres from dorsal surface of sacrum, side of coccyx, sacrotuberous ligament, fascia over gluteus medius
- *Below:* Greater trochanter, gluteal tuberosity.

### Relations

### Superficial

Adipose tissue.

### Deep

- *Bones:* Ilium, sacrum, coccyx, ischial tuberosity, greater trochanter.

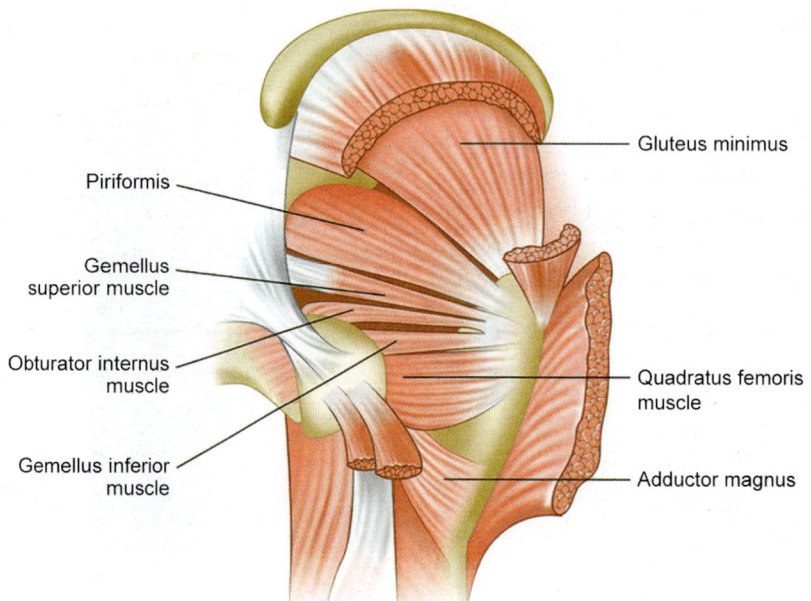

Muscles under the cover of gluteus maximus

- *Muscles:* Gluteus medius, piriformis, gemelli, obturator internus, quadratus femoris, biceps femoris, semi-tendinous, semi-membranous, adductor magnus (all the muscles fan out below the cover of gluteus maximus).
- *Arteries:* Superior and inferior gluteal, internal pudendal, first perforating, medial circumflex femoral.
- *Nerves:* Sciatic, pudendal, muscular branches from sacral plexus.

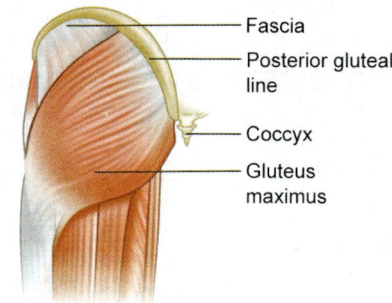

## Nerve Supply

Inferior gluteal nerve L5, S1, S2.

## Action

Extends the flexed thigh (helps in getting up from sitting position and while climbing stairs).

### Q. Hamstrings

**Ans.** String like muscles are present on the back of the thigh namely biceps femoris, semi-tendinosus, semimembranosus. This group of muscles is known as hamstrings.

## Biceps Femoris

### Attachments

- *Above:* As the name suggests it has two heads, ischial tuberosity gives attachment to long head; lateral lip of linea aspera gives attachment to short-head
- *Below:* Head of fibula.

## Semitendinosus

### Attachments

- *Above:* Ischial tuberosity
- *Below:* Upper part of medial surface of tibia.

## Semimembranosus

### Attachments

- *Above:* Ischial tuberosity
- *Below:* Posteriorly into the groove of medial condyle of tibia.

## Nerve Supply

Tibial part of sciatic nerve supplies the long-head of biceps femoris. While the short-head of biceps femoris is supplied by common peroneal part of sciatic nerve.

## Action

The group is the main flexor of the knee.

**Semitendinosus**

**Semimembranosus**

Long-head of biceps femoris

Short-head of biceps femoris

Hamstrings

## Q. Triceps Surae

**Ans.** Gastrocnemius and soleus are together termed triceps surae. They form the belly of the calf.

## Gastrocnemius

### Attachments

- *Above:* Medial head arises from an area behind adductor tubercle and above medial condyle of femur. Lateral head arise from area above lateral condyle.
- *Below:* Unites with tendon of soleus to form tendocalcaneus.

## Soleus

### Attachments

- *Above:* Posterior surface of fibula, soleal line and medial border of tibia, soleal arch
- *Below:* Unites with gastrocnemius to form tendocalcaneus.

## Nerve Supply

Tibial nerve S1, S2.

## Back of Leg

Triceps surae.

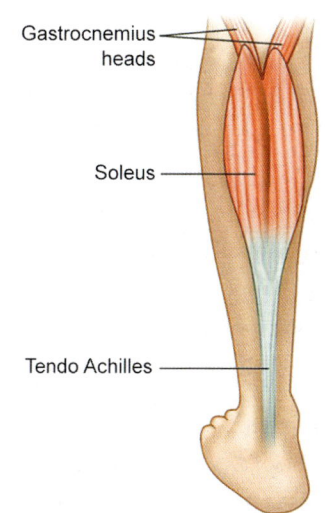

Gastrocnemius heads

Soleus

Tendo Achilles

## Action

Plantar flexion. Plantaris muscle may sometimes be present with triceps surae to contribute in the formation of tendocalcaneus.

### Q. Adductor Hallucis

**Ans.** Adductor hallucis has oblique and transverse heads.

## Attachments

- Oblique head arises from 2nd, 3rd, 4th metatarsal base and sheath of peroneus longus tendon
- Oblique head has medial and lateral part:
  - Medial part joins flexor hallucis brevis and attached to lateral hallucial bone
  - Lateral part joins transverse head and attached to lateral hallucial bone and base of first hallucial phalanx.
- Transverse head arises from plantar metatarsophalangeal ligaments of 3rd, 4th, 5th toes and deep transverse metatarsal ligament.

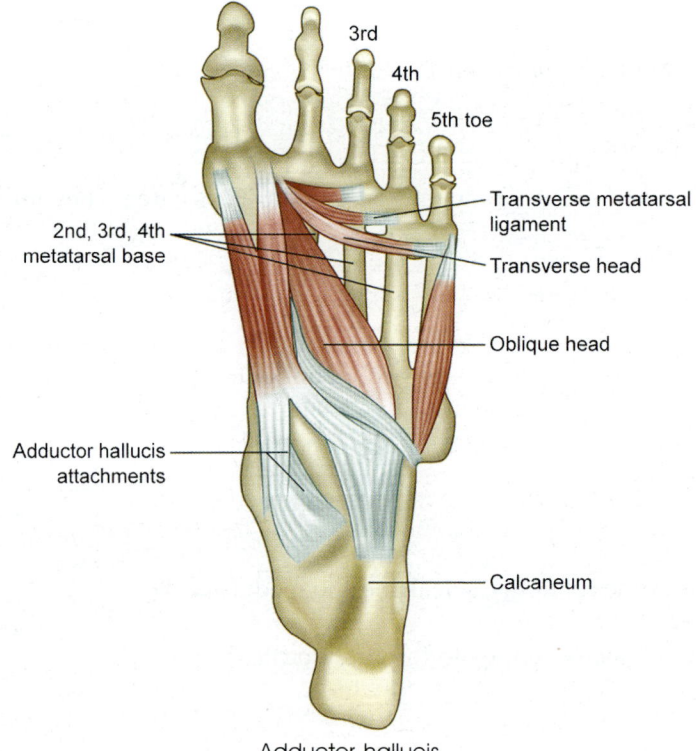

Adductor hallucis

## Nerve Supply

Deep branch of lateral plantar nerve.

## Action

- Adduction of greater toe.
- Maintains transverse arch of foot.

## Q. Muscle Layers of the Foot

**Ans. First Layer**
- Abductor hallucis
- Abductor digiti minimi
- Flexor digitorum brevis (maintains concavity of the sole).

### Second Layer
- Flexor digitorum accessorius
- Lumbricals
- Two tendons namely—flexor digitorum longus and flexor hallucis longus.

### Third Layer
- Flexor hallucis brevis
- Adductor hallucis
- Flexor digiti minimi brevis.

### Fourth Layer
- Dorsal interossei
- Plantar interossei
- Two tendons are tibialis posterior and peroneus longus.

## NERVES

## Q. Lumbar Plexus

**Ans.** The first three lumbar ventral rami and most of the fourth lumbar ventral rami form the lumbar plexus (L1, L2, L3, L4 ventral rami).

### Location

Posterior to psoas major muscle and anterior to transverse process of lumbar vertebra.

### Formation

Ventral rami of L1, L2, L3, L4.
- *L1:*
  - Divides into upper and lower divisions
  - Upper division re-divides into iliohypogastric and ilioinguinal nerves
  - Lower division joins small anterior division of L2 to form genitofemoral nerve.
  *Note:* L2, L3, L4 each divide into anterior and posterior divisions.
- *L2:*
  - Anterior and posterior divisions re-divide into small and large branches
  - Small anterior division joins with a branch of L1 to form genitofemoral nerve
  - Large anterior division joins L3 and L4 anterior division to form obturator nerve
  - Small posterior division of L2 joins the small posterior division of L3 to form lateral cutaneous nerve of thigh

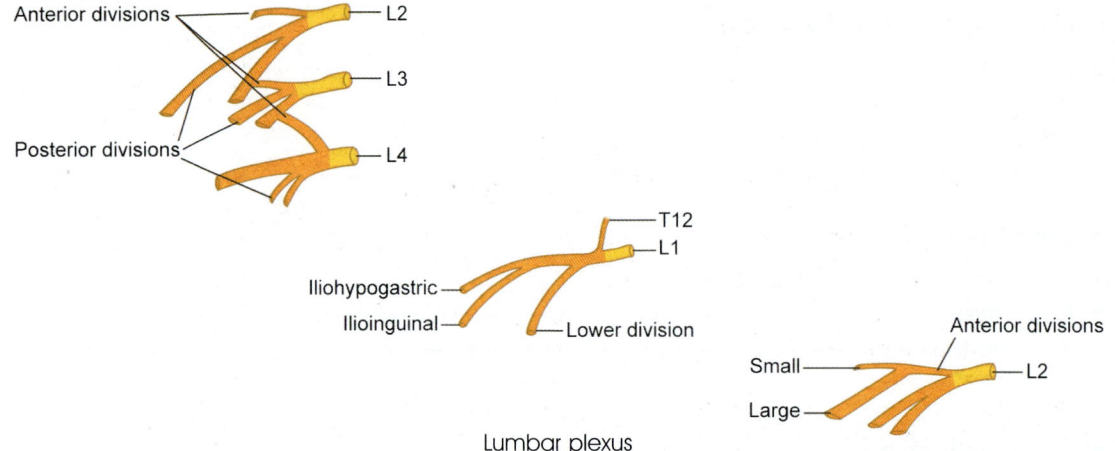

Lumbar plexus

- – Large posterior division of L2 joins large posterior divisions of L3 and L4 to form femoral nerve.
- • *L3:*
  - – Anterior division of L2 joins anterior divisions of L3 and L4 to form obturator nerve
  - – Large posterior division of L2 joins large posterior divisions of L3 and L4 to form femoral nerve.
- • *L4:*
  - – Anterior division contributes to form obturator nerve
  - – Posterior division contributes to form femoral nerve.

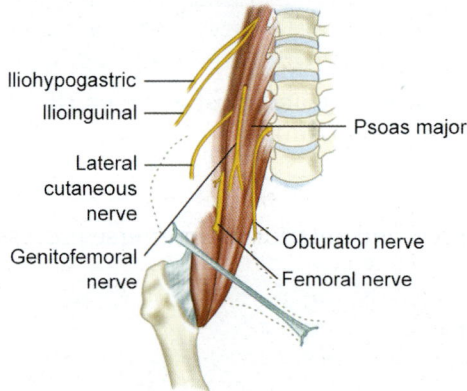

Branches of lumbar plexus

## Genitofemoral

- • Formed by union of small anterior divisions of L1, L2 nerve
- • Dorsal divisions of L2, L3, L4 form femoral nerve
- • Ventral divisions of L2, L3, L4 form obturator nerve.

## Clinical Importance

The major nerves of lower limb begin from lumbar plexus. The lumbosacral trunk may get compressed by pelvic tumors or during pregnancy by fetal head causing severe pain in the lower limb.

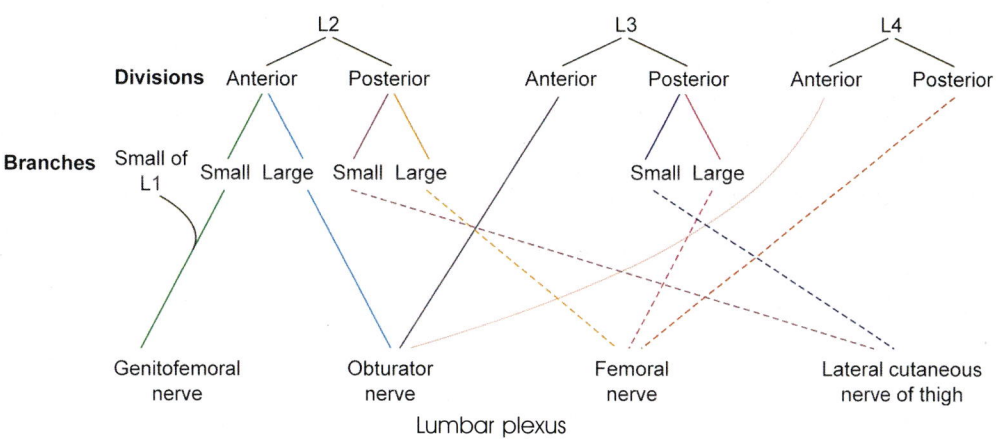

Lumbar plexus

## SACRAL PLEXUS

### Layout of Sacral Plexus

- *Formation:* Pelvic ventral rami of S1, S2, S3, S4. These ventral rami emerge through pelvic sacral foramina.
- *Location:* Ventral rami unite in front of piriformis; on lower part of greater sciatic foramen (S5, C1 pierce sacrococcygeal ligament).
- *Relations:*
  - Between L5, S1 are superior gluteal vessels
  - Below S1 are the inferior gluteal vessels

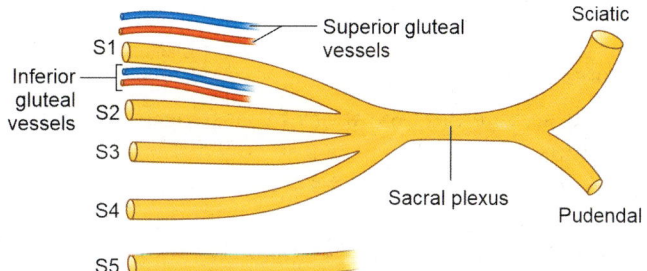

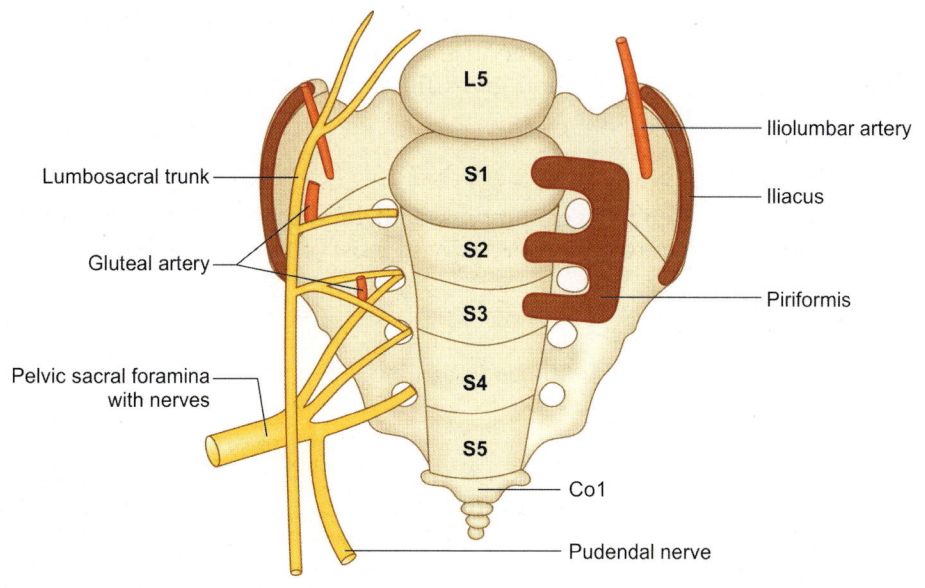

- Posteriorly related to piriformis, sacroiliac joint
- Anteriorly are the internal pudendal vessels.
- **Branches:**
  - Muscular to piriformis, coccygeus, levator ani
  - Pelvic splanchnic S2, S3, S4 to inferior hypogastric plexus
  - Each ventral rami receives gray rami communicans.
- **Terminal branches:**
  - Sciatic nerve
  - Pudendal nerve.

## Q. Femoral Nerve

**Ans.** Femoral nerve is one of the major nerves of lower limb.

### Formation

Dorsal branches of ventral rami of L2, L3, L4.

### Course and Relations

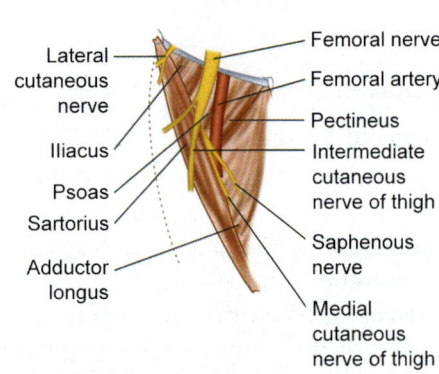

- The nerve enters the thigh by passing behind the inguinal ligament
- Then it emerges from lateral border of psoas major in its lower part
- The nerve descends between psoas major and iliacus muscle
- The nerve lies lateral to femoral artery in femoral triangle
- The nerve ends by dividing into anterior and posterior divisions.

Femoral nerve course and relations in thigh

### Branches

- Chief branches can be conveniently divided into cutaneous, muscular, vascular and articular.
- Anterior division gives fibres to intermediate and medial cutaneous nerve of thigh and a branch to sartorius. Posterior division gives fibres to saphenous nerve and branches to quadriceps femoris and knee joint.

### Clinical Importance

The femoral nerve may sometimes get compressed behind the inguinal ligament leading to paralysis of quadriceps femoris and sensory loss on most of the front of the thigh.

## Q. Sciatic Nerve

**Ans.** Sciatic nerve is thickest nerve in the body around 2 cm broad.

### Formation

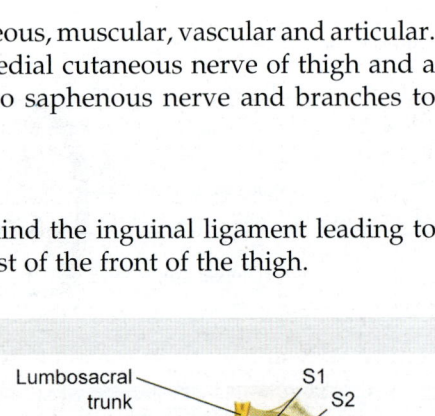

- Ventral rami of L4 (partly), and whole of ventral rami of L5 form lumbosacral trunk
- Ventral rami of S1, S2, S3.

## Course and Relations

*In pelvis:* It lies below levator ani:
- The nerve leaves the pelvis through greater sciatic foramen and is detected below piriformis on back of thigh
- It runs on the back of thigh between hamstrings and obturator internus with gemelli, quadratus femoris with adductor magnus
- It is medially related to posterior femoral cutaneous nerve and inferior gluteal artery
- Usually, the sciatic nerve divides on lower part of back of thigh into tibial and common peroneal nerve (the site of division may be variable).

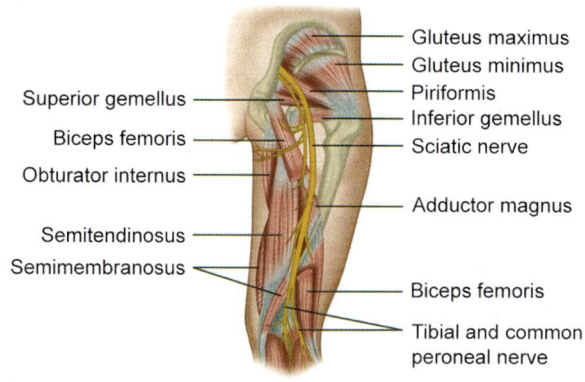

Sciatic nerve on back of thigh

## Branches

- Terminal branches are tibial and common peroneal nerve
- Muscular branches to hamstrings (biceps femoris, semitendinosus, semimembranosus) and ischial part of adductor magnus
- Articular branches to hip joint.

## Clinical Importance

The nerve may get injured in posterior dislocations or fracture of hip joint in which case, muscles distal to the knee and cutaneous sensation is lost (except the area around saphenous nerve).

## Q. Sural Nerve

### Ans. Formation
Sural nerve is a branch of tibial nerve.

### Course and Relations

From its origin approximately in popliteal fossa the nerve runs down on back of leg between the two heads of gastrocnemius.

It pierces the deep fascia in the upper part of leg to become superficial and then join sural communicating branch of common peroneal nerve.

It runs down to lie lateral to tendocalcaneus and then between lateral malleolus and calcaneum. The nerve during this course is closely related to small saphenous vein.

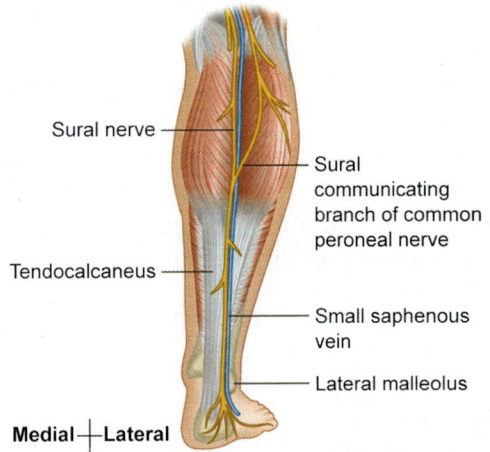

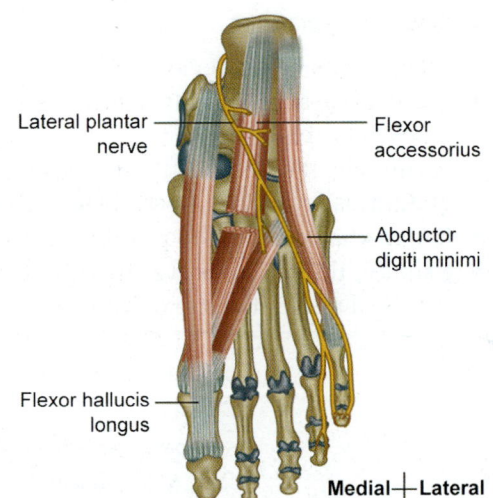

## Connections

Sural nerve joins superficial peroneal nerve on dorsum of foot and in the leg it joins the posterior femoral cutaneous nerve.

## Branches

Cutaneous branches supply posterior and lateral part of distal leg, lateral border of the foot and little toe.

## Clinical Importance

Damage to the nerve may occasionally occur during venesection leading to loss of sensation on lower part of back of leg and lateral part of sole causing pressure sores.

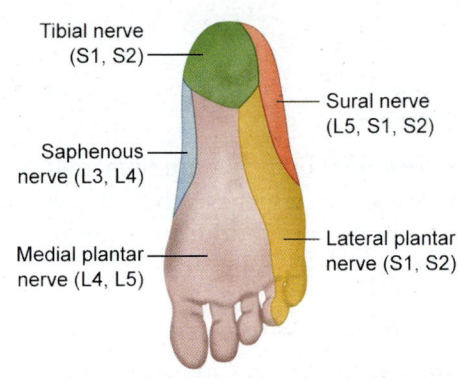

Sciatic nerve on back of thigh

# ARTERIES

### Q. Femoral Artery

**Ans.**

## Origin

External iliac artery continues as femoral artery behind midinguinal point (i.e. between anterior superior iliac spine and pubic symphysis).

## Course and Relations

The artery runs downwards and medially in front of the thigh and crosses two areas namely, femoral triangle and adductor canal.

### In Femoral Triangle

- The initial 3–4 cm of artery is enclosed within femoral sheath
- In front, the artery is covered by skin, superficial fascia, superficial inguinal lymph nodes, fascia lata, femoral sheath, superficial circumflex iliac vein and femoral branch of genito-femoral nerve
- Behind, the artery lies on psoas tendon, femoral sheath
- Femoral vein is medial
- Femoral nerve is lateral.

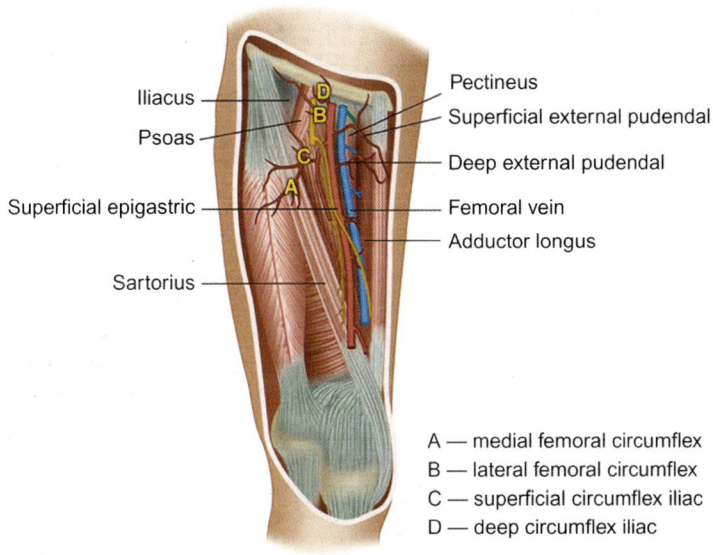

A — medial femoral circumflex
B — lateral femoral circumflex
C — superficial circumflex iliac
D — deep circumflex iliac

### In Adductor Canal

The artery lies under the cover of skin, fascia and sartorius muscle. The saphenous nerve crosses the artery from lateral to medial side. The artery lies on adductor longus muscle.

### Branches

Branches of femoral artery can be classified into superficial and deep.

*Superficial branches*

- Superficial epigastric
- Superficial cirumflex iliac
- Superficial external pudendal

*Deep branches*

- Deep external pudendal
- Muscular
- Arteria profunda femoris

### Clinical Importance

In comatosed patient arterial blood is withdrawn from femoral artery for blood gas analysis. The reference point to withdraw blood is midinguinal point.

### Q. Arteria Profunda Femoris

**Ans. Origin**

Arteria profunda femoris is a deep branch of femoral artery.

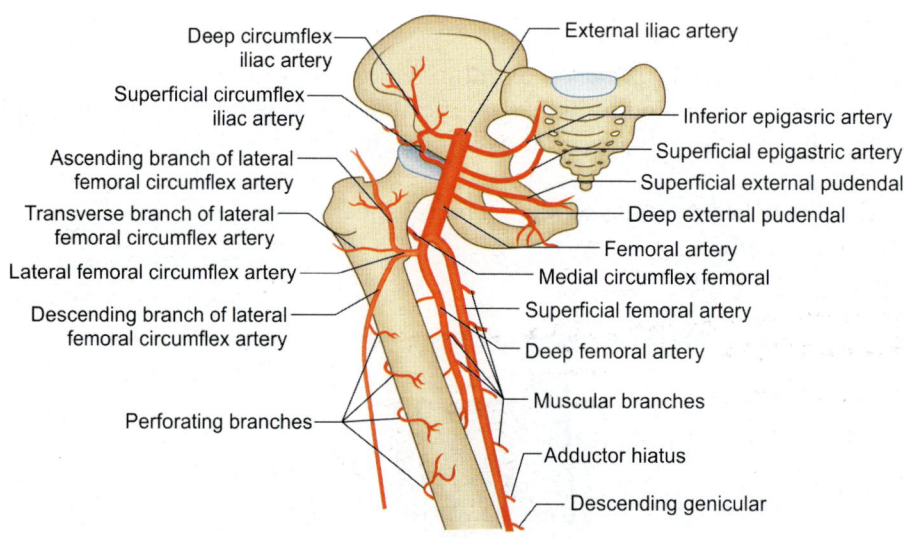

Deep circumflex iliac artery
Superficial circumflex iliac artery
Ascending branch of lateral femoral circumflex artery
Transverse branch of lateral femoral circumflex artery
Lateral femoral circumflex artery
Descending branch of lateral femoral circumflex artery
Perforating branches
External iliac artery
Inferior epigasric artery
Superficial epigastric artery
Superficial external pudendal
Deep external pudendal
Femoral artery
Medial circumflex femoral
Superficial femoral artery
Deep femoral artery
Muscular branches
Adductor hiatus
Descending genicular

## Course and Relations

- It arises from the lateral side of femoral artery and then winds posteriorly to lie between femoral artery and vein medially
- It descends down between pectineus and adductor muscles
- It ends by piercing the adductor magnus and anastomosing with muscular branches of popliteal artery.

## Branches

- Lateral circumflex femoral
- Medial circumflex femoral
- Perforating arteries
- Muscular branches.

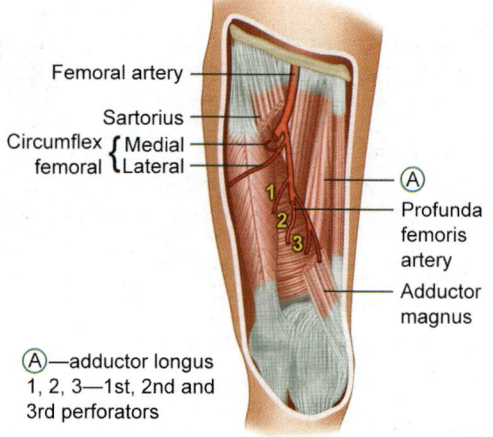

Femoral artery
Sartorius
Circumflex femoral { Medial, Lateral
Profunda femoris artery
Adductor magnus

(A)—adductor longus
1, 2, 3—1st, 2nd and 3rd perforators

## Clinical Importance

If femoral artery is ligated proximal to origin of profunda femoris, a collateral circulation develops between the branches of internal iliac artery and profunda femoris artery.

## Q. Popliteal Artery

**Ans.**

### Origin

Popliteal artery is the continuation of femoral artery in popliteal fossa.

### Course and Relations

Above from opening in adductor magnus the artery runs downwards and laterally toward intercondylar fossa. The artery tilts laterally on back of knee and divides at the lower border of popliteus muscle into anterior and posterior tibial arteries.

## Branches

- Cutaneous
- Muscular
- Genicular.

## Clinical Importance

By virtue of the anastomoses between the branches of popliteal artery branches of the artery a collateral circulation develops in case of blockage in the popliteal artery due to thrombosis.

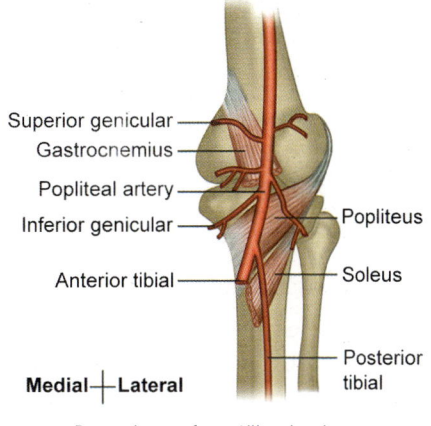

Branches of popliteal artery

### Q. Anastomosis

**Ans.**

## Back of the Thigh

Communicating arterial rings are present on the back of the thigh forming the anastomotic channels extending from gluteal region to popliteal fossa.

*Anastomoses exists between following arteries:*

- Gluteal arteries with medial circumflex femoral artery
- Circumflex femoral with first perforating artery
- Perforating arteries with each other
- Fourth perforating artery with muscular branches of popliteal artery.

## Genicular

This anastomoses exists around the condyles of tibia and femur, and around patella.

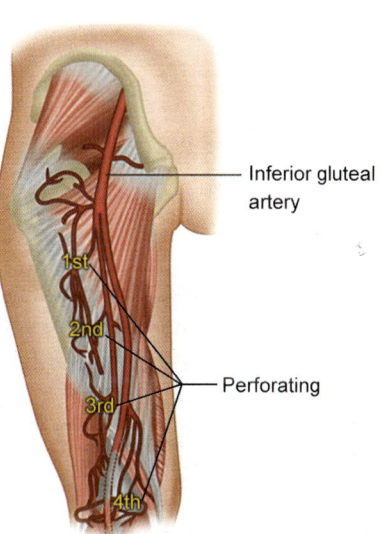

Anastomosis on back of thigh

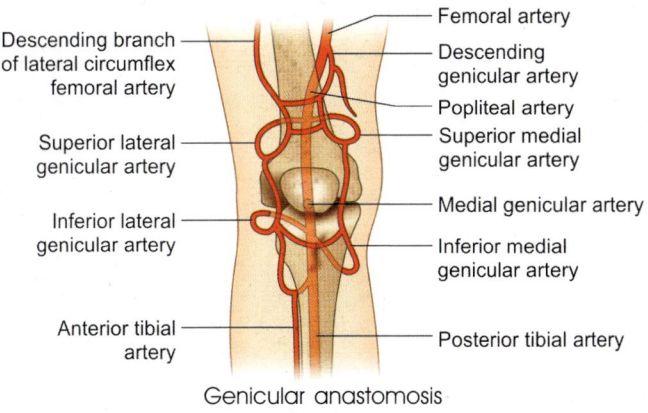

Genicular anastomosis

- Superficial anastomosis exists around the skin and superficial fascia in the region of patella and within the fat, deep to ligamentum patellae.
- Deep anastomoses exists around the articular surfaces of tibia and femur.

*The arteries involved are as follows:*
- Medial, lateral, descending genicular
- Lateral circumflex femoral
- Anterior and posterior tibial recurrent.

### Clinical Importance

Block in any of the major artery is overcome by the collateral circulation, which develops in the anastomoses.

## VEINS

### Q. Femoral Vein

**Ans.**

### Extent

Popliteal vein continues as femoral vein at the level of opening in adductor magnus and ends behind the inguinal ligament to continue as external iliac vein.

### Relations

- In the beginning of adductor canal vein lies posterolateral to femoral artery
- Little above and in lower part of femoral triangle the vein lies posterior to femoral artery
- While towards the base of femoral triangle the vein lies medial to femoral artery.

### Tributaries

- Several muscular veins
- Vena profunda femoris
- Great saphenous vein
- Circumflex femoral veins.

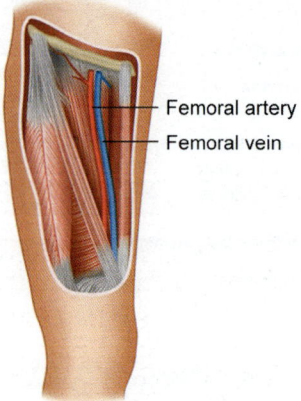

Femoral triangle

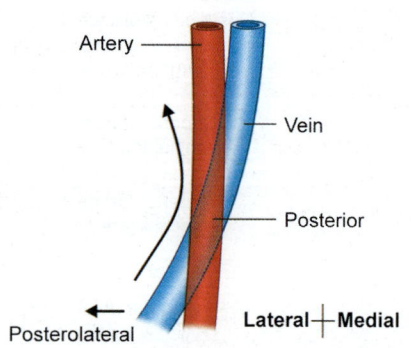

Femoral vein and artery relation

## Clinical Importance

In case of incompetence of valves within the femoral vein there may be backflow of venous blood giving rise to varicose veins.

### Q. Short Saphenous Vein

**Ans. Extent**

Short saphenous vein is a continuation of lateral marginal vein behind lateral malleolus and ends in popliteal vein.

### Course and Relations

In the lower part of the leg the vein lies lateral to tendo-calcaneus just below the skin and superficial fascia.

It ascends medially towards the middle of calf and pierces the deep fascia to lie between two heads of gastrocnemius muscle, where it ends to drain in the popliteal vein.

Sural nerve accompanies the vein on the back of leg.

### Tributaries

- Cutaneous tributaries in the leg.
- Gives out several rami to join great saphenous vein
- Communicating branch to accessory saphenous vein.

There may be 7–13 valves in the vein and one at its termination.

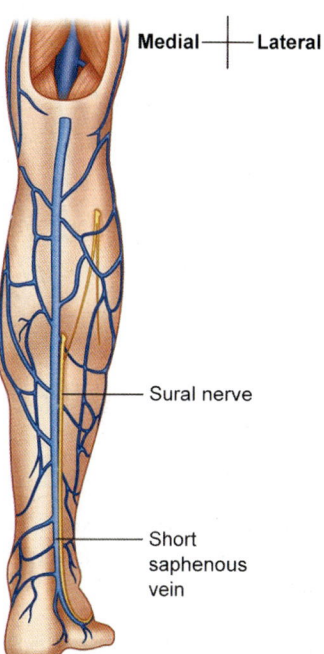

Course of short saphenous vein

### Clinical Importance

Incompetency of the valves may cause reversal of flow of venous blood leading to formation of varicose veins.

## LYMPH NODES

### Q. Inguinal Nodes

**Ans.** Majority of the lymphatic fluid of the lower limb drains into the inguinal nodes. The inguinal lymph nodes are classified into superficial and deep with relation to the deep fascia of the thigh.

### Superficial Inguinal Lymph Nodes

- These nodes are arranged into proximal horizontal group and distal vertical group
- The horizontal group lies under the inguinal ligament and are around five to six in number
- The vertical group lies along the termination of great saphenous vein and are around four to five in number.

*Drainage Area*

Proximal group medially receives lymph from external genitalia (except glans penis or clitoris), anal canal and area around it, lower part of anterior abdominal wall, and round ligament.

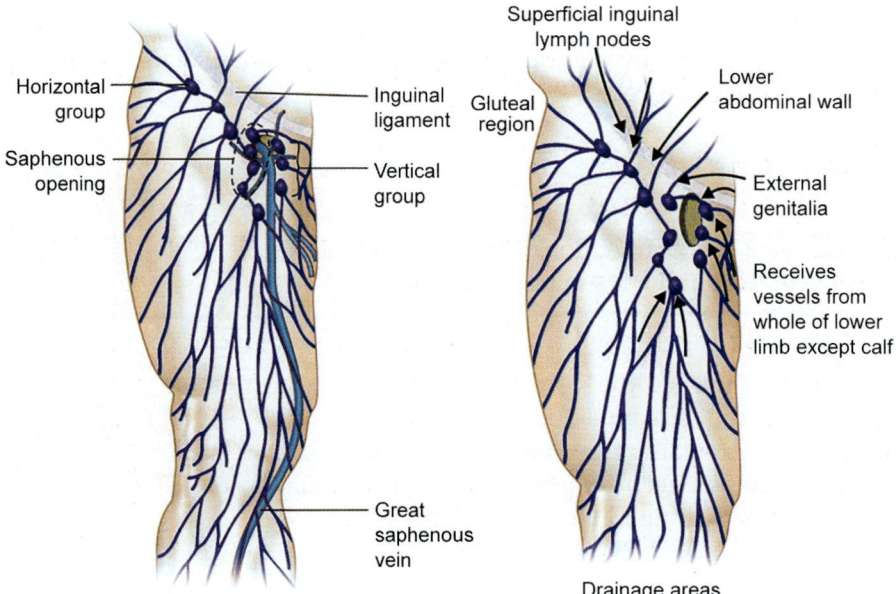

Drainage areas

Proximal group laterally receives lymph from gluteal and lower part of anterior abdominal wall. Distal vertical group receives lymph through superficial vessels from whole of the lower limb except calf.

## Deep Inguinal Lymph Nodes

Located medial to femoral vein. They are three in number, one is close to saphenofemoral junction, another is in the femoral canal and one is close to the femoral ring.

### Drainage Area

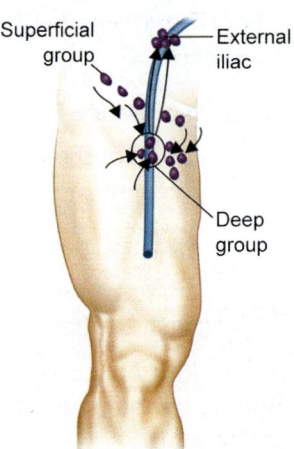

Deep inguinal lymph nodes

- Receives lymph from superficial inguinal lymph nodes and glans penis or clitoris
- All the inguinal lymph nodes drain into external iliac lymph nodes
- Superficial lymphatic vessels of the lower limb drain into superficial inguinal lymph nodes and then into deep inguinal lymph nodes and then into external iliac lymph nodes.

## Drainage Pattern

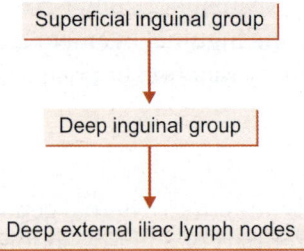

## Clinical Importance

Any lesion like pus collection or cancer in the area of drainage of inguinal lymph nodes leads to enlargement of respective lymph nodes.

# JOINTS

### Q. Ankle Joint

**Ans.** *Type:* Hinge joint, uniaxial joint, synovial joint.

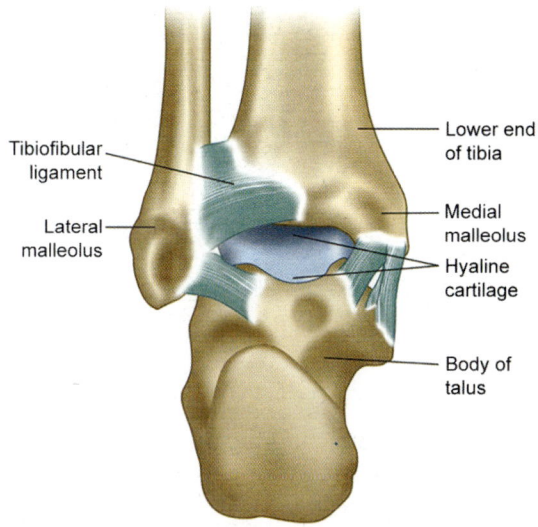

Ankle joint articular surfaces

## Articular Surfaces

*Above*

Lower end of tibia, medial malleolus, lateral malleous of fibula, transverse tibiofibular ligament (all these structures form a socket above).

*Below*

Body of talus.

**Note:** Articular surfaces are covered by hyaline cartilage.

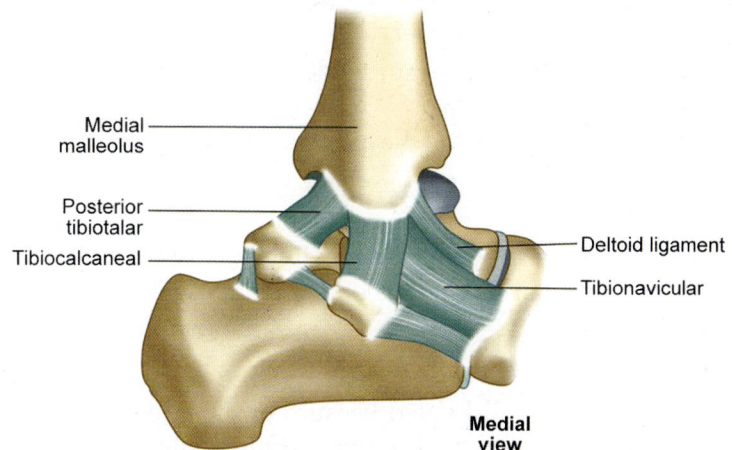

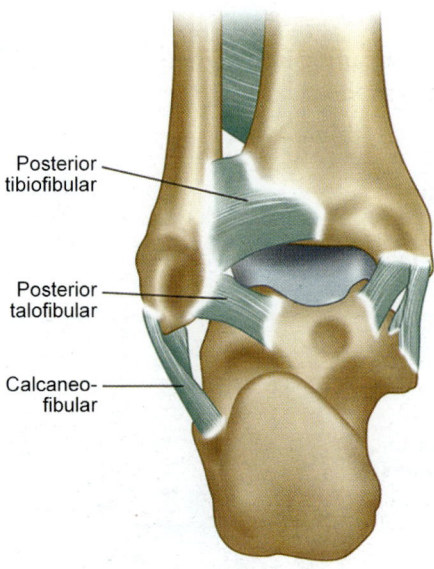

Ankle joint ligaments

## Ligaments

Connects the articular surfaces:

- *Fibrous capsule:* It is thin capsule connecting the articular surfaces
  The ligaments strengthen the capsule.
  *Medial ligament* = Deltoid ligament
  It is a tough triangular band of ligament extending between medial malleolus and calcaneum and talus.
- *Anterior talofibular ligament:* Extends anteromedially from malleolus of fibula to talus.
- *Posterior talofibular ligament:* Runs horizontally between lateral malleolus and talus.

## Relations

- The joint is related in the front by tibialis anterior, extensor tendons, anterior tibial vessels and common peroneal nerve
- Posteriorly related to flexor tendons, tibialis posterior, tibial nerve, posterior tibial vessels and peroneus tendons
- The joint is supplied by the arteries and nerve around it.

## Movements

- Dorsiflexion is brought about by tibialis anterior and assisted by extensors of the leg
- Plantar flexion is brought about by tendo Achilles and assisted by flexors of the leg.

## Clinical Importance

The joint is rarely dislocated because of the structure of articular surfaces. A few fibres of medial ligament may get torn due to sudden movements of foot leading to sprain.

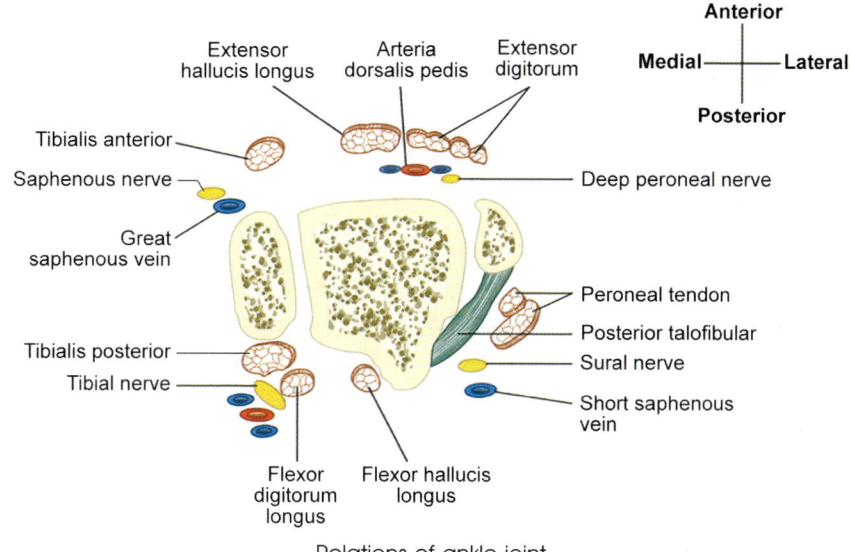

Relations of ankle joint

## Q. Subtalar Joints

**Ans. Definition**

The anterior and posterior talocalcaneal joints are termed subtalar joints.

**Type**

Synovial, multiaxial joint.

**Articular Surface**

- *Above:* Concave inferior surface of talus
- *Below:* Convex superior surface of calcaneum.

**Ligaments**

Connects the articular surface:
- Fibrous capsule
- Lateral, medial and interosseous talocalcaneal ligaments connect the respective sides of articular surfaces
- Cervical ligament connects the area next to sinus tarsi to superior calcaneal surface.

**Movements**

- Inversion is brought about by tibialis anterior and posterior
- Eversion is brought about by peroneus longus and brevis.

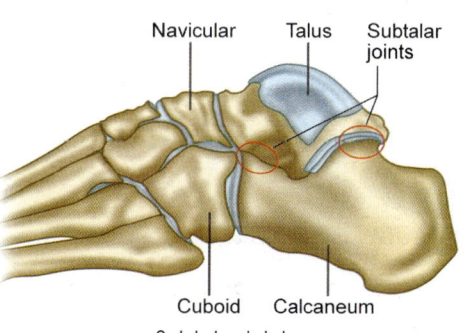

Subtalar joints

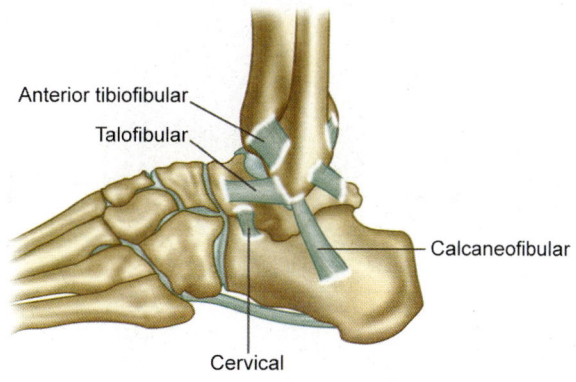

Ligaments of subtalar joint

## Clinical Importance

While walking on uneven surface a sudden movement can lead to injury to ligament causing sprain.

# MISCELLANEOUS

### Q. Femoral Triangle

**Ans.** Femoral triangle is also known as Scarpa's triangle. It is marked by a hollow under the inguinal fold, when thigh is flexed, abducted and laterally rotated.

## Roof

Skin, superficial fascia, superficial inguinal lymph nodes, cutaneous nerves and superficial vessels.

## Boundaries

- *Laterally:* Medial margin of sartorius
- *Medially:* Medial margin of adductor longus
- *Base:* Inguinal ligament.

## Floor

Following muscles from lateral to medial side form the floor:
- Iliacus
- Psoas major
- Pectineus
- Adductor longus.

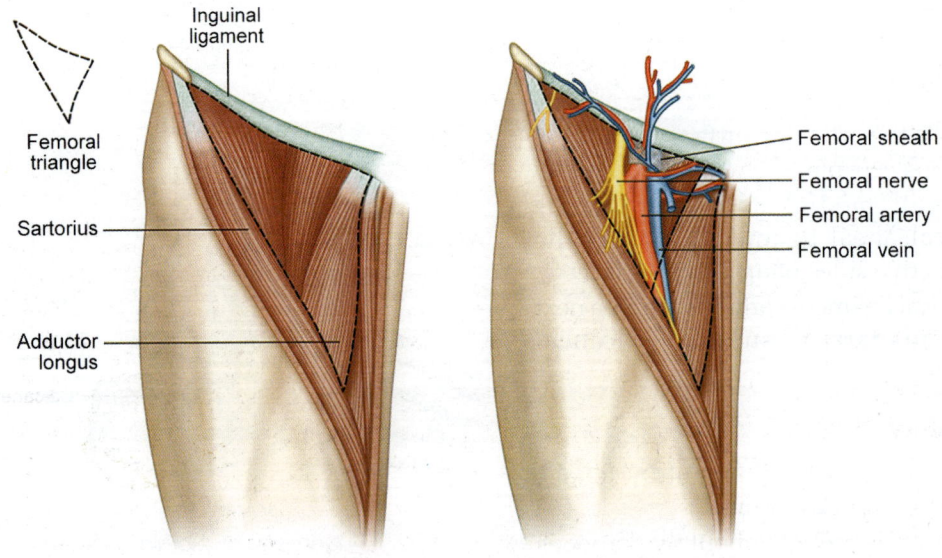

Femoral triangle and its contents

## Contents

Femoral artery, femoral vein, femoral nerve, inguinal lymph nodes and fat.

### Q. Femoral Sheath

**Ans.** Like the half-sleeves of apron, the proximal part of femoral vessels is covered by connective tissue known as femoral sheath (like carotid sheath).
- Anteriorly, it is the extension of transversalis fascia
- Posteriorly, it is the extension of fascia iliaca.

## Contents

There are three compartments namely lateral for femoral artery, middle compartment for femoral vein and medial compartment for deep inguinal lymph nodes.

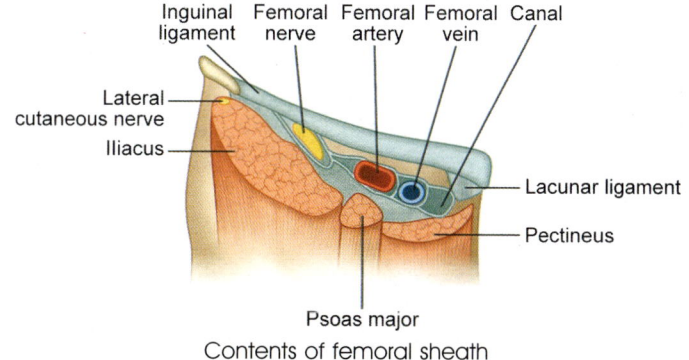

Contents of femoral sheath

The medial compartment is known as femoral canal. The proximal end of the canal is thickened to form femoral ring. The femoral ring is bounded anteriorly by inguinal ligament, posteriorly by pectineus, medially by lacunar ligament and laterally by femoral vein.

### Q. Adductor Canal

**Ans.** Adductor canal is also known as subsartorial canal and proper name is Hunter's canal. It occupies medial side of the thigh, in its middle third and is an aponeurotic tunnel.

### Extent

Adductor canal extends from apex of the femoral triangle to the opening in the adductor magnus.

### Boundaries

Canal is triangular in section:
- *Anterolaterally:* Vastus medialis.
- *Posteriorly:*
  - Adductor longus proximally
  - Adductor magnus distally.

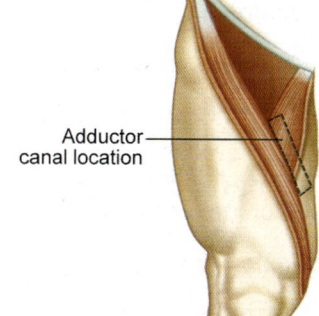

Adductor canal location

Adductor canal location

- *Anteromedially:* Sartorius, aponeurosis extending between adductors and vastus medialis.
- *Anteriorly:* Sartorius.

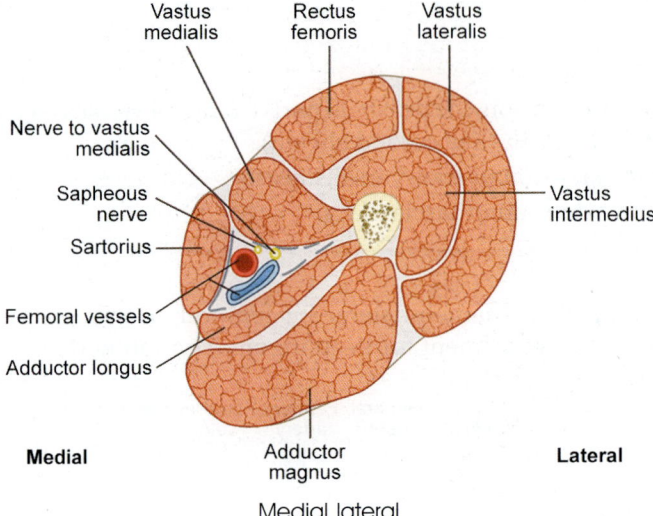

**Medial lateral**

## Contents

- Femoral artery
- Femoral vein
- Saphenous nerve
- Nerve to vastus medialis.

## Clinical Importance

Femoral artery can be approached in adductor canal for ligation in cases of any aneurysm, thrombosis.

### Q. Foot Drop

**Ans.** The common peroneal nerve is very susceptible to injury due to its superficial location around neck of fibula.

## Mode of Injury

Fracture of fibula or pressure on the nerve.

## Consequence of Injury

Injury to the nerve leads to paralysis of dorsiflexors and evertors, i.e. tibialis anterior, extensors of leg and peroneal muscles leading to loss of dorsiflexion. Loss of sensation on dorsum of foot and on outer surface of front of leg.

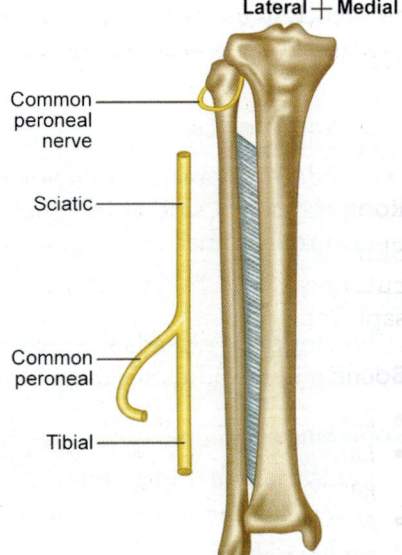

## Attitude of Limb

The ankle is plantar flexed, adducted and inverted.
However second and third phalanx may be extended by interossei, which is supplied by tibial nerve.

## Q. Flexor Retinaculum

**Ans.**

### Attachments

- *Anteriorly:* Tip of medial  malleolus
- *Posteriorly:* Medial calcaneal process
- Structures under the cover of flexor retinaculum from medial to lateral.

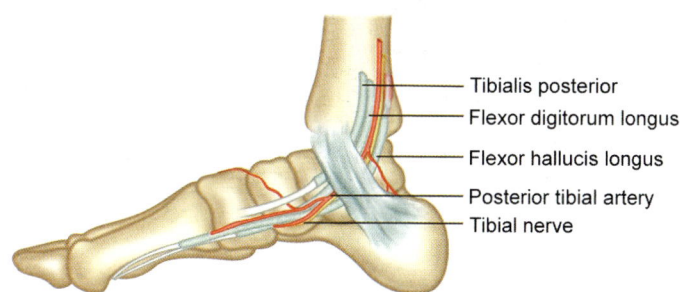

Structures deep to flexor retinaculum

| Mnemonic | Structures |
|---|---|
| "Talented | Tibialis posterior |
| Doctors | Flexor Digitorum longus |
| ARe | Posterior tibial Artery and vein |
| Never | Tibial Nerve |
| Hungry" | Flexor Hallucis longus. |

### Function

The retinaculum holds the tendons in place (like logs of wood tied together).

## Q. Popliteal Fossa

**Ans.** Popliteal fossa is a diamond-shaped area behind the knee joint.

### Roof

Skin, superficial fascia, posterior cutaneous nerve of thigh, short saphenous vein.

### Boundaries

- *Lateral and above:* Biceps femoris
- *Lateral and below:* Lateral head of gastrocnemius, plantaris
- *Medial and above:* Semitendinosus, semimembranosus
- *Medial and below:* Medial head of gastrocnemius.

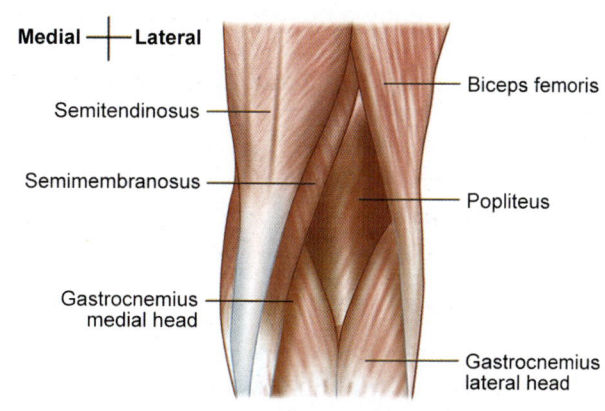

Boundaries of popliteal fossa

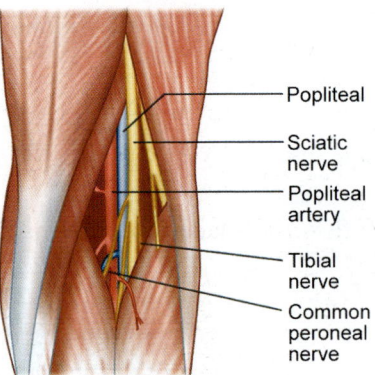

Contents of popliteal fossa

## Floor

- Femoral popliteal surface
- Oblique popliteal ligament
- Popliteus muscle with its fascia.

## Contents

### Superficial

Fat, lymph nodes, posterior cutaneous nerve of thigh, articular branch of obturator nerve.

### Deep

- Popliteal artery and vein
- Tibial nerve and common peroneal nerve.

**Note:** The tibial nerve is most superficial, vein is just below it and popliteal artery is the deepest.

## Q. Deltoid Ligament

**Ans.**
- Deltoid ligament is a medial collateral ligament of ankle joint
- It consists of superficial and deep fibres and is very tough.

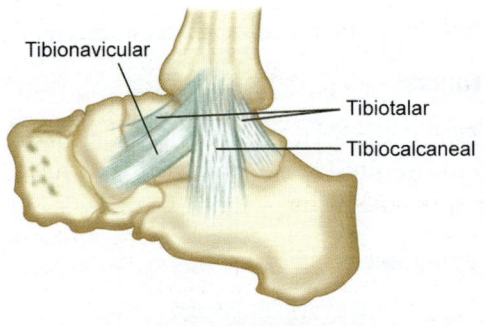

Deltoid ligament

## Attachments

Deltoid ligament is attached to apex and anterior, and posterior borders of medial malleolus.

## Superficial Fibres

- Anterior tibionavicular fibres
- Intermediate vertical tibiocalcaneal fibres, which reach sustentaculum tali
- Posterior tibiotalar.

### Deep Fibres

Anterior tibiotalar.

### Relations

Tendons of tibialis posterior and flexor digitorum longus cross the ligament.

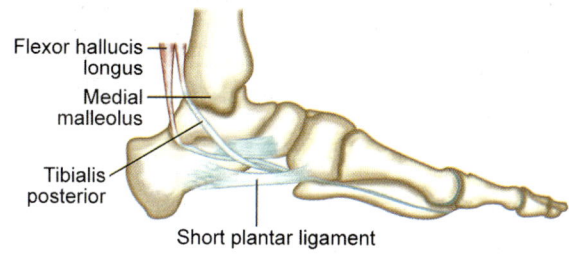

Flexor hallucis longus

Medial malleolus

Tibialis posterior

Short plantar ligament

### Clinical Importance

Since the ligament is very strong, in case of sudden movement or injury on the medial side of ankle, the medial malleolus is first to get affected (avulsion) and then only ligament tear occurs. So sprains are secondary to bony injury.

**Note:** Sprain is injury to ligament.

### Q. Spring Ligament

**Ans.** Spring ligament is plantar calcaneonavicular ligament and is a very strong ligament.

### Attachments

- *Anteriorly:* Navicular bone
- *Posteriorly:* Sustentaculum tali of calcaneum
- *Medially:* A few fibres to deltoid ligament.

### Relations

- *Medial:* Tendon of tibialis posterior
- *Lateral:* Tendon of flexor hallucis longus and flexor digitorum longus.

### Functional Importance

Spring ligament holds the head of talus and maintains the medial longitudinal arch.

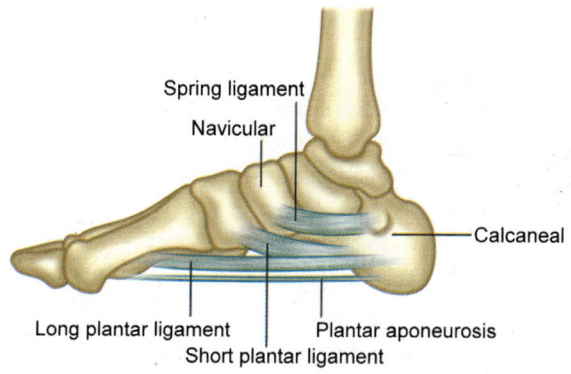

Spring ligament

Navicular

Calcaneal

Long plantar ligament

Plantar aponeurosis

Short plantar ligament

## Q. Cutaneous Innervations

**Ans.**

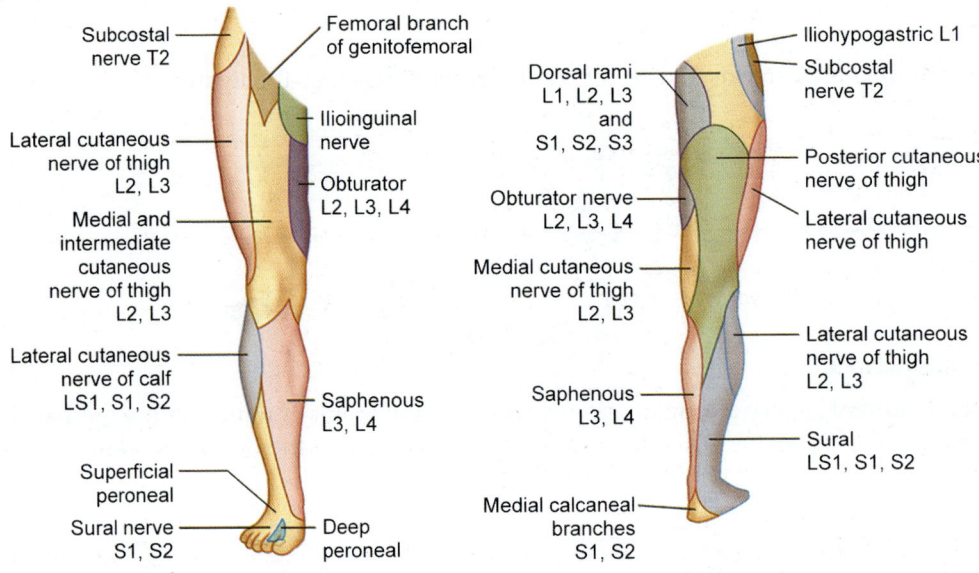

## Q. Bursae Around the Knee Joint

**Ans.** Bursae are fluid filled sac, which reduces the friction between articular surfaces and tendon, and bone. There are many bursae in relation to the knee joint, which facilitate smooth movements at the knee joint.

- *Suprapatellar:*
  - Present between femur bone and tendon of quadriceps
  - It communicates with joint cavity.
- *Popliteal:* Present between popliteus tendon and lateral condyle of tibia.
- *Anserine:*
  - Present between tendons of sartorius, gracilis
  - Semitendinosus, tibia bone and tibial collateral ligament.
- *Medial bursa of gastrocnemius:* It lies deep to medial head of gastrocnemius.

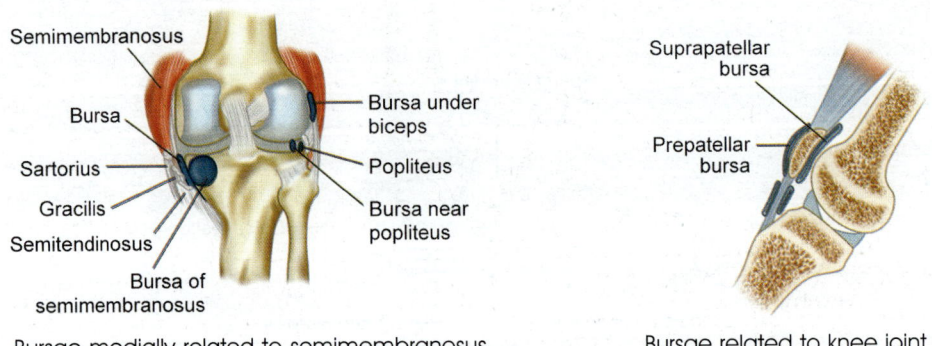

Bursae medially related to semimembranosus          Bursae related to knee joint

- *Semimembranosus bursa:* Present between medial head of gastrocnemius and semimembranosus.
- *Prepatellar:* Lies below the skin and anterior surface of patella.
- *Superficial infrapatellar:* Lies between skin and tibial tuberosity.
- *Deep infrapatellar:* Lies between patellar ligament and anterior surface of tibia.

## Clinical Importance

- *Prepatellar bursitis:* It is also described as housemaid's knee. It is produced due the friction between the skin and patella.
- *Infrapatellar bursitis:* It is also described as clergyman's knee. It is produced due to kneeling on the knee.
- *Baker's cyst:* It is herniation of synovial cavity of knee, with formation of fluid filled sac, which forms a swelling behind the knee and also extends little below the knee.

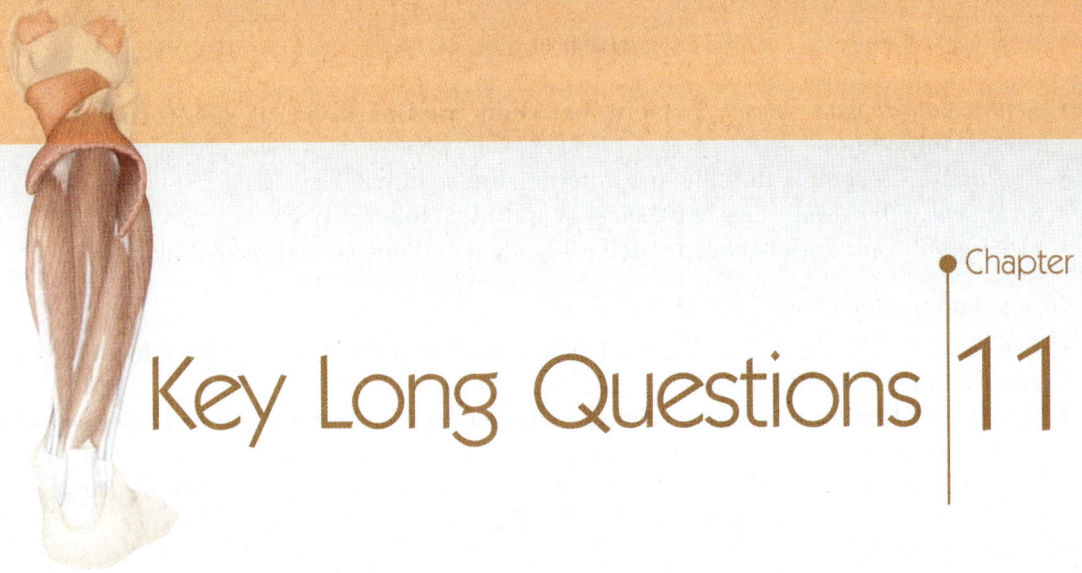

# Key Long Questions | 11

## 11

**Q. Describe the venous drainage of lower limb in detail and add a note on its applied anatomy.**

**Ans.** Venous drainage of lower limb assumes great significance due to the erect posture of human beings. The venous blood has to flow against gravity upwards, which needs a huge mechanical energy like a motor.

This energy is provided by various factors like negative intrathoracic pressure, the valves within the vein, the musculature and thick condensed superficial fascia of lower limb.

## CLASSIFICATION

- Superficial venous system
- Deep venous system
- Perforators.

### Superficial Venous System

The major channels included in this system are great (long) saphenous vein and (small) saphenous vein. These veins run in superficial plane in the form of tunnels of superficial fascia.

*Great saphenous vein:* Great saphenous vein is the longest vein in the body.

*Course*

1. *In leg:* It begins from the medial end of dorsal venous arch of foot ascends upwards in front of medial malleolus (2–3 cm).

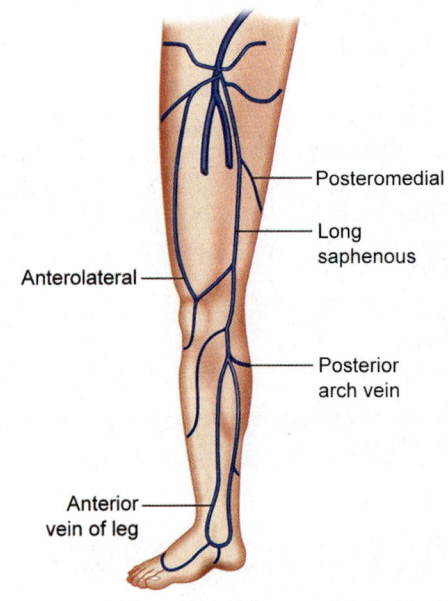

Great saphenous vein with its tributaries

2. The vein further runs straight upwards for short distance in front of leg and then inclines backwards to reach posteromedial side of the knee.

3. *In thigh:* From the backside of the knee the vein again comes in front of the thigh to run obliquely upwards and medially to end in the saphenous opening where it terminates into femoral vein.

### Relations

The saphenous nerve is closely related to the vein. The nerve is in the front of the vein at the level of medial malleolus in most of the cases while it lies posterior to the vein at the level of knee.

### Tributaries

- Posterior arch vein of the leg
- Anterior vein of the leg
- Short saphenous vein through its tributaries
- Posteromedial vein of thigh
- Anteromedial vein of thigh
- External pudendal vein
- Inferior epigastric vein
- Circumflex iliac vein.

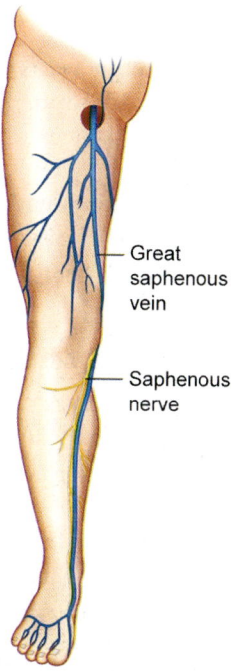

Great saphenous vein

### Clinical Importance

1. In severely dehydrated patients like in cases of burns great saphenous vein can be chosen for pushing intravenous fluids. So while doing venous cut down one has to be careful about the saphenous nerve.

2. Varicosity (tortuous and dilated veins) of great saphenous vein is rarely observed, this is due to the support offered by the condensed fascia around it which helps in venous return. Varicosity is observed in the tributaries of the great saphenous vein.

## Short Saphenous Vein

### Course

It begins from the lateral end of dorsal venous arch of foot and runs behind and below lateral malleolus and ascends upwards on back of the leg, pierces the deep fascia to end in popliteal vein in popliteal fossa in most of the cases. The vein has a short course hence the name.

### Relations

Initially, the vein is lateral to tendocalcaneus and then it lies between the two heads of gastrocnemius. Sural nerve is closely related to the vein on back of the leg.

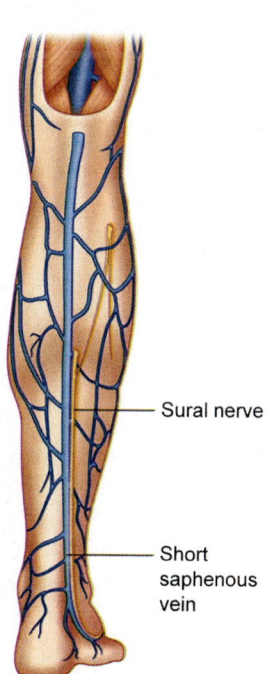

Short saphenous vein

*Tributaries*
- Cutaneous veins of the leg
- Accessory saphenous vein.

*Clinical Importance*

While tackling varicosities if the surgeon ligates the vein subcutaneously there may be recurrence of varicose veins because the vein pierces the fascia of the leg and has a subfascial course. So, the surgeon should ligate (tie) the vein subfascially to avoid recurrence of varicose veins.

## Deep Venous System

The deep venous system comprises of:
- Tibial vein
- Peroneal vein
- Popliteal vein
- Femoral vein.

The veins are supported by the musculature of the lower limb and they accompany arteries of the same name. The interior of the veins has valves except the venous sinuses in soleus muscle. Soleus muscle pumps venous blood from lower limb, and assists in venous return. Thus soleus muscle acts like heart, hence well described as peripheral heart.

*Clinical Importance*

When a patient is bedridden following a major surgery there is a sluggish movement of blood in the veins leading to high chance of thrombus formation, which may eventually lead to pulmonary embolism.

*Perforators*

Perforators are connecting venous channels between superficial veins and deep veins. They are mostly present within the intermuscular septa and have valves.

*Types*
- Direct
- Indirect.

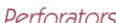

Femoral vein

Popliteal vein

Peroneal vein

Tibial vein

Deep veins

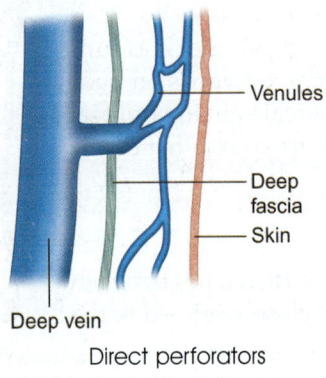

Venules

Deep fascia

Skin

Deep vein

Direct perforators

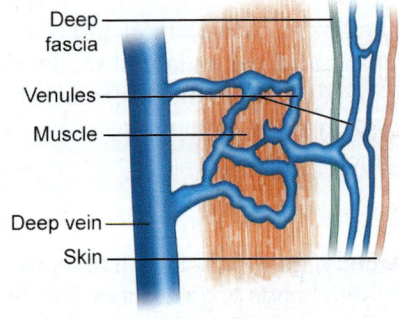

Deep fascia

Venules

Muscle

Deep vein

Skin

Indirect perforators

*Direct:* The superficial veins are directly connected through perforator to deep veins by piercing the deep fascia only (without intervening muscle).

*Indirect:* The superficial veins are first connected to the veins in the muscle and then to the deep veins through the perforators.

### Location of perforators

Certain perforators have constant location:
- Around the medial malleolus there are four perforators namely upper medial, upper lateral, middle and low
- One below the knee
- In the thigh, one in the adductor canal and one at the junction of great saphenous vein and femoral vein.

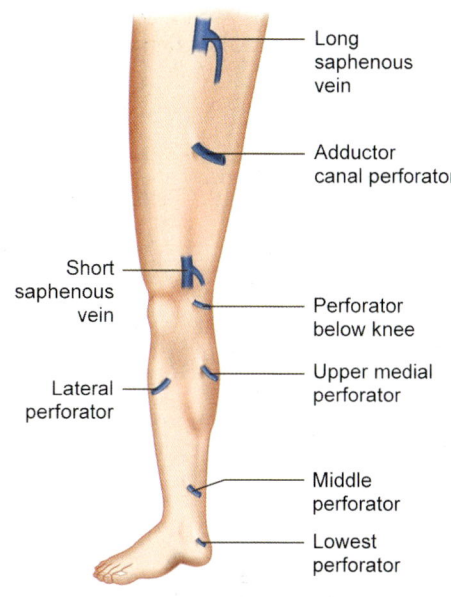

Location of perforators

### Clinical Importance

1. The flow of blood from superficial system to deep system is maintained by competent valves. In case of incompetency (loss of function) of valves the blood may flow in reverse direction leading to varicose veins.
2. The surgical treatment of varicose veins includes removal of incompetent segment.

## DEEP VEIN THROMBOSIS

Thrombosis is predisposed by Virchow's triad:
- Change of vessel wall
- Diminished rate of blood flow
- Increased coagulability of blood
  It is a consequence of prolonged immobility, local trauma, childbirth, operations, etc.

### Q. Discuss hip joint in detail and add a note on its applied anatomy.

**Ans.** Hip joint is one of the ideal ball and socket joint with exceptional strength, stability and also mobility.

### Type

Synovial joint, ball and socket variety.

### Articular Surfaces

- *Above:* Acetabulum of hip bone
- *Below:* Head of the femur.

### Peculiarities

The depth of the acetabulum is increased by fringe like covering around the acetabulum, which increases the depth of acetabulum.

By virtue of the neck-shaft angle of femur, the range of movement at the hip joint increases. However, it also makes it weak by increasing the vulnerability of fracture.

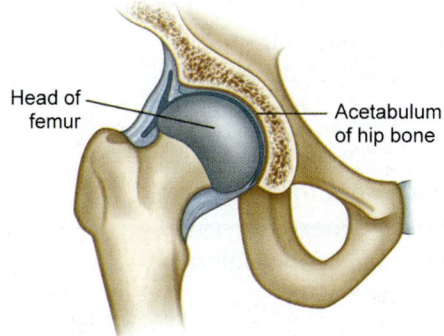

Articulating surfaces of hip bone

## Ligaments

### Fibrous Capsule

The capsule is very strong and surrounds the joint from all sides. It is attached to the margins of acetabulum and its transverse ligament on one side and to the intertrochanteric line on the femur anteriorly. Posteriorly, the capsule is one finger-breadth in front of the intertrochanteric crest.

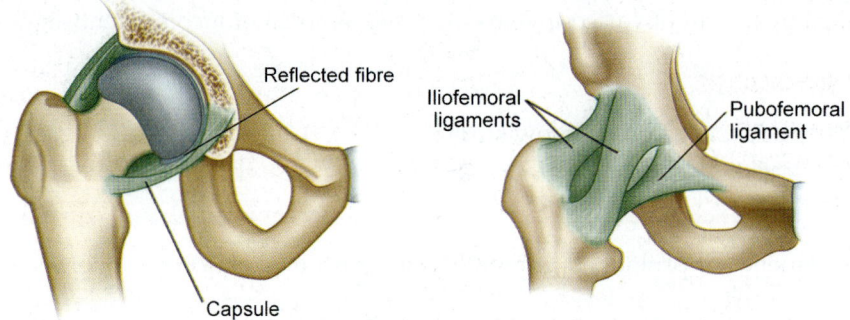

Fibrous capsule

### Iliofemoral Ligament

Iliofemoral ligament is the strongest ligament in the body and is attached above to anterior inferior Iliac spine and below. It fans out to get attached on intertrochanteric line of femur.

### Pubofemoral Ligament

Pubofemoral ligament strengthens the lower and anterior part of fibrous capsule and is attached above to iliopubic eminence and below it blends with iliofemoral ligament.

### Ischiofemoral Ligament

Ischiofemoral ligament is comparatively weak ligament present on the posterior aspect of fibrous capsule. It is attached on one side to a part of ischium posteroinferior to acetabulum and on other side to greater trochanter.

### Ligament of Head of Femur

Ligament of head of femur is also known as round ligament and ligamentum teres. It is attached to the fovea on head of the femur on one side and transverse ligament and margins of acetabular notch on other side.

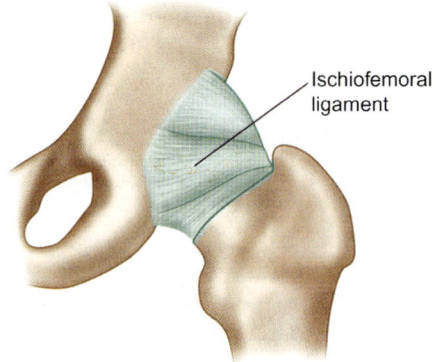

Posterior aspect

It is very weak ligament and hardly supports the joint, but helps to spread the synovial fluid during movement of hip joint.

### Acetabular Labrum

Acetabular labrum is a fibrocartilaginous ring-like structure attached to the margins of acetabulum. It deepens the cavity of acetabulum.

### Transverse Ligament of Acetabulum

Transverse ligament of acetabulum is across the acetabular notch converting it into a foramen for the passage of vessels and nerves.

## Relations

The hip joint is covered all around by muscles.

### Anterior

- Muscles of the floor of femoral triangle (pectineus, psoas major, iliacus)
- Straight head of rectus femoris more laterally.

### Posterior

- Tendon of obturator externus
- Tendon of obturator internus and gemelli.

### Superior

- Rectus femoris (reflected head)
- Gluteus minimus.

### Inferior

- Pectineus (lateral fibres)
- Obturator externus (few fibres).

## Movements

- Flexion and extension around transverse axis
- Adduction and abduction around anteroposterior axis
- Medial and lateral rotation around vertical axis
- Circumduction is combination of above movements.

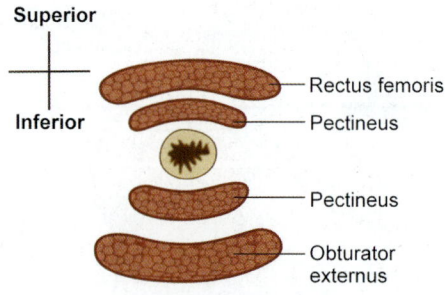

Relations of hip joint

| Movement | Flexion | Extension | Adduction | Abduction | Medial rotation | Lateral rotation |
|---|---|---|---|---|---|---|
| Muscles | Psoas major, iliacus | Gluteus maximus, hamstrings | Adductors of thigh | Glutei medius, minimus | Tensor lata, few fibres of glutei medius, minimus | Quadratus femoris obturators with gemelli |
| Mnemonic | P | G | Adds | Glamor | To | Female gender |

## Arterial Supply

Hip joint receives blood from anastomosis around the neck of femur (circumflex femoral arteries and gluteal arteries).

## Nerve Supply

All the major nerves of the lower limb supply the hip joint:
- Femoral
- Obturator
- Sciatic.

## Clinical Importance

- In cases of joint effusion aspiration of the fluid in the joint can be done by inserting a needle 2 cm lateral to femoral artery and directed posteriorly
- Hip joint can be approached anteriorly, anterolaterally, laterally and posteriorly
- Joint replacement can be done totally by replacing both acetabulum and head of the femur
- Since all the three major nerves of lower limb supply the hip joint, pain in the hip joint can be felt in lower back, knee, calf and around ankle
- The acetabulum can be shallow from birth leading to recurrent dislocations and giving rise to a condition known as acetabular dysplasia.

## INTRAMUSCULAR INJECTIONS (IM) IN GLUTEAL REGION

- In the upper outer quadrant of gluteal region there are no major neurovascular structures (vacant area);  safe area for IM injections.

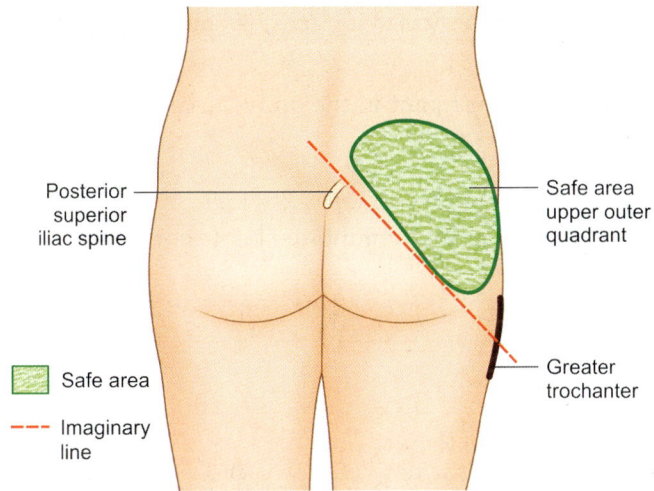

An imaginary line from greater trochanter to posterior superior iliac spine is drawn. Area above this line is safe for IM injections.

## ANATOMICAL BASIS OF TRENDELENBERG'S SIGN

While standing on one leg if pelvis drops on the opposite side; it is positive Trendelenberg's test. It connotes that gluteus medius and minimus, i.e. abductors of hip joint are weak.

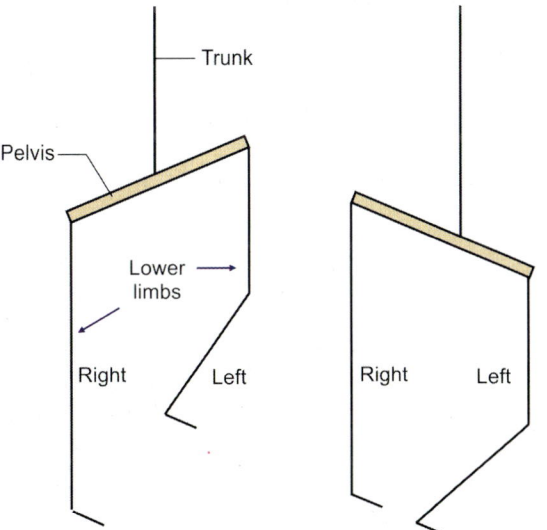

- Fracture neck of femur compromises the blood supply of head of femur causing avascular necrosis.
- Hip dislocation is disruption in joint alignment due to excessive external force, or could be congenital.

- Hip replacement is surgical procedure wherein the hip joint is replaced by prosthetic implant.
- *Osteoarthritis:* It is a degenerative wear and tear process of articular cartilage of joint by and large stress related.

> **Q. Describe knee joint in detail (articular surfaces, ligaments, relations, movements, blood supply and applied anatomy).**

**Ans.** Knee joint is one of the largest joint in the body susceptible to injuries and pathological conditions.

### Type

Synovial joint, of modified hinge variety, compound joint (since more than two bones are involved).

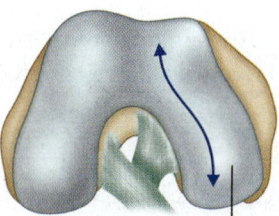

Articular surfaces

### Articular Surfaces

- *Above:* Condyles of femur
- *Below:* Condyles of tibia
- Saddle joint between patella and femur.

### Ligaments

*Fibrous Capsule*

*Attachments on femur*

- *Posteriorly:* Margins of femoral condyles and intercondylar fossa
- *Medially:* Articular margin of femur
- *Laterally:* Proximal to the groove of popliteus tendon
- *Anteriorly:* Blends with patellar retinacula, patellar ligament and patella.

Articular surface of medial condyle of femur

### ATTACHMENTS ON TIBIA

- *Posteriorly:* Margins of tibial condyles and intercondylar area
- *Laterally:* Margins of tibial condyles (laterally-head of fibula also).

### Features

- Capsule is deficient above the level of patella for the passage of suprapatellar bursa

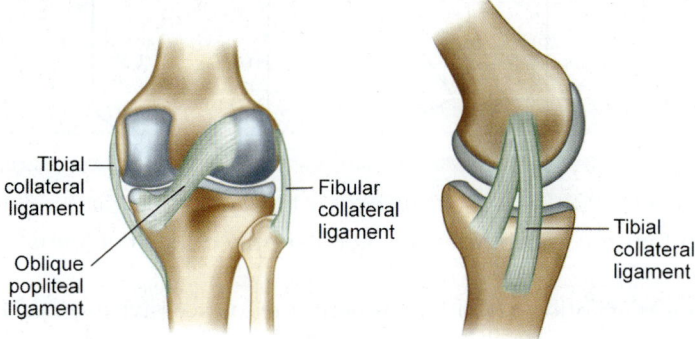

- On the lateral condyle of tibia there is an aperture for the passage of popliteus tendon
- Thickening of the capsule medially is deep part of tibial collateral ligament
- Thin fibres from its deep aspect, i.e. coronary ligaments are attached to both menisci.

### Tibial Collateral Ligament

*Attachments*

- *Above:* Medial femoral epicondyle (just distal to adductor tubercle)
- *Below:* Upper part of medial surface of tibia.

### Fibular Collateral Ligament

*Attachments*

- *Above:* Lateral femoral epicondyle (between the attachment of lateral head of gastrocnemius and tendon of popliteus)
- *Below:* Head of fibula.

**Note:** It is not attached to the capsule and has no connection to the lateral meniscus.

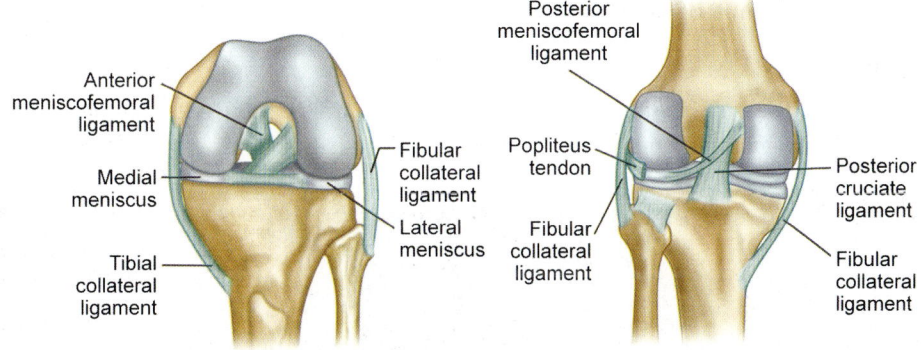

Ligaments of knee joint

### *Oblique Popliteal Ligament*

It is an expansion of tendon of semimembranosus and it merges with the capsule of knee joint and ascends laterally towards intercondylar fossa and lateral femoral condyle.

### *Arcuate Popliteal Ligament*

A Y-shaped thickening of posterior capsular fibre. At one end it is attached to head of fibula, while the medial limb is attached to the posterior edge of the tibial intercondylar area and the lateral limb is attached to the lateral femoral condyle.

### *Cruciate Ligaments*

Cruciate ligaments are intracapsular ligaments between the tibia and femur. There are two ligaments, which cross each other and hence the name.

### Anterior Cruciate Ligament

This is directed upwards and backwards.

*Attachments*

- *On tibia:* Anterior part of intercondylar area between the horns of menisci
- *On femur:* Posteromedial area of lateral femoral condyle.

## Posterior Cruciate Ligament

This is directed upwards and forwards.

*Attachments*

- *On tibia:* Posterior part of intercondylar area between the horns of menisci
- *On femur:* Anteromedial area of medial femoral condyle.

## MENISCI

Menisci are fibrocartilaginous disks on the tibial condyles. They are mostly avascular structures and receive nutrition from the capillaries in the peripheral rim.

### Medial Menisci

Medial menisci is semicircular, in shape having anterior horn and posterior horn, and attached on the intercondylar area of tibia.

### Lateral Menisci

Lateral menisci is almost circular in shape, and has a uniform width. It also has anterior horn and posterior horn, and attached on the intercondylar area of tibia.

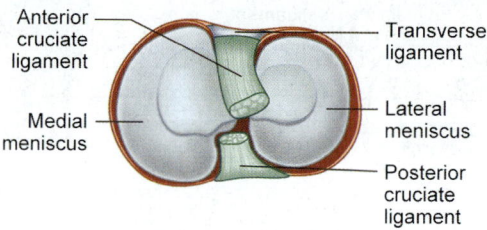

Condylar surface of tibia

## INTERIOR OF THE JOINT

Four cavities coalesce to form the cavity of knee joint. One cavity is between two femoral condyles and another between the tibial condyles. The third is the patella-femoral cavity. And the last is continuous superiorly with the suprapatellar bursa. Synovial membrane lines the cavities except at the articular surfaces, menisci and posterior part of the capsule where it turns forwards to enclose the cruciate ligament.

## Relations

| | |
|---|---|
| Anterior | Ligamentum patellae |
| Posteromedial | Sartorius, gracilis, semitendinosus, semimembranosus, medial head of gastrocnemius |
| Posterolateral | Biceps, common peroneal nerve, lateral head of gastrocnemius posterior popliteal artery, tibial nerve |

| Medial | Tibial collateral ligament |
|---|---|
| Lateral | Fibular collateral ligament, tendon of popliteus lies between the fibrous capsule and lateral meniscus |

## Movements

| Movement | Flexion | Extension | Medial rotation | Lateral rotation |
|---|---|---|---|---|
| Muscles | Hamstrings, gracilis, sartorius, gastrocnemius, popliteus | Quadriceps femoris, tensor fasciae latae | Semimembranosus, semitendinosus | Biceps femoris |

### Locking of the Knee

In fully extended position, i.e. standing position the knee joint is in a locked state and is in a stable position and a person can stand for a long-time without quadriceps fatigue. In this position the tibial tubercles snugly fit into the intercondylar notch, menisci are tightly sandwiched between the tibial and femoral condyles and also the collateral ligaments are taut. This tight situation of the knee joint is known as locking of the knee (medial rotation of femur on tibia in final stages of extension of leg), wherein stability of the knee is maximum, but since there is no movement possible it is vulnerable to injury.

### Unlocking of the Knee

Unlocking of the knee is brought about by popliteus muscle and is lateral rotation of femur on tibia.

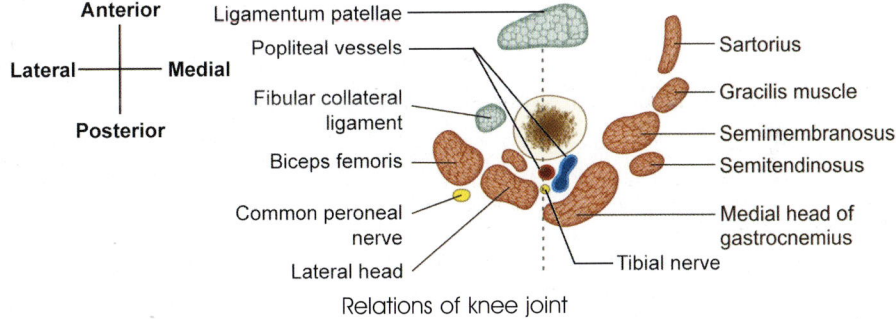

Relations of knee joint

## Arterial Supply

Receives blood from the anastomosis around it through branches of popliteal artery, femoral artery and anterior and posterior tibial arteries.

## Nerve Supply

All the major nerves of the lower limb supply the knee joint.
- Femoral
- Obturator
- Sciatic.

## Clinical Importance
- Knee joint can be surgically approached through anterior vertical midline incision

- The surgeon has to be aware of infrapatellar branch of saphenous nerve, which may get included in the incision
- Posterior approach to knee joint is by giving a 'S'-shaped incision
- Direct examination of the knee joint cavity is known as arthroscopy. An anterolateral approach is adopted by surgeons
- Aspiration of the knee joint is carried out by inserting the needle from the side at the upper lateral margin of the patella
- For injecting any medication in the knee joint directly the joint cavity is approached from the lower border of patella from either side of patellar ligament
- Knee joint is prone for arthritis almost of every kind.

## Q. Describe the arches of the foot in detail.

**Ans.** The entire body weight in erect position is supported by foot. Activities like jumping from a height demand extra strength and resilience to sustain the body weight with extra velocity. This is provided by small individual blocks of bone, which are held in position by ligaments, tendons and muscles.

Impression of wet foot on the ground depicts the pressure points of the foot, i.e. the heel, lateral margin of foot, ball of the foot and pads of distal phalanges. The medial margin of the foot does not produce the impression because it arches upwards.

### Classification

- Longitudinal
- Transverse.

### Longitudinal Arch

Longitudinal arch (rests on calcaneal tuberosity). It is of two types:
1. Medial
2. Lateral.

Foot impression showing pressure points

### Medial longitudinal arch

*Formation:* It is formed by medial part of calcaneum, talus, navicular, three cuneiform bones and inner three metatarsal bones.
**Note:** Talus is the key bone of this arch.

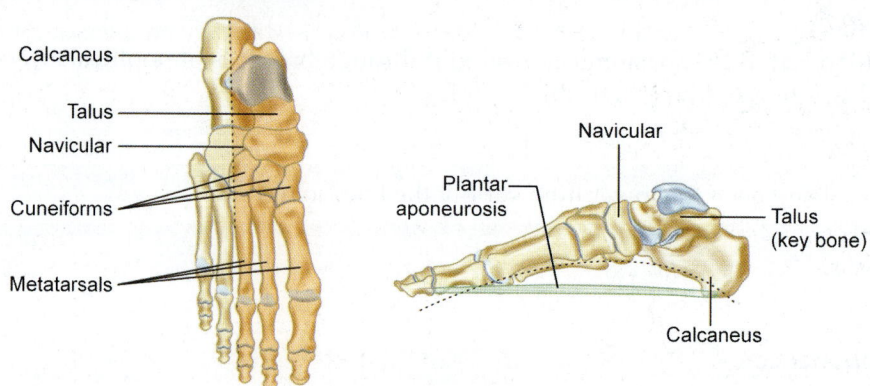

Medial longitudinal arch

*Supports*
- Head of talus supported on sustentaculum tali
- Plantar aponeurosis stretching from the anterior end of the arch to posterior end
- Spring ligament supports the head of talus
- Tendon of flexor hallucis longus along with flexor digitorum longus act as bow strings
- Accessory support is provided by abductor hallucis and medial half of flexor digitorum brevis
- Tibialis anterior and posterior pull the medial border of the arch and maintain the height of the arch
- While the peroneus longus muscle counters the action of tibialis muscle and evert the foot and lower the height of the arch.

### Lateral longitudinal arch
*Formation*
It is formed by lateral part of calcaneus, cuboid, lateral two metatarsals.

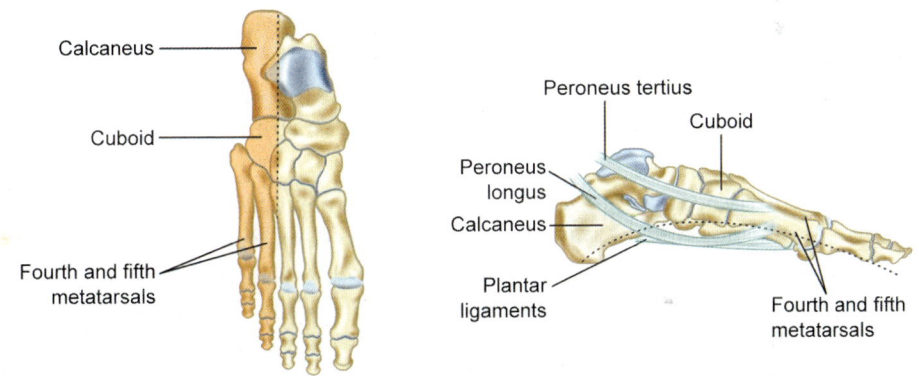

Lateral longitudinal arch

*Supports*
- Lateral part of plantar aponeurosis and plantar ligaments function as bow strings for the arch
- Peroneus longus tendon as it enters the groove of cuboid bone maintains the integrity of the arch
- Other supports include flexor digitorum longus of fourth and fifth toes, lateral half of flexor digitorum brevis.

### Transverse arch
Combination of both feet form a single transverse arch.

*Formation*
It is a combined arch, formed by cuboid, three cuneiforms and bases of metatarsal bones of each foot.

**Note:** Middle cuneiform bone is the key bone of the arch.

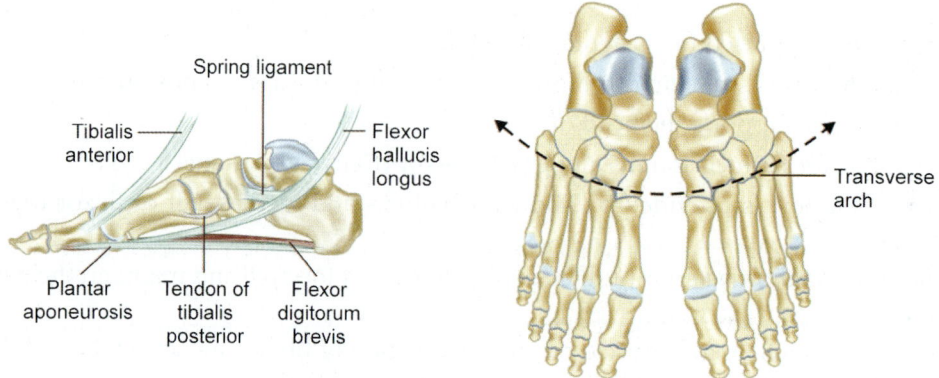

Supports of medial longitudinal arch

*Supports*
- Interosseus ligaments bind the bones in position and maintain the arch
- Peroneus longus tendon approximates medial and lateral borders of the foot.

## Clinical Importance

1. If the medial longitudinal arch touches the ground it is known as flat foot. Normally observed between the age of 1 and 2 years due to which a child has a frequent tendency of falling.

2. Weakness in the intrinsic muscles of the foot may lead to extension at metatarsophalangeal joints flexion at interphalangeal joint. This is known as claw foot.

3. In some newborn babies, the foot may be plantar flexed, inverted and the forefoot in varus (adducted) position. This is known as clubfoot. Anatomically, there is sublaxation of subtalar joint. Treatment of this condition should start immediately after birth and each component of the deformity should be corrected.

4. *Flat foot:* In this condition medial longitudinal arch is reduced so that the medial border of foot is in contact with ground.

5. *Clubfoot:* Foot is adducted, inverted and plantar flexed. Anatomically, there is sublaxation of subtalar joint.

6. *Calcaneum tendon rupture:* Rupture occurs 5 cm above insertion; while running or jumping patient develops excruciating pain, however patient is able to walk. Inevitably plantar flexion is hampered.

7. *Metatarsalgia:* In this condition there is pain in forefoot either due to reduced transverse arch, stress fracture (= March fracture, 2nd or 3rd metatarsal) or plantar digital neuritis.

8. *Plantar fasciitis:* In this condition there is pain under front of calcaneum (anterior part) due to inflammation.

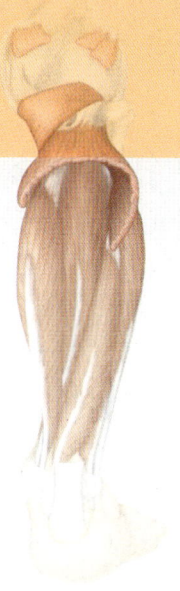

# Key Diagrams with MCQ Tips | 12

## Q. Ischial tuberosity

**Ans.**

- Superolateral side of upper area is for semi-membranosus muscle
- Inferomedial side of upper area is for biceps femoris and semitendinosus
- Medial side of lower area is covered by fat and this area bears the body weight while sitting
- Margin of ischial tuberosity medially provides attachment to sacrotuberous ligament
- Professions, which demand sitting in one place for long-time like tailors are vulnerable to bursitis of ischial tuberosity. This is known as tailor's seat (a bursa is present between ischial tuberosity and gluteus maximus).

Superolateral surface

Upper area

Transverse ridge

Inferomedial surface

Medial area

Lower area

Lateral area

Longitudinal ridge

## Q. Attachments on greater trochanter

**Ans.** Very commonly asked in viva, study the diagram carefully.

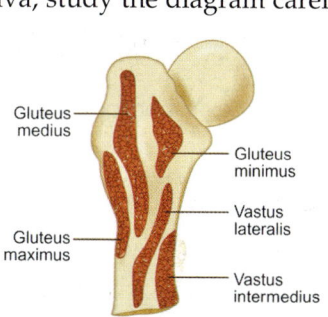

Gluteus medius

Gluteus minimus

Vastus lateralis

Gluteus maximus

Vastus intermedius

**Q. Obturator externus tendon is attached on trochanteric fossa.**

**Q. Quadratus femoris is attached on quadrate tubercle.**

**Q. Gluteal tuberosity when prominent is known is third trochanter.**

**Q. Lesser trochanter anteromedially receives psoas major and iliacus tendon.**

**Q. Proximal articular surface of tibia.**

**Ans.** Study the diagram carefully.

*Mnemonic*

| | |
|---|---|
| "Medical | **Medial** meniscus anterior horn |
| College | Anterior **Cruciate** ligament |
| Lucknow | Anterior horn **Lateral** meniscus |
| Lucknow | Posterior horn **Lateral** meniscus |
| Medical | Posterior horn **Medial** meniscus |
| College" | Posterior **Cruciate** ligament |

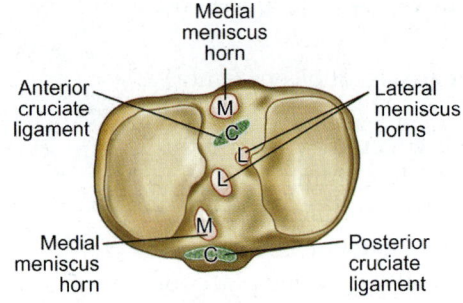

**Q. Nerves related to psoas major muscle.**

**Ans.**

- Lateral border from above downwards is related to iliohypogastric nerve, ilioinguinal nerve, lateral femoral cutaneous nerve and femoral nerve
- Anterolateral surface is related to genitofemoral nerve
- Medial border related to obturator nerve, upper root of lumbosacral trunk.

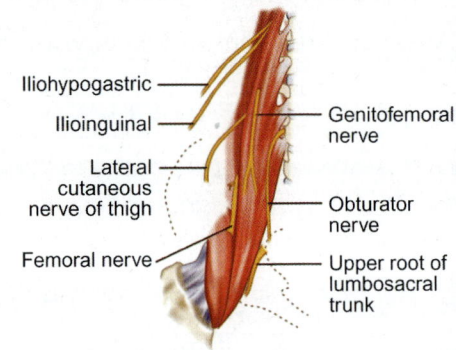

**Q. Gluteus maximus supplied by inferior gluteal nerve and extends the flexed thigh.**

**Q. Gluteus medius and minimus supplied by superior gluteal nerve, and abducts the thigh and also brings about medial rotation of thigh.**

**Q. Femoral triangle boundaries, floor and contents.**

**Ans.**
- Femoral artery is lateral to femoral vein and lies behind the midinguinal point
- Femoral nerve is lateral to femoral artery.

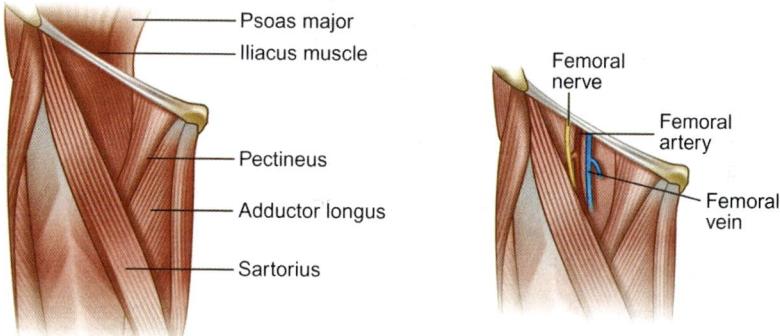

**Q. Femoral sheath**

**Ans.**
- Three compartments—lateral for femoral artery, middle for femoral vein and medial for deep inguinal lymph nodes
- Deep inguinal lymph nodes are also known as gland of Cloquet, which drain glans penis in males and clitoris in females
- Anteriorly, it is the extension of transversalis fascia
- Posteriorly, it is the extension of fascia iliaca.

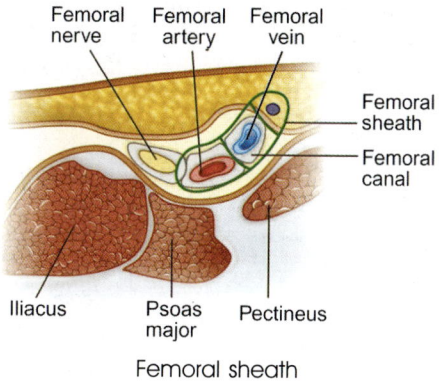

Femoral sheath

## Q. Popliteal fossa contents

**Ans.**

- The tibial nerve is most superficial, vein is just below it and popliteal artery is the deepest
- Sciatic nerve may sometimes divide in popliteal fossa into common peroneal nerve and tibial nerve.

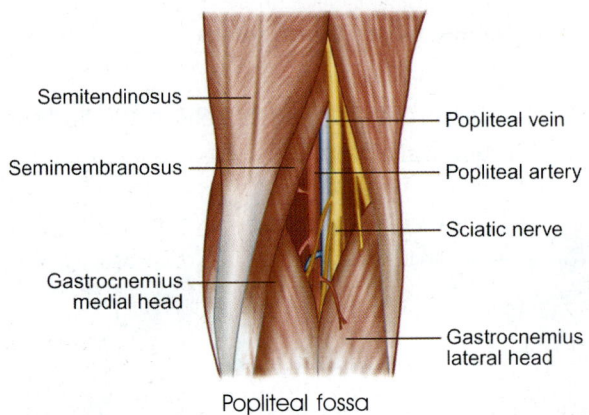

*Popliteal fossa*

## Q. Inguinal lymph nodes

**Ans.**

- Classified into superficial and deep inguinal lymph nodes
- Deep inguinal lymph nodes are known as glands of Cloquet
- Deep inguinal lymph nodes drain glans penis or clitoris.

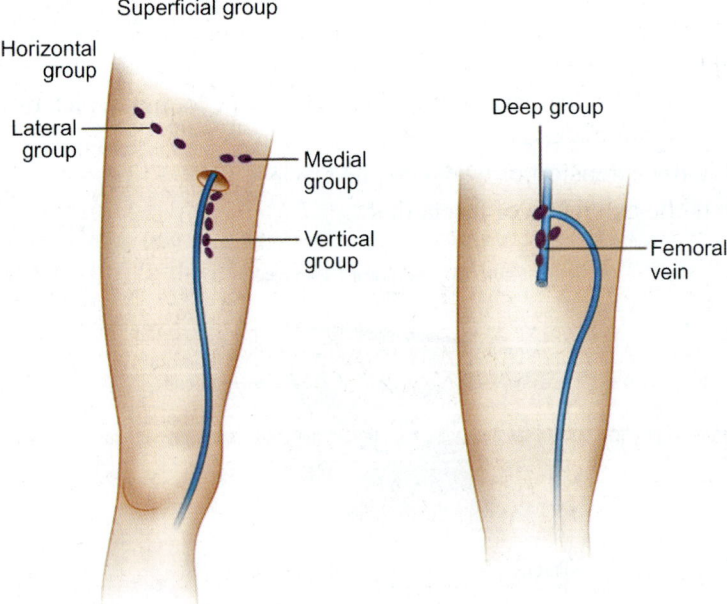

## Q. Veins

**Ans.**

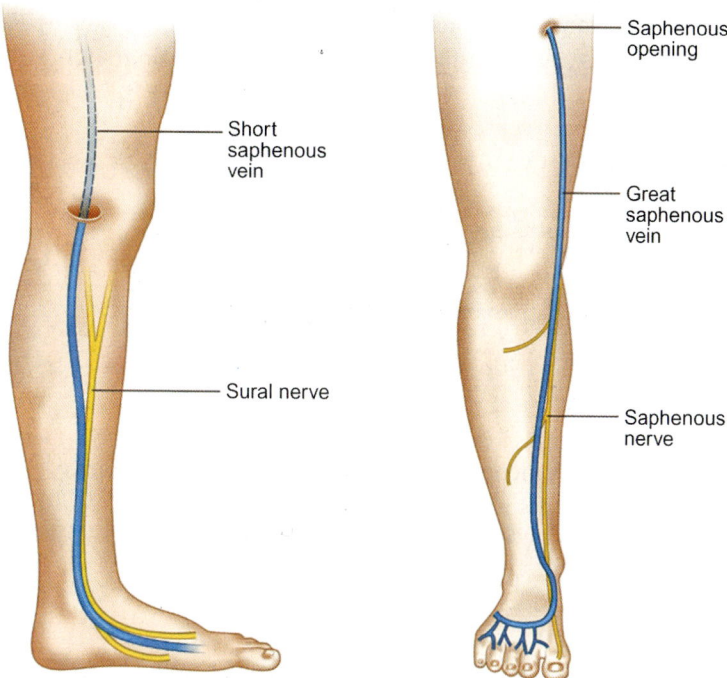

- Great saphenous vein is accompanied by saphenous nerve
- Short saphenous vein is accompanied by sural nerve
- Soleus muscle is known as peripheral heart; since it pumps the venous blood from lower limb.

## Q. Deltoid ligament

**Ans.**
- Deltoid ligament is medial collateral ligament of ankle joint
- It has superficial fibres and deep fibres
- Tendons of tibialis posterior and flexor digitorum longus cross the ligament.

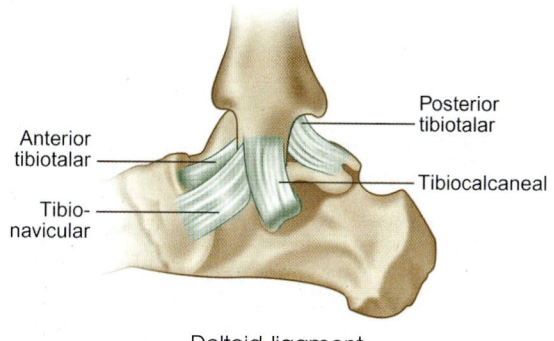

Deltoid ligament

## Q. Spring ligament

**Ans.**
- Spring ligament is plantar calcaneonavicular ligament
- It holds the head of talus and maintains the medial longitudinal arch.

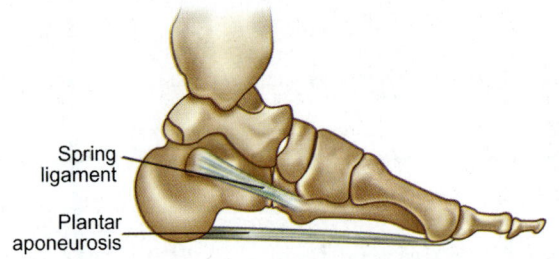

## Q. Subtalar joint

**Ans.**
- Anterior and posterior talocalcaneal joints are termed subtalar joints
- Inversion and eversion occurs at subtalar joint
- Inversion is brought about by tibialis anterior and posterior
- Eversion is brought about by peroneus longus and brevis.

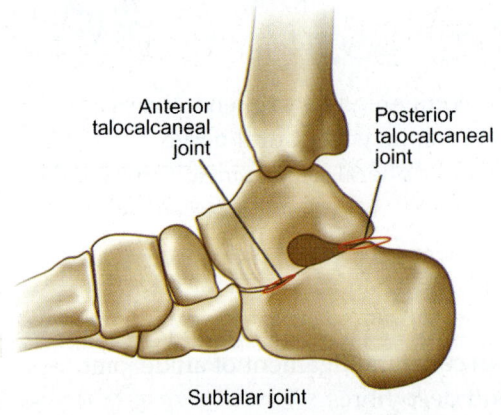

## Q. Flexor retinaculum

**Ans.**

| Mnemonic | Structures |
|---|---|
| "Talented | Tibialis posterior |
| Doctors | Flexor **D**igitorum longus |
| Are | Posterior tibial **A**rtery and vein |
| Never | Tibial **N**erve |
| Hungry" | Flexor **H**allucis longus |

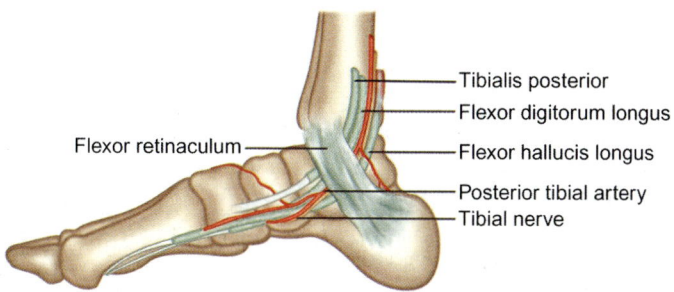

Tibialis posterior
Flexor digitorum longus
Flexor retinaculum
Flexor hallucis longus
Posterior tibial artery
Tibial nerve

## Q. Popliteus muscle

**Ans.**

- Popliteus muscle tendon is within the cavity of knee joint
- Popliteus muscle unlocks the knee.

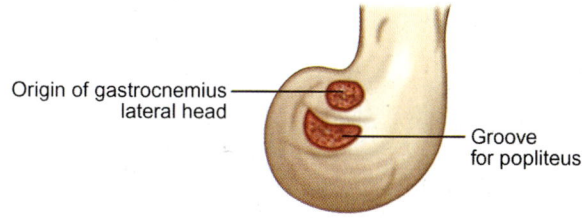

Origin of gastrocnemius
lateral head
Groove
for popliteus

## Q. Ligaments of knee joint

**Ans.**

- Tibial collateral ligament is a degenerated part of adductor magnus tendon
- Fibular collateral ligament is degenerated part of peroneus longus
- Oblique popliteal ligament is expansion of semimembranosus tendon.

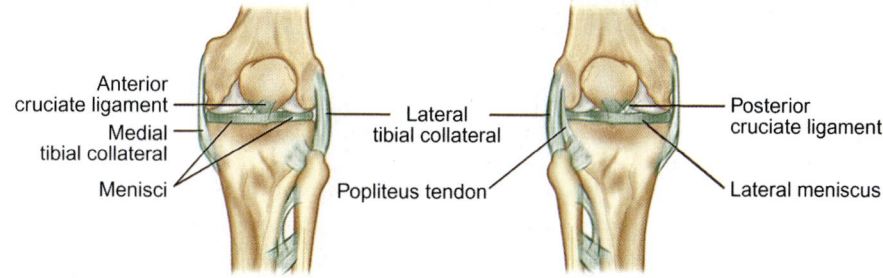

Anterior
cruciate ligament
Medial
tibial collateral
Menisci
Lateral
tibial collateral
Popliteus tendon
Posterior
cruciate ligament
Lateral meniscus

## Q. Bursae around the knee joint

**Ans.**

- Prepatellar bursitis is known as housemaid's knee
- Infrapatellar bursitis is known as clergyman's knee
- Baker's cyst is synovial cavity extension
- Suprapatellar bursa communicates with the knee joint cavity.

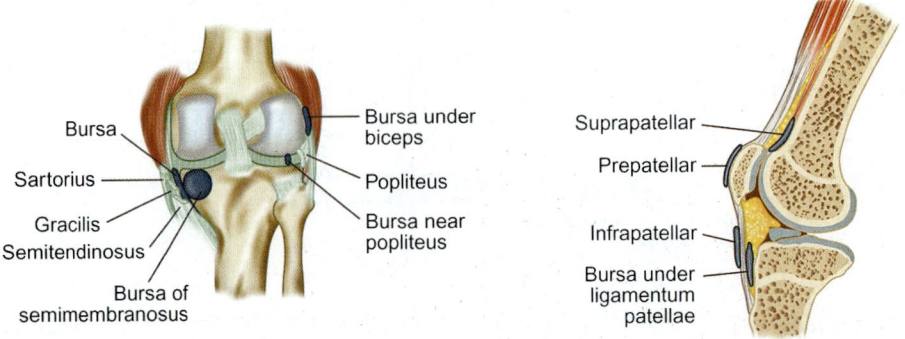

## Q. Arches of foot

**Ans.**

- Talus is key bone of medial longitudinal arch
- Middle cuneiform bone is the key bone of transverse arch.

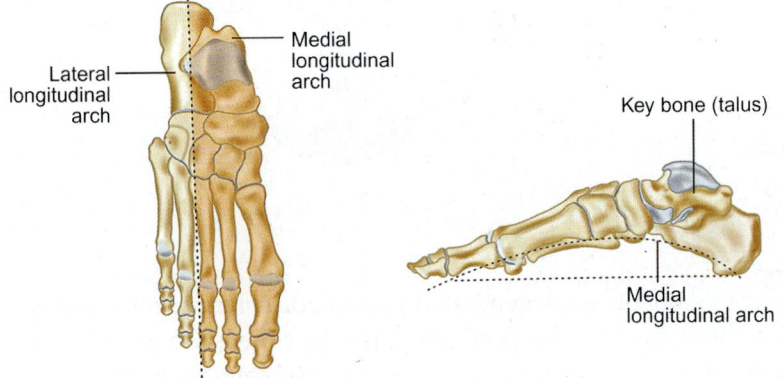

## Q. Dermatomes of lower limb (diagram only).

**Ans.**

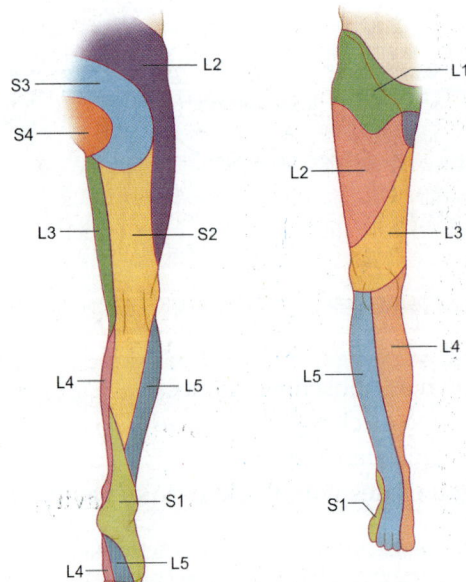

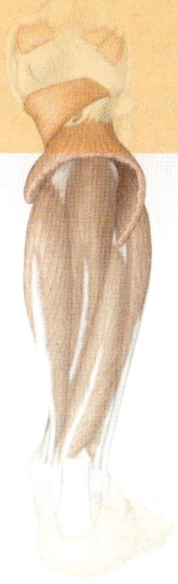

1. **The tubercle of the iliac crest is on the ..................... lip of iliac bone.**

   a. Outer lip

   b. Inner lip

   c. Intermediate area

   d. None

   **Answer: a**

2. **Pubic symphysis is ..................... type of joint.**

   a. Primary cartilaginous

   b. Fibrous

   c. Synovial

   d. Fibrocartilaginous

   **Answer: d**

3. **On the following area of ischial tuberosity hamstrings are attached?**

   a. Above transverse ridge

   b. Below transverse ridge

   c. On transverse ridge

   d. On longitudinal ridge

   **Answer: a**

4. **On the medial area below transverse ridge of ischial tuberosity what is attached?**

   a. Semitendinous

   b. Semimembranosus

   c. Biceps

   d. Fat

   **Answer: d**

5. **Following vessel is related posteriorly to ischial spine .....................**

   a. External iliac

   b. External pudendal

   c. Internal pudendal

   d. Internal iliac

   **Answer: c**

6. **The nerve posterior to ischial spine is** ...................

    a. Femoral nerve

    b. Nerve to obturator internus

    c. Nerve to obturator externus

    d. Pudendal nerve

**Answer: b**

7. **The neck shaft angle of femur is** ...................

    a. 110

    b. 115

    c. 100

    d. 125

**Answer: d**

8. **Following muscle is attached to trochanteric fossa** ...................

    a. Psoas major

    b. Obturator internus

    c. Obturator externus

    d. Iliacus

**Answer: c**

9. **All the following muscles are attached on the lesser trochanter except** ...................

    a. Psoas major

    b. Psoas minor

    c. Adductor magnus

    d. Iliacus

**Answer: b**

10. **Neck shaft angle is** ................... **at birth.**

    a. Widest

    b. Absent

    c. Narrowest

    d. None

**Answer: a**

11. **Following muscle is attached to quadrate tubercle** ...................

    a. Gluteus minimus

    b. Gluteus maximus

    c. Gluteus medius

    d. Quadratus femoris

**Answer: d**

12. **Third trochanter of femur is** ...................

    a. Greater trochanter

    b. Lesser trochanter

    c. Gluteal tuberosity

    d. Quadrate tubercle

**Answer: c**

13. **Following are the major nerves of the lower limb, except** ...................

    a. Femoral

    b. Sciatic

    c. Obturator

    d. Tibial

**Answer: d**

14. **Which muscle is attached to adductor tubercle?**

    a. Adductor longus

    b. Adductor brevis

    c. Adductor magnus

    d. Gluteus maximus

**Answer: c**

15. A 25-year-old male, while playing cricket gets a direct hit on the side of leg by bathe develops severe tingling and numbness over the foot, but still could stand on the foot. On taking X-ray, there was fracture of fibula.

  i. The anatomical basis of the patient could stand on foot is ....................

    a. Tibia not fractured             c. Fibula does not transmit the weight

    b. Metatarsals intact               d. All of the above

**Answer: c**

  ii. Anatomical basis for the tingling and numbness is due to impact on ....................
nerve.

    a. Tibial                          c. Sciatic

    b. Sural                         d. Common peroneal nerve

**Answer: d**

16. Following muscle is attached to talus bone ....................

    a. Peroneus tertius              c. Tibialis anterior

    b. Peroneus longus              d. None

**Answer: d**

17. Sustentaculum tali is present on .................... surface of calcaneum.

    a. Lateral                     c. Medial

    b. Dorsal                    d. Ventral

**Answer: c**

18. Following tendon grooves the inferior aspect of sustentaculum tali ....................

    a. Peroneus longus              c. Peroneus tertius

    b. Flexor hallucis longus       d. Flexor digitorum

**Answer: b**

19. Following muscle fibres are attached to navicular tuberosity ....................

    a. Peroneus longus              c. Tibialis posterior

    b. Peroneus brevis             d. Tibialis anterior

**Answer: c**

20. Fabella is a sesamoid bone in the tendon of .................... muscle.

    a. Gastrocnemius              c. Quadriceps femoris

    b. Soleus                    d. Peroneus longus

**Answer: a**

21. The following is present on the anterolateral surface of psoas major ....................

    a. Obturator nerve              c. Femoral

    b. Genitofemoral               d. Ilioinguinal

**Answer: b**

22. **The largest muscle of the quadriceps femoris group is** .....................
    a. Vastus medialis
    c. Vastus lateralis
    b. Vastus intermedius
    d. Rectus femoris

    **Answer: c**

23. **Literal meaning of patella is** .....................
    a. Cup
    c. Plate
    b. Saucer
    d. Flute

    **Answer: c**

24. **All of the following form, the group of hamstrings except** .....................
    a. Biceps femoris
    c. Semitendinosus
    b. Quadriceps femoris
    d. Semimembranosus

    **Answer: b**

25. **All the muscles of hamstrings are supplied by tibial part of sciatic nerve except** .....................
    a. Semitendinosus
    c. Long-head of biceps
    b. Semimembranosus
    d. Short-head of biceps

    **Answer: d**

26. **Triceps surae muscles are all except** .....................
    a. Lateral head of gastrocnemius
    c. Soleus
    b. Medial head of gastrocnemius
    d. Tibialis posterior

    **Answer: d**

27. **A 75-year-old male slipped and fell down. His leg was rotated externally? On X-ray, there was fracture neck of femur? The external rotation of leg was due to action of** .....................
    a. Gluteus maximus
    c. Psoas minor
    b. Psoas major
    d. Quadratus femoris

    **Answer: b**

28. **Nervus furcalis is ventral rami of** ..................... **nerve.**
    a. L2
    c. L4
    b. L3
    d. L5

    **Answer: c**

29. **Dorsal divisions of ventral rami of L2, L3, L4 form** ..................... **nerve.**
    a. Obturator
    c. Lateral cutaneous
    b. Femoral
    d. Genitofemoral

    **Answer: b**

**30.** Ventral divisions of ventral rami of L2, L3, L4 form .................... nerve.

   a. Femoral
           c. Obturator nerve

   b. Lateral cutaneous nerve
    d. Genitofemoral

**Answer: c**

**31.** The femoral nerve is .................... to femoral artery.

   a. Medial
           c. Posterior

   b. Anterior
         d. Lateral

**Answer: d**

**32.** The terminal divisions of sciatic nerve are ....................

   a. Sural nerve and common peroneal nerve

   b. Common peroneal nerve and tibial nerve

   c. Tibial nerve and sciatic nerve

   d. Tibial nerve and peroneal nerve

**Answer: b**

**33.** The sciatic nerve emerges below the lower border of .................... muscle in the upper part of back of thigh.

   a. Gluteus minimus
      c. Piriformis

   b. Gluteus maximus
     d. Obturator internus

**Answer: c**

**34.** A 45-year-old man suffered a direct injury on back of leg close to short saphenous vein. Patient complains of tingling and numbness over lateral part of the leg. What nerve has got injured?

   a. Saphenous nerve
     c. Lateral femoral cutaneous nerve

   b. Sural nerve
       d. Tibial nerve

**Answer: b**

**35.** The nerve, which crosses the femoral artery from lateral to medial side is ....................

   a. Sural nerve
       c. Femoral nerve

   b. Saphenous nerve
    d. Lateral femoral cutaneous nerve

**Answer: b**

**36.** Femoral artery is a continuation of .................... artery.

   a. External iliac
      c. Popliteal

   b. Internal iliac
      d. External pudendal

**Answer: a**

**37.** Following are the branches of profunda femoris except ....................

   a. Lateral circumflex femoral
   c. Perforating

   b. Medial circumflex femoral
   d. Medial circumflex iliac

**Answer: d**

38. **The popliteal artery divides at the lower borders of** ....................
    
    a. Adductor magnus             c. Soleus
    
    b. Tibialis posterior             d. Popliteus

    **Answer: d**

39. **During the ligation of short saphenous vein, the surgeon has to be careful of the following nerve:**
    
    a. Saphenous nerve             c. Lateral femoral
    
    b. Sural nerve             d. Ilioinguinal

    **Answer: b**

40. **Following is the drainage area of superficial inguinal lymph nodes, except** ....................
    
    a. Gluteal region             c. Glans penis
    
    b. Lower abdominal wall             d. Anal canal

    **Answer: c**

41. **Deltoid ligament is** ....................
    
    a. Lateral ligament of ankle             c. Transverse tibiofibular
    
    b. Medial ligament of ankle             d. Calcaneonavicular

    **Answer: b**

42. **Subtalar joint is** ....................
    
    a. Talocalcaneal             c. Calcaneonavicular
    
    b. Talonavicular             d. Tibiofibular

    **Answer: a**

43. **Inversion and eversion movements occur at** .................... **joint.**
    
    a. Ankle joint             c. Subtalar
    
    b. Inferior tibiofibular             d. All of the above

    **Answer: c**

44. **Following are the boundaries of femoral triangle expect** ....................
    
    a. Adductor longus             c. Psoas major
    
    b. Sartorius             d. Inguinal ligament

    **Answer: c**

45. **Mention the correct statements.**

    Regarding femoral ring boundaries .................... mention   Yes/No.

    | | | |
    |---|---|---|
    | a. Lacunar ligament laterally | Y/ N | Answer: N |
    | b. Lacunar ligament medially | Y/ N | Answer: Y |
    | c. Inguinal ligament superiorly | Y/ N | Answer: Y |
    | d. Inguinal ligament anteriorly | Y/ N | Answer: Y |
    | e. Inguinal ligament posteriorly | Y/ N | Answer: N |

**46.** **Femoral artery is .................... to femoral vein.**

a. Medial      c. Anterior

b. Lateral      d. Posterior

**Answer: b**

**47.** **An 80-year-old male complains of swelling, in the inguinal region and an ulcer, which bleeds on touch on glans penis. Anatomical basis for the swelling in inguinal region is ....................**

a. Superficial inguinal lymph nodes enlargement

b. Deep inguinal lymph nodes enlargement

c. Tumor in inguinal region

d. All of the above

**Answer: b**

**48.** **A 35-year-old diabetic developed a swelling in upper part of the thigh following an injury to big toe, leading to abscess. The reason for the swelling is ....................**

a. Enlargement of inguinal lymph nodes

b. Collection of blood

c. Tumor in upper thigh

d. None of above

**Answer: a**

**49.** **Following are the parts of deltoid ligament except ....................**

a. Calcaneonavicular      c. Tibiocalcaneal

b. Tibionavicular      d. Tibiotalar

**Answer: a**

**50.** **Cervical ligament forms a support to .................... joint.**

a. Inferior tibiofibular joint      c. Subtalar joint

b. Ankle joint      d. Knee joint

**Answer: c**

**51.** **Spring ligament is ....................**

a. Calcaneonavicular      c. Talocalcaneal

b. Tibionavicular      d. Tibiotalar

**Answer: a**

**52.** **The polpliteal fascia forms the .................... of popliteal fossa.**

a. Roof      c. Both

b. Floor      d. None

**Answer: b**

**53. Plantaris forms .................... boundary of popliteal fossa.**

a. Lateral and above       c. Medial and above

b. Lateral and below       d. Medial and below

**Answer: b**

**54. Deltoid ligament is crossed by following tendon ....................**

a. Tibialis anterior       c. Tibialis posterior

b. Flexor hallucis longus       d. Peroneus longus

**Answer: c**

**55. Great saphenous vein is closely related to .................... nerve.**

a. Sural nerve       c. Common peroneal nerve

b. Tibial nerve       d. Saphenous nerve

**Answer: d**

**56. Short saphenous vein is related to .................... nerve.**

a. Sural nerve       c. Common peroneal nerve

b. Tibial nerve       d. Saphenous nerve

**Answer: a**

**57. Strongest ligament of the body is ....................**

a. Pubofemoral       c. Ischiofemoral

b. Iliofemoral       d. All of above

**Answer: b**

**58. Prepatellar bursitis is also known as ....................**

a. Housemaid's knee       c. Baker's cyst

b. Clergyman's knee       d. None

**Answer: a**

**59. Clergyman's knee is .................... bursitis.**

a. Prepatellar       c. Suprapatellar

b. Infrapatellar       d. Synovial cyst

**Answer: b**

**60. Baker's cyst is ....................**

a. Prepatellar bursitis       c. Synovial cavity extension

b. Infrapatellar       d. Suprapatellar bursitis

**Answer: c**

**61. Tibial collateral ligament is a degenerated part of .................... tendon.**

a. Adductor longus       c. Peroneus tertius

b. Peroneus longus       d. Adductor magnus

**Answer: d**

62. Fibular collateral ligament is degenerated part of ....................
    a. Adductor longus
    b. Peroneus longus
    c. Peroneus tertius
    d. Adductor magnus

**Answer: b**

63. A housemaid was complaining of pain and swelling in front of the knee. The most probable reason would be .....................
    a. Infrapatellar bursitis
    b. Prepatellar bursitis
    c. Baker's cyst
    d. Fracture patella

**Answer: b**

64. Oblique popliteal ligament is expansion of .................... tendon.
    a. Semitendinosus
    b. Semimembranosus
    c. Gracilis
    d. Sartorius

**Answer: b**

65. Unlocking of the knee is brought about by .................... muscle.
    a. Semitendinosus
    b. Quadriceps femoris
    c. Popliteus
    d. Biceps femoris

**Answer: c**

66. A traffic police can stand for a long-time, on the road by the virtue of .................... of knee joint.
    a. Strength of quadriceps femoris muscle
    b. Strength of the knee bones
    c. Locking of the knee
    d. All of the above

**Answer: c**

67. Key bone of medial longitudinal arch ....................
    a. Calcaneus
    b. Cuboid
    c. Talus
    d. Navicular

**Answer: c**

68. Single important tendon, which forms key support of lateral longitudinal arch is ....................
    a. Peroneus tertius
    b. Peroneus longus
    c. Abductor digiti minimi
    d. Flexor digitorum brevis

**Answer: b**

69. Following bone is the key bone of transverse arch:
    a. Lateral cuneiform
    b. Medial cuneiform
    c. Middle cuneiform
    d. Cuboid

**Answer: c**

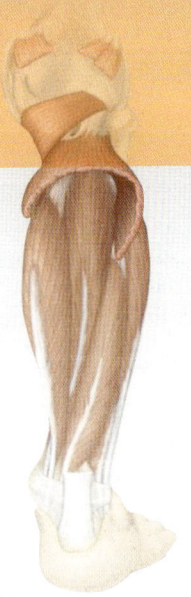

# Dissection | 14

## 1. FRONT OF THIGH (FEMORAL REGION AND ADDUCTOR CANAL)

### a. Incision Markings

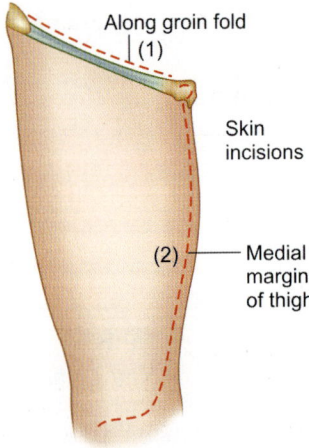

Along groin fold
| (1)

Skin
incisions

(2) —— Medial
margin
of thigh

Skin incisions on thigh

### b. Structures to be Identified

*Femoral Region (Superficial Plane)*

- Reflect the superficial fascia just below the cut, and pass fingers between membranous layer of fascia and aponeurosis of external oblique muscle. Along the fold of groin your fingers will feel a firm resistance along the line of fusion of deep fascia of thigh (fascia lata) and membranous layer of superficial fascia of thigh. This is **Holdens line**.
- Swing the fingers medially along the line of fusion and you will encounter an opening medially leading into perineum. Easily you can get medially into perineum but not laterally into thigh.

- Palpate for the spermatic cord in the male cadaver.

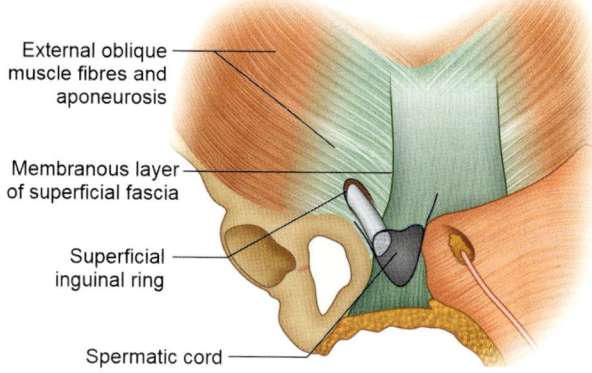

External oblique
muscle fibres and
aponeurosis

Membranous layer
of superficial fascia

Superficial
inguinal ring

Spermatic cord

Superficial dissection of lower part of abdomen

- Now appreciate the great saphenous vein on medial side of thigh, where it pierces deep fascia to drain into the femoral vein. Also look for tiny inconspicuous solid structures, the superficial inguinal lymph nodes.

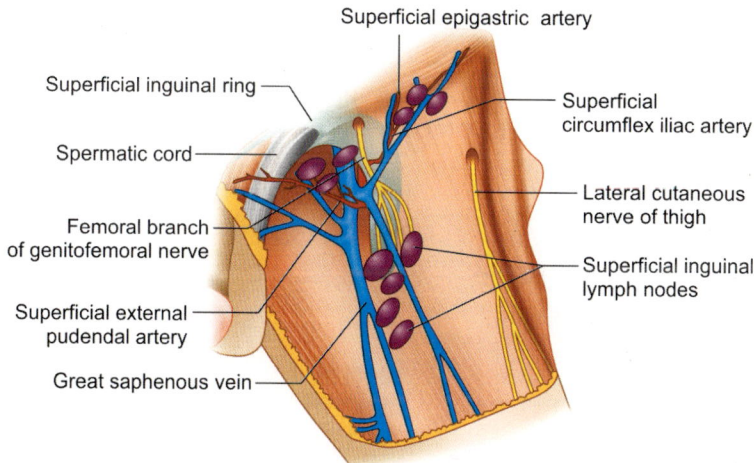

Superficial epigastric  artery

Superficial inguinal ring

Spermatic cord

Femoral branch
of genitofemoral nerve

Superficial external
pudendal artery

Great saphenous vein

Superficial
circumflex iliac artery

Lateral cutaneous
nerve of thigh

Superficial inguinal
lymph nodes

Superficial dissection of proximal part of thigh

- Try to appreciate the superficial veins entering the great saphenous vein, namely—superficial external pudendal vein medially, superficial epigastric running superiorly on anterior abdominal wall, and superficial circumflex iliac in lateral part of groin.
- Identify superficial inguinal ring, which is an opening in the aponeurosis of external oblique muscle, just superolateral to pubic tubercle. Spermatic cord comes out through this ring and locate the ilioinguinal nerve laterally.
- Lift the upper edge of great saphenous vein you will see it turns backwards over a sharp edge of deep fascia, this is the falciform margin of saphenous opening, which leads into cribriform fascia.
- Remove the cribriform fascia to get an access to the femoral sheath. While doing so do not damage the structures piercing the fascia, i.e. superficial external pudendal superficial epigastric vessels and superficial circumflex iliac vessels piercing the fascia lata just lateral to the saphenous opening.

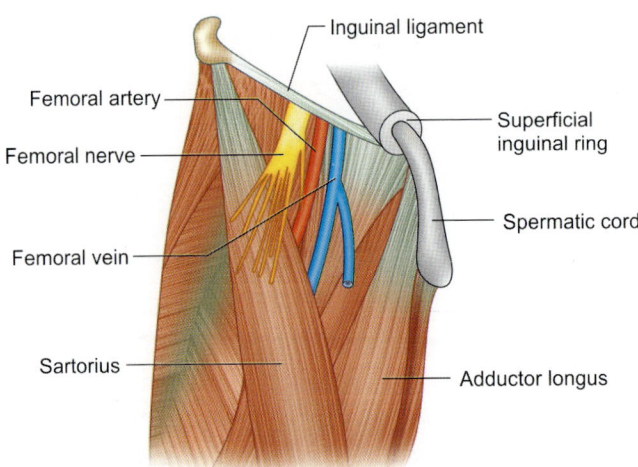

Deep plane

- Expose the femoral vein by tracing the great saphenous vein, where it terminates.

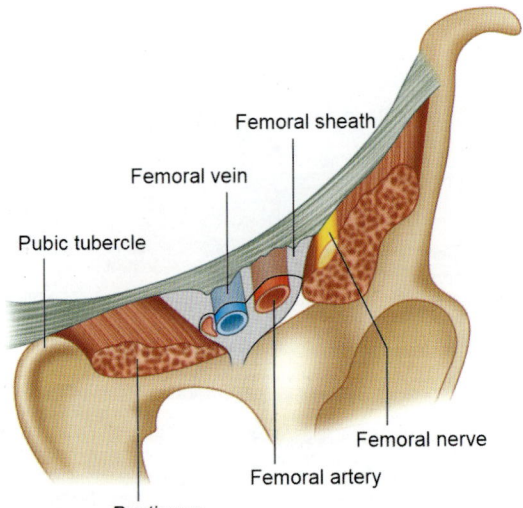

Pectineus
Dissection to show femoral sheath

- Split the femoral sheath medially and laterally to appreciate the fascial compartments within the sheath and its contents.
- Femoral canal is the medial compartment of the sheath and you will be able to enter the abdominal cavity through this canal. Appreciate the lacunar ligament medially inguinal ligament anteriorly, pectin pubis posteriorly at this juncture.
- Place a wooden block below the knee of the cadaver to flex the hip joint and relax the structures in the femoral region. Now, it becomes easy to separate the muscles in the femoral region by doing finger dissection.
- A prominent long muscle running diagonally in front of thigh is the sartorius. Locate a thick nerve, femoral nerve lateral to the femoral artery in a groove between psoas and iliacus muscles. The nerve has a short stem and it bifurcates into several cutaneous and muscular branches. The muscles medially are the adductor muscles.

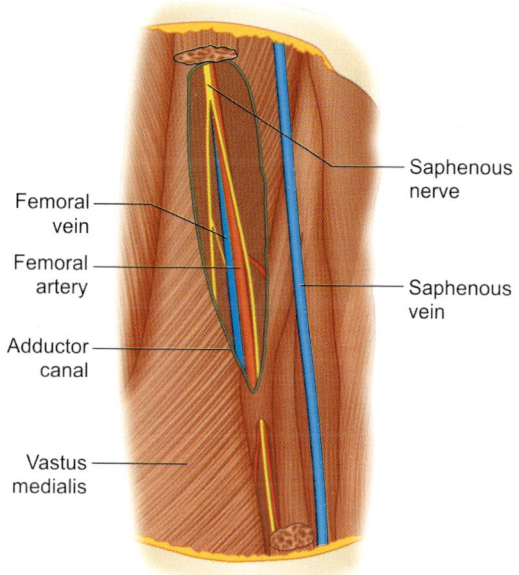

Femoral vein

Femoral artery

Adductor canal

Vastus medialis

Saphenous nerve

Saphenous vein

Adductor canal dissection

- Nerve to pectineus lies medially behind the femoral artery (develop a habit of not damaging the structures while dissecting, this will automatically enhance your operating skills).
- Appreciate the branches of femoral artery, the profunda femoris artery approximately 5 cm below inguinal ligament, on posterolateral surface of femoral artery. Trace the circumflex branches of the profunda femoris arteries.
- Strip the fascia from the anterior surface of iliacus and psoas major and follow the tendon of psoas and press it hard against the bone, the elevation your finger feels on the bone is the lesser trochanter.

### Adductor Canal

- Expose the sartorius medially onto the tibia, make a vertical incision on the deep fascia from the tubercle of iliac crest to lateral margin of patella. Now you can easily separate the four muscles-vastus medialis, rectus femoris, vastus intermedius and vastus lateralis. All these muscles are lateral to sartorius.
- Trace lateral circumflex femoral artery behind sartorius and rectus femoris.

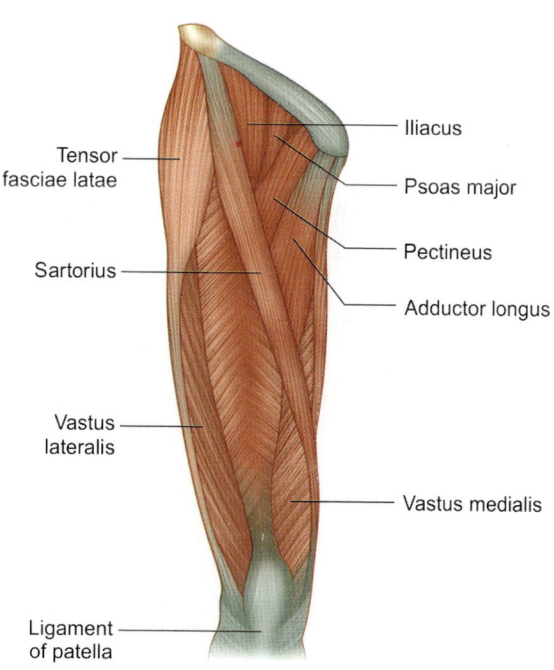

Tensor fasciae latae

Sartorius

Vastus lateralis

Ligament of patella

Iliacus

Psoas major

Pectineus

Adductor longus

Vastus medialis

Front of thigh dissection

- Lift the middle third of sartorius laterally, and you will appreciate the roof of adductor canal between vastus medialis and adductor muscles. Cut through this fascia to study the contents of adductor canal, i.e. femoral vessels, saphenous nerve and nerve to vastus medialis.
- If you remove the vastus lateralis you will appreciate the lateral intermuscular septum.
- Appreciate attachments and nerve supply of all the floor muscles of femoral triangle. Divide the adductor longus 2–3 cm below its origin. Turn the muscle laterally, identify the anterior branch of obturator nerve which supplies adductor longus and gracilis. Study pectineus muscle and try to identify its nerve supply. Also cut the adductor brevis close to its attachment and identify the nerve, anterior branch of obturator nerve. Define the adductor magnus attachments.
- Locate the adductor magnus opening medially and the passage of femoral vessels to and from femoral triangle and adductor canal.

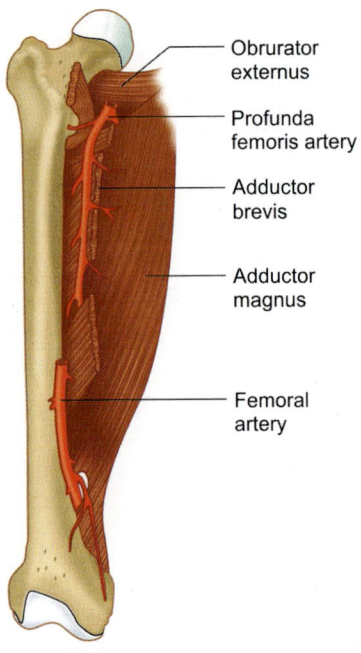

Profunda femoris branches

## c. Vivisection

- As an intern, you will be asked to withdraw arterial blood from femoral artery in comatosed patient, that time you should be able to locate femoral artery, which is lateral to vein in femoral region, and is below mid-inguinal point. Feel for the pulsations and withdraw the blood.
- While operating in this area beware about the relations, i.e. femoral artery is lateral to femoral vein, and femoral nerve is lateral to artery. These are major vessels, a direct continuation of external iliac artery. Any traumatic cut or involvement of the artery due to severe infection will lead to torrential bleeding.
- Variations in the course of arteries is a rule and not an exception. So, while operating for femoral hernia in femoral canal, surgeon has to be aware of the presence of abnormal obturator artery while incising the lacunar ligament.

## d. Viva Questions

- *Femoral triangle: Boundaries*: Laterally sartorius, medially adductor longus, base inguinal ligament, floor formed by iliacus, tendon of psoas major, pectineus adductor longus, femoral artery, femoral vein, femoral nerve are its contents.
- *Femoral sheath:* Covers the upper 1 and 1/2 inch of femoral vessels, anterior wall-formed by fascia transversalis, posterior wall by fascia iliaca. Femoral branch of genitofemoral nerve lies on the anterior wall of the sheath.
- Femoral ring is upper end of femoral canal.
- Femoral canal contains deep inguinal lymph node of Cloquet or Rosenmuller. This node drains the glans in males and clitoris in females.
- Mid-inguinal point lies mid-way between anterior superior iliac spine and pubic symphysis. Femoral artery and head of femur lie beneath it.

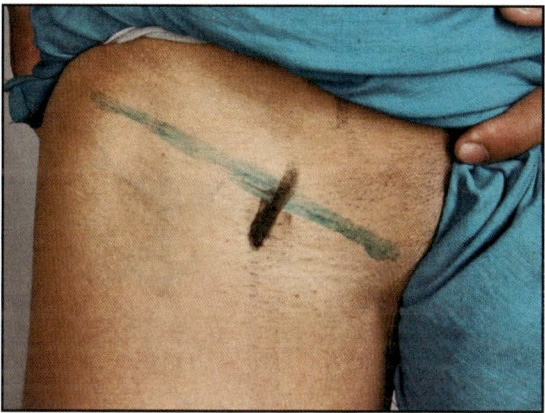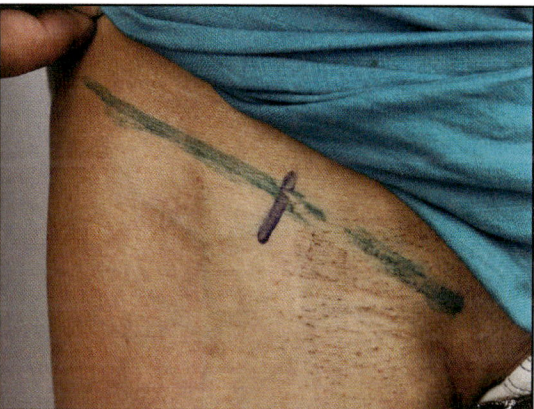

- Mid-point of inguinal ligament is mid-point between anterior superior iliac spine and pubic tubercle.
- Iliotibial tract is a thick band of fascia running vertically on lateral side of thigh. Tensor fascia latae is a thick short muscle in the upper part of the thigh.
- Pectineus is a hybrid muscle supplied by obturator and femoral nerve.

## 2. FRONT OF THE LEG

### a. Incision Markings

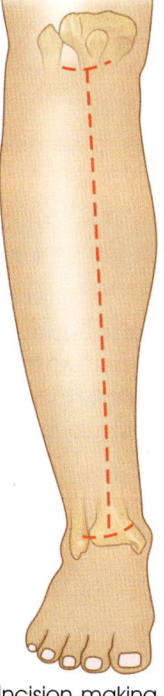

Incision making

## b. Structures to be Identified

### Superficial Plane

- Place a wooden block under the knee and plantar flex the foot.
- Reflect the skin without damaging the superficial fascia, since you have to identify great saphenous vein medially, saphenous nerve along with vein. At this juncture study the course of great saphenous vein; it lies transversely across the metatarsals. Dorsal venous arch laterally continues as small saphenous vein. If you trace the vein till lateral malleolus, you will find a nerve that is named as sural nerve. Superficial peroneal nerve lies on the middle third of leg, laterally.

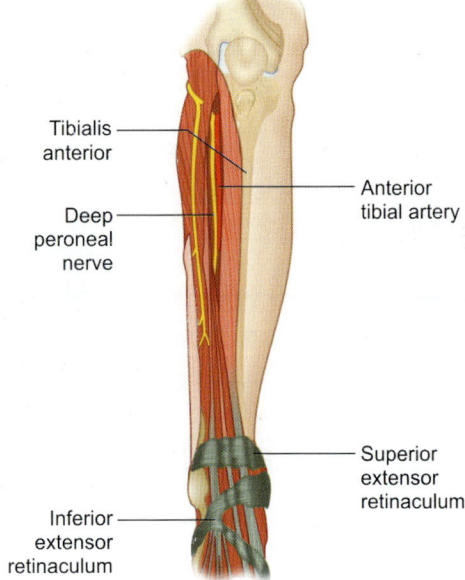

Superficial plane front of leg dissection

### Deep Plane

- Now remove the superficial fascia and cut the deep fascia in front of leg in between tibia and fibula. Do not incise the extensor retinaculum. Pass a blunt probe under the retinaculum and separate the extensor tendons.
- Just next to the shin from medial to lateral side is tibialis anterior, extensor hallucis longus extensor digitorum longus, peroneus tertius peroneus brevis and peroneus longus. Trace the tendons above and below and study their attachments. Dissect the tibialis anterior muscle from other extensor muscles.
- After separating the extensor muscles you will see a glistening interosseous membrane on which lies the anterior tibial vessels and deep peroneal nerve, trace this neurovascular bundle.
- Reflect the peroneus tertius muscle laterally and identify the perforating branch of peroneal artery on the lower. Part of interosseous membrane.

### c. Vivisection

While operating in this area the surgeon should be aware that the anterior border of tibia is subcutaneous, the neurovascular bundle is very deep on the interosseous membrane.

### d. Viva Questions

- You should be able to identify tibialis anterior muscle and define its attachments. It arises from the upper

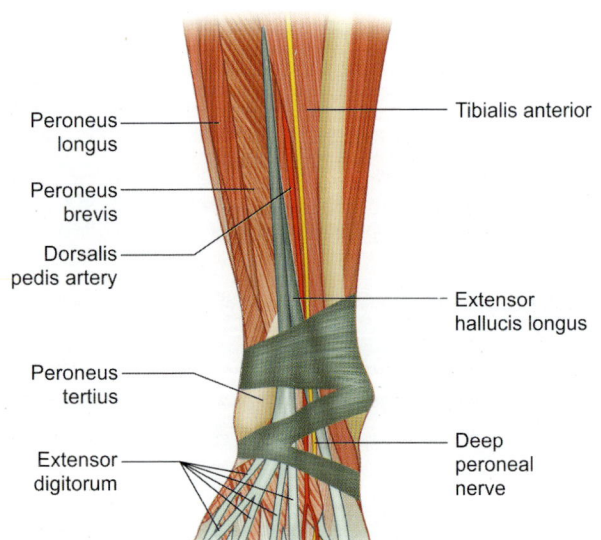

Front of leg dissection

half of lateral surface of tibia and from interosseous membrane and gets attached to medial cuneiform. Supplied by deep peroneal nerve and is dorsiflexor and powerful inverter of foot.

- The neurovascular bundle on the interosseous membrane is deep peroneal nerve and anterior tibial artery.

## 3. DORSUM OF FOOT

### a. Incision Markings

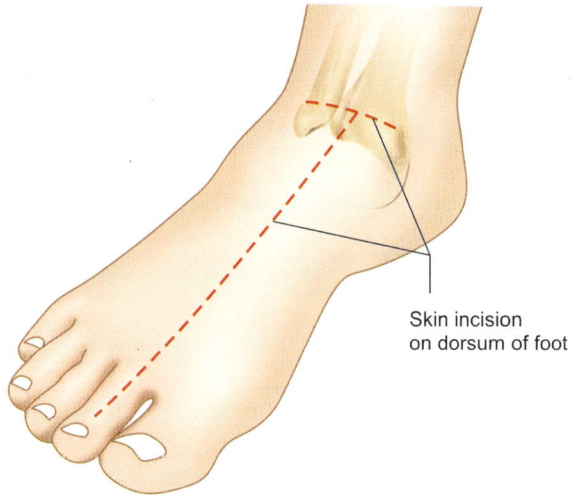

Skin incision on dorsum of foot

Skin incisions on dorsum of foot

### b. Structures to be Identified

*Superficial Plane*

- Reflect the skin and trace the superficial peroneal nerve and its branches, appreciate that the medial branch is medial to the big toe not advancing to the first interdigital cleft. Find the other dorsal digital nerves along the sides of the toes, all these nerves arise from the deep peroneal nerve.
- Appreciate the dorsal venous arch against the metatarsal heads, the medial end of the arch continues as the great saphenous vein and lateral end continues as the short saphenous vein.

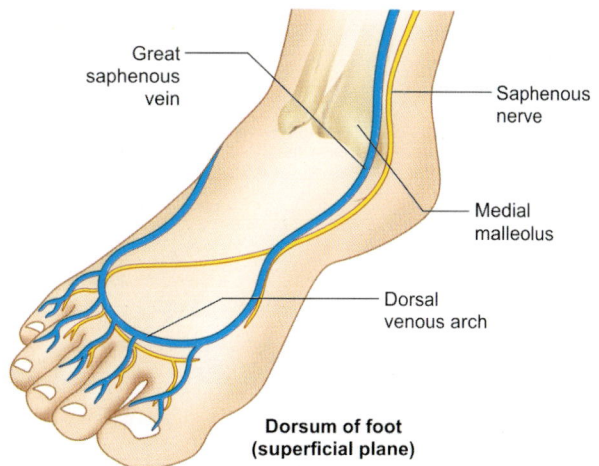

Great saphenous vein

Saphenous nerve

Medial malleolus

Dorsal venous arch

Dorsum of foot
(superficial plane)

*Deep Plane*

- Divide the extensor retinaculum and separate the tendons from medial to lateral side namely—extensor hallucis longus, extensor hallucis brevis, extensor digitorum longus and brevis, peroneus tertius.

- The anterior tibial artery continues on dorsum of foot, now named dorsalis pedis artery.

### c. Vivisection

Beware of the dorsalis pedis artery in this area.

### d. Viva Questions

- Drop-foot is due to the injury to the deep peroneal branch, this nerve supplies all the muscles on the anterior compartment of the leg. Thus, the victim affected cannot dorsiflex the ankle, cannot extend the metatarso-phalangeal joint and also the inversion is weakened.
- Dorsalis pedis artery pulsations can be felt in living person on the dorsum of the foot just lateral to extensor hallucis tendon.
- Great saphenous vein starts from the medial end of dorsal venous arch ascends upwards in front of medial malleolus then on front of leg. For a short distance lies behind the knee then again comes in front of thigh medially to end in femoral vein, the saphenous nerve lies close to great saphenous vein.

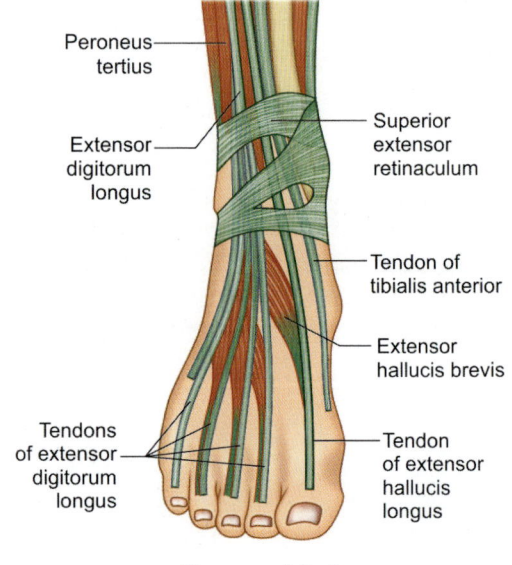

Dorsum of foot

## 4. GLUTEAL REGION

### a. Incision Markings

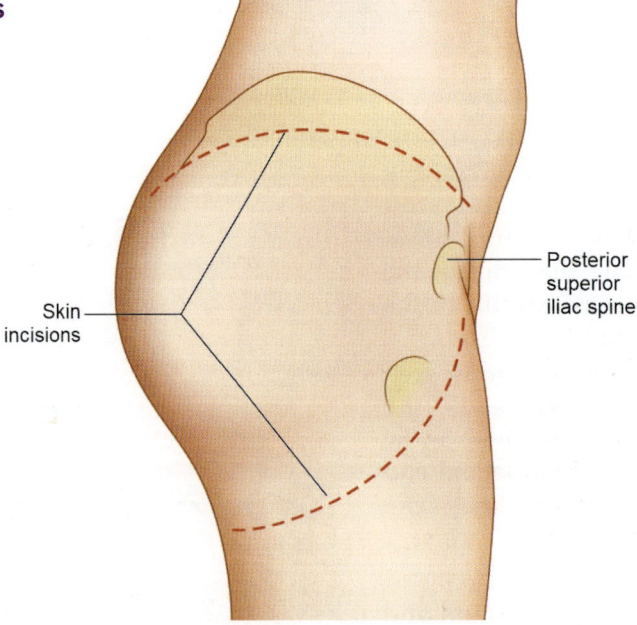

Skin incisions in gluteal region

## b. Structures to be Identified

- While reflecting the skin of gluteal region you will find several cutaneous nerves present haphazard, these are branches of lumbar plexus.
- Bulk muscle of the gluteal region is, gluteus maximus. At its lower border you may be able to locate a branch of posterior cutaneous nerve of thigh. Now remove the deep fascia over the gluteus maximus, and study the attachments of the muscle.
- The next step is to see the structures under the cover of gluteus maximus, for this you need to cut the muscle, but remember the superior and inferior gluteal vessels, and inferior gluteal nerve lie closely pasted to the undersurface of gluteus maximus muscle. So, insert two fingers below the gluteus maximus and then cut the muscle 2–3 cm medial to the femoral insertion and then reflect the muscle from the sacrotuberous ligament.
- Study the structures under the cover of gluteus maximus (commonly asked in exams).
- A prominent, very thick nerve will catch your attention first in this region this is the sciatic nerve. If you trace the nerve upwards you will reach at the lower border of piriformis muscle and downwards up to group of muscles known as hamstrings (= back of thigh muscles). The nerve gives muscular branches to the hamstrings and the vessels accompanying these branches are the branches of medial circumflex femoral vessels.
- Try to palpate ischial spine medial to sciatic nerve and feel the firm resistance offered by the sacrospinous ligament. Find the nerve to obturator internus, internal pudendal vessels and pudendal nerve medial to spine.
- Fan-like muscles encountered are tendon of obturator internus and gamelli. Separate the muscles by doing blunt dissection.
- You will see a horizontal muscle passing from the ischial tuberosity to back of femur, this is the quadratus femoris muscle. Below this is posterior surface of adductor magnus muscle.

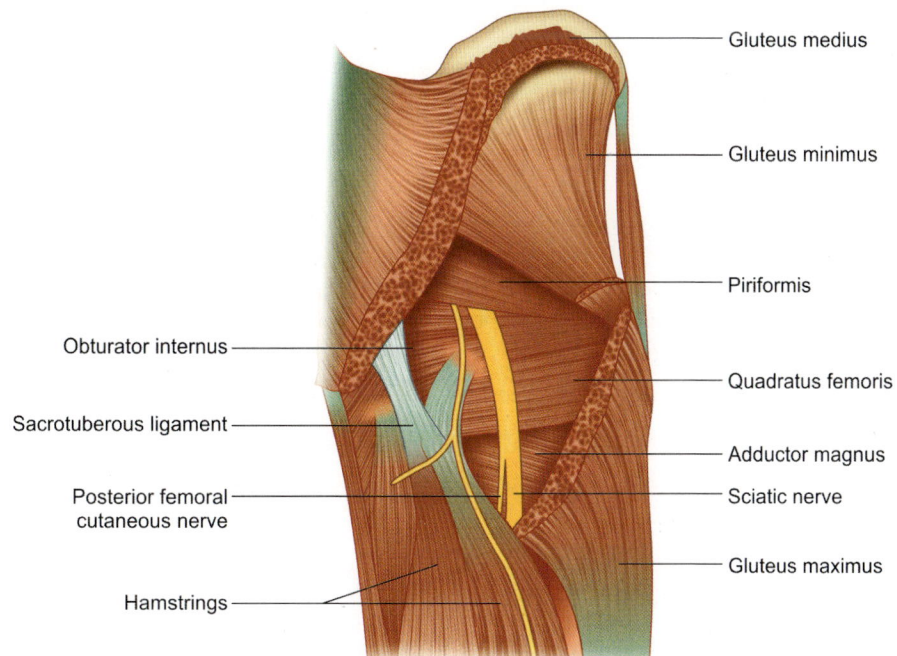

Structures under the cover of gluteus maximus muscle

- You will find branches of medial circumflex femoral vessels above and below quadratus femoris muscle. Identify the nerve to quadratus femoris and by finger dissection separate the muscle from adductor magnus.

### c. Vivisection

- Intramuscular (IM) injections are given in the upper outer quadrant to avoid injury to the neurovascular bundle since this lies in the lower part of the gluteal region. An imaginary line from greater trochanter to posterior superior iliac spine. Area above this line is safe for IM injections.
- Hip replacement is a very common surgical procedure. Approaching hip joint from behind, (posterior approach, Moore or Southern) provides access to the acetabulum and proximal femur for total hip replacement.
- During surgery, while incising the gluteus maximus, surgeon needs to remember the inferior gluteal nerve supplying it and muscle splitting to be stopped once he encounters the first branch of the nerve. Superior gluteal artery supplies the upper part of the muscle while the inferior gluteal artery supplies distal 2/3 rd of muscle.
  - Sciatic nerve can be identified on the posterior surface of quadratus femoris and injury to the nerve can be avoided by extending the hip and flexing knee.
  - Avoid injury to inferior gluteal artery. It leaves the pelvis just below the piriformis.
  - First perforating branch of profunda femoris may get cut during splitting of gluteus maximus insertion.
  - Surgeon needs to remember that superior gluteal artery and nerve leaves the pelvis above the piriformis and enters the deep surface of gluteus medius.
  - Do not retract quadratus femoris vigorously to avoid damage to medial circumflex artery.

### d. Viva Questions

- Identify the muscle, piriformis below which is the thick nerve sciatic nerve.
- You should be able to identify nerve to obturator internus, internal pudendal vessels, and pudendal nerve medial to the upper part of sciatic nerve. These are the PIN structures, i.e. pudendal nerve, internal pudendal vessels, nerve to obturator internus.
- As the sciatic nerve runs downwards it lies typically on 3 horizontally placed muscles namely, superior and inferior gamelli and obturator internus.

### 5. BACK OF THE THIGH

### a. Incision Markings

### b. Structures to be Identified

- After making a vertical incision on back of skin, reflect the skin and superficial fascia from deep fascia by identifying the plane and passing a finger below the superficial fascia. In the superficial plane look for the branches of posterior

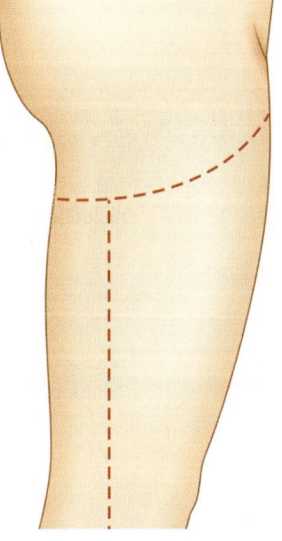

Skin incisions on back of thigh

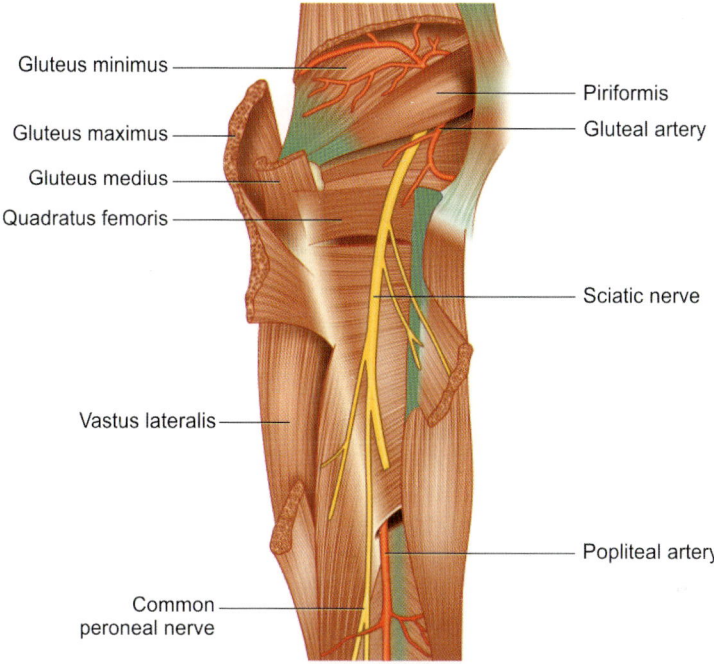

Gluteus minimus

Piriformis

Gluteus maximus

Gluteal artery

Gluteus medius

Quadratus femoris

Sciatic nerve

Vastus lateralis

Popliteal artery

Common
peroneal nerve

Dissected gluteal region and back of thigh

cutaneous nerve of the thigh. Also trace the branches of medial anterior and lateral cutaneous branches of the thigh.

- Divide the deep fascia on the hamstring muscles namely—biceps femoris, semitendinosus, semimembranosus (back of the thigh = Ham, tendons of these muscles= hamstrings) separate the hamstring muscles, trace to their attachments. Identify the muscular branches supplying the hamstrings.
- Cut the hamstrings from the ischial tuberosity this will expose the adductor magnus muscle and short head of biceps.
- Appreciate the division of sciatic nerve into tibial and common peroneal. The site of division may be variable, either back of thigh or back of knee.
- Locate the opening in adductor magnus muscle, and the passage of femoral vessels which go through the opening and later same vessels named popliteal vessels.

## c. Vivisection

Surgeon needs to be aware of the deeply placed popliteal vessels and the sciatic nerve and its division into tibial and common peroneal nerve on back of thigh when operating in this region.

## d. Viva Questions

- Student should be able to identify sciatic nerve, tibial and common peroneal nerve
- You should be able to identify the adductor magnus opening and passage of femoral vessels through it.

## 6. BACK OF KNEE (POPLITEAL FOSSA)

- *Incision markings*

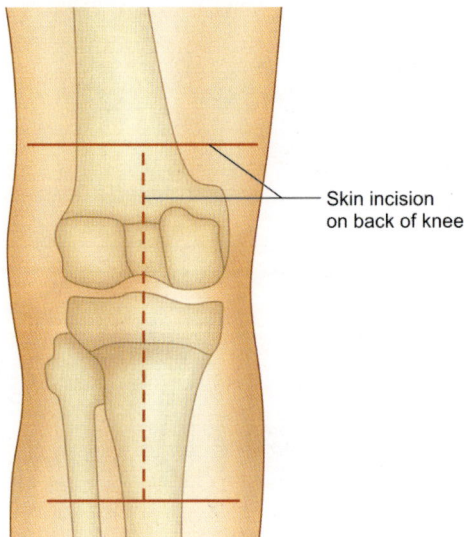

Skin incision on back of knee

### a. Structures to be Identified

- Reflect the skin flaps and try to identify the branches of posterior cutaneous nerve of the thigh, and peroneal communicating nerve. Small saphenous vein and sural nerve should be located in superficial plane
- Divide the fascia over the biceps femoris and expose the muscle, which forms the supero-lateral border of fossa

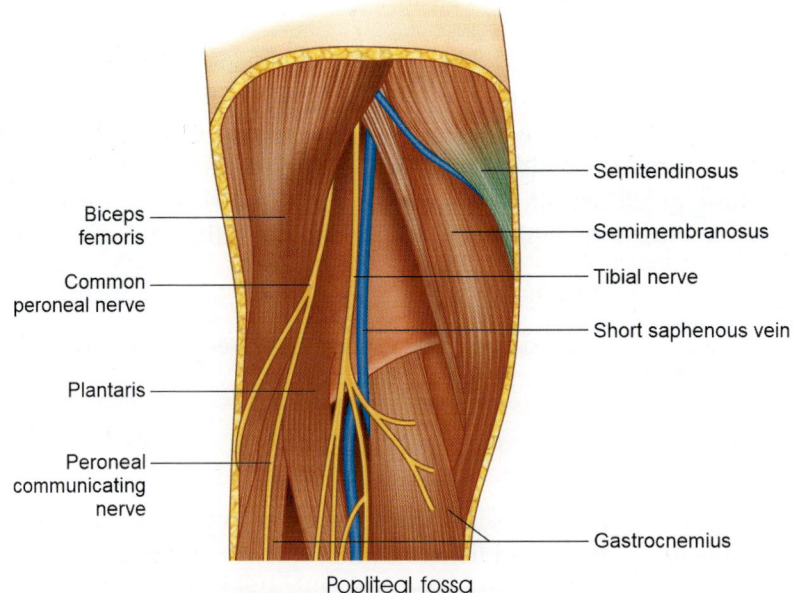

Biceps femoris

Common peroneal nerve

Plantaris

Peroneal communicating nerve

Semitendinosus

Semimembranosus

Tibial nerve

Short saphenous vein

Gastrocnemius

Popliteal fossa

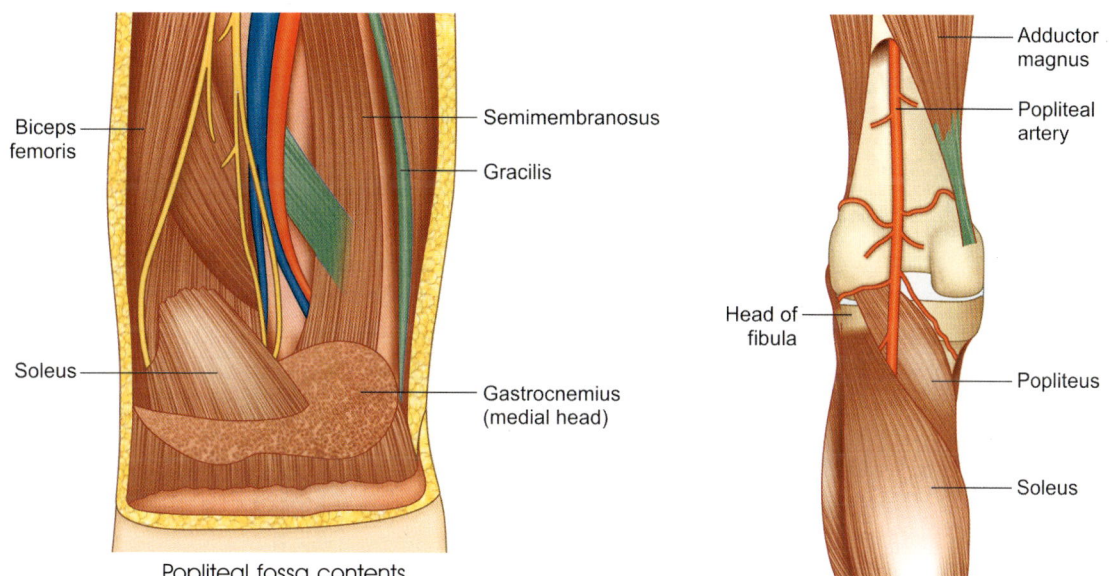

Popliteal fossa contents

Popliteal artery in popliteal fossa (deepest plane)

- Similarly divide the fascia over the semitendinosus, and semimembranosus. This forms the superomedial boundary of the fossa
- Lower boundaries are formed by lateral and medial head of gastrocnemius muscle. A thin shiny plantaris muscle may be present.
- Remove the fat from the fossa to identify the tibial nerve. Common peroneal nerve is just medial to the biceps femoris tendon. Behind the tibial nerve is the popliteal vein and deep to it is popliteal artery.
- If you remove all the structures in fossa leaving behind only the popliteal artery and its branches. Find a diagonally placed muscle closely pasted to the condyles of tibia and femur this is the unlocking muscle of knee, popliteus.

## b. Vivisection

In the posterior approach of knee joint, the same dissection is executed. This approach is used to repair neurovascular bundle in popliteal fossa. A curved S-shaped incision is taken on back of the knee. Appreciate the same structures, after reflecting the skin, small saphenous vein and sural nerve. Then the deep fascia is incised medial to the small saphenous vein. Muscles are retracted and popliteal artery is reached. Surgeon needs to remember that the artery has five branches around the knee, 2 superior, 2 inferior and 1 middle genicular artery.

## c. Viva Questions

- Boundaries of popliteal fossa—superolaterally-biceps femoris, superomedially semi-tendinosus, semimembranosus, inferomedially-medial head of gastrocnemius, and infero-laterally, lateral head of gastrocnemius. Contents—popliteal vessels and tibial nerve
- Popliteal artery lies in a very deep plane, against the bone with its genicular branches
- The sciatic nerve may divide in the popliteal fossa into tibial and common peroneal branch.

## 7. BACK OF LEG

### a. Incision Markings

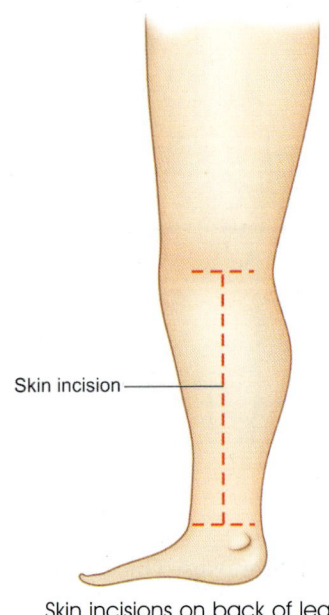

Skin incision

Skin incisions on back of leg

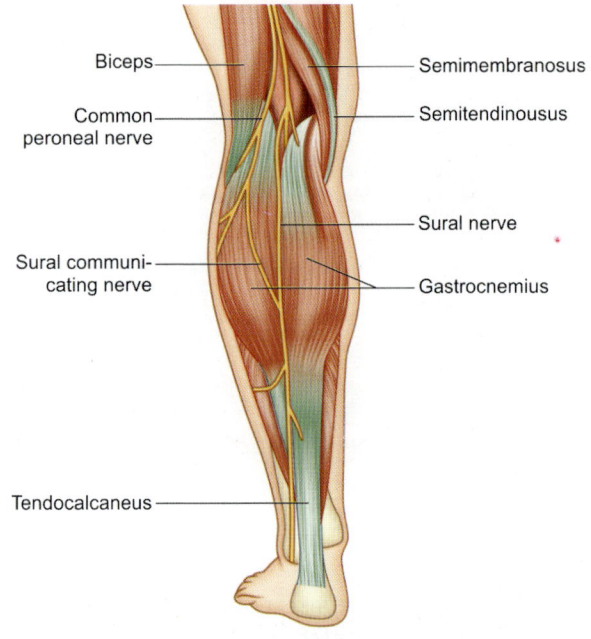

Biceps — Semimembranosus

Common peroneal nerve — Semitendinousus

Sural communicating nerve

Tendocalcaneus — Sural nerve

Gastrocnemius

Dissected back of leg-superficial plane

### b. Structures to be Identified

- After reflecting the skin, in the superficial plane try to identify the sural nerve, small saphenous vein, peroneal communicating nerve. Then divide the deep fascia on muscles.

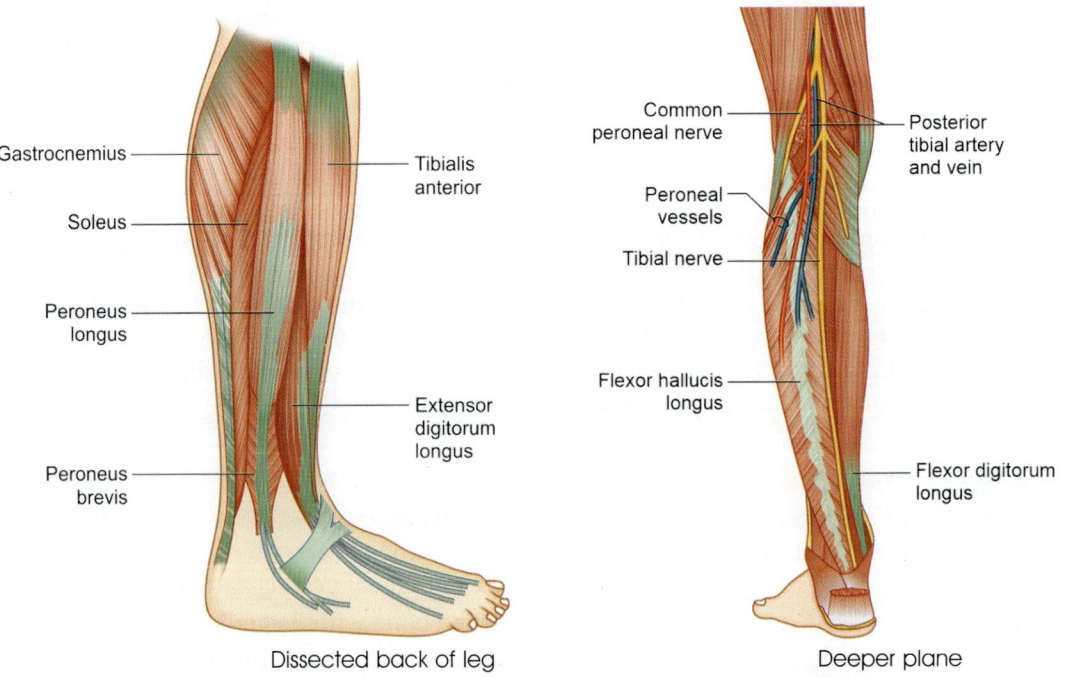

Gastrocnemius — Tibialis anterior

Soleus

Peroneus longus

Peroneus brevis — Extensor digitorum longus

Dissected back of leg

Common peroneal nerve — Posterior tibial artery and vein

Peroneal vessels

Tibial nerve

Flexor hallucis longus — Flexor digitorum longus

Deeper plane

- Muscles on the back of leg are arranged in three layers—superficial is formed by gastrocnemius soleus and plantaris (=Triceps surae) they form a powerful tendon, tendo Achilles near the heel.

  Middle layer is completely separate from superficial muscle layer, one can easily separate it by finger dissection. It consists of flexor hallucis longus and flexor digitorum longus.
- The deepest layer is tibialis posterior lying on interosseous membrane. The fascia covering the tibialis posterior is attached to soleal line above, medial crest on fibula and vertical ridge on tibia. Locate popliteus also.
- Neurovascular bundle on the back of leg is posterior tibial artery and tibial nerve. The popliteal artery divides at the lower border of popliteus into anterior and posterior tibial artery. The anterior tibial artery enters the anterior compartment through the interosseus membrane.

### c. Vivisection

While approaching the back of the leg the surgeon needs to remember the layered arrangement of muscles and the neurovascular bundle.

### d. Viva Questions

Student should be able to identify the popliteus muscle. Viva may proceed to locking and unlocking at this juncture.

Locking is medial rotation of femur on tibia, in terminal stages of extension. While unlocking is lateral rotation of femur on tibia. It is brought about by popliteus muscle.

## 8. MEDIAL SIDE OF THE LEG

### a. Incision Markings

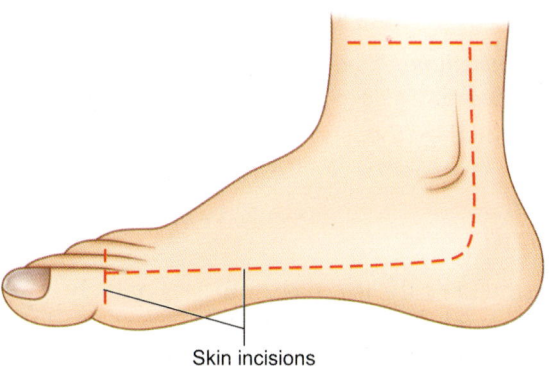

Skin incisions

Skin incisions to be taken on medial side of leg

### b. Structures to be Identified

- Muscle mass of flexor digitorum longus can be appreciated medially.
- In the lower part of medial surface of leg, is a modified band of deep fascia, i.e. flexor retinaculum. Study the structures under the cover of flexor retinaculum—tibialis posterior, flexor digitorum longus, posterior tibial artery, tibial nerve, flexor hallucis longus. Separate the structures.

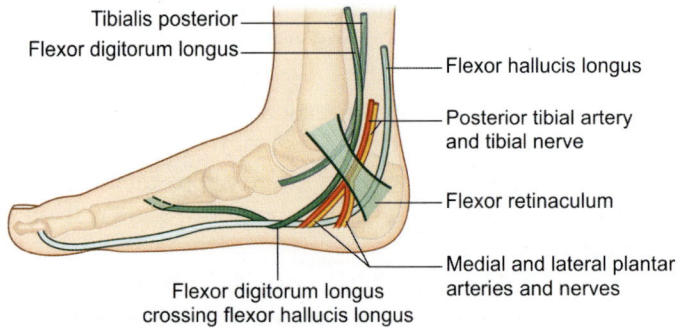

Structures under the cover of flexor retinaculum

## c. Vivisection

The neurovascular bundle in this region is the posterior tibial artery and tibial nerve. Any surgery in this region, surgeon needs to be vigilant about the neurovascular bundle.

## d. Viva Questions

- The structures under the cover of flexor retinaculum are (very commonly asked question):

  *Mnemonic*
  | | |
  |---|---|
  | Talented | Tibialis posterior |
  | Doctors | Flexor hallucis longus |
  | Are | Posterior tibial artery |
  | Never | Tibial nerve |
  | Hungry | Flexor hallucis longus |

- *Attachments of flexor retinaculum:* Anteriorly, medial malleolus of tibia and posteriorly to medial tubercle of calcaneum.
- Tendo Achilles is the formed by the gastrocnemius and soleus. It is the chief plantar flexor of the ankle.

## 9. PERONEAL COMPARTMENT

- It is the lateral compartment of the leg, has 2 muscles namely, peroneus longus and brevis bound in a common synovial sheath.
- Divide the fascia over the muscles and separate the tendons. Trace their attachments.
- You can identify the superior and inferior peroneal retinaculum binding the peroneal tendons.
- Peroneal muscles are evertors of foot, and plantar flexors of ankle joint.

## 10. SOLE OF FOOT

### a. Incision Markings

Skin incisions to be taken on sole of foot.

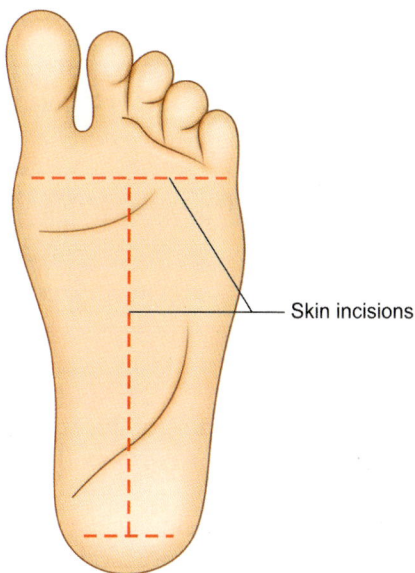

Skin incisions

## b. Structures to be Identified

After cutting longitudinally the skin from the heel to middle toe, reflect the skin and superficial fascia from the deep fascia with a help of knife (skin of sole is very thick).

- You will see that the superficial fascia is very thick and firmly bound to the deep fascia and has fat tightly packed.
- Appreciate the plantar aponeurosis, and the clefts at its distal end through which you will appreciate the plantar nerve and vessels.

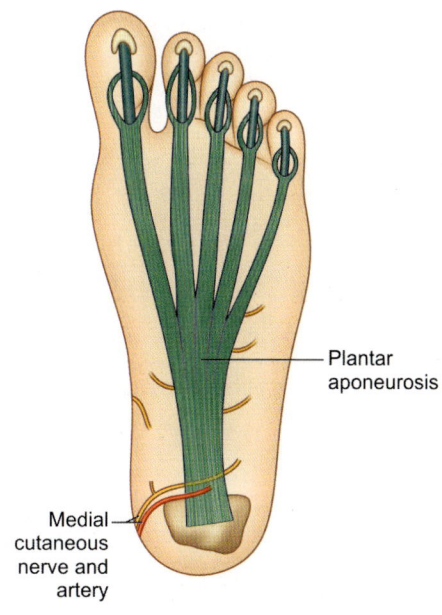

Plantar aponeurosis

Medial cutaneous nerve and artery

Sole of foot-superficial dissection

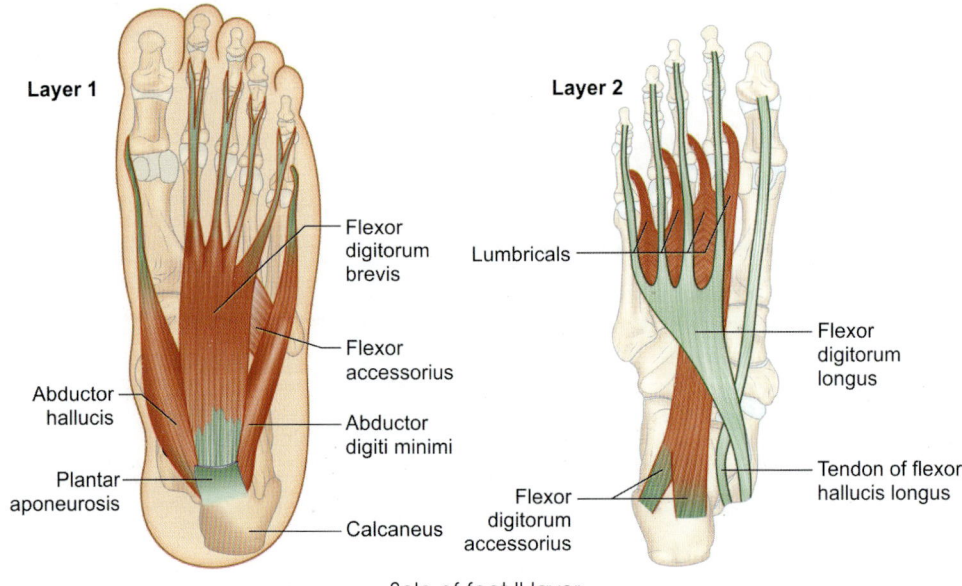

**Layer 1**

Flexor digitorum brevis

Abductor hallucis

Plantar aponeurosis

Flexor accessorius

Abductor digiti minimi

Flexor digitorum accessorius

Calcaneus

**Layer 2**

Lumbricals

Flexor digitorum longus

Tendon of flexor hallucis longus

Sole of foot II layer

• Cut the plantar aponeurosis 2 to 3 cm in front of the heel, and take vertical cut distally. Reflect the aponeurosis from the underlying muscle. Clear cut demarcation is not possible practically but from superficial to deep plane following layers are encountered:
   – *Layer I:* Abductor hallucis, flexor digitorum brevis, abductor digiti minimi.
   – *Layer II:* Flexor hallucis longus, flexor digitorum longus with flexor accessorius, lumbricals
   – *Layer III:* Flexor hallucis brevis, adductor hallucis, flexor digiti minimi brevis.
   – *Layer IV:* Dorsal and plantar interossei, tibialis posterior, peroneus longus.

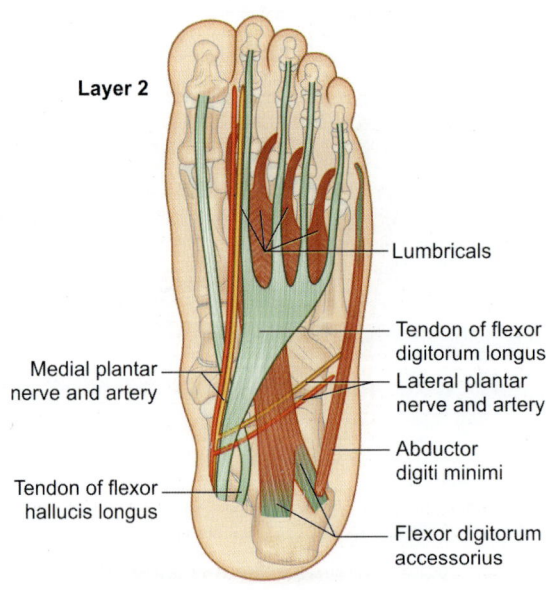

**Layer 2**

Lumbricals

Tendon of flexor digitorum longus

Medial plantar nerve and artery

Lateral plantar nerve and artery

Abductor digiti minimi

Tendon of flexor hallucis longus

Flexor digitorum accessorius

- Reflect layer by layer the muscles of the sole appreciate the nerves and vessels at each layer.

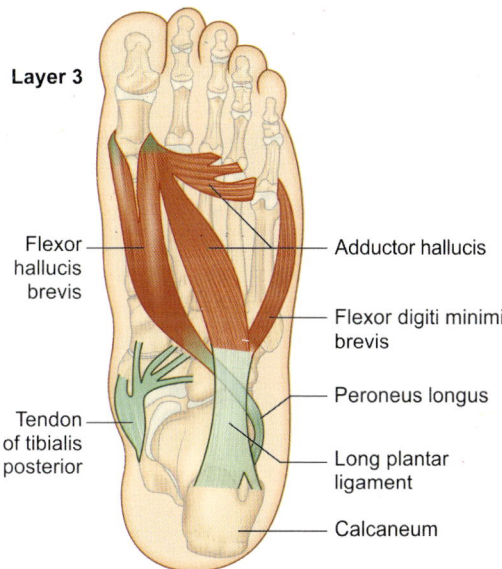

Layer 3

Flexor hallucis brevis — Adductor hallucis

Flexor digiti minimi brevis

Peroneus longus

Tendon of tibialis posterior — Long plantar ligament

Calcaneum

Deep dissection of sole

- Define the attachments of muscles of each layer.

### c. Vivisection

While operating the surgeon should know the layered arrangement of the sole and the plantar nerves and vessels.

### d. Viva Questions

- The students should know the layers of foot
- The viva may proceed to discuss arches of foot which is a very important long question (refer long questions section also).
  - Medial longitudinal arch
  - Lateral longitudinal arch
  - Transverse arch.

### Salient Points

- Phalanges do not participate in arch formation.
- Medial longitudinal arch-anterior end is formed by the of 3 metatarsal heads, and posterior end by medial tubercle of calcaneum, spring ligament (= plantar-calcaneonavicular) is a direct support to head of talus, tibialis posterior and flexor hallucis longus are the sling supports.
- Lateral longitudinal arch—anterior end is formed by the 4th and 5th metatarsal heads, posterior head by lateral tubercle of calcaneum, intersegmental tie is long plantar ligament, short plantar ligament, tie beams are lateral part of plantar aponeurosis, and lateral part of flexor digitorum brevis, slings are the peroneus tendons.

- Transverse arch—most of the tarsal and metatarsal bones help in the formation of this arch, intersegmental ties are the interossei, ligaments between the bones, tie beams are the adductor hallucis, and the sling support is provided by peroneus longus tendon.
- Exaggeration of longitudinal arches of the foot is known as pes cavus.
- Absence of arches causes flat foot, pes planus.
- Club foot is a common deformity in newborns wherein forefoot is adducted, inverted and plantar flexed.
- Inversion and eversion occurs at subtalar joints.

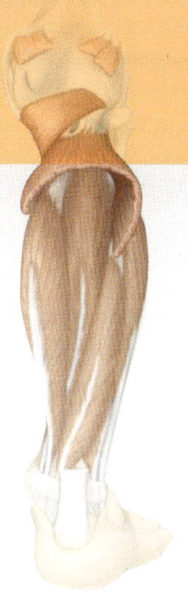

# Osteology 15

## 1. HIP BONE OR INNOMINATE BONE

It is a large, irregular bone and has three parts—ilium, ischium and pubis.

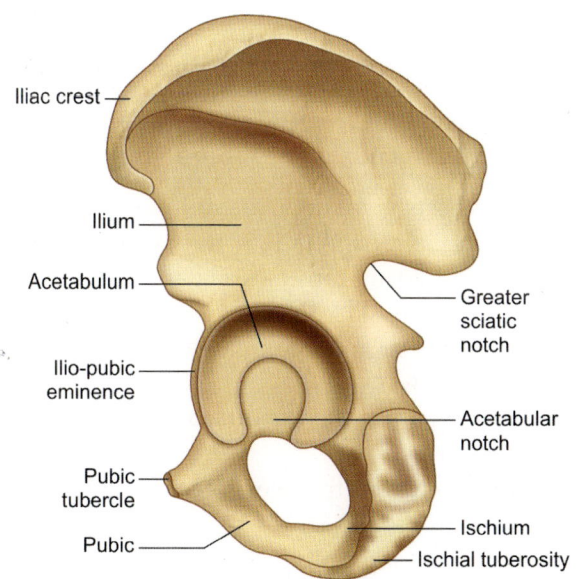

Iliac crest

Ilium

Acetabulum

Ilio-pubic eminence

Pubic tubercle

Pubic

Greater sciatic notch

Acetabular notch

Ischium

Ischial tuberosity

Hip bone (inner side, outer side)

### Side Determination

- Lateral surface has the prominent deep cup-shaped acetabulum
- Anteroinferior to the acetabulum is the obturator foramen
- Ischium is part of lower acetabulum and lies posteroinferior
- Pubis is anterior acetabulum

- Greater sciatic notch is posterior
- Auricular surface is the prominent feature of medial surface of ilium.

## Attachments

- Anterior superior iliac spine gives attachment to the lateral end of inguinal ligament
- Anterior inferior iliac spine gives attachment to rectus femoris, and iliofemoral ligament
- Iliac fossa provides attachment to iliacus

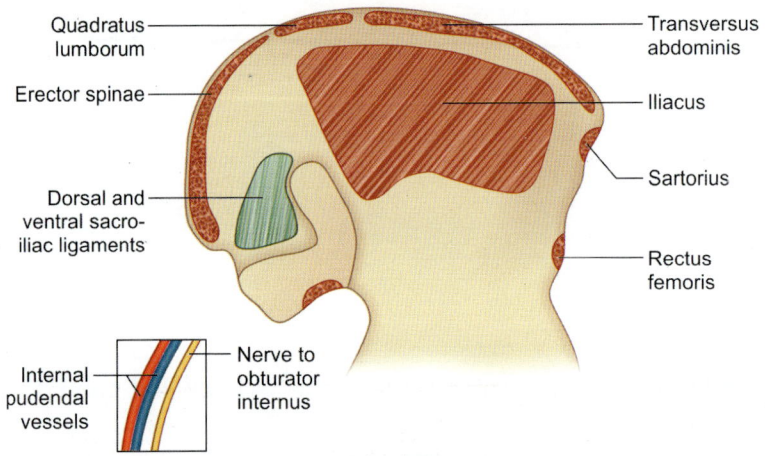

Inner surface of ilium and iliac crest. PIN structures related to ischial spine

- Outer surface of ilium gives attachment to all glutei muscles
- Iliac tuberosity gives attachment to dorsal sacroiliac ligament
- Auricular and preauricular sulcus gives attachment to ventral sacroiliac ligament
- Ischial tuberosity, upper area superolateral part for semimembranosus and inferomedial for biceps femoris and semitendinosus, lower area lateral part gives attachment to adductor magnus, while medial area is covered by fat
- Ischial spine gives attachment to sacrospinous ligament and is crossed by internal pudendal vessels and nerve to obturator internus
- Iliac crest ventral segment outer surface gives attachment iliotibial tract, fascia lata, tensor fascia lata, external oblique fibres
- Inner lip of iliac crest ventral segment transversus abdominis, behind lumbodorsal fascia and quadratus lumborum is attached
- Intermediate area gives attachment to internal oblique.

## Salient Features of Female Iliac Bone

- Preauricular sulcus is more prominent in females
- Obturator foramen is small and triangular in females
- Iliac fossa is deeper in females
- Greater sciatic notch is wider in females
- Ischiopubic rami is not everted in females.

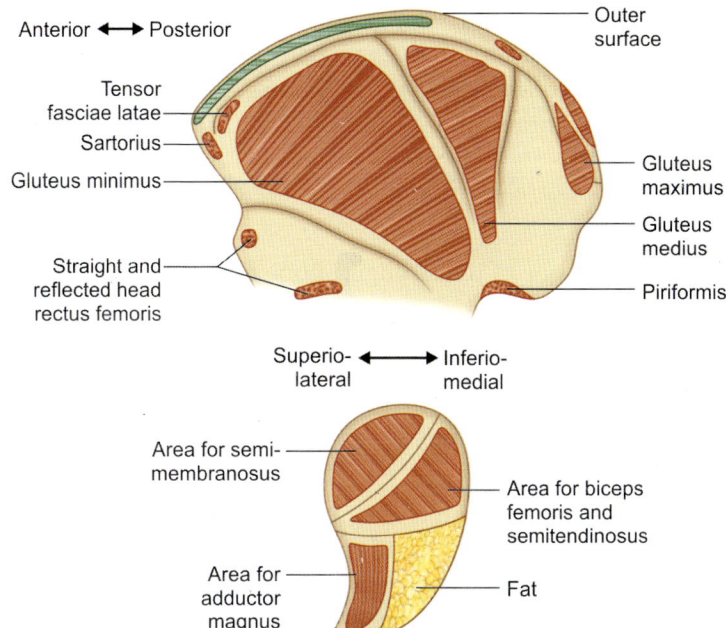

Iliac crest attachments outer surface. Ischial tuberosity attachments

## Ossification

- Three primary centres for ilium, ischium and pubis, for ilium it appears around 8th week of IUL, ischium in its 16 weeks of IUL, and then for pubis around 16 to 20 weeks.
- At the time of birth more than 2/3rd bone is cartilaginous (as shown in figure)

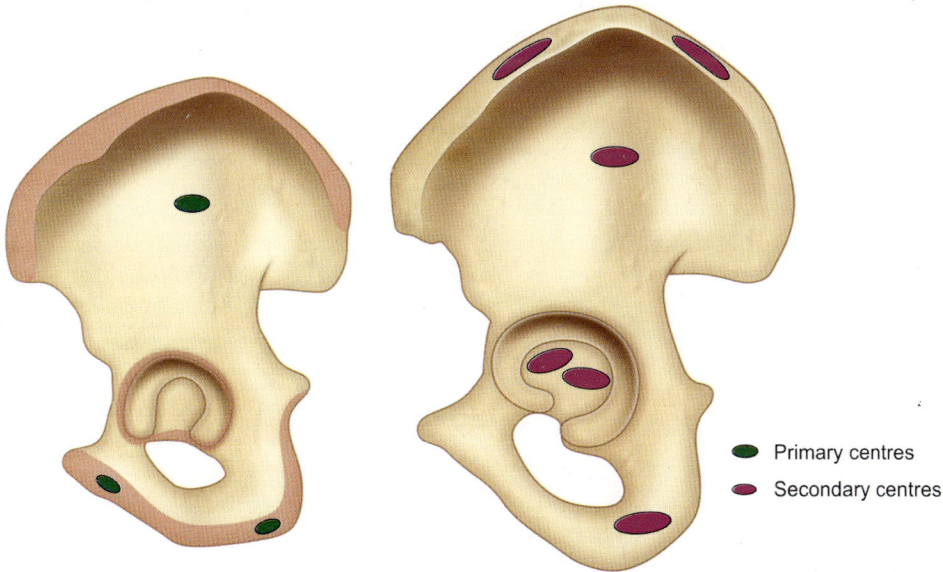

Diagram showing primary centres and secondary centres of hip bone

- Secondary centres are 2 for iliac crest, 2 for acetabular cartilage, 1 for ilium and ischium. All appear around puberty and fuse by 15 to 25 years
- Ischiopubic rami ossifying centres fuse by 7 to 8 years
- There could be additional centres for anterior superior iliac spine, pubic tubercle, crest and symphyseal surface.

## 2. FEMUR

It is a long bone of thigh, and one of the strongest bone in the body.

### Side Determination

- Head of the femur is anteromedially
- Lower end is expanded into condyles
- Medial condyle is more prominent
- Lateral condyle is in line with the shaft
- Anterior surface of the shaft is smooth and convex
- Posterior surface of the shaft is concave and rough

  Suspend the bone on index finger, and the inclination the bone takes automatically is the anatomical position of the bone.

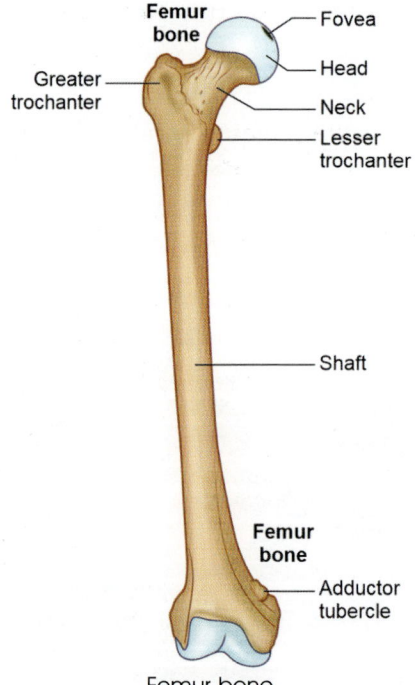

Femur bone

### Attachments

*Greater Trochanter*

- Glutei and vasti muscles are attached. On the greater trochanter (as shown in the figure)
- Trochanteric fossa receives insertion. Of obturator internus and the 2 Gamelli.

### Lesser Trochanter
- Psoas major is attached to its apex. Anteromedial surface
- Base has iliacus

### Quadrate Tubercle
Quadratus femoris

### Gluteal Tuberosity (3rd trochanter)
- Gluteus maximus
- Adductor magnus

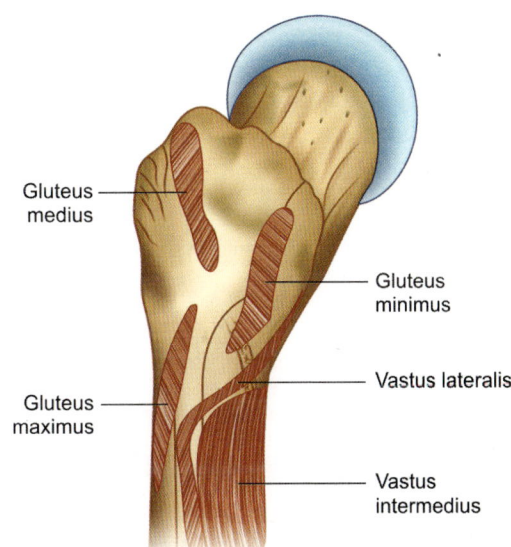

Greater trochanter attachments

### Linea Aspera
- Adductor longus
- Short-head of biceps femoris
- Intermuscular septa
- Vastus medialis
- Adductor magnus
- Vastus lateralis
- Pectineus.

### Lateral Condyle
- Lateral head of gastrocnemius
- Popliteus
- Fibular collateral ligament.

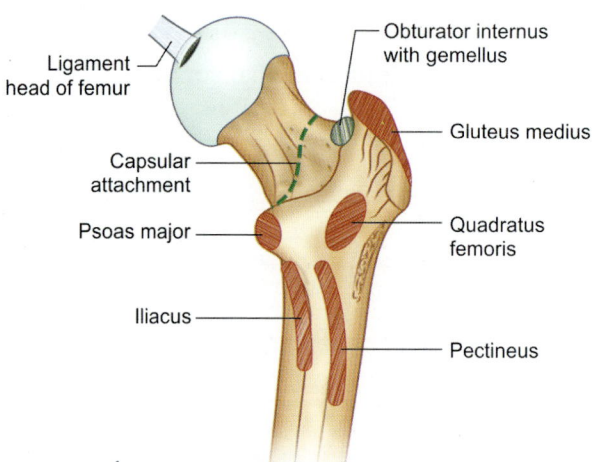

Ligament head of femur

Obturator internus with gemellus

Gluteus medius

Capsular attachment

Psoas major

Quadratus femoris

Iliacus

Pectineus

Upper end of femur—muscle attachments

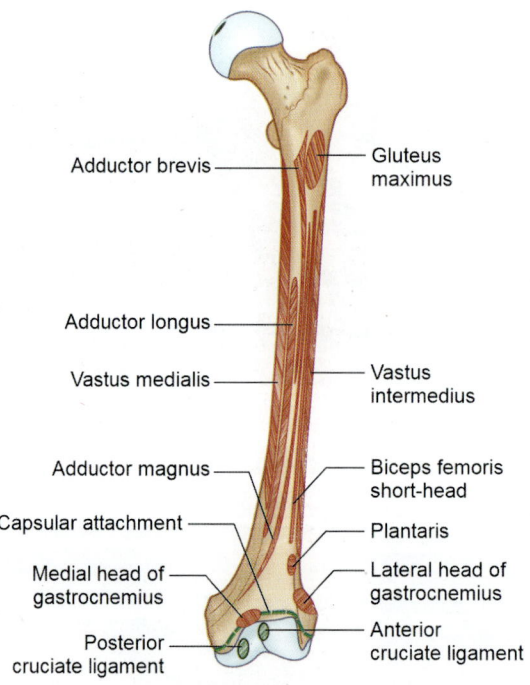

Adductor brevis

Gluteus maximus

Adductor longus

Vastus medialis

Vastus intermedius

Adductor magnus

Biceps femoris short-head

Capsular attachment

Plantaris

Medial head of gastrocnemius

Lateral head of gastrocnemius

Posterior cruciate ligament

Anterior cruciate ligament

Linea aspera attachments

### Medial Condyle

- Medial head of gastrocnemius
- Medial supracondylar line receives adductor magnus fibres. These fibres also extend to adductor tubercle.

### Intercondylar Fossa

Cruciate ligaments

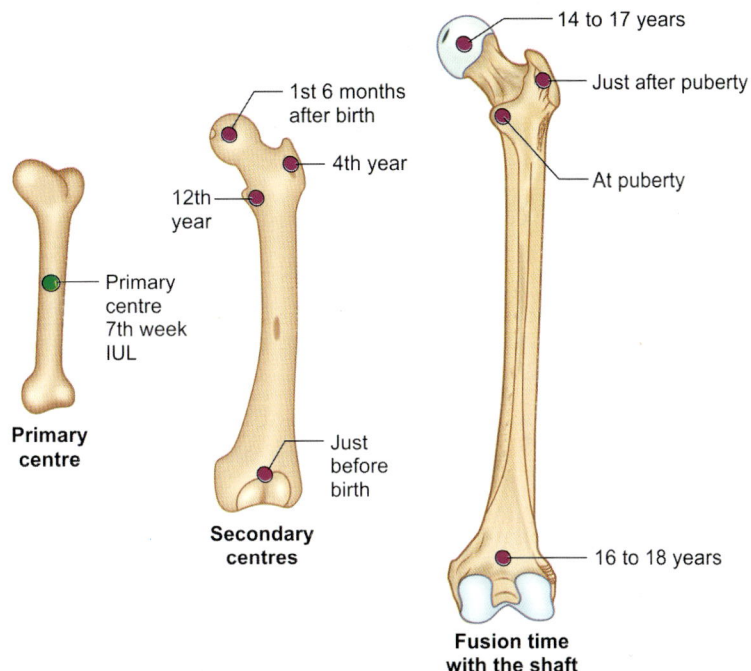

Primary and secondary centres of ossification of femur

## Ossification

- One primary centre for shaft at around 7th week of IUL
- Secondary centre for distal end during 9th month, i.e. just before birth, in the head during first 6 months following birth, greater trochanter at 4th year, lesser trochanter at around 12th and 14th year.
- Lesser trochanter fuses with rest of the bone around puberty, just followed by fusion of greater trochanter, head fuses by 14 to 17 year and lower end fuses with shaft by 16 to 18 years.

## 3. PATELLA

It is the largest sesamoid bone, developed in the tendon of quadriceps femoris, located in front of knee joint and triangular in shape.

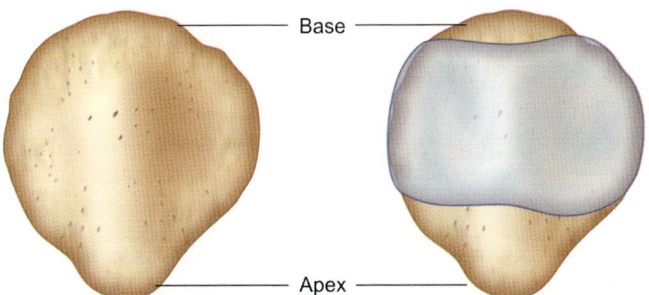

Patella—anterior surface (rough) and posterior surface (smooth)

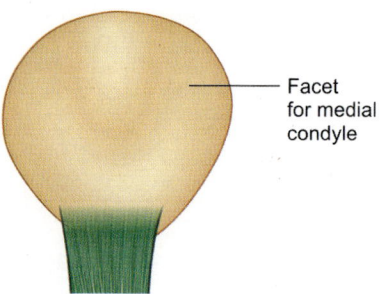

Facet for medial condyle

## Side Determination

- Anterior surface is rough and perforated (for nutrient vessels)
- Posterior surface is smooth, having a faint ridge vertically dividing the surface into lateral and medial facets
- Apex is directed downwards.

## Attachments

- Base posteriorly gives attachment to rectus femoris and vastus intermedius
- Medial and lateral border to vastus medialis and lateralis respectively, extending below as the medial and lateral retinaculi
- Anterior surface and apex is covered by quadriceps tendon which lower down, at the apex gets attached in the form of patellar ligament.

## Ossification

Many secondary centres appear during 3rd to 6th years.

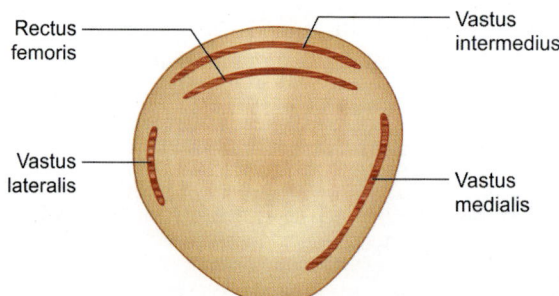

Anterior surface of patella attachments. Muscular attachments

## 4. TIBIA

It is the long bone of the leg placed medially.

## Side Determination

- Upper end of the bone is expanded having the fitting condyles to the femur
- Lower end has a prominence medially known as the medial malleolus
- The most upper part of the shaft has an elevation in front known as the tibial tuberosity.

## Attachments

- Tibial tuberosity: Ligamentum patellae
- Medial upper surface of the shaft in front
  - Sartorius
  - Gracilis
  - Semitendinosus
  - Semimembranosus very few fibres in front
  - Tibial collateral ligament
- Lateral upper surface of the shaft in front
  - Ilio-tibial tract
- Anterior surface of the shaft: Tibialis anterior
- Upper area medially but on posterior aspect: Semimembranosus
- Posterior surface of the shaft
  - Popliteus
  - Soleus
  - Flexor digitorum longus
  - Tibialis posterior

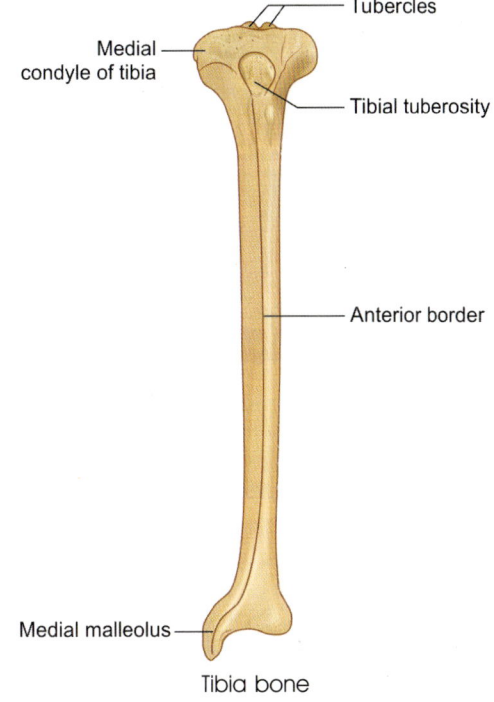

Tibia bone

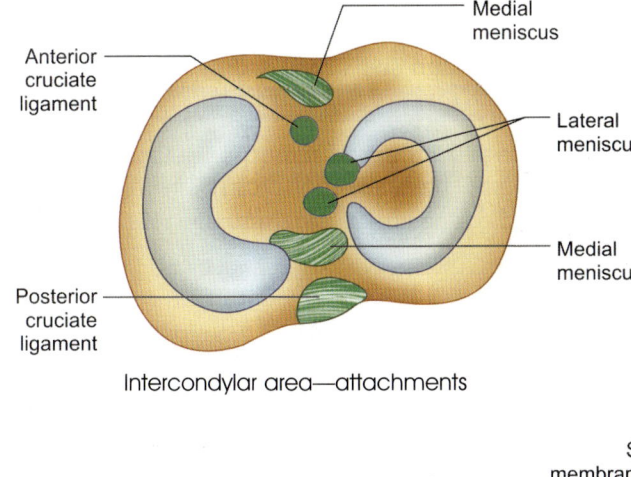

Intercondylar area—attachments

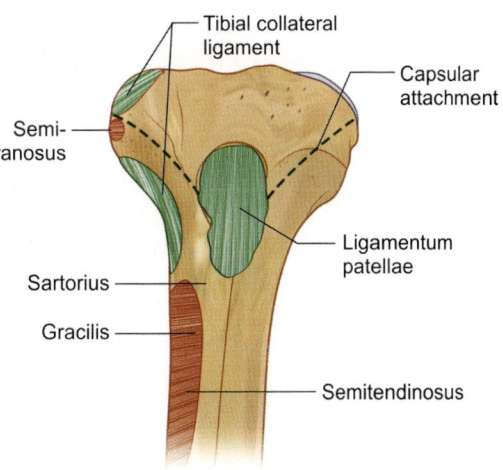

Upper end—anterior surface of tibia

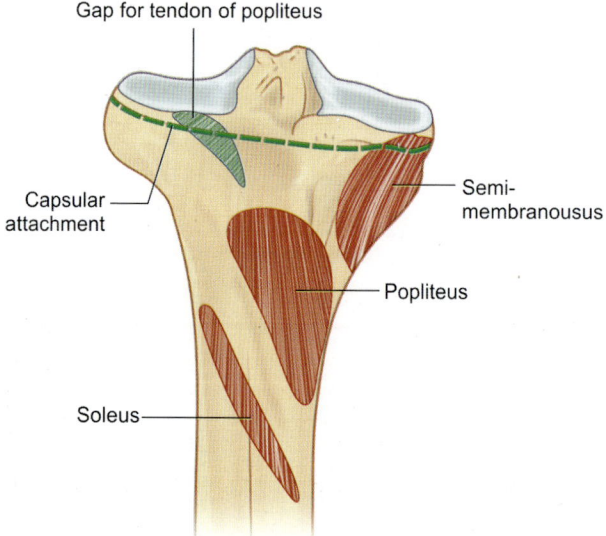

Gap for tendon of popliteus

Capsular attachment

Semi-membranousus

Popliteus

Soleus

Posterior surface of tibia attachments

## Ossification

- Primary centre for the shaft during 7th week of IUL
- Secondary centres for upper end just after birth and it expands by 10 years to form tibial tuberosity, while in distal end the centre appears around end of 1st year
- Upper centre fuses with the shaft by 16 to 18 years and the lower centre fuse by 15 to 17 years
- Medial malleolus is extension of the secondary centre of lower end begins to ossify by 7th year or sometimes may develop from a secondary centre

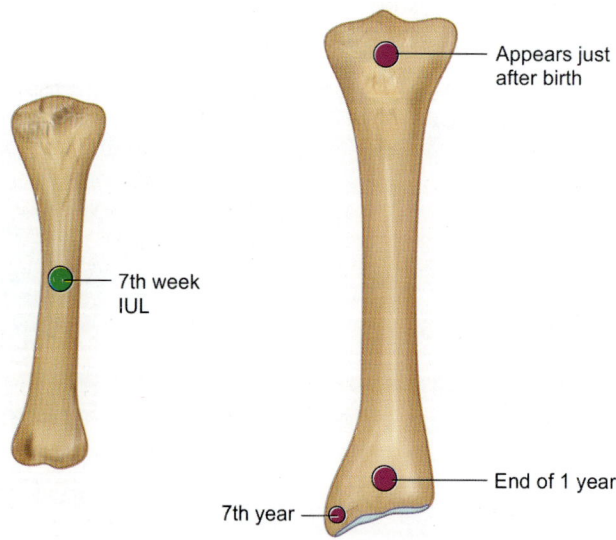

Appears just after birth

7th week IUL

End of 1 year

7th year

Tibia bone showing primary centres and secondary centres of ossification

# 5. FIBULA

It is long bone of the leg placed laterally.

## Side Determination

- Upper end is uniformly expanded (like a flower vas)
- There is a round facet on the medial side of upper end
- A blunt projection, styloid process can be seen from the postero-lateral aspect of upper end
- Medial surface of lower end has triangular facet for talus
- Behind the facet there is malleolar fossa
- Lateral prominence is the lateral malleolus
- Anterior border divides below to include a triangular area
- Interosseous border is sharp and medial
  (be careful in distinguishing upper end from lower end)

## Attachments

### Head

- Common peroneal nerve winds around the neck
- Fibular collateral ligament
- Tendon of biceps femoris.

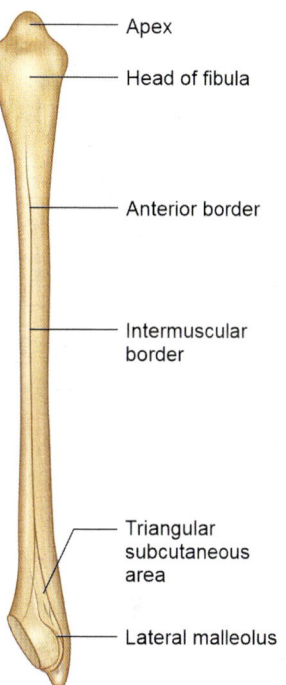

Fibula bone

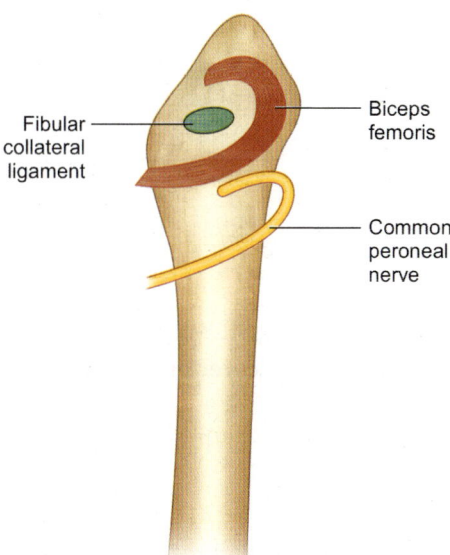

Attachments on head of fibula

### Shaft in Front

- Peroneus longus
- Extensor digitorum longus
- Tibialis posterior

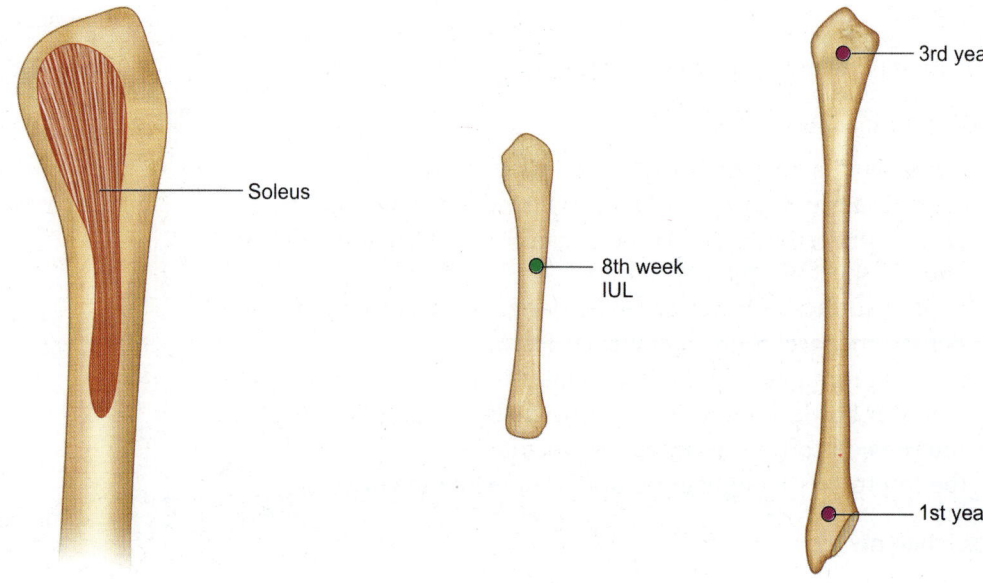

Posterior surface—attachments upper end of fibula

Fibula showing primary centres and secondary centres of ossification

- Peroneus longus
- Peroneus tertius
- Extensor hallucis longus.

*Shaft from Behind*

- Soleus
- Flexor hallucis longus
- Peronius brevis.

## Ossification

- One primary centre for the shaft during 8th week of IUL
- Secondary centre appears first for the lower end during the 1st year of life while for the upper end during the 3rd year of life
- Lower end centre fuses by 15 to 17 years, while the upper end fuses by 17 to 19 years.

## 6. SKELETON OF FOOT

It is made-up of tarsus, metatarsus and phalanges. These bones are naturally very strong and stout to bear the weight of the body.

## Tarsus

- There are 7 tarsus bones, indistinctly divisible into proximal and distal row
- Proximal row is made-up of talus and calcaneum
- Distal row has the 3 cuneiforms and cuboid
- Medially between the talus and medial cuneiform is the navicular bone.

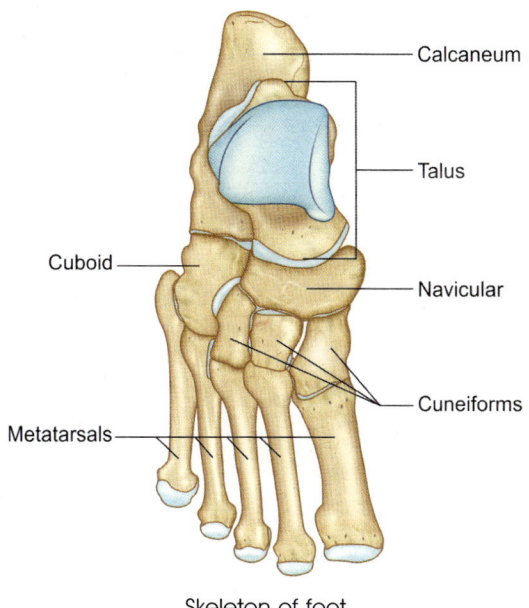

Skeleton of foot

## Talus

It is a block like bone in between the tibia and calcaneum and is an irregular bone.

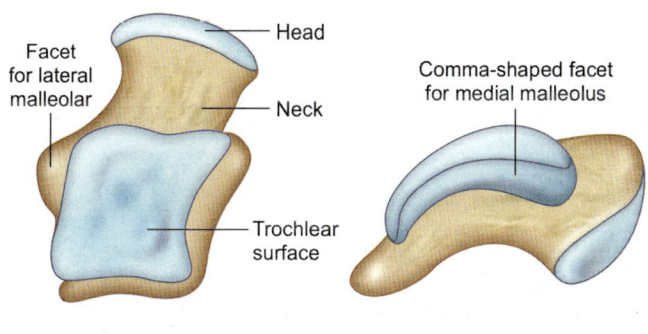

Top view of talus                    Medial view of talus

## Side Determination

- Dorsal surface has the prominent trochlear surface
- A flange-like projection laterally for lateral malleolus
- Head is directed inferomedially
- A comma-shaped facet for medial malleolus medially.

## Attachments

Talus has no muscular attachments: only ligaments are attached connecting the adjacent bones.

## Calcaneum

It is the heel bone and is the largest tarsal bone.

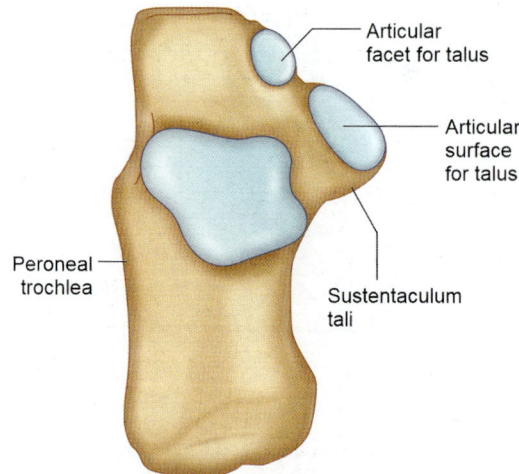

Dorsal aspect of calcaneum

## Side Determination

- Posterior part forms the heel and is the very stout part
- Anterior surface has facets for talar bone
- Medial surface has a typical projection sustentaculum tali
- Lateral surface is flat distally having an elevation peroneal trochlea.

## Attachments

### Dorsal Aspect

Posteriorly is the attachment of tendo Achilles tendon.

### Plantar Aspect

- Abductor hallucis brevis
- Flexor digitorum brevis
- Abductor digiti minimi
- Flexor digitorum accessorius.

### Sustentaculum Tali

Groove below this projection is meant for flexor hallucis longus tendon

### Navicular Bone

It has a prominent tuberosity, 2.5 cm distal and plantar to the medial malleolus, this the navicular tuberosity providing the main attachment of tibialis posterior muscle

### Cuboid

Plantar surface has the groove for the peroneus longus tendon.

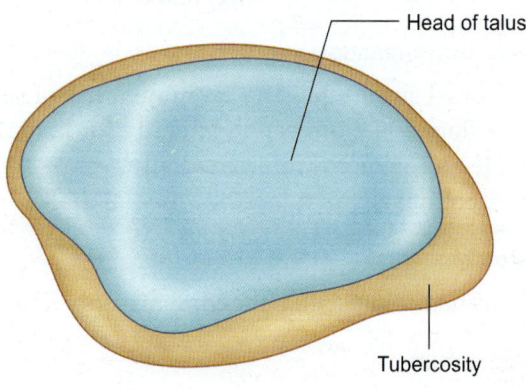

Navicular bone

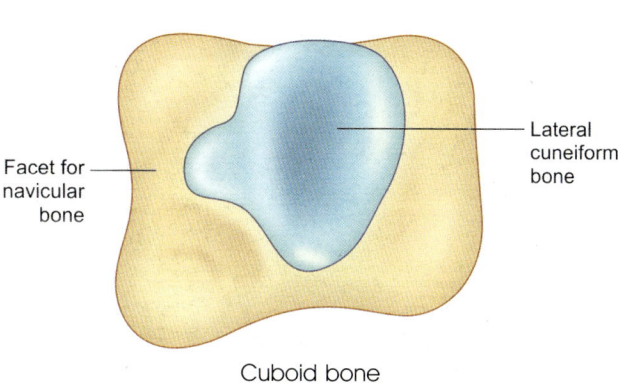

Cuboid bone

## Ossification

- Primary centres are present for calcaneum and talus during 12 to 24 weeks of IUL, cuboid begins to ossify before birth
- Secondary centres are for, lateral cuneiform during 1st year of life, for medial cuneiform, 2 centres during 2nd year, for navicular and intermediate cuneiform centre appears during 3rd year of life
- Calcaneum has a scale-like epiphysis ossifies by 6th year with its completion by 14 to 16 years.

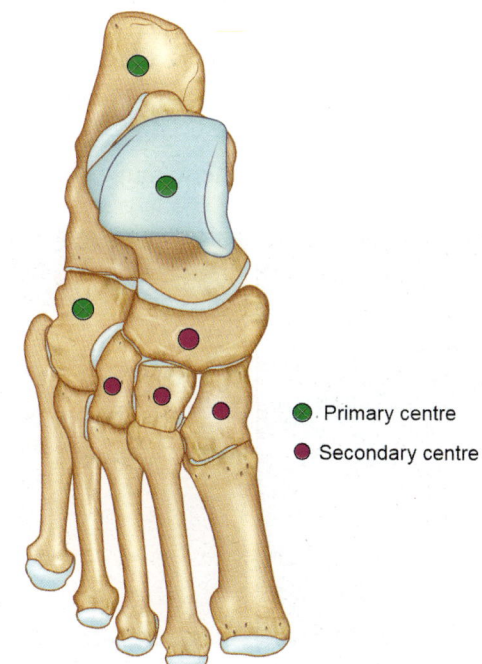

Skeleton of foot showing primary centres and secondary centres of ossification

## Metatarsal Bones

These are short, long bones, having a primary centre for the shaft and secondary centre for the base of 1st metatarsal and appearing in the head of other metatarsals.

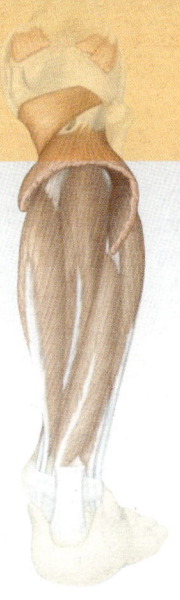

# Surface Anatomy 16

## 1. MID-INGUINAL POINT

- This point lies mid-way between anterior superior iliac spine and pubic symphysis
- Femoral artery lies beneath this point
- On deep palpation, one can feel a bony prominence this is the head of femur.

## 2. MID-POINT OF INGUINAL LIGAMENT

Mid-point of inguinal ligament lies between the anterior superior iliac spine and pubic tubercle.

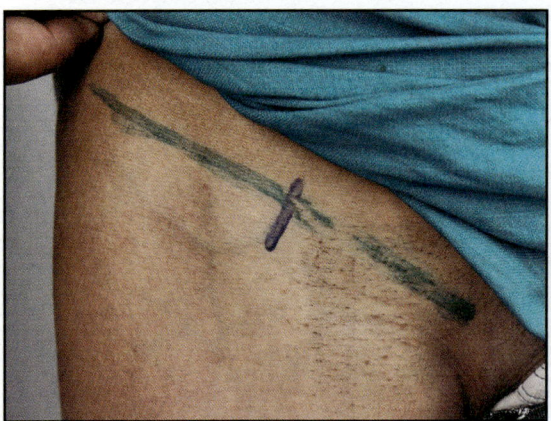

Mid-inguinal point

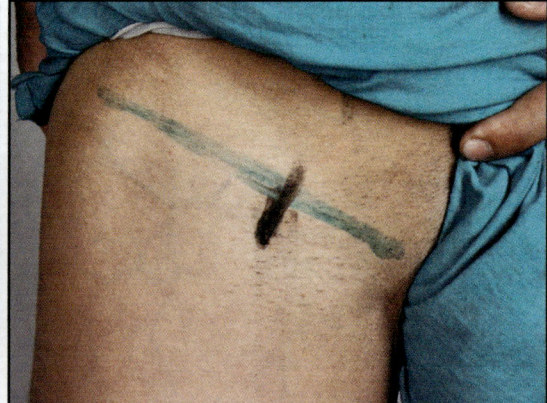

Mid-point of inguinal ligament

## 3. FEMORAL ARTERY

### Position of the Limb

Thigh should be semiflexed, abducted and laterally rotated.

## Points to be Marked

• Mid-inguinal point

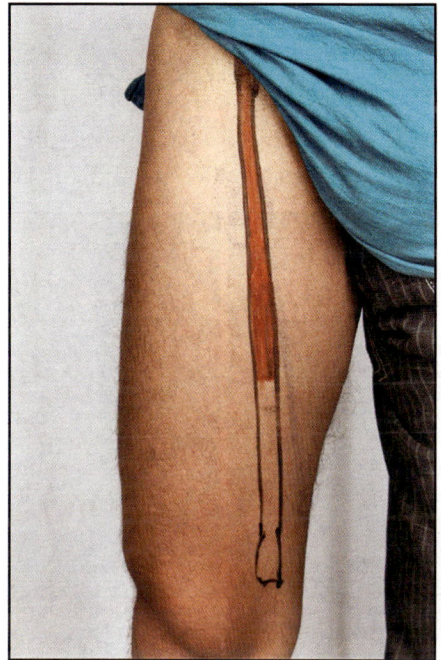

Markings for femoral artery

• Palpate the adductor tubercle (in thin individuals one can easily palpate tendon of adductor magnus) behind the vastus medialis muscle mass medially.

## 4. POPLITEAL ARTERY

### Position of the Limb

Prone position of limb.

### Points to be Marked

• Popliteal artery is the continuation of femoral artery on back of thigh. Thus, end point of femoral artery is the beginning of popliteal artery. The first point lies on lower 1/3rd of thigh medially, 2.5 cm from midline.
• Second point on back of knee in midline.
• Third point diagonally opposite to the tibial tuberosity.

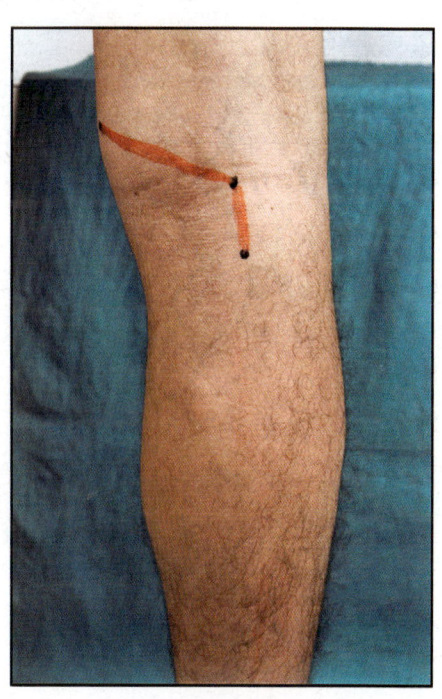

Markings for popliteal artery

## 5. POSTERIOR TIBIAL ARTERY

### Position of the Limb

Prone position of limb.

### Points to be Marked

- At the level of tibial tuberosity in mid-line on back of the calf
- Another point mid-way between medial malleolus and calcaneum.

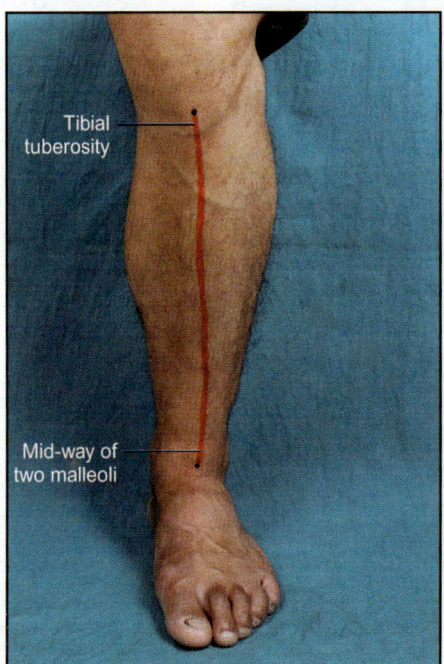
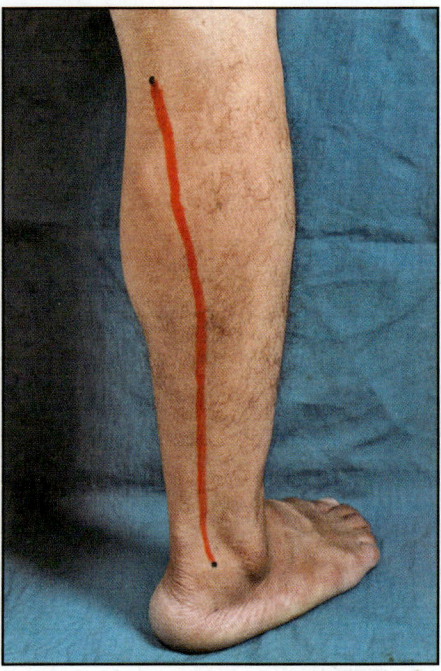

Markings for anterior and posterior tibial artery

## 6. DORSALIS PEDIS ARTERY

### Position of the Limb

Subject can sit on chair with dorsum of the foot at rest on ground.

### Points to be Marked

- A point mid-way between the two malleoli in front of foot
- Second point at the beginning of first intermetatarsal space.
- Feel for the pulsations

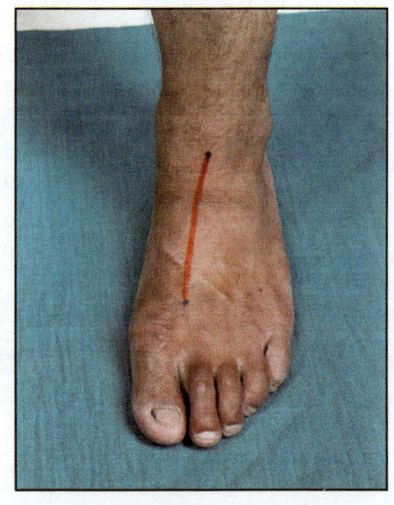

Markings for dorsalis pedis artery

## 7. GREAT SAPHENOUS VEIN (Very commonly asked in viva)

### Position of the Limb

Supine body with legs in natural abduction and laterally rotated position.

### Points to be Marked

- One can easily see the vein on the body, it occupies most of the medial compartment of the leg. First point on the dorsum of the foot, approximately at the base of big toe
- Second 1.5 cm in front of medial malleolus
- Medial side of leg at the junction of upper 2/3rd and lower 1/3rd of leg
- Adductor tubercle
- 4 cm below and lateral to pubic tubercle is the marking of saphenous opening where the vein terminates.

   *Remember:* Saphenous nerve accompanies the great saphenous vein.

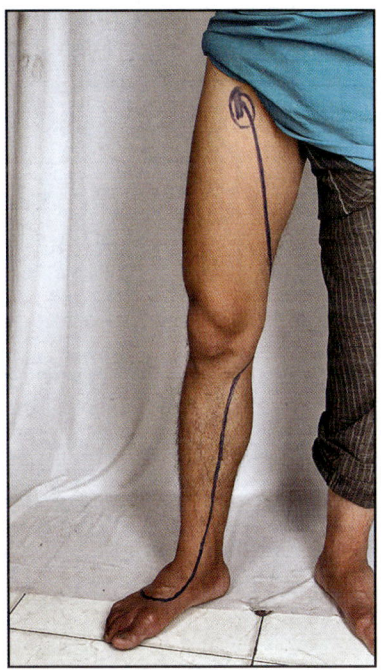

Markings for great saphenous vein

## 8. FLEXOR RETINACULUM

### Position of the Limb

Subject can be seated on a chair with foot resting on ground.

### Points to be Marked

- Medial malleolus
- Calcaneum.

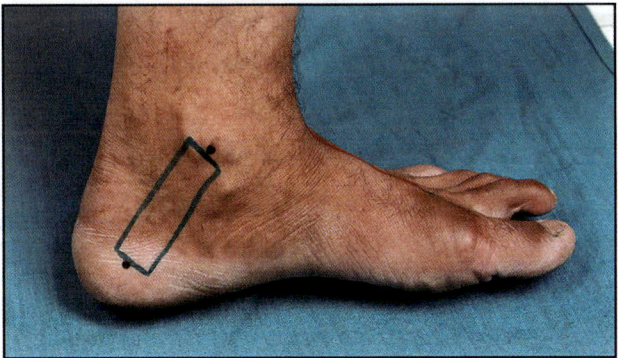

Markings for flexor retinaculum

Student should mark a 2.5 cm band between above points this marks the flexor retinaculum

## TESTING OF LOWER LIMB MUSCLES

### Psoas Major and Hamstrings

Flexion at the hip and knee is tested by asking the patient to lift the hip to abdomen and bending the knee.

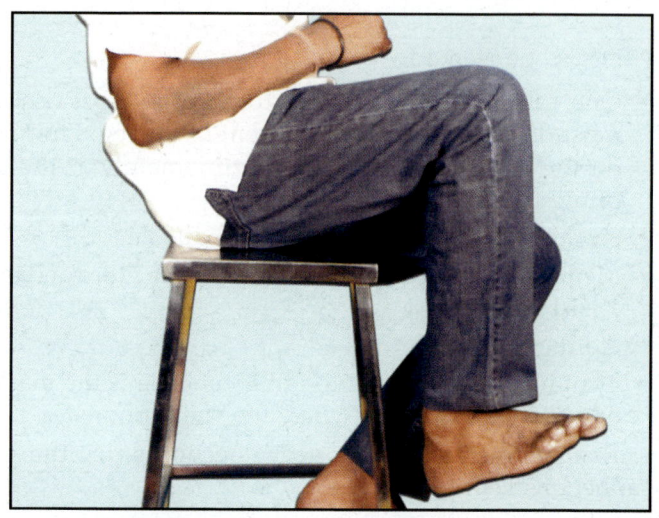

### Gluteus Maximus and Hamstrings

Extension at hip joint

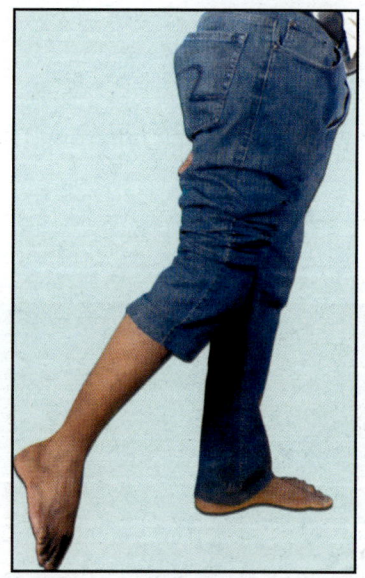

## Dorsiflexion

Tibialis anterior and extensors of leg

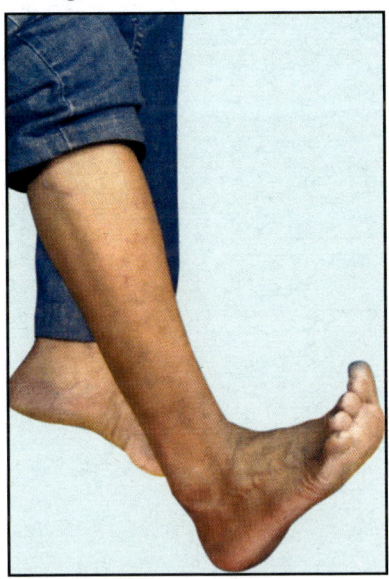

## Plantar Flexion

Tendo Achilles and flexors of the leg

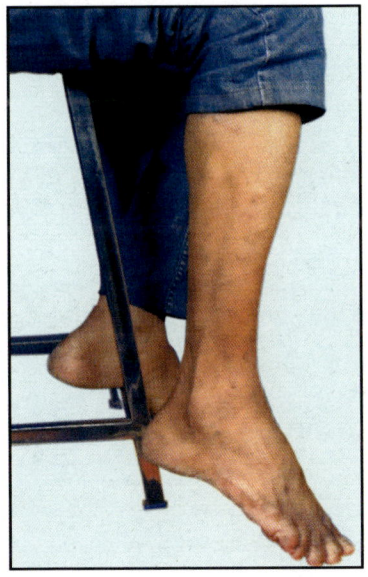

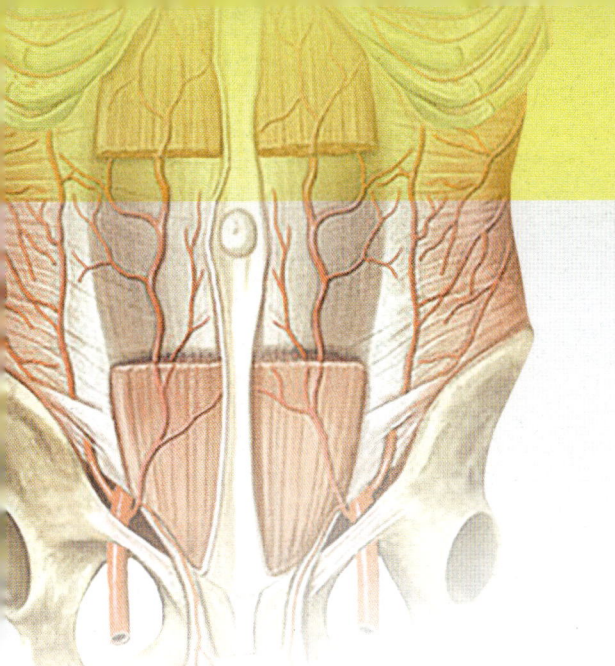

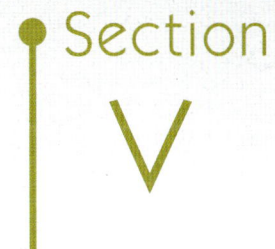
# Abdomen and Pelvis

# Key Osteology Questions | 17

### Q. What are the features of 'typical' lumbar vertebra?

**Ans.** Following are the features of 'typical' lumbar vertebra:
- Body of the vertebra is large, strong and stout
- Transverse diameter is greater than anteroposterior diameter
- Vertebral foramen is relatively large and triangular in shape
- Pedicles are short and strong
- Inferior vertebral notch is deeper than superior vertebral notch
- Laminae are short, thick and broad, and directed backwards and medially
- Spine is in the form of quadrilateral plate
- Transverse processes are thin
- Superior articular process has concave facet facing medially and backwards, and they lie quite apart from each other
- Posterior border of superior articular process has a rough tubercle known as mammillary process
- Inferior articular processes are relatively close to each other.

### Q. Which is the 'atypical' lumbar vertebra?

**Ans.** Fifth lumbar vertebra is the 'atypical' vertebra.

### Q. What do you understand by sacralization of fifth lumbar vertebra?

**Ans.** The fifth lumbar vertebra or its transverse process may be fused with sacrum and this is known as sacralization of fifth lumbar vertebra.

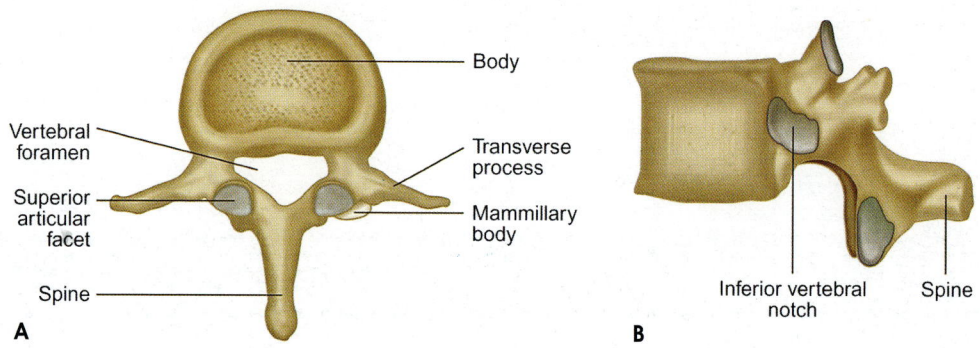

Fifth lumbar vertebra. **A.** Axial view; **B.** Lateral view

## Q. Depict the relations of ala of sacrum.

**Ans.**

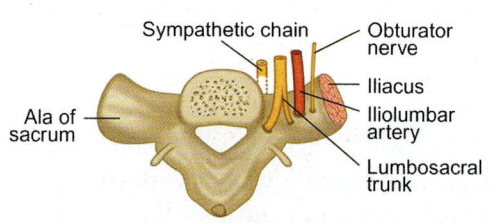

Relations of ala of sacrum

## Q. What are the differences between male and female pelves?

**Ans.**

| Criteria | Male | Female |
|---|---|---|
| Greater sciatic notch | Narrow | Wider |
| Acetabulum | Larger | Smaller |
| Iliac crest | More prominent | Less prominent |
| Iliac fossa | Shallow | Deeper |
| Pubic crest | Shorter | Longer |
| Ischiopubic rami | Everted | Not everted |
| Preauricular sulcus | Less prominent | More prominent |
| Ischial spine | Inturned | Straight, pointed |
| Obturator foramen | Large, oval | Small, triangular |

## Q. What is pelvic brim index?

**Ans.**

$$\text{Pelvic brim index} = \frac{\text{Anteroposterior diameter}}{\text{Transverse diameter}} \times 100$$

### Q. How are the pelves classified depending on pelvic brim index?

**Ans.** The pelves are classified as follows:
- *Platypellic:* Transversely flat
- *Mesatipellic:* Intermediate
- *Dolicopellic:* Anteroposteriorly flat.

### Q. Which ligament is considered strong in female pelvis?

**Ans.** Interosseous sacroiliac ligament is the strongest ligament in female pelvis.

### Q. What are the events occurring at L1?

**Ans.** Following are the events:
- Transpyloric plane passes through L1
- Superior mesenteric artery arises at L1
- Body of pancreas lies at L1
- Pylorus of stomach lies at L1
- First part of duodenum lies at L1
- Superior duodenal flexure lies at L1
- Celiac plexus lies at L1
- Upper part of the hilus of right kidney lies at L1
- Lower part of the hilus of left kidney lies at L1
- Cisterna chyli lies against L1 and L2.

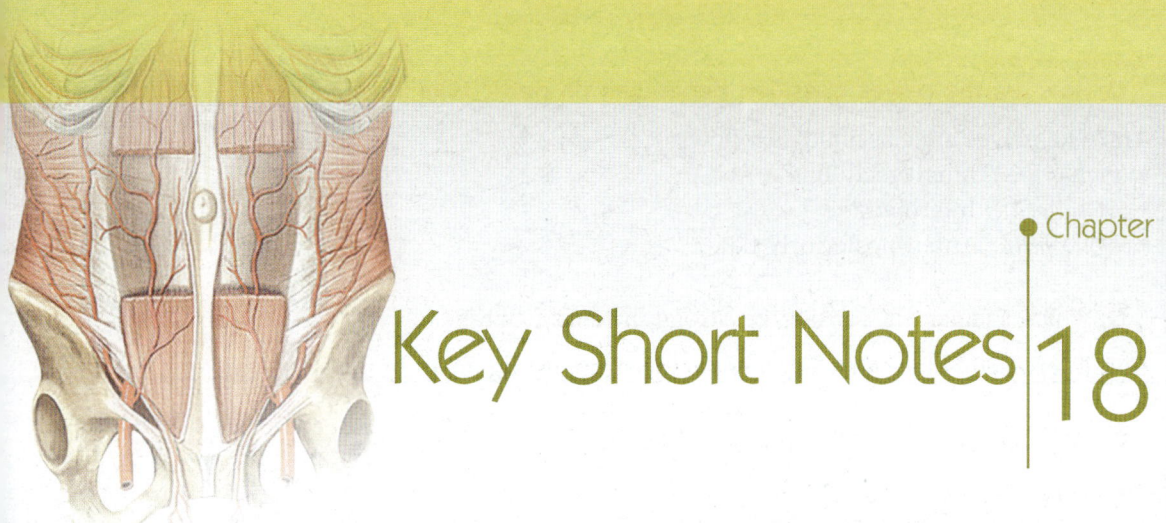

# Key Short Notes | 18

## MUSCLE

### EXTERNAL OBLIQUE MUSCLE

External oblique muscle is the most superficial muscle of the anterolateral side of abdominal wall. The fibres of the muscle are directed downwards, forwards and medially (like hands in pocket).

### Attachments

- Arises from lower eight ribs (upper fibres mingle with serratus anterior and lower fibres mingle with latissimus dorsi).
- Muscle fibres get inserted into anterior 2/3rd of outer lip of iliac crest.

    Aponeurosis gets inserted into xiphoid process, linea alba, pubic symphysis, pubic crest and pectineal line of pubis.

### Nerve Supply

Lower six thoracic nerves.

### Action

- Supports abdominal viscera
- Assists in micturition, defecation, parturition, coughing, sneezing, etc.
- Lateral flexion and rotation of trunk.

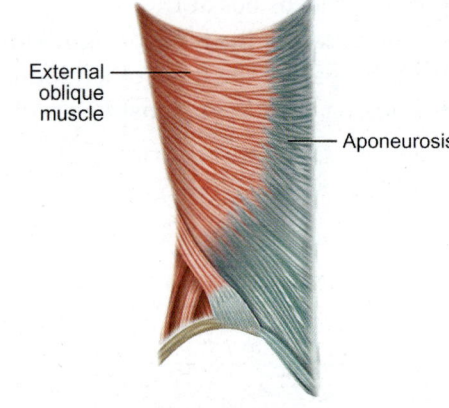

External oblique muscle

## Peculiarities

- Gets inserted in the form of flattened aponeurosis
- Lower edge of the aponeurosis gets folded on itself to form inguinal ligament
- Opening in the aponeurosis is known as superficial inguinal ring.

### Q. Internal oblique muscle

The muscle lies on the anterolateral side of abdominal wall and below external oblique muscle. The fibres of the muscle are directed upwards, forwards and medially (muscle fibres are at right angle to external oblique muscle fibres).

### Attachments

- Arises from lateral two-thirds of inguinal ligament, anterior two-thirds of intermediate area of iliac crest and thoracolumbar fascia
- Gets inserted in the form of broad aponeurosis into 7th, 8th, and 9th costal cartilage, xiphoid process, linea alba, pubic crest, pectineal line of pubis.

### Nerve Supply

Lower six thoracic nerves and first lumbar nerve.

### Action

- Supports abdominal viscera
- Assists in micturition, defecation, parturition, coughing, sneezing, etc.
- Lateral flexion and rotation of trunk.

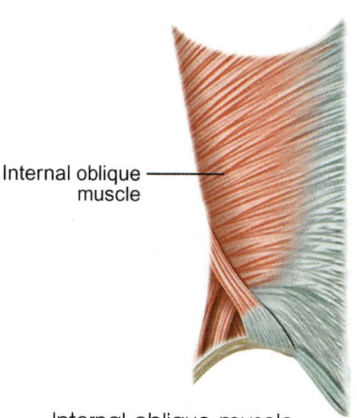

Internal oblique muscle

Internal oblique muscle

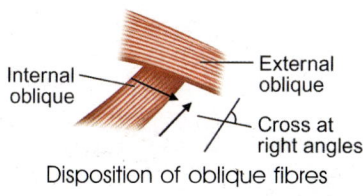

Disposition of oblique fibres

### Q. Transversus abdominis

Transversus abdominis is a deeper muscle on the anterolateral side of the abdominal wall. The fibres run transversely and hence the name.

### Attachments

- Arises from lateral one-third of inguinal ligament, anterior two-thirds of inner lip of iliac crest, thoracolumbar fascia, inner surface of lower six costal cartilages
- Gets inserted in the form of broad aponeurosis into xiphoid process, linea alba, pubic crest, pectineal line of pubis.

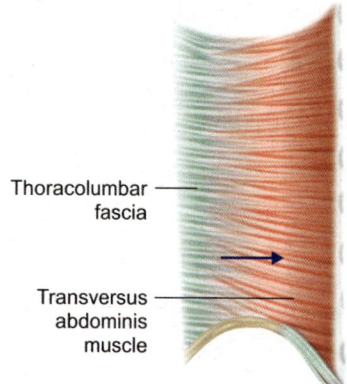

Thoracolumbar fascia

Transversus abdominis muscle

Transversus abdominis

## Nerve Supply

Lower six thoracic nerves and first lumbar nerve.

## Action

- Supports abdominal viscera
- Assists in micturition, defecation, parturition, coughing, sneezing, etc.
- Lateral flexion and rotation of trunk.

## Peculiarities

- Lower fibres of the muscle fuse with fibres of internal oblique to form conjoint tendon.
- Fascia transversalis lines the inner surface of the muscle.
- An oval opening is present in the fascia transversalis, around half inch above mid inguinal point and is known as deep inguinal ring.

### Q. Rectus sheath

**Ans.** Rectus sheath is an aponeurosis of internal oblique muscle, which splits into anterior and posterior layer to enclose rectus abdominis muscle.

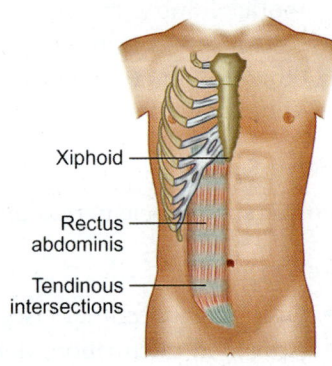

Rectus abdominis muscle

## Peculiarities

- External oblique aponeurosis fuses with anterior layer
- Transversus abdominis aponeurosis fuses with posterior layer
- Below the umbilicus all the three aponeuroses lie in front of rectus muscle

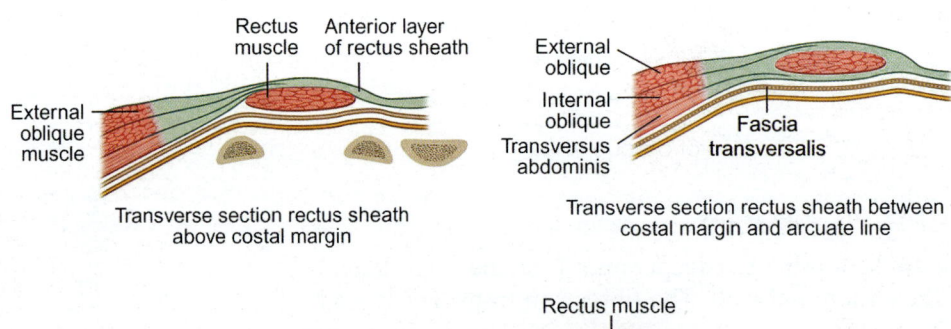

Transverse section rectus sheath above costal margin

Transverse section rectus sheath between costal margin and arcuate line

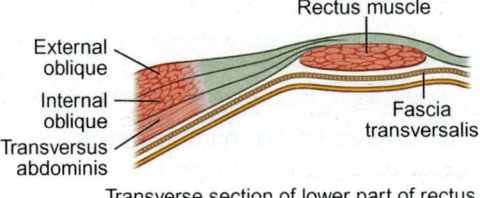

Transverse section of lower part of rectus sheath below arcuate line

Rectus sheath

- Posterior layer of the sheath has a free concave margin known as arcuate line
- Aponeuroses of all the three muscles intersect in the midline to form linea alba
- Linea alba is wide above the umbilicus and narrow below the umbilicus.

## Formation

- Above costal margin only external oblique and its aponeurosis is present
- Between umbilicus and costal margin the rectus muscle is completely enclosed in split internal oblique aponeurosis
- All the three aponeuroses are in front of the rectus muscle below the arcuate line.

## Contents

- Muscles—rectus abdominis and pyramidalis
- Vessels—superior epigastric and inferior epigastric
- Nerves—lower six intercostal nerves.

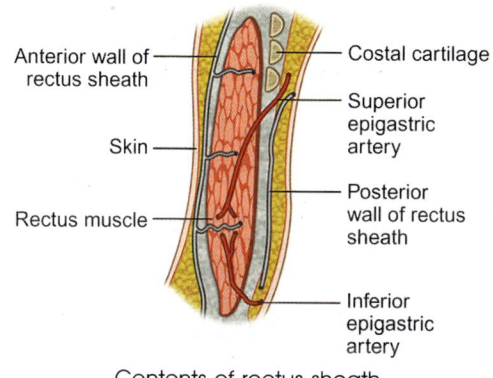

Contents of rectus sheath

## Functions

Maintains the strength of anterior abdominal wall and controls the action of rectus muscle.

## Clinical Importance

- In reconstructive breast surgery, in cases of breast cancer, flap of rectus muscle with its blood supply is used.
- After multiple pregnancies, the linea alba may weaken giving rise to a condition known as divarication of recti
- Supraumbilical median incisions provide bloodless operative field and are safe, but postoperative healing may cause weakness of abdominal wall
- Infraumbilical incisions hardly cause weakness of abdominal wall since natural gap between recti is very less.

### Q. Perineal body

**Ans.** Perineal body is also known as the central tendon of perineum. It provides stability and support to pelvic structures.

## Locations

- Lies at posterior border of perineal membrane
- Located between anal canal and vagina or bulb of penis.

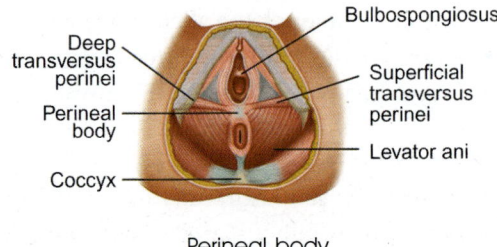

Perineal body

## Formation

Following muscles gain attachment to this midline muscular mass:

- External anal sphincter
- Pubovaginalis (puboprostaticus)
- Levator ani partly
- Bulbospongiosus
- Superficial transversus perinei
- Deep transversus perinei.

## Functions

Perineal body provides stability and support to pelvic structures.

## Clinical Importance

Perineal body may weaken during childbirth giving rise to prolapse (herniation of organs to the exterior due to gravity) of pelvic organs.

### Q. Supports of uterus

**Ans.** Supports of the uterus can be classified into true supports and false supports.

## True Supports

1. *Uterine position:* Angulation of body and fundus of uterus to cervix (angle of anteflexion) and angulation of cervix to vagina (angle of anteversion) itself provides positional support to uterus.

2. *Round ligament of uterus:* It maintains the uterine angulation by virtue of its attachment. It extends from upper part of uterus at the level of attachment of ligament of ovary to deep inguinal ring. It passes through the inguinal canal and gets attached to the fibrofatty tissue of labium majus. It sustains an anterior pull on the uterus.

3. *Uterosacral ligaments:* It counteracts the pull of round ligament, and extends between cervix of uterus to sacrum. In its course backwards it embraces the rectouterine pouch and rectum.

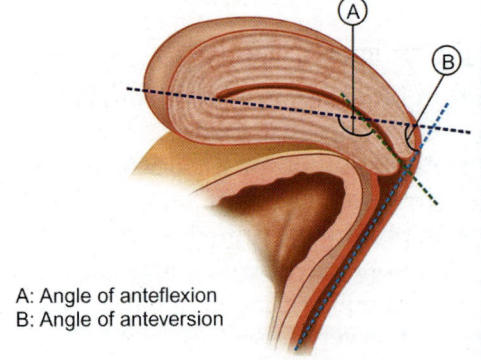

A: Angle of anteflexion
B: Angle of anteversion

Positional support to uterus

4. *Transverse cervical ligament:* Also known as cardinal ligament, Mackenrodt's ligament. It is the condensation of connective tissue between cervix and vaginal fornix to lateral wall of pelvis. It gives lateral support to the uterus and is considered as a cardinal support of uterus.

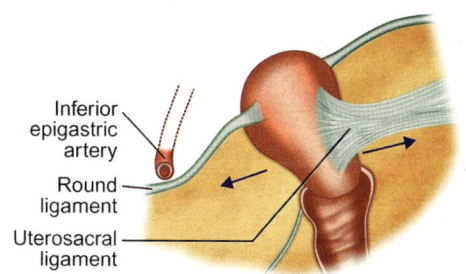

Counteraction of forward and backward pull

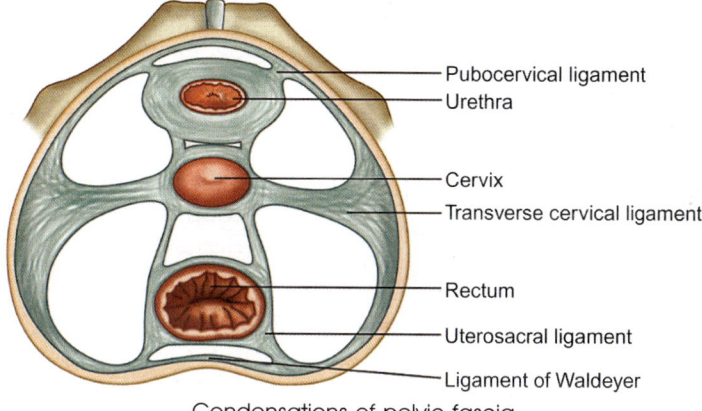

Condensations of pelvic fascia

5. *Pubovaginalis:* This part of levator ani and perineal body with its muscular attachment primarily supports the vagina thus indirectly maintain the position of cervix.

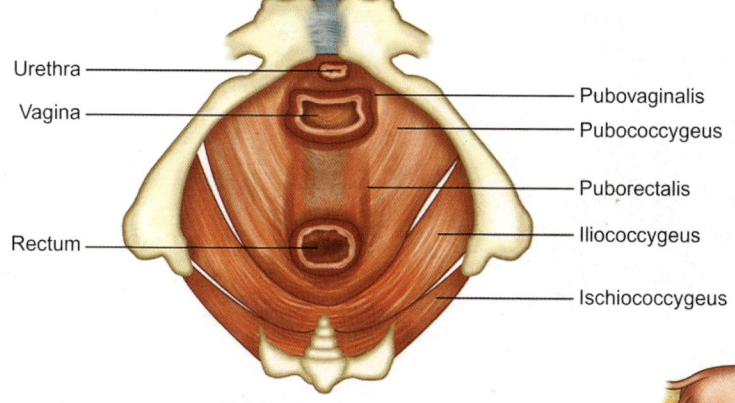

Pelvic diaphragm

## False Supports

1. *Broad ligament:* It is not a true ligament, but a double-layered fold of peritoneum extending between lateral wall of uterus and pelvic wall. The upper free border contains the uterine tube and

Broad ligament

forms the mesosalpinx. The ureter adheres posteriorly while the line of lateral attachment crosses the obturator nerves and vessels.

2. *Anterior ligament:* It is the peritoneal fold reflected onto the bladder from the uterus. Hence known as uterovesical fold.

3. *Posterior ligament:* It is the peritoneal fold reflected from vaginal fornix to the anterior wall of rectum. Hence known as rectovaginal fold.

### Clinical Importance

• Posterior inclination of uterus is known as retroversion wherein the cervix faces forwards
• Sometimes the uterus may have a posterior curvature of the body and this is known as retroflexion
• Due to the weakness of pelvic floor muscles secondary to childbirth the uterus may protrude out of vagina this is known as prolapse of uterus.

### Q. Pelvic diaphragm

**Ans.** The pelvic floor muscles form the pelvic diaphragm. These muscles suspend the pelvic structures like a hammock. It comprises of levator ani group of muscles and coccygeus.

### LEVATOR ANI

The muscle has two parts namely pubococcygeus and iliococcygeus.

### Attachments

• Fibres arise from body of pubis, ischial spine and tendinous arch over obturator fascia
• The fibres get inserted into coccyx and anococcygeal ligament.

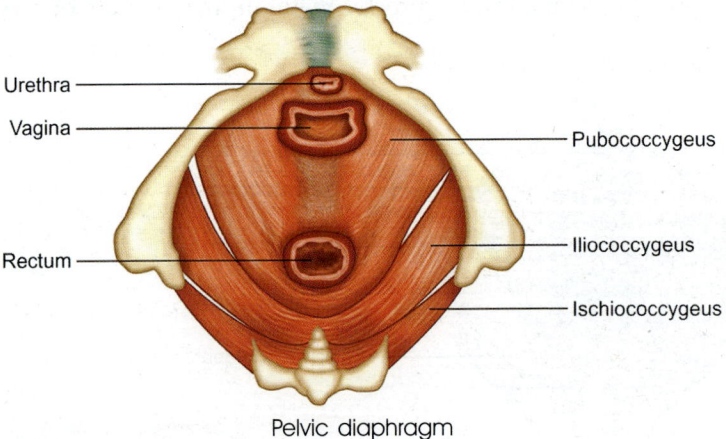

Pelvic diaphragm

### COCCYGEUS

By and large considered as ischiococcygeus.

### Attachments

• Arises from ischial spine
• Gets inserted into side of coccyx and lower part of sacrum.

## Nerve Supply

Chiefly supplied by branches of sacral plexus through S3 and S4.

## Actions

- Supports the pelvic viscera
- Contraction of pelvic floor counteracts the raised intra-abdominal pressure during sneezing, coughing or lifting heavy weights
- Assists during childbirth to expel the head of fetus
- Few fibres assist the urethral sphincter at the end of micturition.

### Q. Anal sphincters

**Ans.** The continence of anus depends on the sphincter mechanism of anus. It comprises of external and internal anal sphincters.

1. Internal anal sphincter is a downward extension of circular muscle layer of rectum.
2. External anal sphincter surrounds the internal muscle and conventionally thought to have deep, superficial and subcutaneous portions. However, it is considered to be a single sheet of muscle variably divided by fibres from longitudinal muscle layer of rectum.

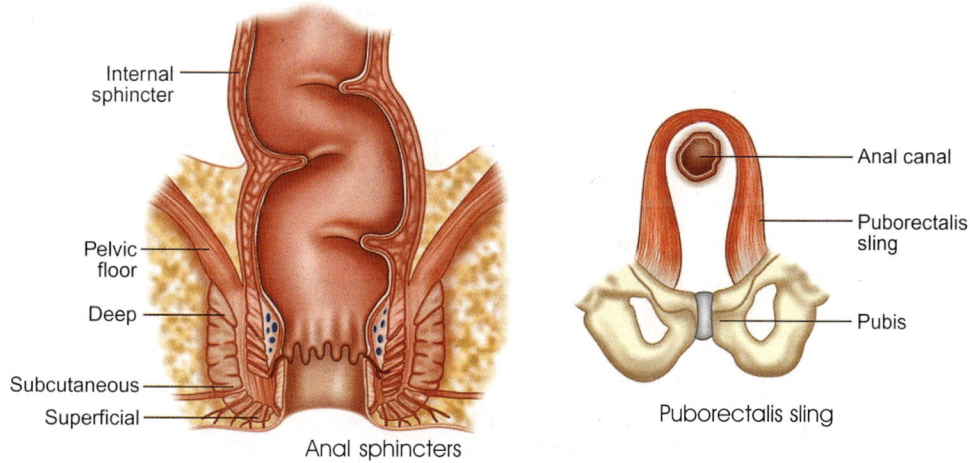

Anal sphincters

Puborectalis sling

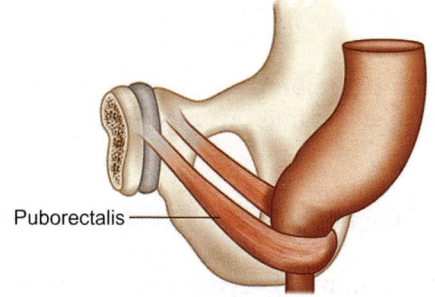

Puborectalis, maintains anorectal angulation and assists continence of anus

## Peculiarities
- Internal anal sphincter is involuntary
- External anal sphincter is under voluntary control.

## Nerve Supply
- Internal anal sphincter receives autonomic innervations
- External anal sphincter supplied by inferior rectal branch of pudendal nerve and perineal branch of S4.

## Clinical Importance
Damage to pudendal nerve during perineal surgeries can cause anal incontinence.

## PERITONEUM

### Q. Greater omentum

**Ans.** Greater omentum is a double fold of peritoneum hanging from the greater curvature of stomach. It is made-up of four layers folded upon itself.

## Architecture
1. Anterior two layers descend from greater curvature of stomach to variable distance over the coils of intestine and then fold upwards to lie in front of transverse colon, where it blends with the peritoneum on transverse colon and transverse mesocolon.

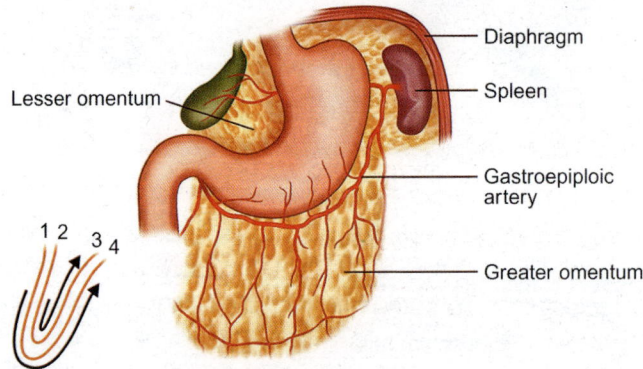

Greater omentum folding pattern

2. The folding is in such a way that the first layer becomes fourth and second layer becomes third.
3. The four layers below transverse colon blend with each other to form a single structure, which contains adipose tissue and numerous macrophages.

## Subdivisions
- The part of greater omentum between stomach and transverse colon is named as gastro-colic omentum
- Double-layered fold of peritoneum between greater curvature of stomach and hilum of spleen is known as gastrosplenic ligament

- Double-layered fold of peritoneum between hilum of spleen and anterior surface of left kidney is known as splenorenal (lienorenal) ligament.

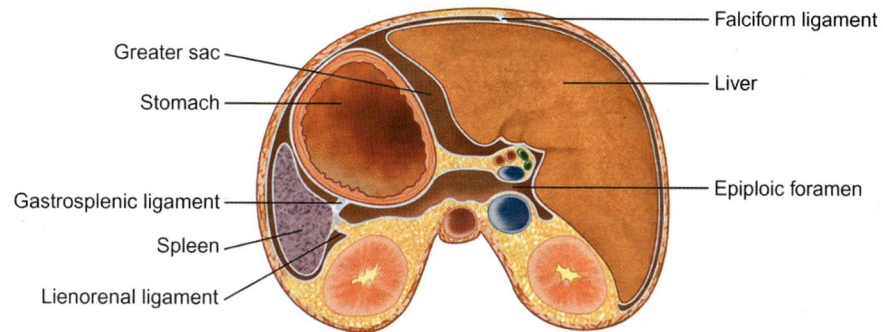

Transverse section of supracolic compartment

## Contents

- Right and left gastroepiploic vessels
- Fat.

## Functions

- Storehouse of fat
- Macrophages in the omentum protect against infection
- It limits the spread of infection by engulfing the site of infection.

## Cilnical Importance

- Lesser sac can be approached through gastrocolic omentum.
- Greater omentum is known as 'Policeman of Abdomen' since it cordons off intraperitoneal infections.

## Q. Lesser omentum

**Ans.** Lesser omentum is a double-layered fold of peritoneum, which can be appreciated in the cadaver by lifting the liver away from stomach.

## Attachments

1. Gastric attachment extends from right side of abdominal esophagus, lesser curvature of stomach and first 2 cm of duodenum.
2. Hepatic attachment is in the form of letter inverted 'L' wherein it is attached to fissure for ligamentum venosum and margins of porta hepatis.

Lesser omentum (attachments and contents)

## Features

- Between the duodenum and the liver is the free margin of lesser omentum where the anterior and posterior layers are continuous
- Free margin forms anterior boundary of epiploic foramen.

## Contents

- Free margin contains hepatic artery, portal vein, bile duct, lymph nodes and nerve plexus
- Along the lesser curvature there are gastric vessels and lymph nodes.

## Clinical Importance

Omental patch can be used for closure of gastric perforation.

## Q. Epiploic foramen

**Ans.** Epiploic foramen is also known as foramen of Winslow or aditus to lesser sac. It is a vertical slit around 2.5 cm in size. The lesser sac communicates with the greater sac through this foramen.

Transverse section at T12 showing epiploic foramen

## Location

Epiploic foramen is located at the right border of the lesser sac and at the level of T12 vertebra.

## Boundaries

- Above: Caudate process of liver
- Below: First part of duodenum
- Behind: Inferior vena cava
- Front: Right free margin of the lesser omentun.

## Clinical Importance

Internal herniation of abdominal organs may occur through this foramen.

## Q. Vertical disposition of peritoneum (diagram only).

**Ans.**

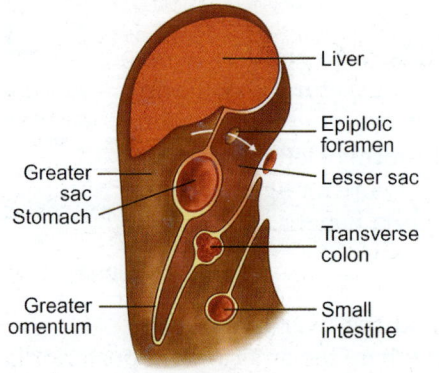

Vertical disposition of peritoneum (sagittal section)

## Q. Horizontal section through supracolic compartment of peritoneum (diagram only).

**Ans.**

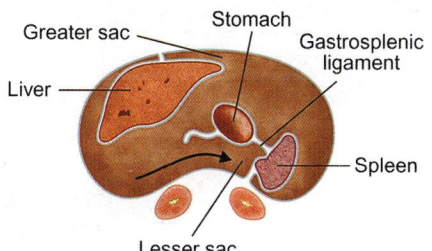

Transverse section of supracolic compartment of peritoneum

## Q. Hepatorenal pouch (Morrison's pouch)

**Ans.**

Hepatorenal pouch is the most dependent space of the supracolic peritoneal cavity in horizontal position.

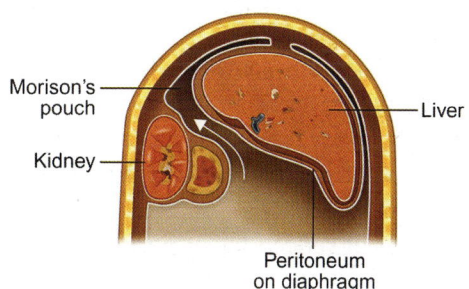

Hepatorenal pouch (Morrison's pouch)

### Location

Hepatorenal pouch is a deep recess located above the upper pole of right kidney lined by peritoneal cavity (right subhepatic space, right posterior space).

### Boundaries

- Front: Inferior surface of liver
- Above: Coronary ligament of liver
- Behind: Peritoneum of diaphragm.

### Clinical Importance

- After surgeries on liver or bile duct fluid may get collected in this pouch due to its position. Thus, the pouch needs to be drained after surgery
- The pus gets collected in this pouch in cases of subphrenic abscess.

## Q. Peritoneal reflections and bare areas on liver

**Ans.** Large surface of liver is covered by peritoneum except few areas, which are not covered are known as bare areas of liver.

### Peritoneal Ligaments on Liver

- Falciform ligament (sickle-shaped)—connects the anterosuperior surface of liver to anterior abdominal wall and under surface of diaphragm
- Left triangular ligament—connects superior surface of left lobe of liver to diaphragm
- Right triangular ligament—connects lateral part of posterior surface of right lobe of liver to the diaphragm
- Coronary ligaments—encloses the bare area on posterior surface of right lobe of liver.

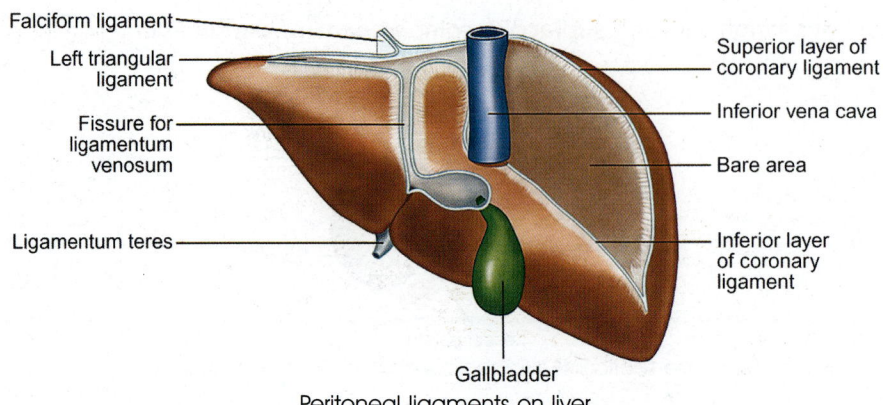

Peritoneal ligaments on liver

## Bare Areas on Liver

- Posterior surface of right lobe of liver between coronary ligament and right triangular ligament
- Groove for inferior vena cava on posterior surface of right lobe of liver
- Fossa of gallbladder on inferior surface of right lobe of liver
- Porta hepatis
- Lines of reflections of peritoneum.

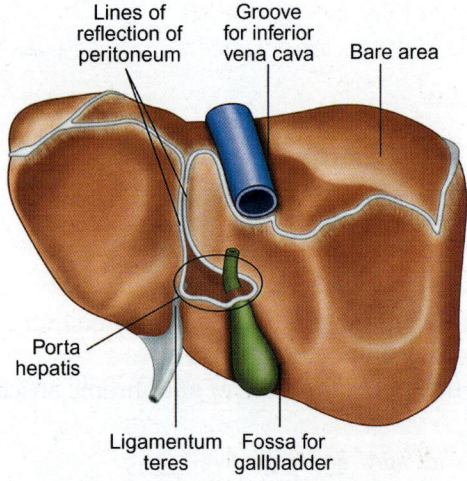

Bare areas of liver (inferior view of liver)

### Q. Mesentery

**Ans.** The coils of jejunum and ileum suspend from the posterior abdominal wall with the help of mesentery.

## Attachment and Disposition

- Root of the mesentery is the fixed portion, disposed obliquely across duodenojejunal flexure to upper part of right sacroiliac joint
- Free border of the mesentery is thrown in folds in the form of fan held in hand.

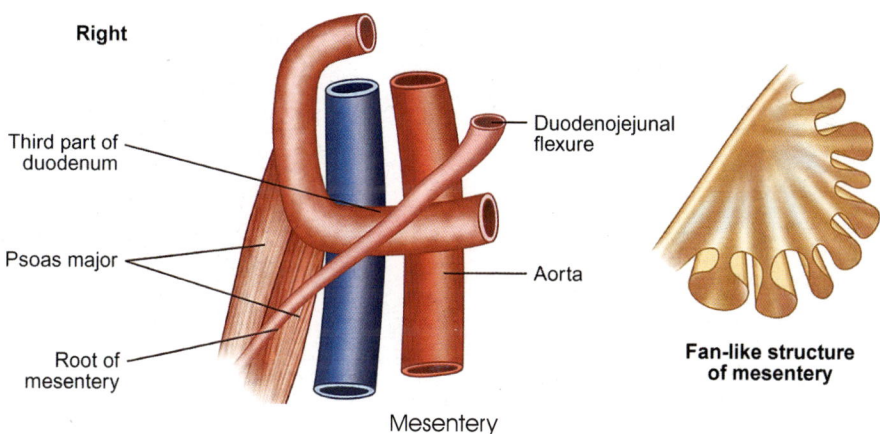

**Right**

Third part of duodenum

Psoas major

Root of mesentery

Duodenojejunal flexure

Aorta

Mesentery

**Fan-like structure of mesentery**

## Relations

Mesentery crosses third part of duodenum, abdominal aorta, inferior vena cava, right ureter and right psoas major.

## Contents

- Fat
- Lymphatics and lymph nodes
- Jejunal and ileal branches of superior mesenteric vessels
- Autonomic nerve plexus.

## Q. Rectouterine pouch (pouch of Douglas)

**Ans.** Rectouterine pouch is the most dependent part of peritoneal cavity in standing position. So, the fluid gets accumulated in this pouch by virtue of gravity.

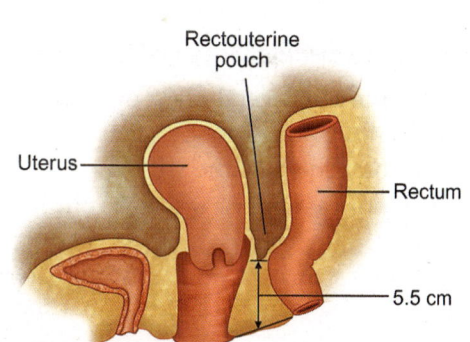

Rectouterine pouch

Uterus

Rectum

5.5 cm

Female pelvis showing rectouterine pouch (sagittal section)

## Boundaries

- *Front:* Uterus and posterior fornix of vagina
- *Behind:* Rectum
- *Above:* Connected to peritoneal cavity
- *Below:* Rectovaginal fold of peritoneum.

## Clinical Importance

- In cases of abscess formation in pelvis the pus may get collected in the pouch
- The pouch can be approached through posterior fornix or rectum
- In per-rectal or pervaginal examination, the pouch can be felt 5.5 cm above anus.

## Q. Duodenal fossae

**Ans.** The peritoneal cavity has pockets of peritoneal folds close to organs like duodenum, cecum and sigmoid colon. Following are the fossae in relation to duodenum.

## Paraduodenal Fossa

It is present on the left side of duodenum, present in 20% of cadavers, other fossae are never present with it.

## Boundaries

- Above—pancreas, renal vessels
- Front—inferior mesenteric vein
- Right—aorta
- Left—kidney.

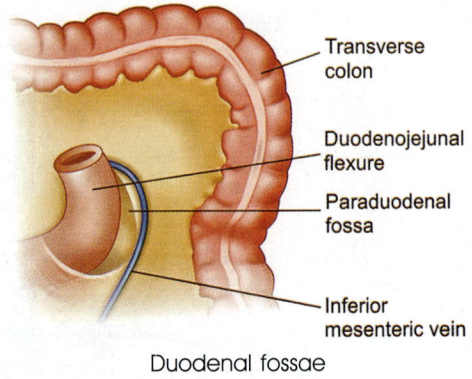

Duodenal fossae

### Clinical Importance

In case of internal herniation, while opening the fossa, surgeon has to be careful of the inferior mesenteric vein in front.

## Superior and Inferior Duodenojejunal Fossa

- These fossae are often present
- They are to the left of duodenum
- Superior fossa looks downwards, is 2–3 cm in depth and is in front of L2 vertebra
- Inferior fossa looks upwards and lies in front of L3.

## Inferior Duodenal Fossa

Inferior duodenal fossa is present below the third part of duodenum.

## Mesentericoparietal Fossa of Waldeyer

- Mesentericoparietal fossa of Waldeyer lies behind the superior mesenteric artery close to beginning of jejunum
- The fossa looks to the left
- Superior mesenteric artery lies in front.

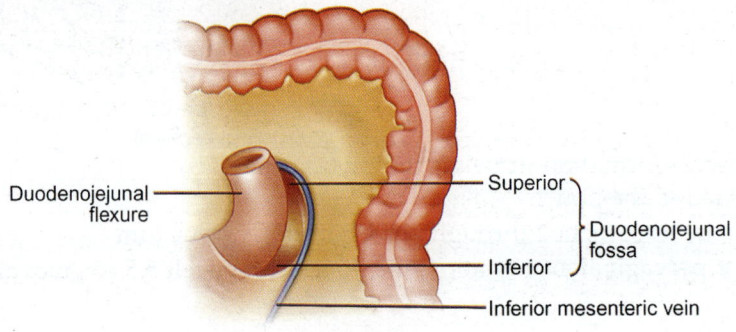

Duodenojejunal fossa

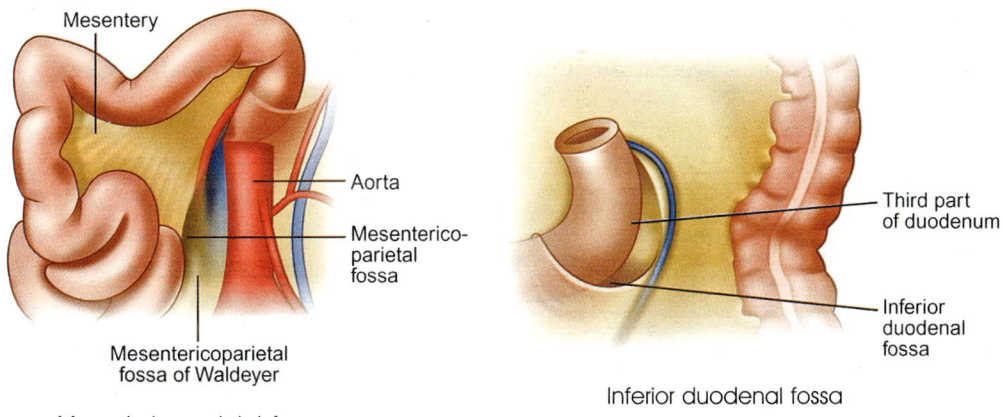

Mesentericoparietal fossa

Inferior duodenal fossa

## Clinical Importance

Surgeon has to be vigilant of superior mesenteric artery, while approaching the fossa.

## TRIANGLES IN ABDOMEN

### Q. Lumbar triangle

**Ans.** Lumbar triangle is also known as Petit's triangle.

### Boundaries

- Laterally—posterior border of external oblique
- Medially—lateral and lower margin of latissimus dorsi
- Base—iliac crest.

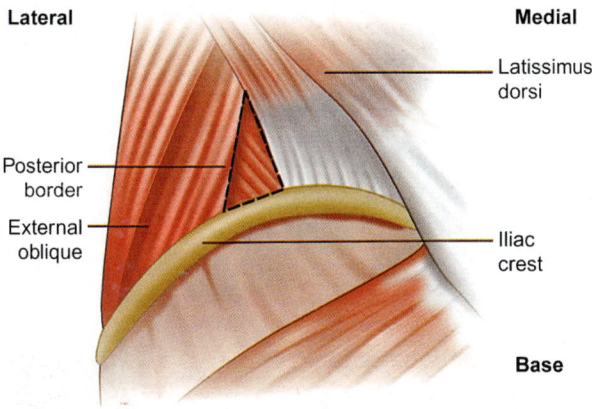

Lumbar triangle

## Clinical Importance

Petit hernia or lumbar hernia may occasionally occur here.

## Q. Hesselbach's triangle

**Ans.** Hesselbach's triangle is seen at the inner surface of anterior abdominal wall.

### Boundaries

- Lateral—inferior epigastric artery
- Medial—outer border of rectus abdominis
- Base—inguinal ligament.

### Divisions

Hesselbach's triangle is divided into medial and lateral parts by obliterated umbilical ligament (lateral umbilical ligament).

### Clinical Importance

Direct inguinal hernia leaves the abdominal cavity through this triangle.

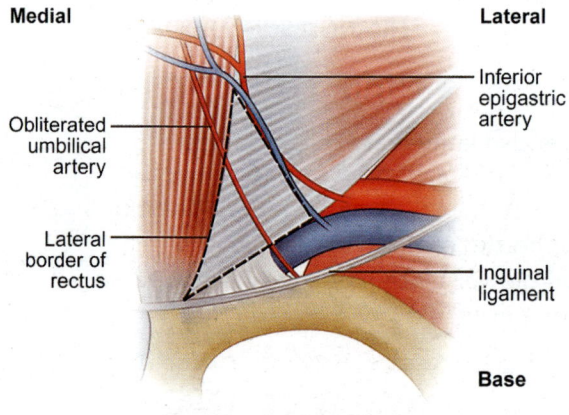

Hesselbach's triangle

## Q. Calot's triangle

**Ans.** A triangle can be identified, while doing cholecystectomy (removal of gallbladder), following are the boundaries of Calot's triangle.

### Boundaries

- Left—common hepatic duct
- Right—cystic duct
- Above—liver.

### Contents

- Cystic artery
- Right hepatic artery.

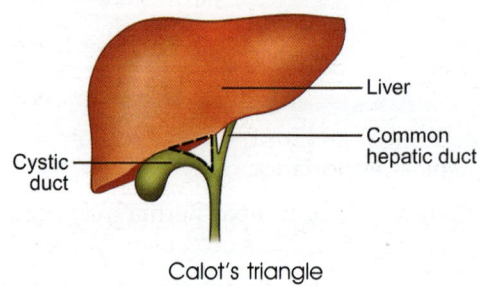

Calot's triangle

## Clinical Importance

- While doing cholecystectomy surgeon has to be aware of the variations of the vessels in Calot's triangle
- While performing cholecystectomy dissection can begin from Calot's triangle.

## ARTERIES

### Q. Celiac trunk

**Ans.** Celiac trunk is the artery of foregut supplying lower part of esophagus, stomach, upper part of duodenum, liver, spleen and pancreas.

## Origin

Arises from front of aorta at the level between T12 and L1 vertebra.

## Main Branches

Celiac trunk is a short trunk, which soon divides into following main branches:
- Left gastric artery
- Common hepatic artery
- Splenic artery.

## Relations

- Surrounded by celiac plexus
- Front—lesser sac, lesser omentum
- Right—right crus of diaphragm, right celiac ganglion, liver
- Left—left crus of diaphragm, left celiac ganglion, stomach
- Inferior—pancreas, splenic vein.

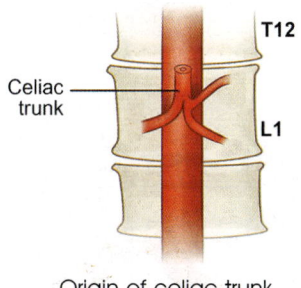

Origin of celiac trunk

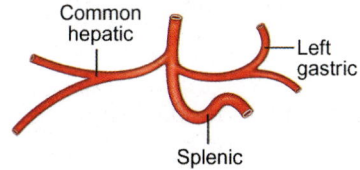

Main branches of celiac trunk

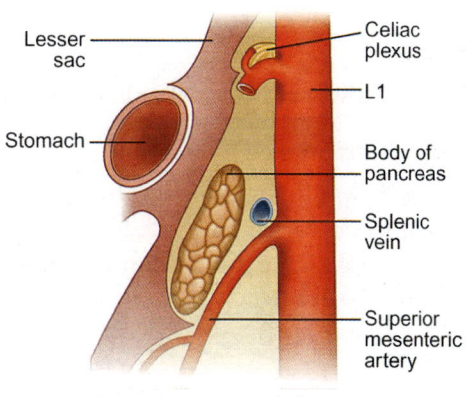

Relations of celiac trunk

## Subdivisions of Main Branches

- Left gastric artery—esophageal branches
- Common hepatic artery—right gastric, gastroduodenal, hepatic artery proper
- Splenic artery—left epiploic, short gastric, arteria pancreatica magna.

## Clinical Importance

Sometimes the origin of celiac trunk may get compressed by median arcuate ligament, giving rise to median arcuate ligament syndrome. Commonly seen in women, wherein blood supply to abdominal viscera may get compromised causing severe epigastric pain following food intake.

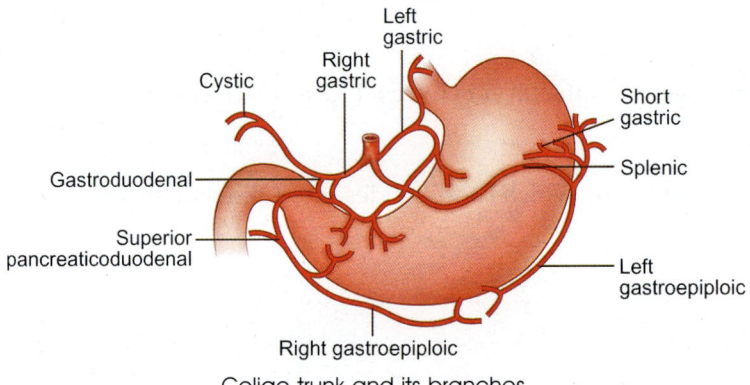

Celiac trunk and its branches

## Q. Superior mesenteric artery

**Ans.** Superior mesenteric artery is the artery of midgut. The artery supplies the portion of the gut from the entrance of bile duct to a level just proximal to splenic flexure of colon.

## Origin

Front of aorta, at the level of L1 vertebra.

## Course

Curved towards the right side (like a sword).

## Clinical Importance

- Pressure of the artery on the renal vein can give rise to left sided varicocele
- Pressure on the duodenum will give rise to symptoms of intestinal obstruction.

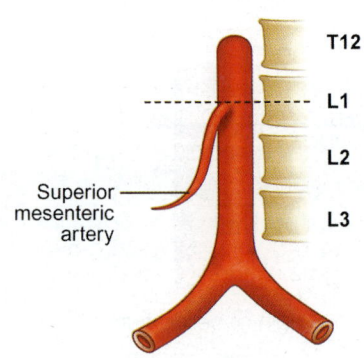

Superior mesenteric artery

## Relations

- Front: Splenic vein, body of pancreas
- Behind: Left renal vein, uncinate process of pancreas, third part of the duodenum

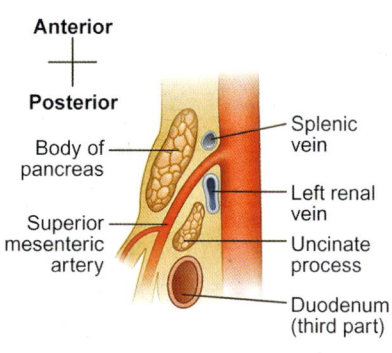

Relations of superior mesenteric artery

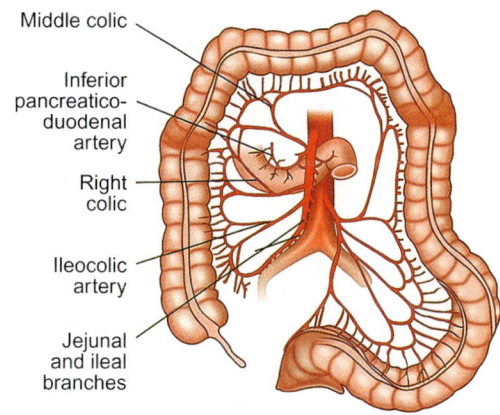

Branches of superior mesenteric artery

- Right: Superior mesenteric vein
- Left: Root of mesentery.

## Branches

- Inferior pancreaticoduodenal
- Jejunal and ileal branches
- Ileocolic
- Right colic
- Middle colic.

### Q. Differences between the vascular arcades of jejunum and ileum

**Ans.** To differentiate between the jejunum and ileum; arrangement and number of vascular arcades (windows) may provide guidance during surgery.

| Parts | Jejunum | Ileum |
|---|---|---|
| Vascular arcades | 1 or 2 | 3–5 |
| Vasa recta | Long and few | Short and many |

*Note:* As you go distally in the gut the number and density of arterial arcades increases.

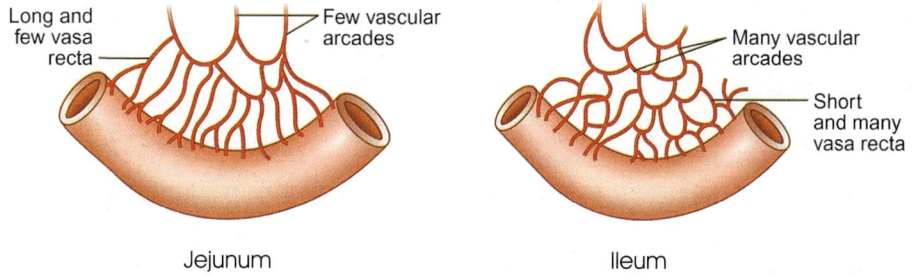

Jejunum  Ileum

## Q. Inferior mesenteric artery

**Ans.** Inferior mesenteric artery is the artery of hind-gut. It supplies the left one-third of transverse colon, descending colon, sigmoid colon and proximal part of anal canal above the pectinate line.

### Origin

- Front of aorta at the level of L3
- Proximal to bifurcation of aorta by 3.8 cm.

### Course

Inferior mesenteric artery runs downwards to the left retroperitoneally.

Origin at L3

T12
L1
L2
L3

Inferior mesenteric artery

### Relations

- Behind—left common iliac artery
- Lateral—ureter, inferior mesenteric vein.

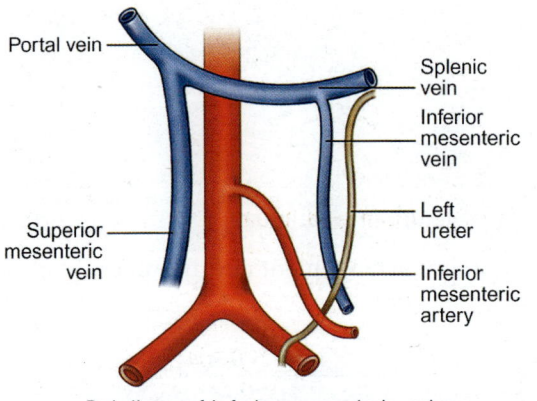

Portal vein
Splenic vein
Inferior mesenteric vein
Superior mesenteric vein
Left ureter
Inferior mesenteric artery

Relations of inferior mesenteric artery

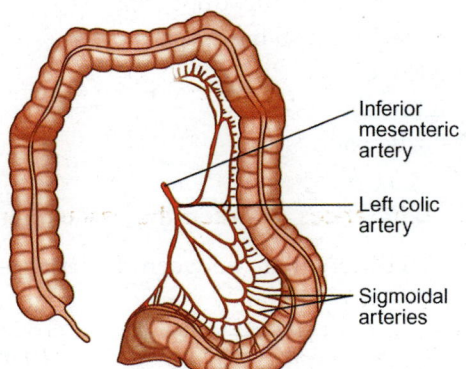

Inferior mesenteric artery
Left colic artery
Sigmoidal arteries

Branches of inferior mesenteric artery

### Branches

- Left colic
- Sigmoids
- Superior rectal
- Inferior mesenteric artery continues as superior rectal artery.

### Clinical Importance

High ligation (to tie) of the artery is indicated in cases of cancer of sigmoid colon or rectum.

## Q. Marginal artery

**Ans.** Marginal artery is a paracolic vessel under the arch of colon, formed by the anastomosis between the branches of colic arteries.

### Extent

Extends from ascending colon to end of pelvic colon.

### Branches

Vasa recta are the terminal arteries to colon forming arterial arcades below the arch of colon.

### Clinical Importance

Integrity of vasa recta may be crucial to maintain blood supply of bowel when the mesenteric arteries are ligated.

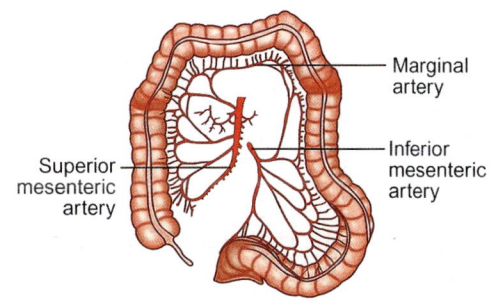

Marginal artery

---

**Q. Branches of internal iliac artery (diagram only)**

**Ans.**

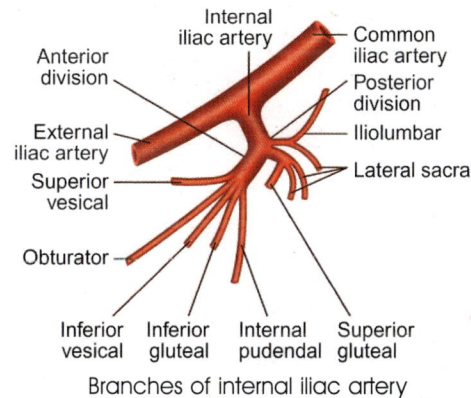

Branches of internal iliac artery

## LYMPHATICS

**Q. Cisterna chyli**

**Ans.** Cisterna chyli is a lymph sac from which the thoracic duct begins.

### Location

Lies in front of L1 and L2.

### Relations

Lies between aorta, right crus of diaphragm and inferior vena cava.

### Tributaries

- Right lumbar trunk
- Left lumbar trunk
- Intestinal trunk.

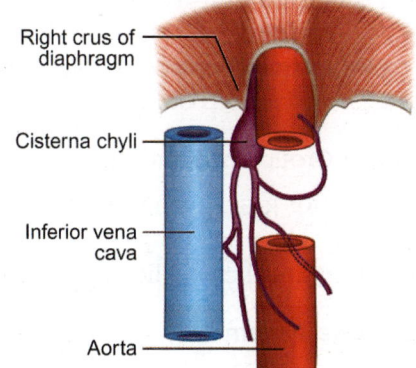

## Drainage Areas
- Lumbar trunks drain the lymph from lower limbs, pelvic viscera, kidney, adrenals and abdominal walls
- Intestinal lymph trunk drains lymph from stomach, pancreas, spleen, most of liver and intestines.

### Q. Lymphatic drainage of stomach

**Ans.** The knowledge of lymphatic drainage of stomach is very important in managing gastric cancer. Stomach is divided into three lymphatic territories similar to the vascular territories of celiac artery.

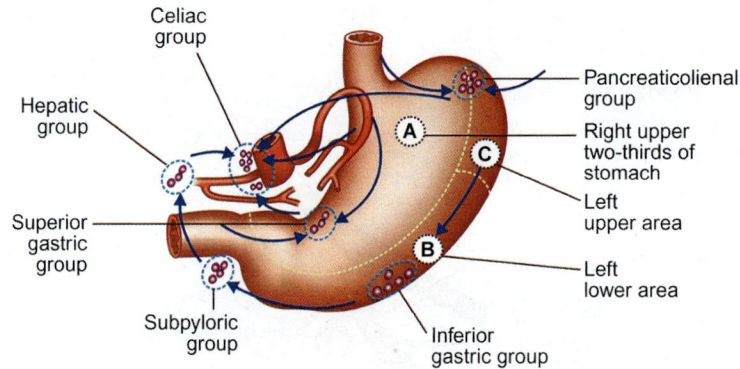

Lymphatic drainage of stomach

## Divisions of Lymphatic Areas
There are three territories identified on the stomach:
- Right: Two-thirds, upper area along the lesser curvature of stomach
- Left: Lower one-third, area along greater curvature of stomach
- Left upper area close to the spleen
- The efferents of all the lymph of stomach goes to celiac group of lymph nodes.

## Lymph Groups of Stomach
- Hepatic group—lies in lesser omentum, receives lymph from liver and gallbladder
- Subpyloric group—lie in the angle between first and second part of duodenum, close to the bifurcation of gastroduodenal artery, receives lymph through inferior gastric nodes draining right two-thirds of lesser curvature of stomach.

## Lymph Groups of Stomach
- Superior gastric group—close to the cardiac end of stomach
- Inferior gastric group—close to the pylorus within the layers of greater omentum
- Pancreaticolienal—lie along the splenic artery.

## Drainage Pattern
- Lesser curvature of stomach is drained by superior gastric nodes and finally celiac nodes

- Region close to pylorus drains into inferior gastric nodes, thence to subpyloric and then to celiac nodes
- Upper gastric area close to the spleen is drained by pancreaticolienal nodes and finally into celiac nodes.

## Clinical Importance

While operating cases of cancer stomach, surgeon has to be aware of the drainage pattern of lymph nodes to clear all those lymphatic areas likely to get involved.

### Q. Lymphatic drainage of rectum

**Ans.** The lymph from the rectum is drained by various lymphatic groups thus cancer can spread in various directions.

## Lymph Groups Involved

- Inguinal group
- Internal iliac group
- Sacral group
- Left common iliac group.

## Efferent Lymph Vessels of Rectum

- Downwards to involve perianal skin, ischiorectal fossa, external anal sphincter
- Laterally involves levator ani muscles, urinary bladder, seminal vesicles (in females involves vagina, cervix and base of broad ligament)

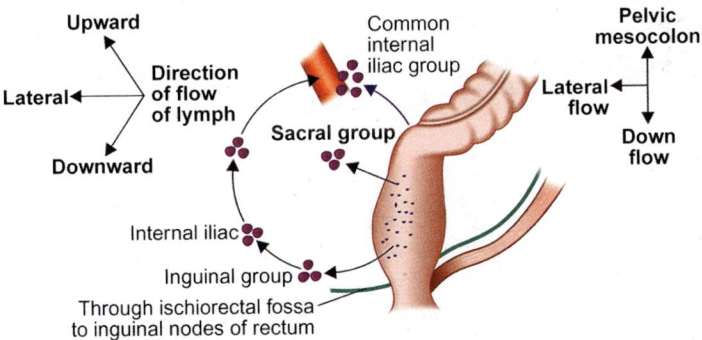

Lymphatic drainage of rectum

- Upwards involves pelvic peritoneum, pelvic mesocolon and nodes close to inferior mesenteric artery.

## Clinical Importance

- Cancer of rectum can spread along these lymphatic channels and secondary involvement can be seen in these areas
- The surgeries in cancer rectum, may mandate removal of pelvic colon with mesocolon, rectum, anus, perianal skin, ischiorectal fossa (fat filled) and levator ani with the fascia.

## NERVES

Autonomic nervous system is concerned with innervations of viscera, glands, blood vessels and smooth muscles.

### Q. Urinary bladder innervation

**Ans.**

### General Features

- The nerves supplying the bladder comprises of sympathetic and parasympathetic components
- These nerves form the vesical plexus
- Both efferent and afferent components are present in sympathetic and parasympathetic fibres.

### Bladder Innervation

- Parasympathetic nerve fibres arise from S2, S3, S4 segments of the spinal cord (nervi erigentes)
- Sympathetic fibres arise from T11, T12, L1 and L2 segments of spinal cord
- Parasympathetic fibres are excitatory to detrusor muscle and inhibitory to sphincter urethrae
- Sympathetic nerves have vice versa function, i.e. inhibitory to detrusor and excitatory to sphincter urethrae
- The pudendal nerve supplies the skeletal muscle, sphincter urethrae.

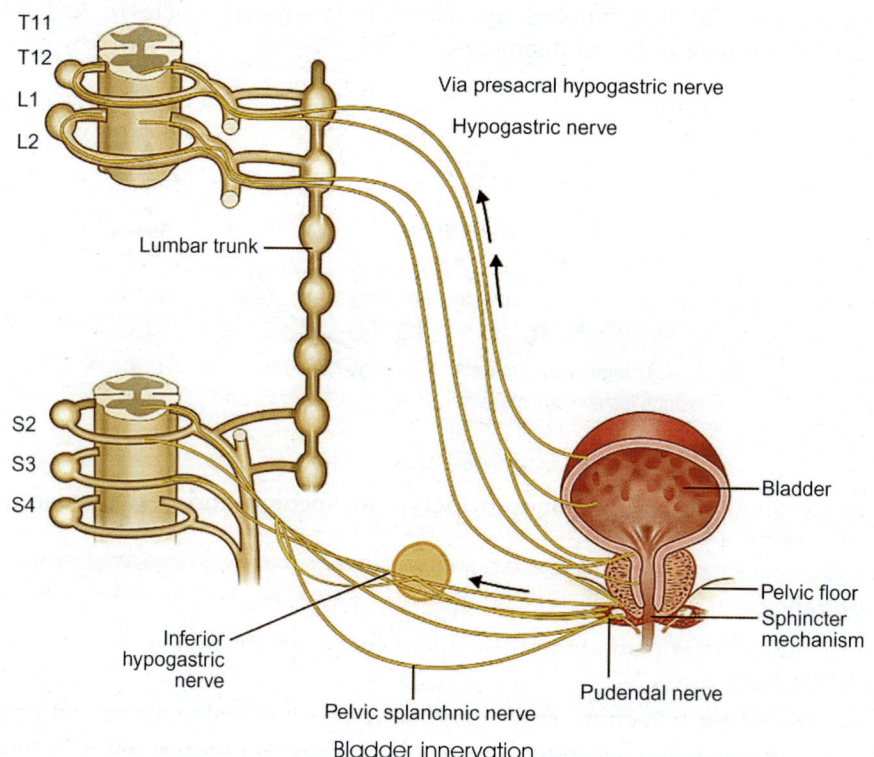

Bladder innervation

## Functional Aspects

1. Normal emptying of the bladder occurs by contraction of detrusor muscle and simultaneous relaxation of urethral sphincter and pelvic floor.
2. Accumulation of urine initially adjusts the tone and then stimulates the stretch receptors, which carry the afferent sensation along pelvic splanchnic nerve to the sacral segments ( S2, S3, S4).
3. Parasympathetic cell bodies when stimulated, efferent impulses flow down through pelvic splanchnic nerve to postganglionic cells within the bladder and cause bladder contraction.
4. This is autonomic stretch reflex.
5. With training, higher centres in brain, i.e. inferior frontal gyrus takes control over the spinal stretch reflex. This centre has an inhibitory activity.

## Clinical Importance

- In spinal cord section above S2, the cortical control is lost and sacral reflex is intact and bladder automatically empties on distension.
- If the sacral segments itself are not functional the detrusor muscle is paralyzed and the bladder distends, but emptying is not possible leading to urinary incontinence.

## SACRAL PLEXUS

### Layout of Sacral Plexus

- *Formation:* Pelvic ventral rami of S1, S2, S3, S4. These ventral rami emerge through pelvic sacral foramina.
- *Location:* Ventral rami unite in front of piriformis; on lower part of greater sciatic foramen (S5, C1 pierce sacrococcygeal ligament).
- *Relations*
  - Between L5, S1 are superior gluteal vessels
  - Below S1 are the inferior gluteal vessels
  - Posteriorly related to piriformis, sacroiliac joint
  - Anteriorly are the internal pudendal vessels.
- *Branches*
  - Muscular to piriformis, coccygeus, levator ani
  - Pelvic splanchnic S2, S3, S4 to inferior hypogastric plexus
  - Each ventral rami receives gray rami communicans.
- *Terminal branches*
  - Sciatic nerve
  - Pudendal nerve.

Labels: Lumbosacral trunk, Superior gluteal artery, Levator ani, S1, S2, S3, S4, Inferior gluteal artery

## Q. Nerve plexuses on posterior abdominal wall (diagram only)

**Ans.**

a. Celiac plexus
b. Left aortorenal plexus
c. Inferior mesenteric plexus

d. Superior mesenteric plexus
e. Inferior hypogastric plexus

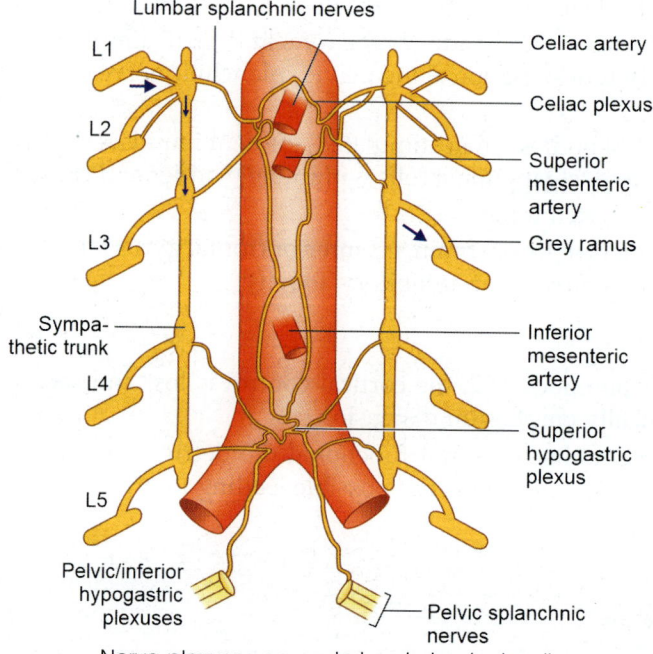

Nerve plexuses on posterior abdominal wall

## MISCELLANEOUS

### COMMON ABDOMINAL INCISIONS

• Mainly two types
  a. Midline
  b. Paramedian

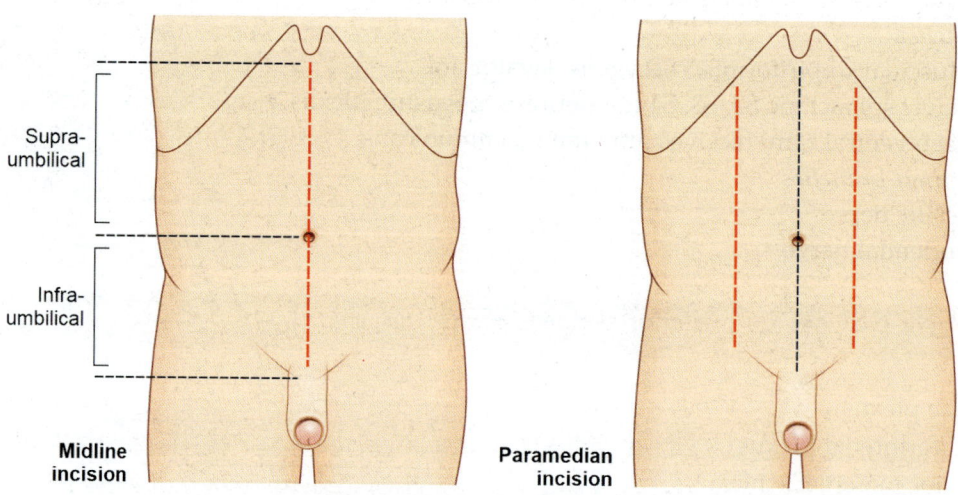

| Midline incision | Paramedian |
|---|---|
| • Divides skin, linea alba, fascia transversalis, extraperitoneal fat peritoneum | • Incision divides skin, anterior and posterior rectus sheath, fascia transversalis, extra-peritoneal fat |
| • Avascular, also nerves do not come in way of incision | • Neurovascular bundle will come in way of incision |
| • Postoperative weakness, wound healing not good (infraumbilical linea alba thick closely intervening, ventral hernia rare) | • Good wound healing and less chance of post-operative weakness |

## Q. Regions of abdomen (diagram only)

Ans.

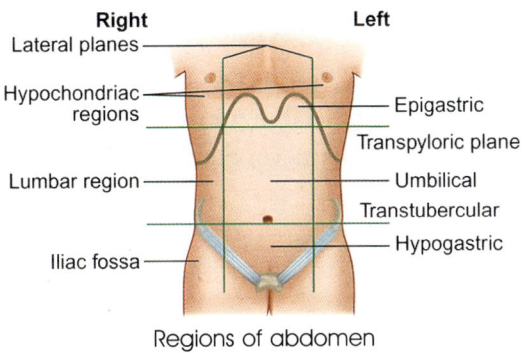

Regions of abdomen

## Q. Inguinal ligament

Ans. The lower border of external oblique aponeurosis folds upon itself to form the inguinal ligament.

### Location

Lies beneath the fold of groin.

### Extent

Anterior superior iliac spine to pubic tubercle.

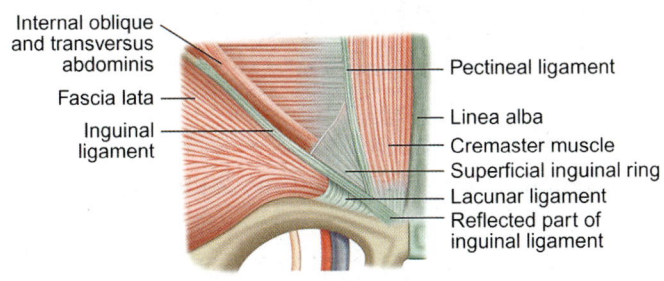

Extensions of inguinal ligament

## Structures Attached to the Ligament

- Fascia lata is attached to outer lower border, thus is convex downwards
- Internal oblique and transversus oblique take origin from its upper surface lateral part
- Cremaster muscle is attached to its middle part.

## Relations

- Medial half forms the floor of inguinal canal
- Spermatic cord in males and round ligament in females is lodged on the superior surface of ligament.

## Extensions

1. *Pectineal part:* It is a triangular extension from the medial part of the ligament, supports the spermatic cord, attached to pubic tubercle medially and laterally supports the inguinal ring.
2. Pectineal ligament (ligament of Cooper): It is the thickening of pectineal fascia and is the extension of lacunar ligament posteriorly.
3. Reflected part of inguinal ligament: It is an extension of lateral crus of inguinal ring medially in front of conjoint tendon and superficial inguinal ring.
4. Lacunar ligament (Gimbernat's ligament), connects inguinal ligament to pectineal ligament close to pubic tubercle.

### Q. Coverings of testis (diagram only)

Ans.

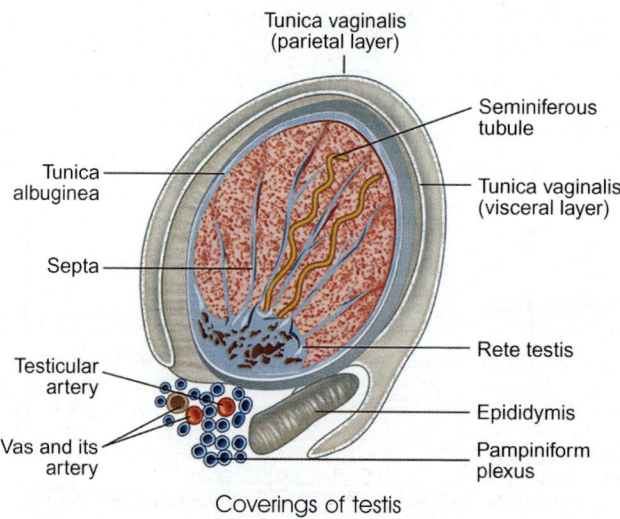

Coverings of testis

### Q. Inguinal canal

Ans. Inguinal canal is an oblique intermuscular slit above the medial half of inguinal ligament, placed horizontally:

- Length: 4 cm
- Extent: Lies between the deep inguinal ring and superficial inguinal ring.

## Boundaries

- Anterior wall-external oblique aponeurosis and assisted laterally by internal oblique muscle

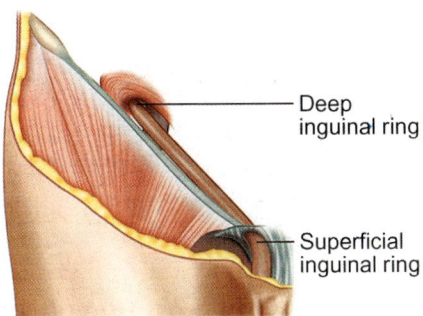

Deep inguinal ring

Superficial inguinal ring

Inguinal canal

- Posterior wall-transversalis fascia, reinforced medially by conjoint tendon
- Floor is the in rolled lower edge of inguinal ligament, strengthened medially by lacunar ligament

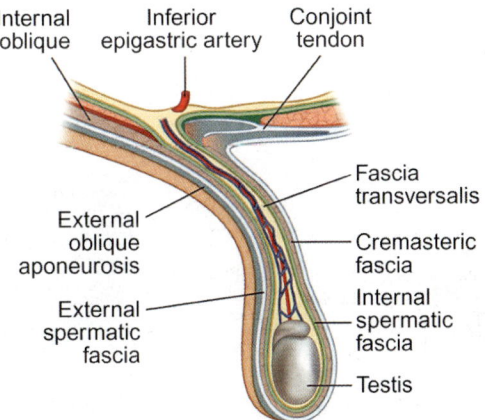

Internal oblique    Inferior epigastric artery    Conjoint tendon

Fascia transversalis

External oblique aponeurosis

Cremasteric fascia

External spermatic fascia

Internal spermatic fascia

Testis

Boundaries of inguinal canal

- Roof arched fibres of internal oblique and transversus abdominis muscle.

## Contents

- *In males:* Spermatic cord, ilioinguinal nerve
- *In females:* Round ligament, ilioinguinal nerve.

## Clinical Importance

- Indirect inguinal hernia occurs through deep inguinal ring lateral to inferior epigastric artery
- Direct inguinal hernia occurs medial to inferior epigastric artery
- Incomplete hernia does not cross superficial inguinal ring.

**Q. Transverse section of penis** (diagram only)

**Ans.**

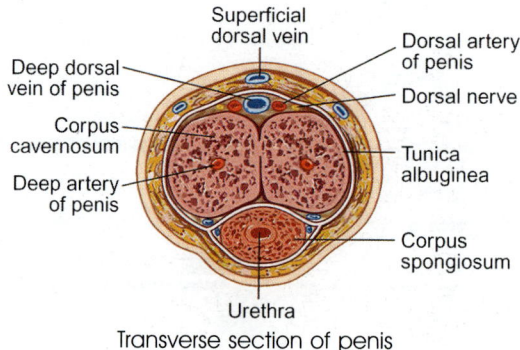

Transverse section of penis

**Q. Spermatic cord**

**Ans.** The spermatic cord lies in the inguinal canal and is well-protected by the coverings around it.

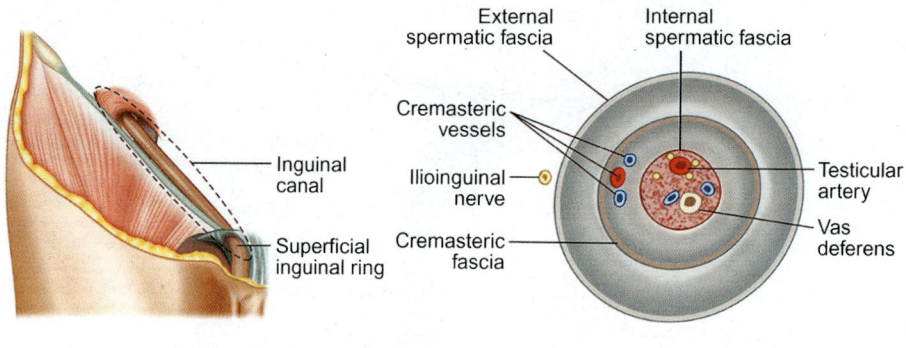

Spermatic cord                    Contents of spermatic cord

Following are the coverings and their derivatives:
- Internal spermatic fascia derived from transversalis fascia
- Cremasteric fascia derived from cremaster muscle
- External spermatic fascia is derived from external oblique aponeurosis.

## Contents
- Vas deferens
- Testicular artery, cremasteric artery, artery to vas
- Pampiniform plexus
- Testicular lymphatics
- Genital branch of genitofemoral nerve
- Processus vaginalis.

## Q. Differences between small and large intestine

**Ans.**

| Features | Small intestine | Large intestine |
|---|---|---|
| Mobility | Freely mobile | More or less fixed |
| Caliber | Large | Small |
| Appendices epiploicae | Absent | Present |
| *Teniae coli* | Absent | Present |
| Sacculations | Absent | Present |
| Villi | Present | Absent |
| Transverse mucosal fold | Permanent | Obliterated |
| Peyer's patches | Present in ileum | Absent |

## Q. Meckel's diverticulum

**Ans.** Normally, the vitellointestinal duct disappears around 6th week of intrauterine life, but if it persists it is known as Meckel's diverticulum.

### Features

- Present in 2% cases
- 2 inches in length
- 2 feet proximal to ileocecal junction
- Present on the antimesenteric border
- Caliber of the diverticulum is equal to ileum
- In 2% cases, accessory pancreatic tissue may be found.

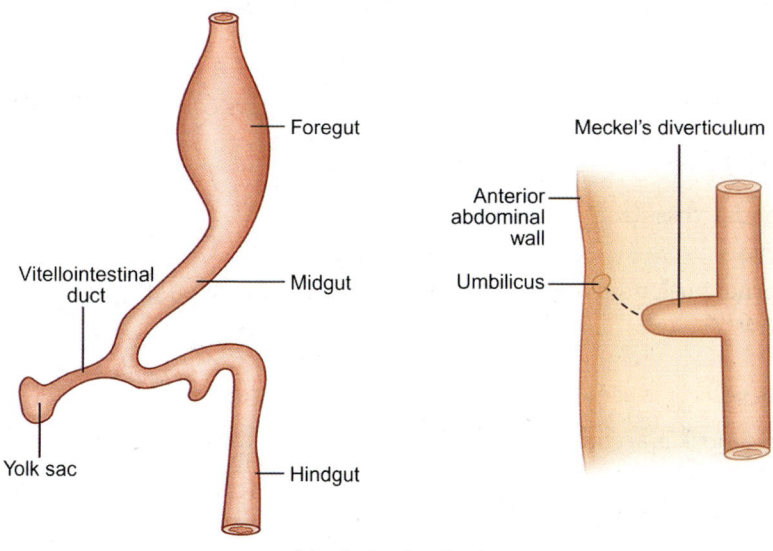

Meckel's diverticulum

## Clinical Importance

- It may cause intestinal obstruction
- Could be site of peptic ulcer
- Acute inflammation may resemble appendicitis
- Tumors may occur in Meckel's diverticulum.

### Q. Pudendal canal

**Ans.** Pudendal canal is also known as Alcock's canal. It runs on the lateral wall of ischiorectal fossa forwards anteriorly.

## Location and Extent

- Pudendal canal is 3.8 cm in length
- Above lower border of ischial tuberosity
- Extends between lesser sciatic foramen posteriorly to perineal membrane anteriorly.

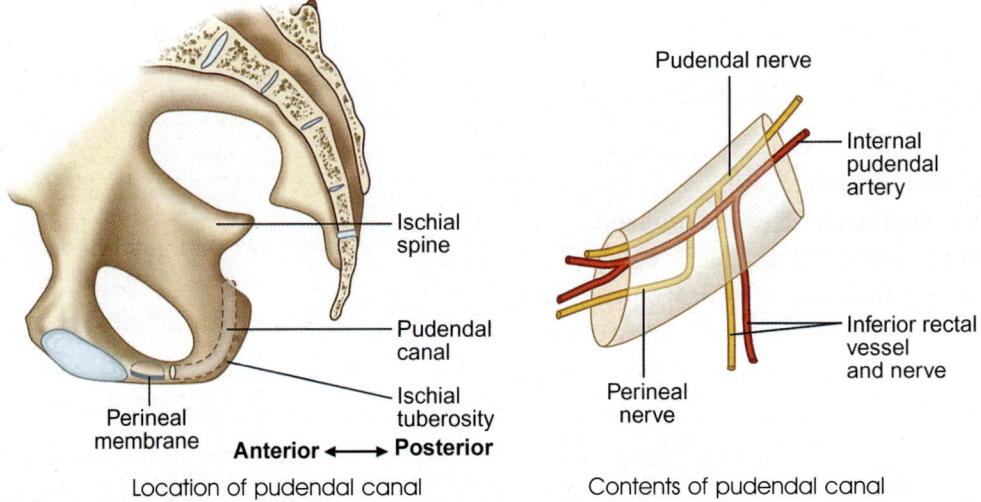

Location of pudendal canal

Contents of pudendal canal

## Contents

- Internal pudendal vessels
- Pudendal nerve
- Branch of internal pudendal artery namely inferior rectal branch (posteriorly) and perineal branch (anteriorly).

## Clinical Importance

- Pudendal nerve block is accomplished by infiltrating local anesthesia where the nerve crosses the ischial spine
- The ischial spine is palpated through vagina.

### Q. Perineal membrane in male (diagram only)

**Ans.** Perineal membrane = inferior fascia of urogenital diaphragm

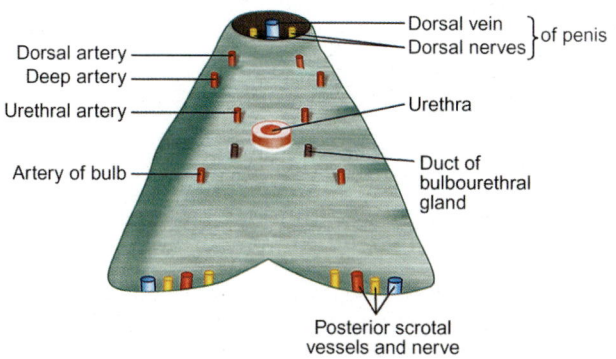

Perineal membrane in male

### PER-RECTAL EXAMINATION

Structures felt in this examination are:

### Common in both Sexes

- Anorectal ring
- Coccyx
- Sacrum
- Ischiorectal fossa
- Ischial spine

*In males:* Anteriorly one can palpate prostate, seminal vesicle, vas deferens
*In females:* Perineal body, cervix

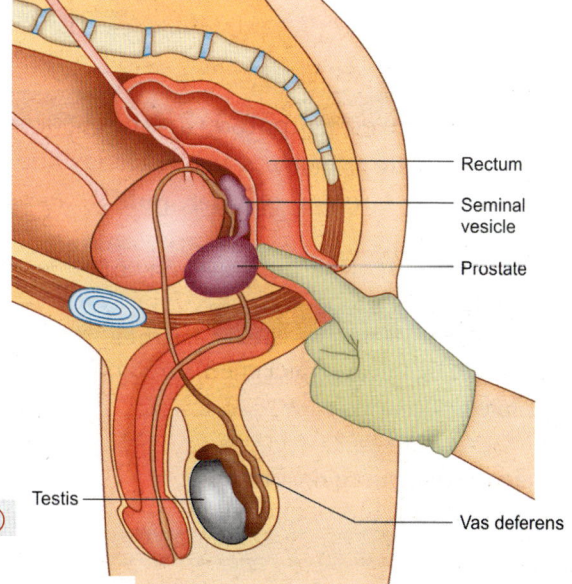

Per-rectal examination

### Q. Perineal membrane in female (diagram only)

**Ans.**

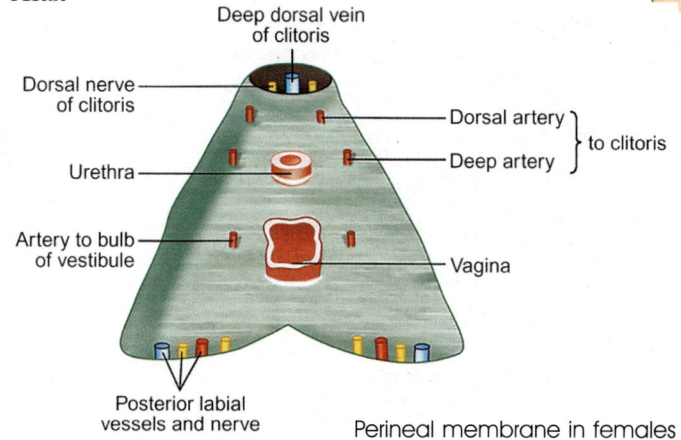

Perineal membrane in females

**Q. Perineal dermatomes (diagram only)**

**Ans.**

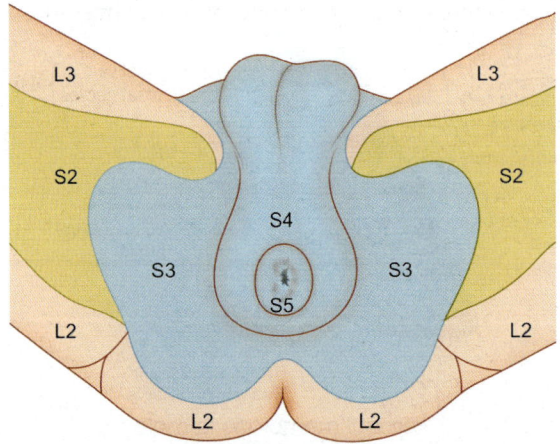

Perineal dermatomes

**Q. Per-vaginal examination**

**Ans.** Structures palpated in this examination are as below:

- Anteriorly: Urethra, bladder, pubic symphysis
- Posteriorly: Rectum, pouch of Douglas
- Laterally: Ovary, uterine tubes, uterine ligaments (thickened), ureters
- *Superiorly:* Cervix.

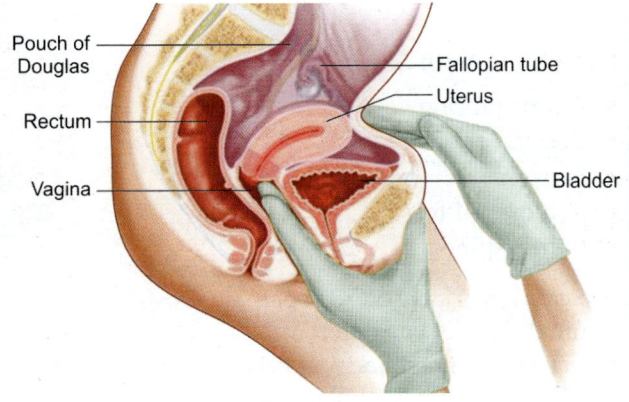

Per-vaginal examination

**Q. Urogenital region of male perineum (coronal section)**

**Ans.**

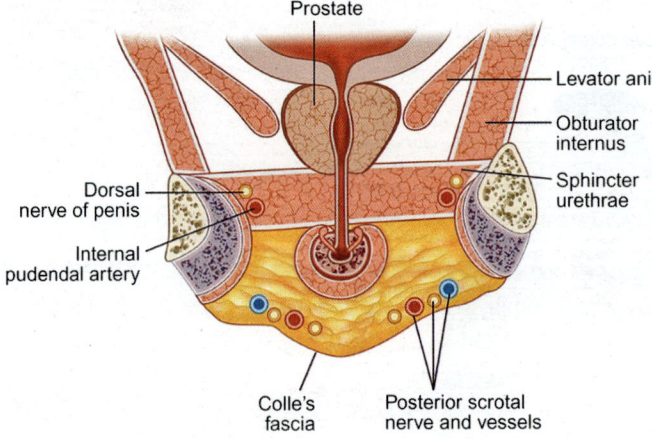

Urogenital region of male perineum

## Q. Urogenital region of female perineum (coronal section)

**Ans.**

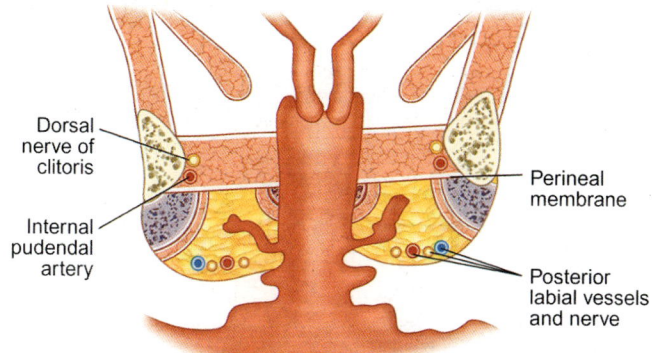

Dorsal nerve of clitoris

Internal pudendal artery

Perineal membrane

Posterior labial vessels and nerve

Urogenital region of female perineum

## Q. Stomach bed

**Ans.** The posterior relations of stomach comprise the stomach bed. Group of structures lying behind the stomach constitutes stomach bed.

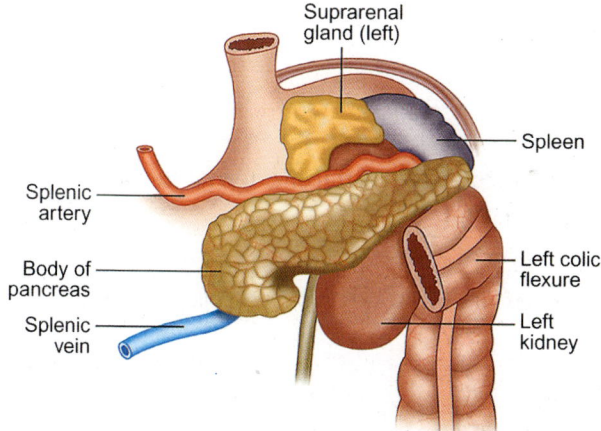

Suprarenal gland (left)

Spleen

Splenic artery

Body of pancreas

Splenic vein

Left colic flexure

Left kidney

Stomach bed

*Following structures form stomach bed:*
- Anterior wall of lesser sac, covers the posterior wall of stomach
- Bed is covered by the lesser sac's posterior wall
- Left crus and dome of diaphragm
- Splenic artery
- Body of pancreas
- Transverse mesocolon
- Upper part of left kidney
- Left suprarenal gland
- Spleen
- Left colic flexure.

## Q. Posterior relations of cecum

**Ans.**

Posterior relations of cecum assume importance due to the surgical cases of appendicitis especially when the appendix is retrocecal.

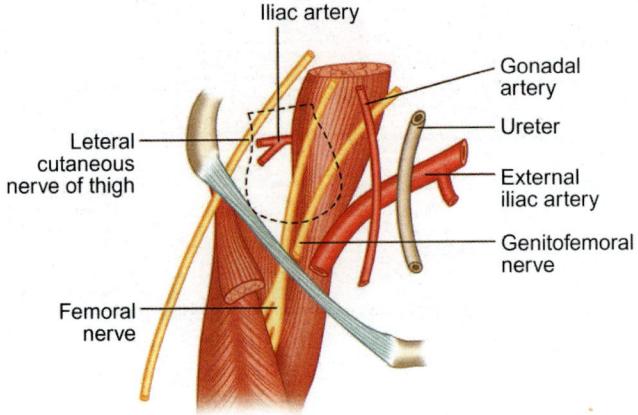

Posterior relations of cecum

- Right psoas and iliacus
- Right genitofemoral nerve
- Right femoral nerve
- Right lateral cutaneous nerve of thigh
- Right gonadal vessels (testicular or ovarian), external iliac artery
- Appendix in retrocecal position.

## Q. Anterior impressions of right and left kidneys (diagram only)

**Ans.**

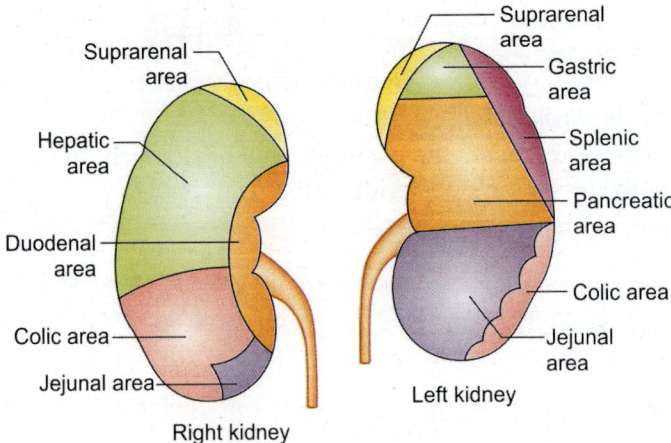

Anterior impressions of right and left kidneys

**Q. Posterior relations of kidney** (diagram only)

**Ans.** The posterior relations of right and left kidney are common.

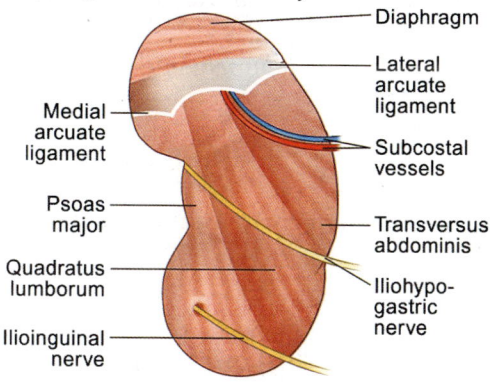

Posterior relations of kidney

**Q. Visceral relations on inferior surface of liver**

**Ans.**

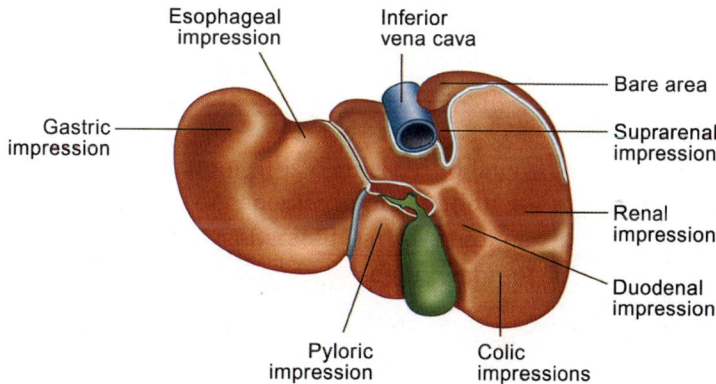

Visceral relations on inferior surface of liver

**Q. Anatomical and surgical importance of pectinate line.**

**Ans.** The dentate line represents the former site of embryonic anal membrane. At the dentate line transverse folds of mucosa form ring of anal valves above which are the anal sinuses. Anal glands open in the anal sinuses wherein anal abscesses and fistula develop.

Following is the anatomical and surgical importance of pectinate line:
- It is an embryological watershed between visceral structures above and somatic structures below.
- Mucosa above has autonomic nerve supply thus insensitive to pain, while skin below is supplied by inferior rectal branch sensitive to pain and other stimuli.
- Venous drainage above is to portal circulation, while below is to systemic venous circulation.
- Lymphatic drainage above the pectinate line goes to iliac group of lymph nodes and below to inguinal group.

- Internal hemorrhoids develop above the dentate line.
- Infection in anal gland may lead to anal abscess formation.
- A midline crack or fissure in the wall of anal canal is associated with severe pain during defecation.
- Stimulation of nerve endings around the dentate line may lead to voluntary changes in the tone of sphincters.

### Q. Holden's line

The superficial fascia of thigh and abdomen are continuous with each other and made-up of two layers. The two layers are:

1. Superficial fatty layer
2. Deep membranous layer.

The membranous layer is loosely attached over the deep fascia of the thigh except in the region of inguinal ligament.

In the region of inguinal ligament, the membranous layer is firmly attached to the deep fascia. This line of firm attachment is known as Holden's line.

#### Clinical Importance

In bladder injuries, extravasation of urine occurs between membranous layer and deep fascia of abdomen, however the urine cannot go down in the thigh due the Holden's line.

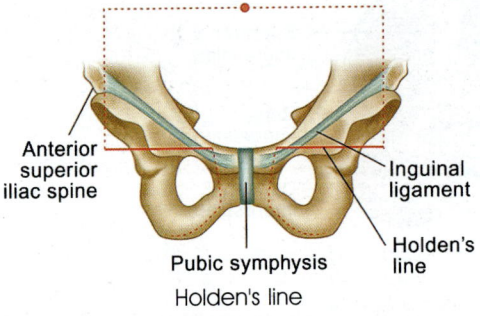

Holden's line

### MCBURNEY'S POINT

- An imaginary line is drawn joining umbilicus to anteriosuperior iliac spine.
- The point lies at the junction of lateral 1/3rd and medial 2/3rd of the line.

#### Clinical Significance

- It is the classical sign of greatest tenderness in appendicitis.
- It is the point which guides the surgeon for taking the grid-iron incision in appendicectomy.

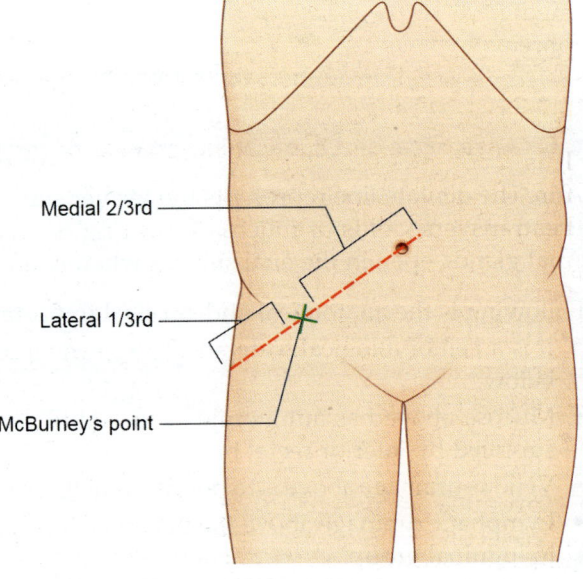

## MURPHY'S SIGN

It is elicited in patients of acute cholecystitis (inflammation of gallbladder). Patient has pain and will catch the breath at the zenith of inspiration in right hypochondrium; while the surgeon is trying to palpate enlarged gallbladder. This is described as Murphy's sign.

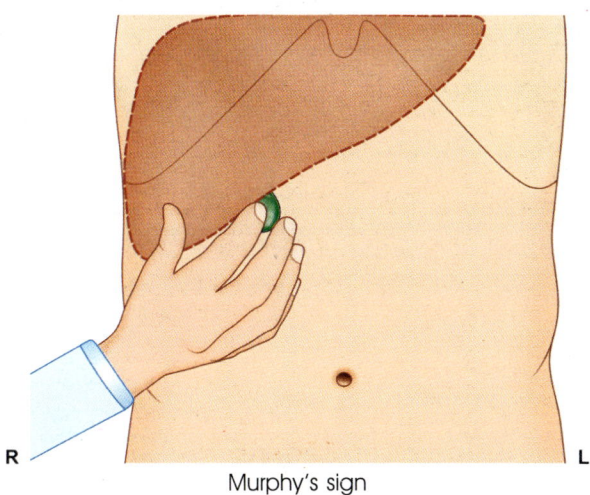

R           Murphy's sign          L

## KEHR'S SIGN

In cases of splenic rupture. Patient feels pain in left shoulder. This is Kehr's sign.

### Anatomical Basis

In splenic rupture, blood lies in contact of under surface of diaphragm. This acts as an irritant to the phrenic nerve supplying motor fibres to diaphragm. Pain is mediated through the afferent fibres of phrenic nerve to the shoulder tip.

## PHIMOSIS

It is a condition characterised by tight foreskin and cannot be pulled back on head of penis.

### Circumcision

- It is a surgical procedure wherein redundant (extra) skin of prepuce is excised.
- Unduly long foreskin of prepuce may lead to pain, swelling and redness of prepuce (= Balanitis); it could be congenital or acquired.

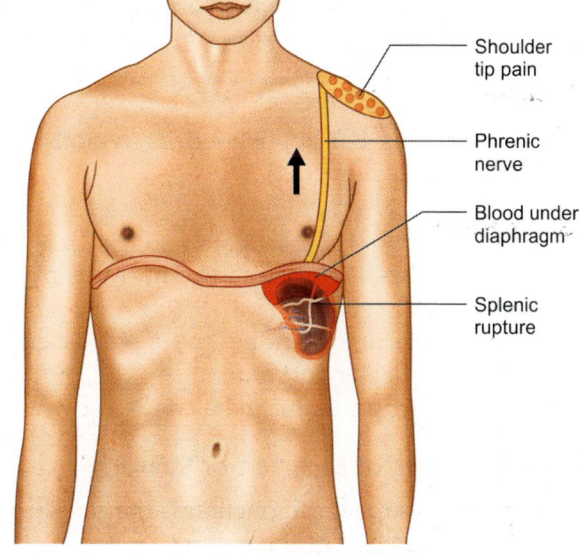

Shoulder tip pain

Phrenic nerve

Blood under diaphragm

Splenic rupture

Kehr's sign

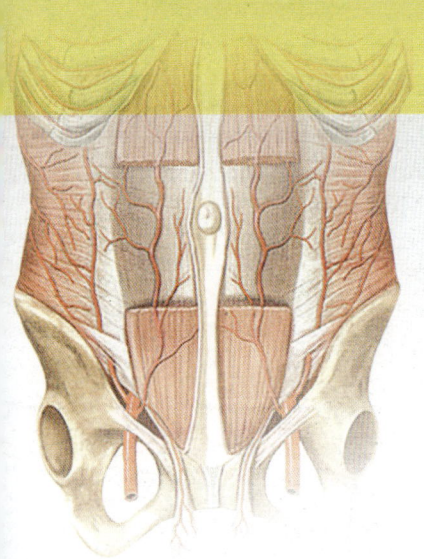

# Key Long Questions 19

## ORGANS

The student should know any organ under following headings—location, gross features, relations, (peritoneal, visceral) blood supply, lymphatic drainage and clinical importance.

### Q. Stomach

**Ans.** Stomach is the most dilated part of the alimentary canal, lying between esophagus and duodenum. The stomach has a variable shape depending upon the volume of fluid or water in stomach. The position of stomach varies depending upon erect or supine position.

### Location

Occupies mainly left hypochondriac region, epigastric and umbilical region.

### Gross Features

- Size 10 inches, approximately 1.5 litres capacity in adult (30 mL at birth)
- Parts: Cardiac end, fundus, body, pyloric end, lesser curvature, greater curvature
- Mucosa of empty stomach has folds known as rugae.

### Salient Features of Each Part of Stomach

- The gastroesophageal junction is the cardia:
    - Most fixed part of the organ
    - Lies 2.5 cm to the left of midline
    - At T10 vertebra
    - Behind seventh left costal cartilage
    - 40 cm from incisor tooth.

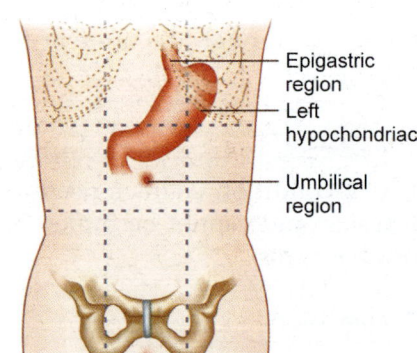

Location of stomach

- The gastroduodenal junction is the pylorus:
  - Fundus is the part of stomach above the cardia of stomach
  - Body is the largest part of stomach lying between fundus and notch along lesser curvature known as angular incisures
  - Greater curvature gives attachment to greater omentum, while, lesser curvature gives attachment to lesser omentum
  - Pylorus extends from angular notch to gastroduodenal junction. It can be subdivided into two parts proximal pyloric antrum and distal pyloric canal. Distal palpable circular muscle on the pyloric canal is known as pyloric sphincter.

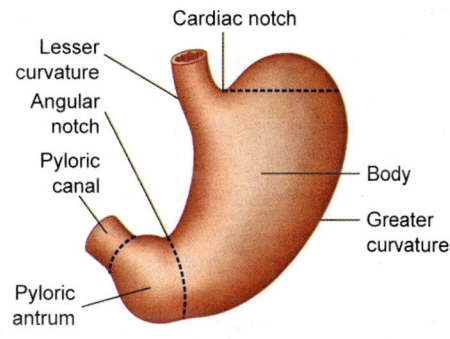

Parts of stomach

## Relations

Relations can be classified into peritoneal and visceral relations.

### Peritoneal Relations

- Stomach is completely invested by peritoneum except near cardiac end
- Double layer of fold, lesser omentum extends between lesser curvature and liver
- Another fold of peritoneum hangs down from the fundus and the greater curvature of stomach as greater omentum.

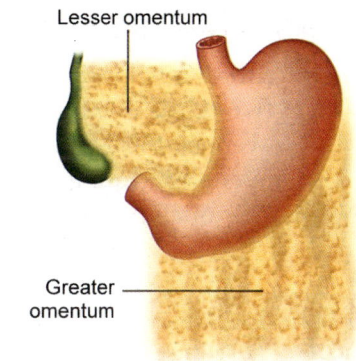

### Visceral Relations

- Anterior surface of stomach is related to liver on the right, diaphragm to the left and anterior abdominal wall in the middle
- Posterior surface is related to the structures that form the stomach bed. Following structures form stomach bed
- Anterior wall of lesser sac covers the posterior wall of stomach
- Bed is covered by the lesser sac's posterior wall
- Left crus and dome of diaphragm
- Splenic artery
- Body of pancreas
- Transverse mesocolon
- Upper part of left kidney
- Left suprarenal gland
- Spleen
- Left colic flexure.

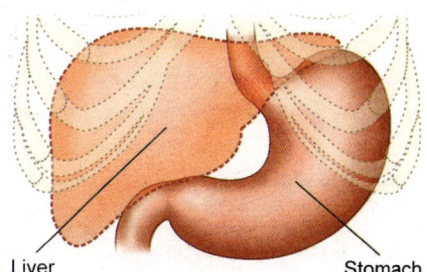

Anterior relations of stomach

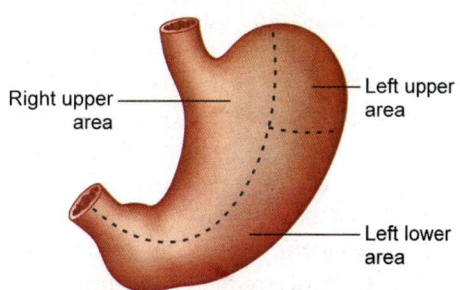

Lymphatic drainage areas

## Blood Supply

1. Stomach receives its blood supply from branches of celiac artery.
2. The branches supplying stomach are right and left gastric arteries, right and left gastroepiploic artery and short gastric arteries.
3. Venous drainage goes to portal vein, superior mesenteric vein and splenic vein.

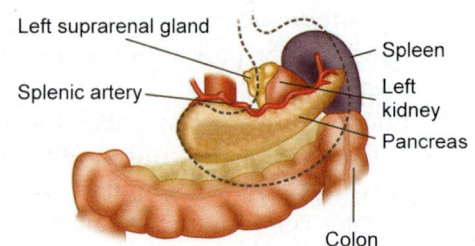

Stomach bed

## Lymphatic Drainage

Stomach is divided into three lymphatic territories similar to the vascular territories of celiac artery.

## Divisions of Lymphatic Areas

There are three territories identified on the stomach:
1. Right two-thirds upper area, along the lesser curvature of stomach
2. Left lower one-third area, along greater curvature of stomach
3. Left upper area, close to the spleen

The efferents of all the lymph of stomach goes to celiac group of lymph nodes.

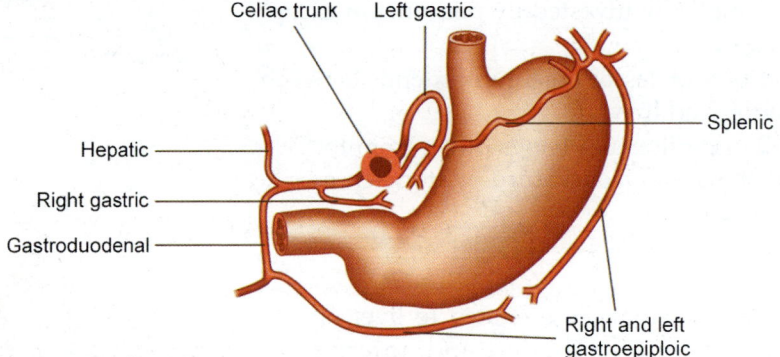

Arterial supply of stomach

## Lymph Groups of Stomach

- *Hepatic group:* Lies in lesser omentum, receives lymph from liver and gallbladder
- *Subpyloric group:* Lies in the angle between first and second part of duodenum, close to the bifurcation of gastroduodenal artery, receives lymph through inferior gastric nodes draining right two-thirds of lesser curvature of stomach
- *Superior gastric group:* Close to the cardiac end of stomach
- *Inferior gastric group:* Close to the pylorus within the layers of greater omentum
- *Pancreaticolienal:* Lies along the splenic artery.

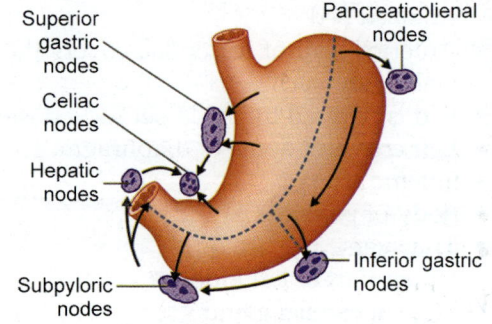

Lymph groups of stomach

## Drainage Pattern

- Lesser curvature of stomach is drained by superior gastric nodes and finally celiac nodes
- Region close to pylorus drains into inferior gastric nodes, thence to subpyloric and then to celiac nodes
- Upper gastric area close to the spleen is drained by pancreaticolienal nodes and finally into celiac nodes.

## Clinical Importance

- Gastric disturbance gives rise to symptoms like anorexia, nausea, vomiting known as dyspepsia.
- Peptic ulcer occurs typically along lesser curvature of stomach.
- Gastric carcinoma occurs along greater curvature of stomach.
- While operating cases of cancer stomach, surgeon has to be aware of the drainage pattern of lymph nodes to clear all those lymphatic areas likely to get involved.
- Hypertrophic pyloric stenosis, causes pyloric obstruction in an infant, which needs surgical intervention wherein the pyloric musculature is incised (Ramstedt's operation).

## Q. Duodenum

**Ans.** Duodenum is the shortest, widest and most fixed part of small intestine, forming a C-shaped curve around the head of pancreas. It extends from the pylorus to duodenojejunal flexure.

## Location

- Duodenum lies above the level of umbilicus
- It is against L1, L2 and L3 vertebrae
- Present on either side of midline.

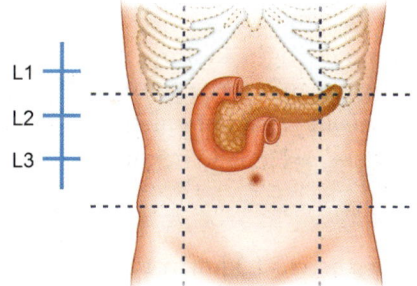

Location of duodenum

## Gross Features

Duodenum is 10 inches long and has four parts:
- First part is 2 inch
- Second part is 3 inch
- Third part is 4 inch
- Forth part is 1 inch.

## Peritoneal Relations

Duodenum is retroperitoneal and fixed.

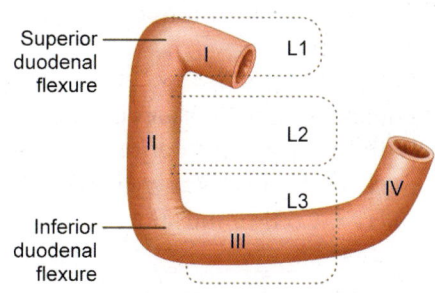

Parts of duodenum

### First Part

- Extends between pylorus and superior duodenal flexure
- Directed backwards, upwards and to the right
- Proximal part has lesser omentum attachment.

### Visceral relations
- *In front:* Quadrate lobe of liver, gallbladder
- *Behind:* Gastroduodenal artery, portal vein and bile duct

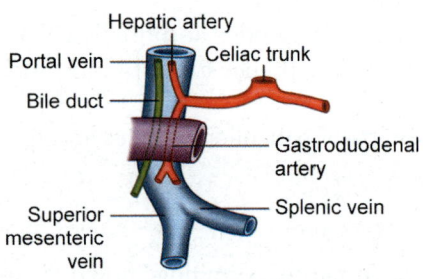

Posterior relations of first part

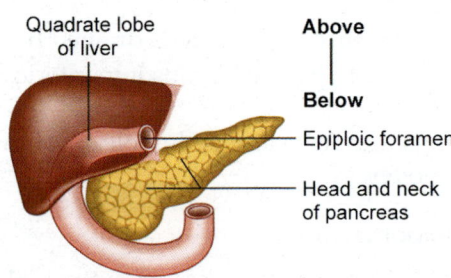

Visceral relations of first part

- *Superior:* Epiploic foramen
- *Inferior:* Head and neck of pancreas.

## Second Part

- Extends between superior duodenal flexure to inferior duodenal flexure
- Major and minor duodenal papillae are present on the inner side.

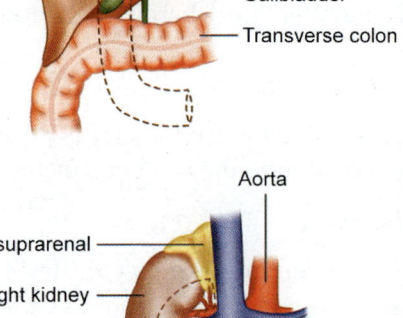

### Visceral relations

- *In front:* Right lobe of liver, transverse colon, coils of intestine
- *Behind:* Right kidney, right renal vessels, right edge of inferior vena cava, right psoas major
- *Medially:* Head of pancreas, bile duct
- *Laterally:* Hepatic flexure of colon.

Visceral relations of second part

## Third Part

- Lies across L3 horizontally
- Extends from inferior duodenal flexure ends in front of aorta.

### Visceral relations

- *In front:* Superior mesenteric vessels, root of mesentery
- *Behind:* Right ureter, right psoas major, right gonadal vessel, inferior vena cava, abdominal aorta with the origin of inferior mesenteric artery
- *Superior:* Head of pancreas with uncinate process
- *Inferior:* Coils of intestine.

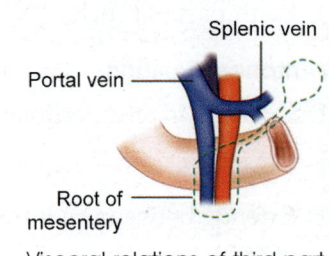

Visceral relations of third part

## Fourth Part

- Runs upwards, left of aorta
- Ends at the upper border of L2, at duodenojejunal flexure.

*Visceral relations*

- *In front:* Transverse colon, transverse mesocolon, lesser sac, stomach
- *Behind:* Left sympathetic chain, left psoas major, left renal vessels, left gonadal vessels, inferior mesenteric vein
- *To right:* Root of mesentery
- *To left:* Left kidney, left ureter
- *Above:* Body of pancreas.

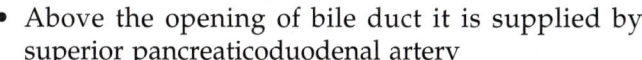

Posterior relations of third and fourth part

## Blood Supply

- Above the opening of bile duct it is supplied by superior pancreaticoduodenal artery
- Below the opening of bile duct it is supplied by inferior pancreaticoduodenal artery
- Right gastric artery
- Supraduodenal artery, a branch of hepatic
- Venous drainage goes to splenic, superior mesenteric and portal vein.

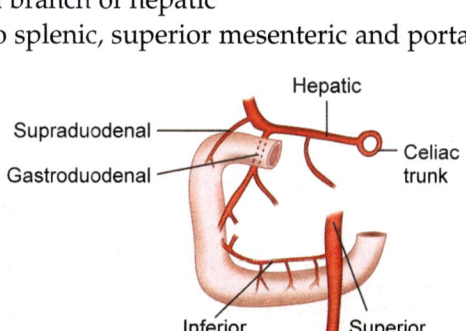

Arterial supply of duodenum

## Lymphatic Drainage

Duodenum drains into pyloric and superior mesenteric nodes.

## Clinical Importance

- First part of duodenum is a common site of peptic ulcer
- Second part of duodenum is commonly involved in congenital stenosis
- Widening of duodenal loop is seen in carcinoma of head of pancreas.

## Q. Spleen

**Ans.** Spleen is a lymphatic organ, functions as a filter of blood and plays vital role in the immune system of the body.

## Location

- Mainly in the left hypochondrium
- Posterior end extends into epigastrium

- Placed between left dome of diaphragm and fundus of stomach
- Related to left 9–11 ribs.

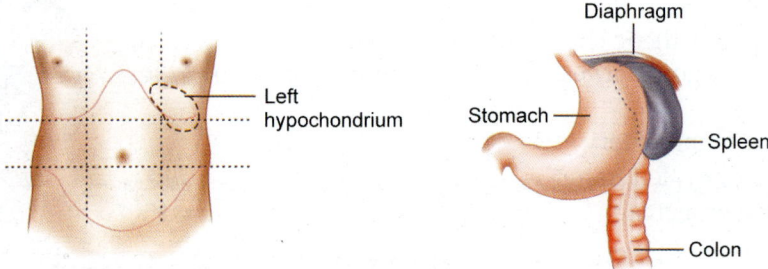

Location of spleen

## Gross Features

- Shape varies depending upon colic impression
- 5 × 3 inches in dimension, 7 ounces in weight
- Directed downwards, forwards and laterally
- Makes angle of 45° with the horizontal

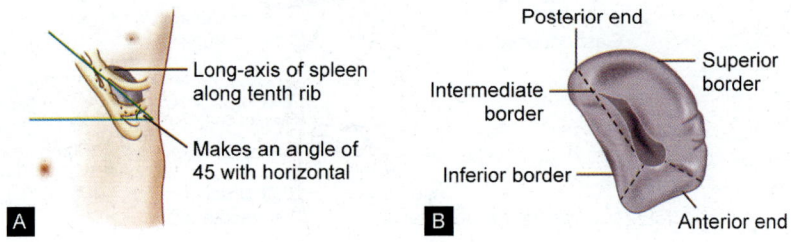

Spleen. **A.** Disposition of spleen; **B.** Gross features

- *Has two ends:* Anterior end (like a border) and posterior end
- *Three borders:* Superior border (has a notch), inferior border, intermediate border
- *Two surfaces:* Diaphragmatic and visceral.

## Peritoneal Relations

Spleen is surrounded by peritoneum and has following ligaments:

- Gastrosplenic ligament between hilum of spleen and greater curvature of stomach
- Lienorenal ligament between hilum of spleen and anterior surface of kidney
- Phrenicocolic ligament supports the anterior end of spleen the ligament extends from splenic flexure of colon and diaphragm.

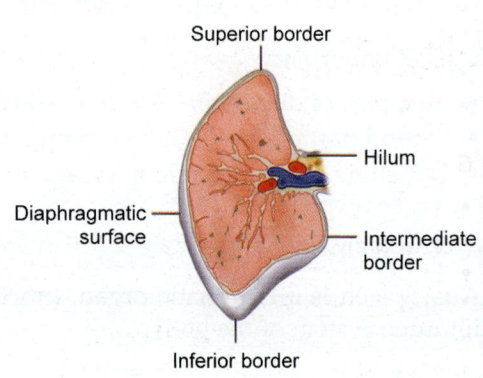

Transverse section of spleen

## Visceral Relations

Following organs create an impression on the visceral surface of spleen:

- Stomach
- Left kidney
- Splenic flexure of colon
- Tail of pancreas.

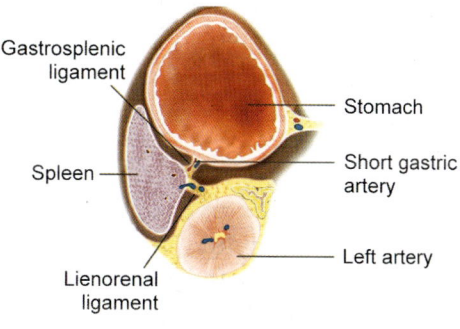

Peritoneal ligaments

## Blood Supply

- Splenic artery, a branch of celiac artery, enters the spleen through the lienorenal ligament
- Splenic vein, drains the spleen.

## Lymphatic Drainage

Lymph drains into pancreaticolienal lymph nodes along the splenic vein.

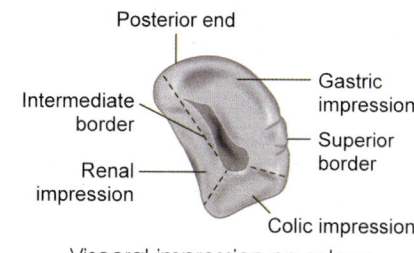

Visceral impression on spleen

## Clinical Importance

- Normally spleen is not palpable
- Splenomegaly is seen in typhoid, hemolytic anemias, Hodgkins's lymphoma
- Splenectomy (removal of spleen) is done in splenic rupture.

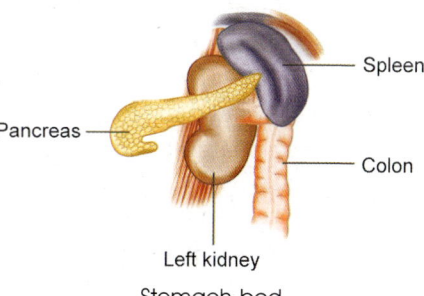

Stomach bed

## Q. Pancreas

**Ans.** Pancreas is a partly exocrine and endocrine gland, secreting digestive enzymes and hormones like insulin and glucagon.

## Location

- Lies horizontally on the upper part of the posterior abdominal wall
- Forms component of stomach bed
- Lies against L1 and L2 vertebra.

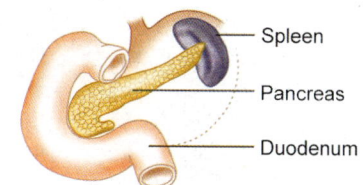

Location of pancreas

## Gross Features

- Weighs 90 g, 6–8 inches long
- Has head, neck, body and tail
- Head has three borders (superior, inferior, right lateral), two surfaces (anterior, posterior) and a uncinate process
- Neck has two surfaces (anterior and posterior)
- Body has three borders (anterior, superior and inferior), three surfaces (anterior, posterior and inferior)
- Pancreatic duct is placed superficially on the posterior surface of the gland
- Accessory pancreatic duct is frequently present.

## Peritoneal Relation

Pancreas is a retroperitoneal organ.

## Visceral Relations

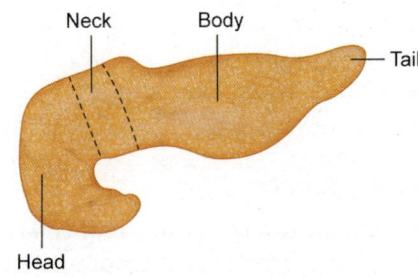

Visceral relations of pancreas

### Head

- Lies within the curve of duodenum
- Anteriorly related to gastroduodenal artery, transverse colon and jejunum
- Posteriorly related to inferior vena cava, renal veins, right crus of diaphragm and bile duct
- Uncinate process is related anteriorly to superior mesenteric vessels and posteriorly to aorta.

### Neck

- Anteriorly is related to pylorus
- Posteriorly to superior mesenteric vein and portal vein.

Parts of pancreas

### Body

- Anterior border gives attachment to root of transverse mesocolon
- Superior border is related to splenic artery
- Anteriorly related to stomach
- Posteriorly related to aorta, left kidney, left suprarenal gland, left crus of diaphragm, left renal vessels
- Inferiorly related to duodenojejunal flexure, left colic flexure.

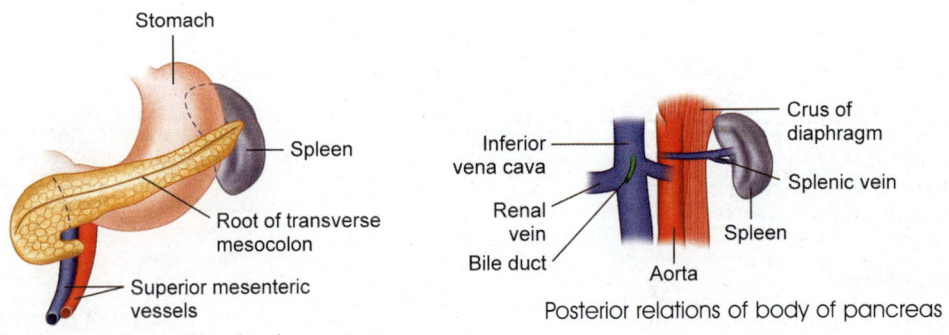

Anterior relations of body of pancreas

Posterior relations of body of pancreas

### Tail

Lies in the lienorenal ligament.

## Blood Supply

- Pancreatic branches of splenic artery
- Superior pancreaticoduodenal artery, branch of celiac artery

- Inferior pancreaticoduodenal, a branch from superior mesenteric artery
- Arteria pancreatica magna, a large branch from splenic artery
- By small veins into splenic vein
- By superior pancreaticoduodenal vein into portal vein
- By inferior pancreaticoduodenal vein into superior mesenteric vein.

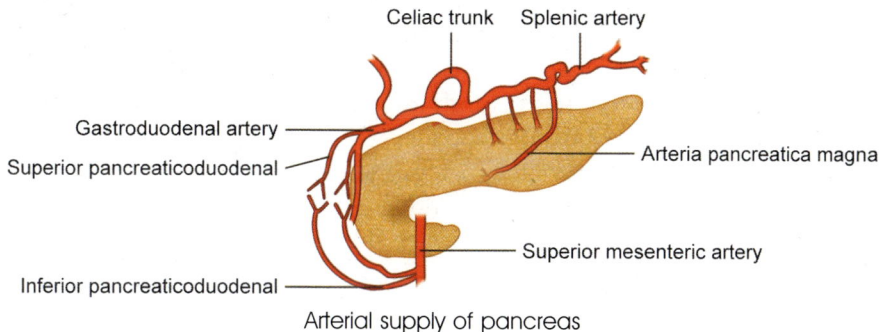

Arterial supply of pancreas

## Lymphatic Drainage

- Pancreaticosplenic group drains area left to neck of pancreas
- Upper part of head drains into celiac group
- Lower part of head and uncinate process drains into superior mesenteric group of pre-aortic nodes.

## Clinical Importance

- The head of pancreas and duodenum can be mobilised by incising peritoneum along the right edge of second part of duodenum and turning duodenum medially known as Kocher's manoeuvre
- Deficiency of insulin causes diabetes mellitus
- Inflammation of pancreas is known as pancreatitis
- Carcinoma of head of pancreas can cause obstructive jaundice
- Pseudocysts of pancreas can follow pancreatitis and can be drained by incising the anterior wall of stomach and opening made through posterior wall of stomach into pseudocyst.

### Q. Extrahepatic biliary apparatus

**Ans.** The extrahepatic biliary apparatus is concerned with the collection, storage and transportation of bile. The components of extrahepatic biliary apparatus are:

- Right and left hepatic ducts
- Common hepatic duct
- Gallbladder
- Cystic duct
- Bile duct.

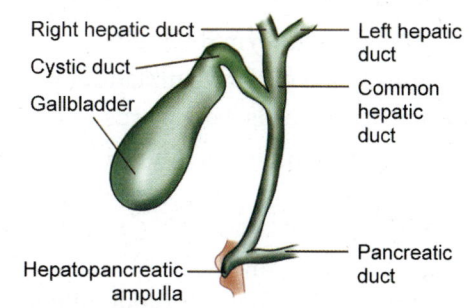

Components of extrahepatic biliary apparatus

## Hepatic Ducts

1. The bile canaliculi within the substance of liver form bile ductules, which in turn form interlobular ducts, these unite to form hepatic ducts.
2. The hepatic ducts emerge from porta hepatis and join each other to form common hepatic duct.
3. At porta hepatis the portal vein lies behind, in between is hepatic artery and in front is hepatic duct.

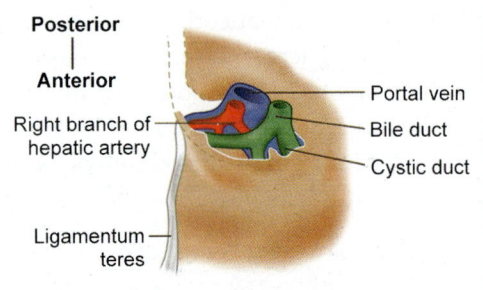

Porta hepatis structures

## Gallbladder

- Gallbladder is a piriform-shaped storage chamber of bile, in a shallow fossa on the right edge of quadrate lobe of liver
- Has three parts—fundus, body and neck
- Fundus protrudes from the inferior margin of liver and touches the anterior abdominal wall
- Fundus and body lie on the first and second part of duodenum
- Posteromedial wall of the neck is dilated to form Hartmann's pouch.

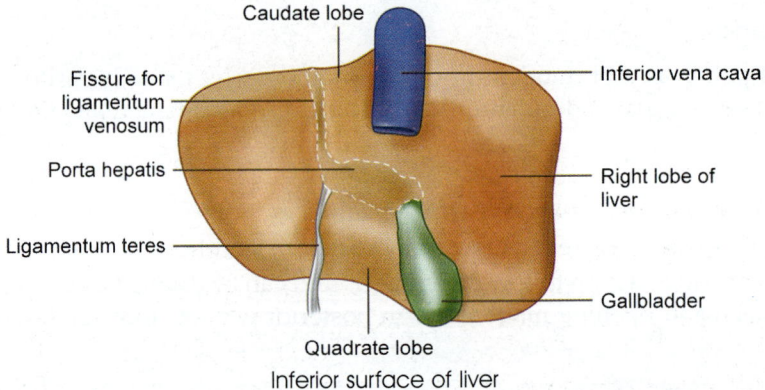

Inferior surface of liver

## Cystic Duct

- On an average 2 cm in length
- Begins at the neck of gallbladder
- Runs downwards, backwards to the left
- Joins common hepatic duct at a variable point to form bile duct.

## Bile Duct

1. Bile duct runs downwards, backwards initially in the free margin of lesser omentum, then behind the first part of duodenum and then behind head of pancreas.
2. Three parts can be identified—supraduodenal, retroduodenal and infraduodenal.

## Visceral Relations

### Supraduodenal Part

- *In front:* Liver
- *Behind:* Portal vein, epiploic foramen
- *To left:* Hepatic artery.

### Retroduodenal Part

- *In front:* First part of duodenum
- *Behind:* Inferior vena cava
- *To left:* Gastroduodenal artery.

### Infraduodenal Part

- *In front:* Groove on posterior surface of pancreas
- *Behind:* Inferior vena cava

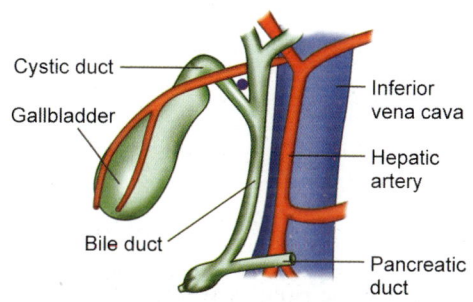

Relations of biliary apparatus

- The union of common bile duct and pancreatic duct forms ampulla of Vater (= hepato-pancreatic duct). There is circular muscle around it known as sphincter of Oddi, which is present at a point where it opens in the second part of duodenum.

## Blood Supply

- Cystic artery is the main source
- Branches from superior pancreaticoduodenal
- Right hepatic artery
- Accessory hepatic artery, branch of common hepatic artery.

Variations in this region, i.e course of hepatic, cystic arteries is a rule not an exception.
- Drains into hepatic veins
- Cystic vein
- Portal vein.

## Lymphatic Drainage

- Cystic nodes
- Hepatic nodes
- Pancreaticosplenic nodes.

## Clinical Importance

- Acute cholecystitis occurs in adult women, presents with sharp agonising pain in right hypochondrium referring to the scapula behind
- Chronic cholecystitis occurs in fat, females above 40 years age
- Variations are very common in the anatomy of biliary apparatus, a surgeon should be aware of the variations, while operating in this region
- A triangle can be identified, while doing cholecystectomy that is known as Calot's triangle; it is bounded by common hepatic duct on left, cystic duct on right and liver above
- Biliary system can be visualised by injecting a radiopaque dye in biliary system a procedure known as cholangiography.

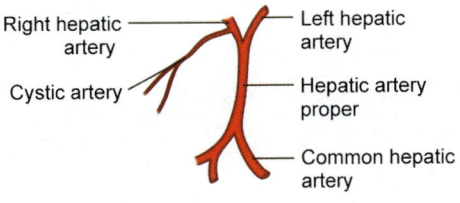

Arterial tree supplying biliary apparatus

## Q. Testis

**Ans.** Testis is the male reproductive organ, suspended by spermatic cord into the scrotum.

### Location

- Suspended in scrotum
- Lies obliquely in a way that upper pole is tilted forwards and laterally and lower pole backwards and medially
- Left testis is lower to right.

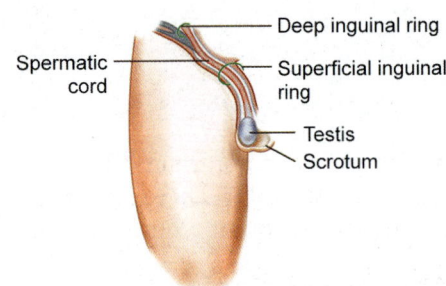

Location of testis in scrotum

### Gross Features

- Testis is oval in shape and is 10–15 g
- Has two poles—upper and lower, two borders— anterior and posterior, two surfaces—medial and lateral, appendix
- Spermatic cord is attached to upper pole, both poles are convex and smooth
- Anterior border—convex and smooth, posterior border is straight
- Epididymis is on the posterolateral surface
- Medial and lateral surfaces are convex and smooth
- Appendix of testis is remnant of paramesonephric duct.

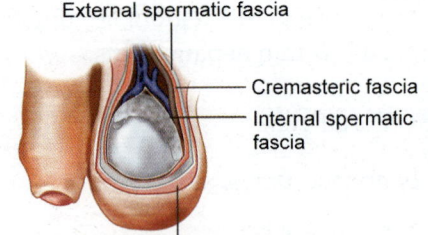

Coverings of testis

### Coverings of Testis

1. Outer covering is tunica vaginalis, it covers whole of the testis except posterior border. Sinus vaginalis is a portion of tunica vaginalis between testis and epididymis.

2. Tunica albuginea is a thick fibrous layer surrounding the testis all around except posteriorly where the testicular vessels and nerves enter the testis.
3. The posterior border is thickened to form a septum, known as mediastinum.
4. Tunica vasculosa is the innermost covering lining the lobules of testis.

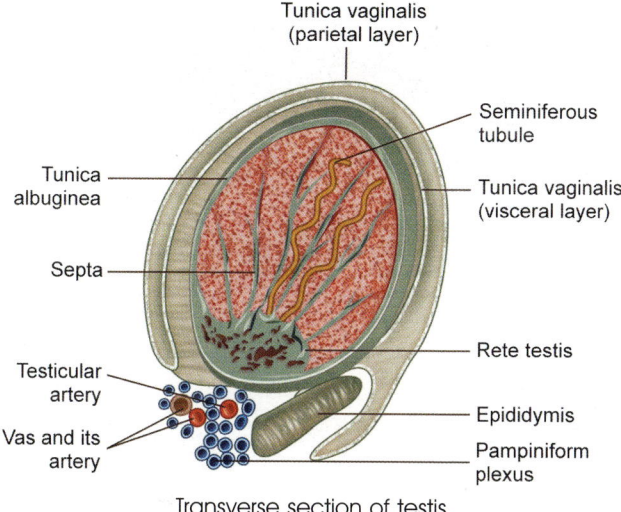

Transverse section of testis

### Blood Supply

- Testicular artery supplies the testis, it is a branch of aorta at L2 level, enters the spermatic cord at deep inguinal ring
- Pampiniform plexus drains the venous blood of testis.

### Lymphatic Drainage

Testis drains into the para-aortic and preaortic group.

### Clinical Importance

1. Sometimes the testis may fail to descend in the scrotum this is known as cryptorchidism. The testis may be located in inguinal, lumbar or upper scrotal region.
2. The testis may be absent known as anarchism.
3. Sometimes testis can be located at abnormal sites like, under skin of lower abdomen, front of thigh, femoral canal, under skin of penis or in perineum.
4. Hydrocele is a condition where the fluid accumulates in the processus vaginalis.
5. Varicocele is dilatation of pampiniform plexus, it commonly occurs on the left side since left testicular vein is longer and drains at a right angle to renal vein. Also crossed by loaded colon giving rise to varicocele formation.
6. Acute orchitis may occur following mumps.

### Q. Urinary bladder

**Ans.** Urinary bladder is a reservoir of urine and is a muscular organ.

## Location

- An empty bladder is present entirely within the pelvis posterior to the pubic bones separated from it by a retropubic space
- When full it extends into the abdominal cavity up to the umbilicus.

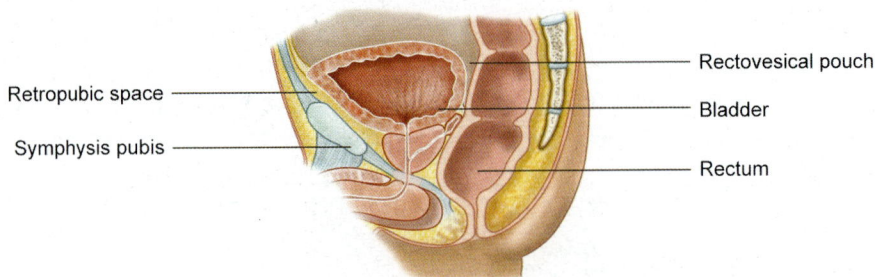

Location of urinary bladder in pelvis

## Gross Features

### Empty Bladder

- Tetrahedral in shape
- Apex directed forwards
- Base directed backwards
- Neck most fixed and lowest part of bladder
- Three surfaces—superior, two inferolateral surfaces
- Four borders—two lateral, one anterior, one posterior.

### Full Bladder

- Ovoid in shape
- Apex directed upwards, towards umbilicus.

Surface of bladder

## Peritoneal Relations

- Apex has remains of urachus, which forms the median umbilical ligament
- Uppermost part of the base between the two vas deferens is covered by peritoneum
- Separated from rectum by rectovesical pouch in males
- Peritoneum is reflected from superior surface of bladder onto the anterior wall of uterus
- Superior surface is covered by peritoneum.

## Visceral Relations

- Base—in females related to uterine cervix and vagina. In males related to rectovesical pouch with coils of intestine within, rectum, in lower part seminal vesicles vas deferens

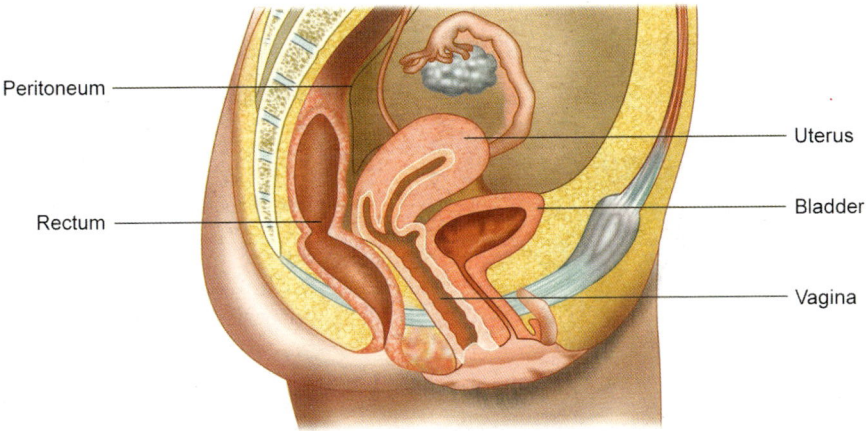

Sagittal section of female pelvis

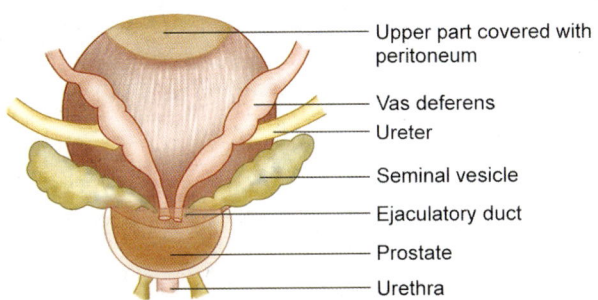

Posterior view of urinary bladder

- Neck—lies 3–4 cm behind pubic symphysis, pierced by internal urethral orifice
- *Superior surface:*
  - In males: Lies in contact with sigmoid colon, coils of ileum
  - In females: Small area near posterior border related to supravaginal part of cervix.

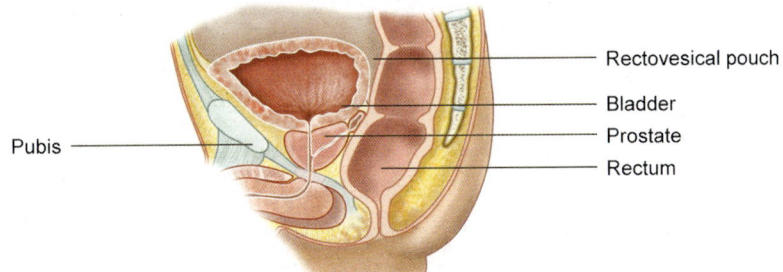

Sagittal section of male pelvis

- *Inferolateral surface:*
  - In males: Puboprostatic ligament, retropubic fat, levator ani, obturator internus
  - In females: Pubovesical ligament, retropubic fat, levator ani, obturator internus.

## Ligaments of Bladder

- Lateral true ligament extends from side of bladder to tendinous pelvic arch

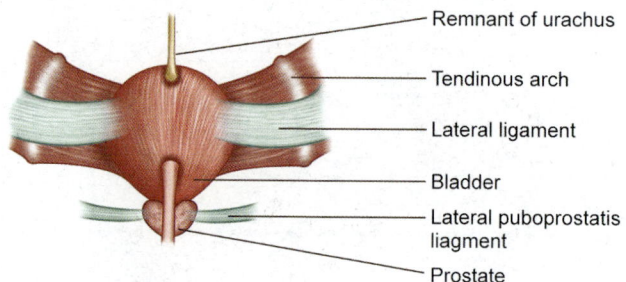

Ligaments of bladder anterior view

- Lateral puboprostatic ligament extends from anterior end of tendinous arch to prostatic sheath, is directed medially and backwards
- Medial puboprostatic ligament extends from pubic bone to prostatic sheath
- Median umbilical ligament is a remnant of urachus
- Posterior ligament of bladder is directed backwards and upwards
- False ligaments include peritoneal folds namely median umbilical fold, medial umbilical fold, lateral and posterior false ligament.

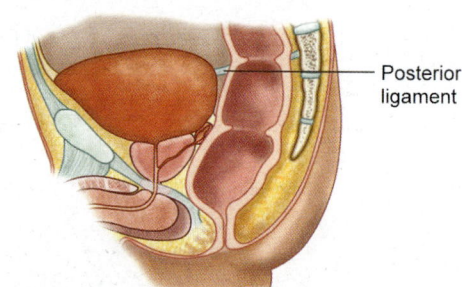

Side view of male pelvis

## Interior of Bladder

1. In empty bladder, mucosa shows irregular folds.
2. In a small area, over the lower part of the base of the bladder the mucosa is smooth due to the firm attachment of the muscular layer. This is known as the trigone of the bladder.
3. Slight elevation is seen posterior to urethral orifice is known as uvula vesicae.
4. Base of the trigone is formed by interureteric ridge.

## Blood Supply

- Superior and inferior vesical arteries branches of internal iliac artery

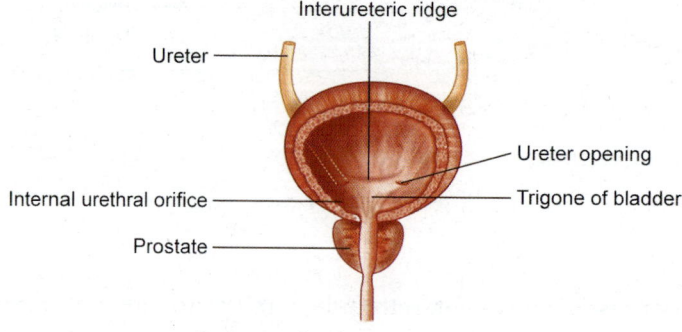

Cystoscopic view of bladder

- Obturator, inferior gluteal arteries (vaginal and uterine arteries in females)
- Vesical venous plexus drains into internal iliac veins.

## Lymphatic Drainage

- Mostly to external iliac nodes
- Few to internal iliac nodes via lateral aortic nodes.

## Clinical Importance

- Distended bladder can rupture by injuries on anterior abdominal wall.
- Interior of bladder can be examined by cystoscopy.
- Chronic obstruction to the outflow of urine can cause hypertrophy of bladder, hydroureter or hydronephrosis.
- *Automatic or reflex neurogenic bladder:* It is characterised by loss of micturition reflex and loss of bladder filling sensation; due to injury or resection of spinal cord above sacral segments.
- *Suprapubic cystostomy:* Surgical opening is done in anterior wall of bladder to relieve urinary obstruction; if conventional catheterisation of bladder is not possible due to acute urethral injury.

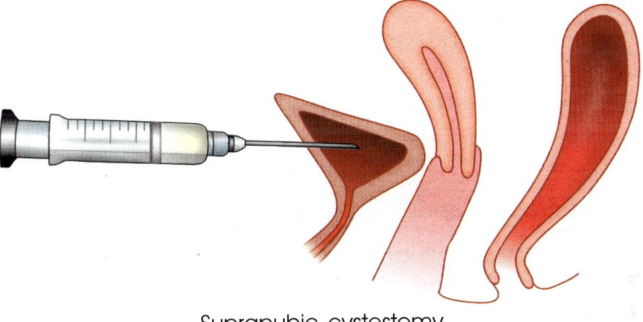

Suprapubic cystostomy

## Q. Ductus deferens

**Ans.** Ductus deferens is a thick walled, muscular tube, which carries the spermatozoa from epididymis to prostatic urethra via ejaculatory duct. It is 45 cm in length.

## Regions the Ductus Traverses

- Scrotum
- Inguinal canal
- Abdominal cavity (extraperitoneal).

## Course

- The duct courses from the posterior border of testis through spermatic cord to the pelvis
- It lies in the posterior part of cord and then traverses the inguinal canal
- The duct leaves the spermatic cord at the deep inguinal ring
- It passes medially, backwards to enter the lesser pelvis and is extraperitoneal
- Runs downwards and backwards in lesser pelvis and takes a sharp turn medially

- Toward its end it runs downwards, forwards and medially behind base of bladder
- The duct is dilated at the base of bladder known as ampulla of vas.

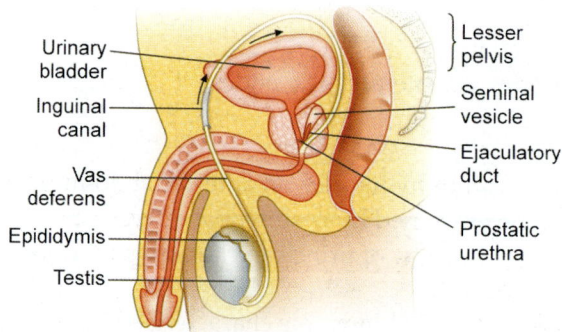

Course of ductus deferens

## Relations

- Begins as a continuation of epididymis
- Lies along posterior border of testis
- Lies on the posterior aspect of spermatic cord
- In pelvis lies lateral to inferior epigastric artery and cross the external iliac vessels
- It is retroperitoneal in pelvis, it crosses the obturator nerve, obliterated umbilical artery and obturator vessels and vesical vessels
- Crosses the ureter runs in the sacrogenital fold of peritoneum
- Lies behind the base of bladder and medial to seminal vesicle
- Ductus deferens joins the duct of seminal vesicle to form ejaculatory duct.

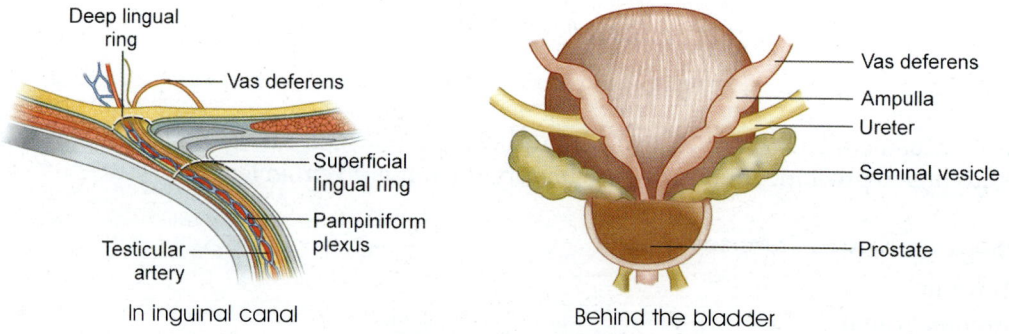

Relations of vas deferens

## Blood Supply

- Artery to vas is a branch of superior or inferior vesical artery
- Vesical venous plexus drains the vas and opens into internal iliac vein.

## Clinical Importance

Vasectomy is a procedure for male sterilisation wherein a part of vas is cut and ligated (tied).

## Q. Male urethra

**Ans.** Male urethra is a passage for discharge of urine and seminal fluid to the exterior.

### Location and Gross Features

- Male urethra extends from neck of the bladder to tip of penis
- Lies between internal urethral orifice to external urethral orifice
- It is 18–20 cm in length
- S-shaped, having two curvatures.

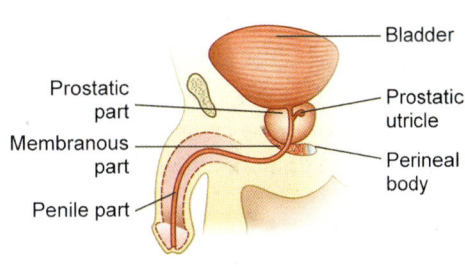

Male urethra

### Parts

- Prostatic urethra as it traverses prostate
- Membranous urethra as it lies surrounded by sphincter urethrae
- Spongy part as it lies within the corpus spongiosum of penis.

### *Prostatic Urethra*

- Widest and dilatable part—3 cm
- Posterior wall has a crest known as urethral crest (verumontanum)
- Middle part of the crest also has another elevation known as colliculus seminalis, which lodges the orifice of prostatic utricle
- On the either side of the utricle are the openings of ejaculatory ducts.

### *Membranous Urethra*

- Lies 2–2.5 cm behind pubic symphysis
- Traverses sphincter urethrae and pierces perineal membrane
- Narrowest and least dilatable part
- Stellate lumen in transverse section
- Bulbourethral glands lie around it and numerous urethral glands open into it.

### *Spongy Urethra (= penile or cavernous)*

- 15 cm in length
- Fixed part runs forwards and upwards in the bulb of penis
- It bends forwards and downwards as the free part
- It is dilated at the commencement as the intrabulbar fossa and at its end as the navicular fossa
- Lumen is oblong horizontally in transverse section
- Ducts of bulbourethral gland open in the proximal part of urethra
- Urethral glands open into it.

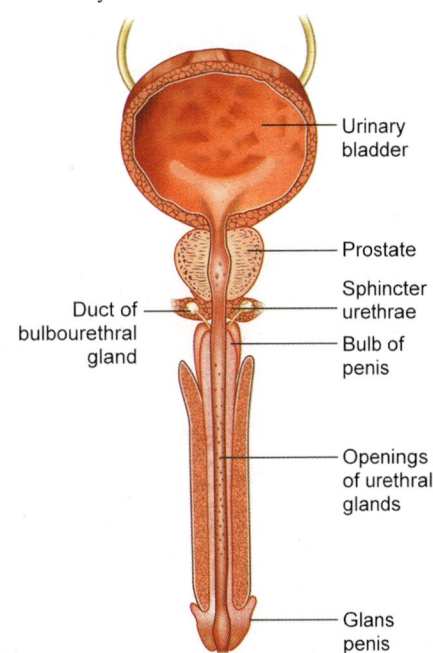

Anterior view of urethra
(schematic representation)

## Sphincters of Urethra

1. Internal urethral sphincter is involuntary in nature lies at the neck of the bladder.
2. External urethral sphincter is voluntary in nature, made-up of striated muscles supplied by perineal branch of pudendal nerve. Voluntary holding of the urine is possible by this sphincter.

## Blood Supply

- Receives branches from inferior vesicle, middle rectal and internal pudendal arteries
- Venous drainage is through internal pudendal vein into the internal iliac vein and vesical veins.

## Clinical Importance

- In retention of urine the urethra is catheterised with rubber tube
- Rupture of urethra is common following pelvic fractures
- External urethral meatotomy can be done to widen the external orifice in cases of obstruction
- Urethritis can occur in infections leading to stricture urethra.

## Q. Prostate

**Ans.** Prostate is a glandular tissue with fibromuscular stroma and is an accessory organ of male reproductive system, which adds to the bulk of seminal fluid.

## Locations

- Surrounds the first 3 cm of urethra
- Lies within the lesser pelvis, below the neck of the bladder
- In front of ampulla of rectum
- Behind lower part of pubic symphysis.

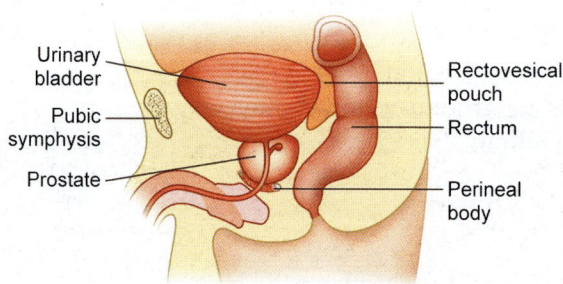

Location of prostate

## Gross Features

- Inverted cone-shaped
- Has apex, base, four surfaces—anterior, posterior and two inferolateral; five lobes—anterior, posterior, median and two lateral lobes
- Anterior lobe—lies in front of urethra and has little glandular tissue
- Posterior lobe—lies behind median lobe

- Median lobe—lies at the neck of the bladder, in between the urethra and ejaculatory ducts, produces an elevation in the lower part of the trigone known as uvula vesicae
- Lateral lobes—lie on either side of urethra, has enough glandular tissue.

## Surfaces

- *Base:* Continuous with neck of bladder
- *Apex:* Rests on upper surface of urogenital diaphragm
- *Posterior:* Rests on rectum
- *Inferolateral:* Lies on levator ani
- *Anterior:* Lies behind symphysis.

## Capsules

- *True:* Formed by condensation of prostatic tissue, deep to false capsules
- *False:* Formed by visceral layer of pelvic fascia. The prostatic venous plexus lies between the two capsules.

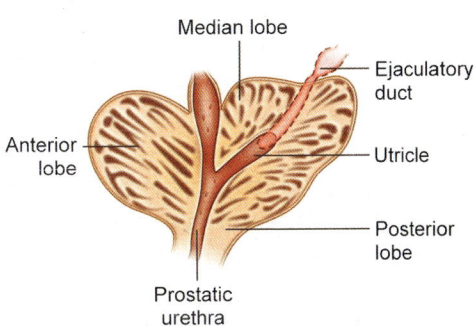

Sagittal section of prostate

## Structures Within the Prostate

- Prostatic urethra
- Prostatic utricle
- Ejaculatory ducts.

## Blood Supply

1. Branches of inferior vesical, middle rectal and internal pudendal arteries supply the gland.
2. Veins form a rich plexus around the gland; it communicates with vesical plexus and internal pudendal vein and then drains into vesical and internal iliac vein.

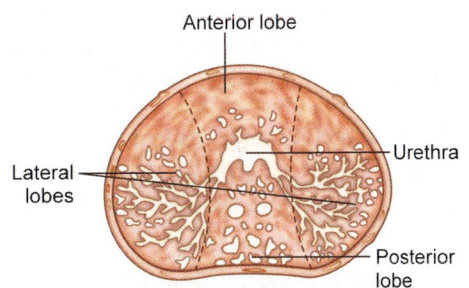

Lobes of prostate in transverse section

## Lymphatic Drainage

- Mainly drains into internal iliac and sacral nodes
- Partly into external iliac.

## Age Changes in Prostate

- At birth it is small in size with only a simple glandular system
- At puberty under the influence of hormones the gland grows in size and stroma condenses
- 20–30 years—marked proliferation of glandular tissue occurs
- 30–40 years—involution begins
- 40–45 years—prostate enlarges causing prostatic hypertrophy or reduces in size causing senile atrophy.

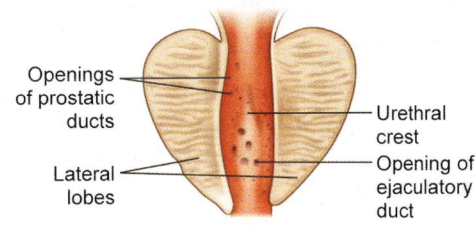

Coronal section of prostate

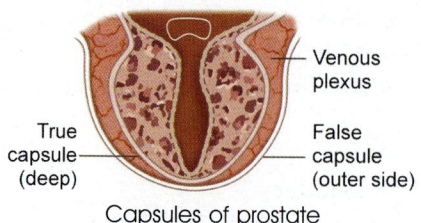

Capsules of prostate

## Clinical Importance

1. Prostatic enlargement can cause urinary retention.
2. Per-rectal examination is clinically useful to detect prostatic enlargement.
3. Prostatectomy can be done by various approaches through bladder, i.e. transvesical through prostatic capsule, i.e. retropubic or through perineum by incising fascia of Denonvilliers', i.e. perineal approach. Both capsules are left behind to avoid damage to venous plexus during prostatectomy.
4. Inflammation of prostate is known as prostatitis, it causes frequency of micturition, pain in perineum and tenderness in prostate.
5. Posterior lobe is the site of beginning of primary carcinoma of prostate.
6. Median lobe is a common site of adenoma or benign hypertrophy.
7. Valveless communication exists between prostatic and vertebral venous plexus leading to the spread of prostatic cancer.

## Q. Ureter

**Ans.** Ureters are thick-walled muscular tubes conveying urine from the kidneys to the bladder.

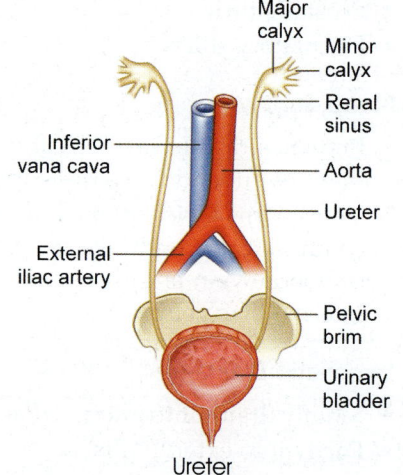

Ureter

### Location and Gross Features

- Ureters are retroperitoneal
- 25 cm in length, upper half lies in the abdomen and lower half in the pelvis
- Has three constrictions—at pelviureteric junction, at brim of pelvis and as it passes through the bladder wall.

### Course and Relations

- Abdominal course
- Pelvic course.

Ureters pass downwards, medially in abdomen and enter the pelvis by crossing the termination of common iliac artery.

### Abdominal Course

- Lies on the medial portion of psoas major muscle (muscle is in between ureter and tip of transverse process)
- Crosses the pelvic brim at the sacroiliac joint

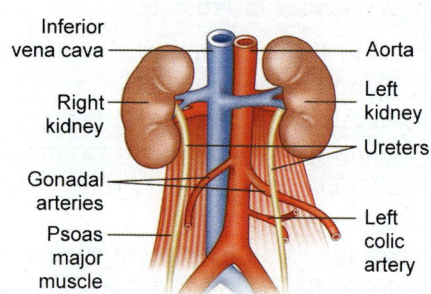

Abdominal course of ureter

- It crosses the genitofemoral nerve
- Gonadal vessels cross the ureter from front Ureter
- Right ureter is covered by second part of duodenum and crossed by right colic and ileocolic vessels
- Left ureter crossed by left colic vessels
- Left ureter lies behind the pelvic mesocolon and its mesentery.

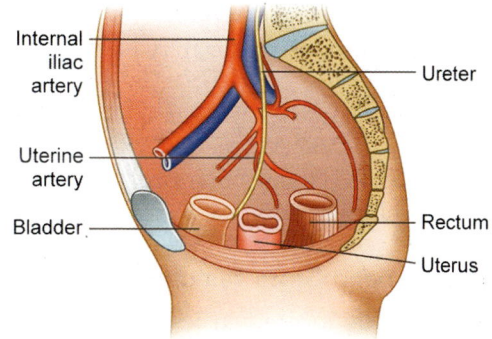

Pelvic course of ureter in females

## Pelvic Course

- Lies in front of internal iliac artery and its anterior division
- At the ischial spine it leaves the pelvic wall by turning medially
- Uterine artery crosses the ureter 2 cm lateral to cervix
- Ureter passes above the lateral fornix of vagina and lies close to the anterior wall of vagina
- Ureter lies behind and below infundibulo-pelvic ligament of ovary.

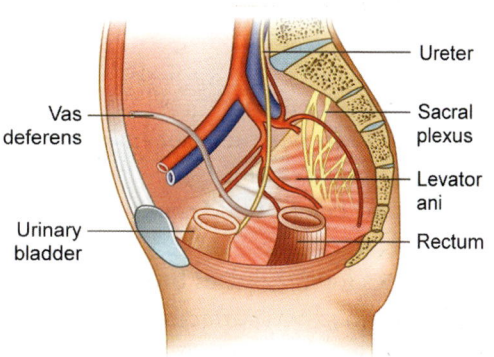

## Blood Supply

- Upper part is supplied by the branches of renal, gonadal or adrenal arteries
- In pelvis it gets blood from internal iliac artery and its branches

Pelvic course of ureter in males

- Arteries from the posterior abdominal wall form a plexus on the ureter
- Arteries enter the ureter from lateral side in the pelvic portion and from the medial side in the abdominal portion
- Similarly, renal, gonadal, adrenal and internal iliac veins drain the ureters.

## Clinical Importance

- While ligating colic vessels during hemicolectomy the ureter may get injured
- During excision of rectum, inferior mesenteric artery ligation is needed ureter may get accidentally injured since it lies close to it
- Ureter lies behind and below infundibulopelvic ligament of ovary, it may get cut, while during ovariectomy
- While ligating uterine artery surgeon needs to remember that ureters are 2.0 cm lateral to the cervix
- Ligation of lateral ligament of rectum can damage ureters
- Application of clamps on the vagina can damage the ureter

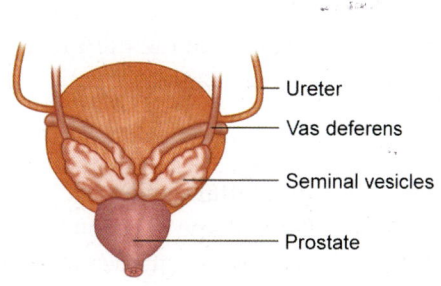

Posterior view of bladder

- Ureteric colic due to kidney stone as it passes through the ureter may cause severe pain
- Sometimes the ureter may be duplicated.

## Q. Uterus

**Ans.** Uterus is a muscular organ, which retains the developing embryo.

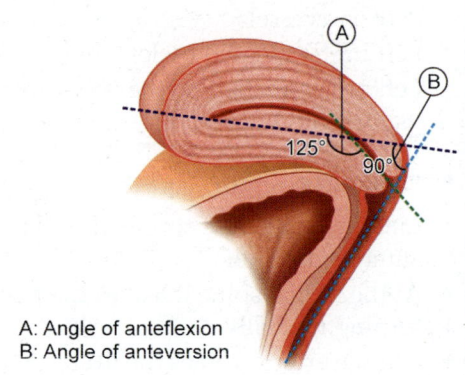

A: Angle of anteflexion
B: Angle of anteversion

### Location and Gross Features

- Uterus is located in lesser pelvis between bladder and rectum
- Parts—fundus, body and cervix
- Constriction between body and cervix is isthmus
- Normal position is of anteversion and anteflexion
- Angulation between cervix and vagina is angle of anteversion
- Forward bend of body on cervix is angle of anteflexion
- 3 inches long, 2 inches broad, 30–40 g weight
- Fundus has two surfaces, anterior and posterior, two lateral borders
- Lower part of the cervix projects into the vagina, dividing the cervix into two parts—supravaginal and vaginal.

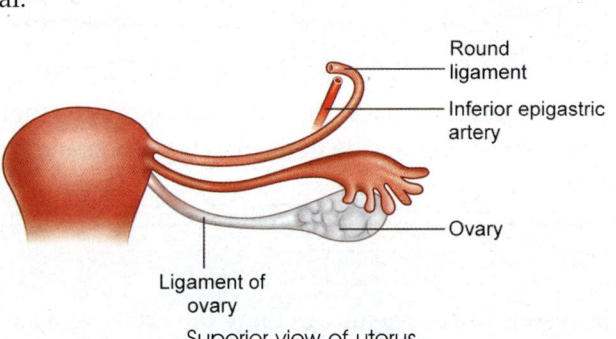

Superior view of uterus

### Communications

- One each side with the uterine tubes
- Below with the vagina.

### Cavity

- Slit like in sagittal section
- Triangular in shape in coronal section
- Internal os is at the site between the body and the cervix
- External os is at the site where the cervical canal opens into the vagina.

## Relations

### Body

- Anterior surface covered by peritoneum and related to bladder
- Posterior surface related to coils of intestine, sigmoid colon, anterior wall of rectouterine pouch
- Lateral border gives attachment to broad ligament, uterus is in its upper part and uterine artery is close to the lateral border between the layers of broad ligament.

### Cervix

- Anteriorly related to bladder
- Posteriorly to rectouterine pouch, coils of intestine and rectum
- On each side to ureter, uterine artery.

## Supports of Uterus

Supports of the uterus can be classified into true supports and false supports.

### True Supports

1. Uterine position angulation of body and fundus of uterus to cervix (angle of anteflexion) and angulation of cervix to vagina (angle of anteversion) itself provides positional support to uterus.

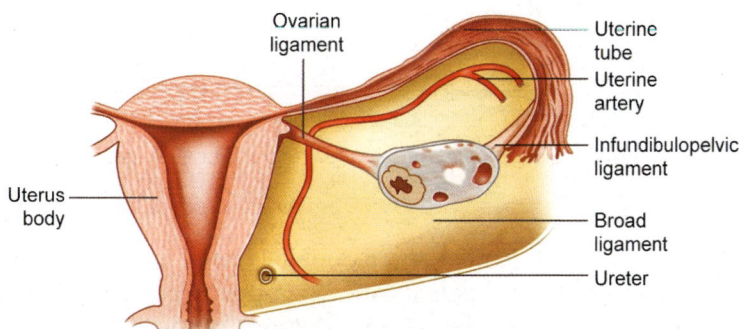

Relations of uterus

2. Round ligament of uterus: It maintains the uterine angulation by virtue of its attachment. It extends from upper part of uterus at the level of attachment of ligament of ovary to deep inguinal ring. It passes through the inguinal canal and gets attached to the fibrofatty tissue of labium majus. It sustains an anterior pull on the uterus.
3. Uterosacral ligaments: It counteracts the pull of round ligament and extends between cervix of uterus to sacrum. In its course backwards it embraces the rectouterine pouch and rectum.
4. Transverse cervical ligament: Also known as cardinal ligament, Mackenrodt's ligament. It is the condensation of connective tissue between cervix and vaginal fornix to lateral wall of pelvis. It gives lateral support to the uterus and is considered as a cardinal support of uterus.
5. Pubovaginalis part of levator ani and perineal body with its muscular attachment primarily support the vagina thus indirectly maintain the position of cervix.

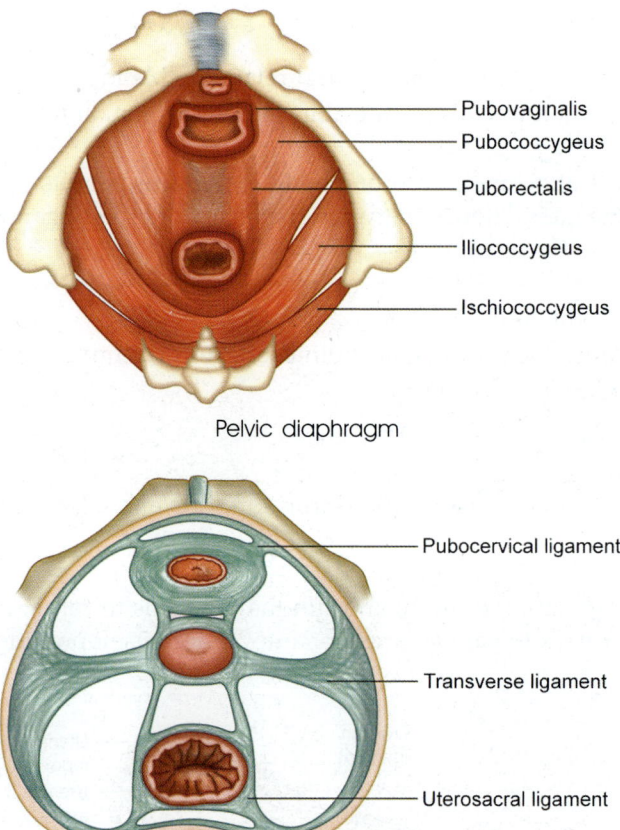

Pubovaginalis
Pubococcygeus
Puborectalis
Iliococcygeus
Ischiococcygeus

Pelvic diaphragm

Pubocervical ligament

Transverse ligament

Uterosacral ligament

Condensation of pelvic fascia forming support of uterus

## False Supports

1. *Broad ligament:* It is not a true ligament, but a double layered fold of peritoneum extending between lateral wall of uterus and pelvic wall. The upper free border contains the uterine tube and forms the mesosalpinx. The ureter adheres posteriorly, while the line of lateral attachment crosses the obturator nerves and vessels.
2. *Anterior ligament:* It is the peritoneal fold reflected onto the bladder from the uterus. Hence known as uterovesical fold.

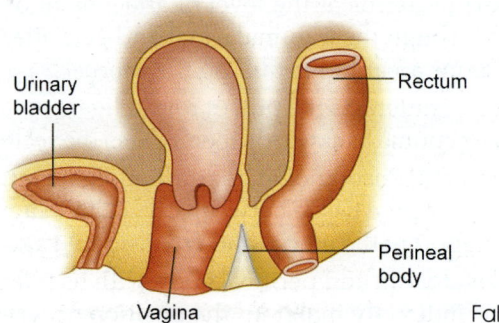

Urinary bladder

Rectum

Perineal body

Vagina

False supports of uterus

3. *Posterior ligament:* It is the peritoneal fold reflected from vaginal fornix to the anterior wall of rectum. Hence known as rectovaginal fold.

## Blood Supply

- Uterine artery, ovarian artery
- Uterine plexus drains via uterine, ovarian and vaginal veins into internal iliac veins.

## Lymphatic Drainage

- Upper part of body, fundus drains into aortic nodes, partly into superficial inguinal lymph nodes through round ligament
- Lower part of body drains into external iliac nodes
- Lymph from cervix drains into iliac nodes and sacral nodes.

## Clinical Importance

- Posterior inclination of uterus is known as retroversion wherein the cervix faces forwards
- Sometimes the uterus may have a posterior curvature of the body and this is known as retroflexion
- Due to the weakness of pelvic floor muscles secondary to childbirth the uterus may protrude out of vagina this is known as prolapse of uterus
- Cancer cervix is a common cancer in Indian women
- Hysterectomy is removal of uterus.

## Q. Uterine tubes

**Ans.** Uterine tubes are tortuous ducts, which carry the ovum from ovary to uterus and sperms from uterus to uterine tubes.

## Location and Gross Features

- Located in the free upper margin of the broad ligament of uterus
- Each tube is 10 cm long
- Parts—intramural part, isthmus, ampulla and infundibular:
  - Intramural part is 1 cm, lies within the wall of uterus, opens through ostium in the uterine cavity
  - Isthmus narrow part, 2–3 cm

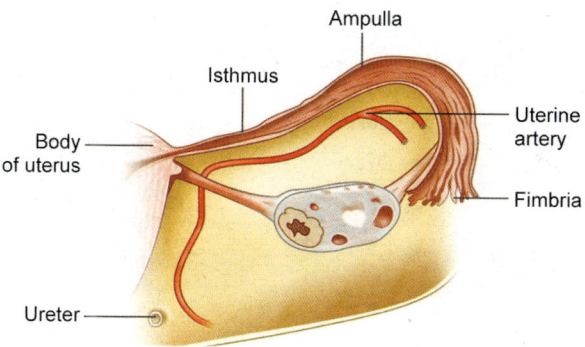

Parts of uterine tube and relations

– Ampulla thin walled, dilated part, 6–7 cm
– Infundibulum funnel-shaped end of tube, which opens in peritoneum.

### Relations

- Isthmus and ampulla are directed posterolaterally in horizontal plane
- Ampulla arches on the ovary and is related to its posterior and anterior borders
- Infundibulum opens in abdominal cavity beyond free border of broad ligament
- Part of broad ligament between mesovarium and uterine tube is mesosalpinx.

### Blood Supply

- Uterine artery supplies the medial two-thirds of tube, while lateral one-third is supplied by ovarian artery
- Tube is drained by pampiniform plexus into uterine veins.

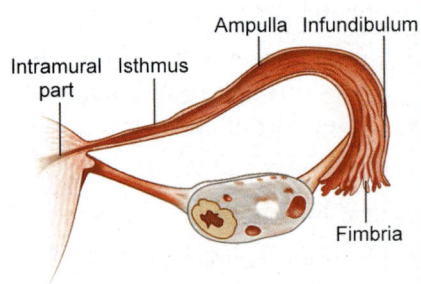

Parts of uterine tube

### Lymphatic Drainage

- Lymph of tube drains into lateral aortic and preaortic nodes
- Lymph from isthmus drains through round ligament into superficial inguinal ligament.

### Clinical Importance

- Inflammation of tube is known as salpingitis. It commonly occurs secondary to tuberculosis leading to fibrosis of the tube causing secondary infertility
- 2–3 cm length of tube is cut and ligated, in tubectomy for sterilisation
- Sometimes the embryo may adhere to the tube instead of uterus giving rise to tubal pregnancy.

### Q. Ovary

**Ans.** Ovaries are pair of female reproductive organs which lie in the pelvis.

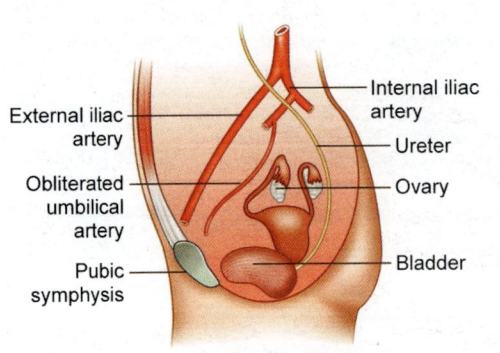

Locations of ovary

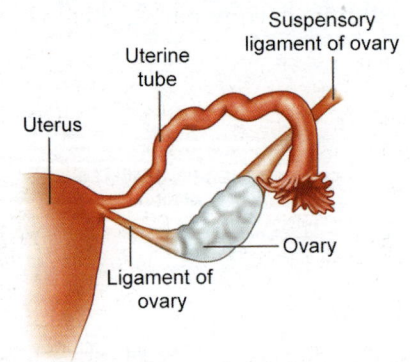

Ligament attachments on ovary (in nulliparous), position of ovary is vertical

## Locations

- Located in the ovarian fossa on the lateral pelvic wall
- Ovarian fossa boundaries—in front by obliterated umbilical artery, and behind by ureter and internal iliac artery.

## Gross Features

- Almond-shaped, grayish pink in colour
- Has anterior and posterior border
- Two surfaces lateral and medial.

## Peritoneal Relations

1. Entirely covered by peritoneum except anterior border where the layers of peritoneum are reflected on posterior layer of broad ligament.
2. Ovary is connected to posterior layer of broad ligament by a fold of peritoneum known as mesovarium.
3. Lateral part of broad ligament of uterus extending from infundibulum to the upper pole forms a fold of peritoneum is known as suspensory ligament of ovary.

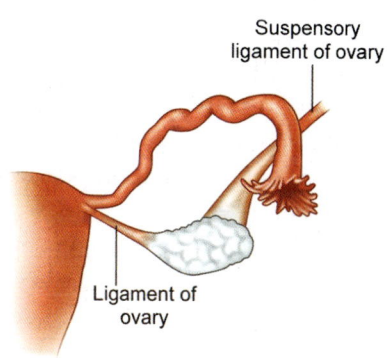

Suspensory ligament of ovary

Ligament of ovary

Ligament of ovary (in multiparous), position of ovary is horizontal

## Visceral Relations

- *Upper pole:* Related to uterine tube, external iliac vein, fimbria and suspensory ligament are attached to upper pole
- *Lower pole:* Related to pelvic floor, it is connected to lateral angle of uterus by ligament of ovary

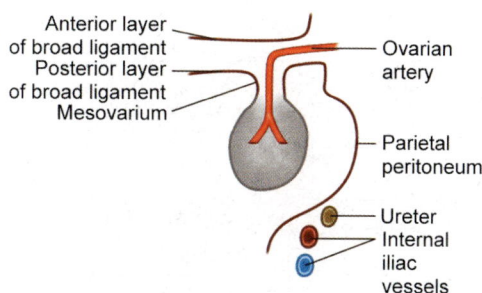

Anterior layer of broad ligament
Posterior layer of broad ligament
Mesovarium
Ovarian artery
Parietal peritoneum
Ureter
Internal iliac vessels

Superior view of ovarian fossa

- Anterior border: Related to uterine tube, obliterated umbilical artery
- Posterior border: Related to uterine tube, ureter
- Lateral surface ovarian fossa, obturator vessels and nerves
- Medial surface covered by uterine tube, peritoneal recess between mesosalpinx and medial surface is known as ovarian bursa.

## Blood Supply

- Ovarian artery, supplies through suspensory ligament
- Uterine artery also supplies the ovary
- Pampiniform plexus of ovary drains into ovarian vein.

## Lymphatic Drainage

Lateral aortic and preaortic.

## Clinical Importance

- Ovulation is detected by recording the basal body temperature, cervical mucus test, endometrial test, etc.
- Ovarian cysts are common
- Stein-Leventhal syndrome comprises of mild hirsutism, hoarse voice, secondary amenorrhea, cystic enlargement of ovaries
- Cancer of ovary is common
- Presence of endometrial tissue in ovary produces endometrial cysts.

### Q. Rectum

**Ans.** Rectum lies between sigmoid colon above and anal canal below. The rectum is not straight as the name suggests, but curved anteroposteriorly and side to side. However, the features of large intestine, i.e. *Teniae coli*, sacculations and appendices epiploicae are absent.

## Locations

- Closely fits into the concavity of sacrum and coccyx
- Lies against S3, S4, S5 and coccyx
- Ends 2–3 cm in front and below coccyx
- It is about 4 cm above the anal verge.

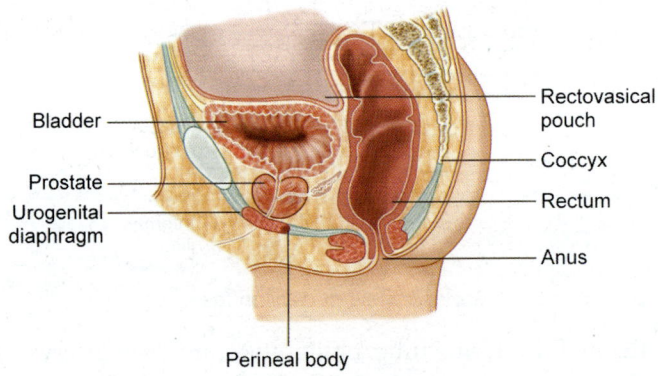

Location of rectum (sagittal section)

## Gross Features

- 12 cm long, lower part dilated to form ampulla
- Runs forwards and downwards, then backwards and downwards
- Two anteroposterior curvatures sacral flexure follows sacral curve, perineal flexure is backward bend
- Three lateral curvatures convex to right, convex to left and lower curve again convex to right.

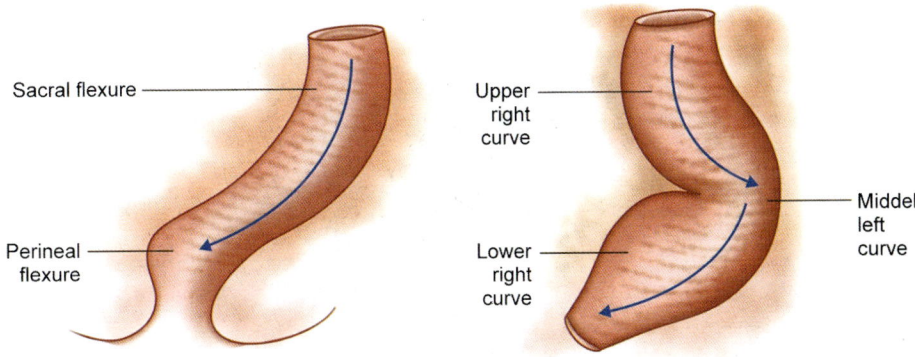

Curvatures of rectum

## Peritoneal Relations

- Upper one-third of rectum is covered in front and sides
- Middle one-third of rectum is covered only in front
- Lower one-third is not covered by peritoneum
- Posteriorly fascia of Waldeyer suspends rectum from the sacrum
- Pelvic fascia condenses laterally to support rectum to form lateral ligaments
- Rectovesical fascia lies between rectum behind and seminal vesicles, prostate and bladder in front.

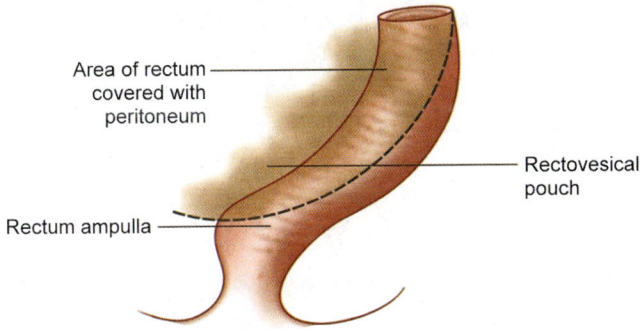

Peritoneal relations of rectum

## Visceral Relations

### Anteriorly

*In males:*
- Upper two-thirds related to rectovesical pouch, coils of intestine, sigmoid colon
- Lower one-third related to base of urinary bladder, ureters, seminal vesicles, vas deferens, prostate.

*In females:*
- Upper two-thirds related to rectouterine pouch, coils of intestine, sigmoid colon
- Lower one-third is related to vagina.

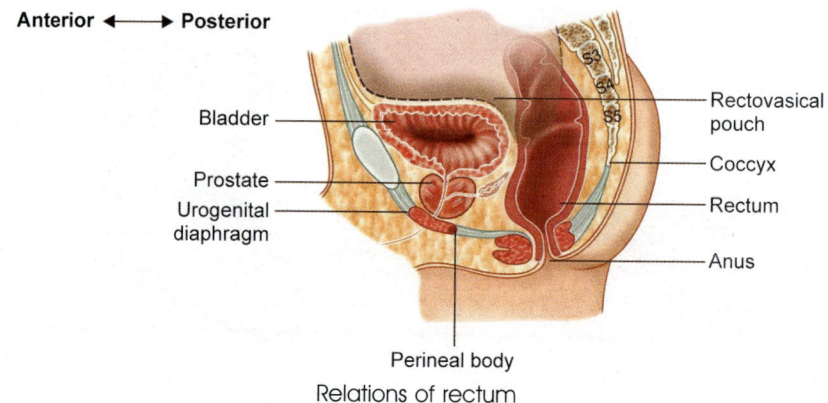

Anterior ←——→ Posterior

Bladder

Prostate

Urogenital diaphragm

Rectovasical pouch

Coccyx

Rectum

Anus

Perineal body

Relations of rectum

## *Posteriorly*

- Sacrum, coccyx, anococcygeal ligament
- Piriformis, coccygeus and levator ani
- Median sacral vessels, superior rectal, lower lateral vessels
- Sympathetic chain, ganglion impar, anterior primary rami of S3, S4, S5
- Lymphatics.

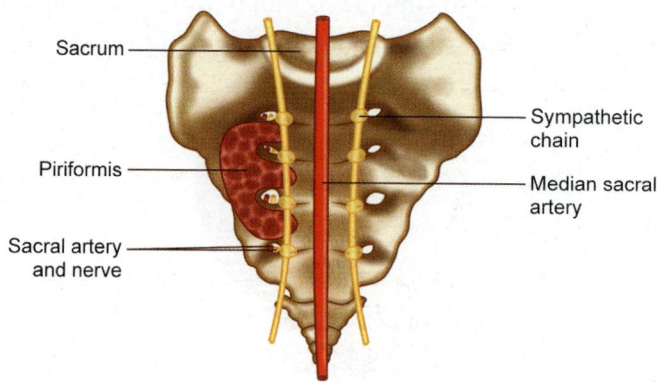

Sacrum

Piriformis

Sacral artery and nerve

Sympathetic chain

Median sacral artery

Posterior relations of rectum

## Mucous Membrane

- Temporary longitudinal folds are present in empty rectum
- Permanent horizontal folds—upper, middle and lower.

## Blood Supply

- Superior rectal artery, is continuation of inferior mesenteric artery is the main supply to rectum, also receives blood from middle rectal and median sacral artery
- Internal rectal venous plexus forms superior rectal vein, which drains into inferior mesenteric vein. Rectum is also drained by middle rectal vein, which opens into internal iliac vein.

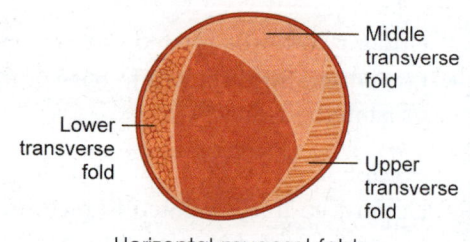

Middle transverse fold

Lower transverse fold

Upper transverse fold

Horizontal mucosal folds

## Lymphatic Drainage

- Upper rectum drains via pararectal and sigmoid nodes to inferior mesenteric nodes
- Lower rectum drains along middle rectal vessels to internal iliac nodes.

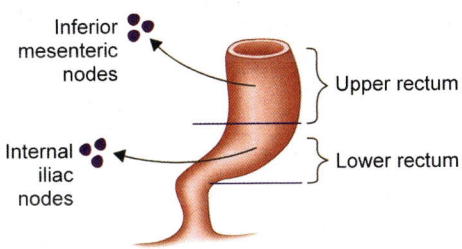

Lymphatic drainage of rectum

## Clinical Importance

- In digital examination of rectum (per-rectal) following structures are felt prostate, seminal vesicles, vas deferens, anorectal ring, sacrum, coccyx (in females, perineal body, cervix can be palpated)
- Direct visualisation of interior of rectum and anal canal is possible by sigmoidoscope and proctoscope
- Violent straining may cause prolapse of rectum.

### Q. Anal canal

**Ans.** Anal canal is a muscular canal, which has a significant sphincter mechanism, present at the distal end of gastrointestinal tract.

## Location and Gross Features

- Length is 4 cm
- Extends from anorectal junction to anus
- Separated posteriorly from tip of coccyx by fibrofatty tissue and anococcygeal ligament
- Ischiorectal fossa on either side of rectum.

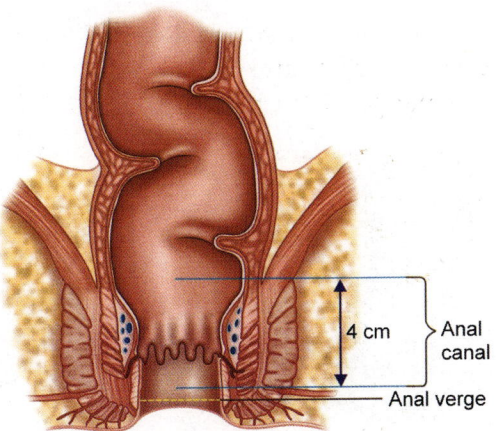

Location and extent of anal canal

## Interior of Anal Canal

### Upper Part

Upper part is 15 mm, lined by columnar epithelium, vertical mucosal folds known as anal columns, with rectal anal valves toward the base of the columns, anal sinuses are pockets above the valves, pectinate line along the attachment of anal valves can be appreciated.

### Middle Part

Middle part is 15 mm, lies between pectinate above and Hilton's line below (lies between the subcutaneous part of external sphincter and lower border of internal sphincter).

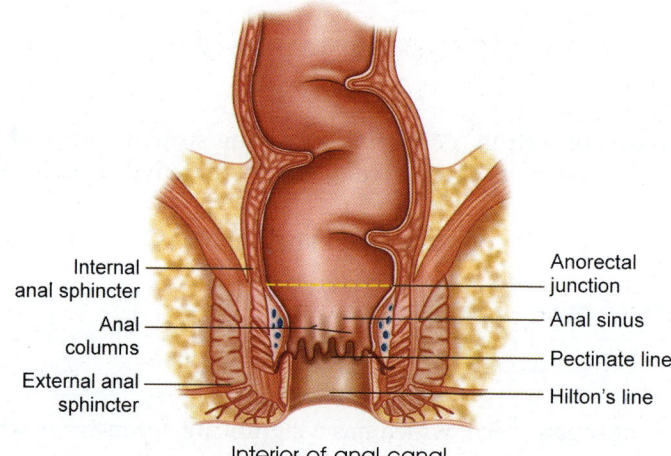

Interior of anal canal

### Lower Part

Lower part is 8 mm, lined by skin (has stratified squamous epithelium, sweat and sebaceous glands).

## Anal Sphincters

### External Anal Sphincter

- Has three parts—subcutaneous, superficial and deep
- Is striated muscle, under voluntary control
- Supplied by inferior rectal, perineal branch of S4

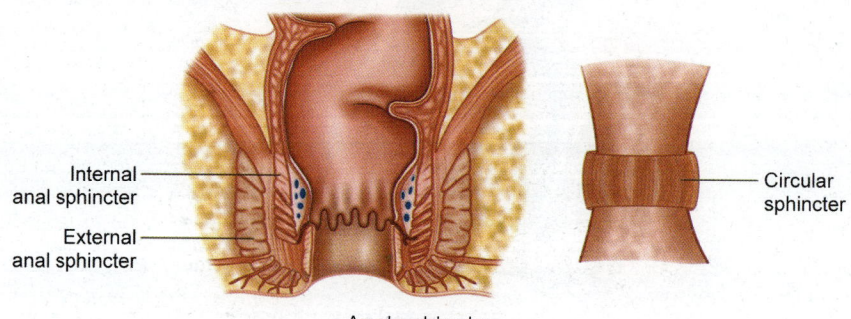

Anal sphincters

- Surrounds the whole length of anal canal
- At the level of anorectal junction it forms a sling of puborectalis muscle.

### Internal Anal Sphincter

- Internal anal sphincter is the downward extension of circular muscle layer of rectum
- It is partly muscular and partly fibrous
- The fibres run down the perianal fat and lower part of external sphincter and get attached to the skin.

## Blood Supply

- Above the pectinate line, it is supplied by superior rectal artery and below the pectinate line is supplied by inferior rectal artery
- Internal rectal venous plexus in the submucosa of anal canal drains into superior rectal vein
- External rectal venous plexus lies outside the muscular layer of anal canal, communicates with internal plexus and drains into internal pudendal vein, internal iliac vein and inferior mesenteric vein.

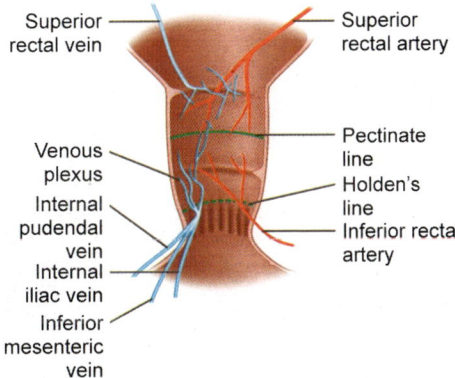

Blood supply of anal canal

## Lymphatic Drainage

- Above the pectinate line drains into internal iliac nodes
- Below pectinate line drains into superficial inguinal lymph nodes.

## Nerve Supply

- Above the pectinate line it is supplied by autonomic nerves
- Below pectinate line it is supplied by somatic nerves
- Internal sphincter is supplied by autonomic nerves
- External sphincter is supplied by somatic nerve.

## Clinical Importance

1. Internal piles are saccular dilatations of internal venous plexus. They occur above pectinate line and are thus painless. Bleed profusely by straining. Occur at 3, 7 and 11 O'clock position. Dilatations at other sites are known as secondary piles.
2. External piles occur below pectinate line and are thus painful. It includes perianal subcutaneous hematoma, tags of skin and anal wall.

3. Anal fissure is a very painful condition caused due to rupture of anal valve following passage of hard stools.
4. Fistula in ano is an abnormal epithelial tract created following drainage of anal abscess.

**MISCELLANEOUS**

### Q. Ischiorectal fossa

**Ans.** Ischiorectal fossa is a conical space around the anal canal with the apex upwards and base downwards. The presence of the space on either side of anal canal allows the dilatation of anus during defecation.

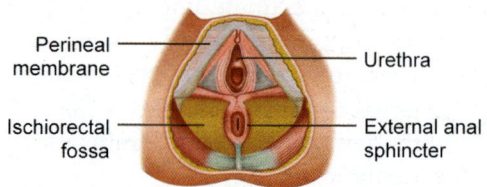

Contents of ischiorectal fossa

### Locations

- On each side of anal canal
- Below the pelvic diaphragm.

### Boundaries

- Base perianal skin
- Apex is the point of meeting of obturator fascia with inferior fascia of pelvic diaphragm
- Anteriorly is posterior boundary of perineal membrane
- Posteriorly lower border of gluteus maximus, sacrotuberous ligament
- Laterally obturator internus, ischial tuberosity
- Medially external anal sphincter, levator ani.

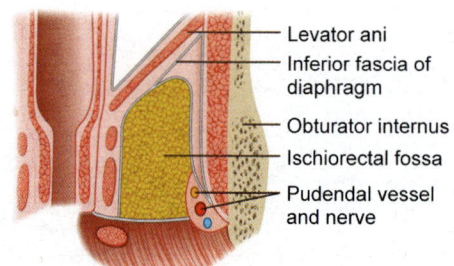

Boundaries of ischiorectal fossa

### Recesses

- Anterior recess is an extra space beyond the boundaries, above the urogenital diaphragm
- Posterior recess is deep to sacrotuberous ligament
- Horseshoe recess connects the two fossae.

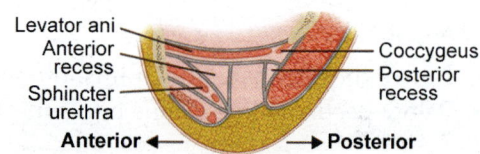

Recesses of ischiorectal fossa (schematic view)

### Spaces Around the Fossa

- Perianal space has subcutaneous fat, tightly arranged in the form of loculi
- Ischiorectal space, fat is loosely arranged
- Pudendal canal is in the lateral wall of fossa.

### Contents

- Fat
- Inferior rectal vessels and nerve
- Posterior scrotal nerves and vessels
- Perineal branch of S4, S2, S3 cutaneous branches.

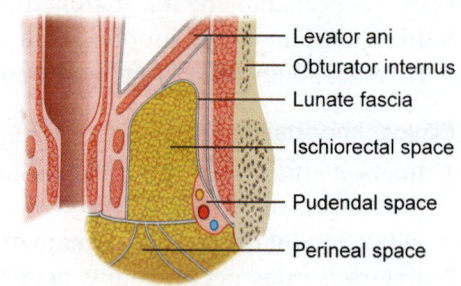

Spaces around ischiorectal fossa

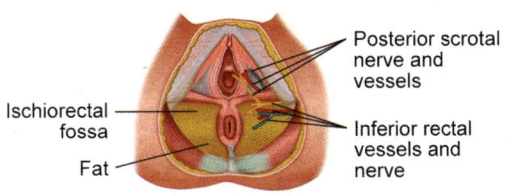

Contents of ischiorectal fossa

## Clinical Importance

1. Ischiorectal abscess is common due to the close proximity of anal canal. Abscess anywhere in the body should be incised and drained and in ischiorectal fossa the drainage can be carried out safely due to less vascularity.
2. Fat in the fossa acts as a support to rectum and anal canal and prevents prolapse of rectum.

### Q. Portal vein and sites of portosystemic anastomosis.

**Ans.** Portal system of vein begins and ends in capillaries. Portal vein is a major vein which collects blood from abdominal organs and carries it to liver. In the liver the portal vein breaks into sinusoids, which drain into hepatic veins and then into inferior vena cava.

## Formation and Course

- Formed by the union of superior mesenteric vein and splenic vein
- Begins behind the neck of pancreas, ascends upwards to the right lying behind first part of duodenum and then in the free margin of lesser omentum
- It ends at the right end of porta hepatis by dividing into right and left branch.

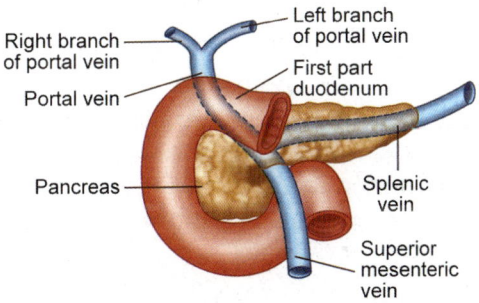

Formation and course of splenic vein

## Parts

- Infraduodenal
- Retroduodenal
- Supraduodenal.

## Relations

### Infraduodenal Part

- In front—neck of pancreas
- Behind—inferior vena cava.

### Retroduodenal Part

- In front—first part of duodenum, common bile duct, gastroduodenal artery
- Behind—inferior vena cava.

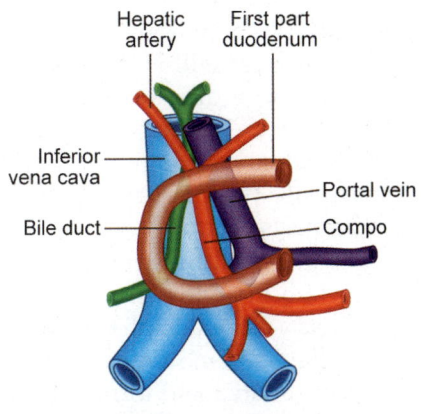

Relations of portal vein

*Supraduodenal Part*

- In front—hepatic artery, bile duct
- Behind—inferior vena cava.
  **(Note; overall portal vein lies in front of IVC)**

## Branches

- Right branch
- Left branch.

## Tributaries

- Gastric veins
- Cystic vein
- Paraumbilical vein
- Superior pancreaticoduodenal vein.

Tributaries of portal vein

## Portosystemic Anastomosis Sites

- At the lower end of esophagus veins of stomach (portal) communicate with esophageal veins (systemic)
- Around umbilicus—veins of liver (portal) communicate with veins around the umbilicus, i.e. epigastric veins (systemic)
- At lower end of rectum. Superior rectal vein (portal) communicates with middle and inferior rectal veins (systemic)
- Bare area of liver—hepatic veins (portal) communicate with phrenic and intercostal veins (systemic)
- Posterior abdominal wall veins of peritoneum, colon (portal) communicate with vessels of kidney (systemic).

## Clinical Importance

1. Normal portal pressure is 7–10 cm of saline and at the junction of hepatic vein and inferior vena cava is 0 cm.
2. In portal hypertension, there is an abnormally high pressure within the portal venous system by and large due to mechanical obstruction. Obstruction can occur in hepatic veins (Budd-Chiari syndrome) or intrahepatic (due to cirrhosis, tumor) or in portal vein (due to thrombosis, tumor).
3. Signs of portal hypertension are ascites (fluid collection in abdomen), enlarged spleen, caput medusa (dilated and tortuous veins around umbilicus) hematemesis due to esophageal varices (dilated and tortuous veins at the lower end of esophagus), bleeding per rectum.

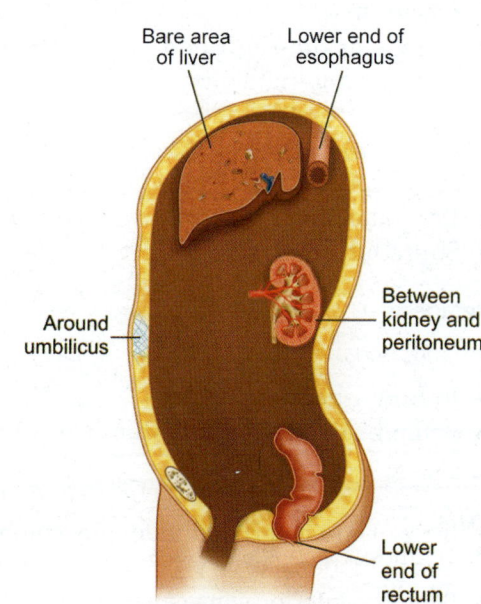

Sites of portosystemic anastomosis (schematic representation)

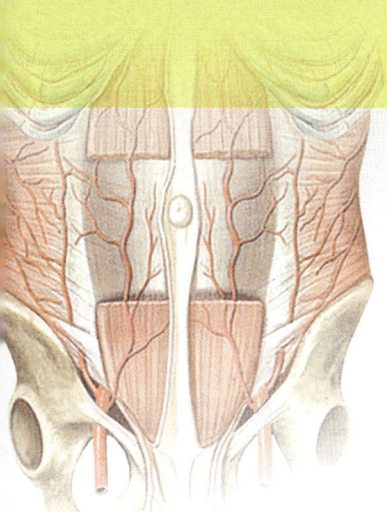

# Key Diagrams with MCQ Tips

## Q. Inguinal ligament of poupart

**Ans.**
- Folded border of external oblique aponeurosis
- Attached to anterosuperior iliac spine and pubic tubercle
- Fascia lata, internal oblique, transversus abdominis, cremaster muscle are attached
- Parts—reflected part, pectineal part, lacunar part.

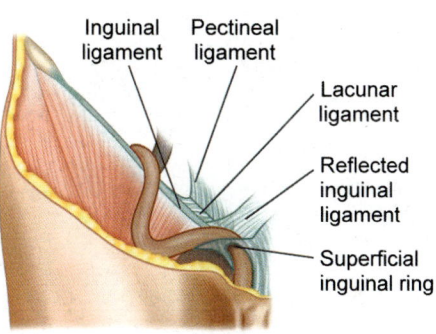

Inguinal ligament

## Q. Hesselbach's triangle

**Ans.**
- Bounded laterally by inferior epigastric artery, medially lateral border of rectus abdominis and base by inguinal ligament
- Divided into two parts by obliterated umbilical artery (lateral umbilical ligament)
- Direct inguinal hernia traverses this triangle.

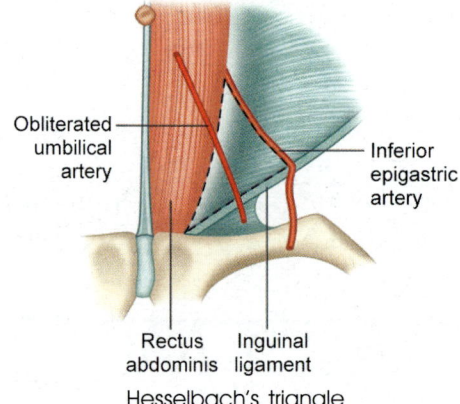

Obliterated umbilical artery

Inferior epigastric artery

Rectus abdominis

Inguinal ligament

Hesselbach's triangle

**Q. Superficial inguinal ring is a triangular gap in the external oblique aponeurosis**

**Q. Deep inguinal ring is an oval opening in the fascia transversalis**

**Q. Transverse section of spermatic cord**

**Ans.**
- Internal spermatic fascia is derived from fascia transversalis.
- Cremasteric fascia is derived from cremasteric muscle.
- External spermatic fascia is derived from external oblique aponeurosis.

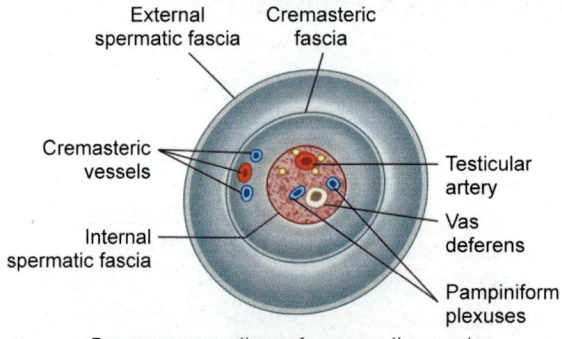

External spermatic fascia

Cremasteric fascia

Cremasteric vessels

Testicular artery

Internal spermatic fascia

Vas deferens

Pampiniform plexuses

Transverse section of spermatic cord

**Q. Rectouterine pouch is pouch of Douglas**

**Q. Hepatorenal pouch is Morrison's pouch**

**Q. Posterior relations of kidney (common for both kidneys)**

**Ans.**
- Muscles—diaphragm, psoas major, quadratus lumborum, transversus abdominis
- Nerves—subcostal, iliohypogastric, ilioinguinal

- Subcostal vessels
- 12th rib on right side, 11 and 12 ribs on left side
- Angle between lower border of 12th rib and outer border of erector spinae is known as renal angle.

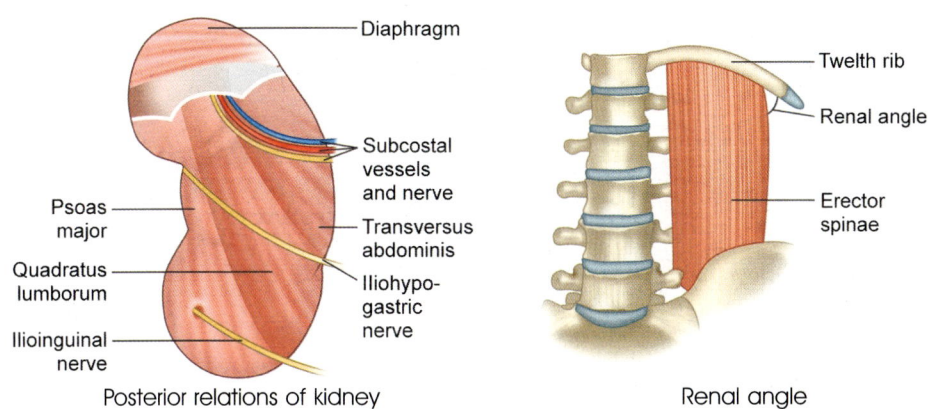

Posterior relations of kidney                              Renal angle

## Q. Mesentery

**Ans.**
- Root of mesentery 6 inches long, directed obliquely to right
- Crosses third part of duodenum, aorta, inferior vena cava, right ureter, right psoas.

## Q. Epiploic foramen

**Ans.**
- Lesser sac communicates with greater sac through epiploic foramen
- Lies at the level of T12

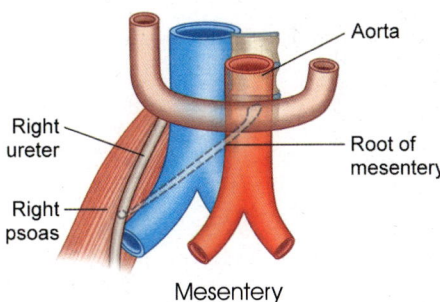

Mesentery

- In front is right free margin of lesser omentum containing portal vein, hepatic artery and bile duct
- Behind is inferior vena cava, right suprarenal gland
- Above—liver; below—first part of duodenum, hepatic artery.

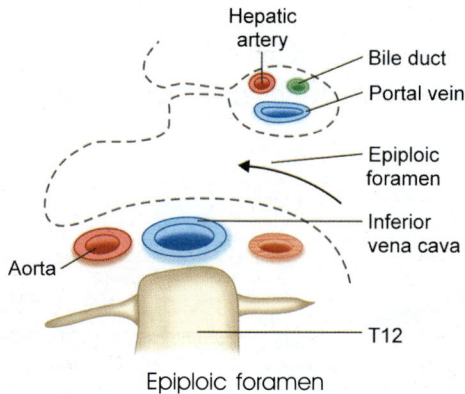

Epiploic foramen

## Q. Branches of abdominal aorta

**Ans.**
- Celiac artery between T12 and L1
- Superior mesenteric artery at L1
- Renal artery between L1 and L2
- Gonadal artery at L2
- Inferior mesenteric artery at L3
- Divides into two common iliacs at L4.

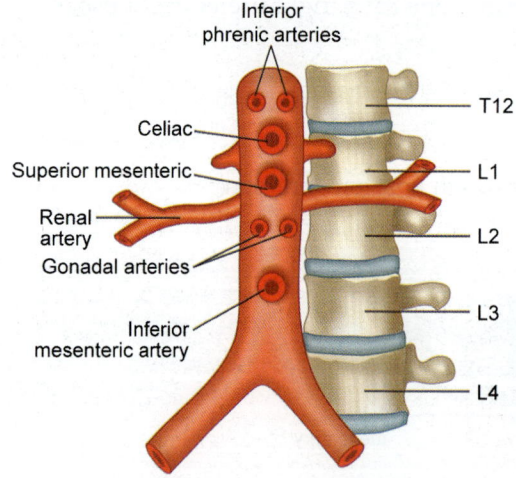

Branches of abdominal artery

## Q. Celiac artery main branches

**Ans.**
- Left gastric artery
- Splenic artery
- Common hepatic artery.

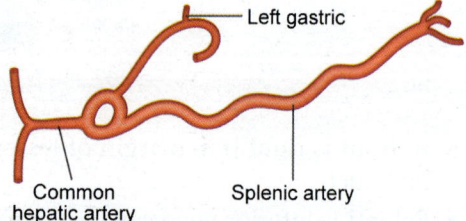

Main branches of celiac trunk

## Q. Superior mesenteric artery branches

**Ans.**

- Inferior pancreaticoduodenal
- Jejunal, ileal
- Ileocolic
- Right colic
- Middle colic.

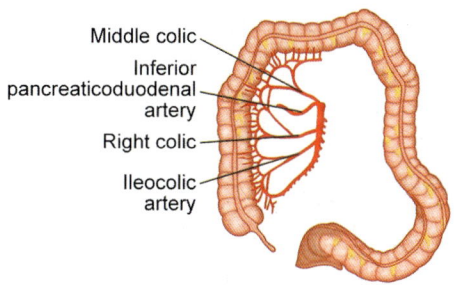

Branches of superior mesenteric artery

## Q. Inferior mesenteric artery

**Ans.**

- Left colic
- Sigmoid
- Superior rectal.

## Q. Posterior relations of cecum

**Ans.**

- *Muscles:* Right psoas, right iliacus
- Nerves: Right genitofemoral, right femoral, right lateral cutaneous nerve of thigh
- Right gonadal vessels
- Appendix if retrocecal.

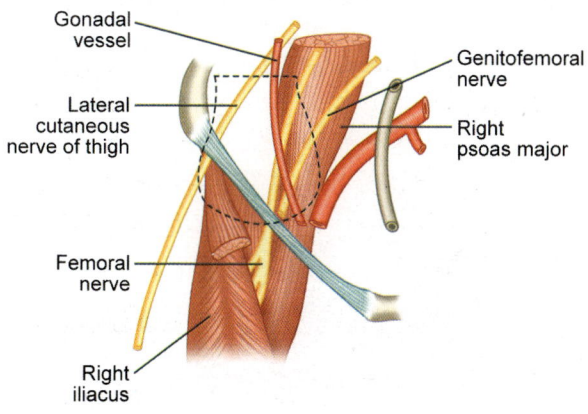

Posterior relations of cecum

**Q. Third part of duodenum is anteriorly related to superior mesenteric vessels**

**Q. Abdominal tonsil means appendix**

**Q. Portal vein**

**Ans.**
- Formed by union of superior mesenteric vein with splenic vein
- At L2
- Behind neck of pancreas.

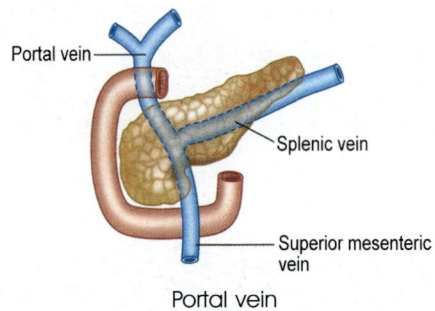

Portal vein

**Q. Gonadal vessels lie in front of ureter**

**Q. Perineal body**

**Ans.**
- 1.25 cm in front of anal margin
- Three paired muscles—superficial and deep transversus perinei, levator ani
- Three unpaired muscles—external anal sphincter, bulbospongiosus, longitudinal muscle coat of rectal ampulla
- Central tendon of perineum, key support of pelvic organs.

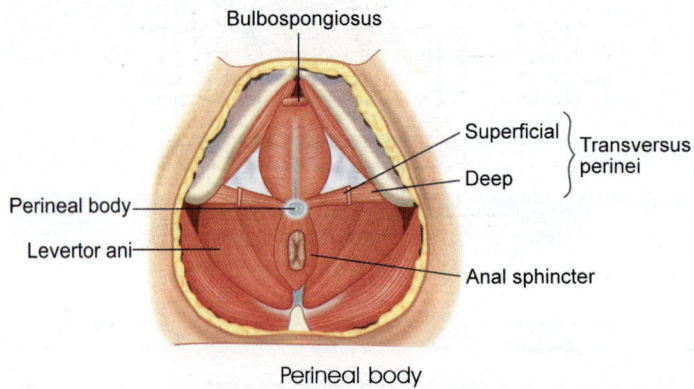

Perineal body

**Q. Pudendal canal is in lateral wall of ischiorectal fossa**

**Q. Forward angulation between cervix and vagina is angle of anteversion, angulation between body and cervix is angle of anteflexion** (diagram only).

**Ans.**

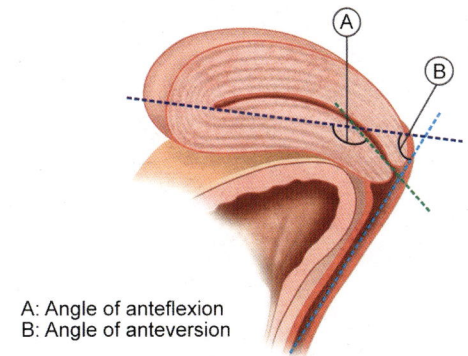

A: Angle of anteflexion
B: Angle of anteversion

Position of uterus

**Q. Uterine artery initially runs medially towards cervix (2 cm lateral to cervix) and, crosses ureter above lateral fornix of vagina (diagram only).**

**Ans.**

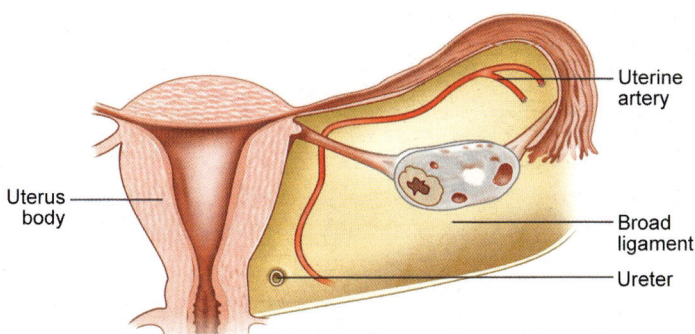

Relation of ureter to uterine artery

**Q. Per-rectal examination**

**Ans.**
- In males—posterior surface of prostate, seminal vesicles, vas deferens
- In females—cervix, perineal body ovaries (sometimes).

**Q. Pectinate line**

**Ans.** Anatomical and surgical importance of pectinate line:
- It is an embryological watershed between visceral structures above and somatic structures
- Mucosa above has autonomic nerve supply thus insensitive to pain while skin below is supplied by inferior rectal branch sensitive to pain and other stimuli

- Venous drainage above is to portal circulation, while below is to systemic venous circulation
- Lymphatic drainage above the pectinate line goes to iliac group of lymph nodes and below to inguinal group
- Internal hemorrhoids develop above the dentate line.

## Q. Branches of internal iliac artery

**Ans.**

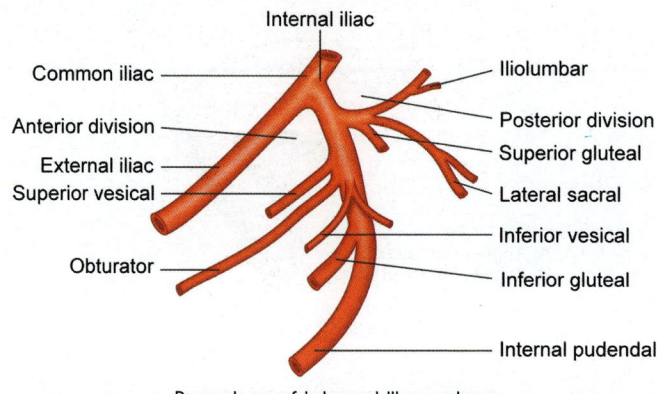

Branches of internal iliac artery

### Anterior Division

- Superior vesical
- Obturator
- Middle rectal
- Inferior vesical/vaginal
- Inferior gluteal
- Internal pudendal.

### Posterior Division

- Iliolumbar
- Lateral sacral
- Superior gluteal.

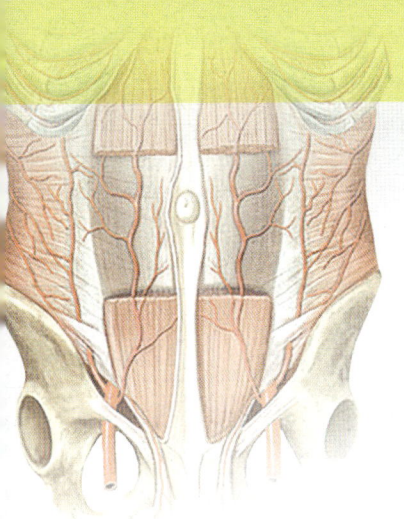

# MCQs 21

1. **Following is the 'atypical' lumbar vertebra:**

    a. L1

    b. L5

    c. L3

    d. L4

    **Answer: b**

2. **Following events occur at L1 except ...................**

    a. Superior duodenal flexure

    b. Celiac plexus

    c. Upper part of the hilus of right kidney

    d. Upper part of the hilus of left kidney

    **Answer: d**

3. **Superficial inguinal ring is an opening in .................... muscle aponeurosis.**

    a. External oblique

    b. Internal oblique

    c. Transversus abdominis

    d. All of the above

    **Answer: a**

4. **Deep inguinal ring is an opening in .................... fascia.**

    a. Fascia iliaca

    b. Cremasteric fascia

    c. Fascia transversalis

    d. None of the above

    **Answer: c**

5. **All of the following are posterior abdominal muscles except ...................**

    a. Psoas major

    b. Quadratus lumborum

    c. Transversus abdominis

    d. Iliacus

    **Answer: c**

6. Following muscles get inserted into the perineal body except ......................

   a. Puborectalis
   b. Pubovaginalis
   c. Transversus perinei
   d. Levator ani

   **Answer: a**

7. Following muscles form the pelvic floor except ......................

   a. Pubococcygeus
   b. Iliococcygeus
   c. Deep transversus perinei
   d. Coccygeus

   **Answer: c**

8. Urogenital diaphragm consists of following muscles ......................

   a. Sphincter urethrae
   b. Deep transversus perinei
   c. Both a and b
   d. None of above

   **Answer: c**

9. Perineal membrane is ......................

   a. Superior fascia of urogenital diaphragm
   b. Inferior fascia of urogenital diaphragm
   c. Obturator fascia
   d. Pelvic fascia

   **Answer: b**

10. The root of mesentery crosses ...................... part of duodenum.

    a. First
    b. Second
    c. Third
    d. Fourth

    **Answer: c**

11. One of the following is not the boundary of Hesselbach's triangle ......................

    a. Linea alba
    b. Rectus muscle
    c. Inferior epigastric artery
    d. Inguinal ligament

    **Answer: a**

12. Following structure divides the Hesselbach's triangle.

    a. Obliterated umbilical vein
    b. Obliterated umbilical artery
    c. Ligamentum teres
    d. Inferior epigastric artery

    **Answer: b**

13. Point out the incorrect statement about the boundaries of Calot's triangle ......................

    a. Right: Cystic duct
    b. Left: Common hepatic duct
    c. Right: Common hepatic duct
    d. Above: Liver

    **Answer: c**

14. Following structure is present in front of paraduodenal fossa ......................

    a. Inferior mesenteric vein
    b. Inferior mesenteric artery
    c. Superior mesenteric artery
    d. Superior mesenteric vein

    **Answer: a**

15. The superior mesenteric artery arises at ..................... level.

    a. L1
    b. L2
    c. L3
    d. L4

    **Answer: a**

16. Following are the main branches of celiac artery except .....................

    a. Left gastric
    b. Common hepatic
    c. Right gastric
    d. Splenic

    **Answer: c**

17. Following structures form the stomach bed .....................

    a. Right crus of diaphragm
    b. Left crus of diaphragm
    c. Transverse mesocolon
    d. Spleen

    **Answer: a**

18. The nerves posterior to the cecum are all except .....................

    a. Right genitofemoral
    b. Left genitofemoral
    c. Right femoral
    d. Right lateral cutaneous nerve of thigh

    **Answer: b**

19. Celiac artery lies at ..................... level.

    a. L1
    b. L2
    c. Between L1 and L2
    d. Between T12 and L1

    **Answer: d**

20. All of the following are the main branches of celiac trunk except .....................

    a. Common hepatic artery
    b. Right gastric artery
    c. Splenic artery
    d. Left gastric artery

    **Answer: b**

21. While doing resection of the small intestine, the surgeon can differentiate between jejunal and ileal segment depending on following criteria mainly .....................

    a. Length of intestine
    b. Diameter of intestine
    c. Vascular arcades
    d. All of the above

    **Answer: c**

22. Following are the branches of inferior mesenteric artery except .....................

    a. Right colic
    b. Left colic
    c. Sigmoidal
    d. Superior rectal

    **Answer: a**

23. While operating, the surgeon has ligated both the mesenteric arteries what maintains the blood supply to the colon in the operating time .....................

    a. Superior mesenteric vein
    b. Inferior mesenteric vein
    c. Vasa recta
    d. Superior rectal artery

    **Answer: c**

24. A 60-year-old male, had a lump in epigastrium, it turned out to be carcinoma stomach. Following lymphatic areas need to be scanned especially except .....................

    a. Hepatic                           c. Subpyloric

    b. Gastric                            d. Diaphragmatic

**Answer: d**

25. A surgeon was operating a case of cancer rectum, following areas need to be excised except .....................

    a. Pelvic colon                     c. Ischiorectal fossa

    b. Anal skin                      d. Mesentery

**Answer: d**

26. Following structures are attached to the inguinal ligament except .....................

    a. External oblique              c. Internal oblique

    b. Fascia lata                   d. Cremaster

**Answer: a**

27. Direct inguinal hernia is ..................... to inferior epigastric artery.

    a. Posterior                    c. Medial

    b. Lateral                      d. Anterior

**Answer: c**

28. Indirect inguinal hernia is ..................... to inferior epigastric artery.

    a. Lateral                      c. Anterior

    b. Medial                     d. Posterior

**Answer: a**

29. Following statements of spermatic cord are true except .....................

    a. External spermatic fascia is derived from internal oblique

    b. Internal spermatic fascia is derived from transversalis fascia

    c. Cremasteric fascia derived from cremasteric muscle

    d. External spermatic fascia is derived from external oblique

**Answer: a**

30. All are features of large intestine except .....................

    a. Appendices epiploicae present       c. Sacculations present

    b. Teniae coli absent                d. Peyer's patch absent

**Answer: b**

31. The anatomical landmark for pudendal nerve block is .....................

    a. Ischial tuberosity               c. Ischial spine

    b. Pubic tubercle                  d. Rectum

**Answer: c**

32. **The structures forming stomach bed ..................... are all except**

    a. Posterior wall of lesser sac         c. Anterior wall of lesser sac

    b. Liver                                     d. Left suprarenal gland

**Answer: b**

33. **The surgeon while doing appendicectomy has to be careful of all nerves except .....................**

    a. Right genitofemoral nerve         c. Right femoral nerve

    b. Left genitofemoral nerve          d. Lateral cutaneous nerve of thigh

**Answer: b**

34. **Following nerves are posterior to kidney except .....................**

    a. Iliohypogastric nerve            c. Subcostal nerve

    b. Ilioinguinal nerve               d. Genitofemoral nerve

**Answer: d**

35. **Mother of a 12-year-old child complained of a lump (swelling) in left hypochondriac region. What organ is likely to be enlarged .....................**

    a. Liver                          c. Stomach

    b. Spleen                       d. Kidney

**Answer: b**

36. **Which vessels lie in front of third part of duodenum?**

    a. Inferior mesenteric            c. Splenic

    b. Superior mesenteric           d. Celiac

**Answer: b**

37. **Vas deferens begins from ..................... border of testis.**

    a. Anterior                     c. Lateral

    b. Medial                       d. Posterior

**Answer: d**

38. **The prostate gland surrounds ..................... of urethra.**

    a. Initial 1 cm                c. Initial 3 cm

    b. Distal 3 cm                d. Distal 3 cm

**Answer: c**

39. **Following are the sites of portosystemic anastomosis except .....................**

    a. Upper end of esophagus         c. Lower end of rectum

    b. Lower end of esophagus         d. Bare area of liver

**Answer: a**

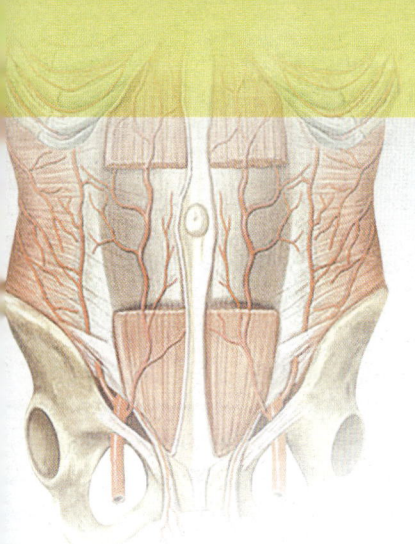

# Dissection | 22

## 1. REGIONS OF ANTERIOR ABDOMINAL WALL

The anterior abdominal wall is divided into 9 regions, by 2 vertical and 2 horizontal lines
- Vertical lines pass through the midinguinal points (lies between anterior superior iliac spine and pubic symphysis)
- Transpyloric plane (of Addison)—passes between jugular notch and pubic symphysis, lies at the tip of 9th costal cartilage

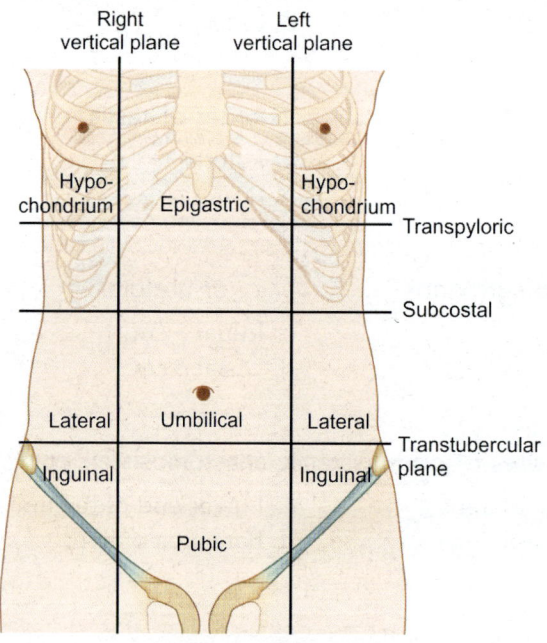

(Regions and planes)
Subdivisions of abdomen and pelvis

- Transtubercular plane—traverses the tubercle of iliac crest (tubercle of iliac crest is on the outer lip, 5 cm behind anterior superior iliac spine).

## 2. ANTERIOR ABDOMINAL WALL (SUPERFICIAL PLANE)

- It has a superficial fatty layer and deep membranous layer, this demarcation is more prominent in the lower half of abdomen
- Incise from anterior superior iliac spine to median plane, raise the lower margin of cut fascia and identify the fatty and membranous layers
- One can easily pass a finger below the membranous layer and loose areolar tissue over the external oblique aponeurosis, except along the inguinal ligament
- Medially one can pass a finger along the spermatic cord, anterior to the body of pubis into the perineum
- Laterally, the membranous fascia is attached to the pubic bone and arch.

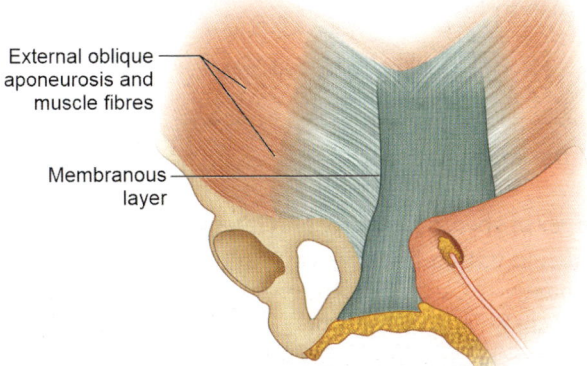

External oblique aponeurosis and muscle fibres

Membranous layer

Lower part of anterior abdominal wall

## 3. INGUINAL REGION

- Locate the superficial inguinal ring supero-lateral to the pubic tubercle, it is a triangular opening in the external oblique aponeurosis.
- Appreciate the spermatic cord (round ligament in females) emerging through the superficial inguinal ring.
- Just superior to the ring try to locate the anterior cutaneous branch of iliohypogastric nerve.

## 4. MUSCLES OF ANTERIOR ABDOMINAL WALL

- External oblique arises from external surface of lower 8 ribs and the fibres run downwards, forwards and medially (like hands in pocket).
- The internal oblique arises from lumbar fascia, iliac crest, lateral two-thirds of

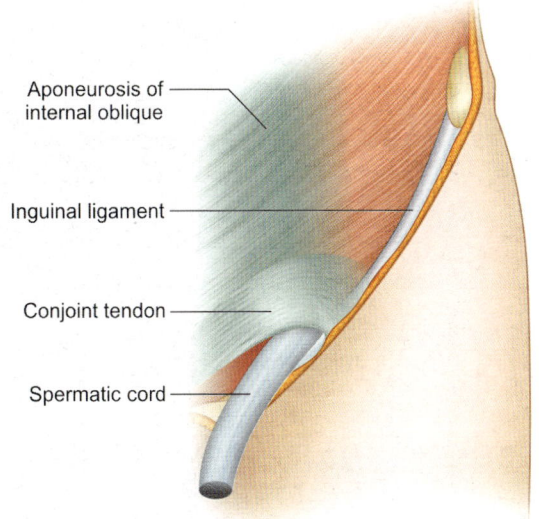

Aponeurosis of internal oblique

Inguinal ligament

Conjoint tendon

Spermatic cord

Dissection of inguinal region

inguinal ligament and runs upwards and forwards.

- The innermost layer is transversus abdominis, runs from internal surface of rib cage, lumbar fascia, iliac crest, lateral third of inguinal ligament to linea alba.
- The deep surface of transversus abdominis is covered by layer of transversalis fascia.
- The aponeurosis of the three muscles fuse in the midline to form the linea alba and also partially enclose the rectus abdominis muscle.
- Lower parallel fibres of internal oblique and transversus abdominis do not intersect at the linea alba but fuse to form conjoint tendon.

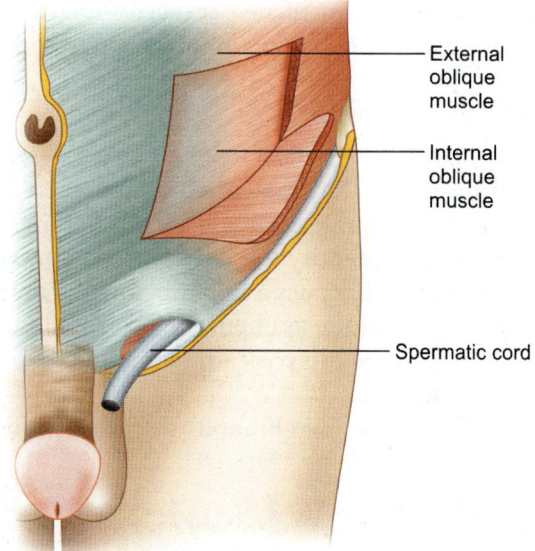

Anterior abdominal wall (deep dissection)

## 5. RECTUS SHEATH

- Take a sharp cut on the anterior layer of sheath
- Reflect the anterior layer of sheath medially and laterally, and cut the tendinous intersections
- Pick-up the rectus muscle with a blunt forceps and identify the intercostals and subcostal nerves entering the sheath
- Cut the rectus abdominis muscle in middle and reflect, identify the superior and inferior epigastric arteries. Define the arcuate line, i.e. the lower curved arch of posterior layer of rectus sheath
- Umbilical hernia occurs as a result of weakness in umbilical scar due repeated pregnancies.

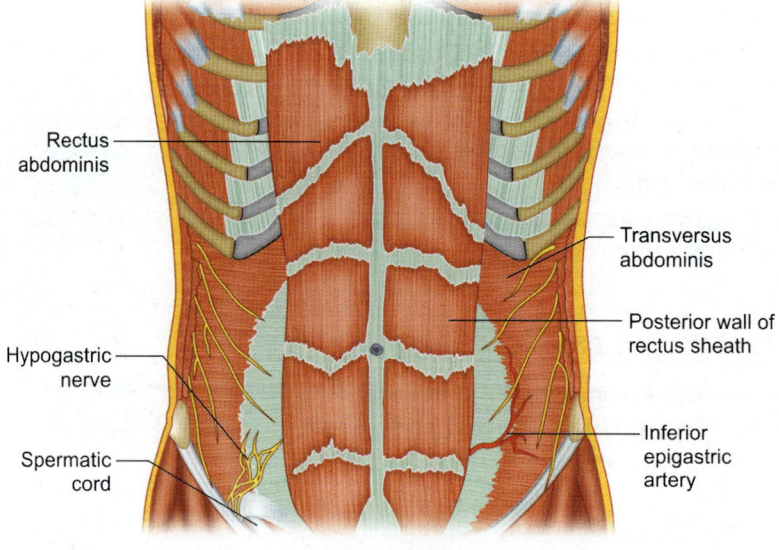

Rectus sheath

## 6. INGUINAL CANAL

### a. Structures to be identified

- It is an intermuscular passage just above the medial half of inguinal ligament
- It begins at the deep inguinal ring, which lies just superior to the midinguinal point, and lies immediately lateral to the inferior epigastric artery.

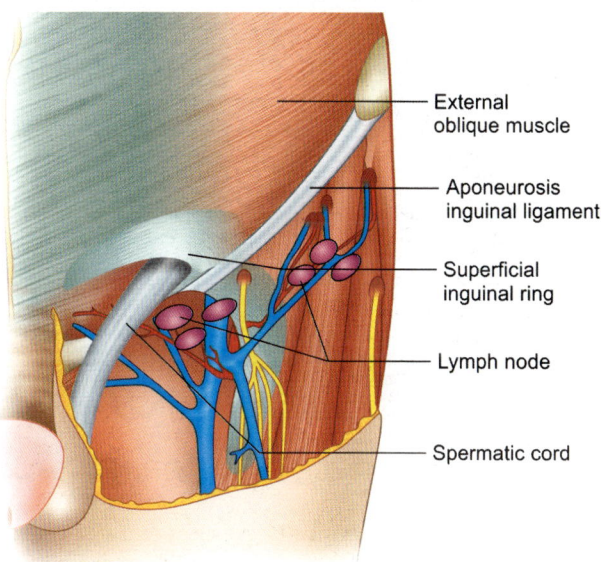

External oblique muscle

Aponeurosis inguinal ligament

Superficial inguinal ring

Lymph node

Spermatic cord

Superficial dissection inguinal region

### b. Viva Questions

- Indirect hernia traverses on the outer side of spermatic cord and is lateral to the inferior epigastric artery. It may be secondary to persistent processus vaginalis
- Direct inguinal hernia is due to weakening of conjoint tendon and is medial to inferior epigastric artery
- Structures passing through the inguinal canal:
  - Spermatic cord in males, round ligament in females
  - Ilioinguinal nerve enters the canal between the external and internal oblique muscles and comes out through the superficial inguinal ring
  - Anterior wall is formed by skin, superficial fascia, external oblique aponeurosis, and its lateral third covered by internal oblique fibres
  - Posterior wall is formed by fascia transversalis, conjoint tendon covers its medial two thirds, medial end formed by reflected part inguinal ligament
  - Roof is formed by arched fibres of internal oblique and transversus abdominis
  - Floor is formed by union of fascia transversalis and lacunar ligament.

## 7. MALE EXTERNAL GENITAL ORGANS

### a. Incisions

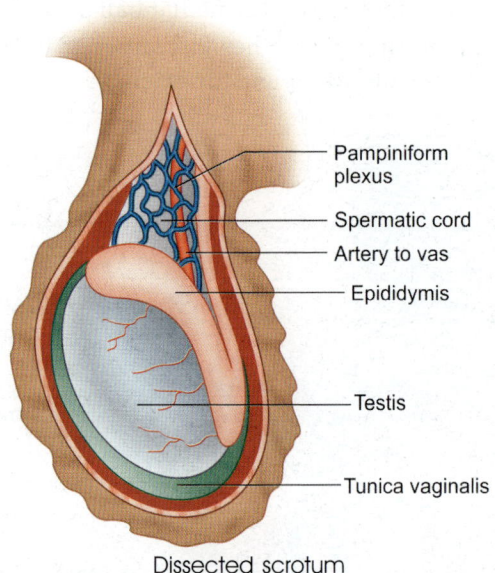

Dissected scrotum

### b. Structures to be Identified

- Carefully reflect the skin from the dartos muscle, and the dartos muscle from the underlying loose areolar tissue
- Lift the testis and spermatic cord from the scrotum
- At the deep inguinal ring, lift the peritoneum away from the extraperitoneal tissue
- Cut the spermatic cord at the superficial inguinal ring and with the testis attached to it place the specimen in the tray
- Incise and reflect the coverings of testis and also study the structures of spermatic cord
- Inject saline through a hypodermic needle to study the extent of tunica vaginalis
- Separate the testis from tunica vaginalis by blunt dissection.

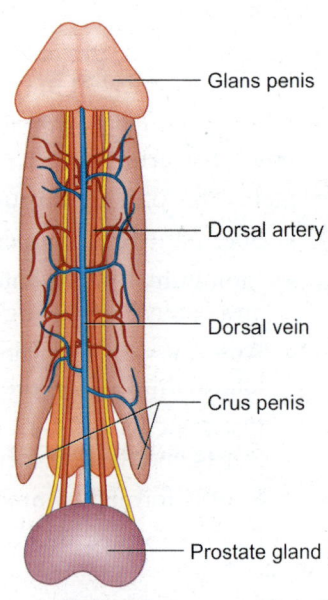

Dorsal surface of penis

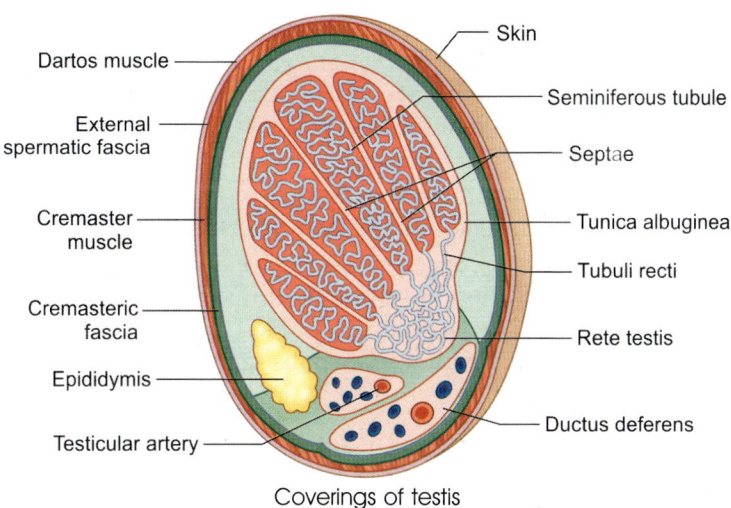

Coverings of testis

Labels: Skin, Dartos muscle, External spermatic fascia, Seminiferous tubule, Cremaster muscle, Septae, Cremasteric fascia, Tunica albuginea, Epididymis, Tubuli recti, Testicular artery, Rete testis, Ductus deferens

## c. Viva Questions

### Contents of Spermatic Cord

Ductus deferens, artery to vas, testicular artery, pampiniform plexus, cremasteric artery, lymph vessels, autonomic nerves supplying the vas.

### Coverings of Testis

External spermatic fascia derived from external oblique aponeurosis
- Cremasteric fascia derived from cremasteric muscle
- Internal spermatic fascia derived from fascia transversalis
- Tunica vaginalis.

### Varicocele

Varicocele is dilatation of veins of pampiniform plexus. It is common on left side since testicular vein enters the renal vein at right angles on left side, left testicular vein is burdened by

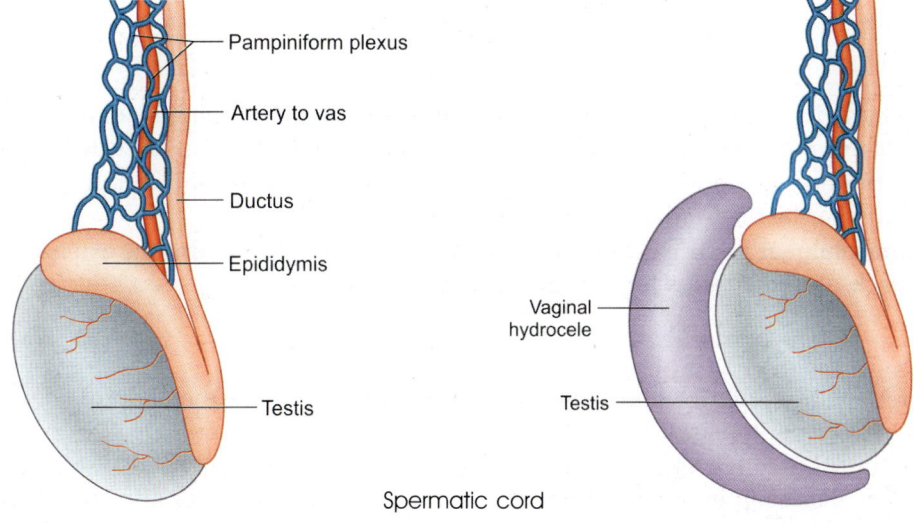

Spermatic cord

Labels: Pampiniform plexus, Artery to vas, Ductus, Epididymis, Testis, Vaginal hydrocele, Testis

descending colon weight, the left renal vein lies between superior mesenteric artery in front and aorta behind, angle between the two arteries may be narrow (like NUTCRACKER) and it may cause compression of left renal vein, left common iliac vein is crossed by the right common iliac artery this increases the pressure in the iliac vein.

- Appendix of testis is remnant of paramesonephric duct
- Appendix of epididymis is remnant of mesonephros
- Epididymis overlies the superior and posterolateral surface of testis
- Dartos is a subcutaneous muscle
- Hydrocele is an abnormal collection of serous fluid in processus vaginalis caused due to defective absorption or excessive secretion of fluid. Treatment includes drainage of the hydrocele fluid and eversion of the tunica vaginalis sac and suturing to underlying layers of testis.

## Penis

- Neurovascular bundle is present on the dorsum of penis
- A transverse cut is taken on the penis. It consists of 3 cylindrical bodies: 2 dorsally placed, corpora cavernosa and corpus spongiosum ventrally

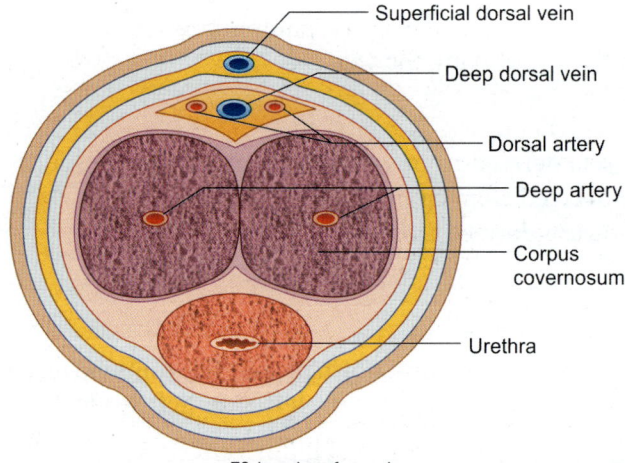

Superficial dorsal vein

Deep dorsal vein

Dorsal artery

Deep artery

Corpus covernosum

Urethra

TS body of penis

## 8. LOIN

- Put the body in prone position, define the inferior border of latissimus dorsi and posterior border of external oblique muscle. The area between these 2 muscles is the lumbar triangle
- Reflect the muscles and you can now see the fibres of internal oblique muscle and thoracolumbar fascia. Medially it splits into 3 layers
- The thoracolumbar fascia extends from the sacrum to neck, it contains the extensor muscles of the back, and quadratus lumborum in lumbar region.

## 9. PERITONEAL CAVITY

- After removal of anterior abdominal wall, without disturbing the abdominal structures appreciate the peritoneum.
- Peritoneum is a tough elastic layer of elastic areolar tissue lined by simple squamous epithelium. Parietal peritoneum lines the internal surface of anterior abdominal wall.

- Open the parietal peritoneum and cut away the greater omentum occupying most of the abdominal cavity in front, now appreciate the disposition of the abdominal organs *in situ*.
- Before cutting the omentum, identify the arterial arcade of gastroepiploic arteries 2–3 cm from the greater curvature of stomach, note that it blends with the greater curvature of stomach and transverse colon.
- Roof of abdominal cavity is formed by dome-shaped diaphragm, anterior and lateral wall is formed by anterior abdominal wall muscle and aponeurosis, and lower part laterally is formed by ilium with iliacus muscle, posterior wall is formed by vertebral column, and muscles attached to it and thoracolumbar fascia.

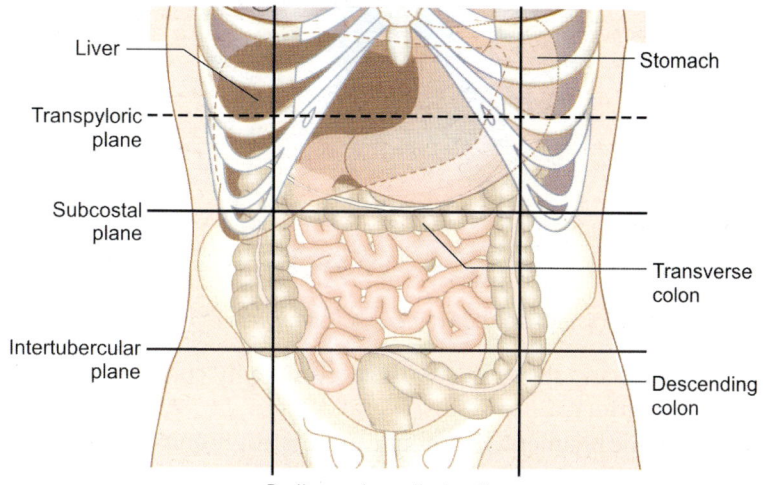

Peritoneal cavity *in situ*

- Small part of the peritoneal cavity lies behind the stomach and posterior abdominal wall. This is the lesser sac or also known as omental bursa.

## 10. LESSER OMENTUM

- Pull the liver superiorly and tilt the inferior border of liver anteriorly, this will make you visualise the lesser omentum

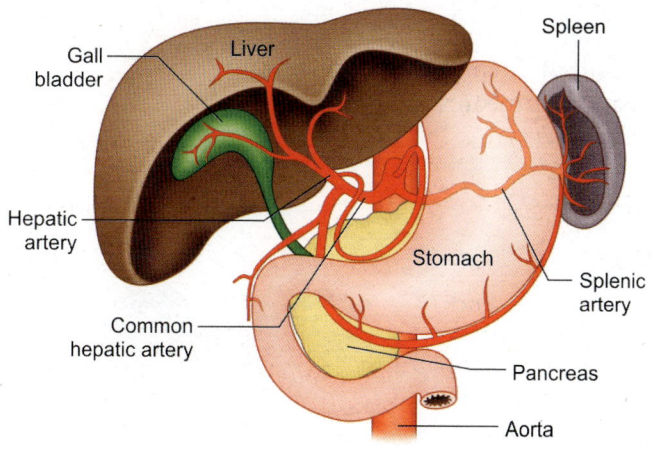

Lesser omentum *in situ*

- Cut the left lobe of liver by cutting to the left of falciform ligament, ligamentum teres and attachment of lesser omentum
- Remove the anterior layer of lesser omentum close to the lesser curvature of stomach trace the left gastric vessels. Appreciate that the gastric vessels curve posteriorly around the esophagus
- Try to locate anterior vagal trunk on anterior surface of esophagus
- Follow the right gastric artery to proper hepatic artery, identify the portal vein, cystic duct common hepatic duct

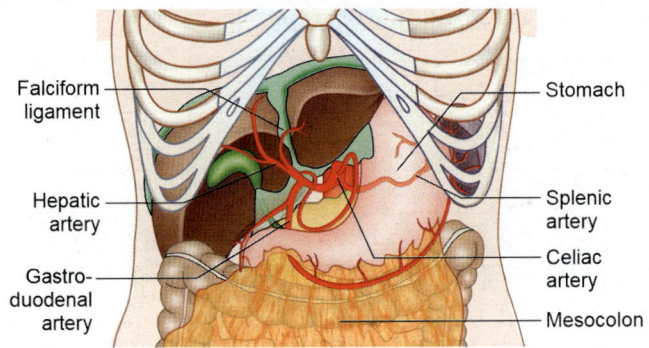

Deep dissection showing celiac artery with its branches

- Identify the celiac trunk and its main subdivisions namely common hepatic artery, splenic artery and left gastric artery
- Identify the gastrosplenic ligament, lienorenal and gastrophrenic ligament and vessels within *in situ.*

### c. Viva Questions

- Branches of celiac trunk—common hepatic, left gastric, splenic, located at T12 and L1
- Lesser omentum attachments—superiorly attached to the lesser curvature of stomach and the upper border of first 2 cm of duodenum and inferiorly attached in the form of inverted L on ligamentum venosum and border of porta hepatis The free border contains the porta hepatis structure (hepatic artery, portal vein, bile duct), and it forms anterior boundary of epiploic foramen which lies at T12

### 11. EVISCERATION OF STOMACH

### a. Steps for Evisceration

- Cut through the esophagus and left gastric vessels close to the diaphragm and then cut the gastrophrenic and gastrosplenic ligaments, and strip the anterior layer of greater omentum.

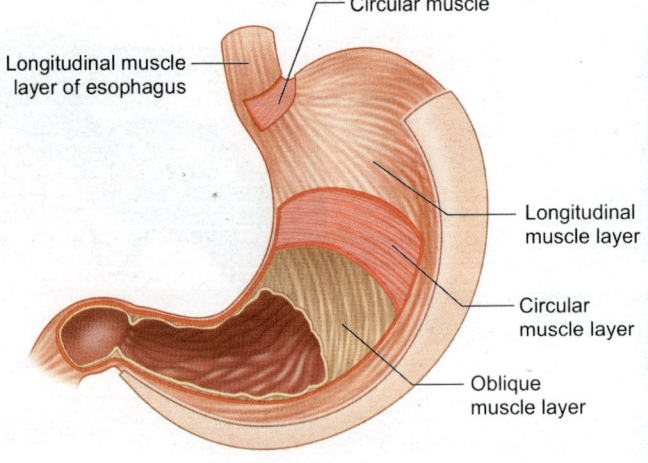

Muscle layers of stomach

• Cut through the pylorus close to the duodenum.

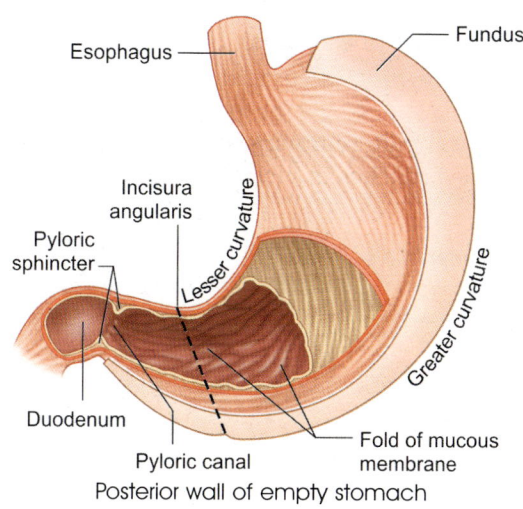

Posterior wall of empty stomach

## b. Study of the Organ

• Open the stomach along the greater curvature of stomach and examine the mucous membrane with the hand lens. Appreciate the mucosal folds rugae, identify gastric pits.

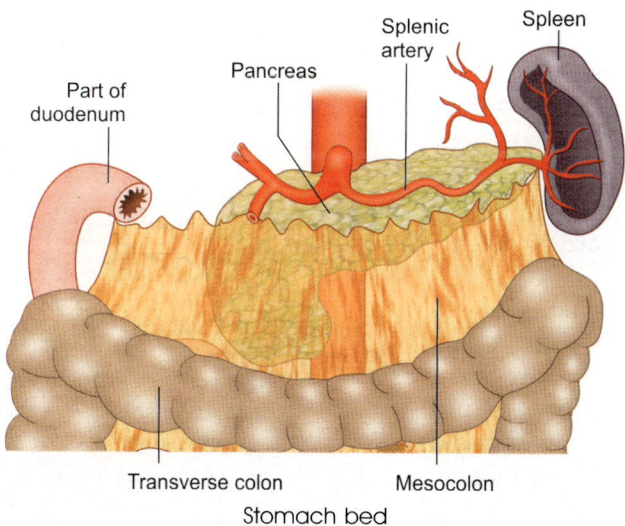

Stomach bed

• Strip the mucous membrane and study the muscle layer of stomach. Pyloric sphincter narrows the canal within.

• After removing the stomach, study the structures under the cover of stomach that constitute the stomach bed separated from it by the omental bursa:
  – Spleen
  – Upper pole of left kidney
  – Left suprarenal gland
  – Diaphragm

- Upper part of pancreas
- Splenic artery
- Mesentery of transverse colon (mesocolon)

## c. Vivisection

Gastric carcinoma is common, while removing the stomach the surgeon has to be vigilant about the celiac artery and the branches in vicinity to stomach.

## d. Viva Questions

- Stomach bed structures:
  - Spleen
  - Upper pole of left kidney
  - Left suprarenal gland
  - Diaphragm
  - Upper part of pancreas
  - Splenic artery
  - Mesentery of transverse colon (mesocolon)
- Celiac artery branches:
  - Left gastric artery
  - Hepatic artery
  - Splenic artery
- Musculature of stomach:
  - It is made-up of 3 layers
  - Outer longitudinal layer—thickest along the curvatures
  - Middle circular layer—thickens along the pyloric region
  - Inner layer—oblique fibres looping around cardiac notch

## 12. STUDY OF SMALL INTESTINE

### a. Steps of Evisceration

- With the pressure of fingers turn the coils of intestine to the left and cut the right layer of peritoneum up to the posterior abdominal wall and separate it from the mesentery.
- Scrape out the fat from the mesentery this will expose the superior mesenteric vessels. Lymph nodes can be appreciated around the vessels and plexus of nerves.
- Identify the branches going to the duodenum, pancreas, colon.

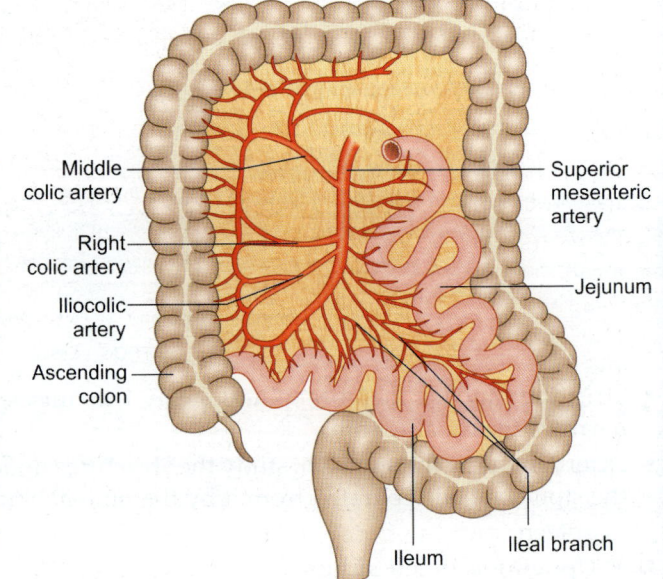

Small intestine with superior mesenteric artery and vascular arcades

Middle colic artery — Superior mesenteric artery — Right colic artery — Jejunum — Iliocolic artery — Ascending colon — Ileum — Ileal branch

- Turn the coils of intestine to the right now and this will expose the inferior mesenteric artery remove the peritoneum in the similar manner as you have done for the superior mesenteric artery. Identify the branches to colon and rectum.

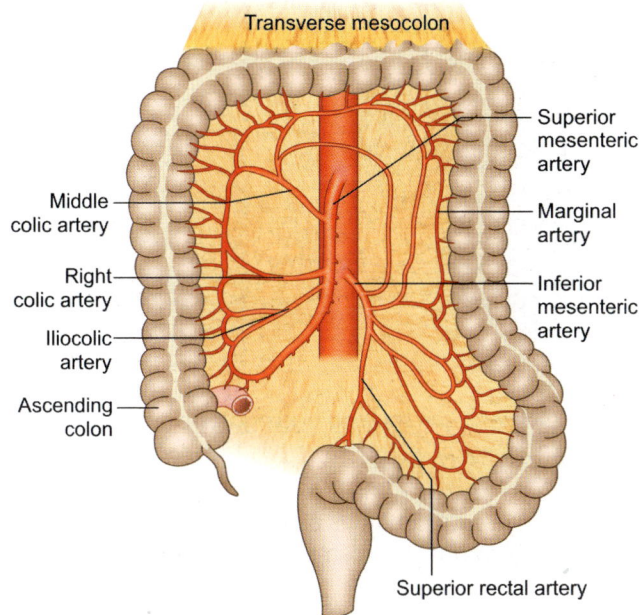

**Mesenteric arteries and marginal artery**

- Tie a thread at the duodenojejunal junction and another around the ileum close to cecum. Cut against the ligatures and remove the intestine and place it in a tray. Wash the intestines with water.
- Study in detail the jejunum, and appreciate that it has a larger diameter, thicker walls, less fat in mesentery, and the lumen is often empty (hence the name).
- Cut longitudinally the jejunal segment and you will prominently see numerous, circular mucosal folds. Use hand lens to see the villi.
- Cut a segment of ileum longitudinally and you will see that the mucosal folds are less numerous. Aggregates of lymph nodes is the peculiar feature of ileum.

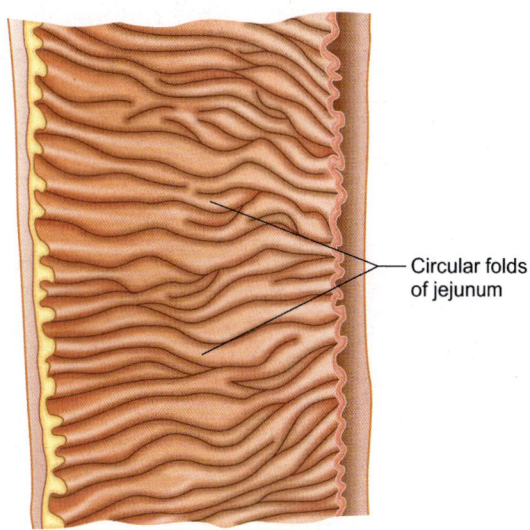

Cut section of jejunum; Mucosal circular folds

## b. Vivisection

- In cases of gangrene of intestine, the surgeon has to define the segment is ileal or jejunal, one has to study the vascular arcades over the mesentery.

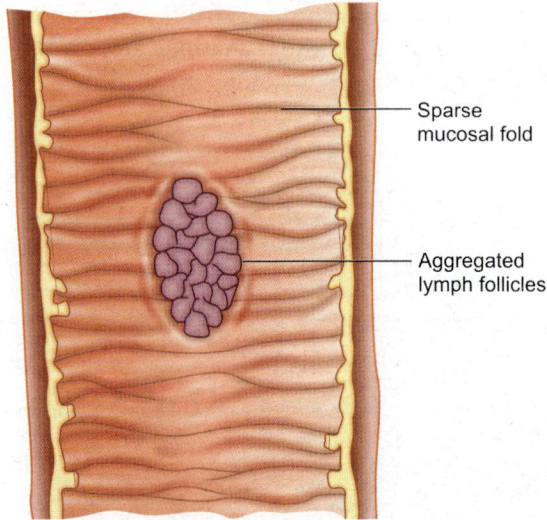

Cut section of ileum showing aggregates of lymphatic tissue

- In jejunum, the number of vascular arcades are few, and the vasa recta are long, while the arcades are numerous in ileum but the vasa recta are short.

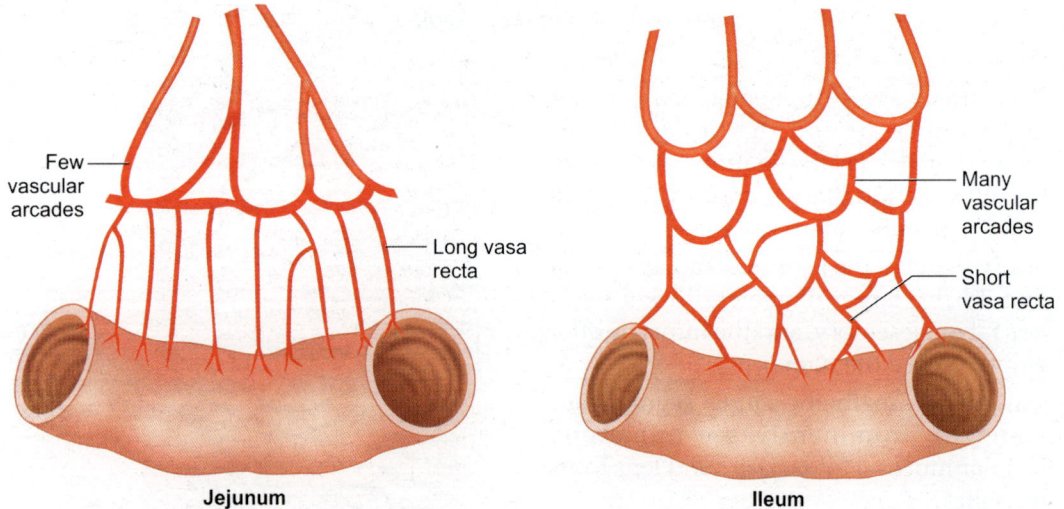

Vasa recta and vascular arcades of jejunum    Vasa recta and vascular arcades of ileum

## c. Viva Questions

- Numerous mucosal folds are present in jejunum while ileum has peculiarity of having aggregation of lymph nodes
- Vascular arcades are less in jejunum and more in ileum, vasa recta are long in jejunum than in ileum.

## 13. CECUM

### a. Study of Cecum

- Identify the cecum, as the most dilated portion of large intestine in right iliac fossa

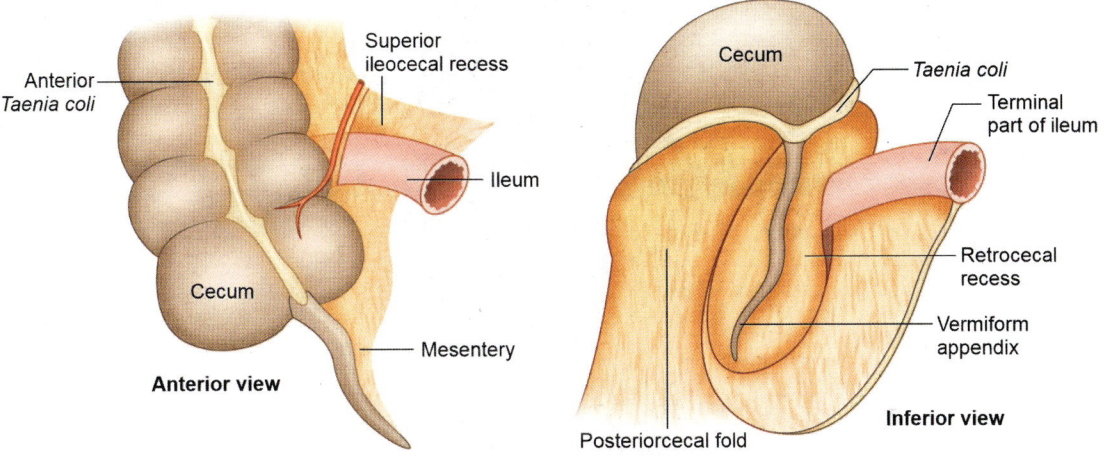

Cecum-gross features

- Cut open the lateral wall of cecum, and identify the ilieal opening and opening of appendix.
- The cardinal feature of large intestine can be appreciated, i.e. *Taenia coli*

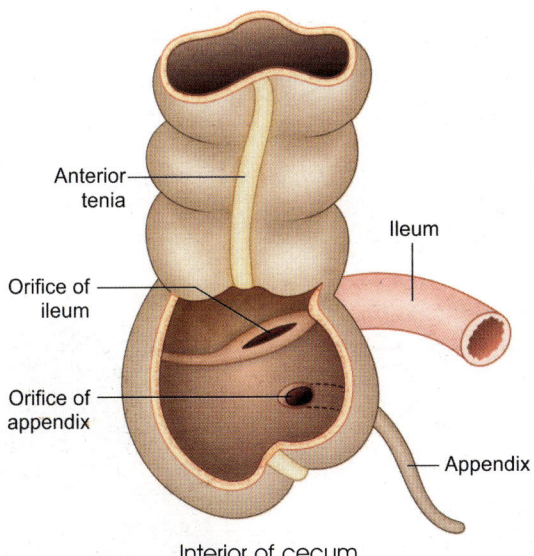

Interior of cecum

- Manually turn the cecum upwards and appreciate the structures posterior to it. Following structures are posterior to it:
  - Iliacus, psoas major
  - Right genitofemoral, right femoral, right lateral cutaneous nerve
  - Gonadal vessels, external iliac artery, appendicular artery
  - Appendix when retrocecal.

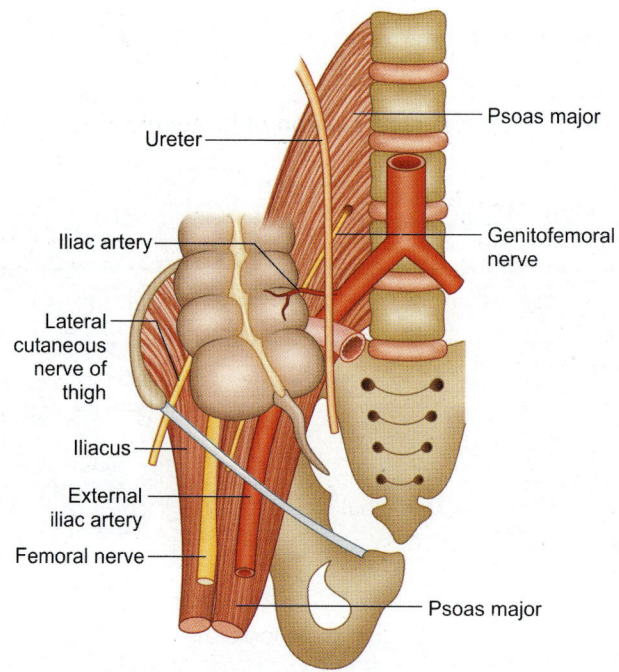

Posterior relations of cecum—cecal bed

## b. Vivisection

While doing appendicectomy, surgeon needs to be vigilant about the neurovascular bundle, i.e. femoral, genitofemoral, lateral cutaneous nerves, gonadal vessels, external iliac vessels.

## c. Viva Questions

- Cardinal features of large intestine—*Taenia coli*, sacculations, appendices epiploicae
- Posterior relations of cecum—right genitofemoral nerve, right femoral nerve, right lateral cutaneous nerve of thigh, right gonadal vessels, external iliac artery, appendix.

## 14. COLON

### a. Evisceration of Colon

- Tie a thread around the ileum and another thread around the junction between the descending and sigmoid colon. Remove the specimen in toto.
- While removing the specimen one needs to cut through the peritoneum and ligate (tie) the vessels supplying the colon (removing the colon exposes the retroperitoneal structures).

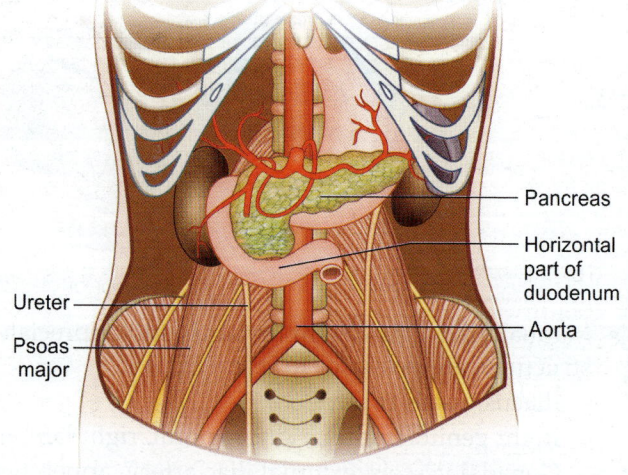

Retroperitoneal structures seen after removing colon

- Wash the lumen of colon, appreciate the external features of colon, i.e sacculations, *Taenia coli*, appendices epiploicae.
- Open the colon longitudinally.

### b. Vivisection

While doing colonectomy, in cases of cancer colon, surgeon needs to ligate the vessels-ascending colon and right flexure of colon are supplied by ileocolic artery and right colic artery, transverse colon by middle colic artery, and descending colon by left colic and sigmoidal arteries.

### c. Viva Question

Cardinal features of large intestine—*Taenia coli*, sacculations, appendices epiploicae.

## 15. RETROPERITONEAL STRUCTURES (DUODENUM, PANCREAS, KIDNEYS)

### a. Steps of Study

- After removal of the coils of intestine, the retroperitoneal structures can be studied, clear off the anterior surface of pancreas, and study the extent.
- Appreciate the extent of the duodenum around the head and neck of pancreas. Turn the descending part of duodenum and head of pancreas to left and locate pancreaticoduodenal vessels and the bile duct.

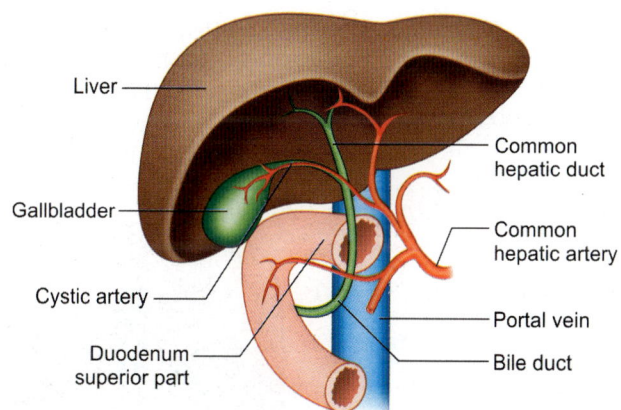

Extrahepatic biliary system

- Cut the peritoneum and remove the fat along the descending and ascending parts of duodenum. By blunt dissection free it from posterior abdominal wall.
- Identify the inferior mesenteric vein lateral to the ascending part of duodenum and superior mesenteric vessels medial to it, left renal vein superiorly.
- You may appreciate the suspensory muscle of duodenum extending from duodenojejunal flexure to right crus of diaphragm. Prominent in child cadaver, extending from esophageal orifice and lies posterior to pancreas and inferior mesenteric vein.
- Cut along the outer side (convex) side of duodenum and flush it with water to appreciate the mucosa.

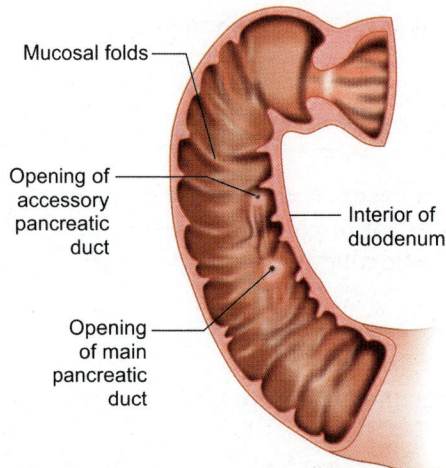

Interior of duodenum

Mucosal folds

Opening of accessory pancreatic duct

Opening of main pancreatic duct

Interior of duodenum

Bile duct

Pancreatic duct

Spleen

Pancreas

Posterior surface of pancreas showing the duct system

- Now approach the tail of pancreas, separate the pancreas from the posterior abdominal wall and identify the splenic vein. Against the neck of pancreas, the splenic vein unites the superior mesenteric vein to form the portal vein, also appreciate that the inferior mesenteric vein drains into the splenic vein. Make a linear cut on posterior surface of pancreas and trace the pancreatic and accessory pancreatic duct.
- Appreciate that the superior mesenteric vessels lie anterior to uncinate process of pancreas and the third part of duodenum.

- Great vessels, i.e. aorta and inferior vena cava lie against the vertebral column.
- Remove the fat and the fascia from the anterior surface of kidneys and suprarenal gland. Displace the kidneys medially and expose the renal vessels. Check for the course of ureter and the muscles posterior to kidney.

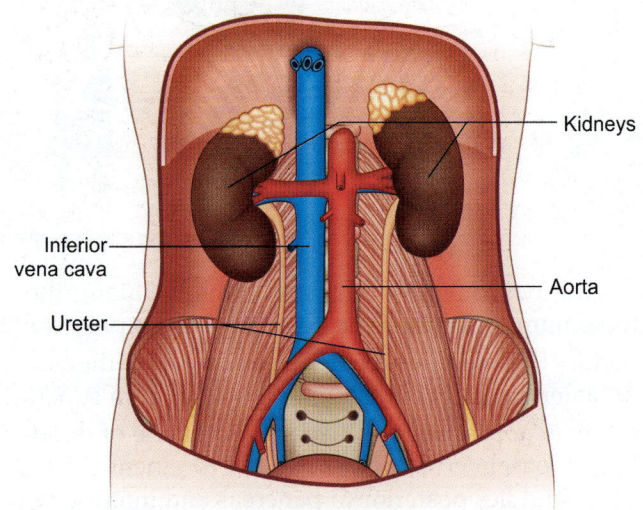

Kidneys

Inferior vena cava

Ureter

Aorta

Posterior abdominal wall—showing great vessels and vertebral column

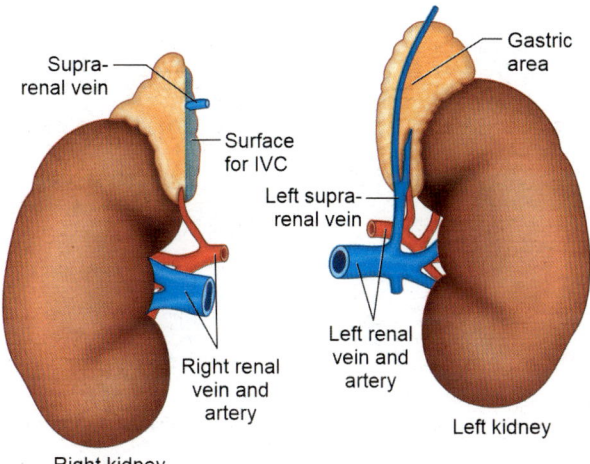

Supra-
renal vein

Surface
for IVC

Left supra-
renal vein

Gastric
area

Right renal
vein and
artery

Left renal
vein and
artery

Left kidney

Right kidney

Right suprarenal gland        Left suprarenal gland

- The muscles on which the kidneys lie are diaphragm superiorly, psoas major medially and quadratus lumborum and transversus abdominis laterally.

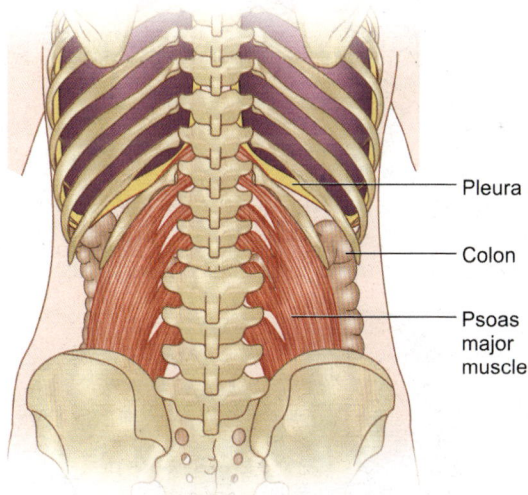

Pleura

Colon

Psoas
major
muscle

Dissection from behind

- Anteriorly, the right kidney is related to duodenum, right colic flexure, and suprarenal gland, while the left kidney is related to suprarenal gland, spleen, pancreas and left colic flexure.

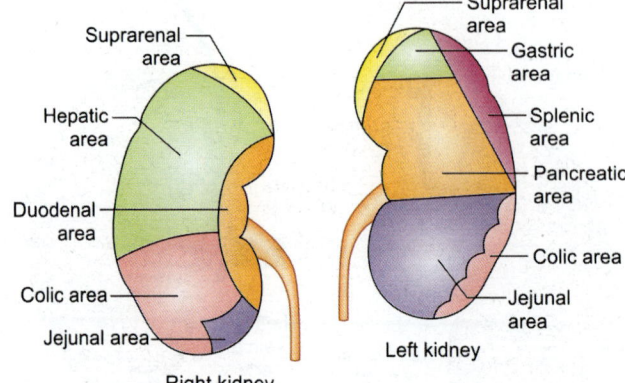

Anterior relations of right kidney     Anterior relations of left kidney

- Slice, the kidney coronally and appreciate the pyramid, papillae, the renal pelvis.

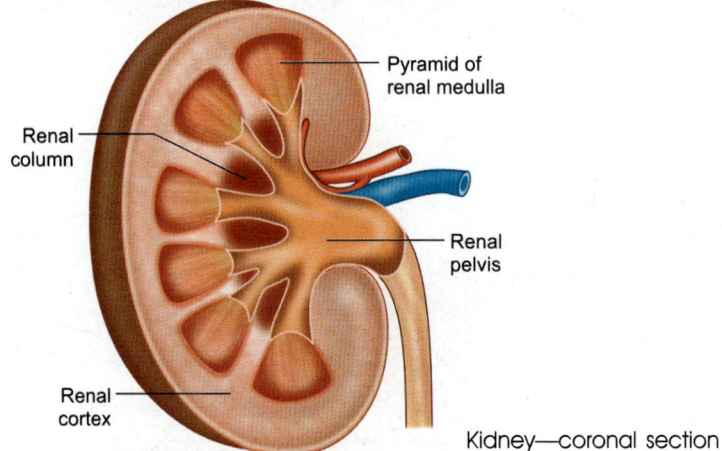

Kidney—coronal section

- Now appreciate the ureters, slit it open and dissect the walls of ureter.

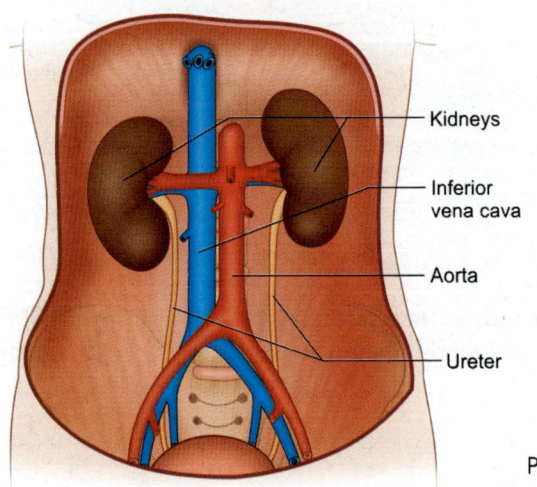

Posterior abdominal wall,
with kidneys, ureter *in situ*

- Abdominal part of ureter is relatively free from the vascular relations while the pelvic part crosses the external iliac vessels in the lower half and in the upper half of pelvic part of ureter is related to gonadal vessels.

### b. Vivisection

- Conveniently kidneys are approached from behind.
- While operating on pelvic organs the course of the ureter has to be kept in mind, otherwise the surgeon may accidentally cut the ureters while ligating the vessels. For instance, while removing the uterus, ureteric injuries are very common.

### c. Viva Questions

- *Relations of kidney:* Anterior relations of right kidney differ from the left, right kidney is related to liver, duodenum, right colic flexure, right suprarenal gland while left kidney is related to spleen, left suprarenal gland, pancreas, left colic flexure. Posterior relations are common for both kidneys, psoas major muscle, quadratus lumborum, transversus abdominis, iliohypogastric and ilioinguinal nerves. The twelfth rib forms renal angle with the kidney.

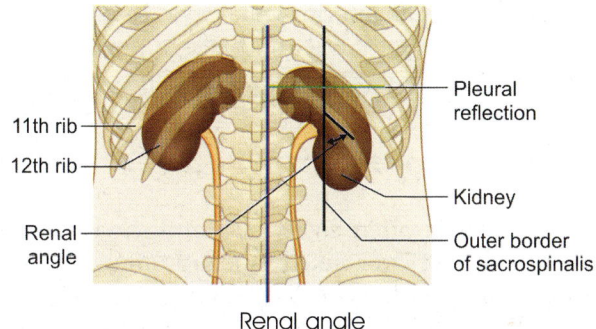

Renal angle

- The third part of duodenum is related to superior mesenteric vessels
- The splenic artery is related to the superior border of the pancreas.

## 16. EVISCERATION OF LIVER

### a. Steps of Evisceration

- Divide the anterior layers of coronary and left triangular ligaments without going too far up to the inferior vena cava.

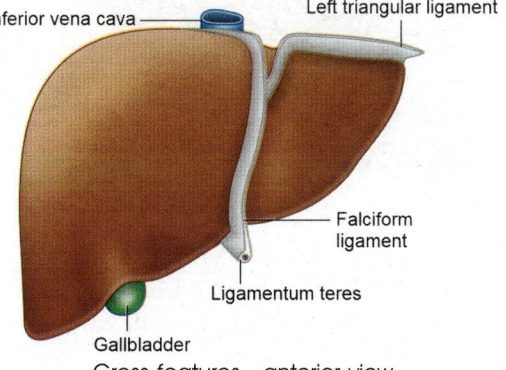

Gross features—anterior view

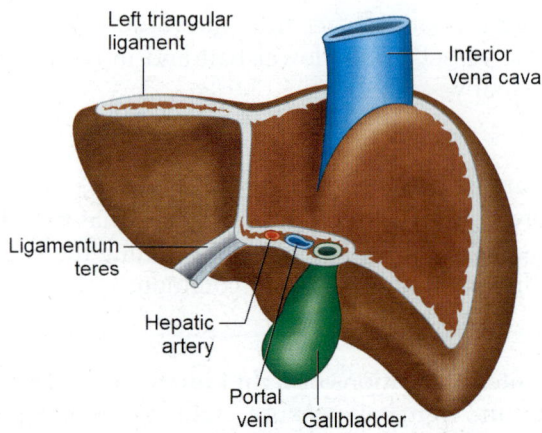

Gross features—posteroinferior view

- Pull the liver downwards, identify the inferior vena cava between liver and diaphragm. Divide the hepatic veins entering the inferior vena cava. Severe the peritoneal attachments of liver. Free it all around and deliver it out and place in the tray.
- Study the surfaces of liver and appreciate the lobes of liver. Identify the cut ends of the ligaments.

## b. Vivisection

- Surgical resection of the liver is often easily accomplished due to the unique internal arrangement of the vasculature of liver (like bronchopulmonary segments of lungs) and a very good regenerating capacity of liver
- Watershed between the surgical right and left lobes is a line passing through the gallbladder fossa and middle hepatic line. This line is known as Cantlie's line.

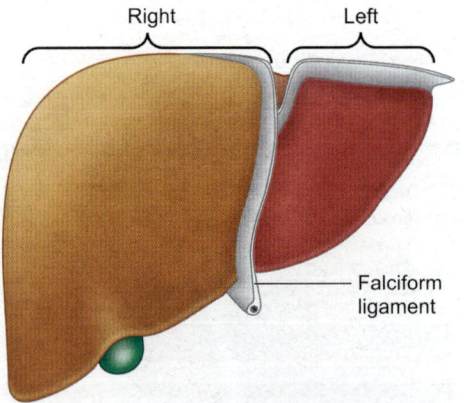

Surgical lobes of liver

- Liver segments to the right (V-VIII) are supplied by right hepatic artery, right branch of portal vein and the bile is drained by the right hepatic duct

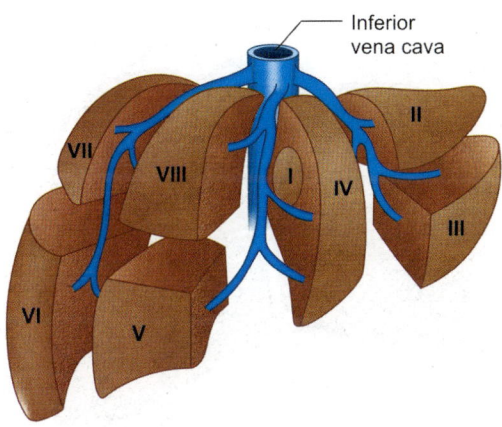

Couinaud's liver segments

- Segments to the left are supplied by left branch of the hepatic artery, left portal vein branch, bile drained by left hepatic duct (compare with bronchopulmonary segments).

### c. Viva Questions

- Students should identify the various lobes of liver, right and left lobe of liver, caudate and quadrate lobe of liver. The H-shaped subdivision between the quadrate and caudate lobe is formed by the fissure for ligamentum venosum, Inferior vena cava fossa, ligamentum teres, and fossa for gallbladder.
- The inverted L-shaped fissure of ligamentum venosum and lips of porta hepatis give attachment to lesser omentum.

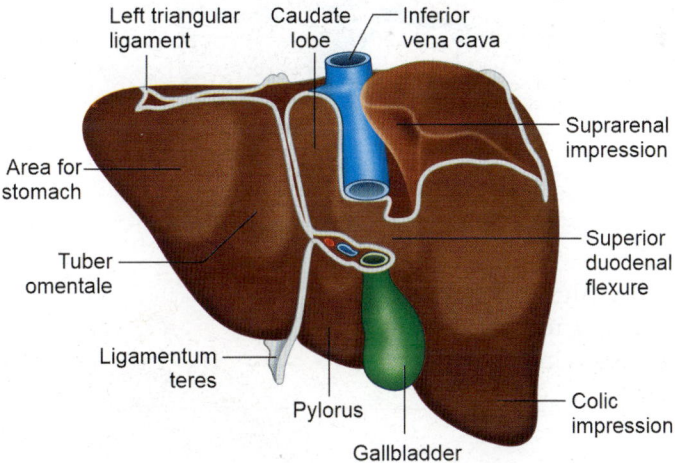

External features of posteroinferior surface of liver

- Posteroinferior surface of liver is related to various organs which create an impression on the liver, i.e. spleen, right kidney, pylorus, duodenum, eosophagus, right suprarenal gland

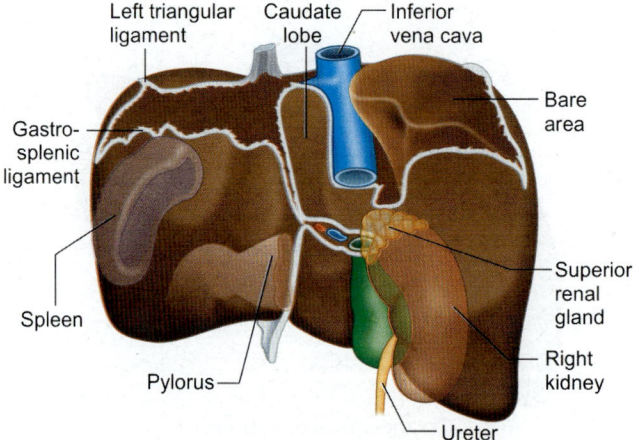

Visceral impressions on posteroinferior surface of liver

## 17. EVISCERATION OF SPLEEN

- Spleen is wedged between the diaphragm and stomach in the left posterosuperior region of supracolic compartment.

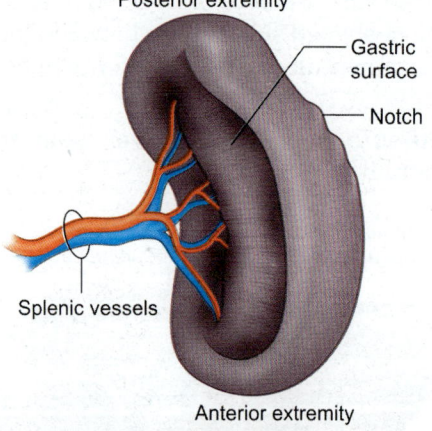

Spleen—location

- Identify the gastrosplenic ligament, lienorenal ligament, and the vessels within severe the vessels in the ligament to remove the spleen.

### a. Vivisection

Splenectomy is done in cases of traumatic rupture of spleen. While doing splenectomy the gastrosplenic vessels are ligated, splenic vessels at the superior border of pancreas are ligated, the spleno-colic ligament, gastrosplenic ligament and

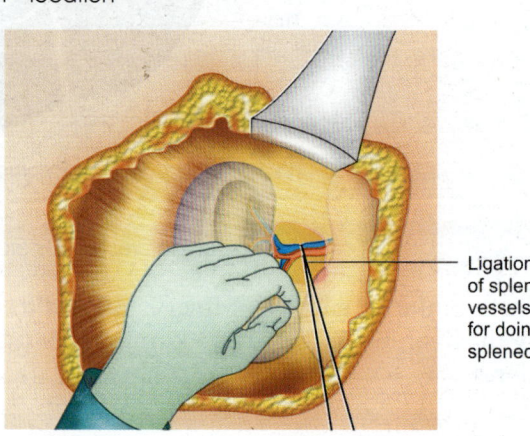

Ligation of splenic vessels for doing splenectomy

lienorenal ligament are severed to deliver the spleen out. While operating the surgeon has to beware of the vessels in and around the spleen, i.e. gastroepiploic vessels, short gastric vessels, splenic artery.

### b. Viva Questions

- Splenic artery is tortuous, other tortuous arteries are lingual, uterine
- Visceral surface of spleen is related to stomach, left kidney, pancreas, left colic flexure.

## 18. DIAPHRAGM

### a. Study of Diaphragm

- Remove the peritoneum of diaphragm and uncover the crura of the diaphragm.

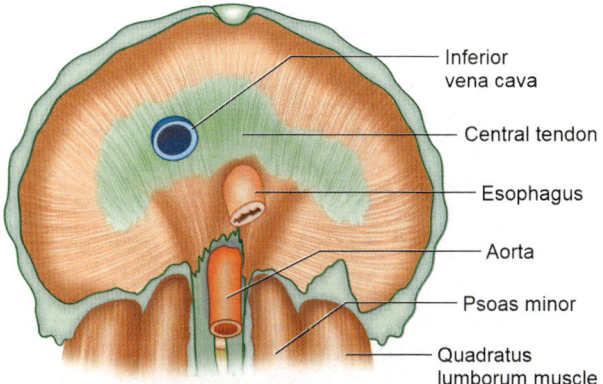

Diaphragm—gross features, *in situ*

- Arch like fascial thickening can be appreciated on the lateral side of each crus, i.e. medial arcuate ligament and a thickening of thoracolumbar fascia is lateral arcuate ligament. Medial arcuate ligament is a tendinous arch in the fascia covering the upper part of psoas major; while lateral arcuate ligament is tendinous arch covering the quadratus lumborum.

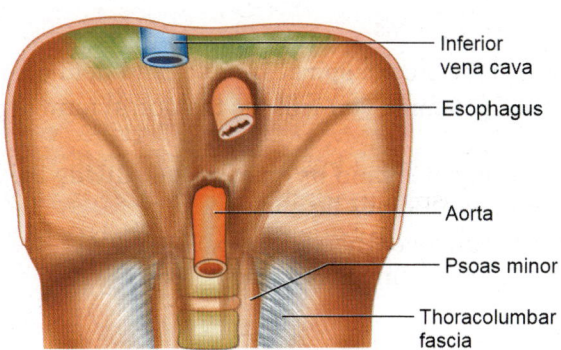

Diaphragm-deep layer

- The large openings of diaphragm are—the inferior vena caval opening, esophageal opening, and aortic hiatus.

### b. Viva Question

Levels of the openings of diaphragm T8-inferior vena caval, T10-esophageal, T12-aorta.

## 19. POSTERIOR ABDOMINAL WALL

### a. Study the Posterior Abdominal Wall

- Appreciate the abdominal aorta and inferior vena cava, and the lymph nodes, the nerve plexus around it
- Try to look for the sympathetic chain on either side of aorta and in front of psoas major muscle
- Between the right crus of diaphragm and aorta is the cysterna chyli and azygos vein trace the gonadal vessels.

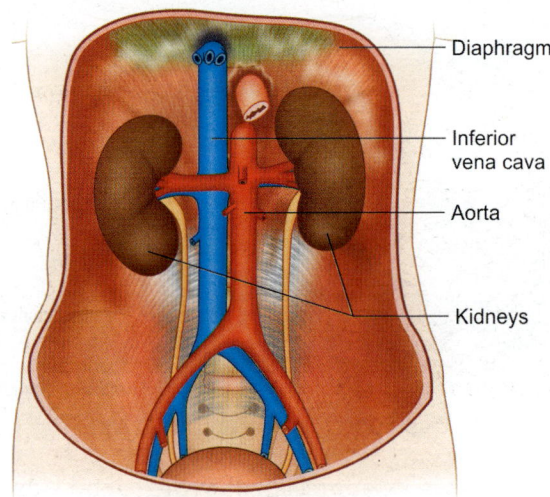

Posterior abdominal wall

## 20. BONY PELVIS

### a. Study of Dorsal View of Bony Pelvis

- Turn the cadaver, remove the erector spinae muscles and define the ligaments
- Uncover the dorsal sacral foramina you will see the dorsal rami of sacral nerves emerging through the foramina
- Define the sacrotuberous ligament and its attachments, divide the ligament and dissect it out from the underlying sacrospinous ligament
- Very importantly locate the pudendal nerve, internal pudendal vessels and nerve to obturator internus curving over the sacrospinous ligament.

### b. Viva Question

Structures on the posterior surface of ischial spine traversing the greater and lesser sciatic foramina are the PIN structures, i.e. pudendal nerve, internal pudendal vessels, and nerve to obturator internus.

## 21. ARRANGEMENT OF PELVIC VISCERA

- Study the male and the female pelvis
- Lift the sigmoid colon from the pelvis, and appreciate the sigmoid mesocolon. The sigmoid colon continues as the rectum at S3
- Rectum follows the curve of sacrum and down it continues as anal canal

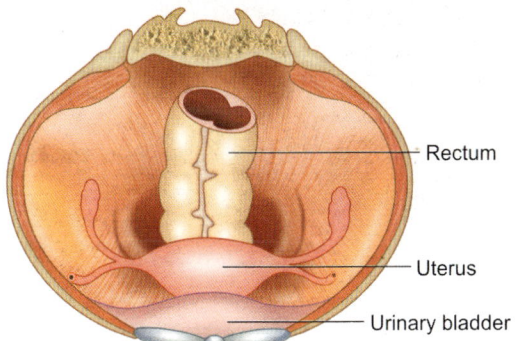

Lesser pelvis in females structures *in situ*

- Urinary bladder lies in the anteroinferior part of the pelvic cavity just behind the pubic symphysis
- There is genital septum between the bladder and rectum
- On either side of genital septum, in males is the ductus deferens, seminal vesicles, and ureter
- Look for the course of ductus in pelvis, from the deep inguinal ring the ductus goes postero-inferiorly in the lateral part of the pelvis then it hooks around the ureter runs medially on posterior surface of bladder above the seminal vesicle
- In female cadaver look for the uterus and the uterine tube, appreciate the ligaments holding the position of the uterus, i.e. round ligament, ligament of ovary and uterosacral ligament
- Put your hand in the rectouterine fold of peritoneum, i.e. pouch of Douglas
- In males appreciate the rectovesicle fold of peritoneum.

## 22. PERINEUM

- Perineum comprises of structures filling the inferior aperture of pelvis. It is a diamond-shaped area between the upper part of thigh and lower part of buttocks.
- Study the female genitalia. During childbirth while doing episiotomy or while catheterising the bladder, one has to be well-versed with the anatomy of perineum. Feel for the perineal body.

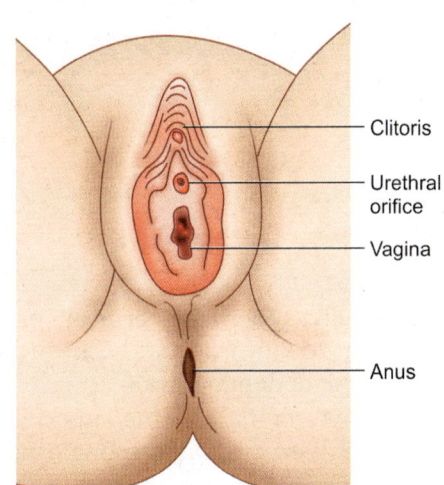

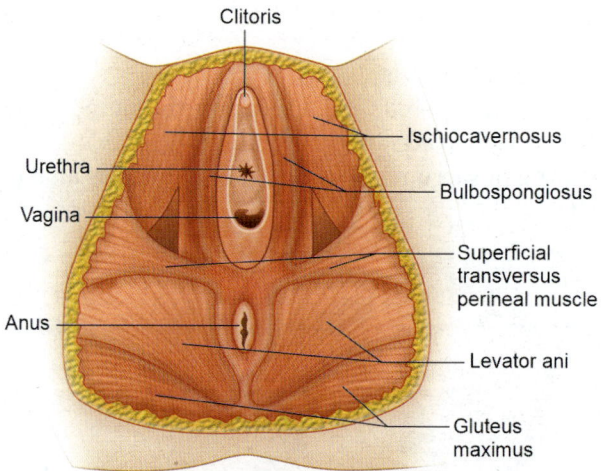

Muscles of female perineum

- The urogenital region has three layers of fascia and superficial and deep perineal space
- The fascia can be well-marked in males, the superficial membranous layer is attached to the ischial tuberosities, and lateral margins of the ischial and inferior pubic rami continuous with the deep fascia of the thigh.
- Make a transverse incision from one ischial tuberosity to another just in front of anus and reflect the skin flaps.

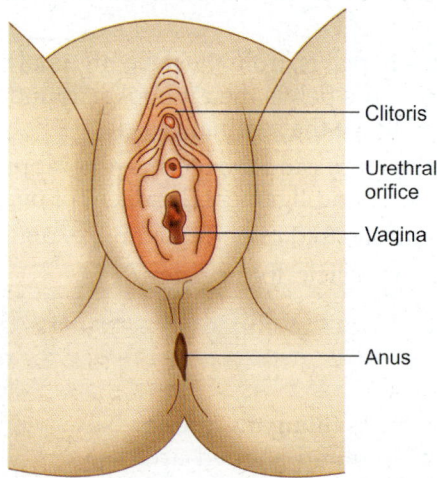

External genitalia (female)

- Enter the superficial perineal space from the anterior abdominal wall by introducing the finger downwards and backwards deep to the membranous layer of superficial fascia of anterior abdominal wall.
- Remove the fat and the superficial fascia from the urogenital region, then identify the ischiocavernous, bulbospongiosus muscle, transversus perinei muscles.
- Identify the posterior scrotal or labial arteries and nerves.

- Hold the urogenital diaphragm in fingers by approaching it through the ischiorectal fossa remove the fat and fascia to study the perineal muscles.

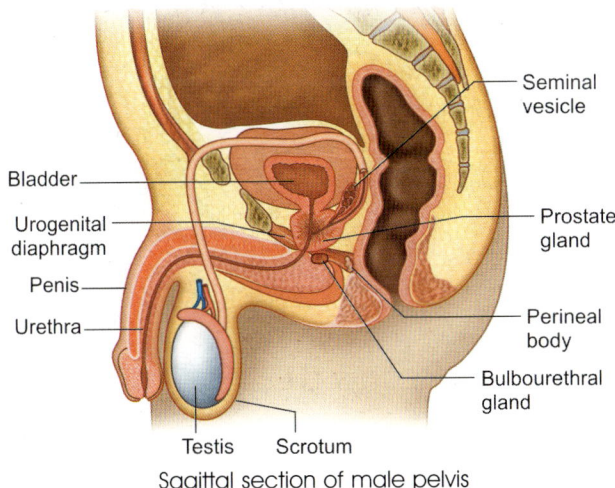

Sagittal section of male pelvis

## 23. PELVIC VISCERA

### a. Study of Pelvic Viscera

- The pelvic viscera and their relations with each other are best studied by taking a sagittal section of the pelvis
- Just behind the pubis is the urinary bladder then uterus in female pelvis and posteriorly is the rectum

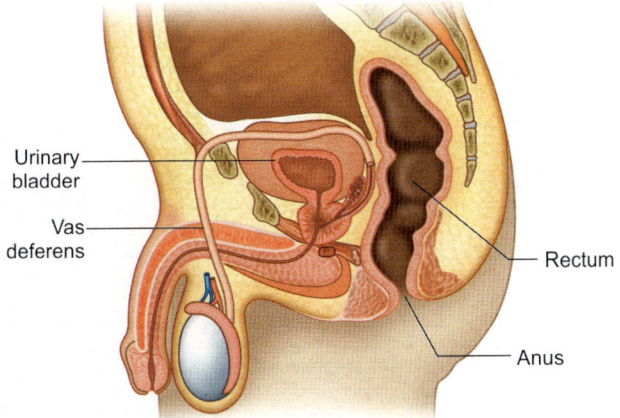

Median section male pelvis

- Study the uterine tube, broad ligament, ovaries. The pelvic ligaments are condensation of pelvic fascia
- The fold of peritoneum between the rectum and uterus is, the rectouterine pouch (pouch of Douglas)

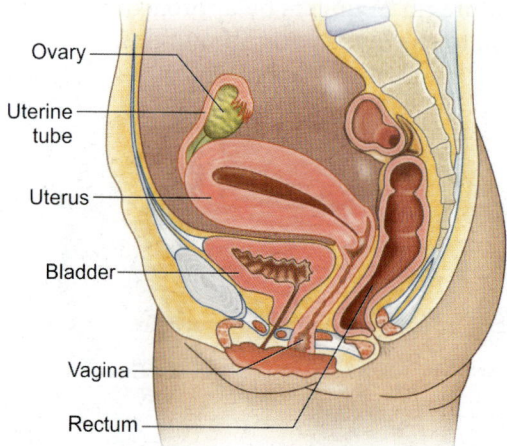

Median section female pelvis

- Study the posterior surface of bladder, feel for the prostate gland in male pelvis at the neck of bladder

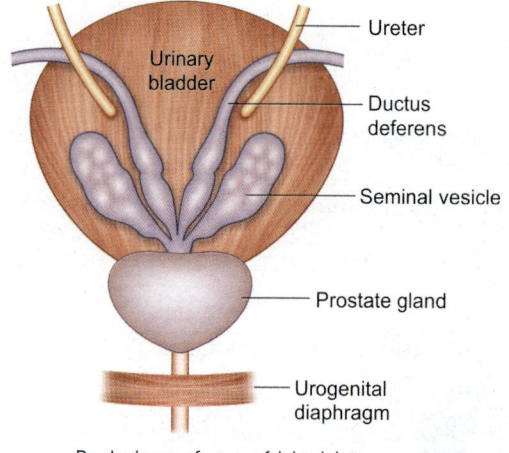

Posterior surface of bladder

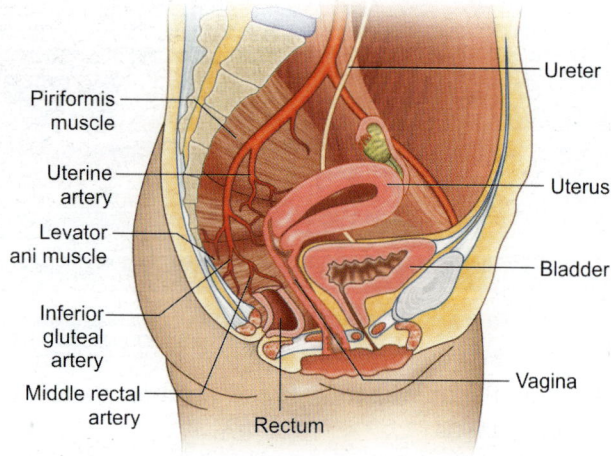

Sagittal section of male pelvis

- Appreciate the internal iliac vessels, the ureter crossed by the uterine artery
- Study the branches of internal iliac artery. The branches supply the pelvic organs. The name of the artery is given according to the organ it supplies.

## b. Vivisection

- Pouch of Douglas is the most dependent portion of pelvic cavity where the pus will tend to gravitate. For draining the abscess, one needs to know the distance of the pouch from the pelvic floor, i.e. 5 cm
- While removing the uterus (hysterectomy), ureteric injuries are very common due to the close proximity to the uterine artery.

## c. Viva Questions

- Student should be able to identify the pelvic organs.
- Define the pouch of Douglas, it is a rectouterine pouch which can be appreciated only in female pelvis. Be sure it is a female pelvis, sometimes the examiner may ask you to show the pouch of Douglas in male pelvis just to check your presence of mind during exams.
- Branches of internal iliac artery
  *Anterior division branches*—superior vesicle artery, obturator artery, inferior vesicle artery, inferior gluteal artery, internal pudendal artery, middle rectal.
  *Posterior division branches*—iliolumbar artery, lateral sacral artery, superior gluteal artery.
- Student should be able to identify the ureter and its relation to uterine artery.

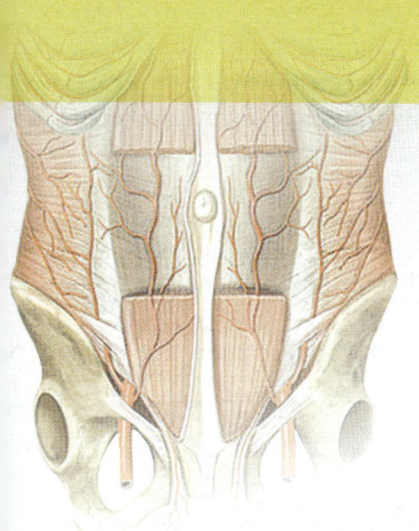

# Osteology | 23

## 1. TYPICAL LUMBAR VERTEBRA

### Identification Points

- Body is strong and stout (to bear the weight of the body)
- Transverse diameter is larger than anteroposterior diameter
- No facets on the side of the body
- Pedicle short and stout
- Spine is horizontal and quadrangular
- Superior articular facet faces medially and has a mammillary process.

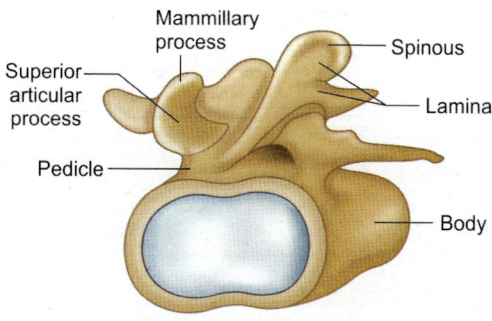

Typical lumbar vertebra

## 2. SACRUM

### Features

- Body is formed by the fusion of 5 vertebrae
- Piriformis and iliacus are attached on its front surface
- Erector spinae and gluteus maximus is attached posteriorly

• Related to ala of sacrum are sympathetic chain behind, iliolumbar artery, obturator nerve and lumbosacral trunk in front.

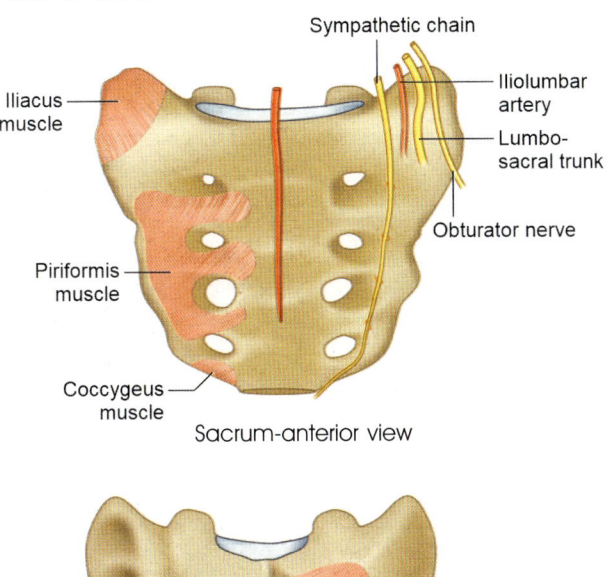

Sacrum-anterior view

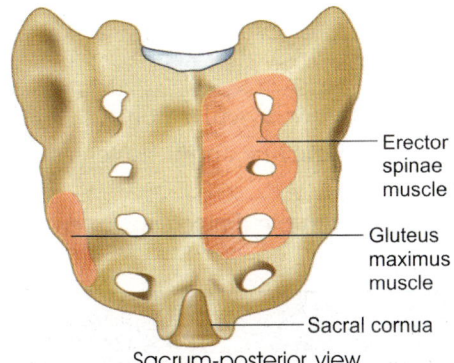

Sacrum-posterior view

## 3. DIFFERENCES BETWEEN MALE AND FEMALE PELVIS

|  | Male pelvis | Female pelvis |
|---|---|---|
| Criteria | Male | Female |
| Greater sciatic notch | Narrow | Wider |
| Acetabulum | Larger | Smaller |
| Iliac crest | More prominent | Less prominent |
| Iliac fossa | Shallow | Deeper |
| Pubic crest | Shorter | Longer |
| Ischiopubic rami | Everted | Not everted |
| Preauricular sulcus | Less prominent | More prominent |
| Ischial spine | In-turned | Straight, pointed |
| Obturator foramen | Large, oval | Small, triangular |

Also refer Key Osteology in section; Abdomen and Pelvis—Chapter 17

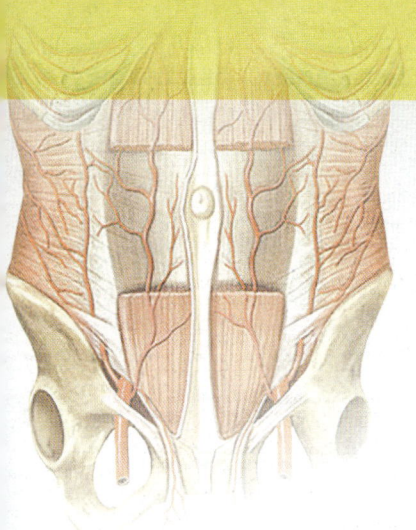

# Surface Anatomy

## 1. PLANES AND QUADRANTS OF ABDOMEN AND PELVIS

- Vertical lines traverse above from midclavicular point to below midinguinal point
- First horizontal line is the transpyloric line and it traverses midway between suprasternal notch and pubic symphysis at L1
- Transtubercular plane passes through the iliac crests on either side at L5

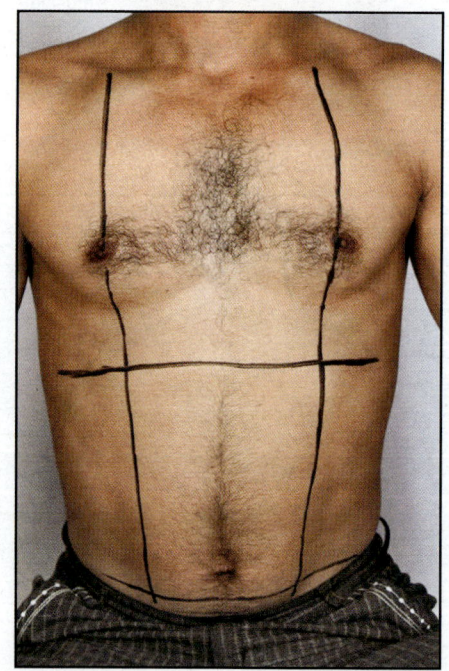

Planes and quadrants of abdomen and pelvis

## 2. STOMACH

- *Position of the subject:* Supine
- *Points to be marked:*
    - 2 cm left of the midline draw 2 lines. This marks the cardiac end of stomach
    - Mark 2 lines apart on transpyloric plane (as the name suggests this marks the pylorus) around 1.5 cm from midline

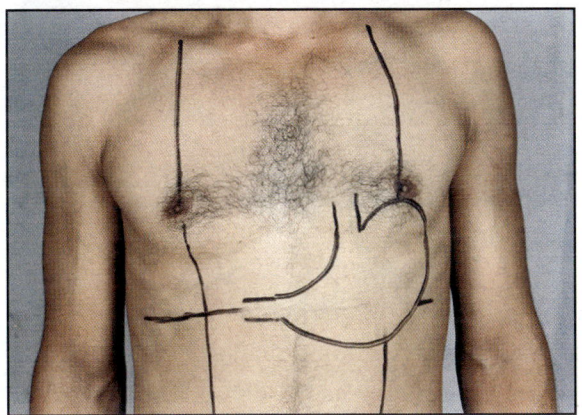

Stomach marking

- Join the above points to get shape of stomach. The lines obtained are the lesser and greater curvature of stomach
- Extend the cardiac end above to just below the left nipple to mark the fundus.

## 3. APPENDIX

- *Position of the body:* Supine
- *Points to be marked:* In right iliac fossa at the point of intersection of right lateral line to the transtubercular line, marks the ileocecal orifice from where 6–8 cm vertical line will indicate the position of appendix.

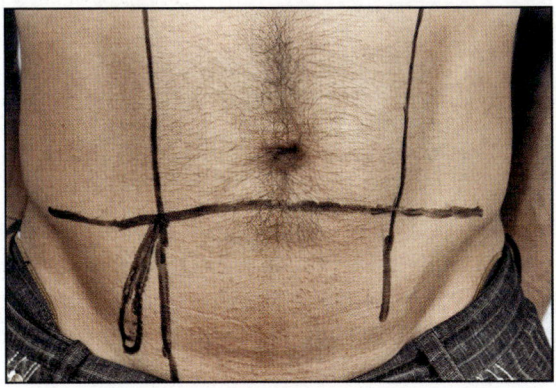

Appendix marking

## 4. INGUINAL CANAL

- *Position of subject:* Supine

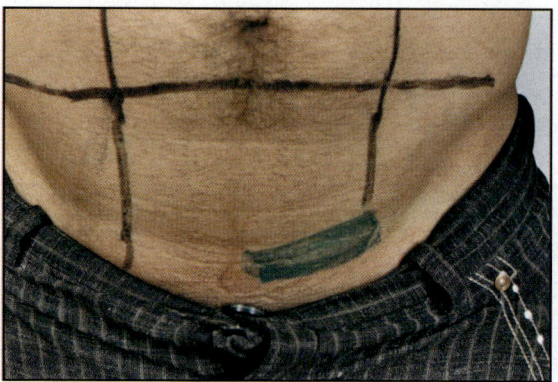

Inguinal canal marking

- *Points to be marked:*
  - This canal lies above the medial half of inguinal ligament
  - Deep inguinal ring is 1 cm above midinguinal point
  - Superficial inguinal ring is just above and lateral to the pubic tubercle
  - Canal is marked by joining the above 2 points with lines 1 cm apart.

## 5. LIVER

- *Position of the subject:* Supine
- *Points to be marked:*

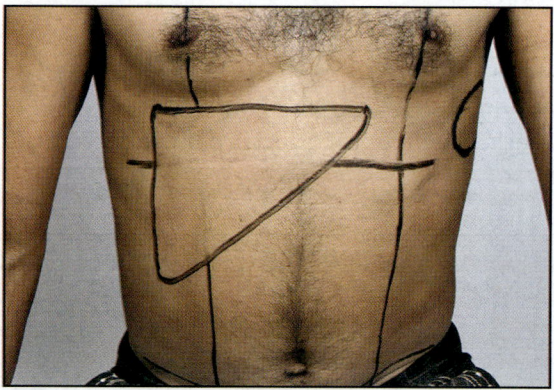

Liver marking (liver is marked as a triangle)

- Upper border of the liver is depicted as a, line crossing the xiphisternal joint, and extending just below right nipple and to the left just inferomedial to left nipple
- Right border line begins from right end of upper border, extend line downwards slightly curved to the right till 1 cm below costal margin at the level of tenth costal cartilage
- Now complete the triangle this marks the inferior border of liver.

## 6. COLON

- *Position of the subject:* Supine

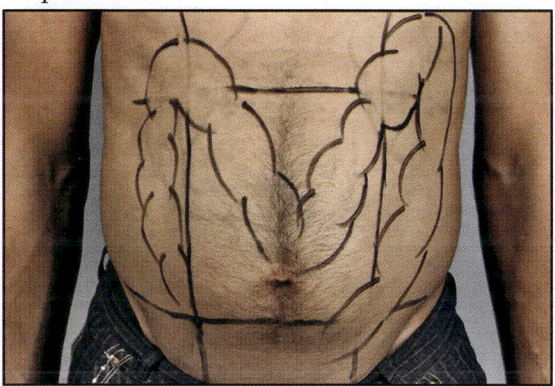

Colon marking

- *Points to be marked:*
  - Ascends lateral to right lateral plane from transtubercular plane to middle of subcostal and transpyloric plane. This marks the ascending colon.
  - Continues from ascending colon end point transversely, first to umbilicus and then to a point superolateral to intersection of left lateral with transpyloric plane, this marks the transverse colon (transverse colon position varies).
  - End-point of transverse colon is beginning of descending colon and it descends just lateral to left lateral line till the inguinal ligament.

## 7. KIDNEYS

- *Position of the subject:* Supine
- *Points to be marked*
  - Hilum of kidney lies along the transpyloric plane 5 cm from midline and medial to the apex of 9th costal cartilage, left kidney is little above the transpyloric plane while right kidney is below.
  - Bean-shaped outline can be marked starting from the hilum 11 cm in vertical dimension and 4.5 cm broad.
  - Upper pole is 2.5 cm from midline, while lower pole is 7.5 cm from midline.
- *Position:* Prone
- *Points to be marked:*
  - Hilum is marked at the level of L1 spine and 5 cm from midline. Make a bean-shaped outline from the hilum.
  - Lower pole is 2.5 cm from the iliac crest.

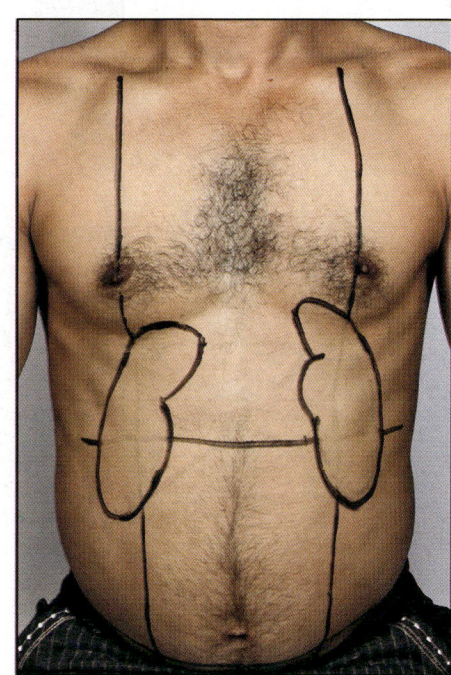

Kidney marking from front

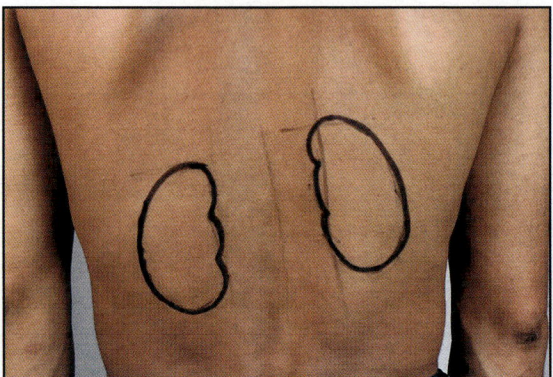

Kidney marking from behind

## 8. SPLEEN

- *Position of the subject:* Left lateral up position
- *Points to be marked:*
  - Dull percussion note over the left upper quadrant will indicate the position of the spleen
  - Spleen can be located against 9 to 11 ribs vertically. Posterior pole does not go beyond midaxillary line.

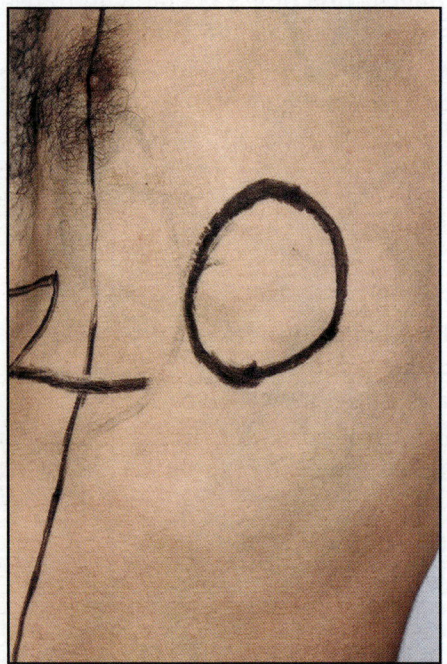

Photo showing marking for spleen

## 9. DUODENUM

- *Position of the subject:* Supine
- *Points to be marked:*
  - I part from pylorus backwards short distance

- II part vertically downwards on right lateral line. 7.5 cm in vertical length
- III part begins from the lower end of II part horizontally for 10 cm crosses the mid-line above the umbilicus
- IV part continues from III part to a point 1 cm below transpyloric plane 3 cm left of median plane.

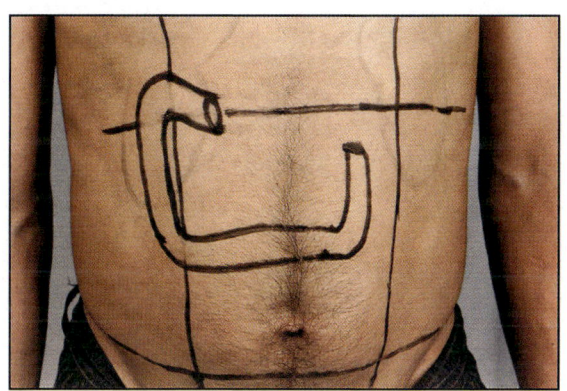

Photo showing markings for all parts of duodenum

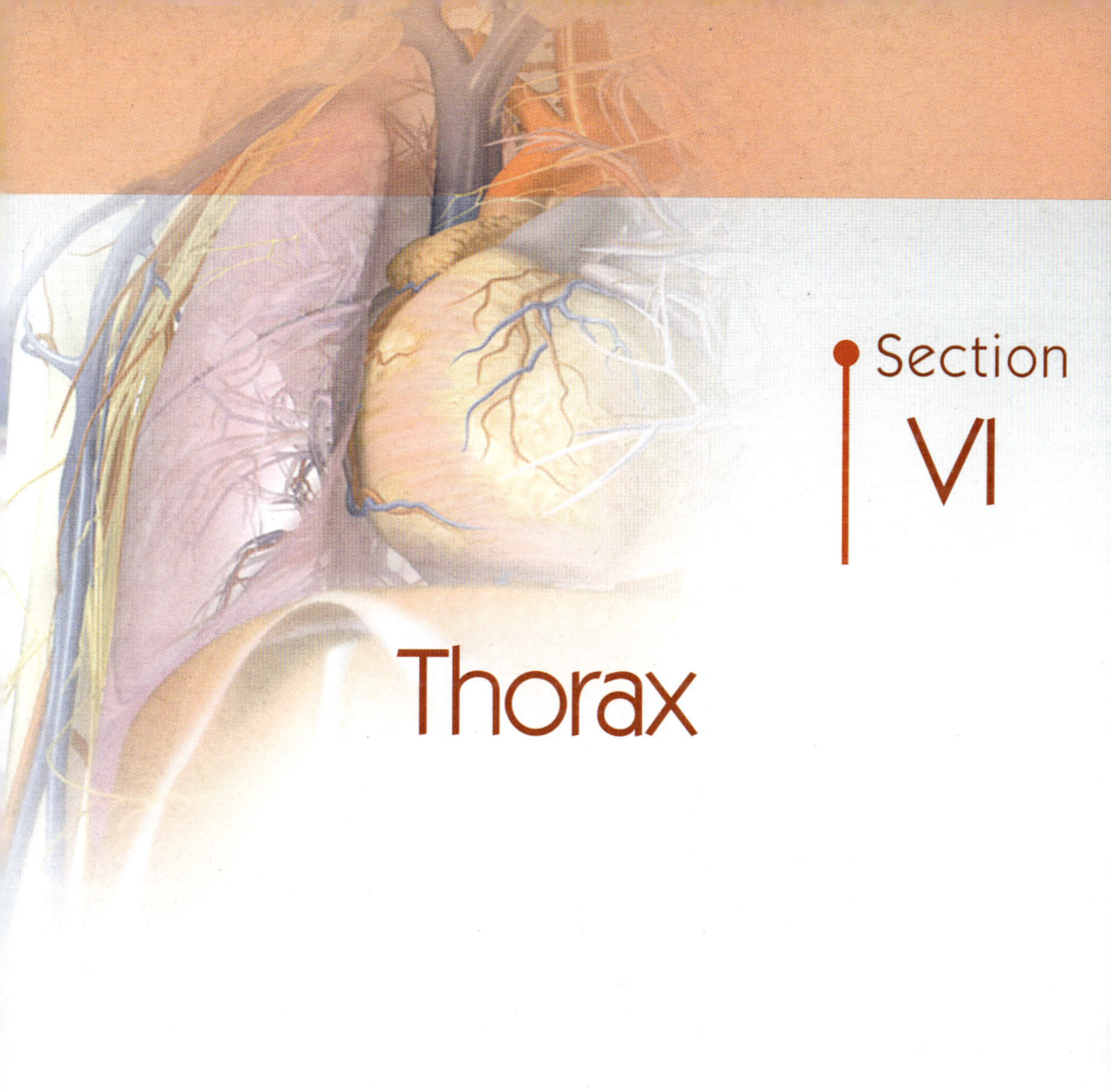

Thorax

# Key Osteology Questions

**Q. How many thoracic vertebrae are there?**

**Ans.** There are 12 thoracic vertebrae.

**Q. How many ribs are there?**

**Ans.** There are 12 pairs of ribs (the number may increase or decrease with the presence of cervical/lumbar rib).

**Q. How are the ribs classified?**

**Ans.** Ribs are classified according to its attachment:
1. True ribs or vertebra-sternal ribs—1–7 ribs are true ribs.
2. Vertebrochondral ribs—cartilage of one rib is attached to next higher cartilage 8th, 9th and 10th ribs.
3. Floating ribs—free ends of 11th and 12th ribs are floating.

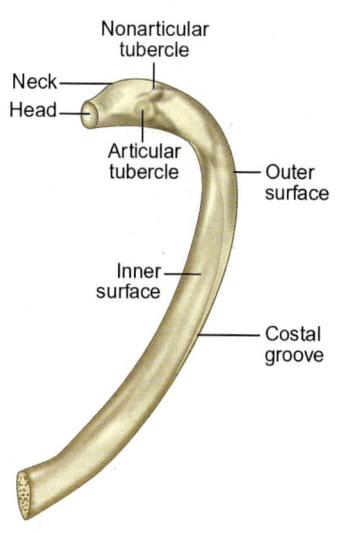

Parts of typical rib

**Q. Which are the atypical ribs?**

**Ans.** The 1st, 2nd, 10th, 11th, 12th are atypical ribs.

**Q. Which of the ribs are typical ribs?**

**Ans.** The 3rd to 9th ribs are the typical ribs.

**Q. What are the features of typical ribs?**

**Ans.** The features of typical ribs are:
1. Each typical rib has anterior end, posterior end and shaft.

2. Anterior end is costal end, oval and concave.
3. Posterior end has head, neck and tubercle.
4. Shaft is flattened, convex upwards, inner surface is smooth and marked by a ridge.
5. There is costal groove between the ridge and inferior border.
6. Upper border is thick and has outer and inner lips.

First rib

### Q. How do you identify first rib?

**Ans.** First rib is identified by the presence of following features:
- It is short, broad and acutely curved
- Shaft is not twisted
- It is flattened from above downwards.

### Q. Draw a diagram to show the superior relations of first rib.

**Ans.**

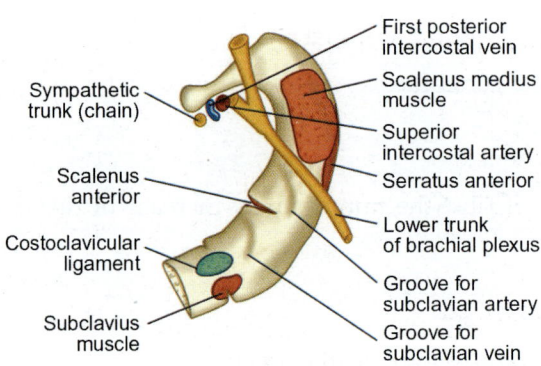

### Q. What are the attachments on the 12th rib (diagram only)?

**Ans.**

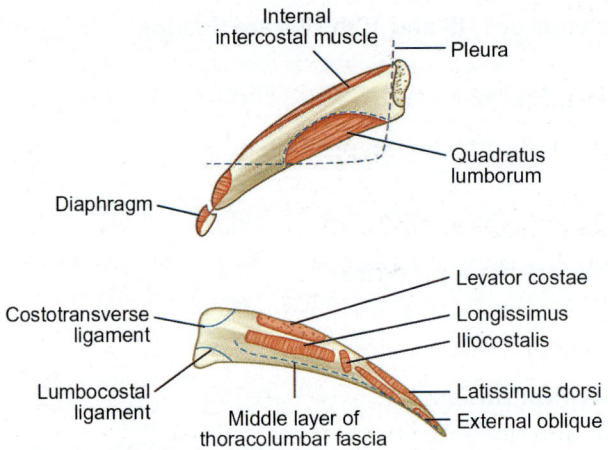

#### Q. What is the 'type' of costal cartilage?

**Ans.** The 'type' of costal cartilage is hyaline cartilage.

#### Q. What is the meaning of sternum?

**Ans.** The meaning of sternum is 'chest'.

#### Q. What are the events occurring at the sternal angle (angle of Louis)?

**Ans.** Following events occur at the sternal angle:
 1. Second costal cartilage and rib lies at this level.
 2. Superior and inferior mediastinum are demarcated.
 3. Ascending aorta ends.
 4. Arch of aorta begins.
 5. Arch of aorta ends.
 6. Descending aorta begins.
 7. Trachea divides into two principal bronchi.
 8. Azygos vein arches over root of right lung.
 9. Pulmonary trunk divides.
10. Thoracic duct crosses from right to left side.
11. Base of heart lies at this level.
12. Cardiac plexus is located at this level.

#### Q. What is the meaning of xiphoid?

**Ans.** Xiphoid means 'sword like'.

#### Q. What are the parts of typical thoracic vertebra?

**Ans.** Parts of typical thoracic vertebra are:
- Rounded body (anteroposterior diameter = transverse diameter)
- On lateral side of body, are costal facets
- Pedicles are short and rounded bars
- Each pedicle continues as lamina
- Laterally are the transverse process
- There are superior and inferior facets.

#### Q. Which are the typical thoracic vertebrae?

**Ans.** The 2nd to 8th are typical thoracic vertebrae.

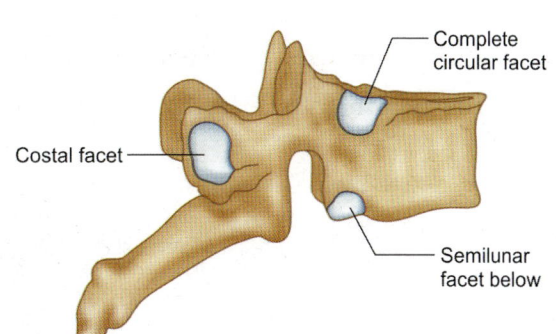

## Q. How do you identify thoracic vertebrae?

**Ans.** Thoracic vertebrae are identified by following features:

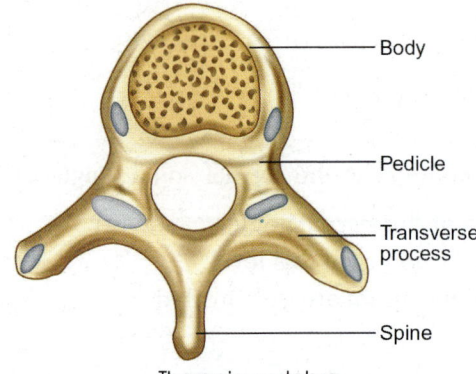

Thoracic vertebra

- Rounded, heart-shaped body (anteroposterior diameter = transverse diameter)
- Presence of costal facets on lateral aspect of the body.

## Q. Morphologically, how is the transverse process of thoracic vertebra formed?

**Ans.** Morphologically, the transverse process has two elements:
- Costal element
- Transverse element.
  Costal element forms the rib in thoracic region.

## Q. What type of joint is manubriosternal joint?

**Ans.** The type of manubriosternal joint is a secondary cartilaginous joint.

## Q. What is the structure of intervertebral disk?

**Ans.** The structure of intervertebral disk is:
- These are fibrocartilaginous in nature
- They have two parts:
  - Central—nucleus pulposus
  - Peripheral—annulus fibrosus.

## Q. What is the 'type' of intervertebral joint?

**Ans.** The 'type' of intervertebral joint is a secondary cartilaginous joint.

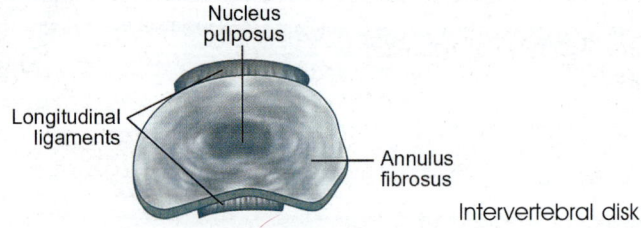

Intervertebral disk

**Q. What is cervical rib?**

**Ans.** Cervical rib is a congenital overdevelopment (bony or fibrous) of the costal process of C7.

**Q. What are the types of cervical rib?**

**Ans.** There are four types of cervical rib as shown below.

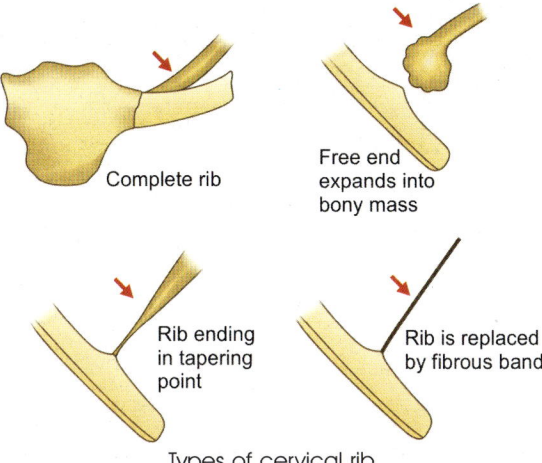

Types of cervical rib

**Q. What is Adson's test?**

**Ans.** On turning the head to the side, where cervical rib is present or on deep breathing, the radial pulse disappears.

**Q. How do you treat cervical rib?**

**Ans.** In 70% of cases, even if cervical rib is not recognised, symptoms are relieved by dividing scalenus anterior.
**Note:** One must excise cervical rib along with its periosteum.

**Q. How many splanchnic nerves are there?**

**Ans.** There are three splanchnic nerves:
- Greater splanchnic nerve
- Lesser splanchnic nerve
- Least splanchnic nerve.

**Q. What are splanchnic nerves?**

**Ans.** Splanchnic nerves are medial branches of thoracic ganglia 7, 8, 9, 10, 11 and 12, relaying into celiac ganglion. They are preganglionic branches of medial branches of thoracic ganglia, as given below:
- Greater—5, 6, 7, 8, 9
- Lesser—10, 11
- Least—12.

# Key Short Notes

## 26

## THORACIC INLET

It is an obliquely truncated, superior opening of thorax where neck continues into thorax and partially obliterated by a membrane on either sides known as Sibson's fascia.

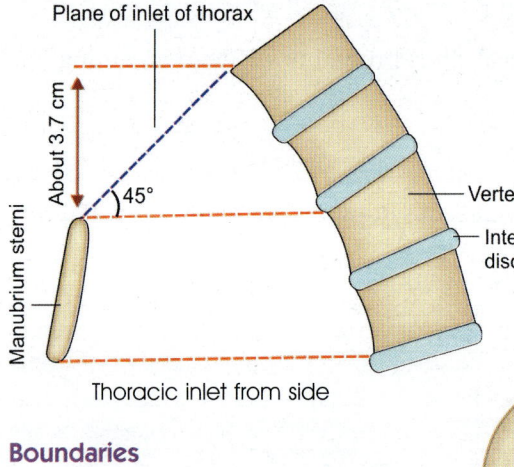

Thoracic inlet from side

### Boundaries

- Anteriorly: Manubrium sterni
- Posteriorly: T1
- On each side: First rib with its cartilage.

### Structures Passing through the Inlet

- *Tubes:* Trachea, esophagus
- *Nerves:* Vagus, phrenic, first thoracic, sympathetic trunks

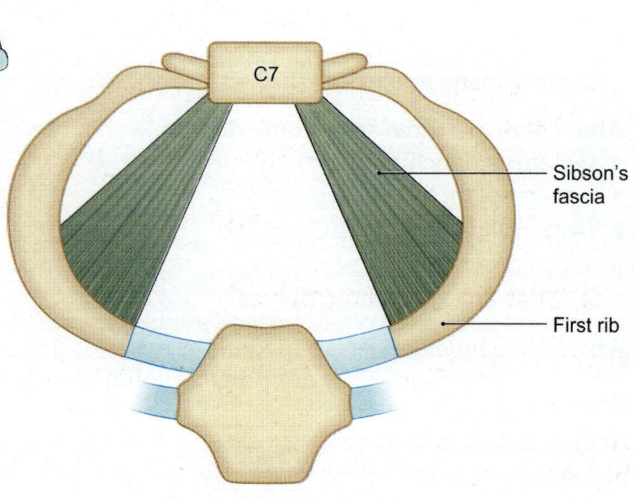

Thoracic inlet from above

- *Arteries:* Right brachiocephalic, left common carotid, left subclavian, internal thoracic, superior intercostals

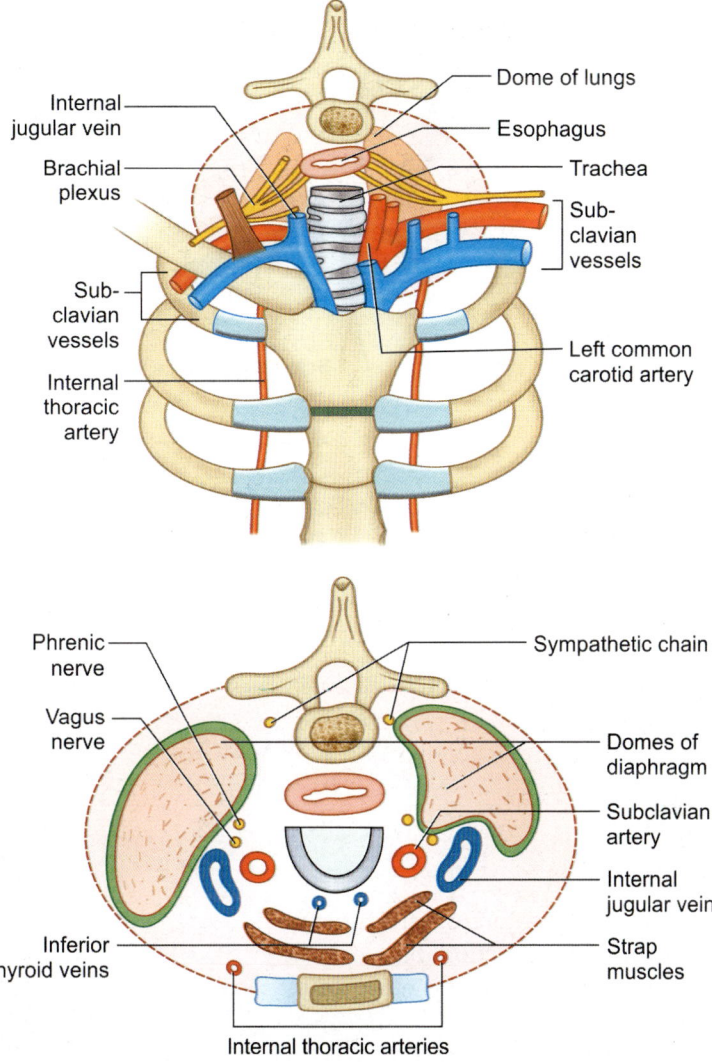

Structures in thoracic inlet and transverse section thoracic inlet

- *Veins:* Brachiocephalic, posterior intercostals, inferior thyroid
- *Muscles:* Sternohyoid, sternothyroid, longus colli.

## Clinical Significance

If there is a cervical rib, subclavian artery and first thoracic nerve which lie above the cervical rib may get compressed by the presence of cervical rib; in which case patient has compromised blood supply to upper limb, tingling and numbness of upper limb (refer Adson's test—in key osteology questions).

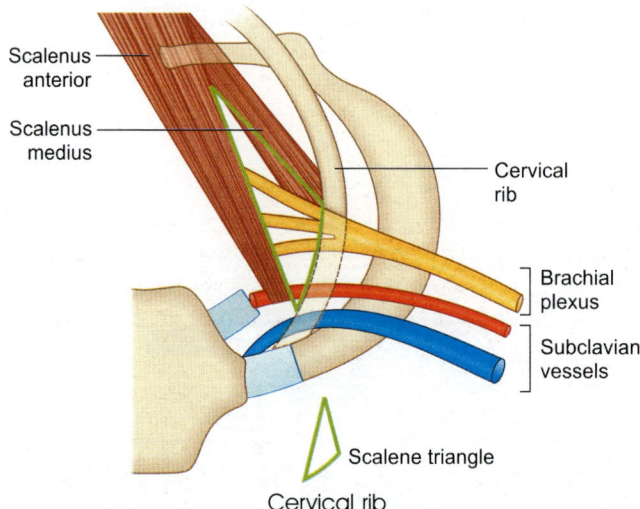

### Q. Intercostal space

**Ans.** The gap between the ribs is the intercostal space. It is filled by intercostal muscles, intercostal nerves, vessels and lymphatics.

## Intercostal Muscles

Intercostal muscles are:

- External intercostal muscle
- Internal intercostal muscle
- Transversus thoracis.

### External Intercostal Muscle

External intercostal muscle extends from the tubercle of the rib to the costochondral junction. Between the costochondral junction and sternum, it is replaced by membrane.

### Internal Intercostal Muscle

Internal intercostal muscle extends from angle of rib to the lateral border of sternum. Fibres run downwards, backwards and laterally.

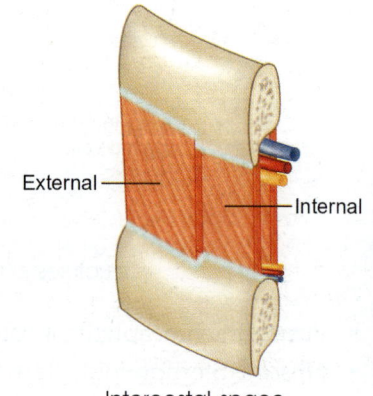

### Transversus Thoracis

Transversus thoracis is made-up of three parts:

1. Subcostalis—posterior part of lower intercostal space.
2. Intercostales intimi—confined to middle two-fourths.
3. Sternocostalis—anterior parts of upper intercostal spaces.

## Intercostal Nerves

Intercostal nerves are anterior rami of thoracic spinal nerve. Upper three intercostal nerves also supply the upper limb and lower five also supply the abdominal wall:
- T4, T5 and T6 are typical thoracic nerves
- T12 is also known as subcostal nerve
- They supply the muscles in the intercostal space, parietal pleura and periosteum of the rib.

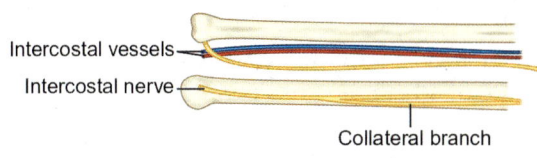

Intercostal vessels
Intercostal nerve
Collateral branch

Intercostal nerve and vessels

## Intercostal Arteries

- Each space has one posterior and two anterior intercostal arteries
- Posterior intercostal arteries are 11 in number
- 1st and 2nd posterior intercostal arteries arise from superior intercostal artery, which is a branch of costocervical trunk
- 3–11 posterior intercostal arteries are branches of descending aorta
- Artery is accompanied by intercostal vein
- Anterior intercostal arteries arises from internal thoracic artery.

**Mnemonic: VAN**
**V**—Vein
**A**—Artery
**N**—Nerve

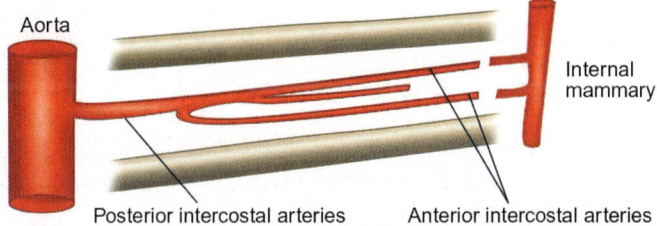

Aorta
Internal mammary
Posterior intercostal arteries
Anterior intercostal arteries

Intercostal artery

*There are two anterior intercostal veins in upper nine spaces:*
1. Upper six drain into internal thoracic vein and remaining veins drain into musculophrenic vein
2. Posterior vein drains into vertebral venous plexus.

## Surgical Significance

The neurovascular bundle lies in the costal groove between internal intercostal and innermost intercostal muscle on the inner side of rib. While doing thoracocentesis, i.e. pleural tap (removing fluid from pleural cavity for diagnostic purpose) surgeon should avoid putting cannula from the inferior side of that particular rib to avoid injury to neurovascular bundle.

## Q. Internal thoracic artery

**Ans.**

### Origin

Internal thoracic artery originates from the first part of subclavian artery opposite to the thyrocervical trunk.

### Cause and Relations

- Internal thoracic artery runs vertically downwards behind the sternal end of clavicle and costal cartilages
- It is anteriorly related to costal cartilages and intercostal space
- Posteriorly to endothoracic fascia and pleura.

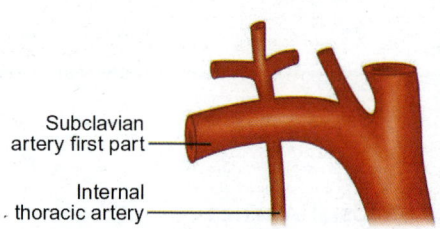

Subclavian artery first part

Internal thoracic artery

Origin of internal thoracic artery

### Termination

- Internal thoracic artery terminates in sixth intercostal space into musculophrenic and superior epigastric
- The artery is accompanied by two venae comitantes.

### Branches

- Pericardiophrenic
- Mediastinal arteries
- Anterior intercostal arteries
- Superior epigastric
- Musculophrenic.

### Applied Anatomy

Internal thoracic artery is used in bypass heart surgeries.

Internal thoracic artery

Superior epigastric

Musculophrenic

Course and branches of internal mammary artery

## Q. Pleural recesses

**Ans.** Pleural recesses are the extra or reserve spaces of parietal pleura, which gives space for the lungs to expand.

### Costodiaphragmatic Recess

- Costodiaphragmatic recess is a space located inferiorly between costal and diaphragmatic pleura
- It is across 8th to 10th ribs along the midaxillary line
- Approximately 5 cm in length.

### Costomediastinal Recess

- Costomediastinal recess lies anteriorly behind the sternum and costal cartilages
- This recess is filled by lung, even during quiet breathing.

## Applied Anatomy

These recesses get filled in cases of pleural effusion.

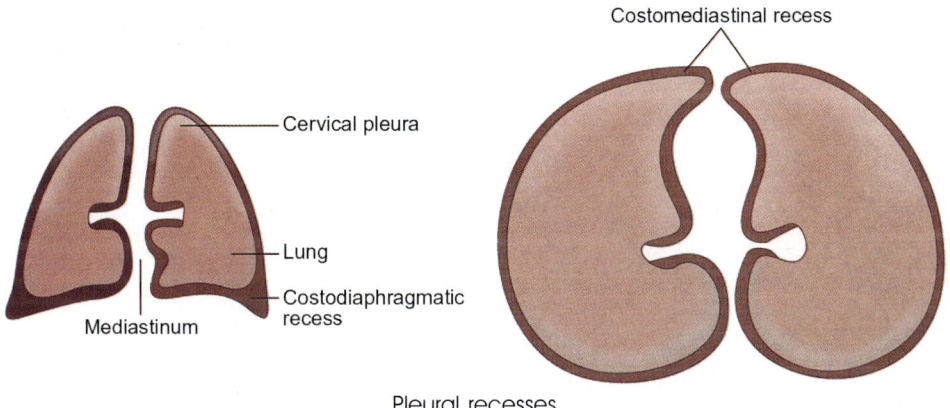

Pleural recesses

## Q. Mediastinal surface of lungs (diagram only)

**Ans.** • Right lung
• Left lung.

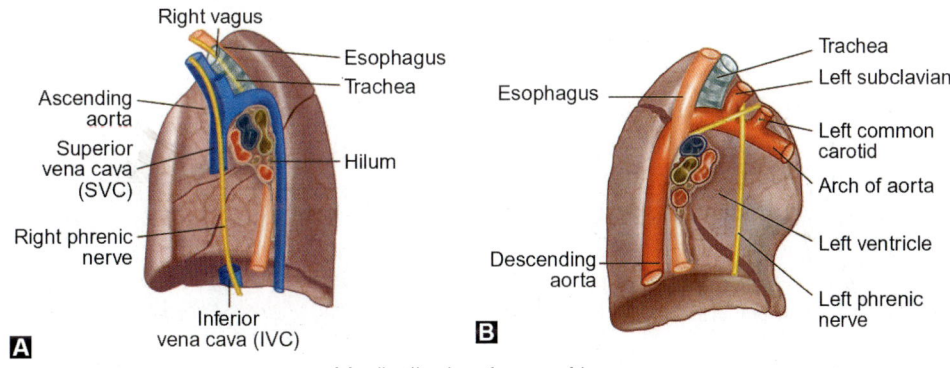

Mediastinal surfaces of lungs

## Q. Hilum of right and left lungs

**Ans.** Hilum is a pedicle of lung, which connects the medial surface of lungs to the mediastinum. It lies against T5, T6, T7 vertebrae.

### Contents

- Principal bronchus
- Pulmonary artery
- Pulmonary veins
- Bronchial arteries
- Bronchial veins
- Anterior and posterior pulmonary plexus
- Lymphatics and lymph nodes.

**Note:** Arrangement of contents varies in right and left side. Terminal part of azygos vein arches over root of right lung, while arch of aorta arches over root of left lung.

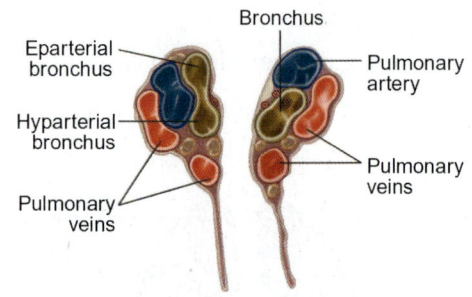

Hilum of right and left lungs

### Q. Pericardium

**Ans.** Pericardium is a covering around the heart and also root of great vessels:
- It is located in the middle mediastinum
- It consists of fibrous and serous pericardium.

### Fibrous Pericardium

- Fibrous pericardium is a fibrous tissue around the heart, it blends with the parietal layer of serous pericardium
- It is connected to sternum with sternopericardial ligaments
- Below, it fuses with central tendon of diaphragm and above with root of aorta.

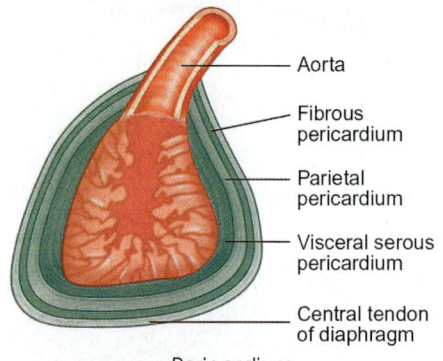

Pericardium

### Serous Pericardium

- Serous pericardium is thin, double-layered serous membrane
- Outer layer is parietal layer, which fuses with fibrous pericardium and inner layer is visceral layer.

### Nerve Supply and Blood Supply of Pericardium

- Internal thoracic, musculophrenic, and descending aorta branches supply the pericardium. (note only the nearby arteries will supply the pericardium).
- Epicardium has autonomic nerve supply thus insensitive to pain while rest of the pericardium receives branches from phrenic nerve which are sensitive to pain.

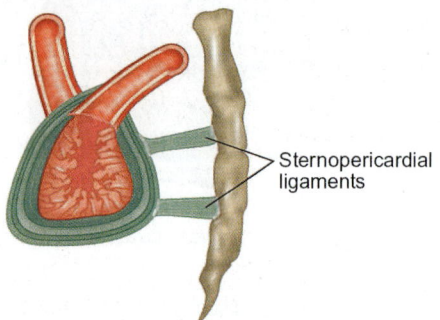

### Applied Anatomy

Pericardial effusion occurs in between the parietal and visceral layer of serous pericardium.

### Q. Fibrous skeleton of heart

**Ans.** Fibrous skeleton of heart lies roughly at the same plane of coronary sulcus, i.e. ventricular base and atrioventricular inflow and arterial outflow. It is a complex framework of dense collagen with intervening membrane. It is a deformable continuum.

## Components

- Mitral annulus
- Aortic valve annulus
- Tricuspid annulus
- Pulmonary valve annulus.

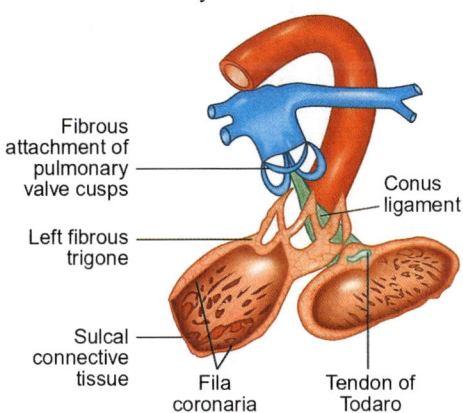

Fibrous attachment of pulmonary valve cusps

Conus ligament

Left fibrous trigone

Sulcal connective tissue

Fila coronaria

Tendon of Todaro

Fibrous skeleton of heart

## Directions

- Mitral and tricuspid valve annuli are in one plane, i.e. coplanar
- Aortic valve annulus faces upwards, forwards (= anterosuperior), right of mitral orifice
- Pulmonary valve is at right angles to aortic valve. The only connection is conus ligament, a fibrous tendon (tendon of infundibulum).

## Functions

- To ensure electrophysiological discontinuity except through conducting system
- Mechanical attachment for ventricular myocardium
- To maintain cardiac portion within the pericardium
- To establish a stable, but deformable base for valvular attachments.

**Q. Cardiac silhouette** (diagram only)

**Ans.**

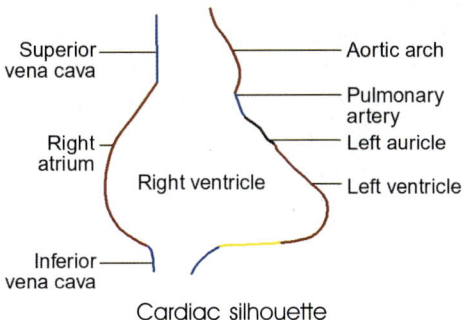

Superior vena cava

Aortic arch

Pulmonary artery

Right atrium

Left auricle

Right ventricle

Left ventricle

Inferior vena cava

Cardiac silhouette

**Q. Sinuses of pericardium**

**Ans.** There are two sinuses of pericardium, namely oblique and transverse:

1. *Transverse sinus:* Passage between arterial end and venous end is the transverse sinus. It lies between ascending aorta and pulmonary trunk in front and superior vena cava (SVC) and left atrium behind.
2. *Oblique sinus:* Between the openings of pulmonary veins is the oblique sinus. It lies between left atrium anteriorly and parietal pericardium posteriorly.

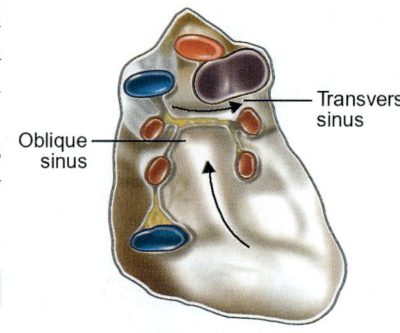

Sinuses of pericardium

### Q. Interior of right atrium

**Ans.** Interior of right atrium has three parts:
1. Smooth posterior part
2. Rough anterior part
3. Septal wall.

### Smooth Posterior Part Features

1. Right atrium is the receiving chamber of the heart. Thus, it has openings of superior and inferior vena cava, coronary sinus and openings of venae cordis minimi
2. Just below the opening of SVC, there is a projection intervenous tubercle of Lower.

### Rough Anterior Part Features

There is vertical crest diagonally below sulcus terminalis known as crista terminalis from where horizontal muscular ridges run on the internal surface of right atrium known as musculi pectinati.

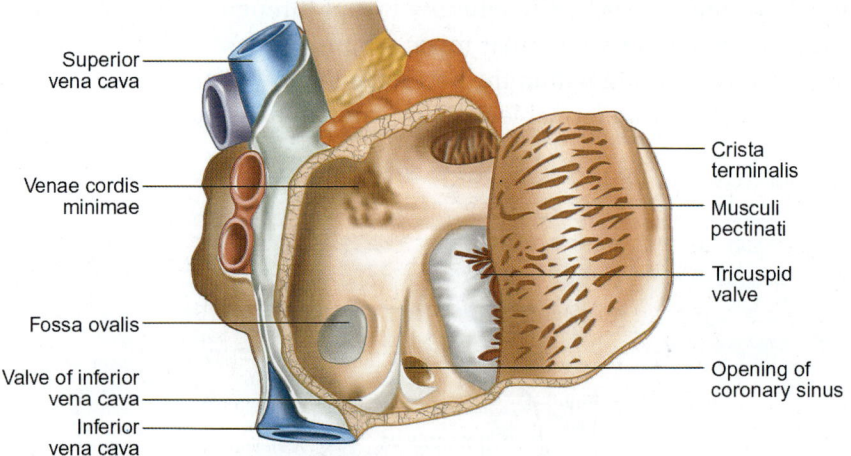

Interior of right atrium

### Septal Wall Features

- Fossa ovalis—remnant of septum primum
- Annulus ovalis—remnant of septum secundum
- Remains of foramen ovale
  All of the above are embryonic remnants.

## Q. Surface projection of heart valves (diagram only)

**Ans.**

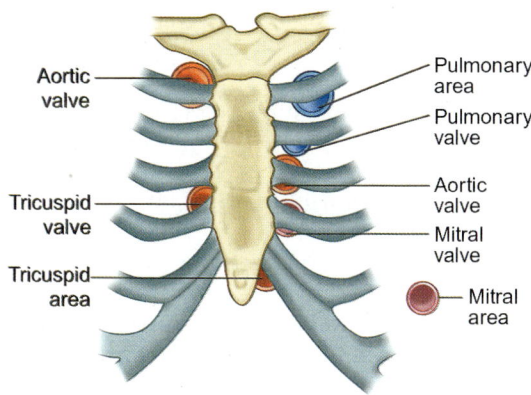

Surface projection of heart valves

## Q. Veins of the heart

Veins draining the heart are grouped as:
- Coronary sinus with its tributaries
- Anterior cardiac vein
- Venae cordis minimae.

### Coronary Sinus

- Coronary sinus is oblong sinus lying posterior on coronary sulcus, i.e. atrioventricular (AV) groove between left atrium and left ventricle.
- Its tributaries are great, small and middle cardiac veins, posterior vein of the left ventricle and oblique vein of left atrium. All veins except that of left atrium have valves.

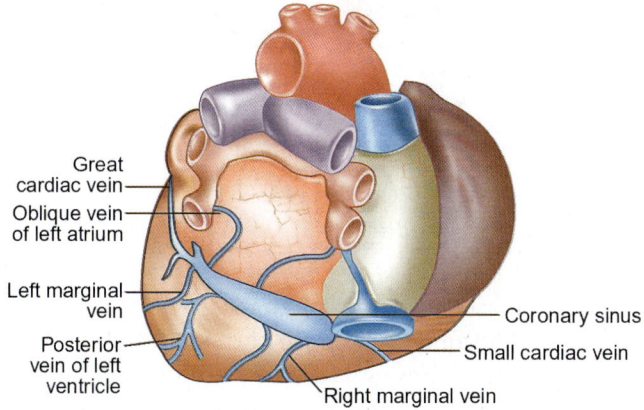

Venous drainage of heart

- Great cardiac vein begins at the cardiac apex and ascends in anterior interventricular sulcus; and it receives blood from left atrium and both ventricles.
- Small cardiac vein lies in posterior atrioventricular sulcus, receives blood from posterior part of right atrium and ventricle.

- Middle cardiac vein is present in posterior interventricular sulcus.
- Oblique vein of left atrium is continuous above with the ligament of left vena cava.

### Anterior Cardiac Vein

Anterior cardiac vein drains the anterior part of right atrium. Right marginal vein courses around the inferior margin draining adjacent parts of left ventricle.

### Venae Cordis Minimae

Venae cordis minimae directly open into right atrium.

### Q. Cardiac plexus

**Ans.** Nerve plexus around the heart is made-up of sympathetic and parasympathetic nerve. Depending upon its plane, it is classified into superficial and deep plexus.

### Superficial Cardiac Plexus

- Superficial cardiac plexus is located in front of arch of aorta
- It is formed by superior cervical cardiac branch of left sympathetic chain and inferior cervical cardiac branch of left vagus.

### Deep Cardiac Plexus

- Deep cardiac plexus is located over bifurcation of trachea
- It is formed by cardiac nerves of cervical and thoracic ganglia.

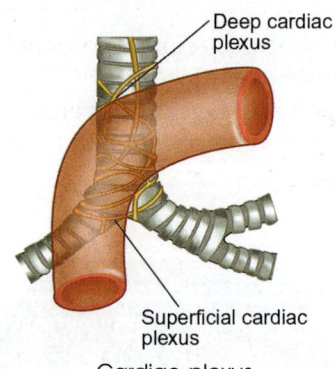

Cardiac plexus

## TYPICAL INTERCOSTAL NERVE

- It is ventral rami of spinal nerve in thoracic region.
- It arises from intervertebral foramen inferior to corresponding vertebra.
- It runs in intercostal space after running laterally, behind sympathetic chain
- By and large lies deep to internal intercostal membrane and superficial to innermost intercostals.

### Branches

- Grey rami (postganglionic) and white rami (preganglionic) communicans to sympathetic chain

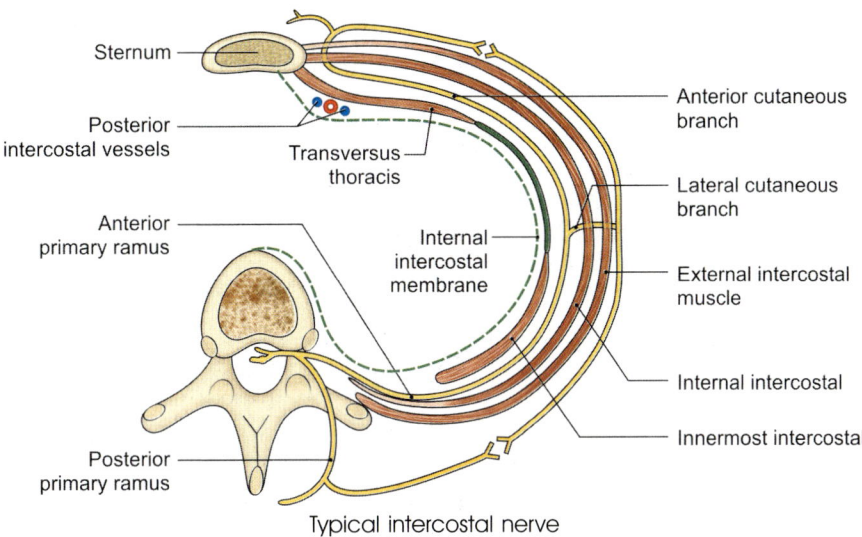

Typical intercostal nerve

- Collateral branches
- Lateral and anterior cutaneous
- Muscular.

## ATYPICAL INTERCOSTAL NERVES

- Greater part of T1 passes up across the neck to join C8. Small thin part is 1st intercostal nerve while T2 ventral rami gives branch to brachial plexus.
- T1 has no cutaneous branch
- T12 also termed subcostal nerve enters abdominal wall along with subcostal artery; it is lateral cutaneous branch crosses iliac crest and supplies skin over the gluteal region.

## PHRENIC NERVE

- *Origin:* C3, C4, C5 ventral rami
- *Relations:* It descends in thorax posterolateral to internal jugular vein, anterior to root of lung and lies medial to mediastinal pleura

### Right Phrenic Nerve

It lies posterolateral to right brachiocephalic vein and superior vena cava, then lies on pericardium; covering the right atrium and runs down to lie anterior to inferior vena cava before reaching the diaphragm.

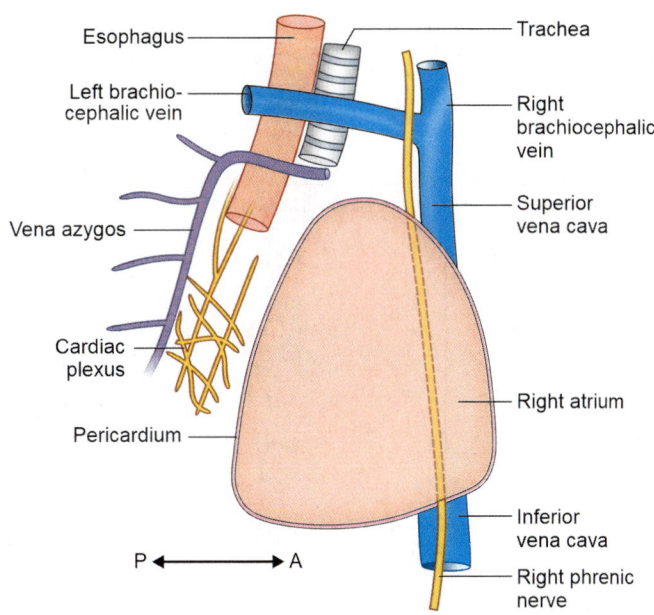

Right side of mediastinum showing right phrenic nerve

## Left Phrenic Nerve

Descends anterior to arch of aorta and lies between common carotid and left subclavian artery.

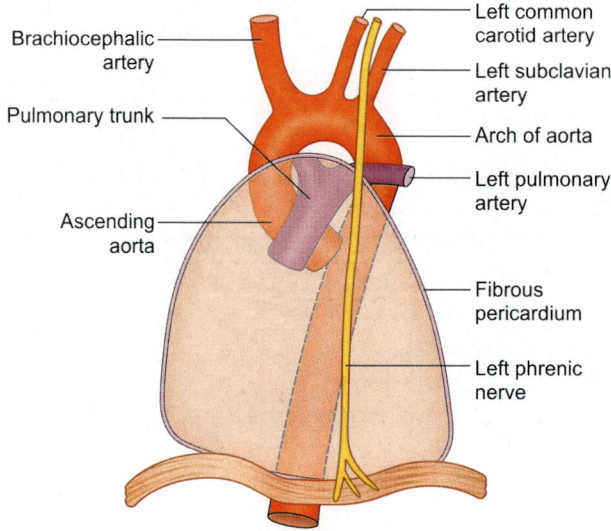

Left phrenic nerve as it descends on heart

The nerve ends by piercing the diaphragm and being motor to it.

## Q. Constrictions of esophagus (diagram only)

**Ans.** Esophagus has four constrictions as shown in the figure.

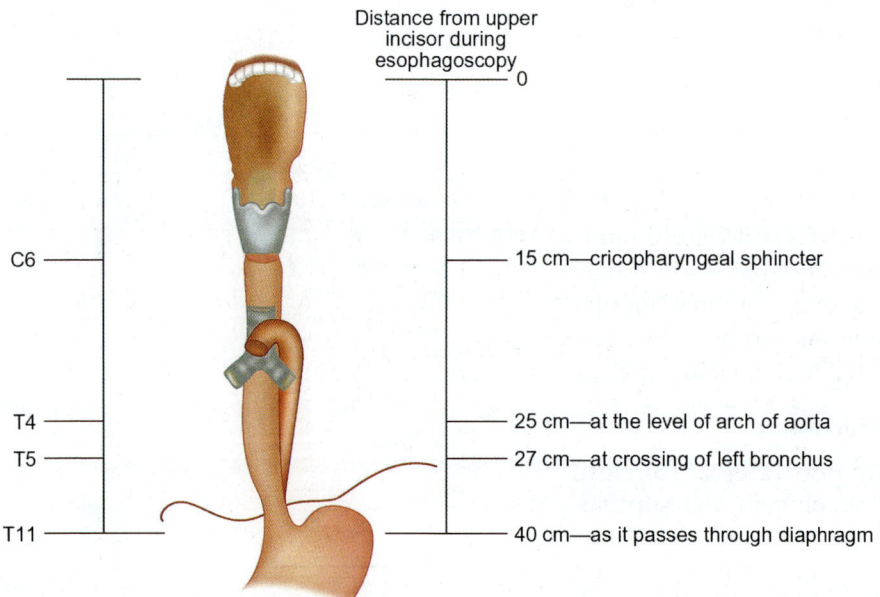

Constrictions of esophagus

## TRACHEA

- *Extent:* Commences from lower border of cricoid cartilage up to sternal angle where it divides into right and left principal bronchi

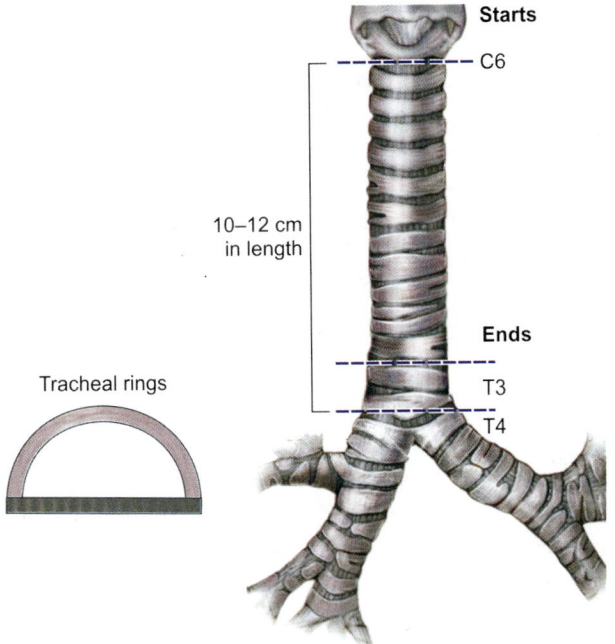

Tracheal ring and trachea—external features

- *Length:* 4–6 inches, appx. 2 cm
- *Parts:* Cervical and thoracic
- *Structure:* U-shaped bars of (hyaline) cartilage, embedded in fibroelastic wall.

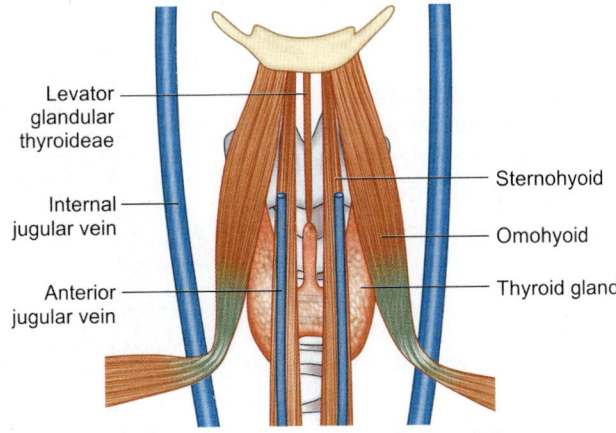

Cervical part of trachea—anterior relations

## Relation

*Cervical part*
- Upper part just below subcutaneous soft tissue.

- *Anteriorly:* Skin, SC tissue, strap muscles in lower part, thyroid gland
- *Posteriorly:* Esophagus

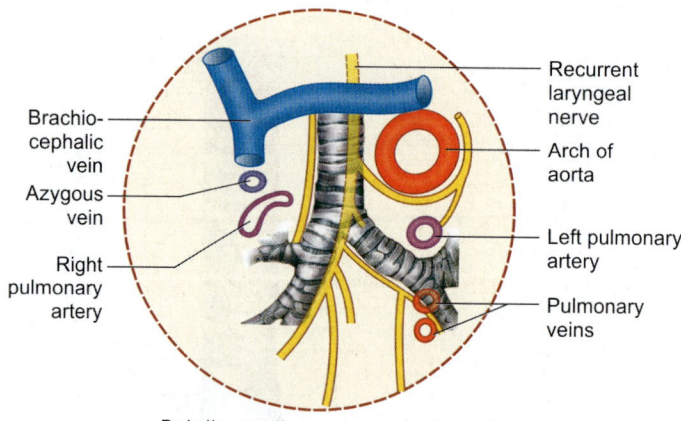

Relations—thoracic part of trachea

### Thoracic part

Mostly surrounded by blood vessels and is in superior mediastinum

- Anteriorly—arch of aorta, brachiocephalic trunk, left common carotid artery
- On each side—pleura, vagus and phrenic nerves.

## Clinical Importance

In event of respiratory obstruction an opening is done 2 finger breath above the jugular notch; this is known as tracheostomy.

## Q. Sibson's fascia

Sibson's fascia is suprapleural membrane. The cervical pleura rises to the neck of first rib, around 4 cm above the level of sternal end of first costal cartilage.

It is protected externally by scalene muscles and lined internally by dense fascia, i.e. the suprapleural membrane (morphologically represents the flattened tendon of Scalenus minimus).

### Attachments

Sibson's fascia spreads out from seventh cervical vertebra to inner border of first rib.

### Functions

- Sibson's fascia gives rigidity to thoracic inlet
- It prevents the cervical pleura from ballooning in and out during respiration.

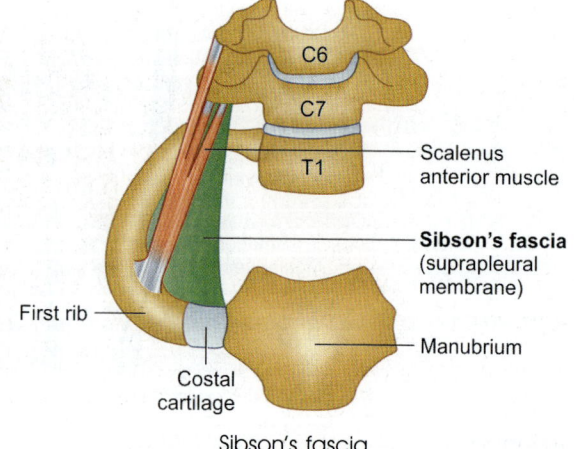

Sibson's fascia

### Q. Triangle of Koch

**Ans.** Triangle of Koch is located in the interior of right atrium.

### Boundaries

Boundaries exist between the base of tricuspid valve's septal leaflet, anteromedial margin of coronary sinus orifice and collagenous subendocardial tendon of Todaro.

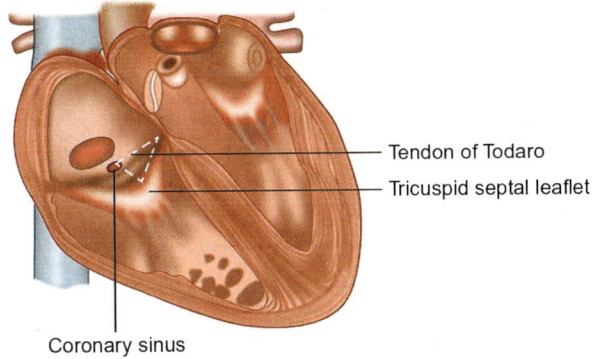

Coronary sinus

*Triangle of Koch*

### Importance

Triangle of Koch is the site of AV node and associated juxta nodal bundles.

### Q. Atrioventricular valves (AV)

**Ans.** There is one pair of atrioventricular (AV) valve, i.e. right and left. Right AV valve is tricuspid valve and has three cusps. Left AV valve is bicuspid valve and has two cusps. It is also known as mitral valve.

### Structure

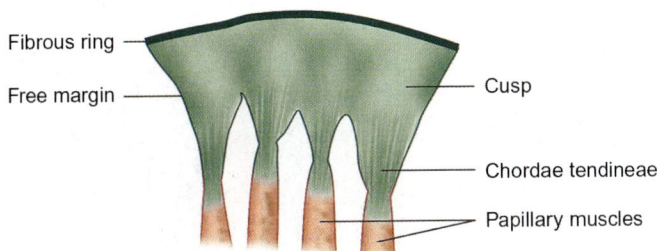

*Structure of atrioventricular (AV) valve*

### Parts

- Fibrous ring
- Cusp has smooth atrial surface and rough ventricular surface
- Free and attached margins
- Free margin gives attachment to chordae tendineae, which in turn is attached to papillary muscle.

## Applied Anatomy

- First heart sound is produced by closure of AV valves
- Valves may get defective either due to narrowing, i.e. stenosis or imperfect closure giving rise to regurgitation.

### Q. Semilunar valves

**Ans.** Aortic and pulmonary valves are semilunar valves. They are termed semilunar, since the cusps are half-moon shaped.

## Structure

Structure of semilunar valve
- Fibrous ring is absent
- Cusps are directly attached to vessel wall
- Free margin has a nodule in the centre, and a flimsy, side margin is known as lunule.

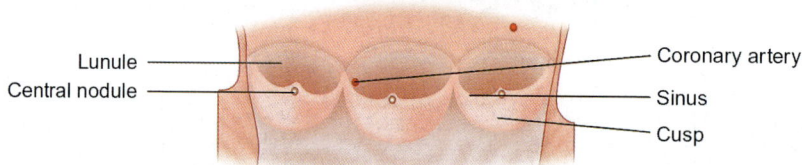

Structure of semilunar valve

## AORTOPULMONARY SPACE

- *Anteriorly:* Ascending aorta
- *Posteriorly:* Pulmonary trunk
- *Laterally:* Mediastinal pleura
- *Medially:* Left principal bronchus.

## Contents

- Lymph nodes
- Ligamentum arteriosum
- Left recurrent laryngeal nerve
- Fat.

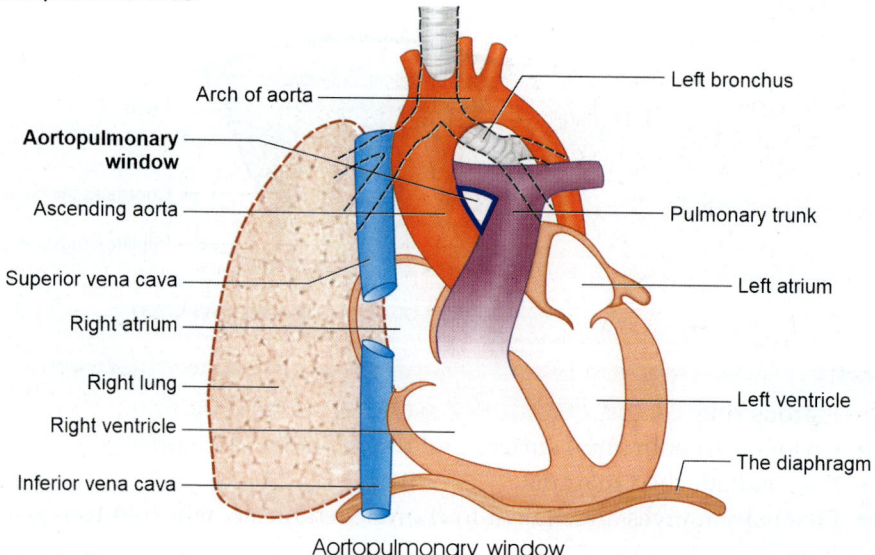

Aortopulmonary window

# Key Long Questions

## 27

**Q. Discuss diaphragm under following headings: Parts, apertures, nerve supply, development and applied anatomy.**

**Ans.** Diaphragm is a musculotendinous partition, which separates thorax from abdomen.

## Parts

- Central tendon
- Costal part
- Sternal part
- Lumbar part (lumbocostal arches and crura).

## Apertures

### Large Apertures (hiatus)

1. *Aortic opening:*
   - Lies at T12.
   - Thoracic duct and azygos vein pass through this opening.
   - Aorta lies within the 2 crus of diaphragm (does not pierce diaphragm) (diaphragm question— can be asked in thorax portions, as well as in abdomen portions).
2. *Esophageal opening:*
   - Lies at T10

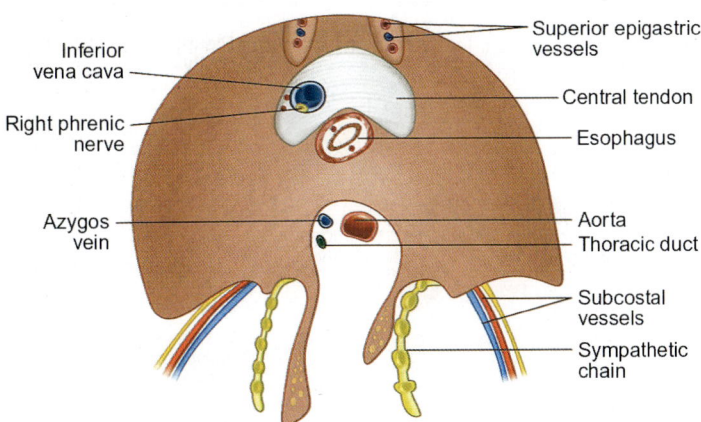

Structures piercing the diaphragm

- Esophagus, vagus nerves and esophageal branches of (L = left) gastric artery and vein pass through it.
3. *Vena caval opening:*
   - Lies at T8
   - It transmits inferior vena cava and branches of left phrenic nerve.

**Mnemonics: Structures**

"Voice      T8: Inferior **V**ena cava

**O**f          T10: **O**esophagus (esophagus)

**A**merica"    T12: **A**orta

## Small Aperture

1. Superior epigastric vessels pass between xiphoid process and 7th costal cartilage. This gap is known as Larry's space or foramen of Morgagni.
2. Musculophrenic vessels pierce the diaphragm at 8th or 9th costal cartilage.
3. Greater and lesser splanchnic nerves piercing the crura.
4. Openings for small veins are common in central tendon.

*Structures closely related to diaphragm are:*
- Sympathetic chain
- Subcostal vessels.

## Nerve Supply

- Motor fibres travel in phrenic nerves
- Lower 6 or 7 intercostal nerves distribute sensory fibers to peripheral diaphragm.

## Development

Following components contribute to the development:
- Septum transversum

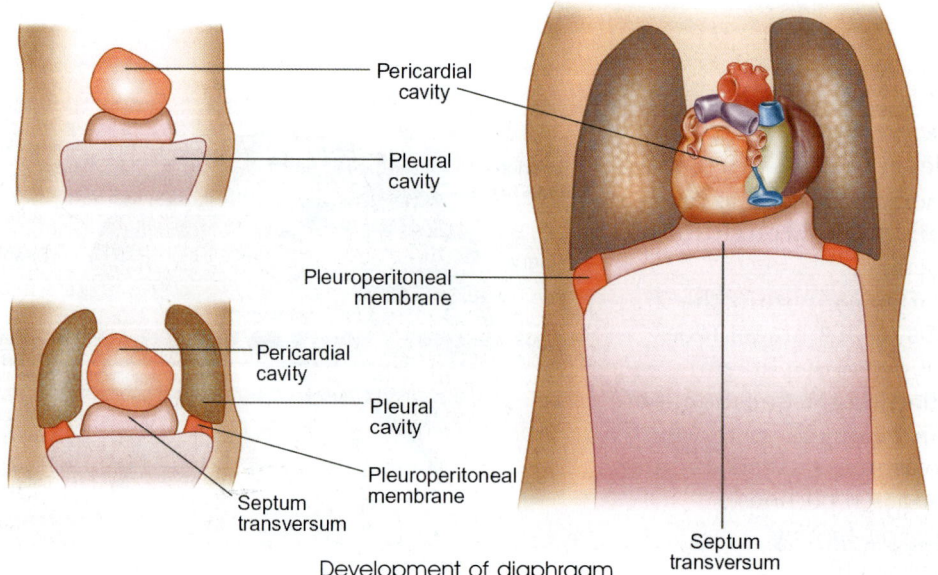

Pericardial cavity

Pleural cavity

Pleuroperitoneal membrane

Pericardial cavity

Pleural cavity

Pleuroperitoneal membrane

Septum transversum

Septum transversum

Development of diaphragm

- Pleuroperitoneal membranes
- Ventral and dorsal mesenteries of esophagus
- Mesoderm of body wall including mesoderm around dorsal aorta.

### Applied Anatomy

When abdominal organs, usually stomach herniate into thorax, i.e. diaphragmatic hernia.

### Q. Describe azygos vein in detail.

**Ans.** Azygos vein is large venous channel draining the thoracic wall and upper lumbar region. It is an important channel connecting superior vena cava to inferior vena cava.

### Formation

Azygos vein is formed by union of right ascending lumbar vein with right subcostal vein.

### Course

Azygos vein ascends upwards and enters the thorax by passing through aortic opening. Then it ascends upwards up to sternal angle, where it arches over the root of right lung. It terminates by joining the superior vena cava.

### Relations

- Anteriorly—esophagus
- Posteriorly—lower eight thoracic vertebra, right posterior intercostal arteries
- To the left—thoracic duct, aorta.

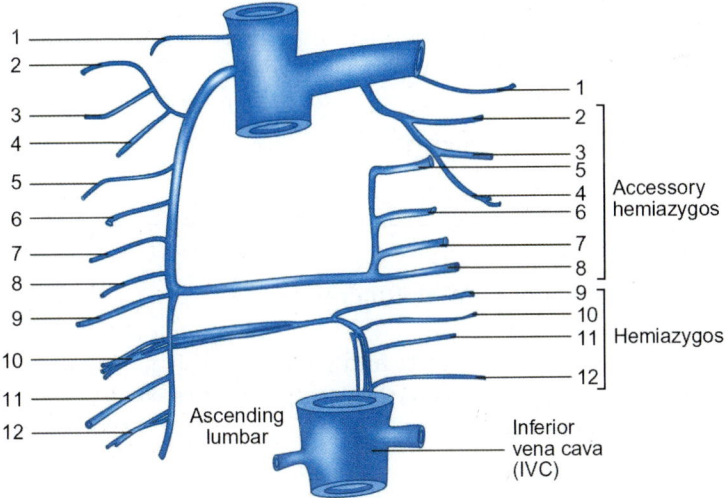

Azygos and hemiazygos veins

### Tributaries

- Right superior intercostal vein
- Intercostal veins 4–11
- Hemiazygos vein

- Accessory hemiazygos vein
- Esophageal, mediastinal and pericardial veins.

### Hemiazygos Vein

Hemiazygos vein is the mirror image of the lower part of azygos vein.

*Formation:* Hemiazygos vein is formed by the union of left subcostal vein and left ascending lumbar vein.

*Course:* Hemiazygos vein pierces the left crus of diaphragm and ascends on the left side of the vertebral column.

*Termination:* At T9, it turns to the right and joins azygos vein.

*Tributaries:* As follows:
- Left ascending lumbar vein
- Left subcostal vein
- Left posterior intercostal veins 9–11.

### Accessory Hemiazygos Vein

Accessory hemiazygos vein is the mirror image of upper part of azygos vein.

*Course:* Accessory hemiazygos vein begins at the medial end of 4th and 5th intercostal space and descends on the left side of vertebral column.

*Termination:* Accessory hemiazygos vein turns to the right at T8.

*Tributaries:* Intercostal veins 5–8.

### Applied Anatomy

In superior vena caval thrombosis, the blood from the upper limb and upper half of the body gets bypassed to inferior vena cava through azygos vein.

### Q. Discuss bronchopulmonary segments.

**Ans.** Each lung has 10 bronchopulmonary segments.

### Peculiarities

- Each segment is an independent unit not merging with adjacent structures
- Each segment has its own bronchus, artery and vein
- Each segment has a constant disposition and relationship to the overlying ribs.

### Right Lung

#### Upper Lobe

The upper lobe has three segments:
1. Apical.
2. Anterior.
3. Posterior.

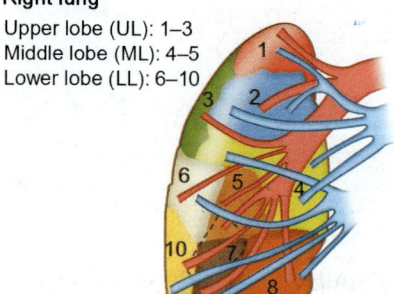

Right lung
Upper lobe (UL): 1–3
Middle lobe (ML): 4–5
Lower lobe (LL): 6–10

Bronchopulmonary segments of right lung

## Middle Lobe

The middle lobe has two segments:
a. 4—Medial.
b. 5—Lateral.

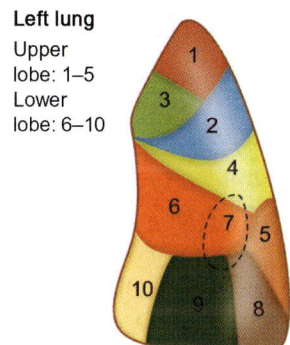

Upper lobe: 1–5
Lower lobe: 6–10

## Lower Lobe

The lower lobe has five segments:
a. 6—Apical.
b. 7—Medial basal.
c. 8—Anterior basal.
d. 9—Lateral basal.
e. 10—Posterior basal.

Bronchopulmonary segments of left lung

# Left Lung

## Upper Lobe

The upper lobe has five segments:
1—Apical.
2—Anterior.
3—Posterior.
4—Superior lingular.
5—Inferior lingular.

## Lower Lobe

The lower lobe has five segments:
1—Apical.
2—Medial basal.
3—Anterior basal.
4—Lateral basal.
5—Posterior basal.

# Surface Projection of the Segments

Lung segments have a constant disposition and relationship to the overlying ribs. Apical portion of lower lobe lies against 4–8 ribs.

# Bronchopulmonary Unit

Each segment has its own bronchial artery, terminal bronchiole and intersegmental vein.

# Applied Anatomy

- Segmental architecture is by and large constant
- Infective or neoplastic processes are located to one or more segments
- Limited resection can be possible, i.e. lobectomy can be done in case of neoplasia restricted to one lobe.

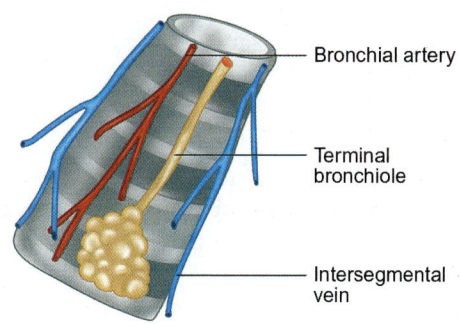

Bronchial artery

Terminal bronchiole

Intersegmental vein

Contents of bronchopulmonary segment

**Ans.** Mediastinum is the median septum between the two lungs.

## Boundaries

- *Anteriorly:* Sternum
- *Posteriorly:* Vertebral column
- *Superiorly:* Thoracic inlet
- *Inferiorly:* Diaphragm
- *On each side:* Pleura.

## Subdivisions

An imaginary line passing through sternal angle divides the mediastinum into superior and inferior mediastinum.

*Inferior mediastinum is subdivided into:*

- Anterior
- Middle
- Posterior.

### Contents of Superior Mediastinum

- Trachea
- Brachiocephalic vein
- Arch of aorta with its branches
- Thymus
- Thoracic duct
- Lymph nodes.

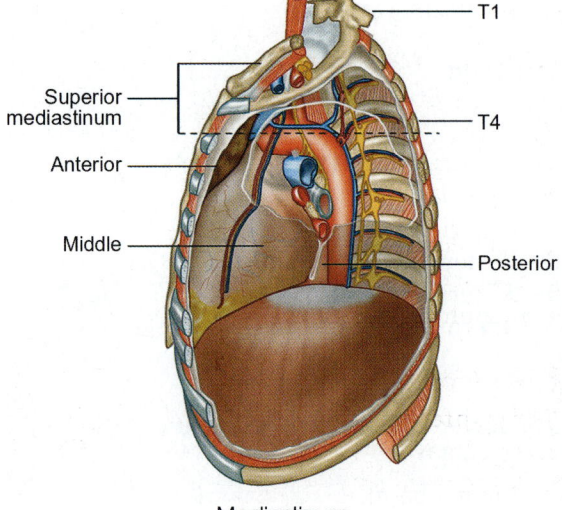

Mediastinum

### Special Features

- Prevertebral fascia extends up to T4. Thus, infection in the neck can track down to superior mediastinum
- Pretracheal fascia also extends up to superior mediastinum, where it blends with arch of aorta.

### Anterior Mediastinum

Anterior mediastinum is a space between sternum in front and pericardium behind. It is continuous with the pretracheal space of the neck above.

*Contents:* As follows:

- Sternopericardial ligaments
- Lymph nodes
- Mediastinal branches of internal thoracic artery
- Lowest part of thymus.

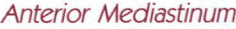

Contents of superior mediastinum

*Middle Mediastinum*

- Heart with its pericardium
- Superior and inferior vena caval openings
- Phrenic nerves and deep cardiac plexus
- Bifurcation of trachea
- Ascending aorta and pulmonary trunk.

Structures in posterior part of superior mediastinum are continuous with the posterior mediastinum.

*Posterior Mediastinum*

Anteriorly bounded by pericardium and posteriorly by vertebral column and intervertebral disk.

*Contents:* As follows:

- Esophagus
- Descending aorta
- Azygos vein, hemiazygos vein, accessory hemiazygos vein
- Right and left vagi
- Splanchnic nerves
- Lymph nodes.

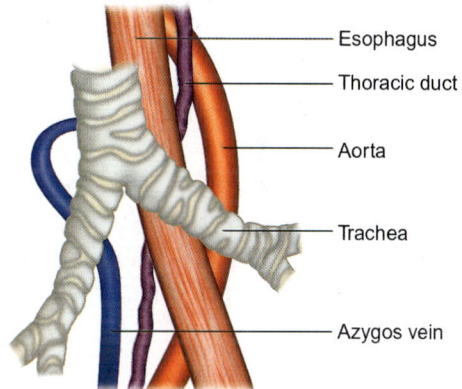

Contents of posterior mediastinum

### Applied Anatomy

Neck infections can track down from retropharyngeal space to posterior part of superior mediastinum.

---

### Q. Discuss thoracic duct.

**Ans.** Thoracic duct is the largest lymphatic channel extending from upper abdomen to the root of the neck. It is about 18 inches long.

### Course

1. It begins from upper end of cisterna chyli and enters the thorax through the aortic opening.
2. Ascends through posterior mediastinum and crosses at the level of sternal angle to end at the junction of left subclavian vein with left internal jugular vein.

### Relations

*In Abdomen*

Thoracic duct lies between azygos vein to the right and aorta to the left all throughout its course.

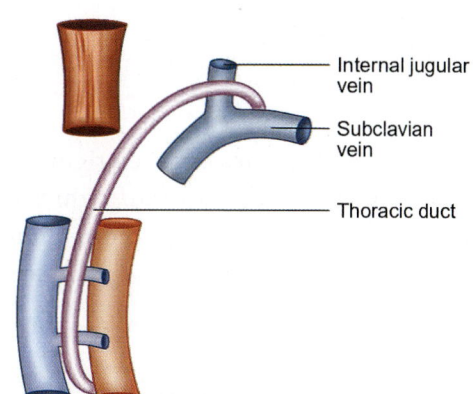

Thoracic duct course and termination

## In Posterior Mediastinum

Anteriorly, it is related to esophagus and posteriorly related to vertebral column.

## In Superior Mediastinum

To the right is esophagus and behind is vertebral column.

## In the Neck

Thoracic duct forms an arch of 3–4 cm above the clavicle.

## Tributaries

1. Receives lymph from both halves of the body below the diaphragm and left half above the diaphragm via left mediastinal trunk.
2. In thorax, it receives lymph vessels from posterior mediastinal nodes.
3. Efferent vessels from nodes in the neck forms left jugular trunk, those from the nodes in the axilla forms left subclavian trunk. These trunks drain into thoracic duct.

## Applied Anatomy

While doing left side neck dissections, the surgeon should be cautious regarding thoracic duct, otherwise there could be lymphatic leak, which needs urgent exploration. On postoperative day one, presence of milky fluid in the drain suggests thoracic duct leak.

## Q. Describe arterial supply to heart in detail.

Heart is supplied by two coronary arteries, which take origin from ascending aorta (coronary = crown like).

## Right Coronary Artery

Like crown

### Origin

Anterior aortic sinus.

### Course

1. At its origin, it lies between right auricle and right pulmonary trunk.
2. It runs downwards toward right in coronary sulcus.
3. It then winds round the inferior border and runs backwards in the posterior coronary sulcus.
4. It ends by anastomosing with left coronary artery.

### Branches

- Marginal
- Posterior interventricular
- Nodal
- Right atrial.

*Areas Supplied*

1. Right atrium.
2. Ventricles:
   a. Most of the right ventricle area except near anterior interventricular groove.

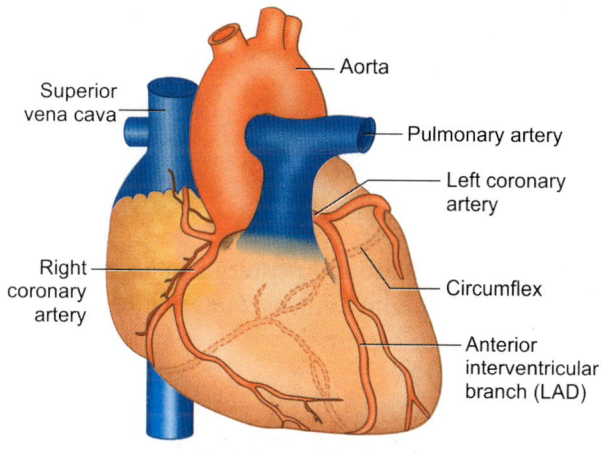

Arterial supply to heart

   b. Left ventricle near posterior interventricular groove.
   c. Posterior part of interventricular septum.
3. Most of the conducting system of heart.

## Left Coronary Artery

*Origin*

Left posterior aortic sinus.

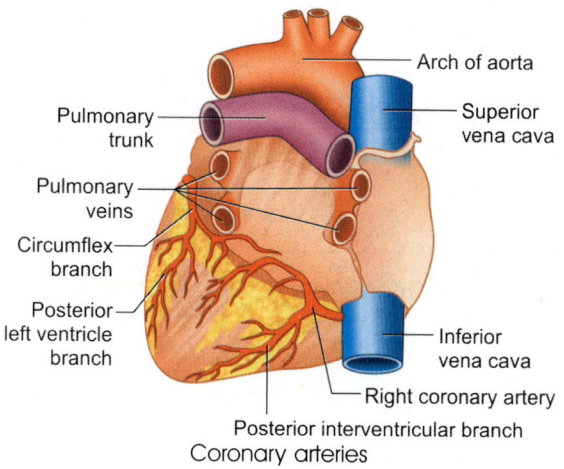

Coronary arteries

*Course*

1. At its origin, it lies between left auricle and left pulmonary trunk.
2. With a short course, it divides into anterior interventricular branch and left circumflex branch.

3. Left circumflex branch winds round the left border of heart and continues in left posterior coronary sulcus.
4. It ends by anastomosing with right coronary artery.

### Branches

1. Anterior interventricular groove.
2. A branch to diaphragmatic surface of heart.
3. Left atrial branch.

### Areas of Distribution

1. Left atrium.
2. Ventricles:
   a. Most of left ventricle except area around posterior interventricular groove.
   b. Small part of right ventricle adjoining anterior interventricular groove.
   c. Anterior part of interventricular septum.

### Applied Anatomy

1. Left anterior descending artery is known as widows artery as it commonly gets blocked.
2. To overcome a block in artery, a by-pass surgery is undertaken.

### Q. Discuss joints of thorax

**Ans.** *Articulating bones*
- Sternum
- Ribs along with costal cartilages

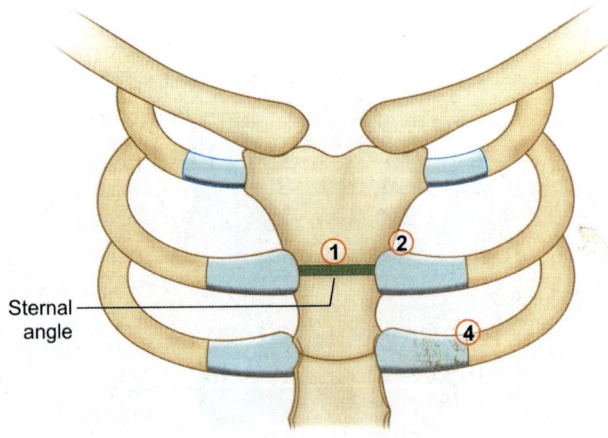

Joints of thorax

- Vertebra (above are the bones forming the rib cage).

### JOINTS

1. Manubriosternal joint
2. Sternocostal

3. Interchondral
4. Costochondral
5. Costovertebral
6. Intervertebral.

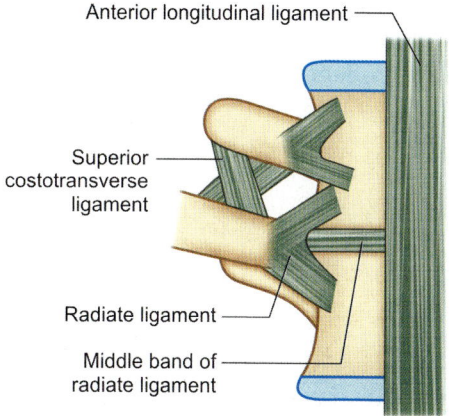

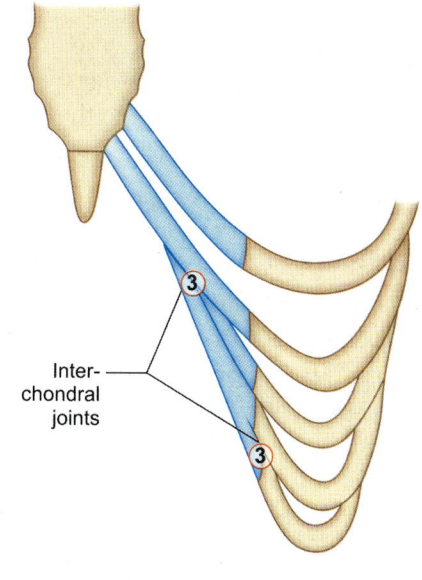

## Manubriosternal Joint

It lies at the level of sternal angle.

*Articulating Bones*

As the name suggests:
- Manubrium sternii
- Body of sternum.

*Type*

Secondary cartilaginous

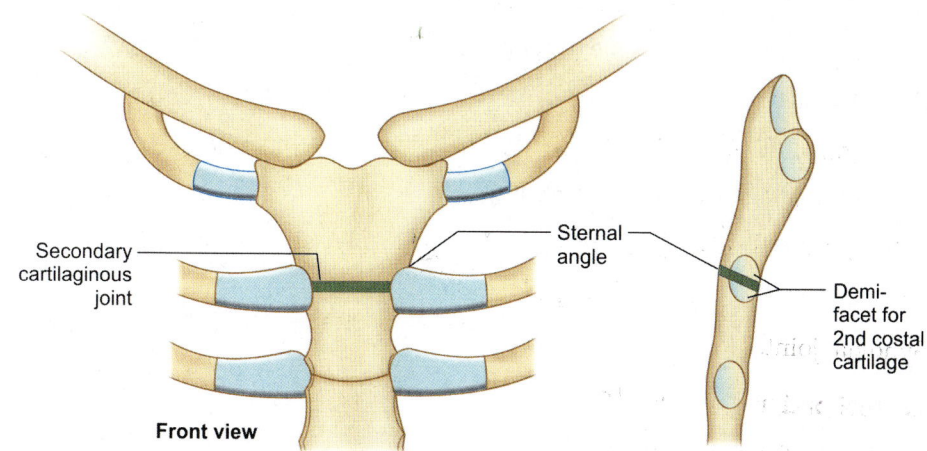

**Front view**

*Structure*

- Articulating surfaces covered by hyaline cartilage
- Joint surfaces held together by the fibrous disc
- Periosteal fibres reinforce the joint surface
  From front and behind

*Peculiarity:* Rarely ossifies

## Sternocostal Joint (=chondrosternal)

- 7 costal cartilages articulate with the side of sternum
  - 1st costal cartilage is fused with sternum
  - 2nd to 7th sternocostal joints
- Type—synovial joint
- Structure—ligaments
  - Fibrous capsule
  - Radiate ligaments
- Peculiarity
  - 2nd sternocostal joint is divided into 2 parts by intra-articular sternocostal ligament.

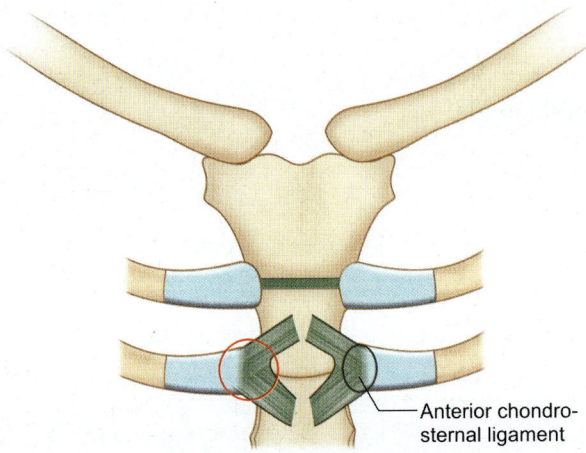

Anterior chondro-
sternal ligament

Sternocostal joint—front view

## Interchondral Joint

*Articulating Cartilages*

Adjacent costal cartilage margins (6th to 9th).

*Type*

Synovial joint.

## Costochondral

*Articulating Surfaces*

Ribs and cartilage of same rib.

### Type
Primary cartilaginous

## Costovertebral Joint

### Articulating Bones
- Rib (head, neck)
- Vertebra (body, transverse process)
- Intervertebral disc.

### Peculiarities
- Head of rib articulates with the same level vertebra, the vertebra above and the intervertebral disc in between
- Articular part of tubercle of rib articulates with the transverse process of vertebra at the same level (= costotransverse joint)
  [Except—head of first and last 3 ribs articulate with only same level vertebra (not adjacent vertebrae while last 2 ribs do not articulate with transverse process of vertebra)]

### Type
- Complex synovial joints (plane type)

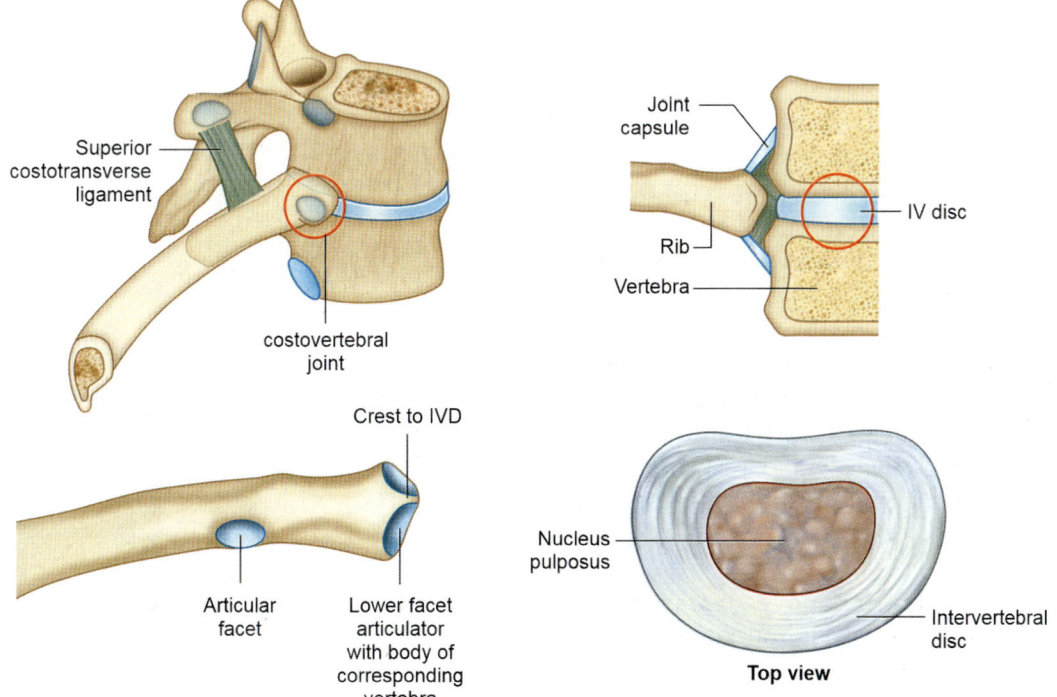

- Ligaments connecting rib with transverse process
- *Fibrous capsule*
- *Lateral costotransverse ligament*. Binds nonarticular part of tubercle to tip of transverse process

- *Costotransverse ligament.* Binds back of the neck of rib to anterior surface of transverse process
- *Superior costotransverse ligament.* Binds crest of the neck of the rib to transverse process (dorsal rami of spinal nerve and dorsal branch of intercostals artery lie above this ligament)
- Head of rib articulates with 2 vertebrae.

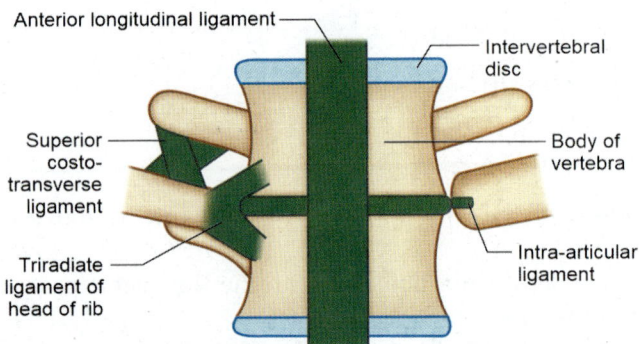

Costovertebral joint from front

## Intervertebral Joint

- Adjacent vertebrae are connected with each other by a median joint and lateral joint between articular processes
- Median joint is secondary cartilaginous
- Lateral articular process joint is synovial.

## MOVEMENTS

- Movements of rib-cage are synchronous with lung expansion and retraction; only minimal movements occur at these joints.
- First 2 ribs and manubrium sternii move as a single unit against 1st thoracic vertebra.
- Peculiar mechanics—1st and 2nd ribs slope downwards and forwards thus raising the manubrium increases the anteroposterior diameter, like pump-handle.
- Rest of the ribs move upwards and outwards increasing anteroposterior (like pump handle) and transverse diameter like bucket handle both actions are executed.

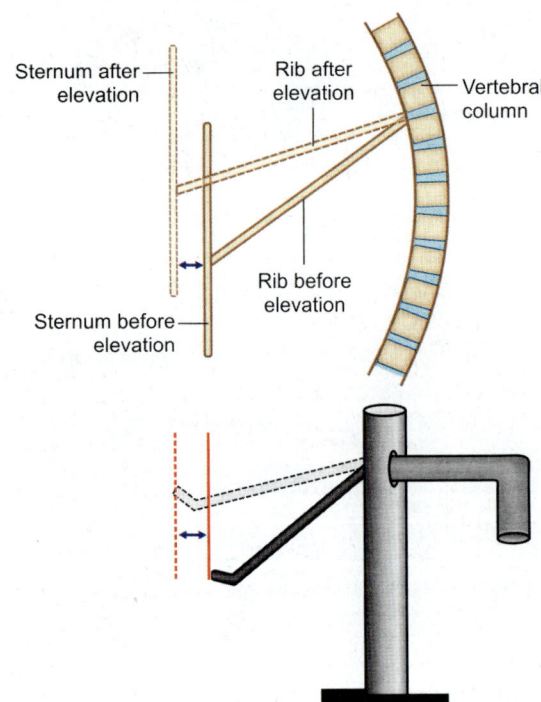

Pump handle —upward movement of rib increasing anteroposterior diameter

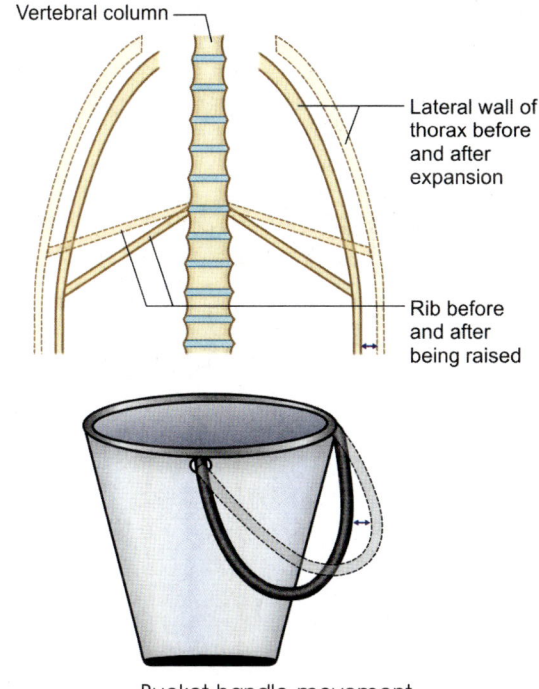

Vertebral column

Lateral wall of
thorax before
and after
expansion

Rib before
and after
being raised

Bucket handle movement

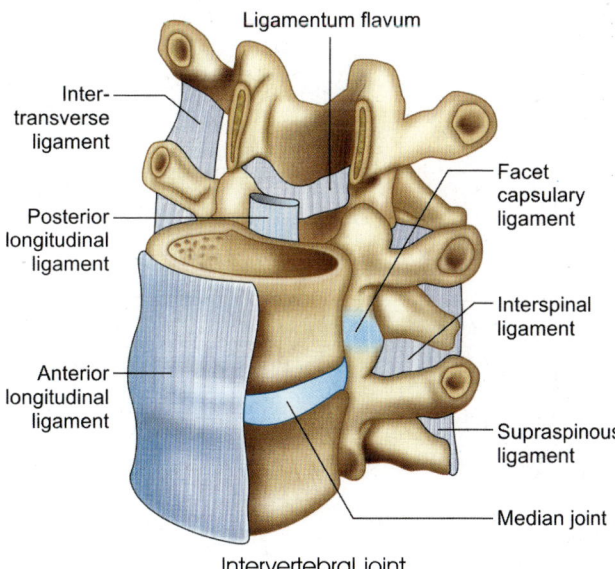

Ligamentum flavum

Inter-
transverse
ligament

Posterior
longitudinal
ligament

Anterior
longitudinal
ligament

Facet
capsulary
ligament

Interspinal
ligament

Supraspinous
ligament

Median joint

Intervertebral joint

- 11th and 12th ribs are held down and stable by abdominal muscles; thus, increasing efficiency of diaphragmatic contraction.

## Q. First rib

**Ans.** *Scalene tubercle:*
- Scalenus anterior muscle is attached
- Lower trunk of brachial plexus is related to first rib.

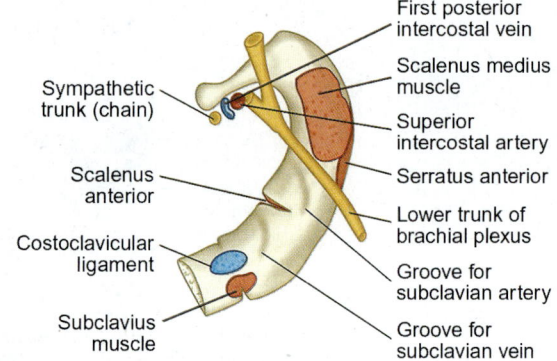

First posterior intercostal vein

Scalenus medius muscle

Sympathetic trunk (chain)

Superior intercostal artery

Scalenus anterior

Serratus anterior

Costoclavicular ligament

Lower trunk of brachial plexus

Groove for subclavian artery

Subclavius muscle

Groove for subclavian vein

## Q. Attachments of 12th rib

**Ans.** Please note that all the attachments can be asked in viva
- Costal cartilage is hyaline cartilage

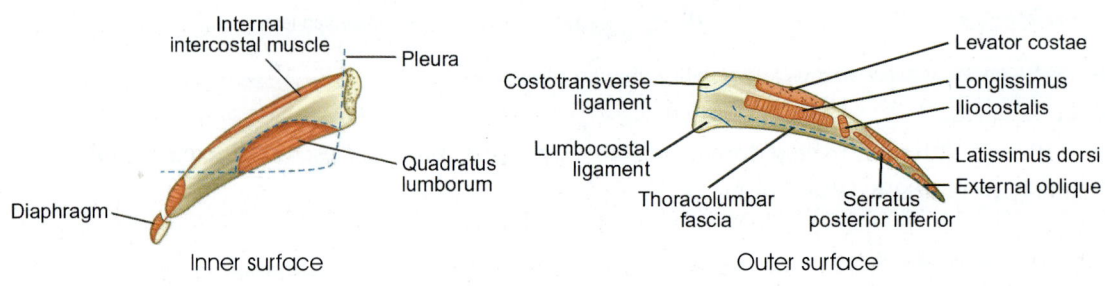

Internal intercostal muscle

Pleura

Costotransverse ligament

Levator costae

Longissimus

Iliocostalis

Lumbocostal ligament

Latissimus dorsi

External oblique

Quadratus lumborum

Thoracolumbar fascia

Serratus posterior inferior

Diaphragm

Inner surface

Outer surface

## Q. Intercostal space

**Ans.**

- There are 11 posterior intercostal arteries are branches of descending aorta.
- While doing thoracocentesis, (= pleural tap) surgeon should bear in mind that the neurovascular bundle is close to the inferior border of rib; thus, the cannula to aspirate fluid should be carefully inserted without damaging the nerves and vessels in the intercostal space.

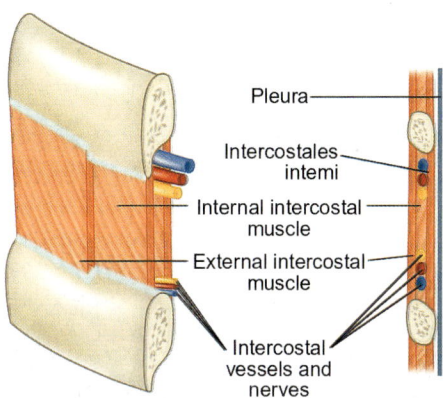

## Q. Internal thoracic artery

**Ans.**

- It is branch of first part of subclavian artery

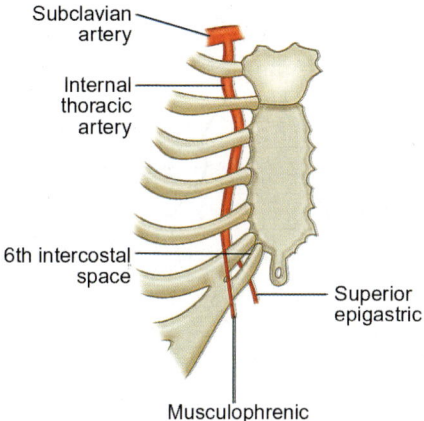

- Internal thoracic artery divides in sixth intercostal space
- Terminal divisions of internal thoracic artery are musculophrenic and epigastric.

## Q. Hilum of right and left lungs.

Ans.

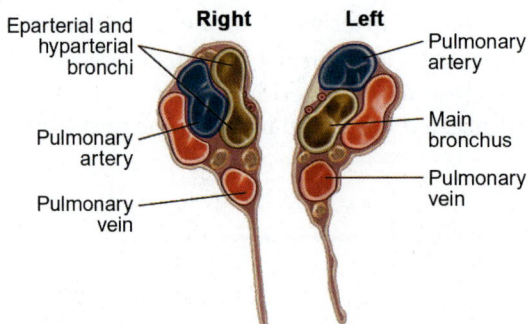

Eparterial and hyparterial bronchi

Pulmonary artery

Pulmonary vein

Right

Left

Pulmonary artery

Main bronchus

Pulmonary vein

## Q. Mediastinal surfaces of right and left lungs.

Ans.

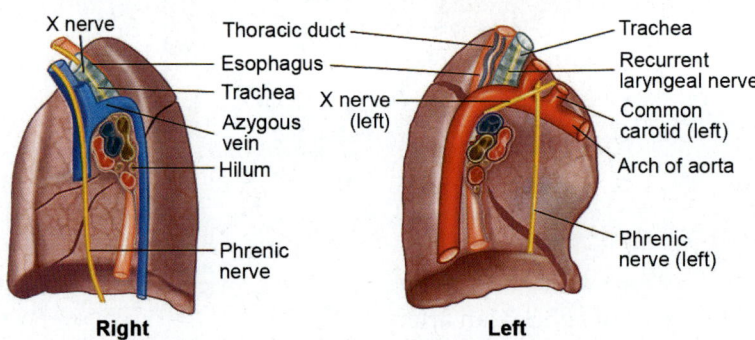

X nerve

Thoracic duct
Esophagus
Trachea
Azygous vein
Hilum

X nerve (left)

Phrenic nerve

Right

Trachea
Recurrent laryngeal nerve
Common carotid (left)
Arch of aorta

Phrenic nerve (left)

Left

## Q. Cardiac silhouette

Ans.

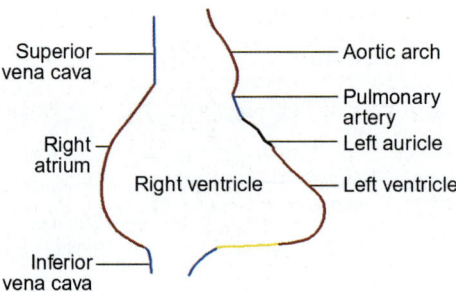

Superior vena cava

Right atrium

Right ventricle

Inferior vena cava

Aortic arch

Pulmonary artery

Left auricle

Left ventricle

## Q. Interior of right atrium

**Ans.**

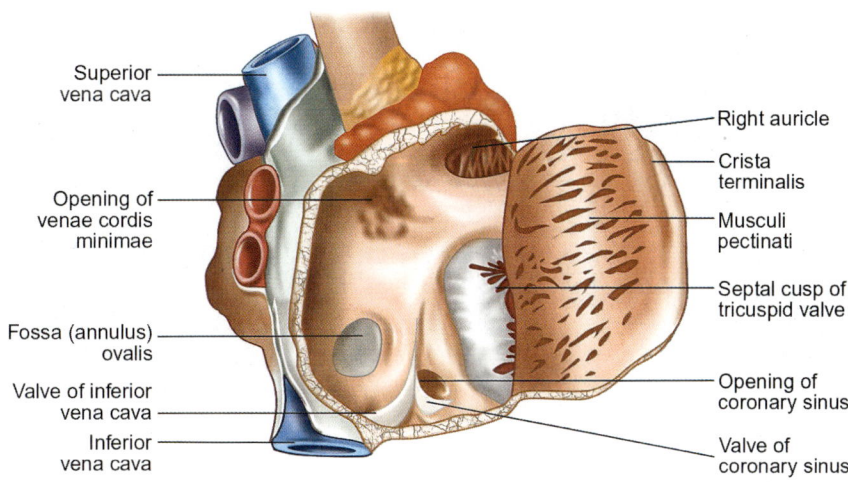

Superior vena cava
Opening of venae cordis minimae
Fossa (annulus) ovalis
Valve of inferior vena cava
Inferior vena cava
Right auricle
Crista terminalis
Musculi pectinati
Septal cusp of tricuspid valve
Opening of coronary sinus
Valve of coronary sinus

## Q. Structures piercing the diaphragm.

**Ans.**

| *Mnemonics* | *Structures* |
| --- | --- |
| "Voice | T8: **I**nferior **V**ena cava |
| **Of** | T10: **O**esophagus (esophagus) |
| **A**merica" | T12: **A**orta |

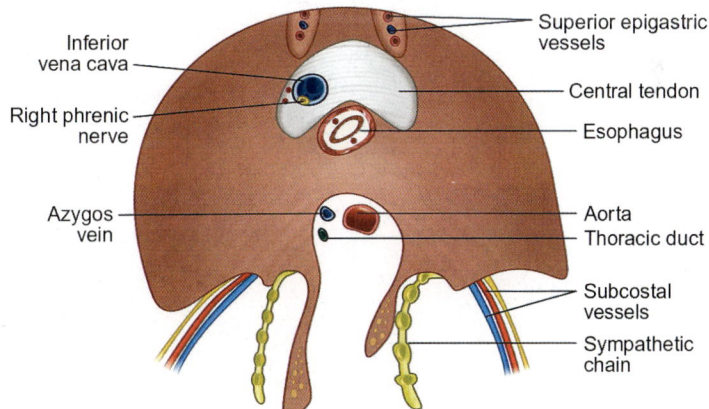

Inferior vena cava
Right phrenic nerve
Azygos vein
Superior epigastric vessels
Central tendon
Esophagus
Aorta
Thoracic duct
Subcostal vessels
Sympathetic chain

## Q. Bronchopulmonary segments

**Ans.**

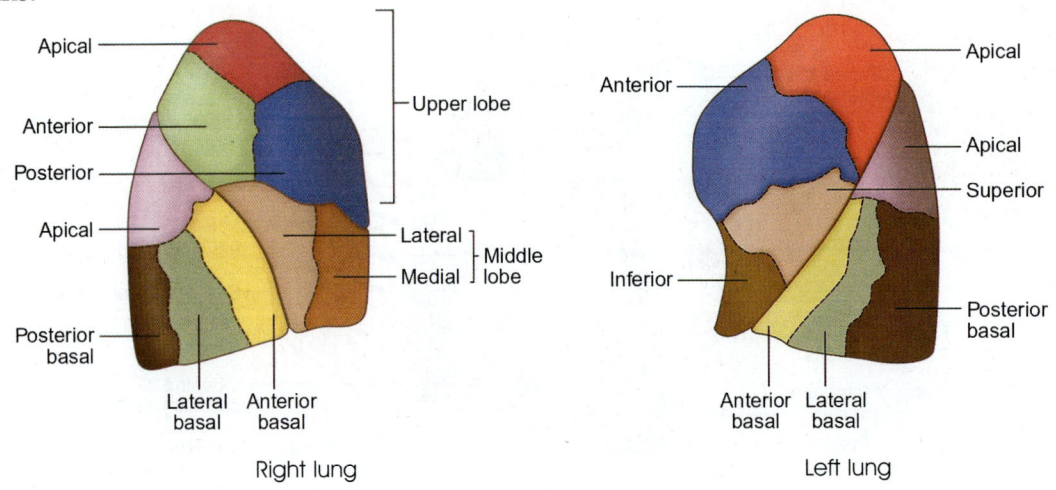

Right lung      Left lung

Segmental resection, is possible of tumor confined to one lobe, since each unit has its own blood and nerve supply, i.e. bronchial artery, terminal bronchiole, intersegmental vein.

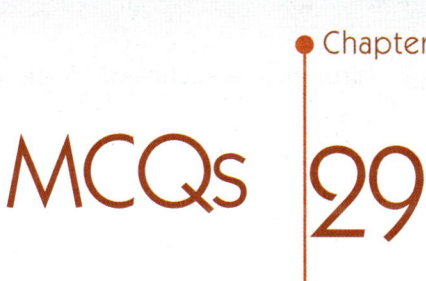

# MCQs

## 29

1. Following are atypical ribs except ....................

   a. 1st
   c. 3rd
   b. 2nd
   d. 12th

   **Answer: c**

2. Following are typical ribs except ....................

   a. 3rd
   c. 4th
   b. 2nd
   d. 7th

   **Answer: b**

3. Subcostal nerve is ....................

   a. T7
   c. T11
   b. T10
   d. T12

   **Answer: d**

4. Posterior intercostal   arteries are .................... in number.

   a. 10
   c. 11
   b. 12
   d. 13

   **Answer: c**

5. Internal mammary artery divides into terminal branches in the .................... intercostal space.

   a. 5th
   c. 4th
   b. 6th
   d. 7th

   **Answer: b**

6. Hilum of lungs line against ..................... thoracic vertebrae.

   a. T3, T4, T5          c. T5, T6, T7

   b. T4, T5, T6          d. T6, T7, T8

   **Answer: c**

7. Left atrium is identified by the openings of ..................... veins.

   a. SVC          c. Pulmonary artery

   b. IVC          d. Pulmonary veins

   **Answer: d**

8. Receiving chamber of the heart is .....................

   a. Left atrium          c. Right ventricle

   b. Right atrium          d. Left ventricle

   **Answer: b**

9. Esophagogastric junction is at the level of ..................... vertebra.

   a. T8          c. T10

   b. T9          d. T11

   **Answer: d**

10. Cricopharyngeal sphincter is ..................... from upper incisor.

    a. 15 cm          c. 27 cm

    b. 25 cm          d. 40 cm

    **Answer: a**

11. Esophagus pierces the diaphragm ..................... from upper incisor.

    a. 15 cm          c. 27 cm

    b. 25 cm          d. 40 cm

    **Answer: d**

12. Arch of aorta crosses the esophagus ..................... from upper incisor.

    a. 15 cm          c. 27 cm

    b. 25 cm          d. 40 cm

    **Answer: b**

13. Left bronchus crosses the esophagus ..................... cm from the upper incisor.

    a. 15          c. 27

    b. 25          d. 40

    **Answer: c**

14. Sibson's fascia is .....................

    a. Cervical fascia          c. Suprapleural membrane

    b. Investing layer          d. Pleura

    **Answer: c**

15. **The boundaries of triangle of Koch are all except** .....................

    a. Posterolateral margin of coronary sinus orifice

    b. Anteromedial margin of coronary sinus orifice

    c. Tricuspid valve septal leaflet

    d. Tendon of Todaro

**Answer: a**

16. **Aortic opening in the diaphragm is at the level of** ................... **vertebra.**

    a. T8                         c. T12

    b. T10                        d. L1

**Answer: c**

17. **Esophageal opening is at the level of** .................... **in diaphragm.**

    a. T8                         c. T12

    b. T10                        d. L1

**Answer: b**

18. **Inferior vena cava pierces the diaphragm at** .................... **level.**

    a. T8                         c. T12

    b. T10                        d. L1

**Answer: a**

19. **Following structure passes through the Larry's space** ....................

    a. Internal mammary vessels       c. Inferior epigastric vessels

    b. Superior epigastric vessels     d. Musculophrenic vessels

**Answer: b**

20. **Azygos vein is formed by the union of** ....................

    a. Intercostal vein with lumbar vein

    b. Renal vein with lumbar vein

    c. Ascending lumbar vein with right subcostal vein

    d. Ascending lumbar vein with left subcostal vein

**Answer: c**

21. **Hemiazygos vein is formed by the union of** ....................

    a. Right subcostal vein with left ascending lumbar vein

    b. Left subcostal vein with left ascending lumbar vein

    c. Left subcostal vein with right ascending lumbar vein

    d. Right subcostal vein with right ascending lumbar vein

**Answer: b**

22. **Hemiazygos vein joins the azygos vein at** .................... **level.**

    a. T7                         c. T9

    b. T8                        d. T10

**Answer: c**

**23. How many bronchopulmonary segments does each lung have?**

a. 8

b. 9

c. 10

d. 11

**Answer: c**

**24. Apical portion of lower lobe of lung lies against .................... ribs.**

a. 3rd to 7th

b. 5th to 9th

c. 7th to 11th

d. 4th to 8th

**Answer: d**

**25. Prevertebral fascia extends up to ....................**

a. T1

b. T2

c. T3

d. T4

**Answer: d**

**26. Thoracic duct enters the thorax through .................... opening in the diaphragm.**

a. Aortic

b. Vena caval

c. Esophageal

d. Foramen of Morgagni

**Answer: a**

**27. Thoracic duct is .................... inches long.**

a. 15

b. 18

c. 20

d. 25

**Answer: b**

**28. Thoracic duct lies in .................... mediastinum in thorax.**

a. Anterior

b. Posterior

c. Superior

d. Middle

**Answer: b**

**29. Right coronary artery takes origin from ....................**

a. Anterior aortic sinus

b. Posterior aortic sinus

c. Right (R) posterior aortic sinus

d. Left (L) posterior aortic sinus

**Answer: a**

**30. Left coronary artery takes origin from ....................**

a. Anterior aortic sinus

b. Posterior aortic sinus

c. Right (R) posterior aortic sinus

d. Left (L) posterior aortic sinus

**Answer: d**

**31. Widows artery is ....................**

a. Right coronary artery

b. Left anterior descending artery

c. Left coronary artery

d. Apical

**Answer: b**

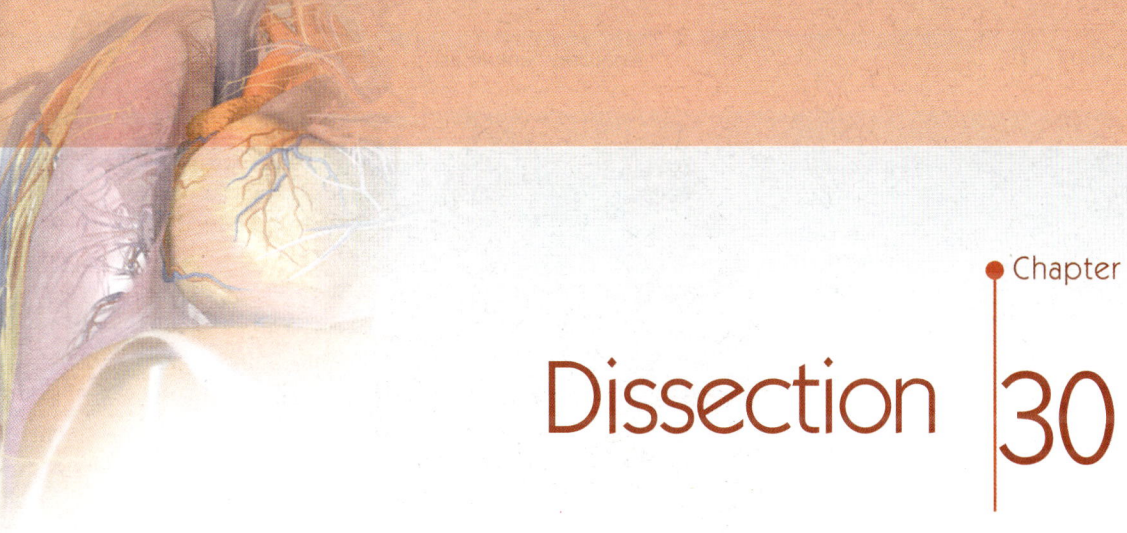

# Dissection

## 30

## Important Vertebral Levels

| Structure | Vertebral level |
|---|---|
| Jugular notch | Disc between T2 and T3 |
| Sternal angle | Disc between T4 and T5 |
| Xiphisternal joint | T9 |
| Lowest part of costal margin | L3 |
| Root of spine of scapula | T3 |
| Inferior angle of scapula | T9 |
| Tip of ninth costal cartilage | L1 |

## 1. ANTERIOR THORACIC WALL

### Structures to be Identified

#### Superficial Plane

- Most of the thoracic wall has upper limb muscles.
    - Identify pectoralis major, attached to the margins of the sternum and adjacent upper six costal cartilages, anterior cutaneous branches of intercostal nerves and branches of intercostal artery can be identified near the sternal end
    - Rectus abdominis is attached to the xiphoid process and cartilages from the seventh to fifth rib
    - Pectoralis minor is attached to third to fifth rib
    - Serratus anterior is attached is on the side of thorax to upper 8 ribs
    - External oblique fibres arise from outer surface of lower 8 ribs
    - Trapezius, rhomboids, latissimus fibres can be appreciated posteriorly.

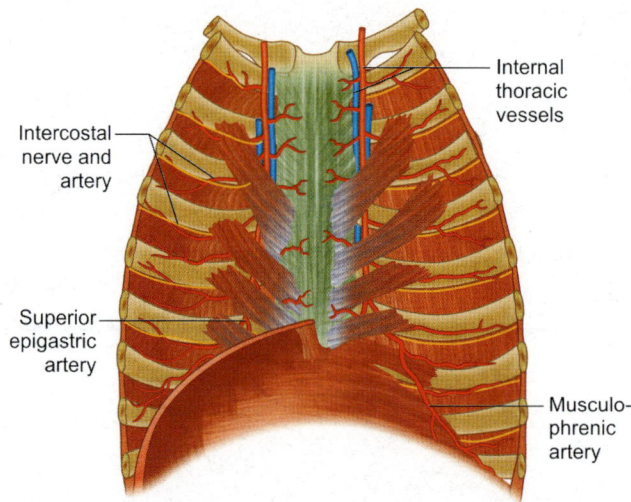

Anterior thoracic wall dissection

- Remove the remains of the upper limb, retaining the cutaneous branches of intercostal nerve.
- Now locate the external intercostal muscle, as you go forwards the muscle is replaced by the membrane.
- Cut through the external intercostal muscle and membrane along the lower border, turn the muscle upwards to expose the internal intercostals muscle. Trace the lateral cutaneous branch of internal intercostal nerve and vessels. Below this is the innermost intercostals.
- Cut the intercostals muscle and membrane anteriorly close to the sternum this will expose the internal thoracic artery and venae comitantes.
- With help of a saw cut the manubriosternal joint, and then cut the parietal pleura in first intercostal space carry this cut posteriorly and repeat the same in each intercostals space.
- Lift the rib cage by blunt dissection and while doing this as the parietal pleura dips in the mediastinum, release from here by taking a sharp cut.
- Expose the transversus thoracis and the internal thoracic vessels.

## 2. MEDIASTINUM

- Mediastinum is a bulky septum between the pleural cavities.
- It is divided by an imaginary line extending from sternal angle to T4, T5.
- Inferior mediastinum is further sub-divided into anterior, middle, posterior.

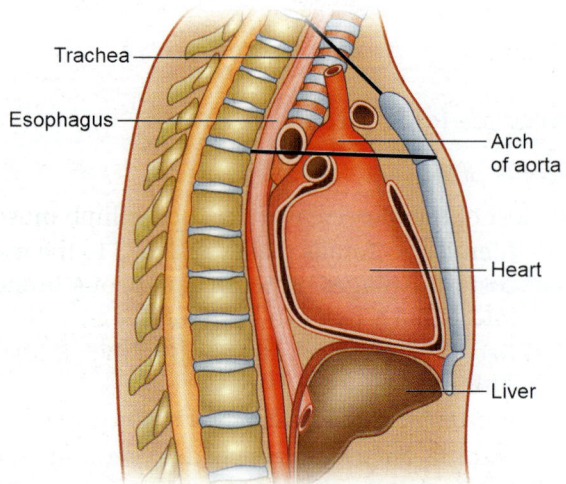

Median section of thorax to show divisions of mediastinum

# 3. LUNGS

## Evisceration of Lungs

- Apply finger pressure on the lungs laterally, and you can see the hilum of lung with its contents
- Take a sharp cut above downwards over the root of lung close to the lungs
- Now deliver the lungs and place it in plastic bag to avoid drying
- After removing the lungs right mediastinum is seen as below

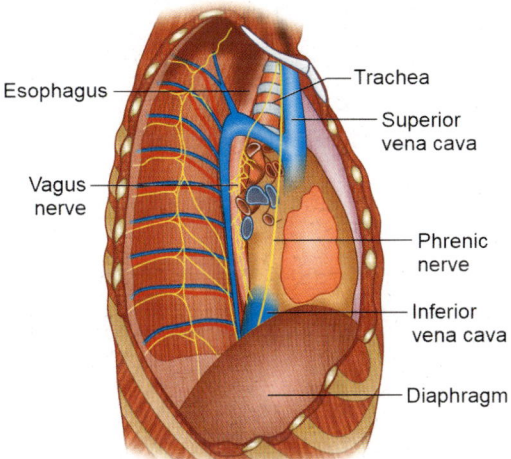

Right side of mediastinum

- Left mediastinum is seen as below
- Remove the pleura covering the phrenic nerve and trace the nerves

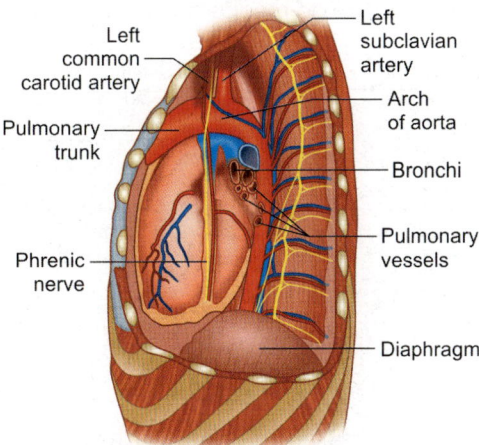

Left side of mediastinum

- Right lung has 2 fissures and 3 lobes, while left lung has 1 fissure and 2 lobes

- Hold right lung in right hand and left lung in left hand

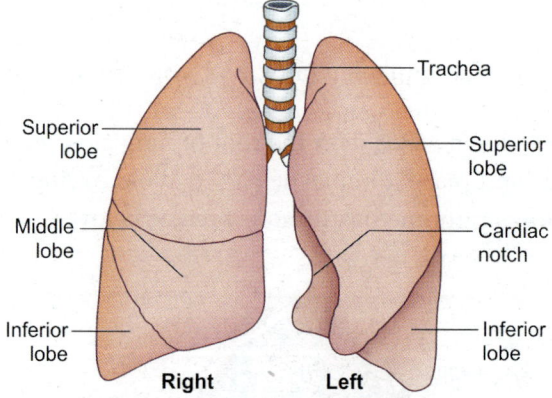

Lungs and trachea specimen

- Mediastinal surface visceral impressions are commonly asked in viva study the given specimens below carefully

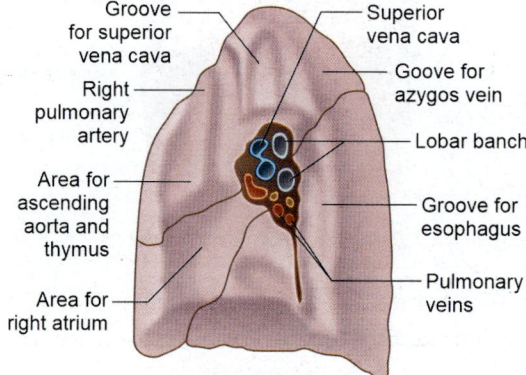

Right lung-mediastinal surface

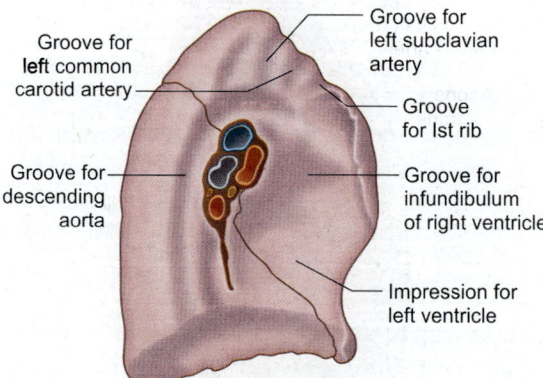

Mediastinal surface of left lung

- Study the hilum of right and left lung and identify the openings
- Pulmonary vein opening is close to the pulmonary ligament which allows its expansion

- Viva may proceed to bronchopulmonary segments

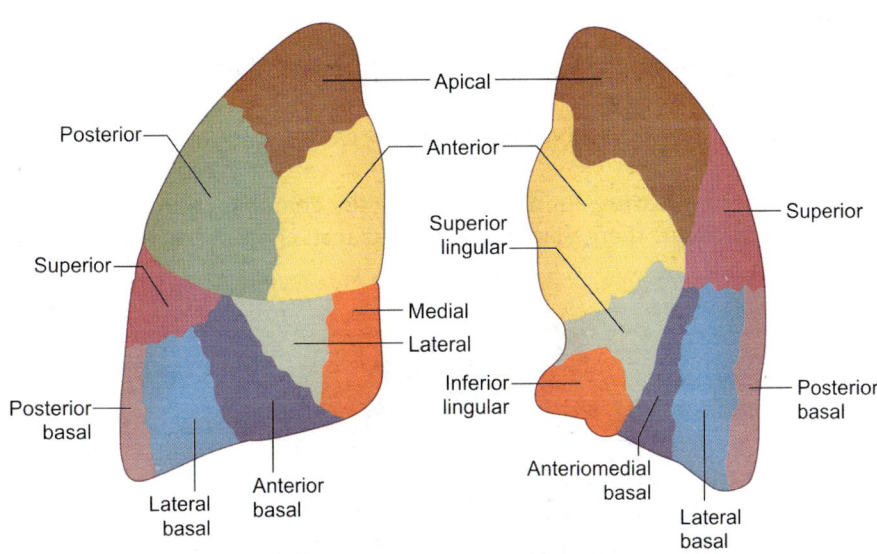

Bronchopulmonary segments

- There are 10 segments in each lung
- These are independent units, which allow the surgeon to resect (cut) only particular segment of lung, without disturbing other lung tissue
- Wash the bronchi with saline and shine a torch within to visualise the openings of other bronchi. A bronchoscope can be introduced in the trachea to visualise the openings of the bronchi, also to remove foreign bodies.

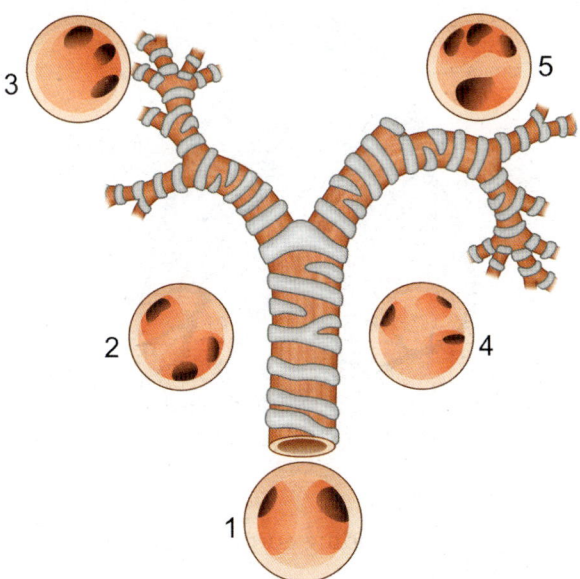

Bronchial tree as seen through the bronchoscope

## 4. HEART

### Evisceration of Heart

- Take a linear cut anterior to the line of phrenic nerve on either side, also take a horizontal cut 1 cm above the diaphragm
- Turn this flap upwards and study the pericardial cavity, and its attachment to the major vessels
- Appreciate the external features of heart, identify the chambers with number of openings, if 4 openings are present, then chamber is left atrium, chamber with 2 large openings is right atrium

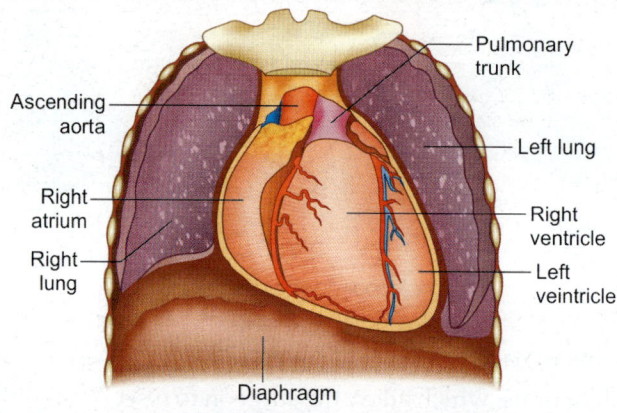

*In situ* thoracic organs

- Strip the visceral pericardium from the anterior surface of the heart
- Remove the fat along the vasculature of heart, and study the blood supply to the heart
- Strip off the myocardium and appreciate the layers of muscle

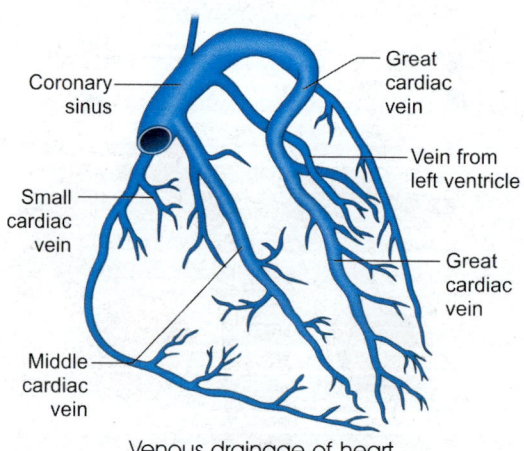

Venous drainage of heart

### Interior of Heart

- Take a coronal cut just in front of ascending aorta, extend the cut to the anterior part of the diaphragmatic surface of the heart
- Hold the knife all along anterior to the pulmonary trunk and right atrium

- Make similar incision on left side of the heart up to the apex passing anterior to left auricle
- Turn the slice of heart downwards on the diaphragmatic surface of heart
- Remove the clots

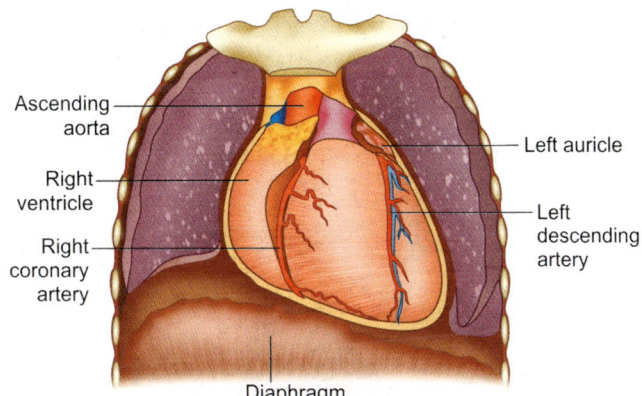

Thoracic organs *in situ*, showing diaphragm and heart musculature

- Study the right atrium, atrioventricular orifice, the atrioventricular valve, right ventricle, infundibulum, pulmonary trunk and the left ventricle.

## Interior of Right Atrium

It is a very important theory question. Try to appreciate all the features—smooth posterior wall showing the huge openings for superior and inferior vena cava, put a forceps and see. A depression known as fossa ovalis, the margins are the limbus ovalis. A rough anterior wall, inner surface shows the comb like elevated muscular ridges the musculi pectinati, which start from linear elevation crista terminalis. Fossa ovalis is a remnant of septum primum, limbus ovalis is remnant of septum secundum, remnants of foramen ovale can be located between the upper part of fossa and limbus.

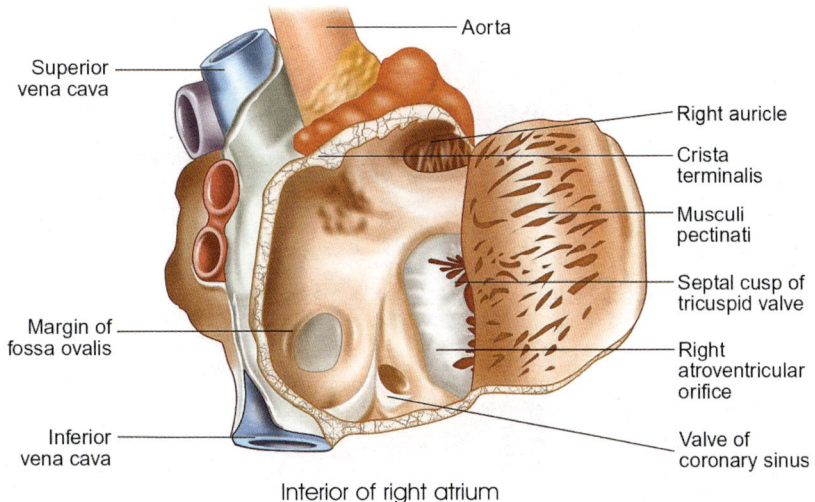

Interior of right atrium

## Interior of Right Ventricle

- The cavity is triangular in shape, demarcate the rough and smooth parts of the cavity
- The smooth part is anterosuperiorly, infundibulum
- Most of the ventricle has rough irregular muscular ridges, the trabeculae carnae
- Appreciate the conical muscles, papillary muscles with the tendinous chorda tendinae
- Study the structure of atrioventricular valve, the cusps and the chorda tendinae.

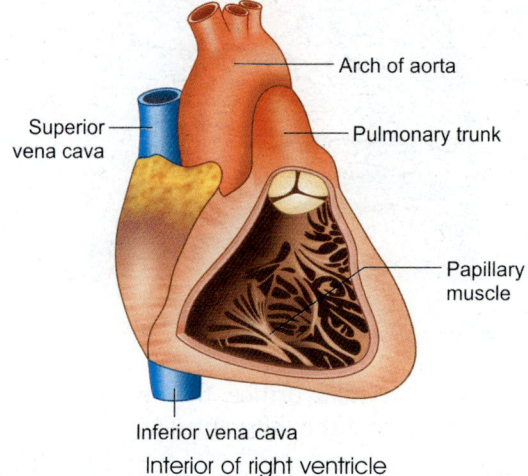

Interior of right ventricle

## Interior of Left Ventricle

- The walls of the left ventricle are strikingly thicker, the cavity is more or less circular
- The muscular ridges, trabecular carnae are more and delicate than right ventricle and prominent towards the apex
- Surface of septum and upper part of anterior wall are smooth
- There are 2 papillary muscles, namely anterior and posterior
- Appreciate the chorda tendinae from the apex of papillary muscle to the cusp of the mitral valve (place the heart on the left palm as it would be in your own body to demonstrate the anatomical position of heart).

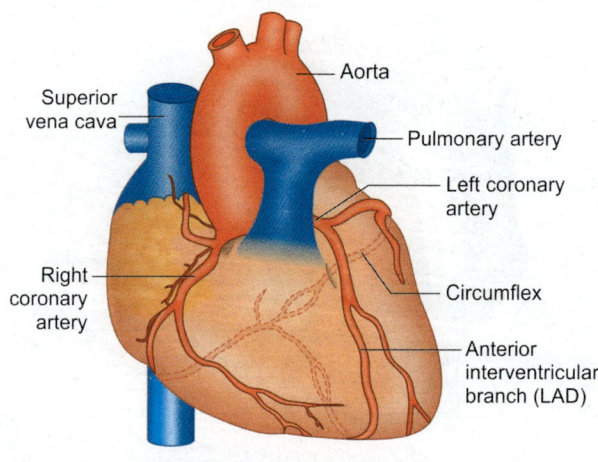

Posterior surface of heart

## Pericardial Sinuses

- There are two pericardial sinuses—namely transverse and oblique
- Transverse sinus is a gap between the arterial and venous end of heart tube. Anteriorly bounded by ascending aorta and pulmonary trunk and posteriorly by superior vena cava and left atrium
- Oblique sinus lies posteriorly on heart and between left atrium and parietal pericardium
- Insert a blunt forceps in the above mentioned gaps to appreciate the sinuses

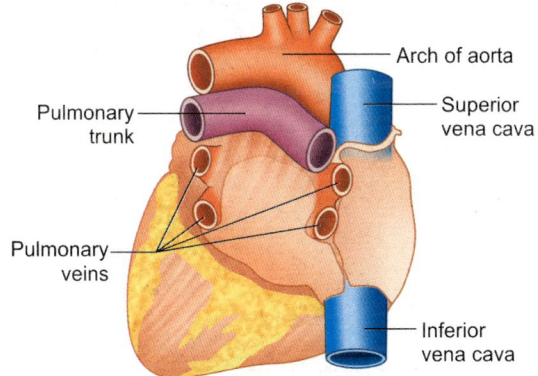

Pericardial sinuses of heart

- Heart blocks are common, hence coronary circulation assumes a great significance
- Angioplasty is a technique of mechanically widening the obstructed coronary artery
- In coronary bypass, a healthy vessel is taken from leg or arm, and connected it to the coronary vessel beyond the block by-passing the existing block.

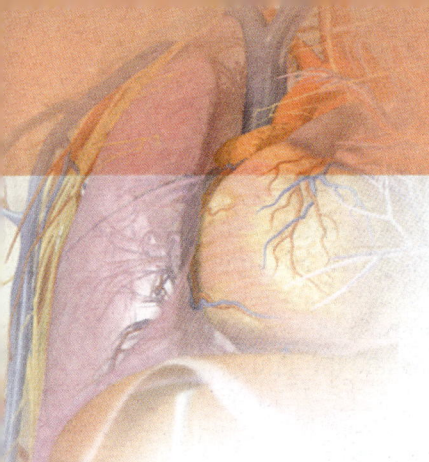

# Osteology | 31

In this section we will deal with sternum and the ribs.

## STERNUM

It is the central bone of the thorax and is a flat bone. It is a very vascular trabecular bone with the medulla containing the red bone marrow.

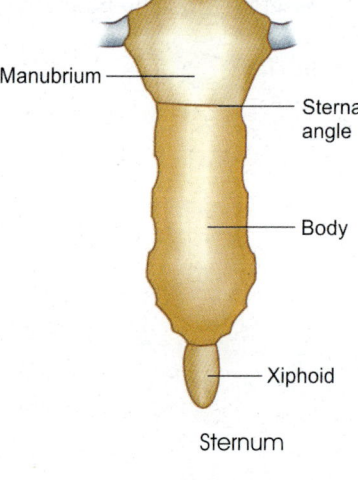

Sternum

### Parts of Sternum

- Manubrium
- Body
- Xiphoid process

### Attachments

- Anterior surface of manubrium
  - Pectoralis major
- Posterior surface of manubrium
  - Sternohyoid
  - Sternothyroid
- Anterior surface of body of sternum
  - Pectoralis major
- Posterior surface of body of sternum

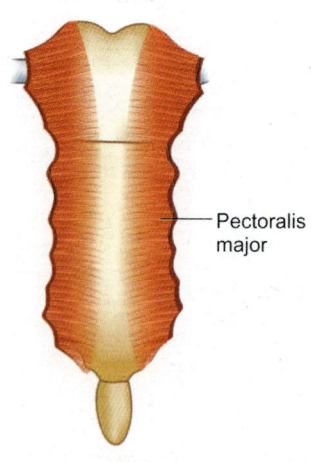

Anterior view

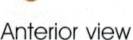

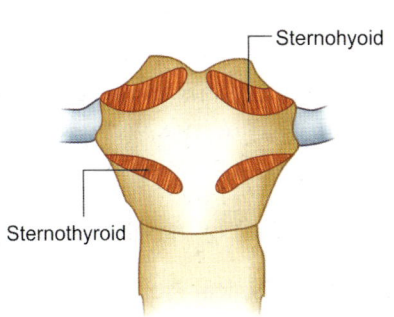

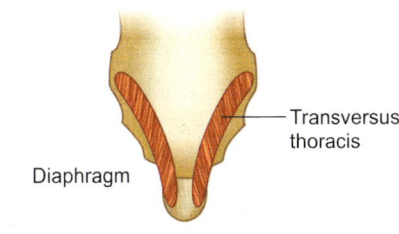

- Transversus thoracis
- Diaphragm
- *Sternal angle:* It is the angle between the manubrium and the body of sternum and can be easily palpable even in obese individuals
- *Following events occur at sternal angle:*
  - Second costal cartilage and rib lies at this level and the 2nd intercostal space below this level
  - Superior and inferior mediastinum imaginary line lies at this level
  - Ascending aorta ends
  - Arch of aorta begins and ends
  - Descending aorta begins
  - Trachea divides into 2 principal bronchi
  - Azygos vein arches over root of right lung
  - Pulmonary trunk divides
  - Thoracic crosses from right to left side
  - Base of heart at this level
  - Cardiac plexus is located at this level.

## Ossification

- Sternum develops by the union of 2 sternal plates, with equal halves on either side of mid-line
- Sternum in developing stage is in the form of segments known as sternebrae
- 1 or 2 primary centres for the manubrium at around 20 weeks IUL, 1st and 2nd sternebrae have 1 primary centre at also around 20 weeks of IUL while the primary centres for 3rd and 4th sternebrae appear around 20 to 24 weeks
- Fusion for all these centres begins during puberty from below upwards and is complete by 25 years
- A separate secondary centre appears for xiphoid process at around 3rd year of life.

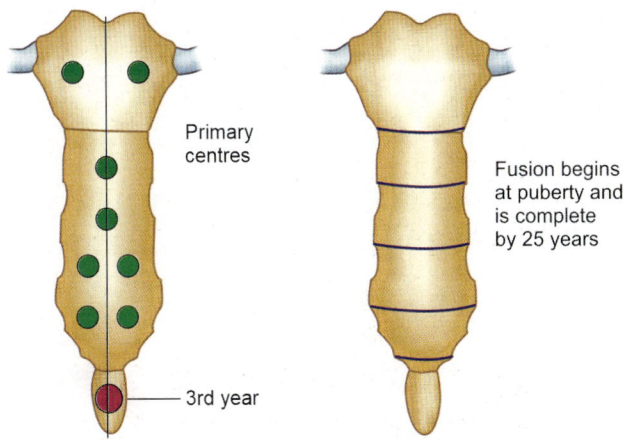

Sternum-showing primary centres and secondary centres of ossification (green colour—primary centre, purple colour—secondary centre)

## RIBS

- There are 12 pairs of ribs forming a bridge between sternum and vertebral column
- First 7 ribs are true, vertebrosternal ribs
- Remaining 5 pairs are false ribs, because 8, 9 and 10 ribs are connected to each other in front, while 11 and 12 have no sternal connection and are known as floating ribs
- Weakest part of the rib is anterior to the angle of rib.

### Features of Typical Rib

Three parts—Head, neck, body
- Head—has 2 articular facets, one for same level vertebra, one for above level
- Neck—has articular tubercle, articulating with transverse process of same level vertebra.

### 1st Rib

*Identification Points*
- It is shortest of all ribs, atypically flat above downwards and sharply curved
- Head, neck are directed upwards and backwards to articulate with the 1st thoracic vertebra
- Superior surface has scalene tubercle and grooves for subclavian vessels on either side
- Inferior surface is smooth.

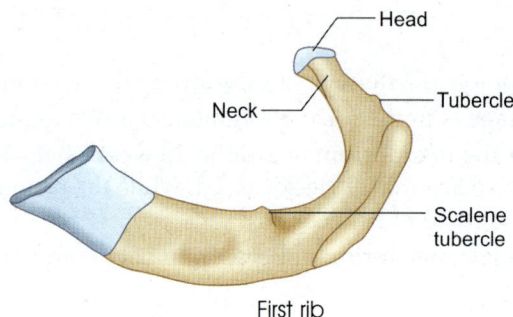

First rib

### Attachments

*Scalene Tubercle*

Scalenus anterior

*Shaft Superior Surface*
- Scalenus medius
- Serratus anterior 1st digitations
- Subclavius.

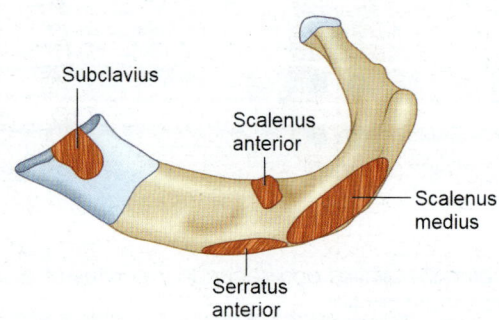

## CRUCIAL RELATIONS

### 12th Rib

*Identification points:*
- It is distinctly atypical rib, sword like 12th rib-external features
- It has no neck, no tubercle only 1 articular facet on the head. Student needs to know all the attachments of the 12th rib as shown in the figure below. Study the figure carefully.

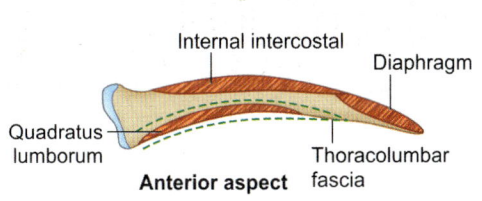
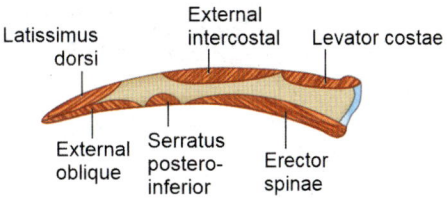

Attachments on anterior aspect 12th rib    Attachments on posterior aspect 12th rib

### Ossification

- All the ribs have 1 primary centre for the shaft (except for 1st, 11 and 12 ribs) which appears around 20 weeks of IUL to begin with for 6th and 7th rib
- Secondary centre for head and tubercle appears around puberty and fuse by 20 years of age.

### 1st Rib

It has 1 primary centre for shaft and secondary centres, each for head and tubercle.

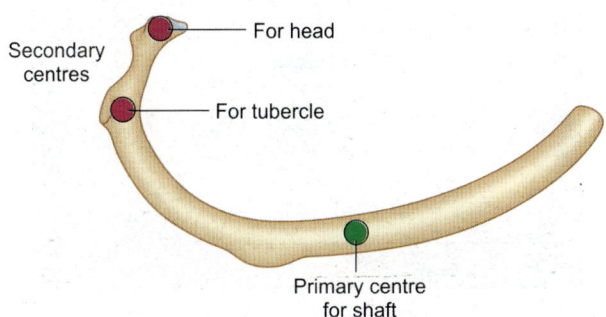

Rib showing primary and secondary centres of ossification

### Typical Thoracic Vertebra

*Identification Points*

- Superior surface of the body is heart-shaped
- Anteroposterior diameter is equal to transverse diameter
- Side of the body has costal facets for articulation with ribs
- Vertebral foramen is small and circular
- Pedicles are stout and short and do not diverge
- Lamina also short, thick and broad
- Spine is blunt and directed downwards (also refer Key Osteology—chapter 25).

# Surface Anatomy

## 32

## 1. STERNAL ANGLE

- Identify the sternal angle (remember the sternal angle can be palpated even in obese individual)

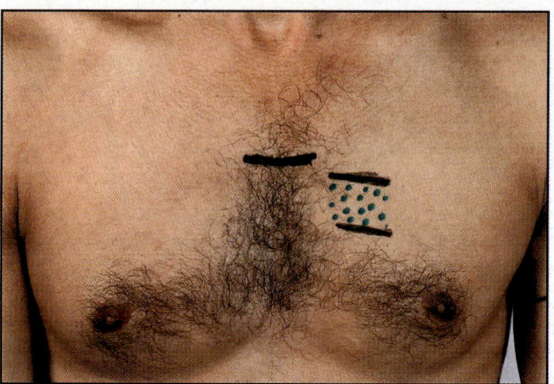

Sternal angle and 2nd intercostal space

- The space below the sternal angle is the second intercostal space, one can start counting the spaces from here
- Male nipple overlies 4th intercostal space.

## 2. PLEURA

- *Position of the patient:* Supine
- *Points to be marked:* Draw a dome over the medial 1/3rd of clavicle with the apex of the dome 1.5 cm above the clavicle
- *Anterior margin markings*
  - Sternoclavicular joint

- Mid-point of sternal angle
- Xiphisternal joint
- On left side to represent the cardiac notch draw a curved line from 4th costal cartilage to 6th costal cartilage.
- Inferior margin
  - Begins from the end of anterior margin
  - 8th rib midclavicular line
  - 10 th rib midaxillary line
  - 12th rib at the lateral border of sacrospinalis muscle

  Remember that the pleura descends at the costoxiphoid and costovertebral angle.
- *Posterior margin:* One point 2 cm lateral to T12, and another point 2 cm lateral to C7 join these lines to obtain the posterior margin.

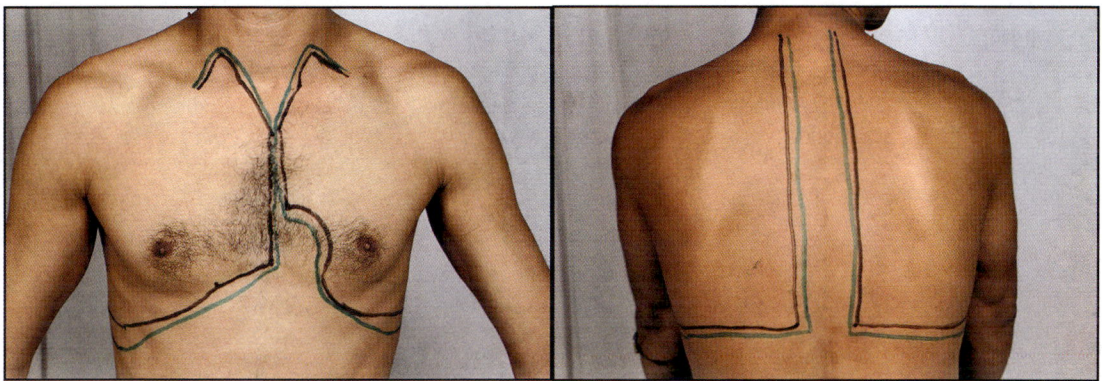

Marking of pleura from front and behind

## 3. LUNGS

- *Position of the subject:* Supine

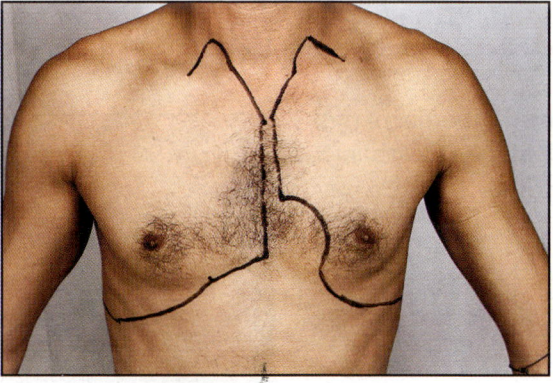

Lung markings from front

- *Points to be marked:* Lung is marked as dome, anterior margin, posterior margin and inferior margin most of the markings are same as for the pleura
- *Dome:* Mark a dome 1.5 cm above the medial half of the clavicle

- *Anterior margin*
  - Sternoclavicular joint
  - Midpoint on sternal angle
  - At the xiphisternal joint in median plane
  - Left side it passes laterally for 3.5 cm from the sternal margin curves downwards around 4 cm from median plane

Area of cardiac notch is dull on percussion; only pleura is present over the pericardium this is known as the area of cardiac dullness.

- *Inferior margin*
  - 6th rib in midclavicular line
  - 8th rib in midaxillary line
  - 10th rib at the lateral border of erector spinae
  - 2 cm lateral to T10.
- *Posterior border:* 2 cm lateral to T10 and 2 cm lateral to C7.

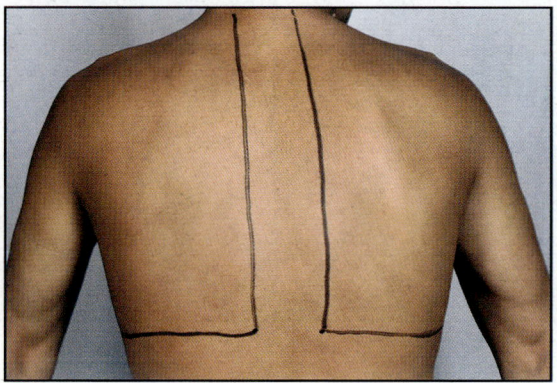
Lung marking from behind

- Oblique fissure
  - 2 cm lateral to T3
  - Midaxillary line on 5th rib
  - 6th costal cartilage 7.5 cm from median plane
- Horizontal fissure
  - One point on the anterior border of right lung at the level of 4th costal cartilage
  - 5th rib midaxillary line.

## 4. HEART

- *Position of the body:* Supine
- Points to be marked
- *Upper border*
  - Lower border of left 2nd costal cartilage 1 cm from the sternal margin
  - Upper border of 3rd costal cartilage 1 cm from sternum, right side

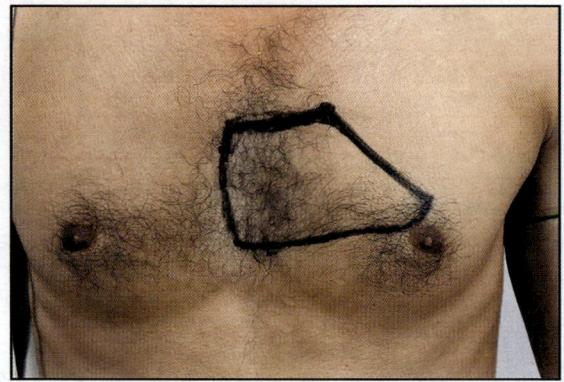
Marking for heart (like trapezium)

- *Lower border:*
  - 6th right costal cartilage
  - Left 5th intercostal space 9 cm from midsternal line.
  Join the upper and lower border vertically with slight curve to give a shape of heart. This area is known as the precordium.

## 5. VALVES OF THE HEART

- *Position of the subject:* Supine
- *Points to be marked*

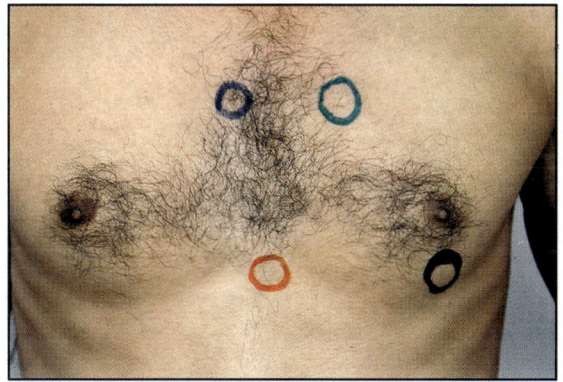

Valves of heart marking

- Aortic area—at 2nd costal cartilage right side
- Pulmonary area—2nd intercostal space left side
- Tricuspid area—Xiphisternal joint area
- Apex beat—mitral valve area.

## 6. INTERNAL MAMMARY ARTERY

- *Position of the subject:* Supine
- Points to be marked
  - 1 cm above the sternal end of the clavicle, 3.5 cm from midline
  - 1.25 cm from the lateral sternal border in the 6th costal cartilage
  - Another point of the termination of the artery in the 6th intercostal space just vertically below the above point

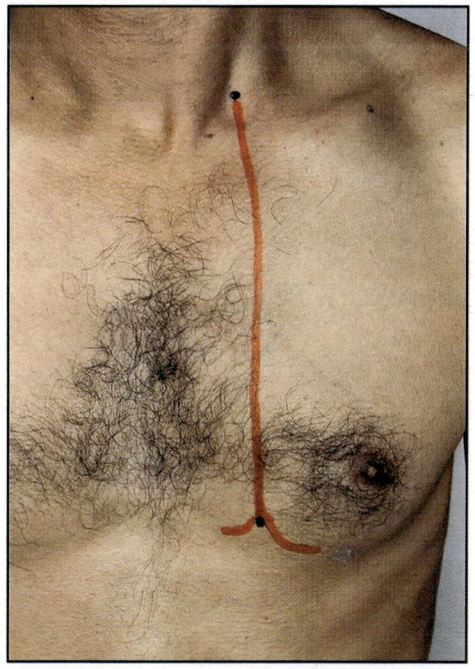

Marking of internal mammary artery

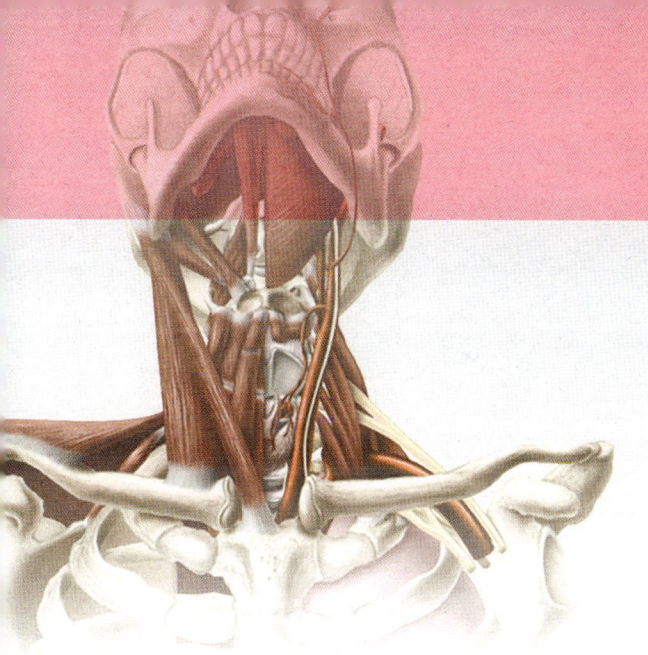

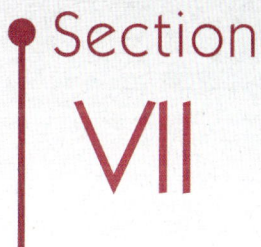
# Head and Neck

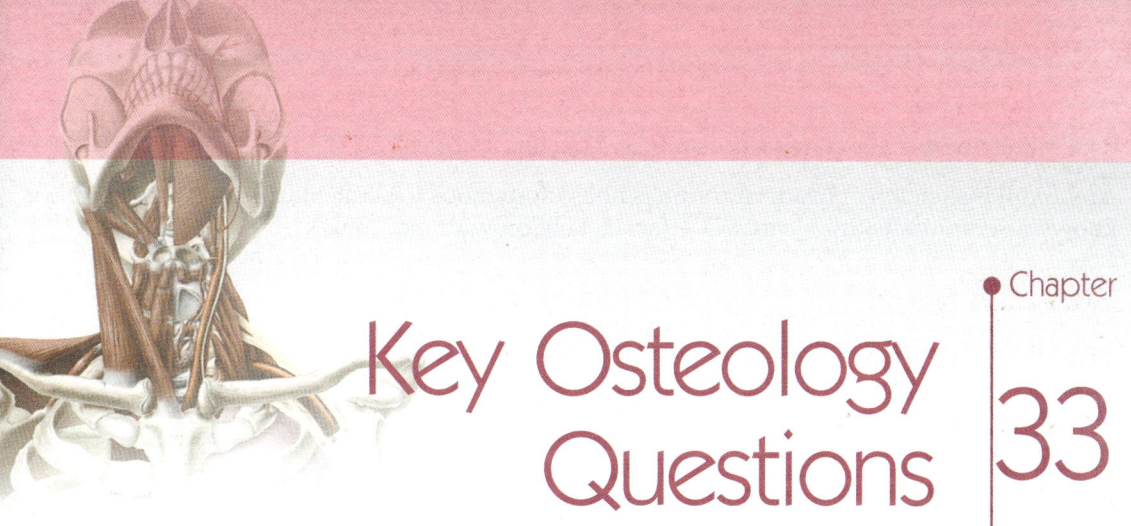

# Key Osteology Questions

## 33

## Q. What is Reid's baseline?

**Ans.** Reid's baseline is an imaginary horizontal line, joining the infraorbital margin to the center of external acoustic meatus (auricular point).

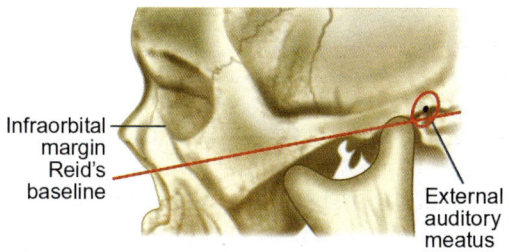

Infraorbital margin
Reid's baseline

External auditory meatus

Reid's baseline

## Q. What is Frankfurt plane?

**Ans.** Frankfurt plane is obtained by joining the infra-orbital margin to the upper margin of external acoustic meatus.

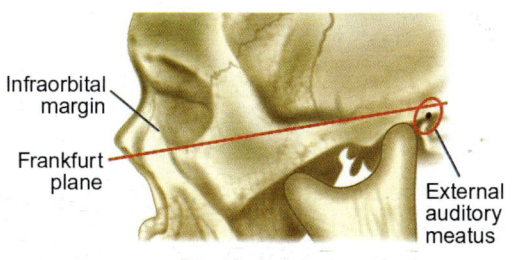

Infraorbital margin

Frankfurt plane

External auditory meatus

Frankfurt plane

**Q. What do you understand by skull? Is cranium synonymous?**

**Ans.** Skull is skeleton of head. Cranium is not synonymous to skull. Skull without mandible is known as cranium (skull = calvaria + facial skeleton with mandible).

**Q. What is vertex?**

**Ans.** Highest point on the sagittal suture is vertex.

**Q. What is bregma? What is lambda?**

**Ans.**
- Junction of coronal and sagittal suture is bregma
- Junction of lambdoid and sagittal suture is lambda.

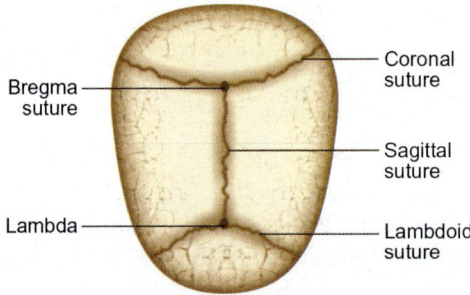

**Q. What is parietal tuber? What is obelion?**

**Ans.**
1. Parietal tuber is the area of maximum convexity of the parietal bone. This is the common site of fracture of skull bone.
2. Obelion is the point on sagittal suture between the two parietal foramina. Some believe that this is the site of pineal (third) eye.

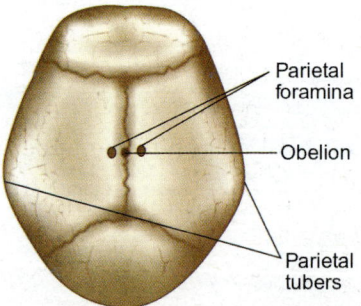

**Q. What is attached to the temporal lines?**

**Ans.** Epicranial aponeurosis and temporalis fascia is attached to the superior temporal line and temporalis muscle is attached to the inferior temporal line.

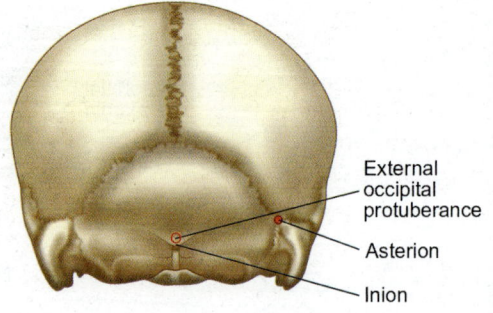

**Q. What is inion?**

**Ans.** The most prominent point on the external occipital protuberance is known as inion.

**Q. What is attached to the superior nuchal line?**

**Ans.** Superior nuchal line gives attachment to the following muscles:
- Medially—trapezius
- Laterally—sternocleidomastoid, splenius capitis.

**Q. What is attached on highest nuchal line?**

**Ans.** Following structures are attached on highest nuchal line:
- *Medially:* Epicranial aponeurosis
- *Laterally:* Occipitalis muscle.

**Q. What is superciliary arch?**

**Ans.** Superciliary arch is a rounded curved elevation, situated just above the medial part of each orbit. It overlies the frontal sinus and is better developed in males. Its medial part gives origin to corrugator supercilii muscle.

**Q. What is glabella?**

**Ans.** Glabella is the median elevation between the two superciliary arches.

**Q. What is gonion?**

**Ans.** The point on the angle of mandible is gonion.

**Q. What is nasion? What is rhinion?**

**Ans.**
- Nasion is the median point at the root of the nose
- Rhinion is the lower point of internasal suture.

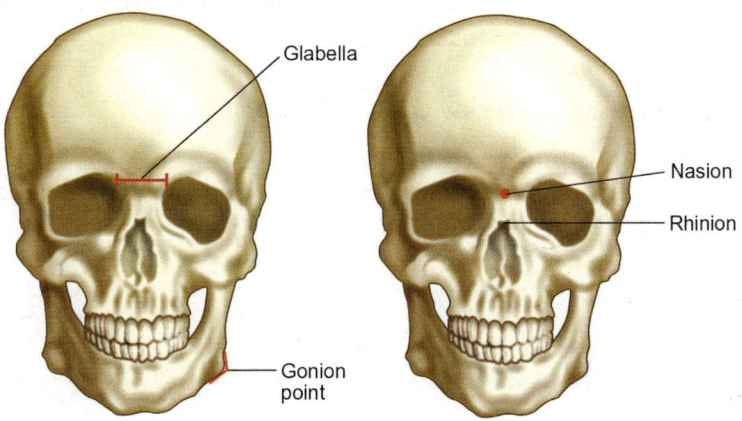

**Q. What are the parts of maxilla?**

Ans.

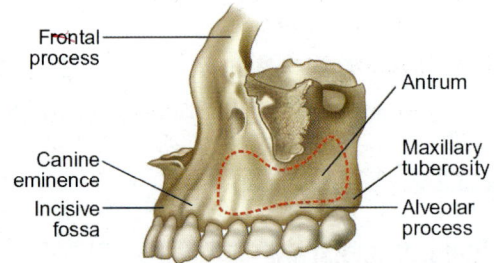

**Q. Where is the maxillary ostium located?**

Ans. Maxillary ostium is the opening of sinus, which is located in the posterior part of middle meatus, at a level higher than floor of the sinus (an unfavourable site for drainage).

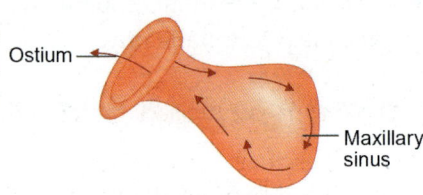

**Q. What do you understand by sinus?**

Ans. Sinus is a blind track leading from the surface down to the tissues.

**Q. What is 'antrum of Highmore'? What are its features?**

Ans. 'Antrum of Highmore' is maxillary sinus.

*Following are its features:*
1. It is pyramidal in shape.
2. It is largest of all the sinuses.
3. It is approximately 15 cc in capacity.
4. Roof is formed by orbital surface of maxilla. Floor is formed by alveolar process of maxilla. Anterior wall is formed by body of maxilla. Posterior wall is a thin plate of bone separating it from pterygopalatine fossa.
5. Ostium lies in the posterior part of middle meatus, near the upper part of sinus cavity.
6. In 30–40% cases, there is accessory ostia.

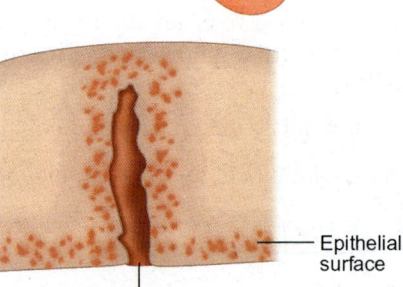

**Q. What do you understand by fistula?**

Ans. Fistula is a communicating track between two epithelial surfaces, commonly between a hollow viscus and skin or between two hollow viscera.

**Q. What is antral puncture?**

Ans. In cases of inadequate drainage of maxillary sinus, another opening is created in maxillary sinus for proper drainage.

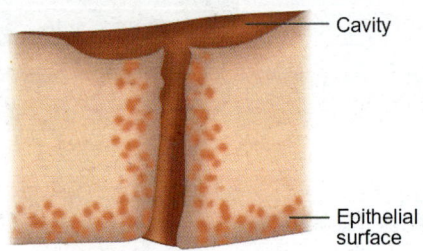

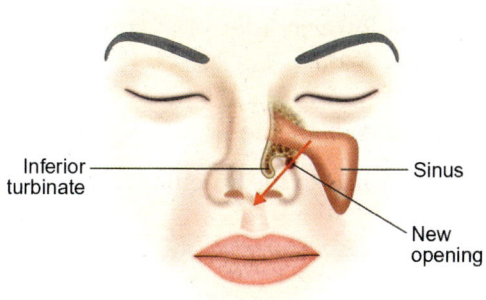

Inferior turbinate — Sinus — New opening

### Q. What is mental point?

**Ans.** Centre of the base of mandible is mental point or gnathion.

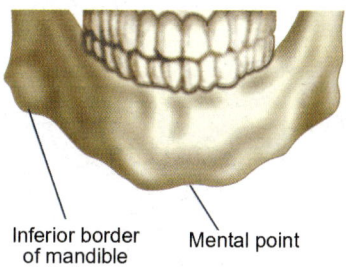

Inferior border of mandible    Mental point

### Q. What lies behind the maxillary antrum?

**Ans.** Pterygopalatine fossa lies behind the maxillary antrum (transantral approach).

### Q. What is jugal point?

**Ans.** Anterior end of the upper border of zygomatic arch is the jugal point.

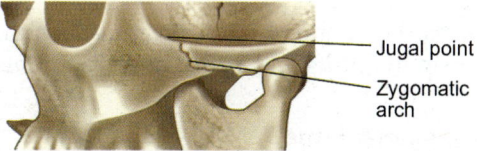

Jugal point — Zygomatic arch

### Q. How is zygomatic arch formed?

**Ans.** Zygomatic arch is formed by temporal process of zygomatic bone (1/3) and zygomatic process of temporal bone (2/3).

### Q. What is attached to zygomatic arch (zygoma)?

**Ans.** Medial surface and lower border gives attachment to masseter and temporalis fascia is attached to the upper border.

**Q. What is articular tubercle?**

**Ans.** Articular tubercle lies on the lower border of zygoma, at the junction of anterior and posterior roots, in front of articular fossa.

**Q. What is attached to the articular tubercle?**

**Ans.** Lateral ligament of jaw is attached to the articular tubercle.

**Q. What is auricular point?**

**Ans.** The central point of external auditory meatus is auricular point through which Reid's baseline passes.

**Q. What is suprameatal triangle (Macewen's triangle)?**

**Ans.** Suprameatal triangle is a small depression posterosuperior to the external auditory meatus.

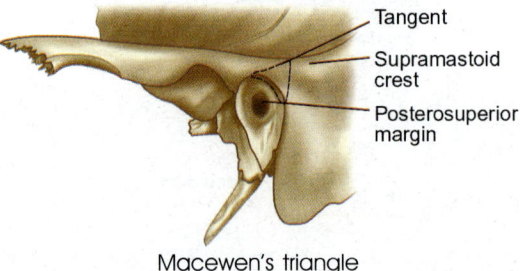

Macewen's triangle

*It is bounded by:*
- Supramastoid crest superiorly
- Posterosuperior margin of meatus anteriorly
- A tangent to posterior margin of meatus posteriorly.

**Q. What is the importance of Macewen's triangle?**

**Ans.** Macewen's triangle forms the lateral wall of mastoid antrum. The antrum lies below it (approximately 12–15 mm deep in adults and 1 mm deep in infants).

**Q. What are the parts of temporal bone?**

**Ans.** There are five parts of temporal bone:
a. Mastoid
b. Styloid
c. Petrous
d. Tympanic
e. Squamous.

**Q. When does the mastoid process ossify?**

**Ans.** Mastoid process ossifies at the end of 2nd year.

### Q. What is entomion?

**Ans.** Entomion is a point near the anterior part of parietomastoid suture.

### Q. What is asterion?

**Ans.** The point, where parietomastoid, occipitomastoid and lambdoid sutures meet is asterion. It is the site of posterior fontanel in infants.

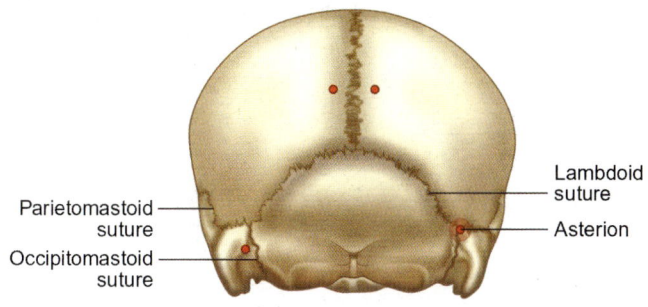

Posterior view of skull

### Q. Where is the tympanomastoid suture located? What does it transmit?

**Ans.** Tympanomastoid suture is placed on the anterior aspect of the base of mastoid process. It transmits the auricular branch of vagus nerve (Arnold's or Alderman's nerve).

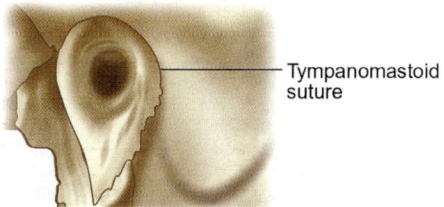

### Q. What structures are attached to the styloid process?

**Ans.** Following structures are attached to the styloid process:
- Three muscles—stylohyoid, styloglossus, stylopharyngeus
- Two ligaments—stylohyoid, stylomandibular.

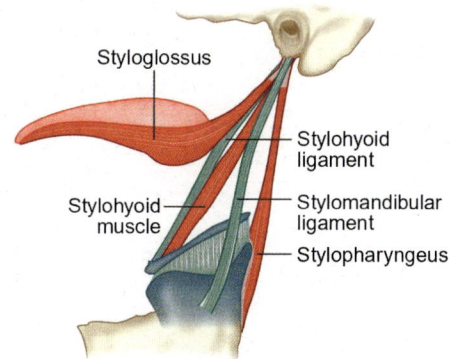

## Q. What are the foramina in the roof of infratemporal fossa?

**Ans.** Roof is pierced by:
- Foramen ovale
- Foramen spinosum.

## Q. What is pterion?

**Ans.** Pterion is an 'H'-shaped suture formed at the junction of frontal, parietal, sphenoid and temporal.

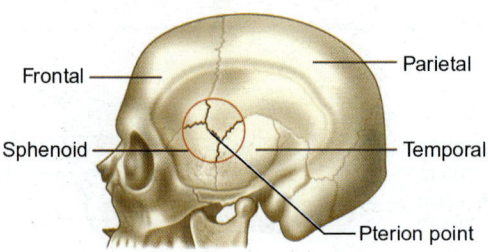

## Q. What is the importance of pterion?

**Ans.** Following structures lie deep to pterion:
- Middle meningeal vein
- Anterior division of middle meningeal artery
- Stem of lateral sulcus of brain.

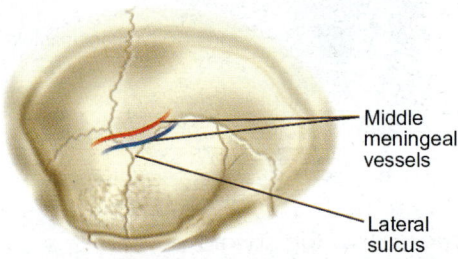

## Q. What are the structures in pterygopalatine fossa?

**Ans.** Structures in pterygopalatine fossa are:
- Maxillary nerves and its branches
- Maxillary artery and its branches
- Fat
- Pterygopalatine venous plexus
- Vidian nerve.

## Q. What is sylvian point?

**Ans.** Stem of lateral sulcus is sylvian point.

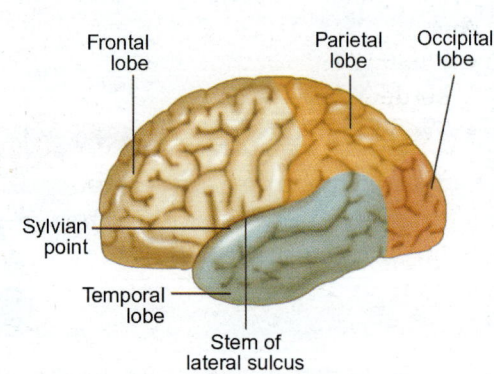

**Q. What is Vidian nerve?**

**Ans.** Also known as nerve of pterygoid canal. It is formed by the union of deep petrosal nerve with greater superficial petrosal nerve.

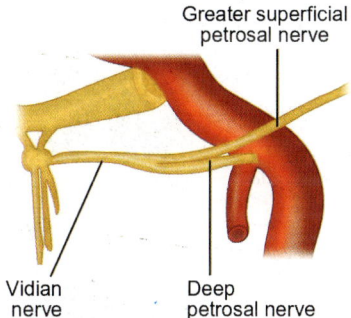

**Q. Which ganglion is present on the roof of infratemporal fossa?**

**Ans.** Otic ganglion.

**Q. What is Arnold's nerve (Alderman's nerve)?**

**Ans.** Auricular branch of vagus nerve is the Arnold's nerve (Alderman's nerve).

**Q. Which muscle takes origin from posterior nasal spine?**

**Ans.** Musculus uvulae muscle takes origin from posterior nasal spine.

**Q. What is nervus spinosus?**

**Ans.** Meningeal branch of mandibular nerve is known as nervus spinosus.

**Q. Where is foramen of Vesalius located?**

**Ans.** Foramen of Vesalius is located between foramen ovale and scaphoid fossa.

**Q. What is palatine crest? What is attached to it?**

**Ans.**
- Palatine crest is a ridge, just in front of posterior border of hard palate
- Tensor palati muscle is attached to it.

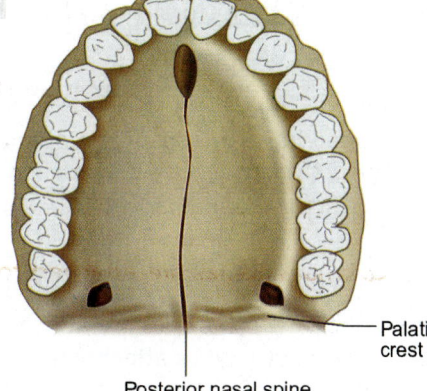

### Q. What is palatovaginal canal?

**Ans.** Vaginal process of medial pterygoid plate gets covered by sphenoidal process of palatine bone and palatovaginal canal formed.

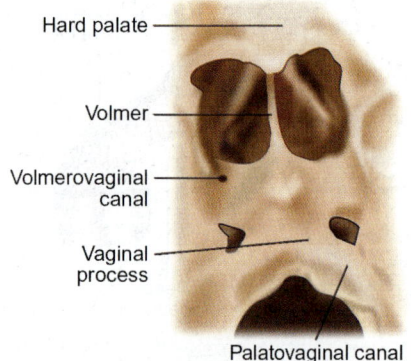

Hard palate

Volmer

Volmerovaginal canal

Vaginal process

Palatovaginal canal

### Q. What is vomerovaginal canal?

**Ans.** Ala of vomer overlaps the vaginal process of medial pterygoid plate, forming the vomero-vaginal canal.

### Q. What is attached to the pharyngeal tubercle?

**Ans.** Uppermost fibres of superior constrictor muscle are attached to pharyngeal tubercle.

### Q. What are the attachments on medial pterygoid plate?

**Ans.** Following are the attachments on medial pterygoid plate:
- Pharyngobasilar fascia is attached to its whole length
- Scaphoid fossa gives origin to tensor palati muscle
- Upper part is notched by auditory tube.

### Q. What is the importance of pterygoid hamulus?

**Ans.** Pterygoid hamulus is infractured during cleft palate surgery, to reduce the tension on suture line and relax the tensor palati muscle.

### Q. What is attached to pterygoid hamulus?

**Ans.** Following is attached to pterygoid hamulus:
- Upper fibres of superior constrictor muscle
- Pterygomandibular raphe.

### Q. What muscles are attached to lateral pterygoid plate?

**Ans.** Following structures are attached to lateral pterygoid plate:
- Lateral surface gives attachment to lateral pterygoid muscle
- Medial surface gives attachment to medial pterygoid muscle.

**Q. Where is auditory tube lodged?**

**Ans.** Auditory tube is lodged in sulcus tubae. Sulcus tubae is a groove between posteromedial margin of greater wing of sphenoid and petrous temporal bone.

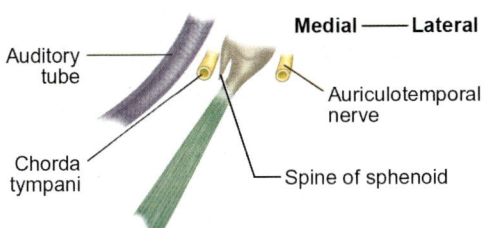

**Q. What are the crucial relations of spine of sphenoid?**

**Ans.** Spine of sphenoid is related laterally to auriculotemporal nerve and medially to chorda tympani nerve and auditory tube.

**Q. What structures pass through foramen lacerum?**

**Ans.** No significant structure passes through foramen lacerum.

**Q. What is tegmen tympani?**

**Ans.** Tegmen tympani is a thin plate of bone, forming the roof of middle ear.

**Q. What ligaments are attached around foramen magnum?**

**Ans.** Anterior and posterior atlanto-occipital membrane and alar ligament.

**Q. What is Gasserian ganglion?**

**Ans.** Trigeminal ganglion is Gasserian ganglion.

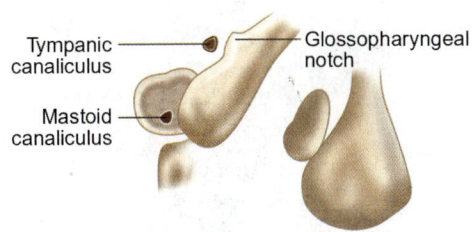

**Q. What structure passes through mastoid canaliculus?**

**Ans.** Auricular branch of vagus nerve passes through mastoid canaliculus.

**Q. What structure passes through tympanic canaliculus?**

**Ans.** Tympanic canaliculus transmits tympanic branch of IX cranial nerve (Jacobson's nerve).

**Q. Where is the glossopharyngeal notch?**

**Ans.** Glossopharyngeal notch is near the medial end of jugular foramen. It lodges the IX cranial nerve ganglion. At its apex, cochlear canaliculus opens and the perilymph drains through it into the subarachnoid space.

**Q. What do the markings on the inner surface of vault signify?**

**Ans.** Markings are produced by meningeal vessels, venous sinuses, arachnoid granulations and gyri.

**Q. What is attached to the frontal crest?**

**Ans.** Falx cerebri is attached to the frontal crest.

**Q. What structures are transmitted through the cribriform plate?**

**Ans.** Olfactory nerves are transmitted through the cribriform plate.

**Q. What is the surface marking of cribriform plate?**

**Ans.** Nasofrontal suture line is the surface marking of cribriform plate.

**Q. What is the location of optic canal?**

**Ans.** Optic canal is located between the two roots of lesser wing of sphenoid.

**Q. Where is the superior orbital fissure located?**

**Ans.** Superior orbital fissure is located between lesser and greater wings of sphenoid.

**Q. Draw a neat labelled diagram of structures passing through the superior orbital fissure.**

**Ans.**

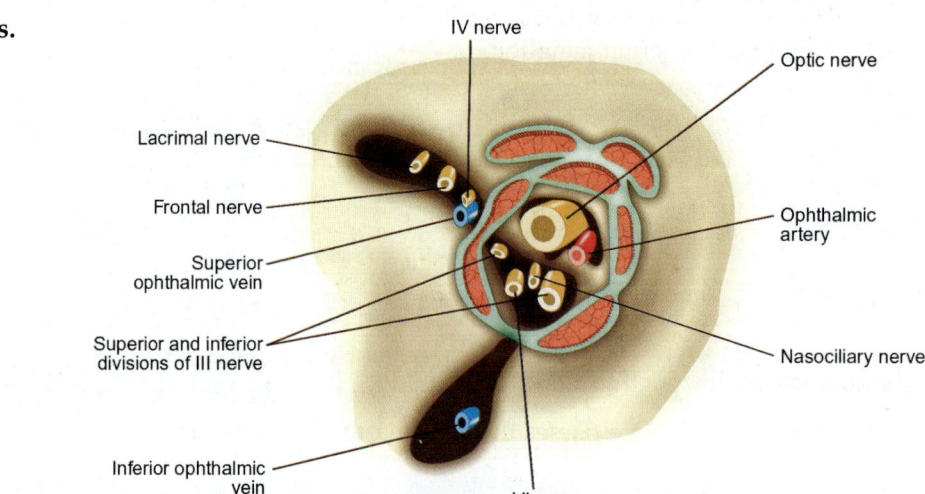

Superior orbital fissure with its contents

**Q. Draw a neat labelled diagram of structures related to cavernous sinus.**

**Ans.**

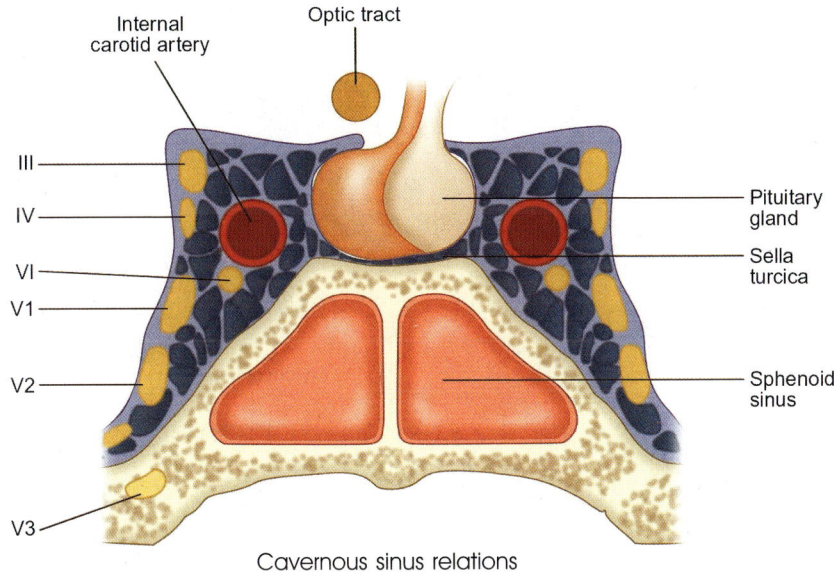

Cavernous sinus relations

**Q. Draw a neat labelled diagram of internal acoustic meatus.**

**Ans.**

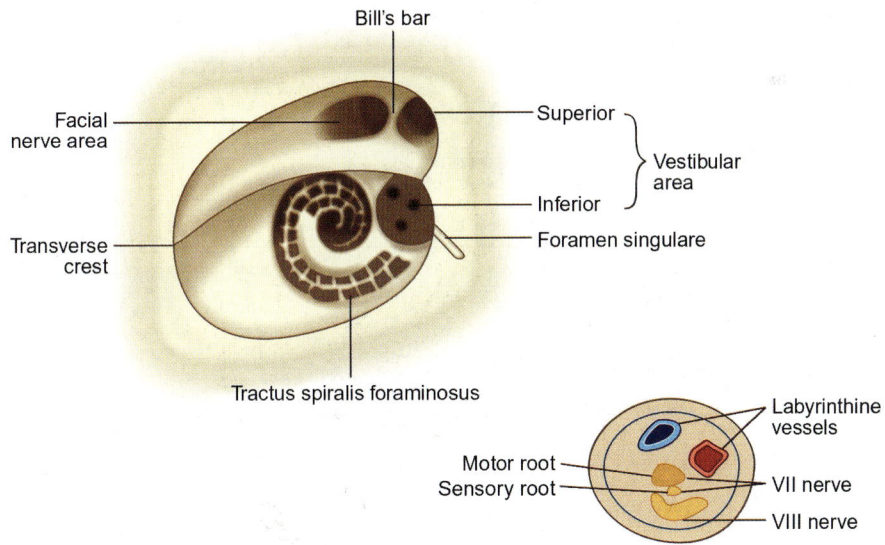

**Q. Which bone ossifies after clavicle?**

**Ans.** Mandible is the bone, which ossifies after clavicle.

**Q. What are the nerves related to mandible?**

**Ans.** Following nerves shown in figure are related to mandible.

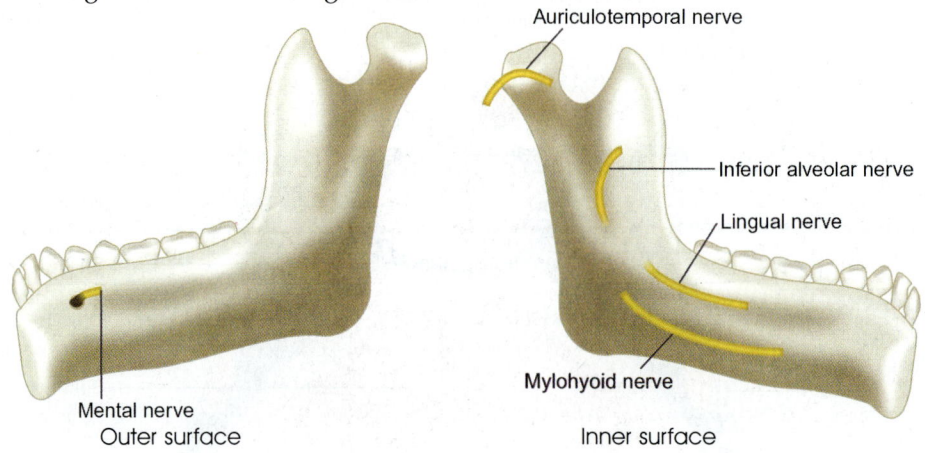

Auriculotemporal nerve

Inferior alveolar nerve

Lingual nerve

Mylohyoid nerve

Mental nerve

Outer surface

Inner surface

**Q. What are the age changes in mandible?**

**Ans.**

| | Child | Adult | Old |
|---|---|---|---|
| Mental foramen site | Near the lower border | Midway | Near the upper border |
| Mandibular angle approximately in degrees | 140 | 110 | 140 |

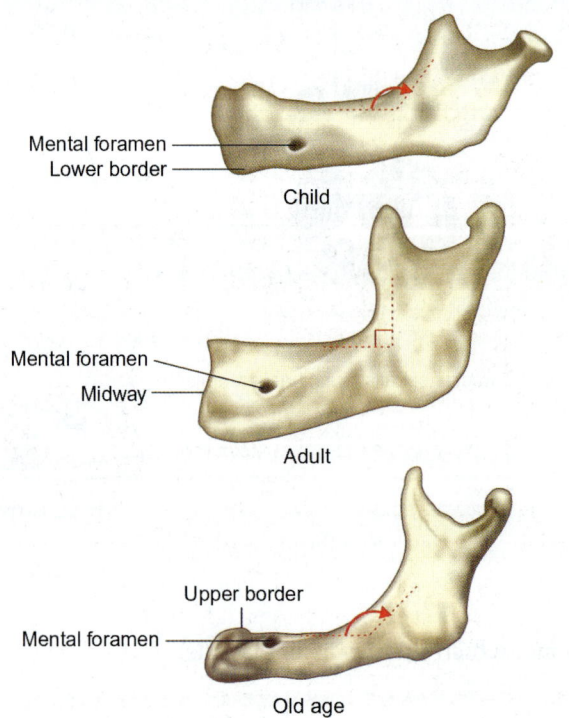

Mental foramen
Lower border

Child

Mental foramen
Midway

Adult

Upper border

Mental foramen

Old age

**Q. Describe the ossification of mandible?**

**Ans.** Ossification of mandible:

- Basic cartilage framework provided is by Meckel's cartilage (1st arch cartilage). Bone is laid over the fibrous membrane of the cartilage.
- Each half of mandible ossifies from a centre appearing near mental foramen around 6th week
- Ossification progresses from the above primary centre to form the body and ramus of mandible
- Later Meckel's cartilage around incisive foramen is surrounded and invaded by bone
- Secondary cartilage appears each for condylar process, anterior border of coronoid process
- One or two cartilaginous nodules appear on each side of symphysis menti, which ossify by 7th month of intrauterine life
- At birth mandible has two halves connected by fibrous tissue at symphysis menti
- Bony union begins below upwards during first year of life and completed by end of first year.

**Q. How are the cervical vertebrae identified?**

**Ans.** Cervical vertebrae are identified by the small size and presence of foramen transversarium.

**Q. What is the other name of first cervical vertebra?**

**Ans.** Cervical vertebra is also known as atlas.

**Q. What is the other name of second cervical vertebra?**

**Ans.** Second cervical vertebra is also known as axis.

**Q. Which vertebra is known as vertebra prominens?**

**Ans.** The seventh cervical vertebra is known as vertebra prominens. Since, its tip can be felt through the skin at the lower end of nuchal furrow.

**Q. What events occur at the transverse process of sixth cervical vertebra?**

**Ans.** Following events occur at the transverse process of sixth cervical vertebra:

- First part of vertebral artery ends
- Second part of vertebral artery begins
- Pharynx continues as esophagus
- Trachea begins
- Jugular vein crosses and terminates in subclavian vein
- Middle cervical ganglion lies at this level.

### Q. How does the cervical vertebra ossify?

**Ans.** A typical cervical vertebra ossifies from three primary centres and six secondary centres:
1. There are two primary centres for the two halves of neural arch and one for the centrum. They fuse by 1–3 years.
2. There are two secondary centres for annular epiphyseal disks, two for the transverse processes, two for the spine. All fuse by 25 years.

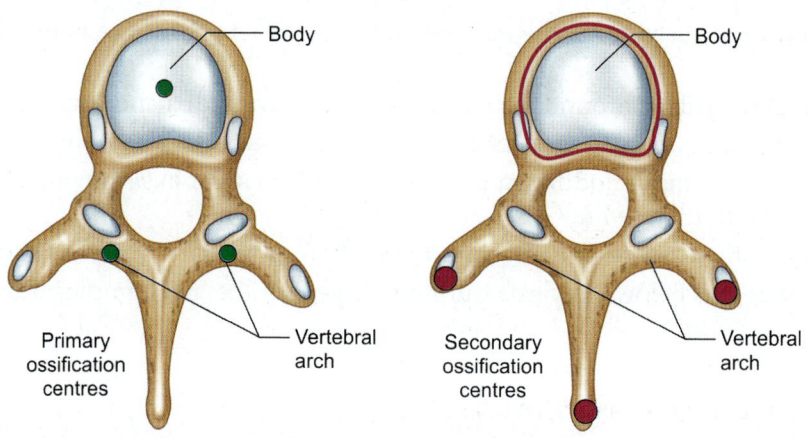

### Q. How does a fetal skull differ from adult skull?

**Ans.** Fetal skull has following features:
- Skull is large in size
- Fetal skull has membranous gaps between suture lines known as fontanelle.
- Facial skeleton is small compared to the calvaria due to rudimentary status of facial bones and small size of sinuses
- Base of the skull is short
- Frontal and parietal tuber are prominent
- Glabella, superciliary arches and mastoid processes are not developed
- Stylomastoid foramen is exposed.

### Q. What structure of fetal skull is of adult size?

**Ans.** Middle and internal auditory parts are of adult size in fetal skull.

### Q. What is cephalic index?

**Ans.** Cephalic index expresses the shape of the head and is the proportion of breadth to the length of the skull.

$$\text{Cephalic index} = \frac{\text{Breadth}}{\text{Length}} \times 100$$

### Q. When does the anterior fontanelle close?

**Ans.** Anterior fontanelle closes by 18th months (1½ year).

**Q. When does the posterior fontanelle close?**

**Ans.** Posterior fontanelle closes by 2–3 months.

**Q. What is metopic suture?**

**Ans.** When two halves of frontal bone fail to fuse in midline, a metopic suture develops, 3–8% of individuals with racial variations have metopic suture.

**Q. What is sella turcica?**

**Ans.** The upper surface of the body of sphenoid is hollowed out in the form of Turkish saddle. This is known as sella turcica.

**Q. What are Le Fort fractures? How are they classified?**

**Ans.** Central variety of middle third facial fractures are Le Fort fractures.

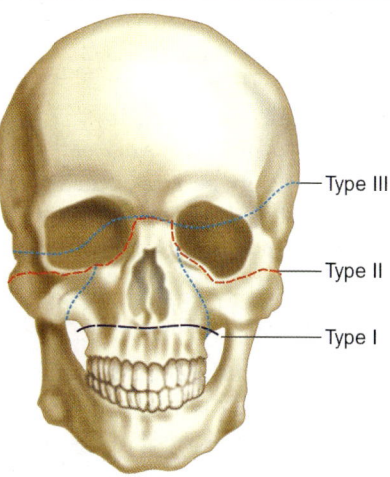

*There are three types of Le Fort fractures:*
Type 1: Transverse fractures of maxilla involving palate only
Type 2: Fracture en bloc of palate and middle third of face
Type 3: Complete disruption of facial skeleton from the cranium.

Le Fort fracture lines

**Q. What is the status of paranasal sinuses at birth?**

**Ans.** All the paranasal sinuses are rudimentary at birth except frontal, which is absent.

**Q. How is the lateral wall of the nose divided?**

**Ans.**

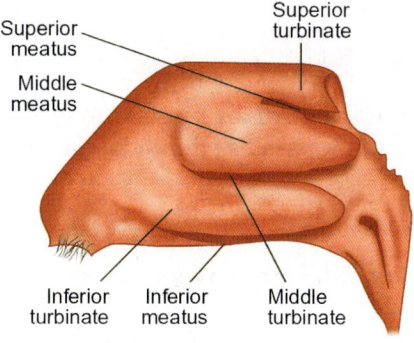

Lateral wall of nose

1. The lateral wall of the nose is divided by bony elevations namely superior, middle and inferior turbinates (conchae). Due to which the lateral wall space gets divided into superior, middle and inferior meatus below the respective turbinates.

2. Superior and middle conchae are parts of ethmoid bone.
3. Inferior conchae is a separate bone.

### Q. What are the parts of ethmoid bone?

**Ans.** Ethmoid bone has a horizontal—perforated cribriform plate, a median—perpendicular plate and on each side lateral—labyrinth.

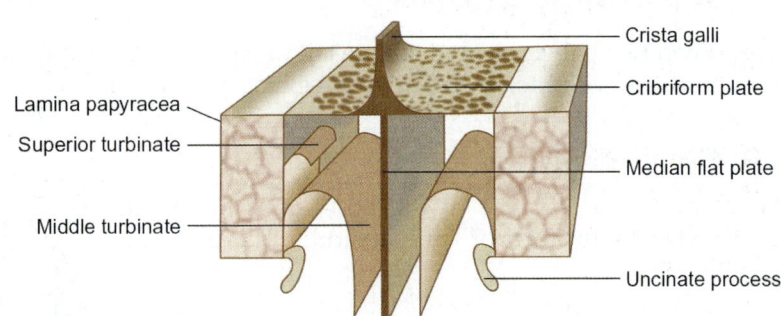

Ethmoidal labyrinths consist of thin-walled ethmoidal air cells (anterior, middle and posterior) between two vertical plate. The lateral vertical plate is lamina papyracea, which forms part of the medial orbital wall. The medial vertical plate forms part of lateral nasal wall. Superior middle turbinate and uncinate process are parts of ethmoid bone.

### Q. How is the middle turbinate attached?

**Ans.** Middle turbinate has three planes of attachment:
- Anterior attachment is in sagittal plane to frontonasal process of maxilla
- In coronal plane and horizontal plane it is attached to lamina papyracea.

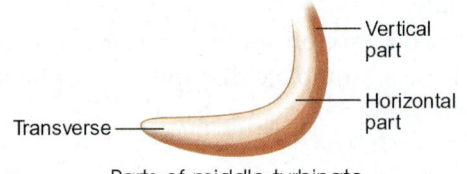

Parts of middle turbinate

### Q. What is ground lamella (basal lamella)?

**Ans.** Middle turbinate turns laterally to get attached in coronal plane to the lamina papyracea. This area of attachment is ground lamella. It separates the anterior ethmoidal cells from the posterior ethmoidal cells.

### Q. What are the boundaries of ethmoidal air cells?

**Ans.** Ethmoidal air cells are bounded medially by superior and middle turbinate and laterally by paper-thin lamina papyracea. It separates ethmoidal air cells from orbit.

### Q. Which arteries pierce ethmoid labyrinth?

**Ans.** Anterior and posterior ethmoidal artery pierce ethmoid labyrinth.

### Q. What is the relation of optic nerve to ethmoidal arteries?

**Ans.** Anterior ethmoidal artery enters the orbit 4 cm behind the medial ligament of orbit and posterior ethmoidal artery is 2 cm behind anterior ethmoidal artery and optic nerve is just 1 cm or even less than 1 cm behind posterior ethmoidal artery.

### Q. What is FESS?

**Ans.** FESS means functional endoscopic sinus surgery.

### Q. What is osteomeatal complex?

**Ans.** The various openings in the middle meatus as seen endoscopically is known as osteo-meatal complex. It is divided into anterior and posterior parts by ground lamella.

### Q. What are the age changes in maxilla?

**Ans.** *At birth:*
- Transverse and sagittal dimensions are greater than vertical (small body)
- Frontal process is prominent
- Alveoli reach the orbital floor
- Maxillary sinus is rudimentary.

*In adults:*
- Vertical dimension is greater than transverse and sagittal dimensions
- Maxillary sinus is well-developed.

*In old age:*
- Height reduces
- Alveolar process gets absorbed.

### Q. What are the boundaries and contents of scalene triangle?

**Ans.** Scalene triangle is bounded by:
- *Anteriorly:* Scalenus anterior
- *Posteriorly:* Scalenus medius
- *Base:* Subclavian artery
- *Contents:* Trunks of brachial plexus.

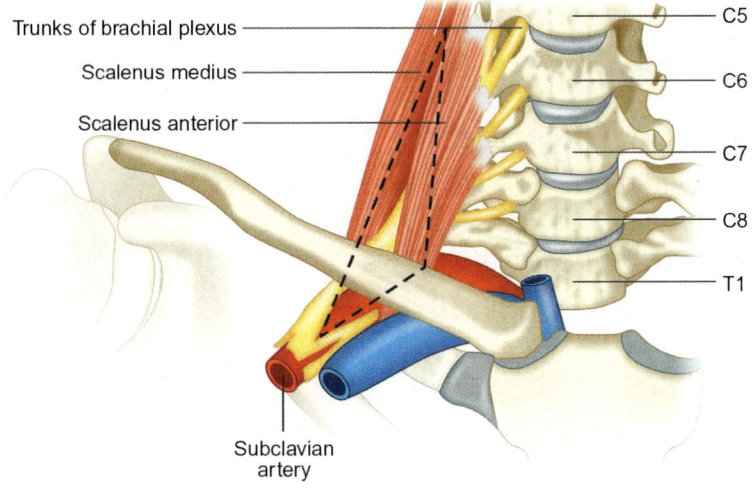

## Q. What are the boundaries of Joll's triangle?

**Ans.** Following are the boundaries of Joll's triangle:
- *Laterally:* Upper pole of thyroid with superior thyroid vessels
- *Superiorly:* Attachment of strap muscles
- *Medially:* Midline.

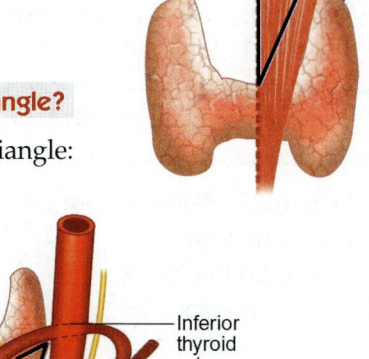

Attachment of strap muscle

Superior thyroid vessels

Midline

## Q. What are the boundaries of Beahrs' triangle?

**Ans.** Following are the boundaries of Beahrs' triangle:
- *Superiorly:* Inferior thyroid artery

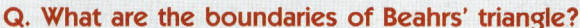

Recurrent laryngeal nerve

Inferior thyroid artery

Common carotid artery

- *Medially:* Recurrent laryngeal nerve
- *Laterally*: Common carotid artery.

**Note:** Surgeon should be vigilant about this triangle, while operating on thyroid gland to avoid inadvertent injury to recurrent laryngeal nerve.

## Q. What are the parts of sphenoid bone?

**Ans.** Following are the parts of sphenoid bone:
- Body
- Greater wing
- Lesser wing
- Medial pterygoid process
- Lateral pterygoid process.

## Q. What is the meaning of 'sphenoid'?

**Ans.** Literal meaning of sphenoid is 'wing like'.

## Q. What are the parts of palatine bone?

**Ans.** Following are the parts of palatine bone:
- Horizontal plate
- Perpendicular plate
- Pyramidal process
- Orbital process
- Sphenoidal process.

### Q. What are the parts of lacrimal bone?

**Ans.** Following are the part of lacrimal bone:
- Lateral orbital surface
- Lacrimal crest
- Lacrimal hamulus
- Lacrimal fossa.

### Q. Sphenopalatine notch is present on which bone?

**Ans.** Sphenopalatine notch is present on palatine bone between orbital and sphenoidal process.

### Q. Which is the artery of epistaxis?

**Ans.** Sphenopalatine artery is the artery of epistaxis.

### Q. What is Inca or Goethe's ossicle?

**Ans.** Goethe's ossicle is a sutural bone in lambda.

### Q. Important foramina and its corresponding structures.

**Ans.**

| Foramina | Structures |
|---|---|
| Anterior canal | Anterior ethmoidal artery, vein and nerve |
| Canaliculus innominatus | Lesser petrosal nerve |
| Carotid canal | Internal carotid artery with its venous and sympathetic plexus |
| Condylar canal | Emissary vein connecting sigmoid sinus to suboccipital venous plexus |
| Cochlear canaliculus | Aqueduct of cochlea |
| Foramen ovale (mnemonic: **MALE**) | **M:** Mandibular nerve<br>**A:** Accessory meningeal artery<br>**L:** Lesser petrosal nerve<br>**E:** Emissary vein (connecting cavernous sinus to pterygoid plexus of veins) anterior trunk of middle meningeal vein |
| Foramen spinosum | Middle meningeal artery meningeal branch of mandibular nerve (nervous spinosus) |
| Foramen rotundum | Maxillary nerve |
| Foramen lacerum | Meningeal branch of ascending pharyngeal artery emissary vein from cavernous sinus (in fetal life only cartilage is present) |
| Foramen magnum | Lower part of medulla, tonsils of cerebellum, meninges, spinal accessory nerve, vertebral arteries with its sympathetic plexus, anterior and posterior spinal arteries, apical ligament of dens, membrana tectoria |
| Foramen of Vesalius | Emissary vein (connecting cavernous sinus to pterygoid plexus of veins) |
| Foramen cecum | A vein from the nose to the superior sagittal sinus |
| Foramina in cribriform plate | Olfactory nerves |

*Contd...*

*Contd...*

| Foramina | Structures |
|---|---|
| Greater palatine foramen | Greater palatine artery and vein anterior palatine nerve |
| Hypoglossal canal | Hypoglossal nerve, ascending pharyngeal artery (meningeal branch), emissary vein connecting sigmoid sinus with internal jugular vein (IJV) |
| Internal acoustic meatus | Facial nerve, vestibulocochlear nerve, labyrinthine vessels |
| Inferior orbital fissure | Maxillary nerve |
| Jugular foramen | IX, X, XI cranial nerves; ascending pharyngeal and occipital arteries, (meningeal branch), internal jugular vein, inferior petrosal nerve |
| Lesser palatine foramen | Middle and posterior palatine nerves |
| Mastoid foramen | Meningeal branch of occipital artery, emissary vein (connecting sigmoid sinus with posterior auricular vein) |
| Mastoid canaliculus | Auricular branch of vagus nerve (Arnold's or Alderman's nerve) |
| Mental foramen | Mental artery, vein and nerve |
| Mandibular foramen | Inferior alveolar artery, vein and nerve |
| Optic canal | Optic nerve with its meningeal sheath, ophthalmic artery |
| Parietal foramen | Emissary vein from superior sagittal sinus |
| Palatovaginal canal | Pharyngeal branch of maxillary artery, pharyngeal branch from pterygo-palatine ganglion |
| Petrotympanic fissure | Chorda tympanic nerve, anterior tympanic artery |
| Posterior ethmoidal canal | Posterior ethmoidal artery and vein |
| Stylomastoid foramen | Facial nerve, stylomastoid branch of posterior auricular artery |
| Superior orbital fissure | Lacrimal nerve, frontal nerve, trochlear nerve, superior ophthalmic vein, meningeal branch of lacrimal artery, oculomotor nerve (upper and lower division), nasociliary nerve, abducens nerve, inferior ophthalmic vein |
| Supraorbital foramen | Supraorbital artery, vein and nerve |
| Tympanic canaliculus | Glossopharyngeal nerve (tympanic branch) |
| Vomerovaginal canal | Pharyngeal artery, vein and nerve |

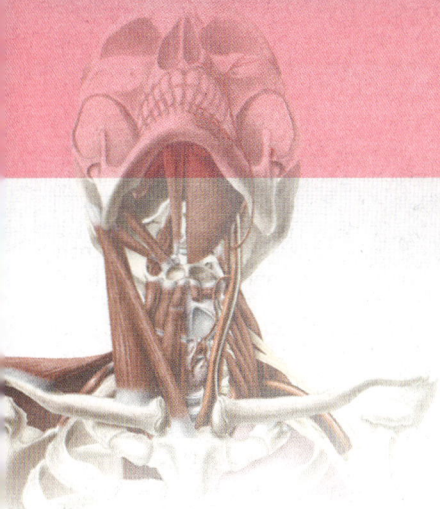

# Key Short Notes

## 34

## MUSCLE

### Q. Facial muscles

**Ans.** Facial muscles differ from other skeletal muscles in following ways:

- Subcutaneous muscles
- Control the orifices on face (like sphincters)
- Have fine control on movement
- Exhibit facial expression
- Develop from second branchial arch.

### Classification

*Muscles around the eye:*
- Orbicularis oculis
- Corrugator supercilii
- Levator palpebrae superioris.

*Muscles around the mouth:*
- Orbicularis oris
- Levator labii superioris alaeque nasi
- Levator labii superioris
- Levator anguli oris
- Zygomaticus major and minor
- Depressor anguli oris and labii inferioris
- Mentalis
- Risorius
- Buccinator.

*Muscles around the nostril:*
- Procerus
- Compressor naris
- Dilator naris
- Depressor septi
- Occipitofrontalis
- Platysma.

## Nerve Supply

Facial nerve.

## Function

- Primarily regulates the facial openings
- Frontalis causes wrinkling of forehead
- Orbicularis oris—whistling
- Orbicularis oculis—helps in tight closure of eyes
- Platysma—draws the angle of mouth downwards.

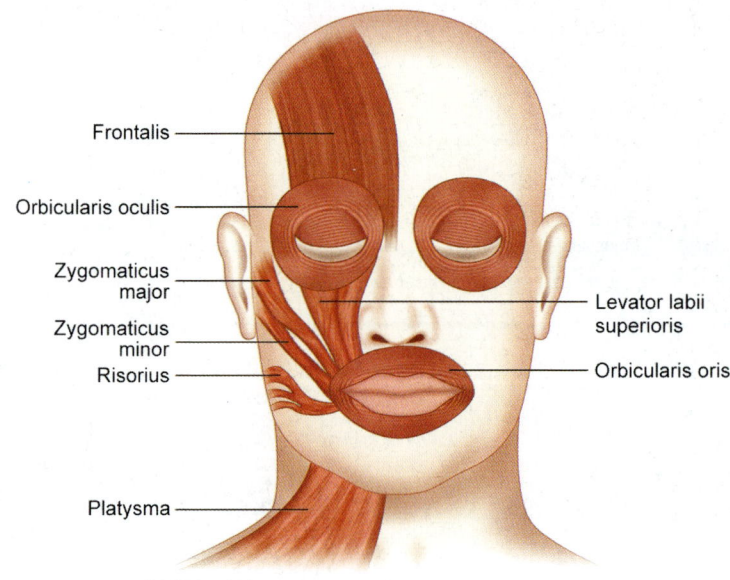

Facial muscles

## Common Facial Expressions

- Smiling and laughing—zygomaticus major
- Sadness—levator labii superioris, levator anguli oris
- Grief—depressor anguli oris
- Frowning—corrugator supercilii and procerus.

## Applied Anatomy

Facial nerve injury will affect facial muscles and lead to facial asymmetry.

### Q. Sternocleidomastoid muscle

**Ans.** Sternocleidomastoid muscle is considered as a key muscle of the neck, surgically dividing the region into anterior triangle and posterior triangle.

## Attachments

Superior attachment is to the mastoid process, while inferiorly it has two heads—clavicular and sternal by virtue of which it gets attached to clavicle and sternum respectively. Both attachments are tendinous.

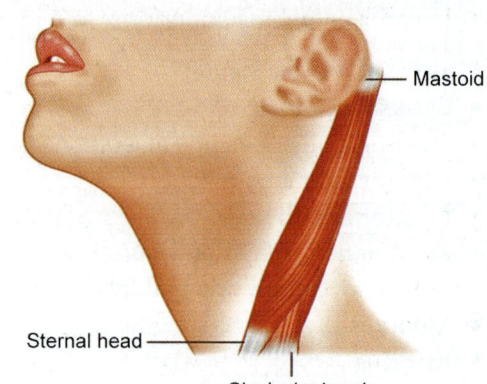

## Relations

### Superficial

- Skin, platysma
- External jugular vein, great auricular nerve and transverse cervical nerve
- Superficial lamina of deep cervical fascia
- In upper part, it is overlapped by parotid gland.

### Deep

Great vessels of the neck (carotid sheath).

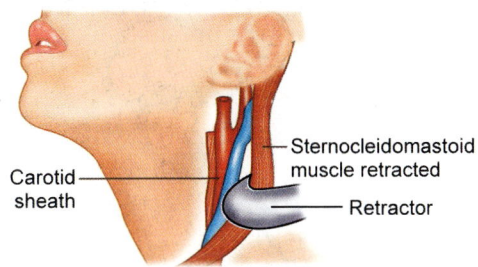

Sternocleidomastoid muscle

## Nerve Supply

Accessory nerve and ventral rami of C2, C3, C4, spinal nerves.

## Action

Acting alone, the muscle tilts the head toward the ipsilateral shoulder turning the face to opposite side.

## Applied Anatomy

Torticollis is due to permanent contraction of sternocleidomastoid.

### Q. Extraocular muscles

**Ans.** There are seven voluntary and three involuntary extraocular muscles.

*Voluntary muscles are:*
- Four recti—superior, inferior, medial, lateral
- Two obliques—superior, inferior
- One—levator palpebrae superioris.
  All have short tendons of origin and long tendons of insertion.

*Involuntary muscles are:*
- Superior tarsal (i.e. deeper portion of levator palpebrae superioris)
- Inferior tarsal
- Orbitalis.

## Origin

1. All the four recti originate from common tendinous ring of Zinn. Lateral rectus has additional tendinous head, which arises from orbital surface of greater wing of sphenoid.

2. Superior oblique arises from body of sphenoid.
3. Inferior oblique arises from orbital surface of maxilla.

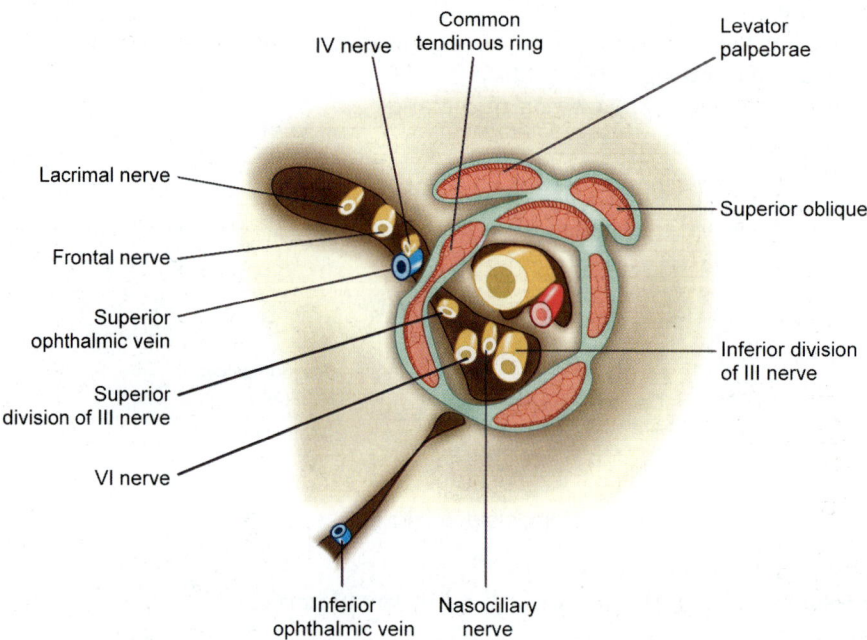

## Insertion

- The recti are inserted into the sclera, a little posterior to the limbus on an average 6–7 mm
- The obliques are inserted on the sclera behind the equator of eyeball
- Superior lamella of levator muscle is inserted into anterior surface of tarsus and skin of upper lid
- Inferior lamella of levator muscle is attached onto the upper margin of superior tarsus.

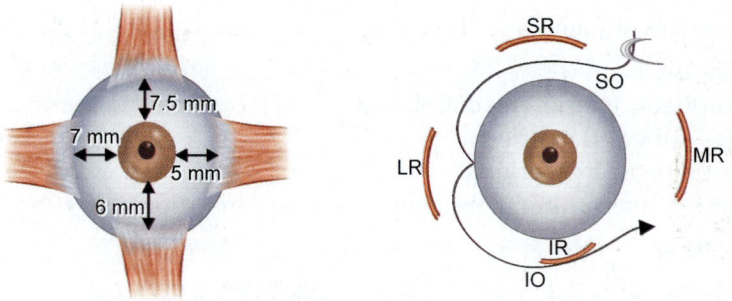

Extraocular muscles

## Nerve Supply

- Superior oblique—trochlear nerve ($SO_4$)
- Lateral rectus—abducens nerve (LR6).
  Rest all the extraocular muscles are supplied by oculomotor nerve.

## Action

*Movements occur around:*

- Transverse axis—elevation and depression
- Vertical axis—medial and lateral rotation
- Anteroposterior axis—intorsion and extortion.

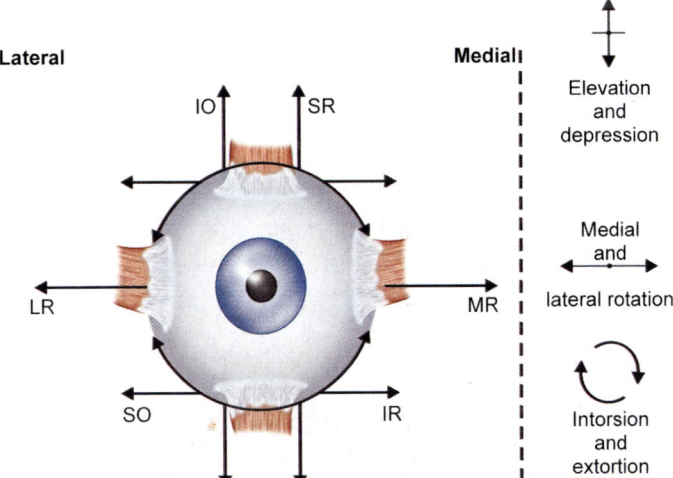

*Movements can be best demonstrated on ball:*

- Superior rectus—upward rotation, medial rotation, intorsion
- Medial rectus—medial rotation
- Inferior rectus—downward rotation, medial rotation, extortion
- Lateral rectus—lateral rotation
- Superior oblique—downward rotation, lateral rotation, intorsion
- Inferior oblique—upward rotation, lateral rotation, extortion.

### Applied Anatomy

- Paralysis of extraocular muscles causes squint
- Nystagmus is characterised by involuntary, rhythmic, oscillatory movements.

### Q. Lateral pterygoid muscle

**Ans.** Lateral pterygoid muscle is a muscle of mastication, which divides the maxillary artery into three parts.

### Attachments

*From*

- Upper head—infratemporal surface and greater wing of sphenoid
- Lower head—lateral surface of lateral pterygoid plate.

*To*

- Pterygoid fovea
- Articular disk and capsule of temporomandibular joint.

## Relations

- It is closely related to maxillary artery and branches of mandibular nerve
- Buccal nerve lies between the upper and lower head
- Lingual nerve and inferior alveolar nerve are along the lower border of the muscle
- Pterygoid plexus of veins lies around it.

## Nerve Supply

Mandibular nerve (anterior division).

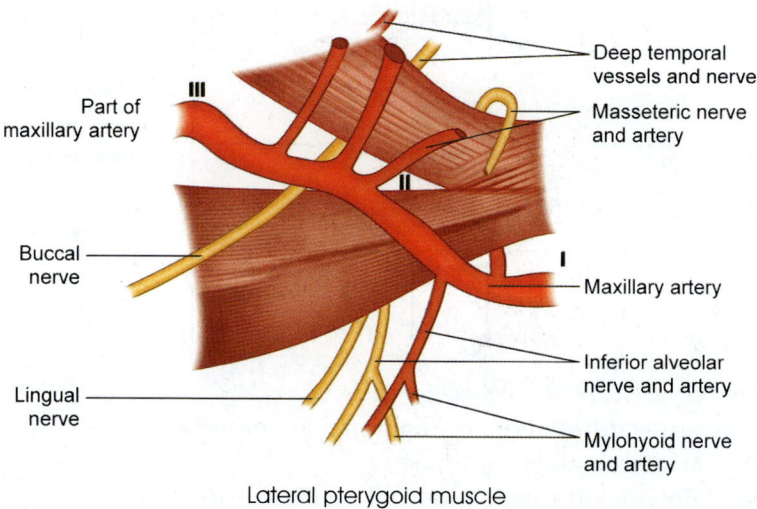

Part of maxillary artery

Buccal nerve

Lingual nerve

Deep temporal vessels and nerve

Masseteric nerve and artery

Maxillary artery

Inferior alveolar nerve and artery

Mylohyoid nerve and artery

Lateral pterygoid muscle

## Action

- Opens the mouth
- Along with medial pterygoid muscles protrudes the mandible and brings about grinding movements.

### Q. Soft palate

**Ans.** Soft palate is movable, muscular fold separating the nasopharynx from oropharynx. It is made up of:

- Tensor palati
- Levator palati
- Musculus uvulae
- Palatopharyngeus
- Palatoglossus.

## Tensor Palati

*Attachments*

*From*

- Auditory tube (lateral side) sphenoid (scaphoid fossa, spine and greater wing)

- The muscle forms a tendon, which winds around pterygoid hamulus. (= hook like projection at the lower extremity of medial pterygoid plate).

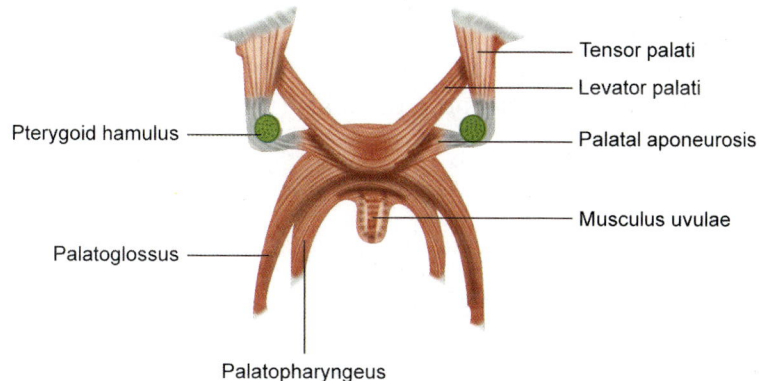

*To:* Hard palate (posterior border and inferior surface).

### Action

- Tightens soft palate
- Opens auditory tube.

## Levator Palati

### Attachments

*From*

- Inferior surface of petrous temporal and auditory tube
- Upper part of carotid sheath.
  Muscle enters pharynx by passing over the upper border of superior constrictor.

*To:* Upper surface of palatine aponeurosis.

### Action

- Elevates soft palate
- Opens auditory tube.

## Musculus Uvulae

### Attachments

*From*

- Posterior nasal spine
- Palatine aponeurosis.
  Palatine aponeurosis splits to enclose the muscle.

*To:* Mucous membrane of uvula.

### Action

Pulls up the uvula.

## Palatopharyngeus

*Attachments*

*From*
- Hard palate (posterior border)
- Palatine aponeurosis.
  Muscle has two fasciculi—anterior and posterior.

*To*
- Lamina of thyroid cartilage
- Median raphe of pharynx.

### Action

Pulls up and shortens pharynx during swallowing.

## Palatoglossus

*Attachments*

*From:* Palatine aponeurosis (oral surface). Descends in palatoglossus arch.

*To:* Side of tongue.

### Action

Pulls up root of the tongue and closes the oropharyngeal isthmus.

### Nerve Supply

All the muscles of soft palate are supplied by pharyngeal plexus except tensor palati muscle, which is supplied by mandibular nerve.

### Applied Anatomy

- Diphtheria may produce paralysis of soft palate resulting in regurgitation of fluids, nasal intonation and flattening of palatal arch
- Oral cavity in a newborn should be carefully examined otherwise a soft palate cleft may be missed easily.

### Q. Constrictors of pharynx

**Ans.** Pharynx is a muscular tube made-up of three muscles; (arranged like glass in one another) They are:
- Superior constrictor
- Middle constrictor
- Inferior constrictor.

### Superior Constrictor

*Attachments*

*From*
- Pterygoid hamulus, medial pterygoid plate
- Pterygomandibular raphe

- Mylohyoid line
- Side of tongue.

*To:* Pharyngeal tubercle and raphe.

## Middle Constrictor

*Attachments*

*From*
- Stylohyoid ligament
- Lesser and greater horn of hyoid bone.

*To:* Pharyngeal raphe.

## Inferior Constrictor

*Attachments*

*From*
- Oblique line of thyroid cartilage (thyropharyngeus)
- Side of cricoid (cricopharyngeus).
  (Inferior constrictor has two parts thyropharyngeus and cricopharyngeus).

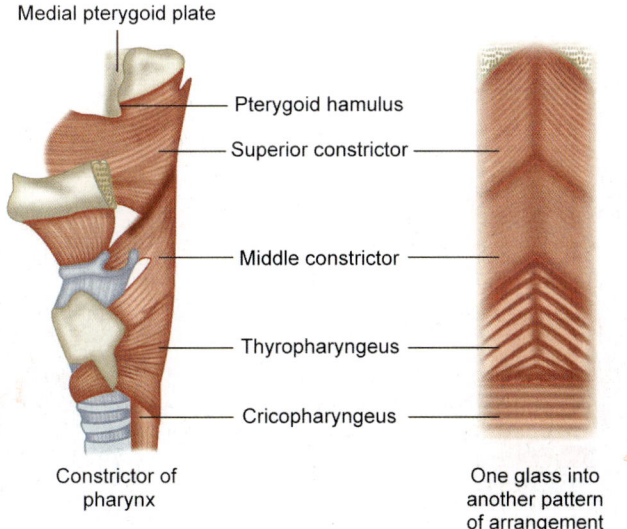

Medial pterygoid plate

Pterygoid hamulus

Superior constrictor

Middle constrictor

Thyropharyngeus

Cricopharyngeus

Constrictor of pharynx

One glass into another pattern of arrangement

*To:* Pharyngeal raphe.

## Action

All the constrictors help in deglutition.

## Nerve Supply

All the constrictors are supplied by pharyngeal plexus.

## Applied Anatomy

1. The lower part of thyropharyngeus is a single sheet of muscle, not overlapped internally by middle constrictor. This part is limited below by cricopharyngeal sphincter. This weak area is known as Killian's dehiscence. Pharyngeal diverticulum is an outpouching of this dehiscence.

2. Paralyses of constrictors lead to dysphagia.

### Q. Scalenus anterior muscle

**Ans.** Scalenus anterior muscle is a key muscle of the lower part of posterior triangle of the neck.

## Attachments

*From:* Anterior tubercles of transverse processes of 3, 4, 5, 6 cervical vertebra

*To:* Scalene tubercle of first rib.

## Relations

*Anteriorly:*

- Phrenic nerve
- Prevertebral fascia.

## Nerve Supply

Ventral rami of C4, C5, C6 nerves.

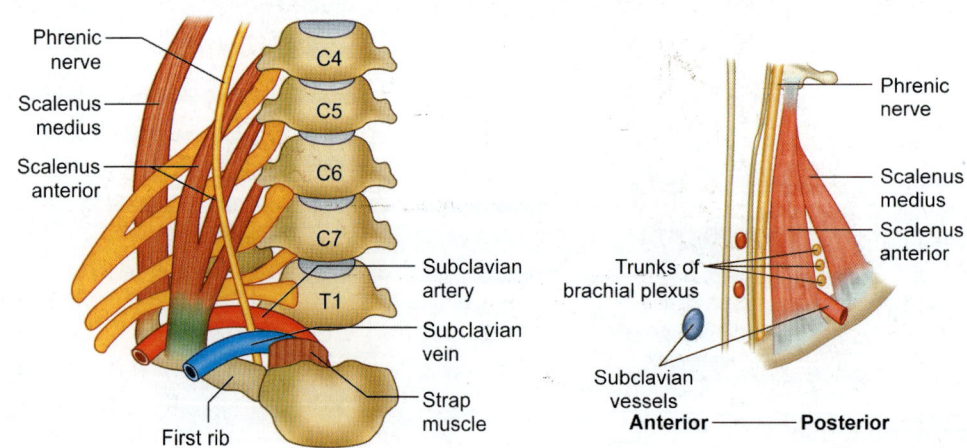

Scalenus anterior (muscle relations)

## Action

- Flexion and rotation of cervical spine
- Elevates first rib during inspiration.

## Q. Intrinsic muscles of larynx

**Ans.** These are the muscles whose attachments are within the cartilages of larynx. Following are the intrinsic muscles of larynx:

- Cricothyroid
- Posterior cricoarytenoid
- Lateral cricoarytenoid
- Transverse arytenoid
- Oblique arytenoid and aryepiglottic
- Thyroarytenoid, vocalis and thyroepiglottic.

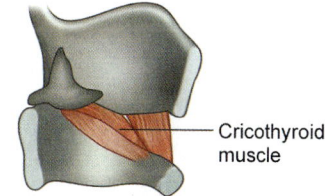
Cricothyroid muscle

### Attachments

Name of the muscles itself denotes its attachments.

Arytenoid is the key cartilage to receive muscular attachments. It has a vocal process and a muscular process.

### Nerve Supply

All intrinsic muscles of larynx are supplied by recurrent laryngeal nerve except cricothyroid, which supplied by external laryngeal nerve.

### Action

1. Cricothyroid is tensor of vocal cord.
2. Posterior cricoarytenoid—opens the glottis; it is known as the 'safety muscle of larynx' because it maintains the patency of airway:

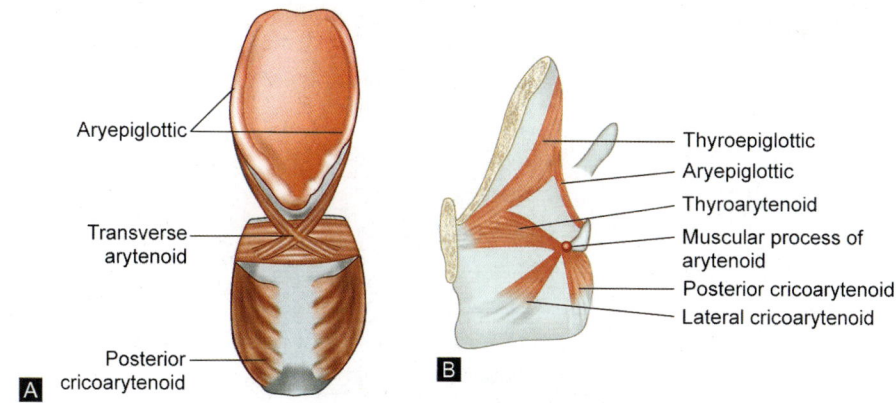

Intrinsic muscles of larynx

- Lateral cricoarytenoid—close the glottis
- Transverse arytenoid—close the glottis
- Oblique arytenoid and aryepiglottic—close the inlet of larynx
- Thyroarytenoid, vocalis—relax the vocal cord.

## Applied Anatomy

- External laryngeal nerve injury will result in loss of tension of vocal cord giving rise to weak voice
- Laryngeal nerve injuries could be due to different causes like infection (diphtheria), cancer, diabetes.

<u>NERVE</u>

### Q. Secretomotor pathway to parotid gland.

**Ans.** Following is the secretomotor pathway to parotid gland:

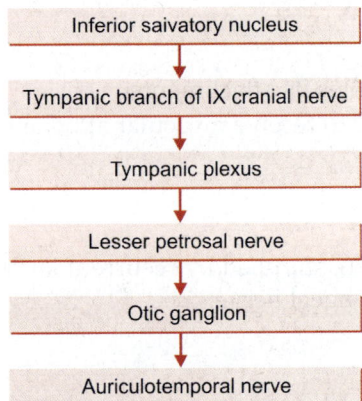

### Q. Secretomotor pathway to submandibular gland.

**Ans.** Following is the secretomotor pathway to submandibular gland:

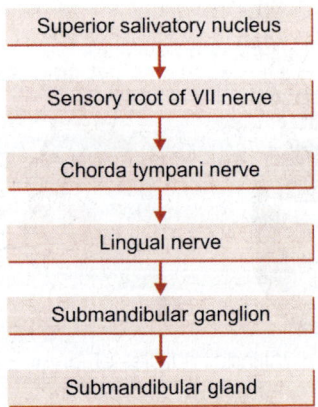

## Q. Secretomotor pathway to lacrimal gland.

**Ans.** Following is the secretomotor pathway to lacrimal gland:

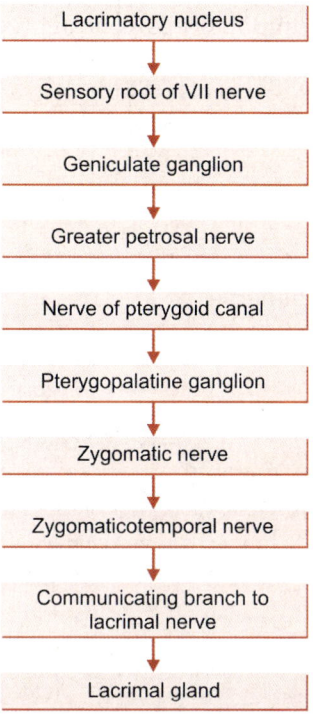

Lacrimatory nucleus

↓

Sensory root of VII nerve

↓

Geniculate ganglion

↓

Greater petrosal nerve

↓

Nerve of pterygoid canal

↓

Pterygopalatine ganglion

↓

Zygomatic nerve

↓

Zygomaticotemporal nerve

↓

Communicating branch to
lacrimal nerve

↓

Lacrimal gland

## Q. Trigeminal ganglion

**Ans.** Trigeminal ganglion is also known as semilunar or Gasserian ganglion. This is the sensory ganglion of V cranial nerve, which is homologous with the dorsal root ganglion.

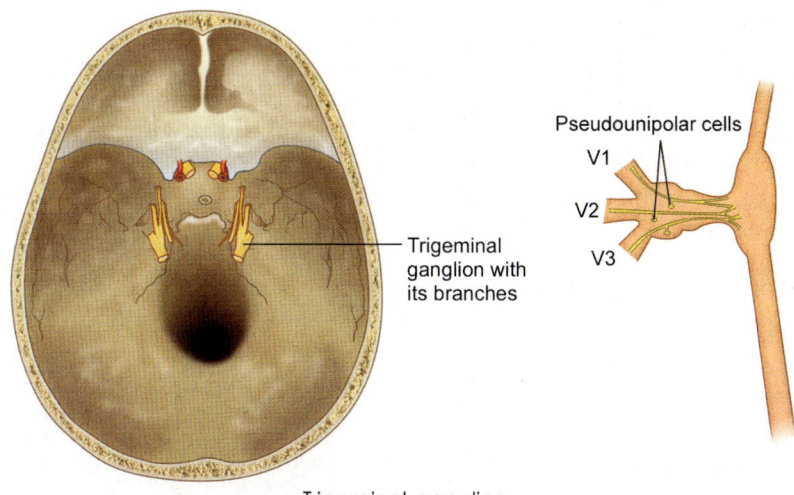

Trigeminal ganglion with its branches

Pseudounipolar cells

V1

V2

V3

Trigeminal ganglion

## Location

The ganglion lies on trigeminal impression, which is on the anterior surface of the apex of petrous temporal bone. It is enclosed in a dural pocket known as Meckel's cave.

Ganglion comprises of pseudo-unipolar cells, central processes of which form sensory root, which is attached to pons and peripheral processes form the three principal divisions of the trigeminal nerve (ophthalmic, maxillary, mandibular).

## Relations

- *Medially:* Internal carotid artery
- *Laterally:* Middle meningeal artery
- *Superiorly:* Parahippocampal gyrus
- *Inferiorly:* Motor root of V cranial nerve.

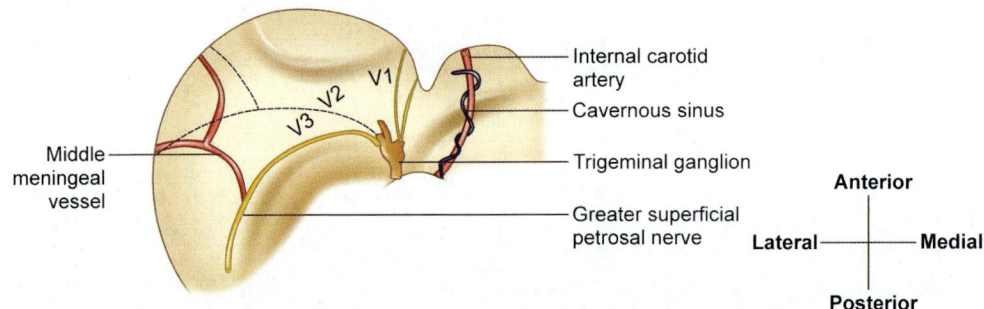

## Arterial Supply

Ganglion is supplied by adjacent arteries, i.e. internal carotid artery and middle meningeal artery.

## Applied Anatomy

Ganglion lies at a depth of 5 cm from preauricular point, which needs to be approached in cases of intractable trigeminal neuralgia for injecting alcohol.

### Q. Otic ganglion

**Ans.** Otic ganglion is peripheral parasympathetic ganglion, which serves to relay the secretomotor fibres to parotid gland.

Located close to mandibular nerve, but functionally connected to IX cranial nerve.

## Size and Location

Otic ganglion is 2–3 mm in size and is located in infratemporal fossa, just below foramen ovale.

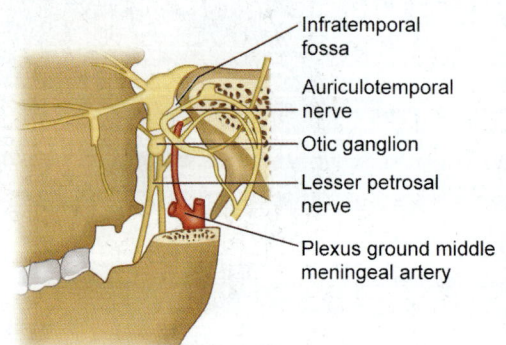

## Connections

- Motor root of the ganglion is lesser petrosal nerve

- Sympathetic root is derived from the plexus on the middle meningeal artery
- Sensory root comes from auriculotemporal nerve.

## Branches

- Mainly supplies the parotid gland the auriculotemporal nerve
- Some fibres only traverse the ganglion without relaying; these are motor nerves to medial pterygoid, tensor palati and tensor tympani
- One branch connects to chorda tympani nerve and another to the nerve of pterygoid canal.

## Relations

- *Laterally:* Mandibular nerve
- *Medially:* Tensor palati muscle
- *Posteriorly:* Middle meningeal artery
- *Anteriorly:* Medial pterygoid muscle.

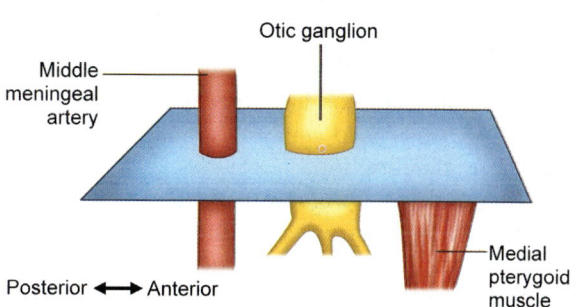

## Q. Pterygopalatine ganglion

**Ans.** Pterygopalatine ganglion is also known as Meckel's ganglion. This ganglion is connected with maxillary division of V cranial nerve and is the parasympathetic relay station between superior salivatory nucleus in pons and lacrimal gland and mucous glands of the palate, nose and paranasal sinuses.

## Location

Pterygopalatine ganglion is located in the upper part of pterygopalatine fossa.

## Roots

1. *Motor roots:* The fibres leave the brainstem in nervus intermedius join the VII nerve and deviate from the geniculate ganglion as greater superficial petrosal nerve.
2. *Sympathetic roots:* The cell bodies are in superior cervical ganglion from which nerve fibres pass to the internal carotid plexus. It leaves the plexus as deep petrosal nerve and joins the greater superficial petrosal nerve to form nerve of pterygoid canal (Vidian nerve).
3. *Sensory root:* Comes from maxillary nerve.

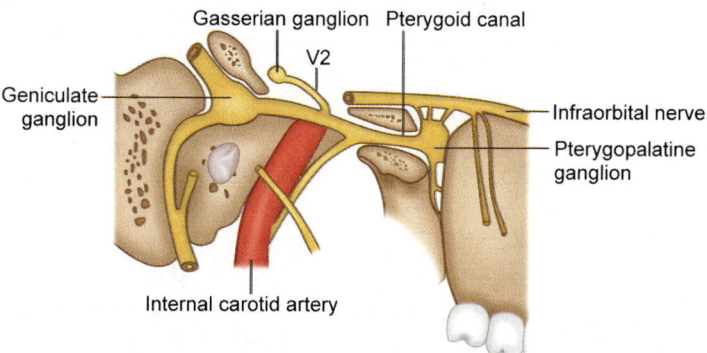

Connections of pterygopalatine ganglion

## Branches

Branches to lacrimal gland through zygomaticotemporal branch of maxillary nerve and lacrimal branch of ophthalmic nerve:
• Orbital branches to periosteum of orbit
• Palatine nerves to the roof of mouth, soft palate, tonsil and nasal mucosa
• Nasal branches to anterior part of hard palate
• Pharyngeal branch to nasopharynx.

### Q. Stellate ganglion

**Ans.** Stellate ganglion is a large ganglion formed by the fusion of lower two cervical segmental ganglion with first thoracic ganglion.

When not receiving contribution from thoracic mass it is known as inferior cervical ganglion.

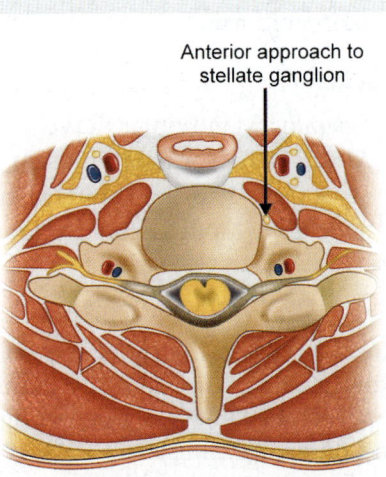

Anterior approach to stellate ganglion

### Relations

• Stellate ganglion lies behind vertebral artery between first rib and transverse process of C7
• It is separated from cervical pleura by suprapleural membrane.

### Branches

• It gives rise to gray rami communicantes to C7, C8, T1
• Contributes to the plexus around the subclavian artery and sympathetic supply to head and neck.

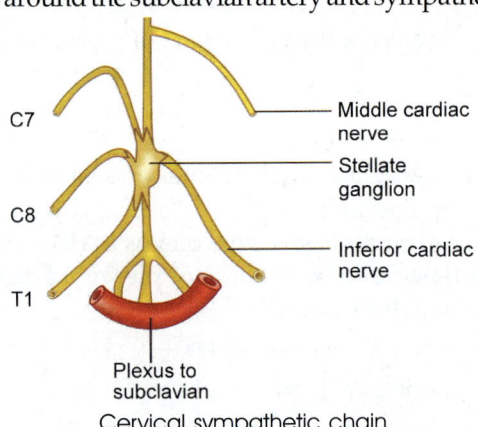

Cervical sympathetic chain

### Applied Anatomy

Stellate ganglion block can be given by anterior approach. Stellate ganglion block will produce temporary Horner's syndrome.

### Horner's Syndrome

It is characterised by dramatic appearance of the face-ptosis (drooping of eyelids), miosis (constriction of pupils), anhydrosis (lack of sweating) enophthalmos (retracted eyeball) and absent ciliospinal reflex.

## Q. Submandibular ganglion

**Ans.** Submandibular ganglion is size of pinhead. It is situated on outer surface of hyoglossus muscle; suspended from lingual nerve.

### Relations

- *Lateral:* Submandibular gland
- *Medial:* Hyoglossus muscle
- *Above:* Lingual nerve
- *Below:* Submandibular duct.

### Roots

- Motor from chorda tympani
- Sensory from lingual
- Sympathetic from plexus around facial artery.

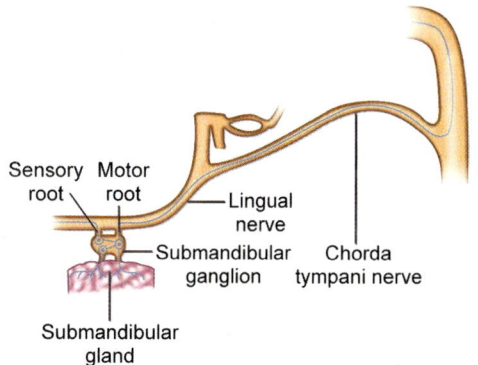

### Branches

Submandibular ganglion hangs from the lingual nerve by two filaments and distributes fibers to submandibular gland and duct, to the sublingual gland, to the mucous membrane of mouth and tongue.

## Q. Acoustic pathway

**Ans.** Acoustic pathway is as follows:

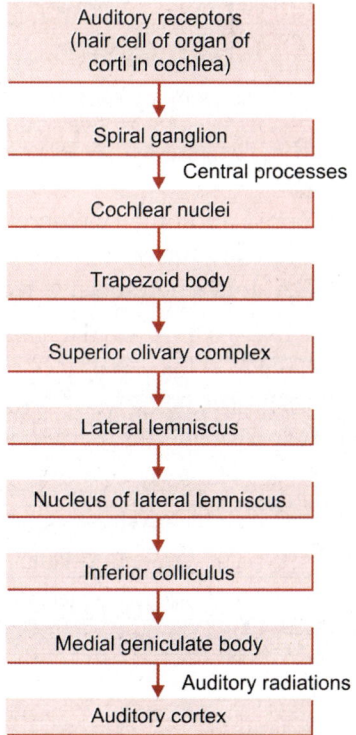

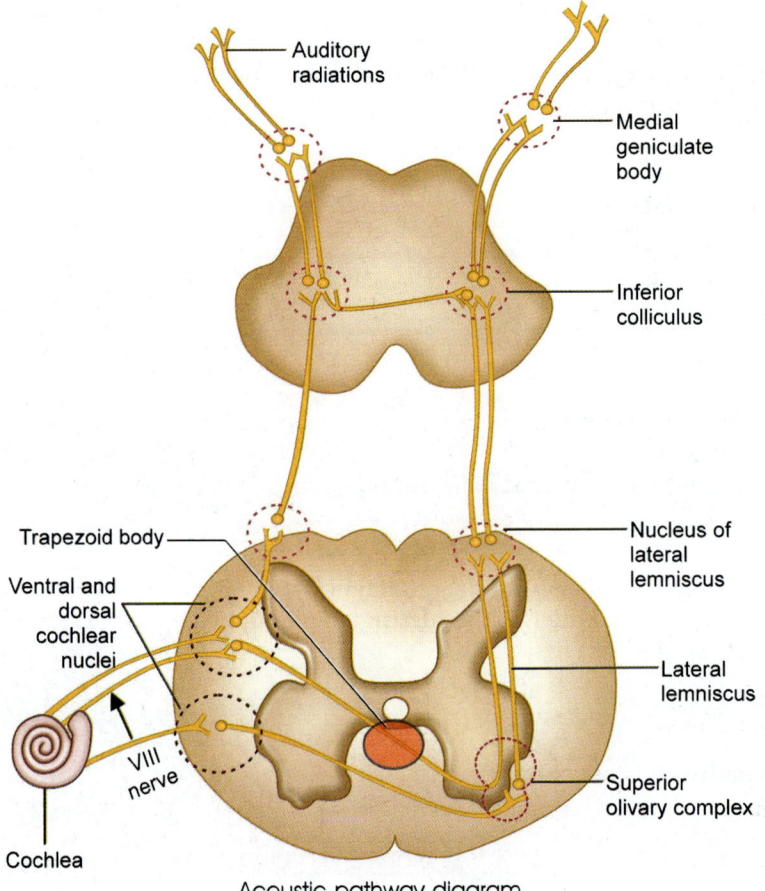

Acoustic pathway diagram

## Applied Anatomy

BERA means brainstem evoked response audiometry wherein electrical responses in cochlear nuclei and central connections are recorded for early detection of deafness.

Seven waves are recorded in BERA. It is a noninvasive technique to detect the integrity of auditory pathway.

| Waves | Site |
|-------|------|
| I | Vestibulocochlear nerve |
| II | Cochlear nuclei |
| III | Superior olivary complex |
| IV | Lateral lemniscus |
| V | Inferior colliculus |
| VI | Medial geniculate body |
| VII | Auditory radiations |

## Q. Galen's anastomosis

**Ans.** The internal branch of superior laryngeal nerve ends by anastomosing with an ascending branch of recurrent laryngeal nerve. This loop is Galen's anastomosis and is purely sensory.

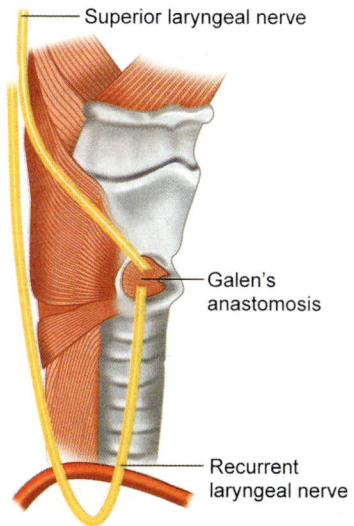

## Q. Frey syndrome

**Ans.** Frey syndrome is also known as auriculotemporal nerve syndrome. In this condition, there is redness and sweating of the skin over the parotid region, while having food.

It follows parotid surgeries or temporomandibular joint surgeries or direct injury.

### Anatomical Basis of Frey Syndrome

After injury, during regeneration auriculotemporal nerve gets aberrantly connected to branches from superior cervical ganglion, i.e. a parasympathetic nerve gets connected to sympathetic nerve.

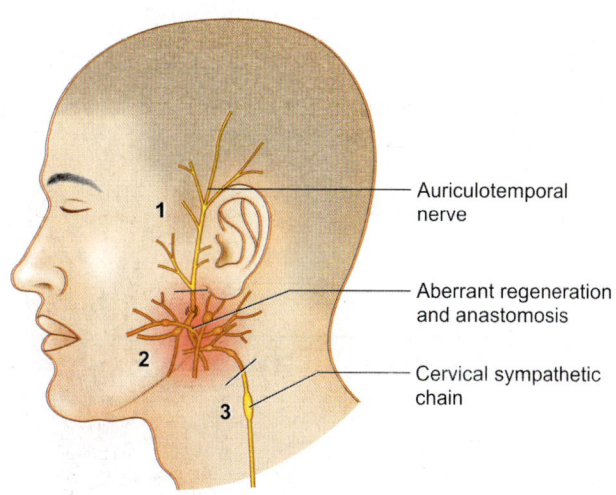

Thus, whenever parasympathetic component, i.e. secretomotor pathway gets stimulated during mastication sympathetic fibres also gets stimulated. Hence, the patient complains of sweating and redness on face, while chewing.

## Q. Ansa cervicalis

**Ans.** It is a loop (handle of neck) of nerves connected to cervical plexus; (ventral rami of C1, C2, C3) lying in front of carotid sheath, and supplying infrahyoid muscles.

## Parts
- Superior root
- Inferior root
- Loop.

## Formation
- Superior root
  - C1 spinal nerve, as it leaves XII nerve
  - It crosses occipital artery
- Inferior root: C2, C3 spinal nerve
- Loop: Formed by the combination of above nerves.

## Branches
- Superior root supplies superior belly of omohyoid.
- Loop and inferior root supplies sternohyoid. Sternothyroid and inferior belly of omohyoid muscles.

## ARTERY

### Q. Facial artery

**Ans.** Facial artery is one of the tortuous artery, of the body others being uterine artery, lingual artery and splenic artery. It is tortuous to adapt to the movements of pharynx during swallowing and on the face to adapt to the movements of mandible, lips and cheeks.

### Origin
Facial artery is a branch of external carotid artery given off above the tip of greater horn of hyoid bone in the carotid triangle.

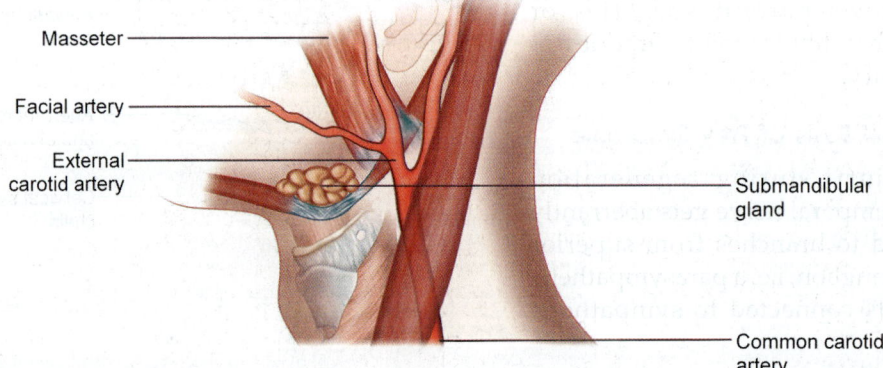

### Course and Termination
- From its origin it arches upwards and forms a loop around the submandibular gland posteriorly, lying midway between mastoid tip and angle of mandible
- It winds the inferior margin of mandible after crossing the submandibular region to lie, at anteroinferior angle of masseter
- It runs upwards ½ inch lateral to angle of mouth, by the side of the nose to terminate at the medial angle of eye.

## Relations

1. In the neck, the artery is quite in a superficial plane covered only by skin, platysma and crossed by hypoglossal nerve.
2. As it ascends upwards it gets related to submandibular gland posteriorly, lies deep to digastric and stylohyoid muscle.
3. It lies very superficial along the inferior border of mandible, where it can be easily palpated.
4. On the face it is covered by skin, fat of the cheek and facial muscles. Buccinator and levator anguli oris lie deep to it.
5. At its termination, it lies embedded in levator labii superioris alaeque nasi.
6. The facial vein lies posterior to the artery and has a straight course, while the branches of the facial nerve crossover the artery.

## Branches

The branches of facial artery can be broadly divided into cervical and facial.

| Cervical | Facial |
|---|---|
| Ascending palatine | Inferior labial |
| Tonsillar | Superior labial |
| Glandular | Lateral nasal |
| Submental | |

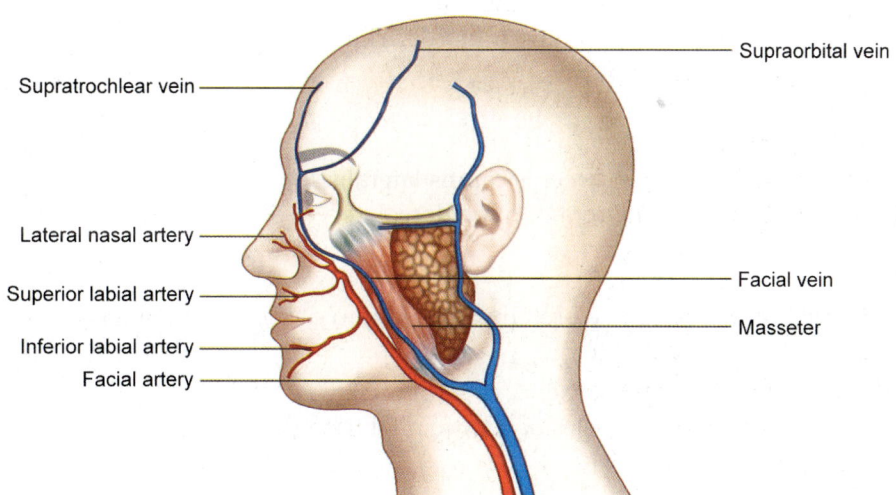

## Applied Anatomy

- Rich vascularity of face causes blushing
- Wounds of the face bleed profusely, but also heal rapidly due to rich blood supply of the face.

## Q. Vertebral artery

**Ans.** Vertebral artery is one of the principal arteries supplying the brain.

## Origin

Vertebral artery is a branch of first part of subclavian artery.

## Course

Vertebral artery is divided into following four parts:
Part I—from its origin to C6
Part II—from C6 to C1, in foramen of transverse process
Part III—it lies on the posterior arch of atlas in suboccipital triangle
Part IV—it extends from suboccipital triangle to lower border of pons.

## Relations

*Part I:*
- Anteriorly related to carotid sheath, vertebral vein, inferior thyroid artery, thoracic duct on the left side
- Posteriorly transverse process of C7, stellate ganglion, ventral rami of C7, C8.

*Part II:*
- Ventral rami of C2-C6 lie posterior to the artery
- II part traverses through the foramina transversarium
- It is accompanied by venous plexus.

*Part III:*
- Anteriorly lateral mass of atlas
- Posteriorly semispinalis capitis, rectus capitis lateralis.

*Part IV:* It ascends in front of the root of hypoglossal nerve.

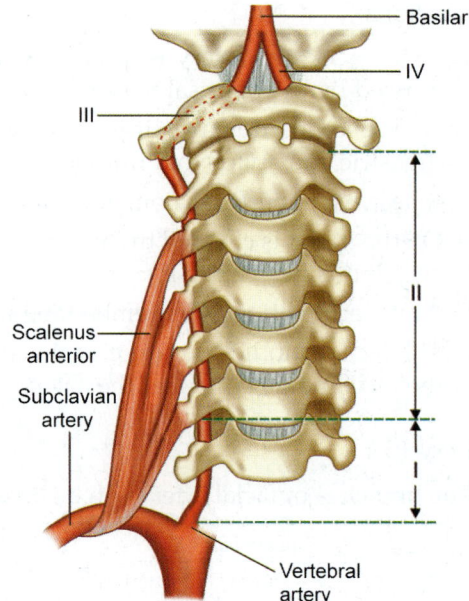

## Branches

Branches of vertebral artery can be broadly divided into cervical and cranial branches:
1. Cervical branches are divided into:
    - Spinal supplying the spinal cord
    - Muscular supplying the muscles of suboccipital triangle.
2. Cranial branches include:
    - Meningeal
    - Anterior and posterior spinal
    - Posteroinferior cerebellar
    - Medullary.

## Applied Anatomy

Thrombosis of vertebral artery causes medial medullary syndrome characterised by contralateral hemiplegia (sparing face), contralateral loss of deep sensation and ipsilateral hypoglossal paralysis.

## Q. External carotid artery

**Ans.** External carotid artery (ECA) is one of the terminal branches of common carotid artery and supplies the structures in front of the neck and face.

### Origin

Common carotid artery gives rise to external carotid artery at the level of upper border of thyroid cartilage in carotid triangle.

### Course and Relations

- From its origin it runs upwards under the cover of sternocleidomastoid and crossed superficially by VII and XII cranial nerves
- Above it lies within the parotid gland sandwiched between retromandibular vein and facial nerve
- It terminates behind the neck of the mandible into superficial temporal and maxillary arteries.

| Anterior | Posterior | Terminal |
|---|---|---|
| • Superior thyroid | • Occipital | • Maxillary |
| • Lingual | • Posterior auricular | • Superficial temporal |
| • Facial | | |

| Mnemonics | Branches |
|---|---|
| Sister | Superior thyroid |
| Lucy's | Lingual |
| Powdered | Posterior auricular |
| Face | Facial |
| Often | Occipital |
| Attracts | Ascending pharyngeal, (medial branch) |
| Medical | Maxillary |
| Students | Superficial temporal |

- Superior thyroid branch is given off just below the level of greater cornu of hyoid bone
- Lingual branch is given off opposite to the tip of greater cornu of hyoid bone
- Facial branch is given off just above the tip of greater cornu of hyoid bone
- Occipital and posterior auricular branches are related to posterior belly of digastric.

### Applied Anatomy

The ECA ligation is done in cases of severe tonsillar bleeding and severe epistaxis.

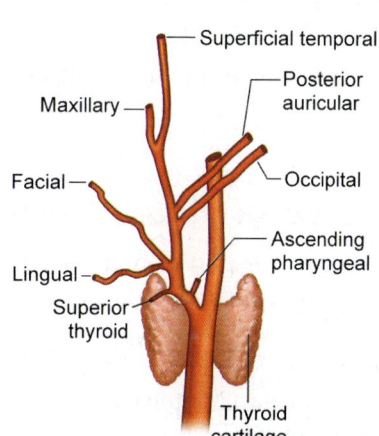

### Q. Central artery of retina

**Ans.** Central artery of retina is a classic example of end artery.

### Origin

Central artery of retina is a branch of ophthalmic artery.

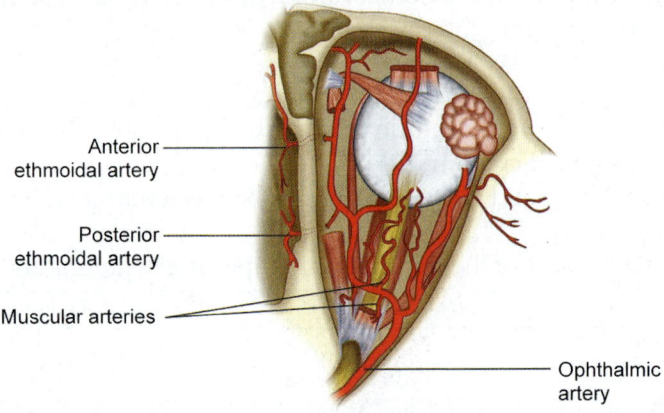

Anterior ethmoidal artery

Posterior ethmoidal artery

Muscular arteries

Ophthalmic artery

### Course and Relations

- It is the first and small branch of ophthalmic artery, which begins below the optic nerve and is within its dural sheath
- About 1.25 cm behind the eye it enters the nerve and then lies at the inferomedial surface and runs toward the retina.
  The central retinal artery occupies the aperture in lamina cribrosa.

### Branches

Central retinal artery divided into two equal branches—superior and inferior, which further divide into superior and inferior nasal, and superior and inferior temporal branches. The arteries supply the respective quadrants of retina.

### Applied Anatomy

- Central retinal vessels can be visualised by doing ophthalmoscopy
- Blockage in the retinal artery causes loss of vision, since it is an end artery.

## VEIN

### Q. Venous drainage of the face (danger area of face).

**Ans.** Lower part of nose, philtrum and upper lip are considered as the 'danger area of face' because infections in these regions lead to cavernous sinus thrombosis.

### Anatomical Basis

Venous blood of the face finally drains into cavernous sinus. Following is the venous drainage of the face.

Supratrochlear and supraorbital vein unite to form angular vein, which continues below as facial vein, to join below with anterior division of retromandibular vein.

## Deep Connections of Facial Vein

- It communicates with superior ophthalmic vein through supraorbital vein to cavernous sinus
- Deep facial vein drains into pterygoid plexus of veins, which in turn drains into cavernous sinus.

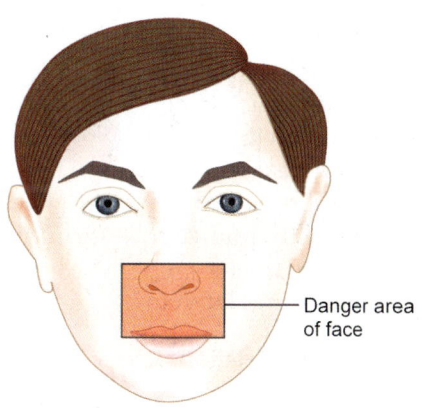

Danger area of face

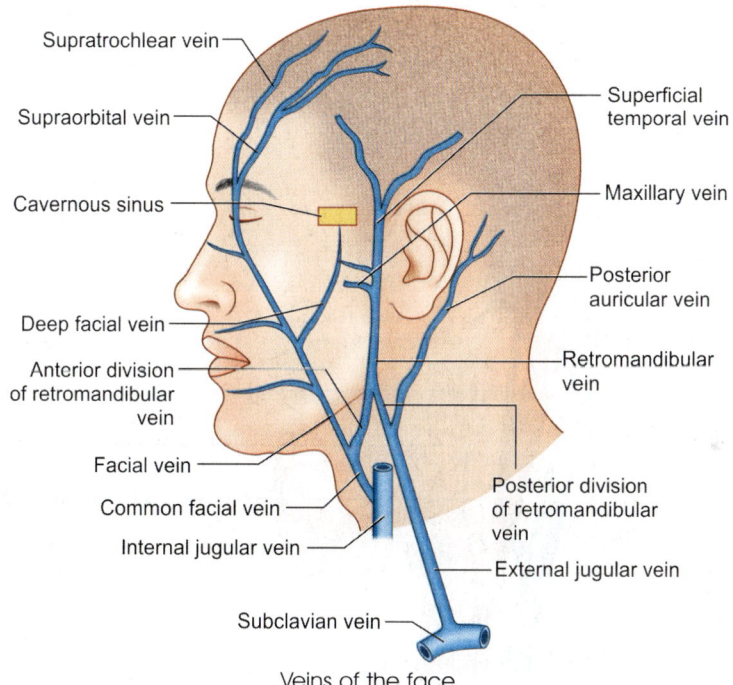

Veins of the face

## Applied Anatomy

Furunculosis in the danger area of face should be treated aggressively with antibiotics to avert cavernous sinus thrombosis.

### Q. Internal jugular vein

**Ans.** Internal jugular vein (IJV) is the prime venous channel in the neck within the carotid sheath.

## Origin

Internal jugular vein is the direct continuation of sigmoid sinus at the jugular foramen. The origin is marked by 'superior bulb', which lies in the jugular fossa.

## Tributaries

- Inferior petrosal sinus
- Common facial vein
- Lingual vein
- Pharyngeal veins
- Superior thyroid vein
- Middle thyroid vein
- Thoracic duct
- Oblique jugular vein.

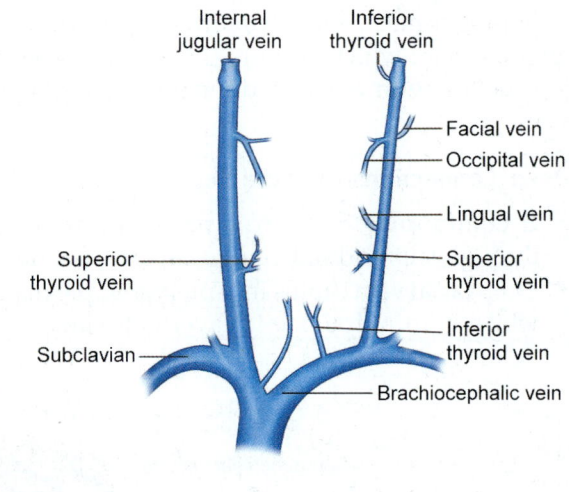

## Course and Relations

- Internal jugular vein courses vertically downwards behind the sternocleido-mastoid up to the sternal end of clavicle
- It lies in front of the scalene muscles, rectus capitis muscles and first part of subclavian artery
- Carotid artery and vagus nerve lie medial to it.

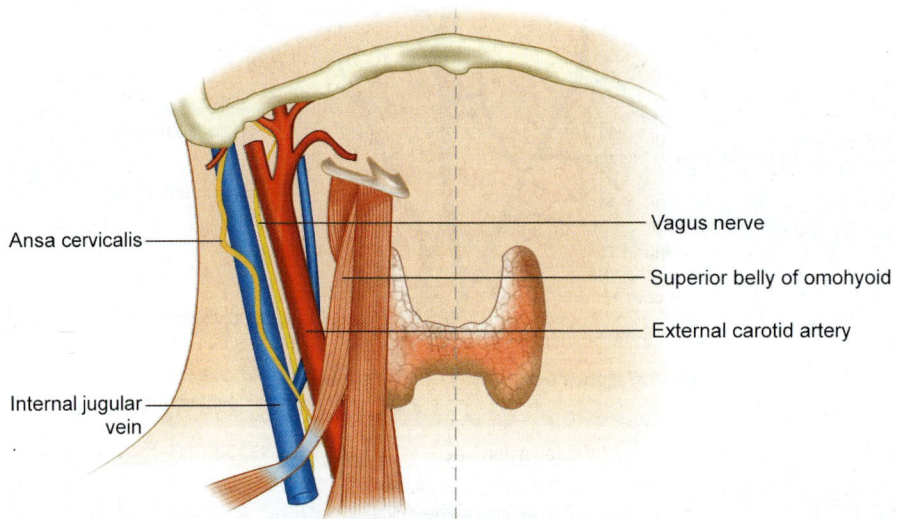

Tributaries of internal jugular vein

## Termination

Internal jugular vein terminates behind the sternal end of clavicle by joining the subclavian vein to form brachiocephalic vein. It is marked by 'inferior bulb'.

## Applied Anatomy

- It is used for recording venous pulse tracings.
- In cardiac failure IJV is markedly dilated and engorged.
- Jugular venous thrombosis may occur secondary to sigmoid sinus thrombosis in long-standing and neglected ear infections.
- In radical neck dissection IJV is removed along with sternocleidomastoid and XI cranial nerve.

## Q. Cavernous sinus (diagram only)

**Ans.**

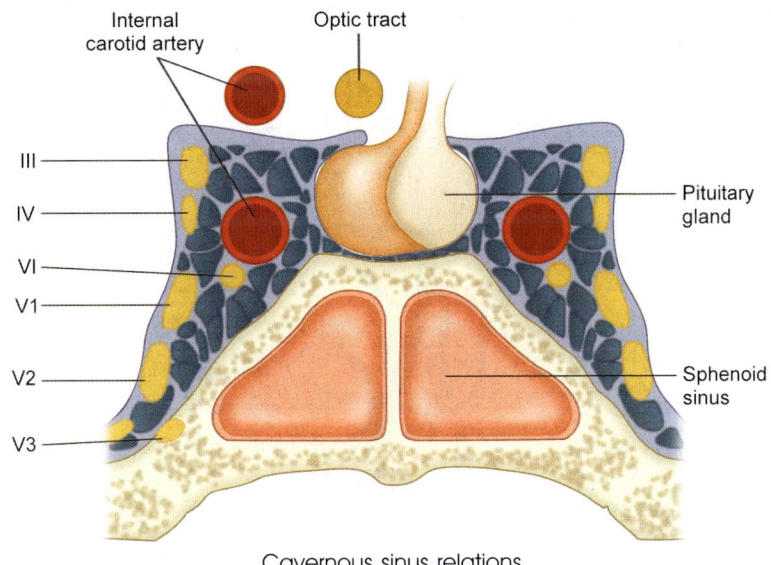

Cavernous sinus relations

## Q. External jugular vein

**Ans.** External jugular vein (EJV) by and large drains the scalp and the face.

### Formation

External jugular vein is formed by the union of posterior division of retromandibular vein and posterior auricular vein near the mandibular angle.

### Course and Relations

- It runs obliquely and superficial to sternocleidomastoid up to the subclavian triangle to end in subclavian vein.
- It is covered by skin, superficial fascia and platysma and lies in front of deep cervical fascia.
- It lies parallel with the great auricular nerve, ascending posterior to its upper half.

### Tributaries

- Retromandibular vein
- Posterior auricular vein
- Posterior external jugular vein
- Transverse cervical vein
- Suprascapular vein
- Anterior jugular vein

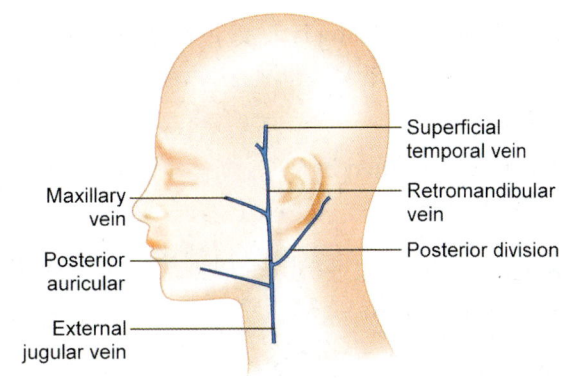

- Internal jugular vein
- Occipital vein (sometimes).

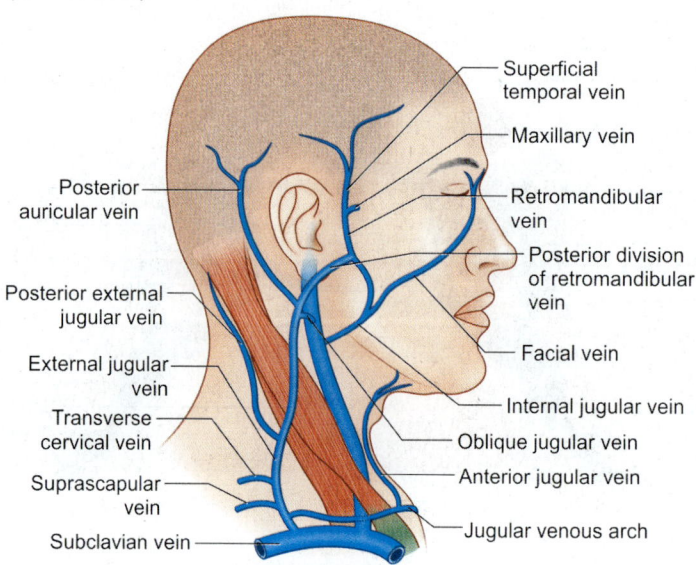

Superficial temporal vein

Maxillary vein

Posterior auricular vein

Retromandibular vein

Posterior division of retromandibular vein

Posterior external jugular vein

External jugular vein

Transverse cervical vein

Suprascapular vein

Subclavian vein

Facial vein

Internal jugular vein

Oblique jugular vein

Anterior jugular vein

Jugular venous arch

## Peculiarities

- Size of the vein is inversely proportional to other veins in the neck
- It has valves at its termination into subclavian vein
- It is dilated 4 cm above the clavicle and is known as sinus
- The valves do not prevent regurgitation.

## Applied Anatomy

- EJV gets distended by expiring against resistance (Valsalva maneuver)
- Division of EJV may give rise to air embolism and death, since the vein lies outside the axillary sheath and prevented from retraction.

## LYMPH NODES

### Q. Waldeyer's ring

**Ans.** Waldeyer's ring is an aggregation of lymphoid tissue at the junction of upper respiratory and upper digestive tract.

## Formation

The ring is formed by:
- Adenoids
- Tubal tonsils
- Palatine tonsils
- Lingual tonsils.

Waldeyer's ring differs from other lymphatic tissue in following ways:

| Waldeyer's ring | Lymph nodes |
|---|---|
| Situated at the junction of upper aerodigestive tract | Grouped according to the region |
| No afferent channels | Both afferent and efferent channels |
| No capsule | Capsulated |
| Crypts present | Crypts absent |
| Growth curve present | Growth curve absent |
| No division into cortex and medulla histologically | Divided into cortex and medulla histologically |

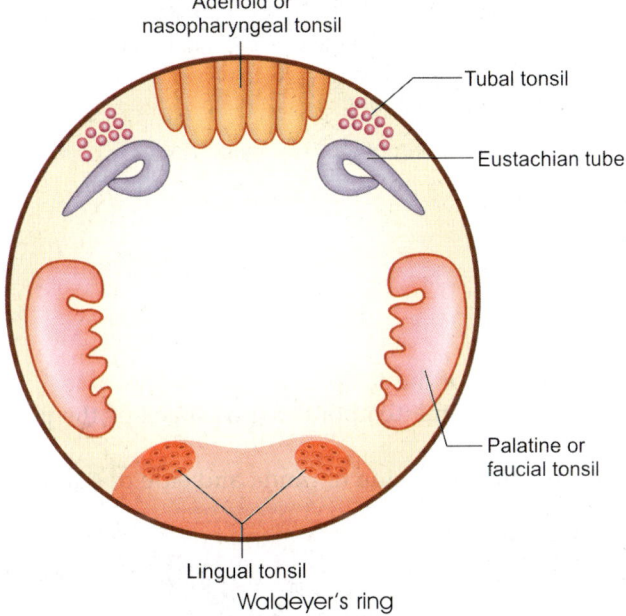

Waldeyer's ring

## Functions

- Helps in maintaining body immunity
- Protects the lower respiratory tract.

### Q. Superficial cervical lymph nodes.

**Ans.** There are approximately 800 lymph nodes in the body out of which 300 are in the neck.

Superficial cervical lymph nodes are classified according to the region they are present in the form of circular chain as follows:

- Occipital
- Posterior auricular
- Preauricular
- Parotid
- Facial

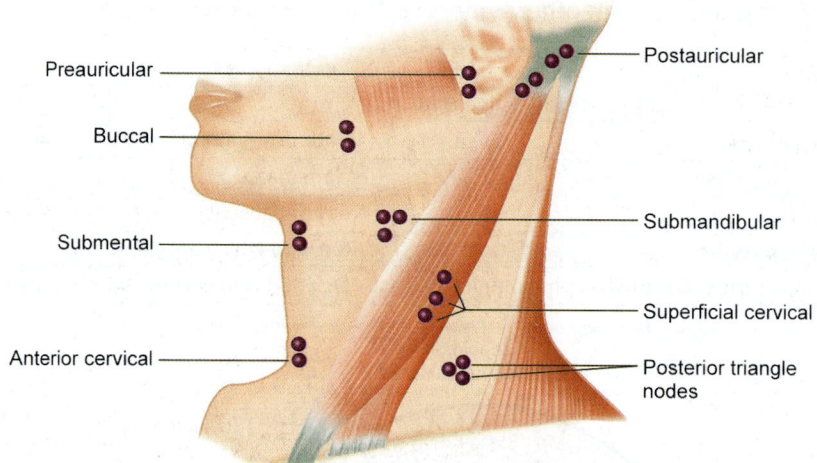

Grouping of cervical lymph nodes

- Submandibular
- Submental
- Superficial cervical
- Anterior cervical.

## Drainage Area

1. Occipital nodes drain the back of the scalp.
2. Posterior auricular nodes drain the temporal region, back of the pinna, external auditory meatus.
3. Preauricular nodes drains the outer side of pinna and side of scalp.

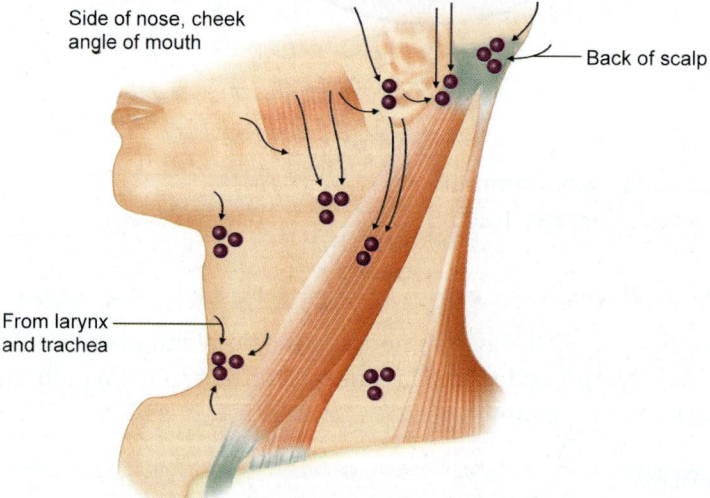

Drainage areas of cervical lymph nodes

4. Parotid nodes located in the substance of the gland drain the eyelids, front of scalp, external auditory meatus and tympanic cavity, while the nodes deep to the gland drain the nasopharynx and nose.

5. Superficial facial nodes receive lymph from conjunctiva, eyelids, nose and cheek. Deep facial nodes drain the temporal fossa, infratemporal fossa, back of the nose and pharynx.
6. Submandibular nodes drain the side of the nose, cheek, angle of eye and mouth, upper lip, gums and side of tongue.
7. Submental nodes drain the central part of the lower lip and floor of the mouth.
8. Superficial cervical nodes drain the parotid region and the lower part of the ear.
9. Anterior cervical nodes drain the larynx and thyroid.
   All the superficial lymph nodes drain into deep cervical lymph nodes.

## Applied Anatomy

1. Malignancies are staged according to the involvement of the lymph nodes.
2. In radical neck dissections lymph nodes are cleared according to the level of involvement. Following are the levels of lymph nodes:
   - Level I—submental and submandibular nodes
   - Level II—upper cervical nodes
   - Level III—middle cervical nodes
   - Level IV—lower cervical nodes
   - Level V—posterior triangle nodes
   - Level VI—pretracheal and prelaryngeal nodes
   - Level VII—mediastinal nodes.

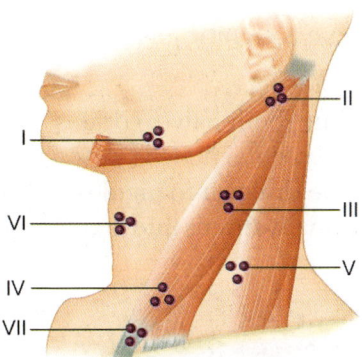

Levels of lymph nodes (surgically)

## Q. Deep cervical lymph nodes.

**Ans.** All the deep cervical lymph nodes receive lymph from superficial cervical lymph nodes.

## Location

Deep cervical lymph nodes form a vertical chain along the internal jugular vein.

## Classification

Deep cervical lymph nodes are grouped as jugulodigastric, jugulo-omohyoid and supraclavicular lymph nodes.

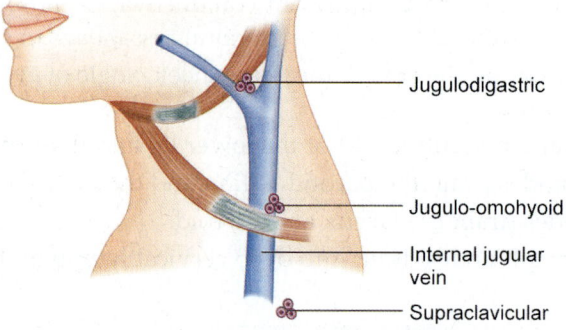

Deep cervical lymph nodes

## Drainage Area

- Jugulodigastric nodes mainly drains the tonsils.
- Jugulo-omohyoid mainly drains the tongue.
- Supraclavicular lymph nodes receive the lymph from preceding nodes. Additionally, left side receives lymph from pelvic viscera (ovaries, testis) and breast.

## Applied Anatomy

Enlarged left supraclavicular lymph nodes are known as Virchow's nodes.

### Q. Lymphatic drainage of tongue.

**Ans.** Lymphatic drainage of tongue is significant since cancer tongue is common in India.

*Following is the lymphatic drainage of tongue:*
- Anterior two-thirds of the tongue (both halves) drains into submandibular nodes
- Tip of the tongue drains into submental nodes
- Posterior one-third of the tongue drains into jugulo-omohyoid nodes bilaterally.

All the lymph from the tongue finally drains into jugulo-omohyoid node. Hence, it is known as lymph node of the tongue.

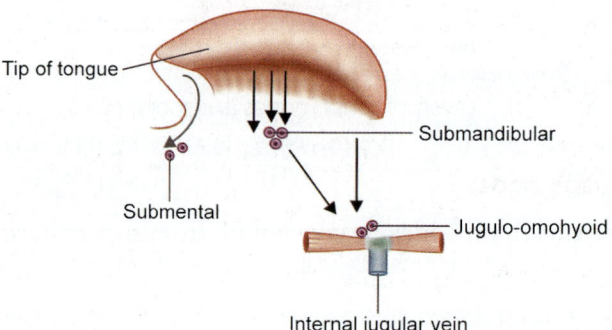

## Applied Anatomy

- Commonest site of cancer tongue is lateral side of the tongue next common site is posterior one-third of tongue
- Cancer tongue is best treated by radiotherapy

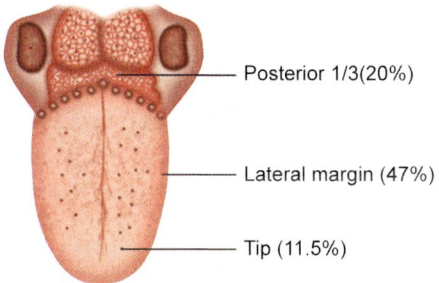

Posterior 1/3(20%)

Lateral margin (47%)

Tip (11.5%)

- Cancer of posterior one-third of tongue is more dangerous due to bilateral lymphatic drainage.

## JOINT

### Q. Atlanto-occipital joint

**Ans.** Types of atlanto-occipital joint synovial joint, ellipsoid variety.

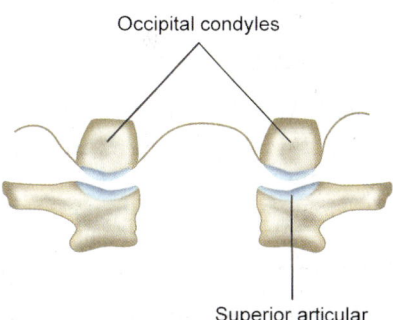

Occipital condyles

Superior articular facets of atlas

Articular surface

### Articular Surfaces

- From above—occipital condyles
- From below—superior articular facets of atlas vertebra.

### Ligaments

*Fibrous capsule:* It surrounds the articular surfaces. It is thick posterolaterally and thin anteromedially.

*Anterior atlanto-occipital membrane:* It extends from anterior margin of foramen magnum above to the upper border of anterior arch of atlas. It is reinforced anteriorly by anterior longitudinal ligament.

*Posterior atlanto-occipital membrane:* It extends from posterior margin of foramen magnum above to the upper border of posterior arch of atlas.

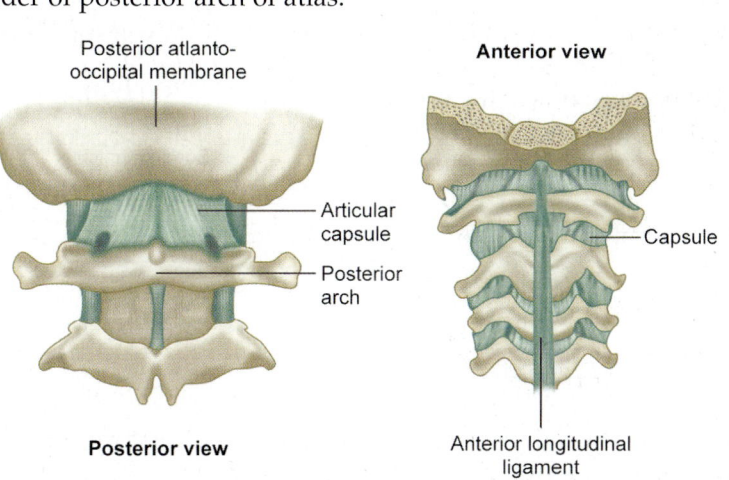

Posterior atlanto-occipital membrane

Anterior view

Articular capsule

Posterior arch

Capsule

Posterior view

Anterior longitudinal ligament

### Nerve Supply

First cervical spinal nerve.

### Blood Supply

Vertebral artery.

### Action

'Yes' movement, i.e. flexion and extension occurs at this joint:
- *Flexion:* Longus capitis, rectus capitis anterior
- *Extension:* Rectus capitis posterior major and minor, superior oblique, semispinalis capitis, splenius capitis.

### Applied Anatomy

Cervical vertebrae may be fractured or dislocated by a fall on the head with acute flexion of neck.

### Q. Atlantoaxial joint

**Ans.** Atlantoaxial joint comprises of paired lateral joints and a median single joint:
1. Lateral joints lie between inferior facets of atlas and superior facets of axis; they are plane joints.
2. Median joint lies between the dens, anterior arch and transverse ligament of atlas.

### Ligaments

Lateral joint is covered by capsule all over, anterior longitudinal ligament and ligamentum flavum.

Median joint also covered by capsule and reinforced by transverse ligament.

*Ligaments supporting atlantoaxial and atlanto-occipital joints are:*
1. Membrana tectoria: It is an upward continuation of posterior longitudinal ligament.
2. Cruciate ligament: It is an extension of transverse ligament.
3. Apical ligament of dens: It is in the centre.
4. Alar ligament: It is on the sides.

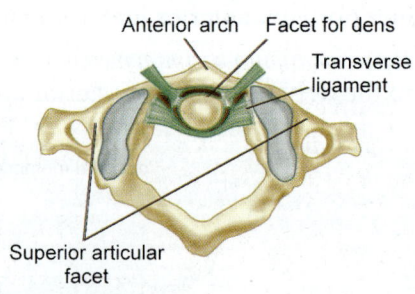

### Nerve Supply

First and second cervical spinal nerve.

### Blood Supply

Vertebral artery.

### Action

'No' movement, i.e. rotatory movements ocurs at these joints. Rotatory movements are brought about by obliquus capitis inferior, rectus capitis posterior major and splenius capitis.

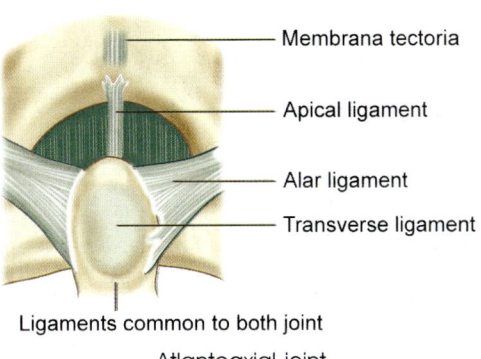

Membrana tectoria

Apical ligament

Alar ligament

Transverse ligament

Ligaments common to both joint

Atlantoaxial joint

## Applied Anatomy

- Death by hanging is due to dislocation of dens following rupture of transverse ligament
- Neck abscesses can cause attritional changes in transverse ligament causing dislocation of atlas or axis (Grisel's syndrome)
- Cervical spondylosis leads to degenerative changes in intervertebral disk, causing disk prolapse.

### Q. Sphenomandibular ligament

**Ans.** Sphenomandibular ligament is an accessory ligament of temporomandibular joint. It is a remnant of Meckel's cartilage.

## Attachments

- *Above:* Spine of sphenoid
- *Below:* Lingula of mandibular foramen.

## Relations

- *Laterally:* Lateral pterygoid, auriculotemporal nerve, maxillary artery, inferior alveolar nerve and vessels
- *Medially:* Medial pterygoid, chorda tympani nerve, pharynx. It is pierced by mylohyoid nerve and vessels.

### Q. Stylomandibular ligament

**Ans.** Stylomandibular ligament is also an accessory ligament of temporomandibular joint. It represents the thickened portion of deep cervical fascia and separates parotid gland from sub-mandibular gland.

## Attachments

- Above: Lateral surface of styloid process
- Below: Ramus of mandible.

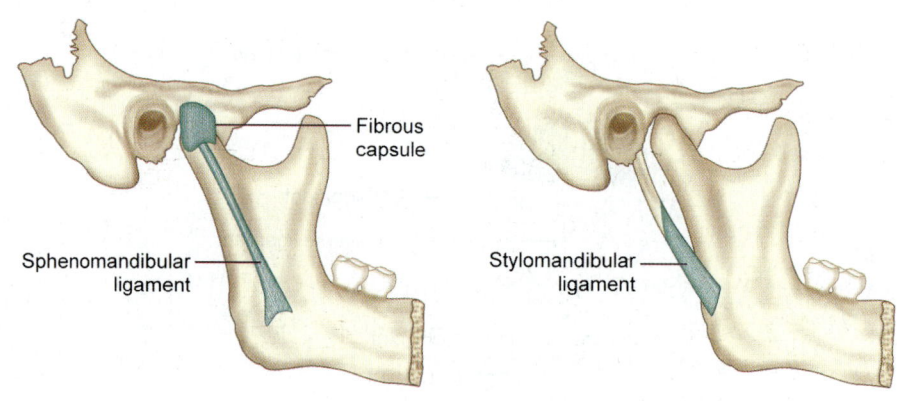

Fibrous capsule

Sphenomandibular ligament

Stylomandibular ligament

## MISCELLANEOUS

**Q. Auricle** (diagram only)

**Ans.**

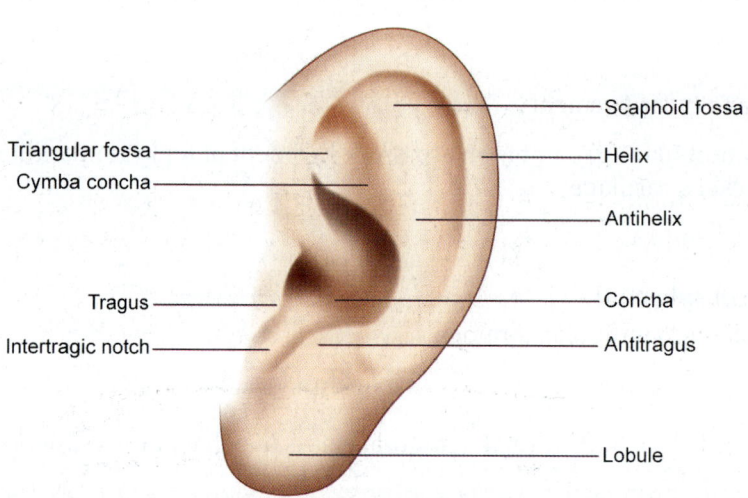

Triangular fossa

Cymba concha

Tragus

Intertragic notch

Scaphoid fossa

Helix

Antihelix

Concha

Antitragus

Lobule

## Q. Formation of the triangles of the neck.

**Ans.** For study purposes, the neck region is divided into triangular areas. Sternocleidomastoid is the key muscle of the neck region dividing it into anterior and posterior triangles.

### Anterior Triangle

Anterior triangle is in front of sternocleidomastoid and subdivided into four triangles:
1. Submental
2. Digastric
3. Muscular
4. Carotid.

## Posterior Triangle

Posterior triangle is behind sternocleidomastoid and subdivided into two triangles:
1. Occipital
2. Supraclavicular.

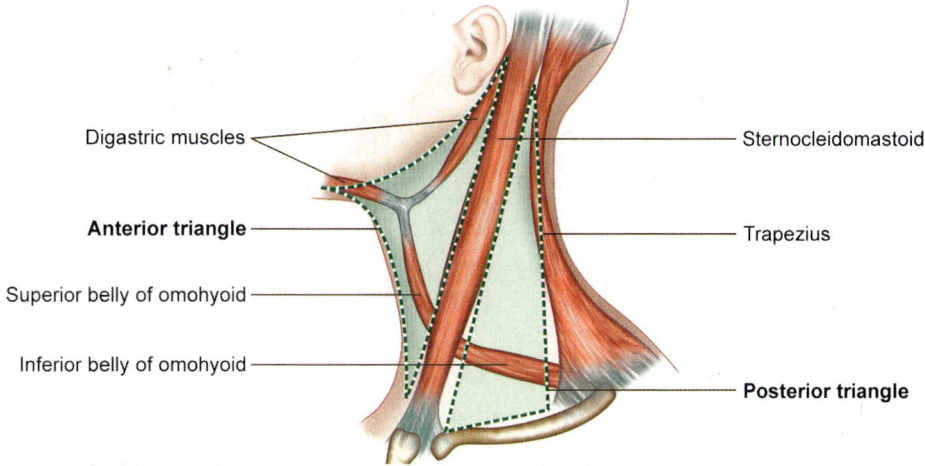

## Q. Carotid sheath

**Ans.** Carotid sheath is a condensation of fibroareolar tissue around the great vessels of the neck. It is derived from all the three layers of deep cervical fascia (investing layer, pretracheal layer and prevertebral layer).

## Contents

Carotid sheath encloses the following structures:
- Common carotid artery with its bifurcation
- Internal jugular vein
- Vagus nerve.

## Relations

- Anteriorly—ansa cervicalis
- Posteriorly—sympathetic chain.

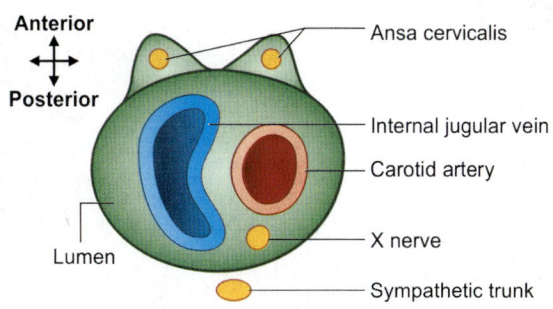

## Surgical Significance

Common carotid bifurcates at the upper border of thyroid cartilage. For external carotid artery ligation, surgeon has to dissect the sheath.

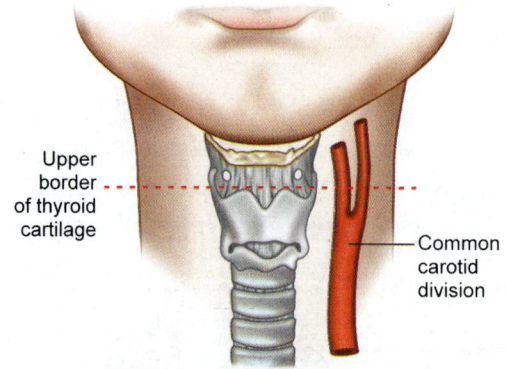

## Q. Carotid triangle

**Ans.** Carotid triangle is an area on the lateral side of the neck.

### Boundaries

- *Superiorly:* Posterior belly of digastric
- *Anteroinferiorly:* Superior belly of omohyoid
- *Posteriorly:* Anterior border of sternocleidomastoid.

### Roof

Skin, superficial fascia with platysma, cervical branch of facial nerve, transverse cutaneous nerve of the neck. Investing layer of deep cervical fascia.

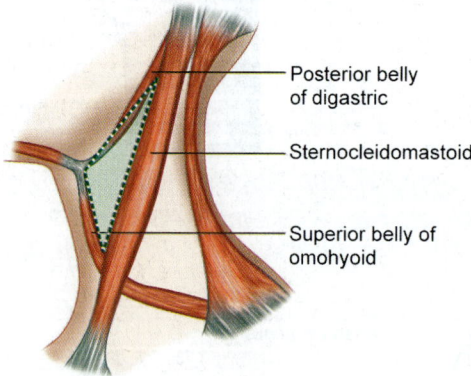

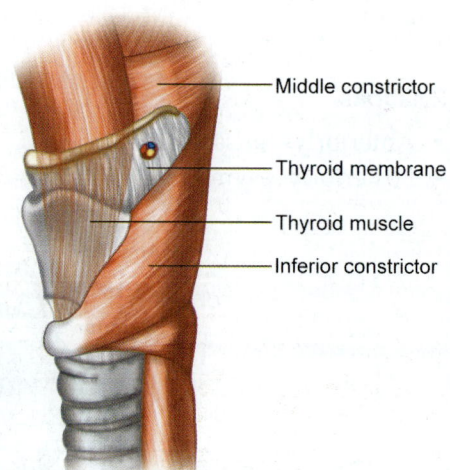

### Floor

Constrictors of pharynx, thyrohyoid membrane and muscle, hyoglossus muscle.

Floor of carotid triangle

## Contents

Carotid artery with bifurcation and its five branches (facial, lingual, ascending pharyngeal, superior thyroid, occipital).

Internal jugular vein with its tributaries (common facial vein, superior thyroid vein and lingual vein) and X, XI, XII nerves.

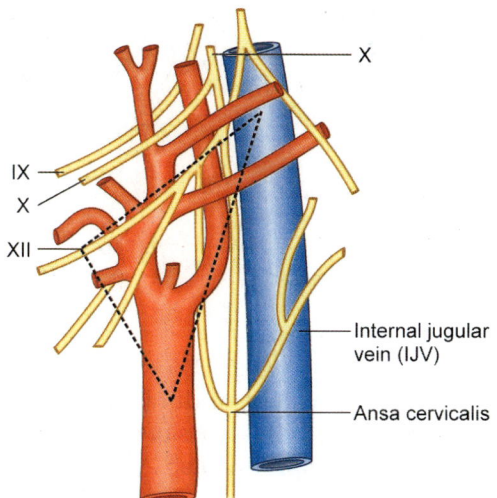

## Surgical Significance

Carotid artery should be protected in any patient whose skin wound is likely to get infected; like in patients who are poorly nourished, diabetics. Carotid artery can be protected by rotating the levator scapulae muscle.

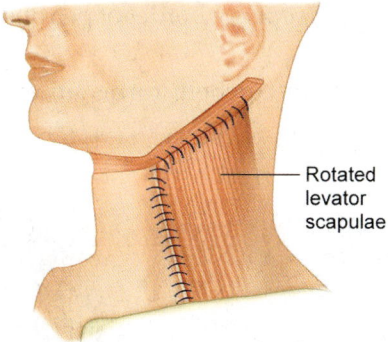

### Q. Falx cerebri

**Ans.** Meningeal layer of dura mater folds within the cranial cavity and divides it into different chambers. Falx cerebri is one of the folds, which lies in median longitudinal fissure and divides the cranial cavity in two halves between the two cerebral hemispheres.

## Attachments

- Anterior end is attached to crista galli
- Posterior end is broad and is attached along the median plane to the upper margin of tentorium cerebelli

- Upper margin is attached to the lips of sagittal sulcus and encloses superior sagittal sinus
- Lower margin is free and encloses inferior sagittal sinus.

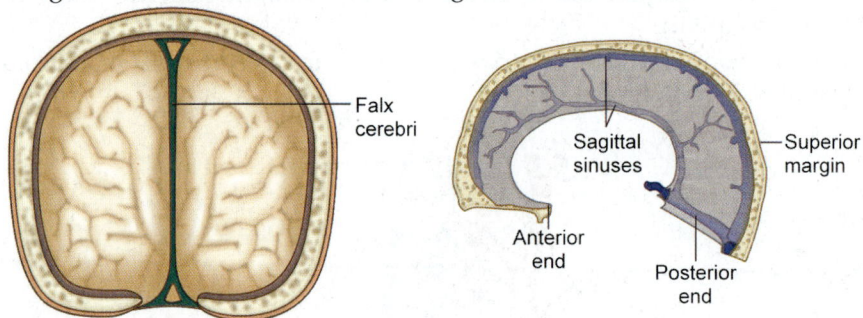

### Relations

Surfaces are related to cerebral hemispheres.

### Q. Tentorium cerebelli

**Ans.** Tentorium cerebelli is a tent-shaped fold of dura mater covering the posterior cranial fossa. It separates the cerebellum from occipital lobes of cerebrum. It divides the cranial cavity into supratentorial and infratentorial compartments.

### Attachments

*Anterior margin:* It is free and concave, with its anterior most end attached to anterior clinoid process. It bounds tentorial notch and occupies the midbrain.

*Outer margin:* It is convex and attached to the lips of transverse sulcus of occipital bone and posteroinferior angle of parietal bone, superior border of petrous temporal bone and to posterior clinoid process.

*Inferior layer:* This layer of tentorium cerebelli forms an extra recess over the trigeminal impression known as Meckel's caves.

### Surfaces

- Superior surface is convex and sloping. Along the line of attachment of falx cerebri it encloses straight sinus
- Inferior surface is concave
- At the junction of free and attached margins, it is pierced by III and IV cranial nerves.

### Applied Anatomy

Lesions in the infratentorial compartment should be attended at the earliest, as it may cause pressure on the brainstem and coning of medulla causing death.

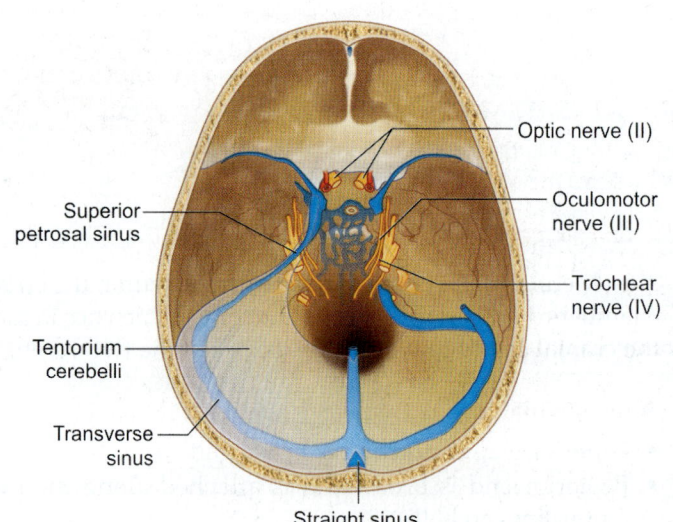

## Q. Midline structures of the neck.

**Ans.** Midline is the central region, extending from the chin to the sternum. Midline structures of the neck can be divided into suprahyoid and infrahyoid regions.

### Peculiarities

Skin covering this region is freely movable over deeper structures:
- *Superficial fascia:* It contains platysma, anterior jugular vein, lymph nodes and transverse cutaneous nerve
- *Deep fascia:* It is a single layer, up to cricoid, but below cricoid it splits to form suprasternal space of burns.

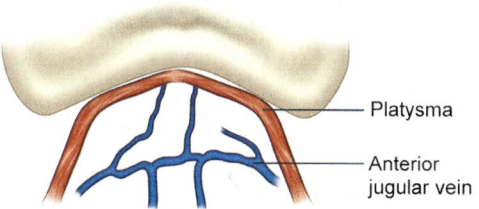

### Suprahyoid Region

Suprahyoid region has mylohyoid muscle, forming the oral diaphragm and on either sides are the anterior bellies of digastric.

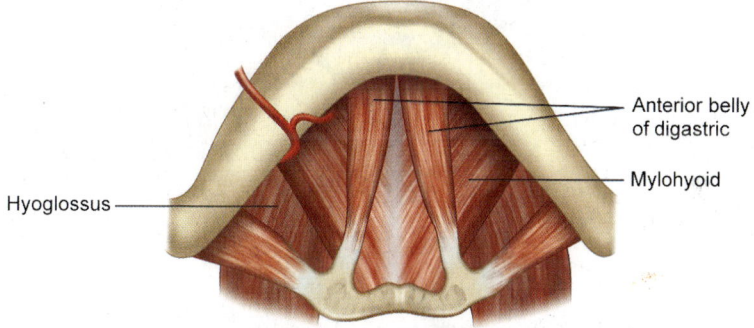

Suprahyoid region

### Infrahyoid Region

1. Strap muscles cover the infrahyoid region. These are ribbon-like muscles namely, thyrohyoid, sternothyroid, sternohyoid, omohyoid.
2. Deep structures are thyrohyoid membrane, between hyoid and thyroid cartilage, cricoid cartilage, thyroid gland and tracheal rings.
3. Superior laryngeal vessels and internal laryngeal nerve pierce the thyrohyoid membrane.
4. Cricothyroid is the deep muscle in midline, which is the tensor of vocal cord.

### Applied Anatomy

- Common midline swellings are thyroid enlargement known as goiter. Other swellings are thyroglossal cyst, lymph node enlargement, etc.
- Tracheostomy is a life-saving procedure done about two finger breath above jugular notch.

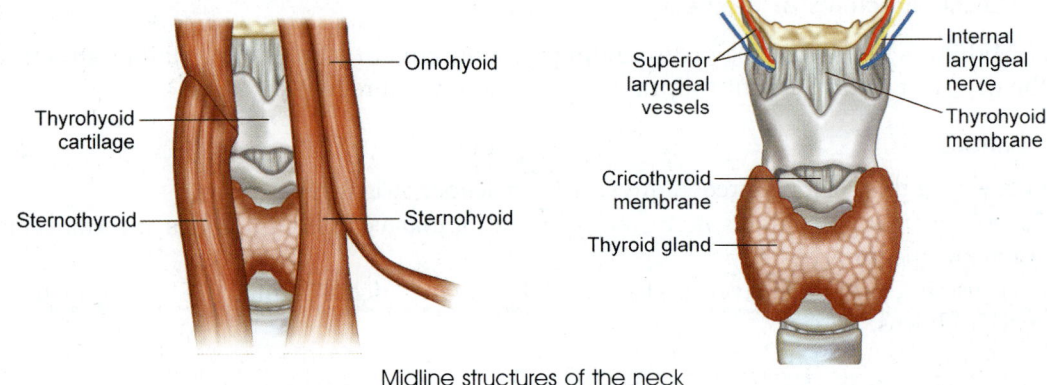

Midline structures of the neck

**Q. Superior orbital fissure** (diagram only).

**Ans.**

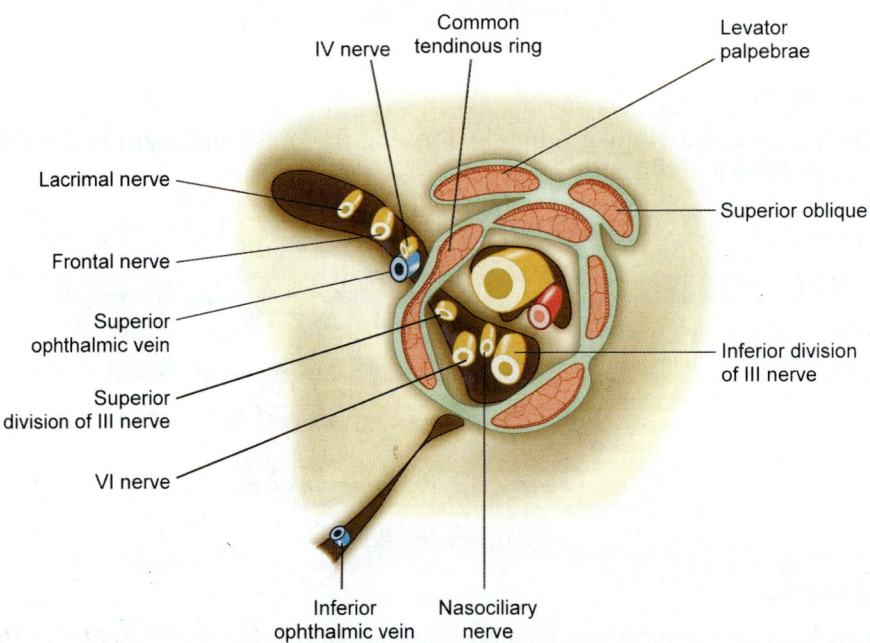

## Q. Styloid apparatus

**Ans.** Styloid process is slender bony projection from the temporal bone between parotid gland laterally and internal jugular vein (IJV) medially. Styloid process with its attachments is known as styloid apparatus.

### Attachments

Styloid apparatus gives attachments to three muscles and two ligaments. These have diverse embryological origins.

## Embryological Basis

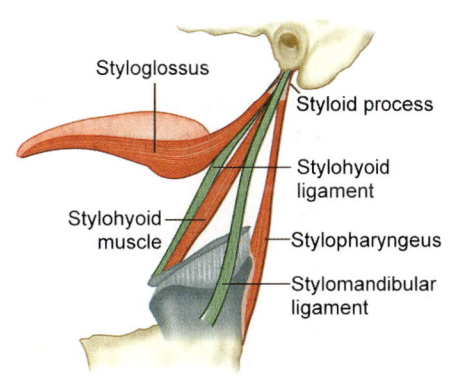

- Styloid process, stylohyoid ligament and stylohyoid muscle take origin from second branchial arch
- Stylopharyngeus from third branchial arch
- Styloglossus from occipital myotomes
- Stylomandibular ligament is a part of deep cervical fascia
- Stylohyoid muscle runs parallel to posterior belly of digastric; controls movement of hyoid bone
- Styloglossus muscle pulls the tongue upwards and backwards
- Stylopharyngeus muscle helps to lift the larynx during swallowing
- Stylomandibular ligament separates the parotid gland from the submandibular gland and is thickening of investing layer of deep cervical fascia between the two glands
- Stylohyoid ligament is between tip of styloid process to lesser cornu of hyoid bone.

## Applied Anatomy

Elongated styloid process is known as Eagle's syndrome, wherein the patient presents with continuous nagging pain in the neck. This is detected by taking X-ray of skull and comparing the lengths on both sides. Best detected by CT scan base of skull, It is treated surgically by doing styloidectomy by transtonsillar approach.

### Q. Palatine tonsillar bed

**Ans.** Palatine tonsils are lodged in tonsillar fossa (between palatoglossus and palato-pharyngeus muscles), which form the tonsillar bed.

Lateral surface of tonsil is separated from superior constrictor by lax connective tissue.

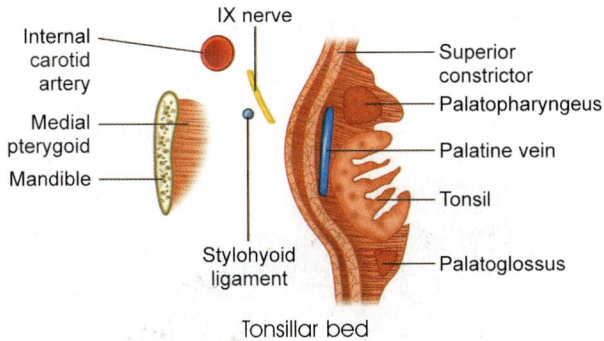

Tonsillar bed

*Structures deep to the superior constrictor are:*

- Ascending palatine artery
- Tonsillar artery
- IX cranial nerve
- Stylohyoid ligament
- Internal carotid artery (ICA) lies 2.5 cm behind and lateral to the tonsil
- Palatine vein.

## Applied Anatomy

- Quinsy is a peritonsillar abscess
- Styloidectomy can be done through tonsillar fossa in cases of elongated styloid process
- Surgeon should remember the relation of internal carotid artery to tonsillar fossa, while doing tonsillectomy.

### Q. Auditory tube (eustachian tube)

**Ans.** Auditory tube is a cone-shaped passage connecting middle ear space with nasopharynx; lodged in sulcus tubae over the base of skull.

## Gross Features

Auditory tube is about one and a half inch long and directed forwards and medially.

## Parts

Auditory tube has two parts:

1. *Bony part*
   - Lateral end of bony part ends into anterior wall of middle ear cavity and medial end gives attachment to cartilaginous part
   - Superiorly, it is related to tensor tympani, medially to carotid canal, laterally to chorda tympani and spine of sphenoid.
2. *Cartilaginous part*
   - It is a triangular part of cartilage, which curls to form superior and medial walls
   - Anterolaterally, it is related to tensor palati, mandibular nerve and its branches, otic ganglion, chorda tympani, middle meningeal artery and medial pterygoid plate
   - Levator palati is attached to its inferior surface.

## Blood Supply

Auditory tube receives arterial blood through ascending pharyngeal and middle meningeal artery and drains into pharyngeal plexus of veins.

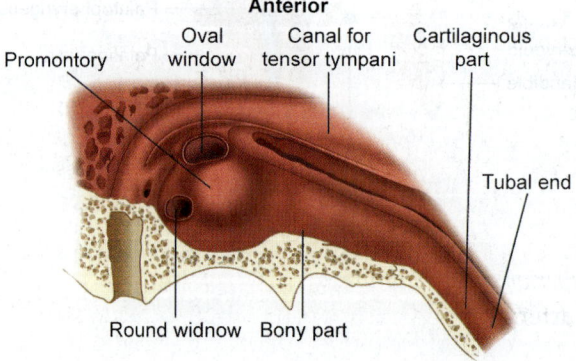

Auditory tube parts and middle ear connection

## Nerve Supply

Pharyngeal plexus of nerves.

## Function

Auditory tube maintains atmospheric pressure in the middle ear cavity. Thus, air pressure on both sides of tympanic membrane is equalised.

## Applied Anatomy

- Inflammation of auditory tube secondary to common cold gives rise to middle ear effusion, which is common in children
- Throat infections may be transmitted by the tube to middle ear cavity causing otitis media.

### Q. Nasal septum

**Ans.** Nasal septum is a median osseocartilaginous partition between the two halves of nasal cavity and is covered by mucous membrane.

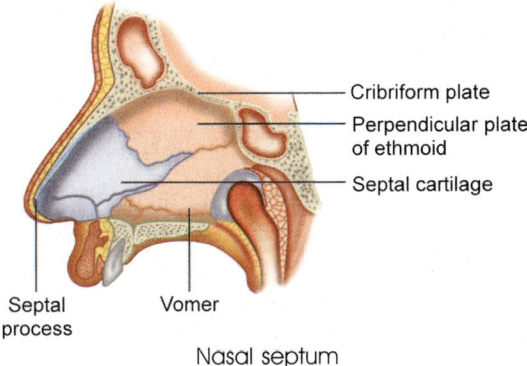

Nasal septum

## Parts

Nasal septum is made-up of three parts:
1. *Bony components:*
   - Vomer
   - Perpendicular plate of ethmoid.
2. *Cartilaginous:*
   - Septal cartilage
   - Septal process of inferior nasal cartilage.
3. Cuticular part:
   - Formed by fibrofatty tissue covered by skin
   - Nasal septum has four borders and two surfaces.

## Borders

- Anterior
- Posterior
- Superior
- Inferior.

## Surfaces

Right and left.

## Blood Supply

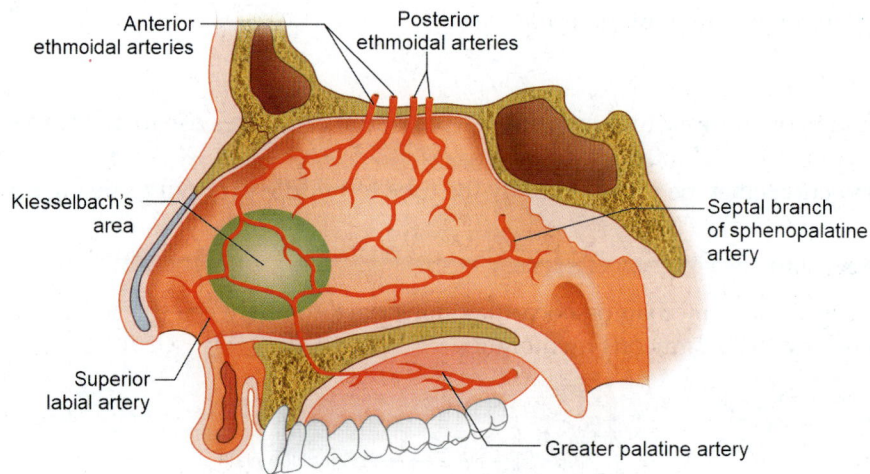

Blood supply of nasal septum

1. Anterosuperior part is supplied by anterior ethmoidal artery and superior labial branch of facial artery.
2. Posteroinferior part is supplied by sphenopalatine artery.

   Venous plexus is present over the lower part of septum, which drains into facial vein anteriorly and pterygoid plexus of veins posteriorly.

## Nerve Supply

- Anterosuperior part is supplied by anterior ethmoidal nerve
- Posteroinferior part is supplied by nasopalatine branch of pterygopalatine ganglion.

## Lymphatic Drainage

Anterior half to submandibular nodes, posterior half to retropharyngeal and deep cervical nodes.

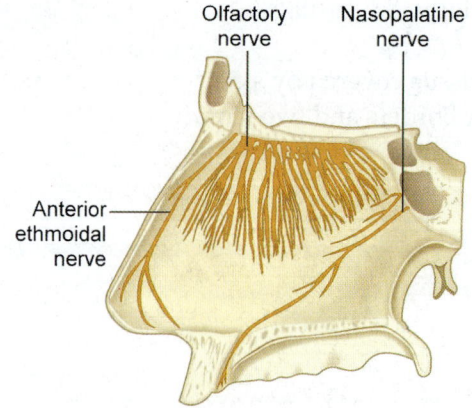

Nerve supply of nasal septum

## Applied Anatomy

1. Nasal septum is deviated in most of the individuals. However, in a few cases the septum is grossly deviated giving rise to symptoms of nasal obstruction and headache. This is known as deviated nasal septum (DNS) and it can be corrected by surgeries like septoplasty, submucous resection.
2. Anterior ethmoidal nerve syndrome is also known as Sludger's syndrome.
3. Little's area is a common site of bleeding through the nose. It is at the anteroinferior part of septum and contains anastomosis between septal ramus of superior labial branch, anterior ethmoidal artery, sphenopalatine artery and greater palatine artery.
4. Sphenopalatine artery is the artery of epistaxis.

### Q. Cavity of larynx

**Ans.** The cavity of larynx is divided into compartments by mucosal folds as described below.

### Extent

The cavity of larynx extends from inlet of larynx to lower border of cricoid cartilage.

### Boundaries

- *Anteriorly:* Epiglottis
- *Posteriorly:* Interarytenoid fold of mucous membrane
- On each side aryepiglottic fold.

### Compartments

There are two folds of mucous membrane within the cavity of larynx:
1. Upper fold is vestibular fold.
2. Lower fold is vocal fold.

*Above folds divide cavity into three parts:*
1. *Upper part:* Vestibule.
2. *Middle part:* Sinus (ventricle).
3. *Lower part:* Infraglottic.

*Areas of importance are:*
1. Area between two vestibular folds is known as rima vestibuli.
2. Area between two vocal folds is known as rima glottidis.
3. Area between vestibular fold and vocal fold is known as sinus of larynx.

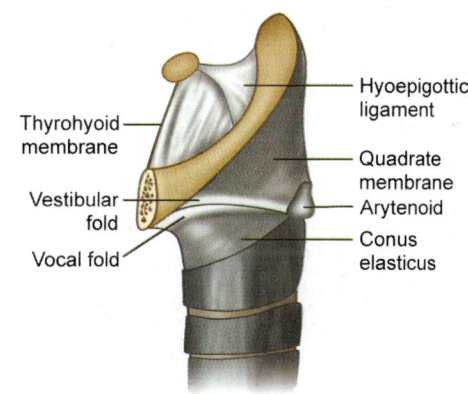

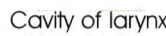

Cavity of larynx

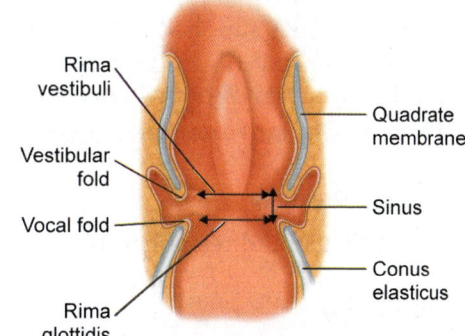

### Applied Anatomy

Surgically, the cavity of larynx is divided into supraglottic, glottic and infraglottic parts:
- *Supraglottic:* Above the vestibular folds

- *Glottic:* Between the vocal and vestibular fold
- *Infraglottic:* Below vocal fold up to the level of cricoid cartilage.

### Q. Tympanic membrane (eardrum)

**Ans.** Tympanic membrane (TM) is a thin translucent partition between external acoustic meatus and middle ear.

### Gross Anatomy

Tympanic membrane is oval in shape, 9 × 10 mm in size, placed obliquely at 55 degrees to the floor of meatus and facing downwards, forwards and laterally.

Circumference of TM is thickened forming the tympanic sulcus all around except superiorly, where it is deficient and attached to the notch of Rivinus. From the notch, two bands namely anterior and posterior malleolar folds arise to the lateral process.

#### Surfaces

- Outer surface is free and concave
- Inner surface is convex and provides attachment to the handle of malleus, the point of maximum convexity at the tip of handle is called umbo.

#### Parts

- Pars flaccida
- Pars tensa.

#### Layers

- Outer cuticular
- Middle fibrous
- Inner mucosal.

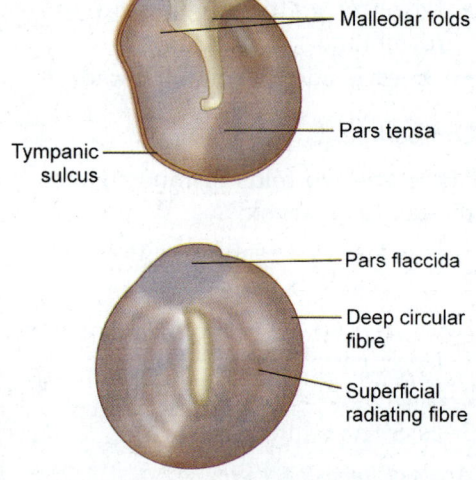

Tympanic membrane

### Blood Supply

- Outer surface is supplied by deep auricular branch of maxillary artery
- Inner surface is supplied by anterior tympanic, a branch of maxillary artery and posterior tympanic, a branch of posterior auricular artery
- Blood drains into external jugular vein.

### Lymphatic Drainage

To preauricular and retropharyngeal lymph nodes.

### Nerve Supply

- Lateral surface in front supplied by auriculotemporal nerve and behind by auricular branch of vagus
- Medial surface is supplied by chorda tympani nerve.

## Applied Anatomy

Myringotomy is a radial or curvilinear, incision taken on TM for middle ear effusion.

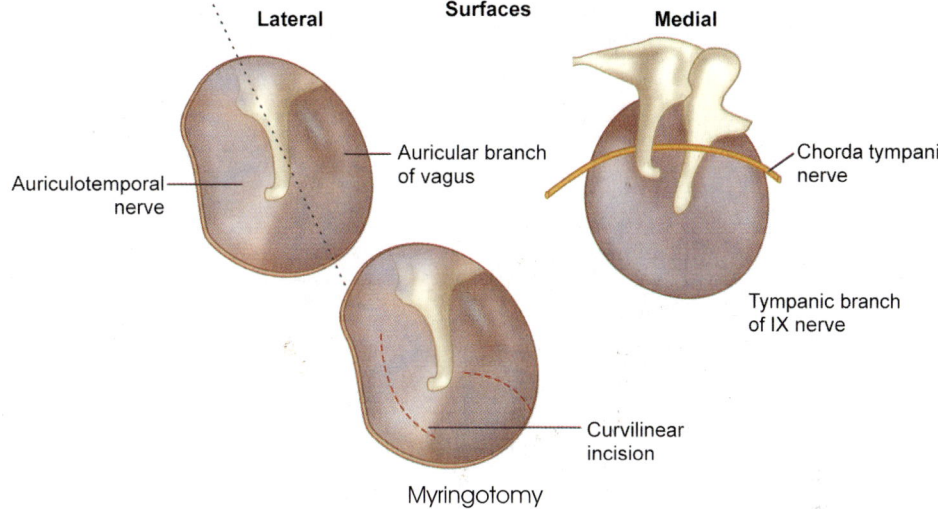

Myringotomy

## Q. Prussak's pouch

**Ans.** The mucous membrane lines the bony walls of the tympanic cavity and extends to cover the ossicles and their supporting ligaments; in much the same way as the peritoneum covers the viscera in the abdomen.

The mucosal folds divide the middle ear space into compartments. Prussak's pouch is a part of epitympanic region.

## Boundaries

- *Above:* Lateral malleolar fold
- *Below:* Neck of malleus
- *Laterally:* Pars flaccida.

## Applied Anatomy

Unsafe middle ear disease begins from Prussak's pouch commonly.

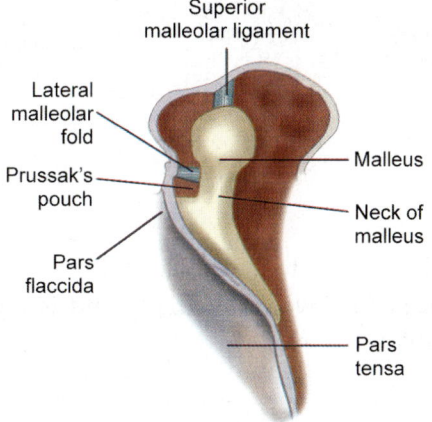

**Q. Eyeball** (diagram only)

Ans.

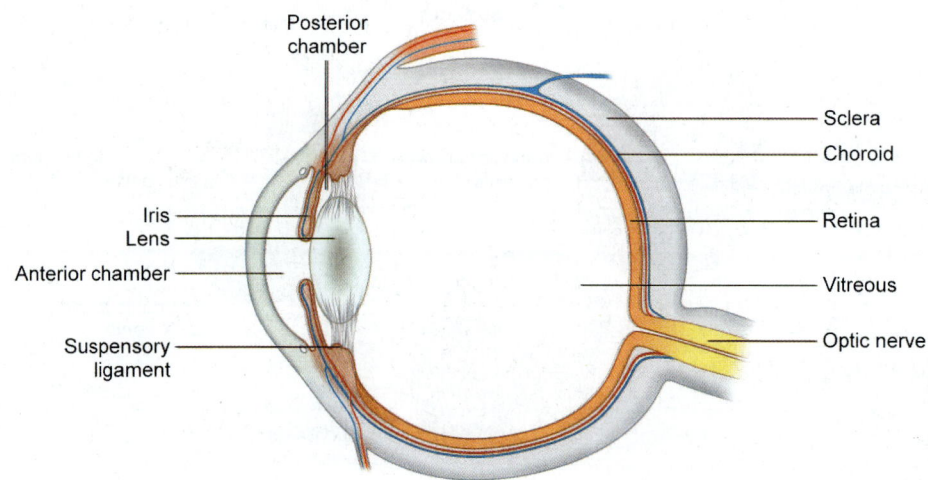

**Q. Ear ossicles**

**Ans.** Ear ossicles are the smallest bones in human body. There are three ossicles in the middle ear cavity namely malleus, incus and stapes.

### Malleus

- Derived from Meckel's cartilage
- It is a largest ossicle located close to TM
- It has following parts—head, neck, anterior process and lateral process, and handle
- Head lies in attic and articulates posteriorly with incus
- Neck lies against pars flaccida and related medially to chorda tympani
- Anterior process has anterior ligament getting attached to petrotympanic fissure

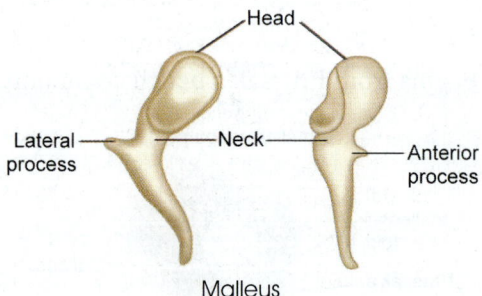

Malleus

- Lateral process provides attachment to malleolar folds
- Handle extends downwards, backwards medially and is attached to TM. The point of attachment is known as umbo.

## Incus

- Derived from second arch
- It has body, short process in fossa incudis, long process parallel to handle of malleus.

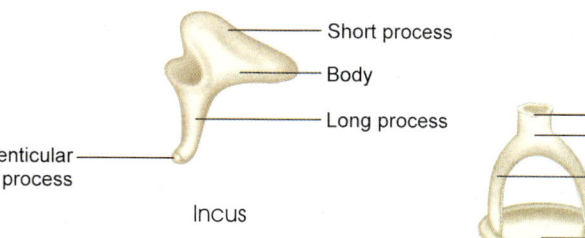

Incus

## Stapes

- Derived from second arch
- It has head, neck, crura and footplate.

Stapes

## Joints

- Incudomalleolar joint is saddle joint
- Incudostapedial joint is a ball and socket joint.

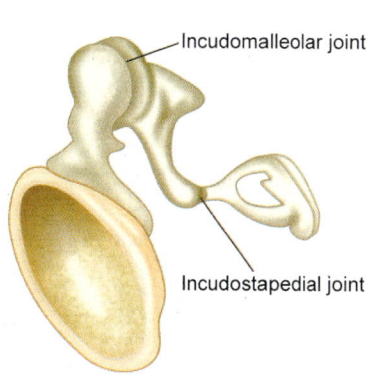

## Muscles of Ossicles

- Tensor tympani is a muscle for malleus, it arises from the walls of auditory tube and gets inserted into the upper part of handle of malleus
- Stapedius arises from pyramid and inserts on the neck of stapes.

Joints

## Applied Anatomy

- Deafness behind intact TM may be due to ossicular chain fixity or stapes footplate fixation known as otosclerosis
- Stapedectomy is done in otosclerosis.

**Q. Cochlear section** (diagram only)

**Ans.**

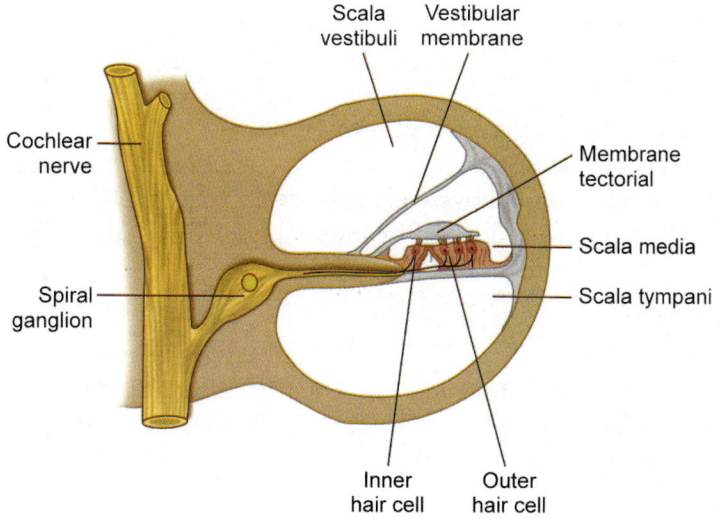

### Q. Sclerocorneal junction

**Ans.** The junction between sclera and cornea is the sclerocorneal junction, which is marked by canal of Schlemm.

### Circulation of Aqueous Humor

The aqueous humor is secreted by ciliary process and it enters the posterior chamber. It then passes forward through the pupil to anterior chamber, where it leaves the eye by way of trabecular meshwork canal of Schlemm, aqueous veins and mixes with the blood in episcleral vessels.

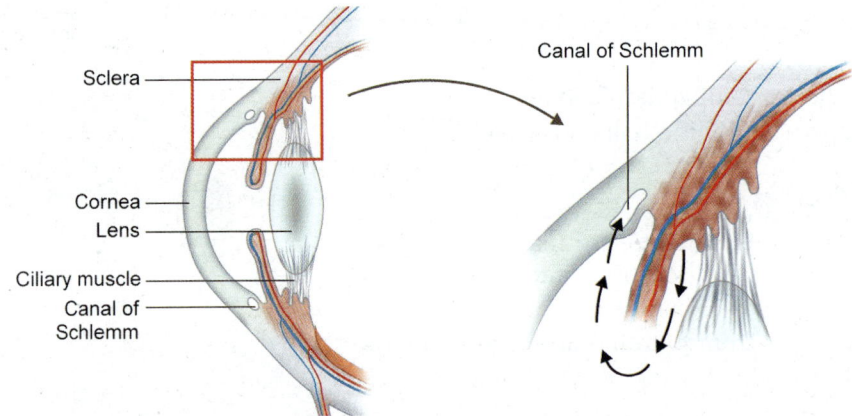

Circulation of aqueous humor

### Applied Anatomy

*Glaucoma occurs due to following reasons:*
- Commonly, when there is resistance to the flow of aqueous at any level during its pathway
- Rarely, when more of aqueous is produced.

### Q. Pyriform fossa boundaries

**Ans.** • *Classified* as part of hypopharynx
- *Boundaries*
  - *Medially:* Aryepiglottic fold
  - *Laterally:* Thyroid alae and thyrohyoid membrane
  - *Anteriorly:* Glossoepiglottic fold
- Fossa is continuous below and above with postcricoid part of retropharynx
- Mucosa of floor of the fossa is supplied by internal branch of superior laryngeal nerve.

### Q. Killian's dehiscence

- It is a potential gap between oblique fibres of thyropharyngeus muscle and transverse fibres of cricopharyngeus muscle.
- In event of weakness of muscle fibres; the pharyngeal mucosa may bulge and get herniated in this space resulting into pharyngeal diverticulum or pharyngeal pouch, i.e. Killian's dehiscence.

## Q. Surgeon's graveyard

**Ans.** While examining the head and neck region for early detection of cancer, one can miss out certain areas. These are the hidden areas, where cancer can begin from.

*Following are the hidden sites:*
- Retromolar region
- Floor of mouth
- Pyriform fossa
- Tonsillolingual sulcus
- Vallecula
- Fossa of Rosenmüller (area around auditory tube opening in nasopharynx).

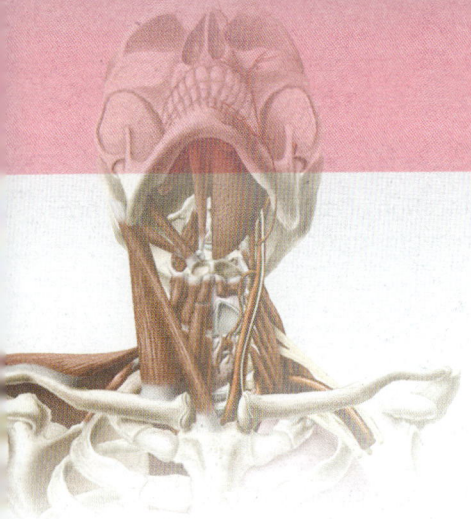

**Ans.** Soft tissues covering the upper part of skull form the scalp.

### Boundaries

- Anteroposteriorly it extends between the supraorbital margin and external occipital protuberance and superior nuchal lines
- On either side, superior temporal lines form the boundary (thus forehead is included in scalp).

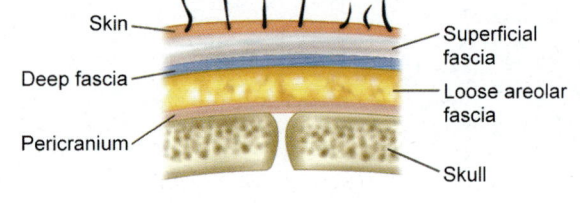

Skin — Superficial fascia
Deep fascia — Loose areolar fascia
Pericranium — Skull

### Layers

The following are the five layers:
1. Skin.
2. Superficial fascia.
3. Deep fascia (aponeurosis).
4. Loose areolar tissue.
5. Pericranium.

*Here scalp stands for:*
**S**—Skin
**C**—Connective tissue
**A**—Aponeurosis
**L**—Loose areolar tissue
**P**—Pericranium

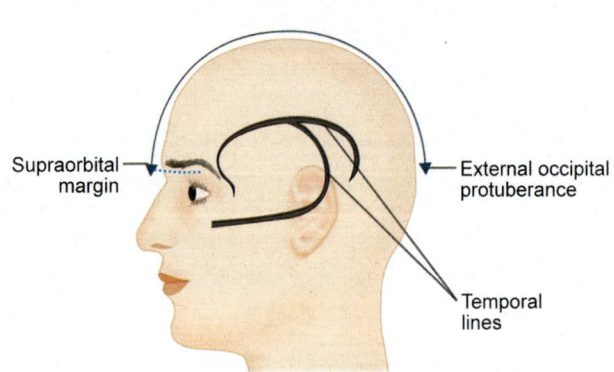

Supraorbital margin — External occipital protuberance

Temporal lines

Extent of scalp

*Skin*

- Thick and hairy
- It is adherent to epicranial aponeurosis through dense superficial fascia.

*Superficial Fascia*

- It is very fibrous and dense (central portion is more dense than periphery)
- Neurovascular bundle traverses this layer to reach the skin
- Occipitofrontalis muscle is present in this layer.

*Deep Fascia*

- It is adherent to the skin of scalp above, but freely movable from below
- It provides insertion for the occipitalis and temporalis muscle
- On each side it is attached to the superior temporal lines.

*Loose Areolar Tissue*

Extends anteriorly into the eyelids posteriorly to the superior nuchal lines and on each side temporal line.

*Pericranium*

Pericranium is loosely attached to the surface of the bone except at the suture lines, where it is firmly attached.

## Blood Supply

Scalp has a rich blood supply derived from both internal and external carotid arteries (ICA and ECA):

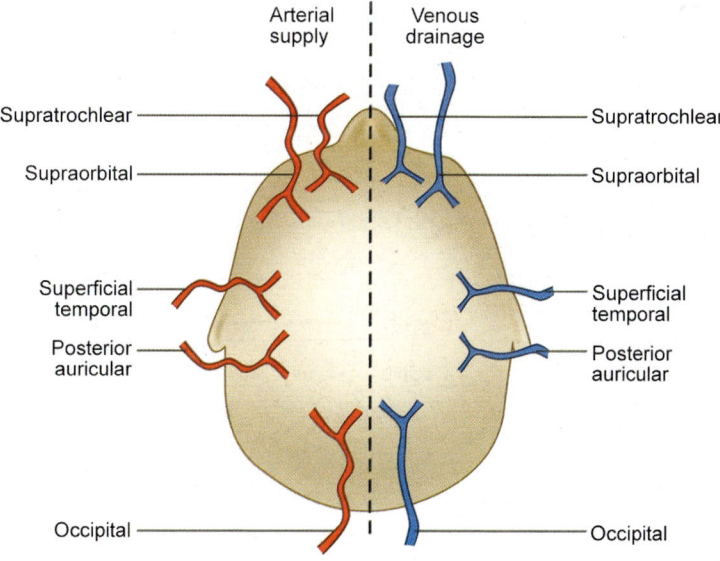

Blood supply of scalp

1. In front, scalp is supplied by:
   - Supratrochlear

- Ophthalmic artery—a branch of ICA
- Supraorbital
- Superficial temporal—a branch of ECA.

2. From behind scalp is supplied by:
- Occipital—branches from ECA
- Posterior auricular.

Veins run close to the arteries and have the same nomenclature.

## Lymphatic Drainage

Scalp drains anteriorly into preauricular lymph nodes and posteriorly into posterior auricular and occipital lymph nodes.

## Nerve Supply

Scalp is supplied by three sets of nerves; they are V nerve, VII nerve and cervical plexus:

1. *In front supplied by:*
- Supratrochlear
- Supraorbital
- Zygomaticotemporal
- Auriculotemporal
- Temporal branch of VII nerve.

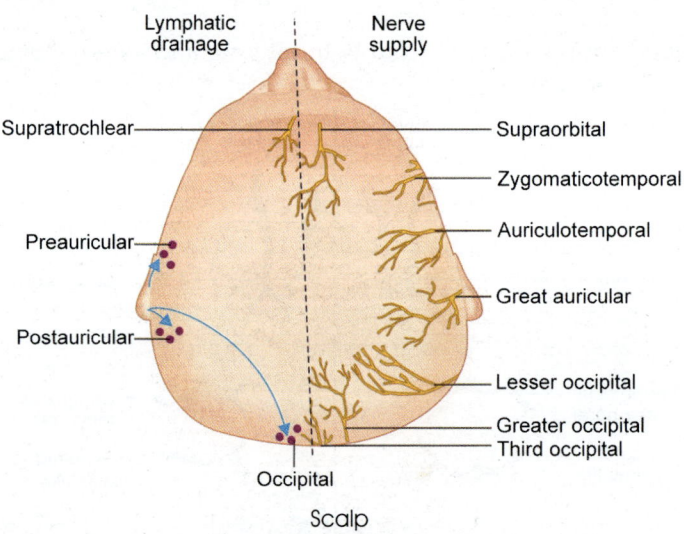

Scalp

2. *From behind supplied by:*
- Great auricular
- Lesser occipital
- Great occipital
- Third occipital
- Posterior auricular branch of VII nerve.

## Applied Anatomy

1. Sebaceous cysts are very common in scalp.
2. In cases of head injury, scalp wounds bleed profusely because the fibrous nature of superficial fascia inhibits the injured blood vessels from retracting. Scalp also has rich blood supply.
3. Loose areolar layer (IV layer) of scalp is known as danger area of scalp, because infection from the scalp may traverse through the emissary vein to the cranial venous sinuses.
4. Hematoma in loose areolar layer may easily spread to the eyelids giving rise to the formation of black eye.
5. From the surgical standpoint, the skin, connective tissue, aponeurosis is intimately united and should be regarded as single layer attached to the bone posteriorly and skin anteriorly. One can easily peel off the first three layers from the pericranium with the intervening loose connective tissue in between.
6. Veins of the scalp are in subcutaneous plane and intravenous infusions can be given through them.

### Q. Discuss sensory innervation of face.

**Ans.** Trigeminal nerve and cervical plexus carry the sensation from the face. It also supplies the nasal cavity, paranasal sinuses, eyeball, oral cavity, dura mater of anterior and middle cranial fossa. Trigeminal nerve has three divisions:

1. Ophthalmic
2. Maxillary
3. Mandibular.

The above branches innervate the face.

## Ophthalmic Division

Ophthalmic division gives five branches to supply upper part of face and scalp up to the vertex. The branches are:

- Supratrochlear
- Supraorbital
- Lacrimal
- External nasal
- Infratrochlear.

## Maxillary Division

Maxillary division gives three branches to supply middle part of face. The branches are:

1. Infraorbital
2. Zygomaticofacial
3. Zygomaticotemporal.

## Mandibular Division

Mandibular division supplies the lower part of face. The branches are:

- Auriculotemporal

- Buccal
- Mental.

## Cervical Plexus

The branches of cervical plexus supply the angle of jaw. The branches are:
- Great auricular nerve
- Transverse cutaneous nerve
- Lesser occipital nerve.

## Applied Anatomy

1. Headache is a common symptom in common cold, sinusitis or dental caries by virtue of common innervation.
2. Trigeminal neuralgia (tic douloureux) is a condition, wherein patient complain of lancinating pain incited by trivial factors like washing the face.

Surgery is required in the form of thermocoagulation or cryotherapy or direct section of roots of V nerve.

### Q. Discuss 'Lacrimal Apparatus'. Add a note on applied anatomy.

**Ans.** Lacrimal apparatus consists of structures involved in production and secretion of tear fluid. The components are:
- Lacrimal gland and its duct
- Conjunctival sac
- Lacrimal puncta and lacrimal canaliculi
- Nasolacrimal duct.

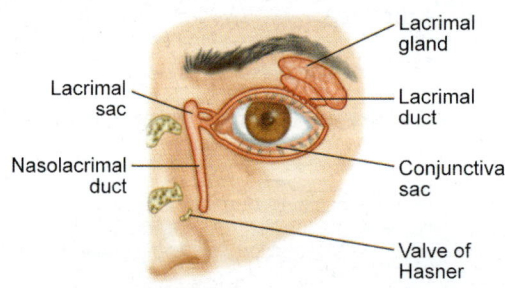

Components of lacrimal apparatus

## Lacrimal Gland

Lacrimal gland is a serous, exocrine gland located in the lacrimal fossa. It is 'J'-shaped, being indented by the tendon of levator palpebrae superioris muscle. Thus, it has two parts as orbital and palpebral. Ducts of the lacrimal gland open in the conjunctival sac. Gland is supplied by lacrimal nerve and lacrimal branch of ophthalmic artery.

## Conjunctival Sac

Conjunctival sac is a mucous membrane covering the inner surface of eyelids (palpebral part) and front of the eyeball (orbital part):

- Palpebral part is thick, opaque and highly vascular
- Bulbar part has two parts—one covering the sclera, which is thick, transparent and loosely attached to eyeball and another covering the cornea, which is thin and firmly attached.

Ophthalmic artery and lacrimal artery supply the sac. Supratrochlear and supraorbital nerves supply the upper part and infraorbital nerve supply the lower part of eyelid.

### Lacrimal Puncta and Canaliculi

Puncta is a small opening in the conjunctival sac, which leads into canaliculus. Canaliculus has a vertical and horizontal part, with the dilated part ampulla at the bend. Both the canaliculi open into lacrimal sac.

### Lacrimal Sac

Lacrimal sac is a membranous sac, lodged in lacrimal groove just behind the medial palpebral ligament. It opens below into the nasolacrimal duct.

### Nasolacrimal Duct

Nasolacrimal duct is membranous passage approximately 1.5 cm in length directed downwards, backwards and laterally and opens into inferior meatus and guarded by valve known as valve of Hasner.

### Applied Anatomy

1. Conjunctivitis is one of the commonest diseases of eye.
2. Inflammation of lacrimal sac is known as dacryocystitis. It causes excessive watering of eyes and pus discharge on pressing the sac. Long-lasting ailment is treated by dacryocystorhinostomy (DCR), endoscopic method is in vogue (endoscopic DCR).
3. Syringing is an OPD procedure to check the patency of canaliculi and sac.

**Q. Describe the arrangement of deep cervical fascia and the various neck spaces.**

**Ans.** Deep fascia of the neck has three layers:
1. Investing layer
2. Pretracheal layer
3. Prevertebral layer.

### Investing Layer

As the name suggests, it invests the structures on its way (resembles a polo neck T-shirt).

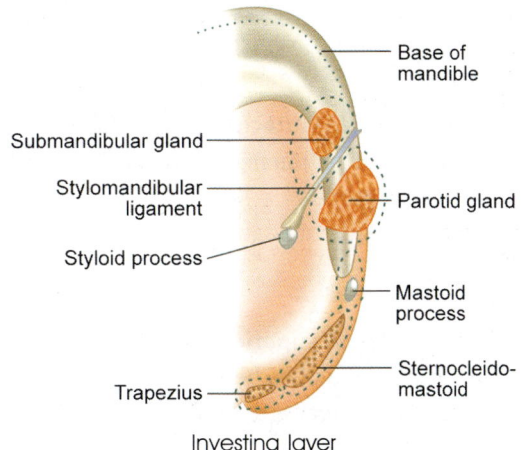

Investing layer

*Attachments*

- *Superiorly:* External occipital protuberance, superior nuchal line, mastoid process, base of mandible
- *Inferiorly:* Spine of scapula, acromion process clavicle, manubrium
- *Anteriorly:* Symphysis menti, hyoid bone
- *Posteriorly:* Spine of C7 vertebra.

*Special Features*

- It forms two extra spaces, suprasternal and supraclavicular
- It forms two extra pulleys to bind the tendon of digastric and omohyoid
- It encloses two muscles, trapezius and sternocleidomastoid muscles
- It encloses two glands, parotid and submandibular gland.

## Pretracheal Fascia

Pretracheal fascia encloses the thyroid gland.

*Attachments*

- *Superiorly:* Hyoid bone, oblique line of thyroid cartilage and cricoid cartilage
- *Inferiorly:* It blends with adventitia of inferior thyroid veins and aorta
- *On each side:* It blends with carotid sheath.

*Special Features*

- On either side of the thyroid gland the fascia is thick, forming the so-called suspensory ligament of Berry
- Thyroid gland moves during deglutition by virtue of its attachment to hyoid bone, thyroid cartilage superiorly and inferiorly to the adventitia of great vessels.

## Prevertebral Fascia

Prevertebral fascia lies in front of muscles of vertebra and forms the floor of posterior triangle of the neck.

*Attachments*

- Superiorly, it is attached to the base of skull
- Inferiorly, it is attached to the body of third and fourth thoracic vertebra
- On either side, it is attached deep to trapezius.

*Special Features*

- It continues in superior mediastinum
- Brachial plexus lies behind the fascia
- Subclavian artery is covered by fascia known as axillary sheath.

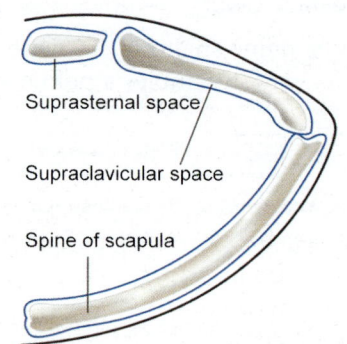

Suprasternal space

Supraclavicular space

Spine of scapula

Investing layer of deep cervical fascia

## Applied Anatomy

1. Parotitis is very painful because the parotid fascia is thick and unyielding in nature and also it sends thick septa into substance of gland.
2. Neck infections are very common; secondary to dental infections. Since, the spaces are inter-connected and extend up to mediastinum, a dental infection may spread into mediastinum and lead to death.
3. Division of external jugular vein may lead to air embolism and death, since vein lies outside the axillary sheath and prevented from retraction.

## Neck Spaces

The arrangement of deep cervical fascia is such that it gives rise to 11 potential spaces. These spaces communicate with each other as a result of which infection in one space can spread to another. Few important spaces are discussed below.

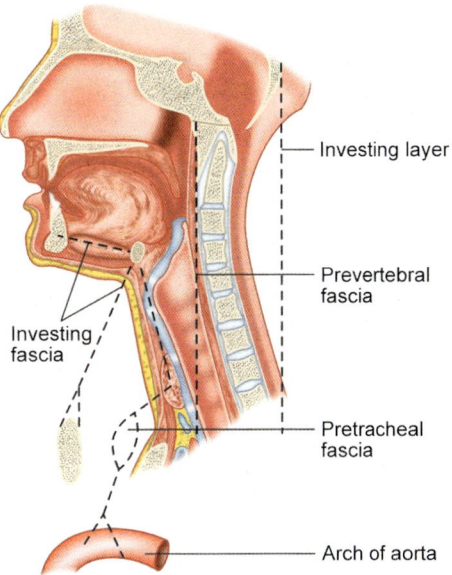

Layers of deep fascia of the neck

## Parapharyngeal Space

Parapharyngeal space (lateral pharyngeal space, pterygomaxillary space, pterygopharyngeal space). This space is located above the hyoid bone (suprahyoid space). It extends from base of skull to lesser cornu of hyoid bone. Important posterolateral relation is carotid sheath.

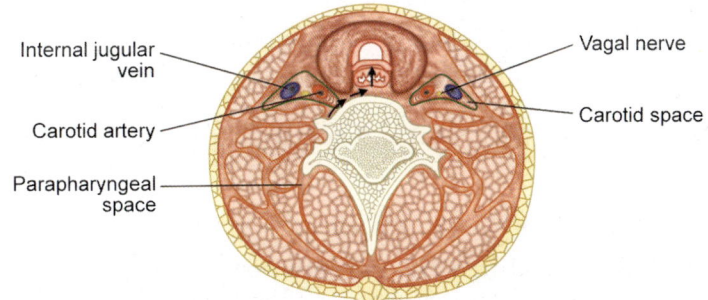

Transverse section of parapharyngeal space

### Communications

- Anteriorly communicates with submaxillary and submandibular space
- Posteriorly communicates with retropharyngeal space and hence to prevertebral space.

### Parotid Space

1. It lies between superficial and deep capsules of parotid gland.
2. The superficial capsule is thick and adherent to underlying parotid gland. There are multiple septae running from lateral capsule into gland itself. Medial capsule is thin and cuts around the lateral pharyngeal space.
3. Infection tends to spread medially into lateral pharyngeal space.

## Submandibular Space

Mylohyoid muscle splits the submandibular space into sublingual and submaxillary.

**Communications**

Submandibular space communicates with parapharyngeal space.

## Masticator Space

Masticator space is formed by splitting of superficial layers of deep cervical fascia. It encloses mandible and muscles of mastication.

**Communications**

Masticator space communicates superiorly with deep temporal space.

Temporalis muscle

Superficial temporal space

Parapharyngeal space

Sublingual space

Submaxillary space

Mylohyoid muscle

## Retropharyngeal Space

1. It lies between prevertebral fascia and buccopharyngeal fascia. An ancillary portion of deep cervical fascia divides it into danger space, i.e. prevertebral space proper and retropharyngeal space.
2. It extends from skull to second thoracic vertebra, i.e. posterior mediastinum. It is divided into two lateral compartments by median raphe.

**Communications**

Retropharyngeal space communicates with prevertebral and parapharyngeal space.

## Applied Anatomy

- Deep neck space infections are secondary to dental infections most commonly
- A neck infection can spread to mediastinum by virtue of its communications.

> **Q. What are the boundaries, floor, roof and contents of posterior triangle of neck? What is its clinical significance?**

## Divisions of Triangle of the Neck

**Ans.** Side of the neck is divided into anterior and posterior triangles by the key muscle-sternocleidomastoid. Area in front of it is anterior triangle and behind it is posterior triangle.

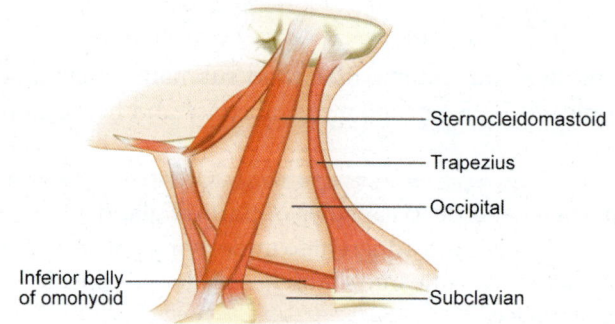

Sternocleidomastoid

Trapezius

Occipital

Inferior belly of omohyoid

Subclavian

Divisions of triangles of the neck

## Boundaries

- *Anteriorly:* Posterior border of sternocleidomastoid
- *Posteriorly:* Anterior border of trapezius
- *Base:* Middle one-third of clavicle
- *Apex:* Meeting of sternocleidomastoid and trapezius.

## Roof

Roof is formed by the investing layer of deep cervical fascia. Following structures are present in the roof:

1. Skin, platysma, cutaneous nerves namely:
   - Lesser occipital nerve
   - Great auricular nerve
   - Anterior cutaneous nerves
   - Supraclavicular nerves.
2. Cutaneous arteries
3. External jugular vein
4. Lymphatics.

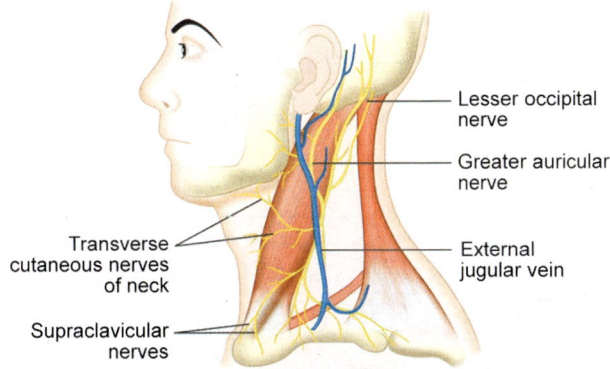

Nerves innervating the roof of posterior triangle

## Floor

The floor is formed by muscles covered by prevertebral fascia. Following structures form the floor.

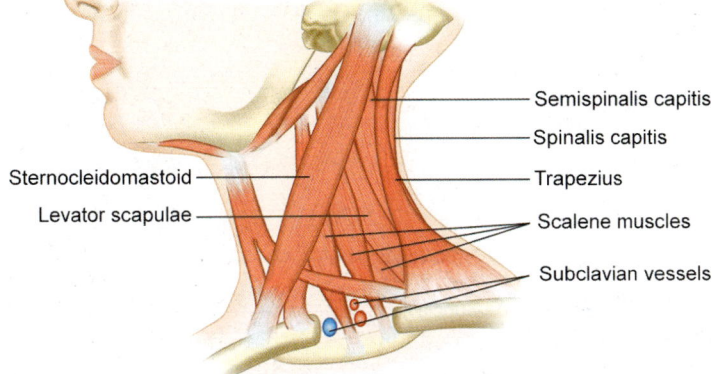

Muscles of the floor of posterior triangle

*Muscles*

- Semispinalis capitis
- Scalenus medius
- Splenius capitis
- Levator scapulae.

*Nerves*

- Spinal accessory
- Nerve to subclavius
- Nerve to trapezius
- Nerve to rhomboids
- Trunks of brachial plexus
- Nerve to serratus anterior
- Suprascapular.

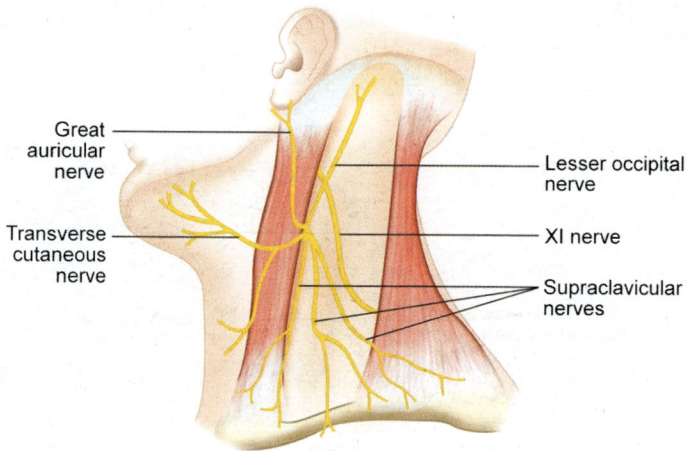

Nerves in posterior triangle

*Vessels*

- Transverse cervical
- Suprascapular
- Occipital
- Subclavian.

*Lymph Nodes*

Posterior triangle nodes.

### Applied Anatomy

1. Left-sided supraclavicular lymph nodes are enlarged in malignancies of stomach, testis known as Virchow's nodes.

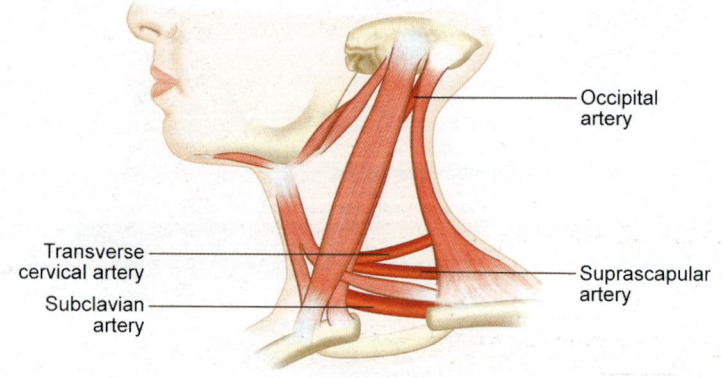

Vessels in posterior triangle

2. Spasm of sternocleidomastoid is known as wryneck.
3. In neck dissections for malignancies, certain groups of lymph nodes are removed. Spinal accessory nerve may get injured, while removing the nodes. Injury to this nerve may lead to drooping of shoulder and requires postoperative rehabilitation.

### Q. What are the boundaries, floor, roof and contents of suboccipital triangle of neck? What is its clinical significance?

Suboccipital triangle is a muscular space in the deepest plane of nape of the neck. To reach the triangle, one needs to expose the following layers from outside:

- Skin
- Superficial fascia
- Trapezius
- Splenius capitis
- Semispinalis capitis.

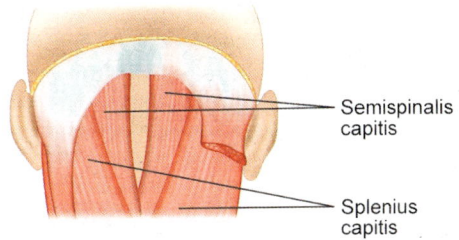

Muscles covering the suboccipital triangle

### Boundaries

- Superomedially—rectus capitis posterior minor and major
- *Superolaterally:* Superior oblique
- *Inferiorly:* Inferior oblique.

### Roof

- Semispinalis capitis medially
- Longissimus capitis laterally.

### Floor

- Posterior arch of atlas
- Atlanto-occipital membrane.

### Contents

- Dorsal ramus of C1
- Third part of vertebral artery
- Suboccipital plexus of veins.

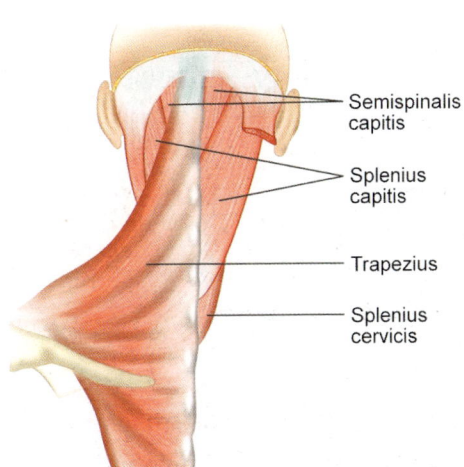

Suboccipital triangle

*Surgical Significance*

Posterior cranial fossa can be approached via suboccipital triangle for cisternal puncture.

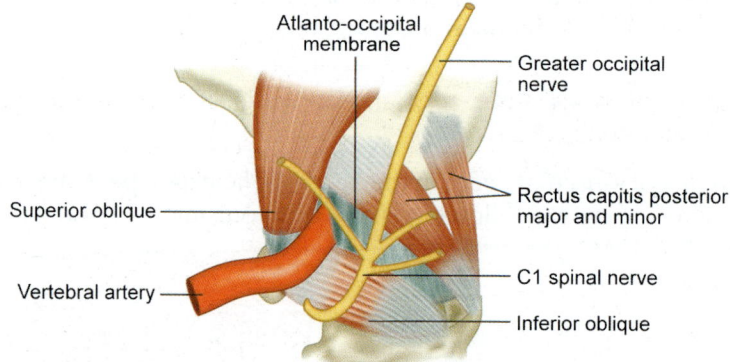

Contents of suboccipital triangle

**Ans.** Venous sinuses are the venous spaces between two layers of dura mater. Unlike veins they have no valves and no muscular coat.

## Classification

Venous sinuses can be classified as paired and unpaired sinuses.

*Paired Sinuses*

- Cavernous
- Superior petrosal
- Inferior petrosal
- Transverse
- Sigmoid
- Sphenoparietal.

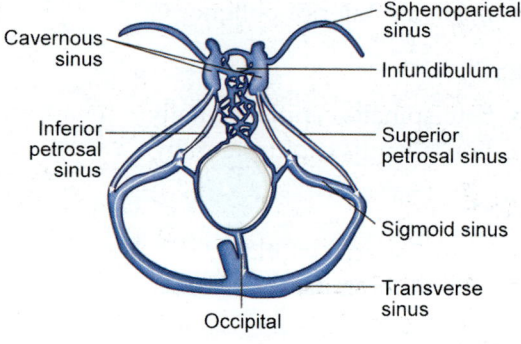

Paired venous sinuses

*Unpaired Sinuses*

- Superior sagittal
- Inferior sagittal
- Straight
- Occipital
- Anterior intercavernous
- Posterior intercavernous.

## Arrangement of Sinuses and Drainage Pattern

Arrangement and drainage pattern are shown in the figure below.

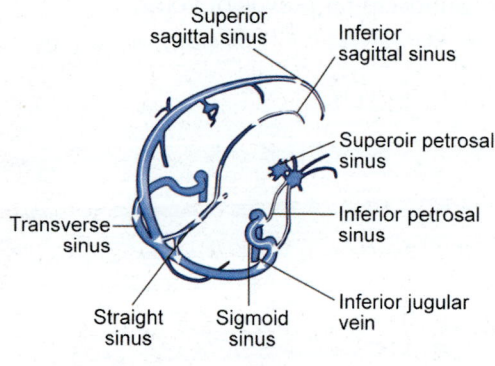

Unpaired venous sinuses

## Cavernous Sinus

Cavernous sinus is a large venous sinus located on either side of pituitary fossa, forming a very crucial location.

*Extent:* Anteriorly, it extends up to the medial end of superior orbital fissure and posteriorly, it extends up to the petrous temporal.

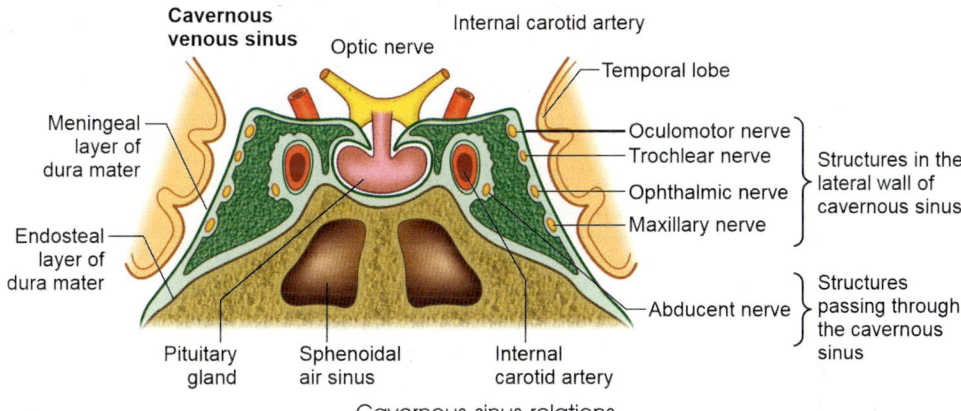

Cavernous sinus relations

*Relations*
- *Superiorly:* Optic tract, internal carotid artery
- *Inferiorly:* Foramen lacerum
- *Medially:* Hypophysis cerebri and sphenoidal air sinus
- *Laterally:* Temporal lobe
- *Anteriorly:* Superior orbital fissure
- *Posteriorly:* Apex of petrous temporal.
  Structures in the lateral wall and the cranial nerves are shown in the figure above.

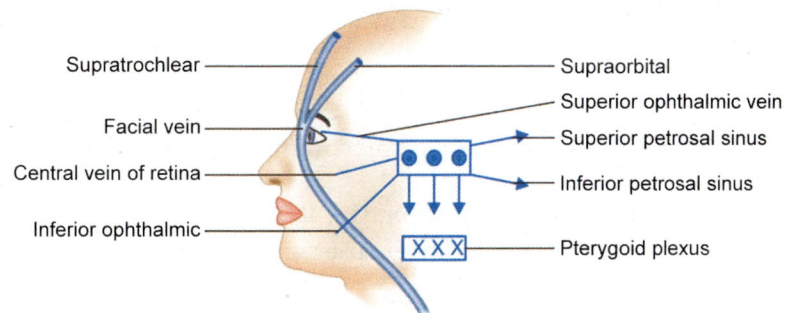

Tributaries of cavernous sinus

*Draining channels and communications of cavernous sinus*
1. Cavernous sinus receives the superior ophthalmic vein, central vein of retina, inferior ophthalmic vein, sphenoparietal sinus.
2. It drains into transverse sinus, internal jugular vein, pterygoid plexus of veins, facial vein.
3. The two sinuses communicate with each other anteriorly and posteriorly.
4. All the communications are valveless and the blood can flow in either directions.

## Superior Sagittal Sinus

Superior sagittal sinus is located on the superior border of falx cerebri.

### Extent

Superior sagittal sinus begins at crista galli, here it communicates with veins of frontal sinus and veins of nose. It ends at internal occipital protuberance by turning to the right and becomes continuous as right transverse sinus.

### Communications

Superior sagittal sinus communicates with superior cerebral veins, and veins from the nose and parietal emissary veins.

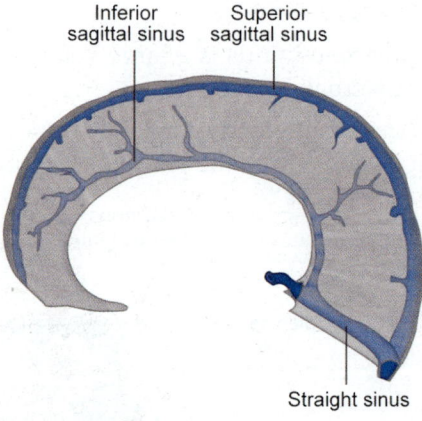

Superior, inferior and straight sinuses

## Inferior Sagittal Sinus

Inferior sagittal sinus lies on the concave free margin of falx cerebri. It ends at the middle of anterior free margin of tentorium cerebelli by ending in great cerebral vein to form straight sinus.

## Straight Sinus

Straight sinus is formed by the union of inferior sagittal sinus with great cerebral vein.

## Transverse Sinus

Right transverse sinus is a continuation of superior sagittal sinus and left is the continuation of straight sinus.

## Sigmoid Sinus

Sigmoid sinus is the continuation of transverse sinus and extends from posteroinferior angle of the parietal bone to the jugular foramen, where it continues as internal jugular vein.

### Applied Anatomy

- Thrombosis (block) of sigmoid sinus occurs most commonly secondary to otitis media or mastoiditis
- Cavernous sinus thrombosis may occur secondary to infection in 'danger area of face'
- During mastoid operations one should not expose sigmoid sinus.

> **Q. Describe the gross anatomy of parotid gland, its relations, blood supply, nerve supply and lymphatic drainage. Add a note on its applied anatomy.**

**Ans.** Parotid gland is the largest of the salivary gland located below external acoustic meatus and between ramus of mandible and sternocleidomastoid.

### Gross Features

Gland resembles inverted pyramid and has following parts:
- Apex

- Base
- Surfaces—superficial, anteromedial and posteromedial
- Borders—anterior, posterior, medial
- Parotid capsule—gland is covered by the investing layer of deep cervical fascia, which is thick and adherent.

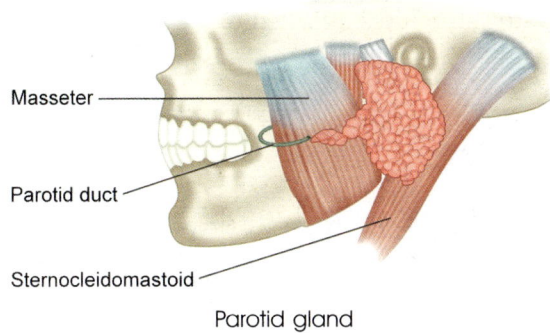

Parotid gland

## Relations

### Apex

Apex is related to posterior belly of digastric muscle, cervical branch of VII nerve and retromandibular vein.

### Base

Base lies just below external auditory meatus:
- Related to temporomandibular joint
- Superficial temporal vessels
- Auriculotemporal nerve.

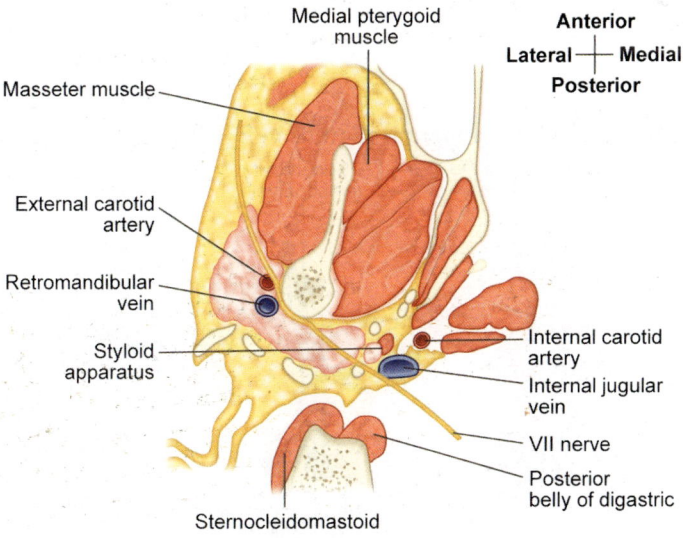

Cross-sectional relations of parotid gland

## Surfaces

*Superficial surface:* It is covered with skin, superficial fascia, deep cervical fascia, lymph nodes.

*Anteromedial surface:* It is related to mandible and thus related to the muscles attached.

*Posteromedial surface:* It is related to mastoid and styloid process and thus, the structures attached to it.

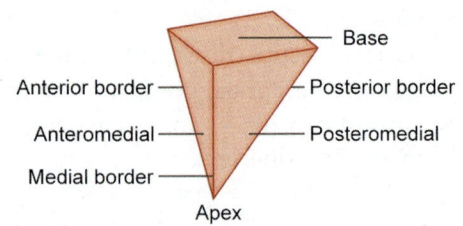

Surfaces of parotid gland (as seen from medial side)

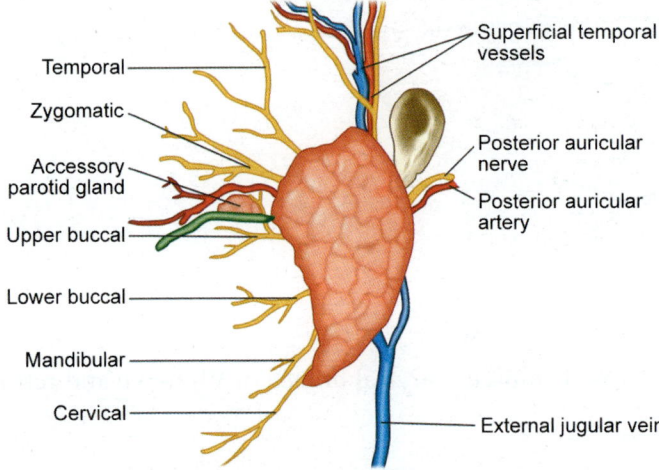

Neurovascular relations of parotid gland

### Structures Within the Parotid Gland

The structures within the parotid gland are as follows:
- External carotid artery (it enters the gland through the posteromedial surface)
- Retromandibular vein
- Facial nerve.

### Blood Supply

External carotid artery (ECA) and external jugular vein (EJV).

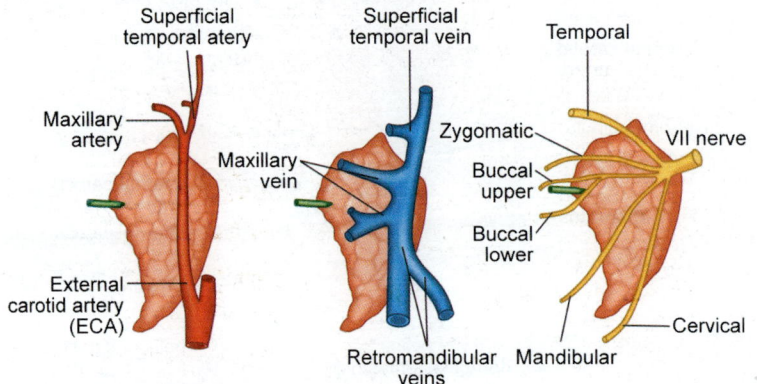

Structures piercing the parotid gland

## Lymphatic Drainage

Drains into parotid nodes within the substance of the gland and then to the upper deep cervical nodes.

## Nerve Supply

Parasympathetic nerves are secretomotor to gland:
- Sympathetic nerve-derived from plexus around ECA
- Sensory nerve-derived from auriculotemporal nerve and great auricular nerve
- Angle of mandible is supplied by great auricular nerve.

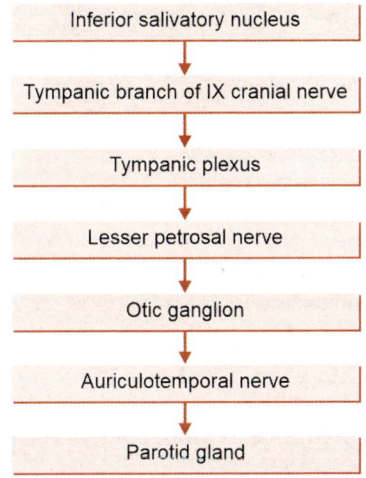

Secretomotor pathway to parotid gland

## Applied Anatomy

- Parotid swellings, i.e. parotitis is extremely painful due to thick and adherent parotid fascia
- Conley's cartilaginous pointer—by pulling the pinna backwards, tragus points at a place from where the facial nerve is 1–1.5 cm deep
- Frey's syndrome—in cases of injury to auriculotemporal nerve, the nerve grows aberrantly to anastomose with superior cervical ganglion fibres (it is an anastomosis between sympathetic and parasympathetic fibres).
  In this condition, while chewing there is redness and sweating over the parotid region.

### Q. Discuss cervical lymph nodes and add a note on its clinical significance.

There are approximately 800 lymph nodes in the body out of which 300 are in the neck.

## Superficial Cervical Lymph Nodes

Superficial cervical lymph nodes are classified according to the region they are present in the form of circular chain as follows:
- Occipital
- Submandibular
- Posterior auricular
- Submental

- Preauricular
- Superficial cervical
- Parotid
- Anterior cervical
- Facial.

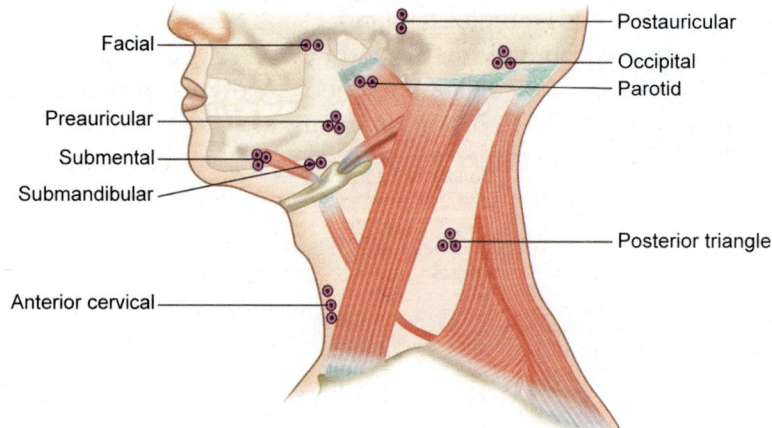

Superficial cervical lymph node grouping

*Drainage Area*

1. Occipital drains the back of the scalp.
2. Posterior auricular drains the temporal region, back of the pinna, external auditory meatus.

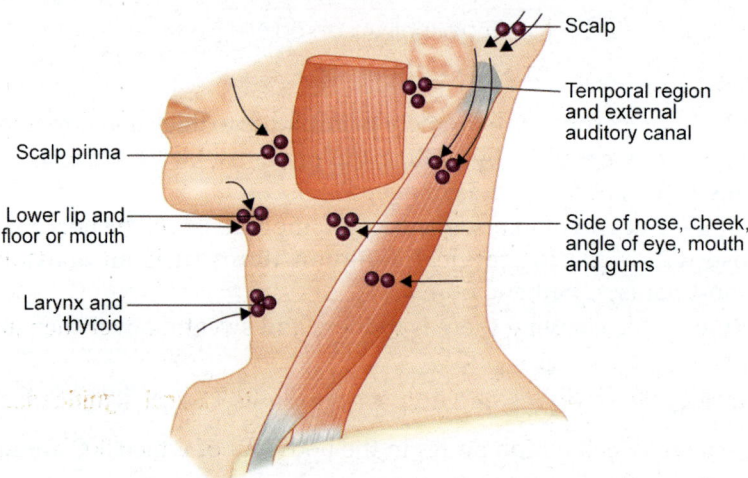

Drainage areas of superficial cervical lymph nodes

3. Preauricular nodes drains the outer side of pinna and side of scalp.
4. Parotid nodes located in the substance of the gland drain the eyelids, front of scalp, external auditory meatus and tympanic cavity, while the nodes deep to the gland drain the nasopharynx and nose.
5. Superficial facial nodes receive lymph from conjunctiva, eyelids, nose and cheek. Deep facial nodes drain the temporal fossa, infratemporal fossa, back of the nose and pharynx.

6. Submandibular nodes drain the side of the nose, cheek, angle of eye and mouth, upper lip, gums and side of tongue.
7. Submental nodes drain the central part of the lower lip and floor of the mouth.
8. Superficial cervical nodes drain the parotid region and the lower part of the ear.
9. Anterior cervical nodes drain the larynx and thyroid.
   All the superficial lymph nodes drain into deep cervical lymph nodes.

## Applied Anatomy

1. Malignancies are staged according to the involvement of the lymph nodes.
2. In radical neck dissections, lymph nodes are cleared according to the level of involvement.

*Following are the levels of lymph nodes.*
Level I: Submental and submandibular nodes.
Level II: Upper cervical nodes.
Level III: Middle cervical nodes.
Level IV: Lower cervical nodes.
Level V: Posterior triangle nodes.
Level VI: Pretracheal and prelaryngeal nodes.
Level VII: Mediastinal nodes.

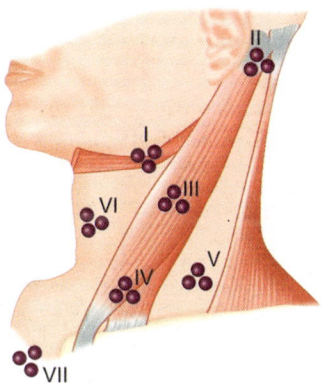

Superficial divisions of cervical lymph nodes

## Deep Cervical Lymph Nodes

All the deep cervical lymph nodes receive lymph from superficial cervical lymph nodes.

### Location

Deep cervical lymph nodes form a vertical chain along the internal jugular vein.

### Classification

Deep cervical lymph nodes are grouped as jugulodigastric, jugulo-omohyoid and supraclavicular lymph nodes.

### Drainage Area

1. Jugulodigastric nodes mainly drain the tonsils.
2. Jugulo-omohyoid mainly drains the tongue.

3. Supraclavicular lymph nodes receive the lymph from preceding nodes. Additionally, left side receives lymph from pelvic viscera (ovaries, testis) and breast.

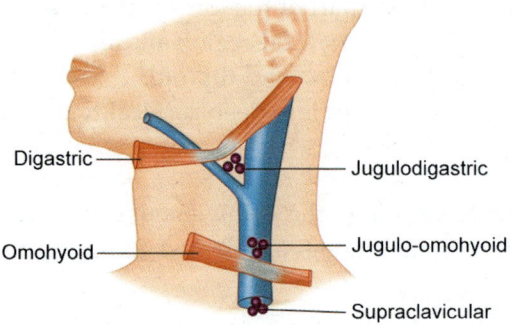

*Applied Anatomy*

Enlarged left supraclavicular lymph nodes are known as Virchow's nodes.

---

**Q. Describe facial nerve in detail (functional components nuclei, course, branches and applied anatomy).**

**Ans.** Facial nerve is the VII cranial nerve, which supplies the muscles of the face, salivary glands (submandibular and sublingual) and lacrimal gland and carries sensation of taste from anterior two-thirds of tongue.

Embryologically facial nerve is the nerve of second branchial arch.

## Nuclei

There are four nuclei of facial nerve, located in lower pons are as follows:
- Motor nucleus
- Superior salivatory nucleus
- Lacrimatory nucleus
- Nucleus of tractus solitarius.

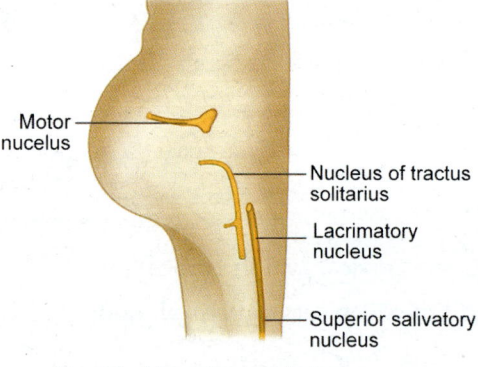

Nuclei of facial nerve in lower pons

## Functional Components

- Special visceral afferent—for taste
- General visceral efferent—secretomotor for glands
- General somatic afferent—proprioception and general sensation from external auditory canal
- Branchial efferent—for facial muscles.

## Course

The course of the facial nerve is divided into three parts:
1. Intracranial
2. Intrapetrous (intratympanic part)
3. Extracranial.

## Intracranial Part

The nerve begins at lower pons from two distinct roots—motor and sensory. The motor root winds the abducent nerve nuclei and emerges from lower border of pons to lie in the cerebellopontine angle.

It runs laterally and forwards to reach the internal acoustic meatus (IAM). In the meatus, motor root lies over the auditory nerve with intervening sensory root; accompanied by labyrinthine vessels.

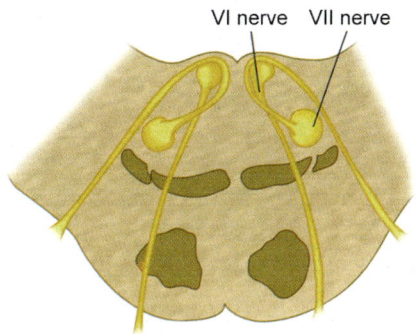

VI nerve    VII nerve

Transverse section at lower pons

## Intrapetrous Part

In the intrapetrous part, the nerve runs in the bony canal known as fallopian canal with a sigmoid course. It has three parts:

1. One part is on top of vestibule-labyrinthine part A
2. Another part is closely related to the middle ear cavity-tympanic part B
3. The third part is vertically related to mastoid cavity-mastoid part C.

The point at which the nerve takes a sharp turn posteriorly lies the geniculate ganglion.

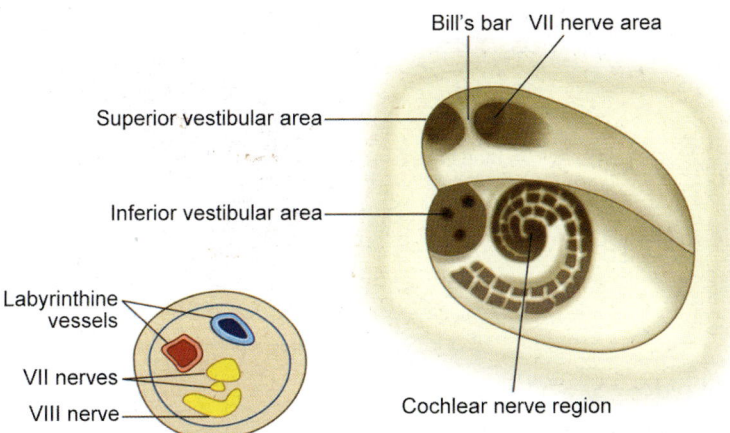

Bill's bar   VII nerve area

Superior vestibular area

Inferior vestibular area

Labyrinthine vessels

VII nerves

VIII nerve

Cochlear nerve region

Internal acoustic meatus (IAM) with its structure

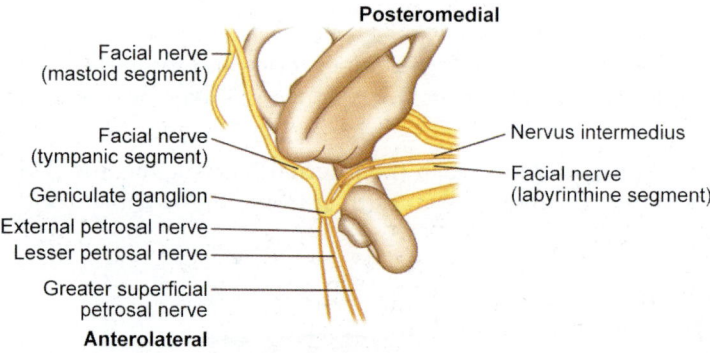

**Posteromedial**

Facial nerve (mastoid segment)

Facial nerve (tympanic segment)

Geniculate ganglion

External petrosal nerve

Lesser petrosal nerve

Greater superficial petrosal nerve

**Anterolateral**

Nervus intermedius

Facial nerve (labyrinthine segment)

Intratemporal part of VII nerve

## Extracranial Part

Extracranial part leaves the skull through stylomastoid foramen; crosses laterally, the base of styloid process, enters the posteromedial surface of parotid gland, crosses the retromandibular vein and external carotid artery and divides behind the neck of mandible into five terminal branches.

## Branches

- Greater superficial petrosal nerve
- Branch to stapedius
- Chorda tympani nerve
- Posterior auricular

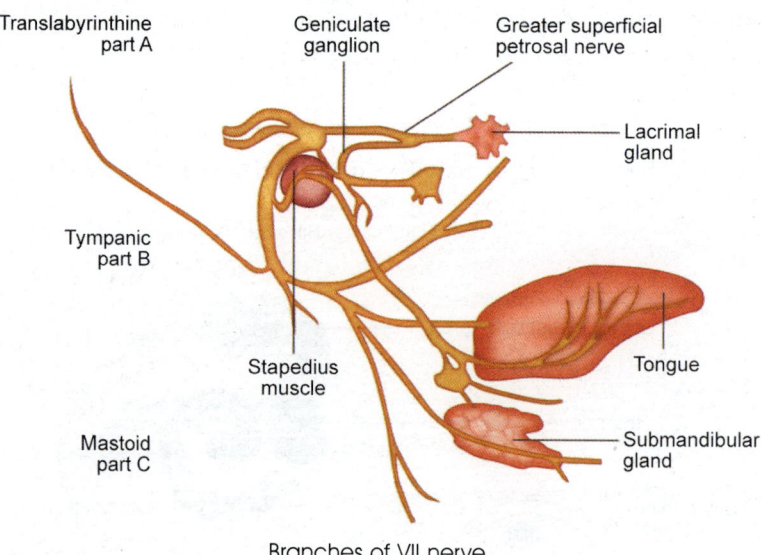

Translabyrinthine part A

Geniculate ganglion

Greater superficial petrosal nerve

Lacrimal gland

Tympanic part B

Stapedius muscle

Tongue

Mastoid part C

Submandibular gland

Branches of VII nerve

- Nerve to stylohyoid
- Nerve to digastric (posterior)
- Temporal, zygomatic, buccal, mandibular, cervical.

## Applied Anatomy

- Lesion of VII nerve in middle ear does not affect lacrimation, but affects stapedial reflex, submandibular gland secretion and taste function.
- Lesion in vertical course of VII nerve in mastoid segment, will cause decreased taste sensation and submandibular secretion however, lacrimation and stapedial reflex would be normal.

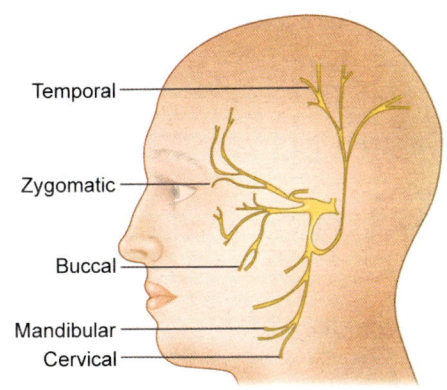

Extracranial branches of VII nerve

**Q. What are the muscles of mastication? Describe their attachments, nerve supply and action.**

**Ans.** There are four pairs of muscles of mastication, which bring about jaw movements. They are as follows:
1. Masseter
2. Temporalis
3. Lateral pterygoid
4. Medial pterygoid.

### Masseter

*Attachments*

*From*
Zygomatic arch.

*To*
Lateral surface of ramus mandible and coronoid process.

*Nerve Supply*
Masseteric nerve.

*Action*
Closes the mandible.

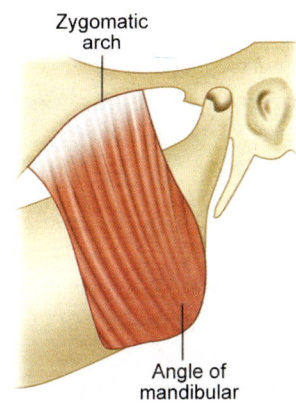

Masseter muscle attachment

### Temporalis

*Attachments*

*From*
Temporal fossa and temporalis fascia.

*To*
Coronoid process of mandible.

*Nerve Supply*
Mandibular nerve.

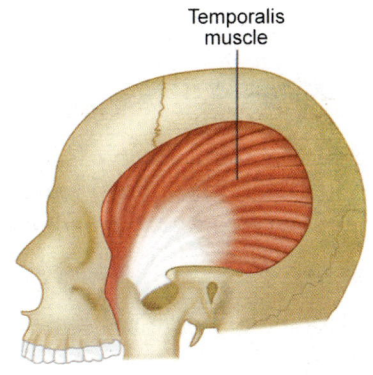

Temporalis muscle attachment

*Action*
Closes the jaw, retracts the mandible behind and helps in side-to-side chewing movements.

## Lateral Pterygoid

*Attachments*

*From*
Greater wing of sphenoid and lateral surface of lateral pterygoid plate.

*To*
Pterygoid fovea, articular disk and capsule of temporomandibular (TM) joint.

*Nerve Supply*
Mandibular nerve.

*Action*
Opens the mouth.

## Medial Pterygoid

*Attachments*

*From*
Tuberosity of maxilla medial surface of lateral pterygoid plate.

*To*
Medial surface of angle and ramus of mandible.

*Nerve Supply*
Mandibular nerve.

*Action*
Elevates the mandible.

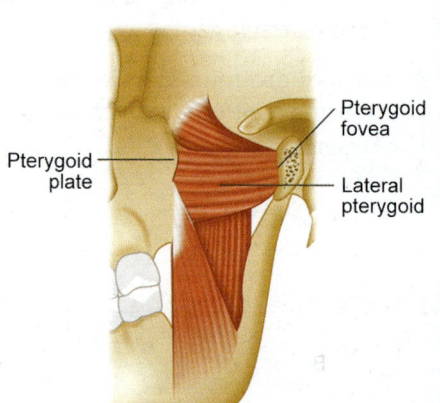

Pterygoid muscle

## Applied Anatomy

Trismus may occur due to fibrosis of muscles of mastication giving rise to dysphagia.

### Q. Describe mandibular nerve.

**Ans.** Mandibular nerve is largest of the three divisions of trigeminal nerve. It supplies teeth, gums, skin in temporal region, auricle, lower lip, lower part of face, muscles of mastication and mucosa of tongue and oral floor.

## Roots

Mandibular nerve has two roots, i.e. sensory and motor.

## Relations

- Motor root lies deep to sensory root
- Both unite just distal to foramen ovale

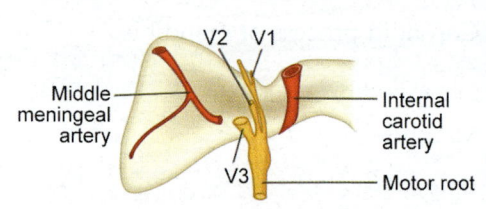

Root of mandibular nerve

• After emerging from foramen ovale, the nerve lies between tensor veli palatini and lateral pterygoid muscle.

## Branches

### From the Trunk

• Meningeal branch (also known as nervous spinosus) supplies dura mater of middle cranial fossa
• Nerve to medial pterygoid.

### From Anterior Trunk

All are muscular branches namely masseter, deep temporal, nerve to lateral pterygoid except buccal nerve, which is sensory.

### From Posterior Trunk

• Auriculotemporal
• Lingual nerve

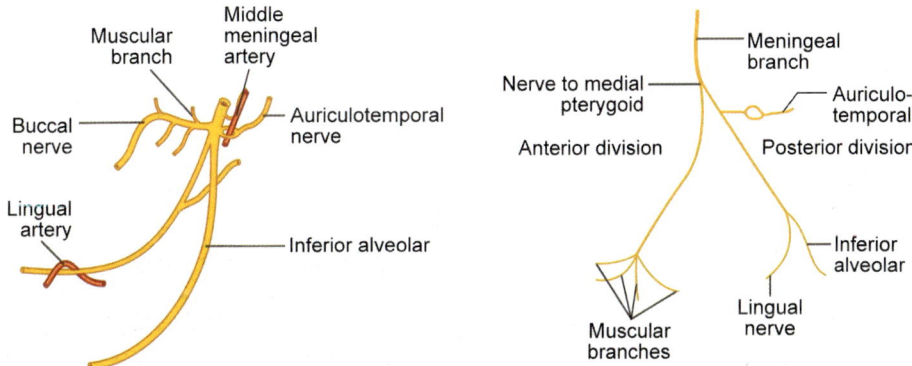

Branches of mandibular nerve

• Inferior alveolar.
  Auriculotemporal nerve forms a loop around middle meningeal artery.

## Applied Anatomy

In cases of cancer tongue, pain is referred to ear over the area of distribution of auriculotemporal nerve.

> **Q. What is the origin, course, relations and branches of maxillary artery. Mention its surgical importance.**

**Ans.** Maxillary artery is one of the terminal branches of external carotid artery at the neck of the mandible.

## Course

For simplicity, the artery is divided into three parts as follows:
*I part:* Horizontal part, which is proximal to lateral pterygoid

*II part:* It lies sometimes superficial or deep to lateral pterygoid

*III part:* It lies between the two heads of lateral pterygoid muscle and enters pterygopalatine fossa through pterygopalatine fissure.

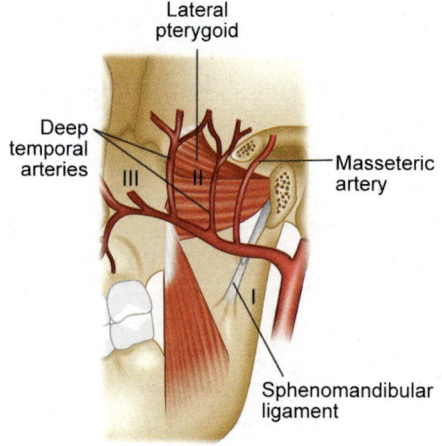

Parts of maxillary artery

## Relations

*I part:* It lies between neck of mandible and sphenomandibular ligament

*II part:* It lies either above or below lateral pterygoid

*III part:* It lies in front of pterygopalatine ganglion.

## Branches

*I part:*
- Deep auricular
- Anterior tympanic
- Middle meningeal
- Accessory meningeal
- Inferior alveolar.

*II part:*
- Deep temporal
- Pterygoid
- Masseteric
- Buccal.

*III part:*
- Posterior superior alveolar
- Infraorbital
- Greater palatine
- Pharyngeal
- Artery of pterygoid canal
- Sphenopalatine artery.

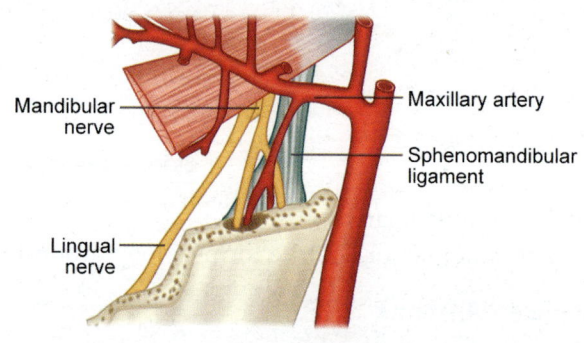

Maxillary artery

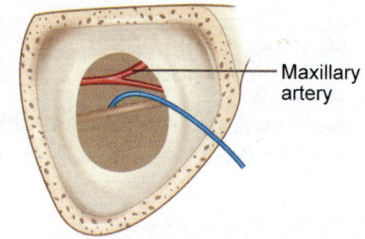

Transantral approach to maxillary artery

## Surgical Aspects

- Maxillary artery can be approached transantrally
- Maxillary artery ligation is indicated in transantral approach to maxillary artery (tie) cases of recurrent epistaxis (bleeding through nose).

**Q. Discuss temporomandibular joint in detail.**

### Ans. Types

- Synovial joint, condylar
- Complex variety (disc divides the joint cavity into 2 parts)

## Articular Surfaces

- *Above:* Anterior part of mandibular fossa
- *Below:* Head of mandible.

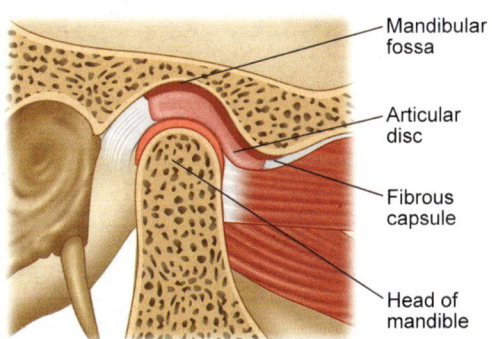

Articulating surfaces of temporomandibular joint

## Ligaments

1. *Fibrous capsule:* It is attached above around mandibular fossa and squamotympanic fissure, below to the posterolateral aspect of the neck of the mandible.
2. Fibrous capsule is thickened laterally to form lateral ligament; attached above to the zygomatic process of temporal bone and articular tubercle and below to lateral side of neck of mandible (inverted triangle in shape).
3. *Articular disc:* It is a fibrous plate dividing the joint into upper and lower compartment and is fused with capsule.
4. *Sphenomandibular ligament:* Attached superiorly to the spine of sphenoid and inferiorly to lingula of mandible.
5. *Stylomandibular ligament:* It is a thickened portion of deep cervical fascia (above ligaments 4, 5 hardly contribute to the strength of joint).

   Strength of the joint is maintained by the muscles of mastication.

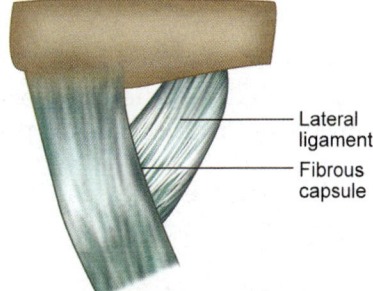

Ligaments of temporomandibular joint

## Relations

Temporomandibular joint is surrounded by parotid gland externally and internally related to spine of sphenoid.

This spine is related laterally to lateral pterygoid muscle, auriculotemporal nerve, maxillary artery; medially to medial pterygoid muscle and chorda tympani nerve.

## Actions

- Depression is brought about by lateral pterygoid and other strap muscles assist depression
- Elevation is brought about by medial pterygoid, masseter and temporalis
- Protrusion is brought about by pterygoids
- Retraction is brought about by temporalis
- Side-by-side movement brought about by pterygoids.

## Nerve Supply

- Auriculotemporal nerve
- Masseteric nerve.

## Blood Supply

Superficial temporal and maxillary artery.

## Applied Anatomy

Temporomandibular joint arthritis may cause difficulty in opening the mouth, i.e. trismus.

---

**Q. Describe the gross anatomy of submandibular gland, its relations, blood supply, nerve supply and lymphatic drainage. Add a note on its applied anatomy.**

**Ans.** Submandibular gland is a relatively small (half the size of parotid gland) mixed salivary gland, located below the mandible (hence the name).

## Gross Anatomy

Submandibular gland is divided into two parts by mylohyoid muscle:
- Superficial part
- Deep part.
  Superficial part lies between body of mandible and mylohyoid muscle. The deep part lies deep to mylohyoid muscle and superficial to hyoglossus.

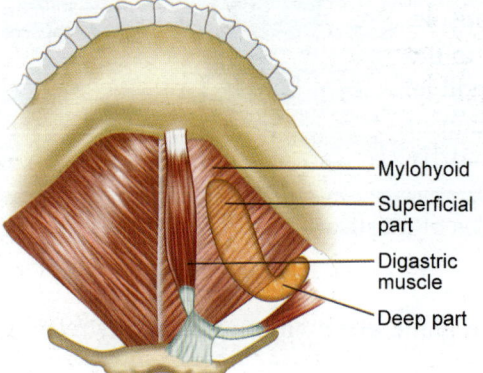

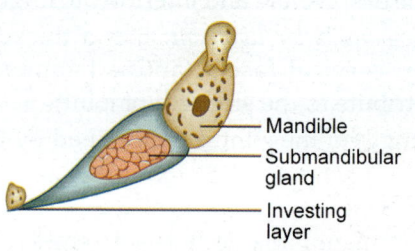

*Superficial Part Surfaces*

Inferior surface, lateral surface and medial surface.

*Deep Part Surfaces*

Lateral surface, medial surface.

### Relations of Superficial Part

- It is partially enclosed between two layers of investing cervical fascia
- *Inferior surface:* Skin, platysma, cervical branch of facial nerve, deep fascia, facial vein and lymph nodes
- *Lateral surface:* Posteriorly to medial pterygoid muscle, and facial artery and anteriorly mandible
- *Medial surface:* Mylohyoid muscle and intervening mylohyoid nerves and vessels.
  Facial artery grooves the posterosuperior part of gland loops anteroinferiorly to lie between the gland and medial pterygoid to be felt at inferior border of mandible.

### Relations of Deep Part

- *Lateral surface:* Mylohyoid muscle
- *Medial surface:* Hyoglossus muscle, lingual nerve, XII nerve, submandibular ganglion. (Remember lingual artery is deep to hyoglossus muscle)

Wharton's duct (= submandibular duct)

*Course*

- It arises from deep part of gland and lies between side of tongue and mylohyoid muscle, runs anterosuperiorly to open below the tongue, in floor of mouth
- Lingual nerve winds the duct.

### Blood Supply

Submandibular gland is supplied by facial artery and drains in common facial vein.
  Lymphatics pass to submandibular nodes.

### Nerve Supply

Chorda tympani nerve conveys secretomotor fibres, lingual nerve carries sensory fibre, sympathetic innervation comes from plexus around facial artery.

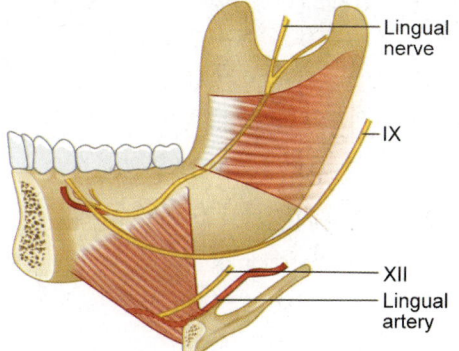

Deep part of submandibular gland neurovascular relations

*Secretomotor Pathway*

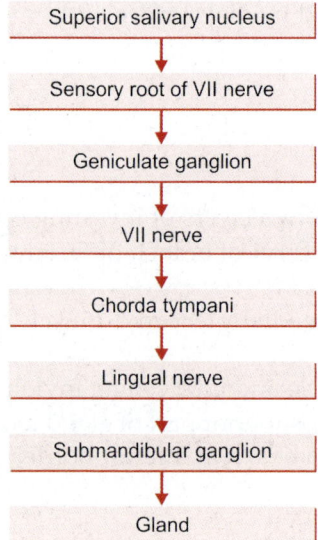

Superior salivary nucleus

↓

Sensory root of VII nerve

↓

Geniculate ganglion

↓

VII nerve

↓

Chorda tympani

↓

Lingual nerve

↓

Submandibular ganglion

↓

Gland

## Applied Anatomy

- Submandibular gland is commonly excised in patients having calculi in submandibular duct
- It is palpable bimanually
- While operating the surgeon has to be vigilant about the facial artery on the posterosuperior aspect of superficial part of the gland.

**Q. Describe the gross anatomy of thyroid gland, its relations and blood supply. Add a note on its applied anatomy.**

**Ans.** Thyroid gland is an endocrine gland, located in lower part of the neck. It undergoes physiological changes during pregnancy and menstruation.

## Gross Anatomy

- It is butterfly-shaped gland, located against C5, C6, C7 vertebrae
- Gland weighs approximately 25 g
- Gland has two lobes connected by isthmus.

## Capsule

Thyroid gland has two capsules:
- True capsule is condensation of connective tissue of gland
- False capsule is derived from pretracheal fascia
- Capillary plexus lies deep to true capsule.

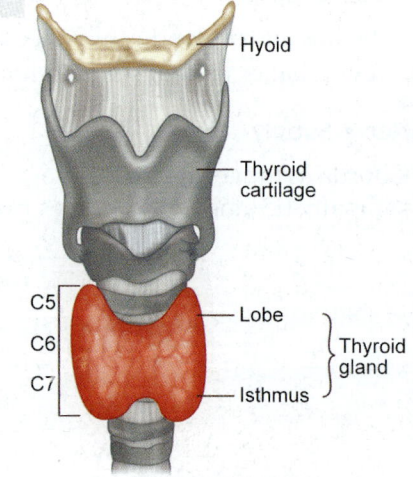

Location of thyroid gland

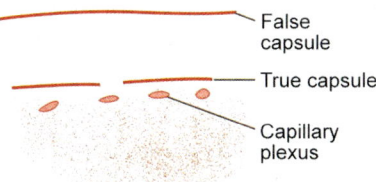

Capsule of thyroid gland

## Relations

- Lateral surface of the lobes is related to strap muscles
- Medial surface is related to trachea and esophagus
- Posterolateral surface is related to carotid sheath.

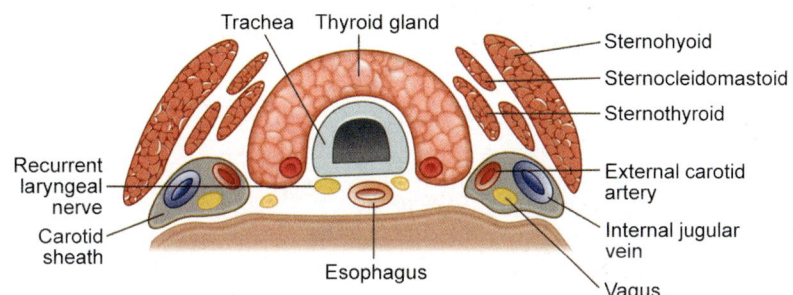

Transverse section showing relations of thyroid gland

### Crucial Neurovascular Relations

1. External laryngeal nerve lies in close relation to superior thyroid artery. The distance between 2 structures is more, i.e. more widely spaced, close to the gland. So, artery should be ligated close to the gland.
2. Recurrent laryngeal nerve is related to inferior thyroid artery. The distance between 2 structures is more, i.e. widely spaced away from the gland. So, the artery should be ligated away from the gland.
3. Recurrent laryngeal nerve lies in the tracheoesophageal groove.

## Blood Supply

1. Superior and inferior arteries supply the gland (sometimes thyroidea ima artery arises from brachiocephalic trunks).
2. It is drained by superior and inferior thyroid vein, which finally drains into internal jugular vein.

## Applied Anatomy

- Enlargement of thyroid gland is known as goitre
- Hyperthyroidism and hypothyroidism are conditions associated with the functional status of the gland

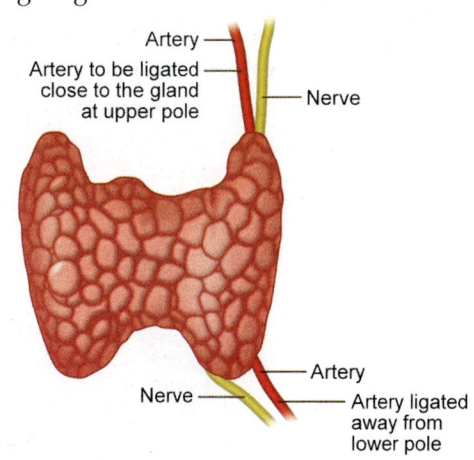

- During thyroidectomy, surgeon needs to be cautious regarding the surgical relations of vessels, nerves and parathyroid glands
- Enlargement of thyroid can cause pressure symptoms on trachea and esophagus.

### Q. Discuss larynx in detail.

**Ans.** Larynx is 'voice box', an organ, which produces voice, maintains the airway and acts as a guard for lower respiratory passage.

### Gross Anatomy

Larynx is a midline structure in neck lying against C3, C4, C5, C6 vertebrae. In children and female, it lies at a higher level. Differences between infant and adult larynx are shown in Table.

| Features | Infant | Adult |
| --- | --- | --- |
| Position | C3, C4 | C4, C6 |
| Epiglottis | Folded and narrow | Leaf like |
| Narrowest part | Subglottis | Glottis |
| Cartilage | Soft | Rigid |
| Adam's apple | Less prominent | More prominent |

The framework of larynx is made-up of cartilages and membranes connecting the cartilages. Following form the skeleton of larynx:

- Three unpaired cartilages—epiglottis, thyroid, cricoid
- Three paired cartilages—arytenoid, corniculate, cuneiform.

### Thyroid Cartilage

Thyroid cartilage is a shield-like cartilage, splaying apart and forming a angular prominence in front of the neck as Adam's apple (more evident in males).

### Cricoid Cartilage

Cricoid cartilage is a ring-shaped cartilage, narrow in front and broad behind.

### Epiglottic Cartilage

Epiglottic cartilage is a leaf-shaped cartilage with upper free end projecting behind tongue, while lower end attached to thyroid cartilage.

Arytenoid, corniculate, cuneiform, cartilages are on the posterior aspect of larynx.

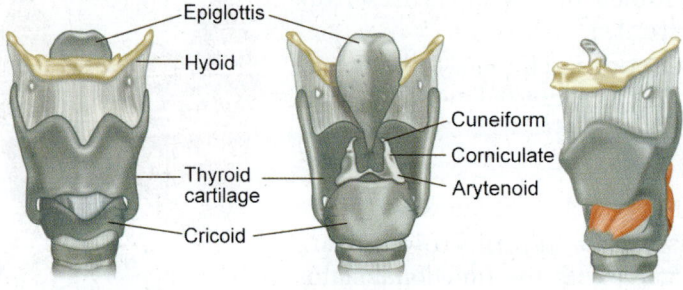

Laryngeal framework

## Ligaments and Membranes

Ligaments connecting the adjacent cartilages are: thyrohyoid membrane, hyoepiglottic ligament.

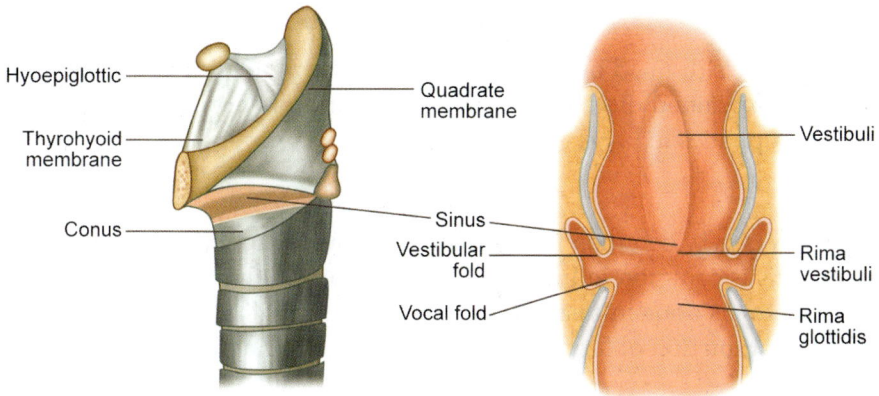

## Interior of Larynx

- Interior of larynx is lined by fibroelastic membrane, which is not continuous due to presence of 'sinus'. The membrane above the sinus is quadrate membrane and lower part is conus elasticus.
- Area between vestibular and vocal fold is sinus of larynx
- Area between 2 vestibular fold is rima vestibuli
- Area between 2 vocal fold is rima glottidis.

## Muscles of Larynx

There are two varieties of muscles—the muscles within laryngeal framework are intrinsic muscles, while extrinsic muscles attach larynx to surrounding structures.

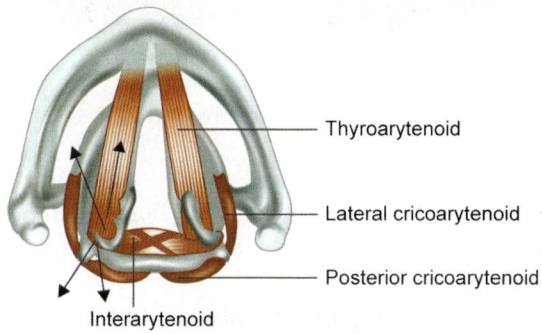

Intrinsic muscles of larynx

## Salient Features

- Name of the muscle depicts the attachment of the muscles.
- Cricothyroid is the only intrinsic muscle located on external surface.
- All the intrinsic muscles of larynx are supplied by recurrent laryngeal nerve except cricothyroid, which is supplied by external laryngeal nerve.

- Cricothyroid is the tensor of vocal cord.
- Posterior cricoarytenoid is the safety muscle of larynx since it abducts the vocal cord and maintains the patency of the airway.

## Drainage

- Supraglottic larynx is drained by upper deep cervical lymph nodes
- Infraglottic larynx drained directly into pretracheal and prelaryngeal (Delphian) nodes
- There are no lymphatics in vocal cords.

## Applied Anatomy

- Cancer of larynx is very common in India due to tobacco chewing and smoking habits
- Carcinoma glottis is common in India, however cervical metastasis is rare
- Total laryngectomy is done in cases of cancer larynx
- Laryngitis is inflammation of larynx due to infection, swelling or trauma.

**Q. What are the relations of middle ear? Mention its surgical significance.**

**Ans.** Middle ear space is a narrow space situated in the petrous part of temporal bone.
- Tympanic cavity is a biconcave space with vertical and anteroposterior diameter of about 15 mm and transverse diameter of 2–6 mm respectively
- Middle ear has six walls—roof, floor, anterior and posterior wall, medial and lateral wall
- Middle ear space is divided as epitympanum, mesotympanum, posterior tympanum, hypotympanum.

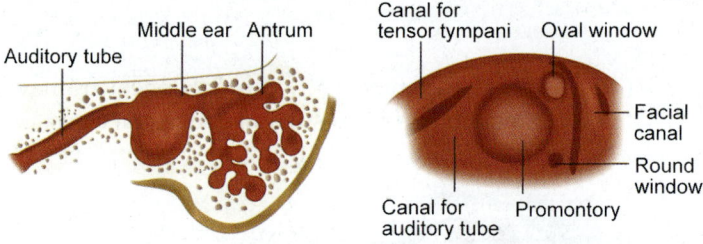

Communications and relations of middle ear

## Relations

1. Roof is also known as tegmen tympani. It is a thin plate of bone separating middle ear cavity from cranial fossa.
2. Floor is related below to jugular bulb.
3. Lateral wall is formed mainly by tympanic membrane and partly above by bone (scutum).
4. *Anterior wall has three important relations:*
   a. Canal for tensor tympani.
   b. Eustachian tube orifice.
   c. Wall of carotid canal.
5. *Medial wall has following features:*
   a. A bulge produced due to the basal turn of cochlea-promontory.
   b. Above and behind is fenestra ovalis (oval window) closed by footplate of stapes.

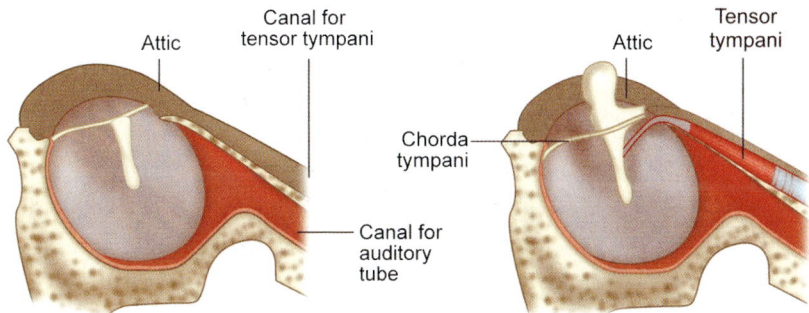

Inner side of tympanic membrane and anterior connections of middle ear cavity

c. Above oval window is fallopian canal with facial nerve.

d. Below and behind is fenestra rotunda (round window) closed by secondary membrane.

6. *Posterior wall:* It presents an opening, which leads to mastoid antrum (= aditus ad antrum)

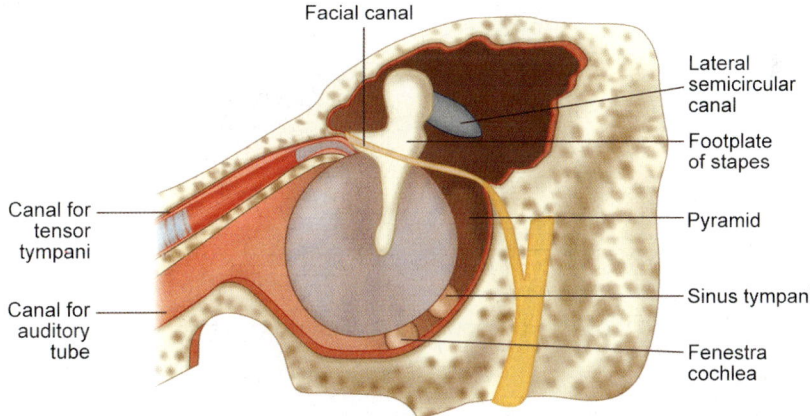

## Applied Anatomy

- The surgeon should be aware of the middle ear relations, while analyzing symptoms of complications associated with untreated ear infections.
- During ear surgery, while working in middle ear, surgeon should be vigilant about the facial nerve.

### Q. Discuss lateral wall of nose, and its blood and nerve supply. Add a note on its surgical anatomy.

**Ans.** Lateral wall of nose is an uneven area, which separates nose from orbit, maxillary sinus and nasolacrimal duct.

## Bony Skeleton of Lateral Wall

Bony skeleton is made-up of (front to behind) nasal bone, frontal process of maxilla, lacrimal, ethmoid with superior and middle concha, perpendicular plate of palatine bone, medial pterygoid plate.

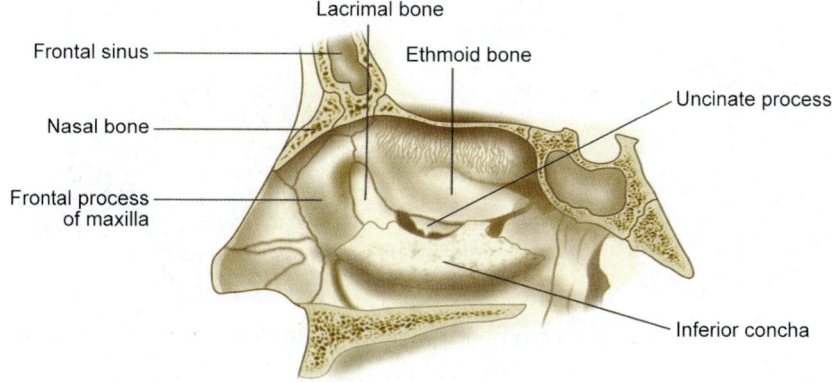

Bony framework of lateral wall of nose

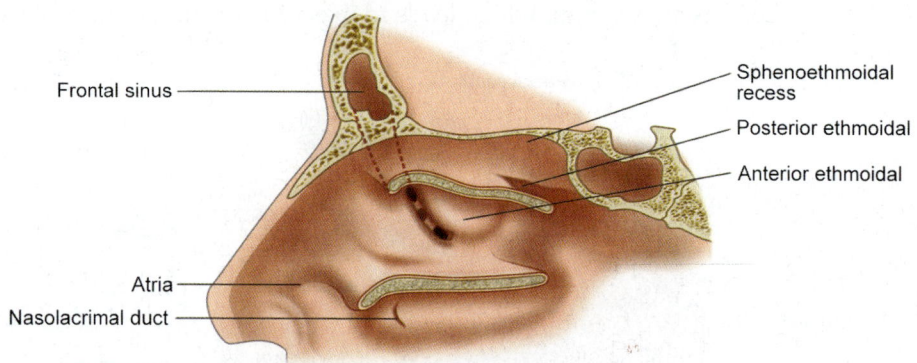

Lateral wall showing openings of sinuses

## Features

1. Nasal conchae are shelf-like projections on lateral wall of nose:
   a. Superior and middle concha are part of ethmoid bone.
   b. Inferior concha is a separate bone.
2. Meatus of nose—area below each concha is known as meatus:
   a. Inferior meatus is underneath inferior concha. Nasolacrimal duct opens in it.
   b. Middle meatus lies below middle concha. It presents openings of middle and ethmoidal cells, frontal sinus and maxillary sinus. Openings of ethmoidal cells in the middle meatus produces bulge called ethmoidal bulla. Linear space between bulla and uncinate process is known as hiatus semilunaris.
   c. Superior meatus lies below superior concha and receives opening of posterior ethmoidal cells.
   d. Atria is a shallow depression in front of middle meatus and above nasal vestibule.
   e. Sphenoethmoidal recess, space above superior concha, receives sphenoidal sinus opening.

## Blood Supply

- Anterosuperior area is supplied by anterior and posterior ethmoidal arteries
- Anteroinferior area is supplied by facial and greater palatine artery

- Posterosuperior quadrant by sphenopalatine artery
- Posteroinferior quadrant by greater palatine artery
- Veins drain into facial vein anteriorly and pterygoid plexus posteriorly.

## Nerve Supply

- Anterosuperior quadrant is supplied by anterior ethmoidal nerve
- Anteroinferior quadrant by anterosuperior alveolar nerve
- Posterosuperior and posteroinferior quadrant by branches from pterygopalatine ganglion.

## Lymphatics

Drain into submandibular nodes, retropharyngeal and deep cervical nodes.

## Endoscopic Anatomy

Middle meatus with the openings of sinuses is known as osteomeatal complex.
Endoscopically lateral wall of nose is broadly divided into two areas—osteomeatal complex anterior and osteomeatal complex posterior.

## Applied Anatomy

- Maxillary sinusitis is the commonest affection following common cold
- In antral puncture an accessory ostia is created at a lower level to improve the drainage of maxillary sinus
- Endoscopic sinus surgery involves improving drainage and aeration of sinuses by widening the natural ostia with the use of endoscopes.

### Q. What are the boundaries, communications and contents of pterygopalatine fossa?

Pterygopalantine fossa is cul de sac (blind sac, purse) behind maxilla. This fossa serves as a distribution channel for nerves and vessels to face, nose and palate.

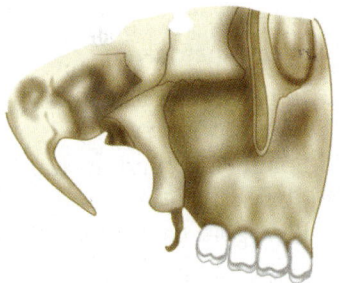

## Boundaries

1. It lies between maxilla in front and pterygoid extension of sphenoid behind.
2. Laterally, it is open.
3. Medially, it is closed by vertical plate of palatine bone (the vertical plate of palatine bone bifurcates into short sphenoidal process and orbital process. The bifurcation is closed from above by body of sphenoid).

## Communications

Pterygopalantine fossa opens into the apex of the orbit via inferior orbital fissure. It communicates medially into nasal cavity via sphenopalatine foramen and laterally through pterygomaxillary fissure to infratemporal fossa.

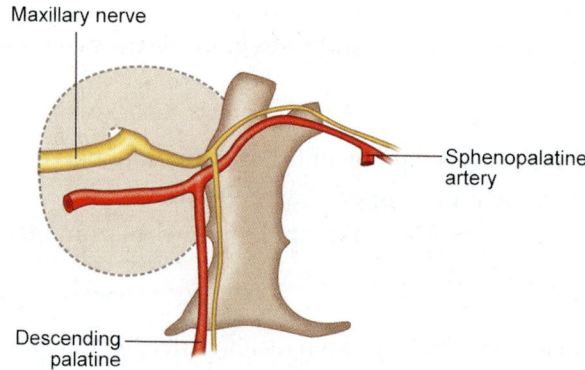

Pterygopalatine fossa with its contents

## Contents

- Maxillary artery
- Maxillary nerve
- Pterygopalatine ganglion
- Vidian nerve
- Fat.

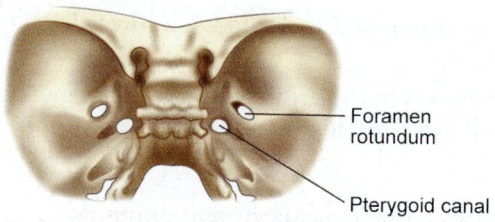

Foramen rotundum in pterygoid palatine fossa

## Surgical Anatomy

1. In the sphenoid wall of the fossa there are two foramen namely—foramen rotundum and pterygoid canal.
2. Foramen rotundum transmits maxillary nerve and marks the upper limit of dissection of pterygopalatine fossa.
3. Pterygoid canal is 1 cm long, placed anteroposteriorly and lies inferolateral to sphenoid sinus.

## Applied Anatomy

- Pterygopalatine fossa can be approached transantrally
- Vidian neurectomy is done in vasomotor rhinitis.

### Q. Discuss parathyroid glands.

**Ans.** Parathyroid glands are endocrine glands in vicinity to thyroid gland. They may vary from two to six in number, but in 80% cases they are four in number. Total weight of all the glands is 200 mg.

## Development

- The upper parathyroid arise from fourth branchial pouch and come to lie in close association with the upper part of lateral lobes of thyroid. This position is constant.
- Lower parathyroid are derived from third branchial pouch in association with thymus and descend with thymus; and thus, inferior parathyroid may be found anywhere from upper pole of thyroid to the mediastinum.

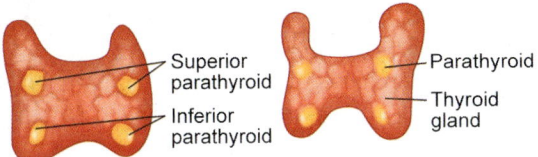

## Gross Anatomy

- Glands are size of split pea
- Pink or brown in colour, but covered by fat making them difficult to recognise
- Superior glands lie on the posterior surface of the middle third of thyroid gland, usually above inferior thyroid artery
- Inferior glands are found on posterior surface of thyroid gland within 1 cm of lower lobe of thyroid gland
- Parathyroid glands are located within the surgical false capsule of thyroid gland.

## Blood Supply

- For upper parathyroid gland, artery comes from inferior thyroid artery
- For lower parathyroid gland, artery comes from either inferior thyroid artery or anastomosing artery joining superior and inferior thyroid artery.

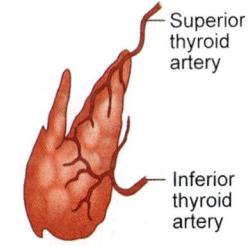

Blood supply of parathyroid gland

## Endocrine Function

Parathyroid glands are controlled by calcium levels in the blood.

Parathormone is secreted by parathyroid glands and calcitonin is secreted by parafollicular cells of thyroid gland.

## Applied Anatomy

- Lower parathyroid artery is a guide to the gland, if it lies below the lower margin of thyroid
- During thyroidectomy, parathyroid glands should be salvaged
- Parathyroid gland adenoma may cause hypercalcemia; it is surgically treated by excising the gland.

### Q. Describe pharyngeal muscles with its applied anatomy.

**Ans.** Pharynx is a muscular tube made-up of three muscles (like one glass into another):
1. Superior constrictor
2. Middle constrictor
3. Inferior constrictor.

## Superior Constrictor

*Attachments*

*From*

- Pterygoid hamulus, medial pterygoid plate
- Pterygomandibular raphe
- Mylohyoid line
- Side of tongue.

*To*

Pharyngeal tubercle and raphe.

## Middle Constrictor

*Attachments*

*From*

- Stylohyoid ligament
- Lesser and greater horn of hyoid bone.

*To*

Pharyngeal raphe.

## Inferior Constrictor

*Attachments*

*From*

- Oblique line of thyroid cartilage (thyropharyngeus)
- Side of cricoid (cricopharyngeus).
   Inferior constrictor has two parts—thyropharyngeus and cricopharyngeus.

*To*

Pharyngeal raphe.

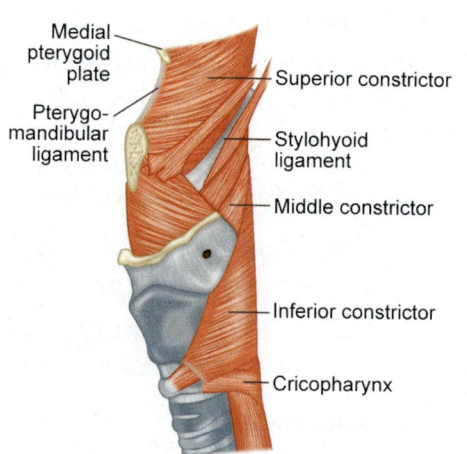

Pharyngeal musculature

*Action*

All the constrictors help in deglutition.

## Nerve Supply

All the constrictors are supplied by pharyngeal plexus.

## Applied Anatomy

1. The lower part of thyropharyngeus is a single sheet of muscle, not overlapped internally by middle constrictor. This part is limited below by cricopharyngeal sphincter. This weak area is known as Killian's dehiscence.
2. Paralyses of constrictors leads to dysphagia.

### Q. Discuss innervation of tongue and its embryological basis.

**Ans. Development**

- The tongue develops in relation to pharyngeal arches in the floor of developing mouth
- Medial most parts of mandibular arches proliferate to form two lingual swellings

- In between the lingual swelling is another swelling-tuberculum impar
- Another midline swelling appears in relation to II, III, IV arches called hypobranchial eminence
- Another two-thirds of tongue is formed by fusion of tuberculum impar and lingual swelling, in relation to I arch
- Posterior one-third of tongue develops from cranial part of hypobranchial eminence
- Posteriormost part is derived from IV arch.

*With this embryological backdrop:*
- Anterior two-thirds is supplied by lingual nerve, branch of mandibular nerve and chorda tympani
- Posterior one-third is supplied by IX nerve, which is nerve of III arch
- Posteriormost part by superior laryngeal nerve which is nerve of IV arch
- Muscles of tongue develop from occipital myotomes, supplied by XII nerve, which is the nerve of these myotomes.

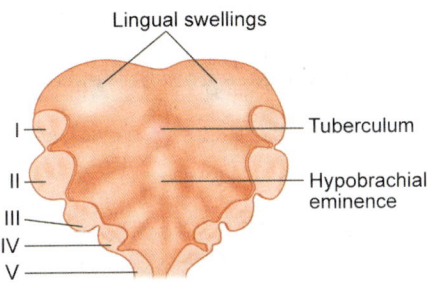

Pharyngeal arches

## Applied Anatomy

- Taste is checked objectively by using galvanic current and subjectively by placing different solutions of salt, sugar
- In ear surgeries like tympanoplasty, chorda tympani may be stretched or severed giving rise to altered sensation or loss of taste.

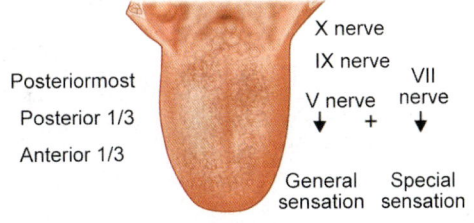

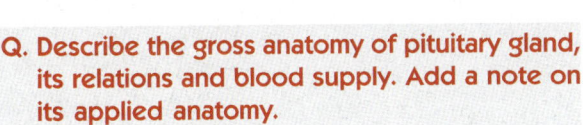

**Q. Describe the gross anatomy of pituitary gland, its relations and blood supply. Add a note on its applied anatomy.**

Pituitary gland is also known as master gland since it produces trophic hormones, which control the secretions of other glands.

## Location

Pituitary gland is lodged in pituitary fossa (sella turcica), which is roofed by diaphragma sella. Stalk of pituitary gland perforates the sella and is attached above to the third ventricle.

## Dimension and Weight

Pituitary gland is 8 × 16 mm in dimensions and weighs around 500 mg.

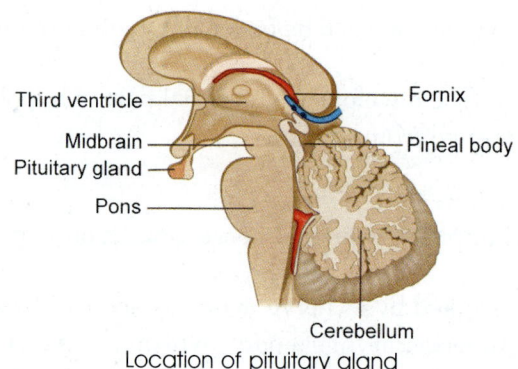

Location of pituitary gland

## Parts of Pituitary Gland

The gland has two main parts, which differ from each other embryologically, morphologically and functionally.

Adenohypophysis develops from Rathke's pouch. Neurohypophysis develops as a down growth from floor of diencephalon.

### Subparts of Adenohypophysis

- Anterior lobe
- Intermediate lobe
- Tuberal lobe.

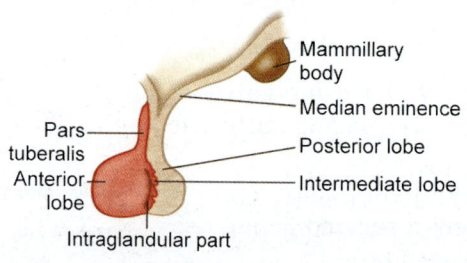

Parts of pituitary gland

### Subparts of Neurohypophysis

- Posterior lobe
- Infundibular stem
- Median eminence.

## Relations

- Superiorly—diphragma sella, optic chiasm
- Inferiorly—sphenoidal air sinus
- On each side—cavernous sinus.

## Blood Supply

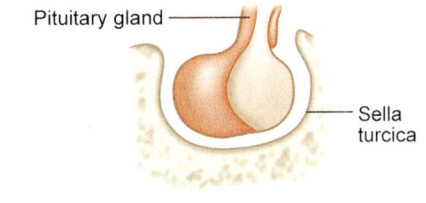

Pituitary gland
Sella turcica

### *Arterial Supply*

- Superior hypophyseal artery—branch of internal carotid artery
- Inferior hypophyseal artery—supplies the gland.

### *Portal System*

Anterior lobe is supplied by portal vessels arising from capillary tufts formed by superior hypophyseal artery.

Long portal vessels drain median eminence and infundibulum, short portal vessels drain lower infundibulum. Portal vessels carry the hormone-releasing factors.

Anterior lobe receives blood from portal system, while posterior lobe receives the blood from superior and inferior hypophyseal artery.

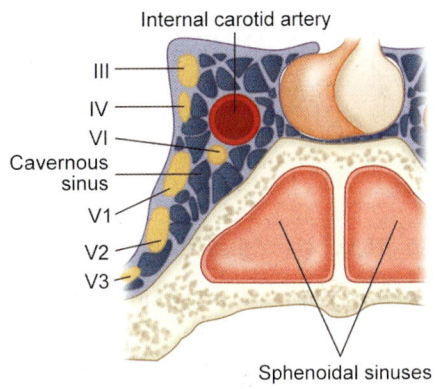

Internal carotid artery
III
IV
VI
Cavernous sinus
V1
V2
V3
Sphenoidal sinuses

Relations of pituitary gland

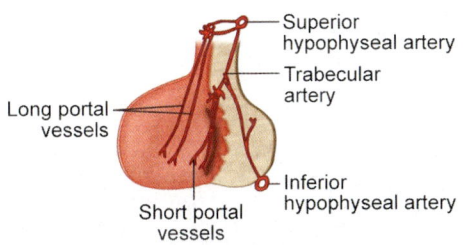

Superior hypophyseal artery
Trabecular artery
Long portal vessels
Short portal vessels
Inferior hypophyseal artery

Blood supply of pituitary gland

### *Hormones Secretion*

1. *Anterior lobe:*
   - Growth hormone
   - Lactogenic hormone
   - Adrenocorticotropic hormone (ACTH)
   - Thyroid-stimulating hormone (TSH), follicle-stimulating hormone (FSH), luteinising hormone (LH).
2. *Inferior lobe:* Melanocyte-stimulating hormone (MSH).
3. *Posterior lobe:*
   - Antidiuretic hormone (ADH)
   - Oxytocin.

## Applied Anatomy

1. Pituitary tumor gives rise to general symptoms due to pressure on surrounding structures and due to hormonal imbalance. For example, posterior lobe tumor causes diabetes insipidus.
2. Hypophysectomy, i.e. removal of pituitary gland can be done by transfrontal route or by trans-sphenoidal route, endoscopically.

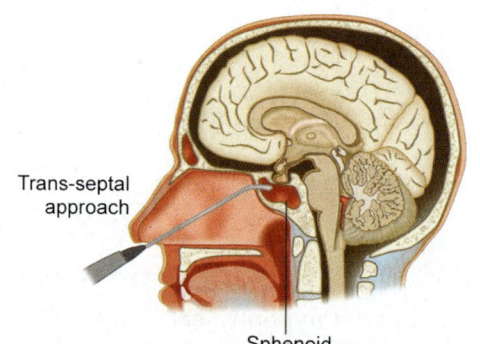

Trans-septal approach

Sphenoid

Hypophysectomy through trans-sphenoidal route

## Q. Discuss internal ear in detail.

**Ans.** Internal ear lies in the petrous part of temporal bone. It consists of bony labyrinth and membranous labyrinth.

The membranous labyrinth is filled with endolymph and surrounded by perilymph.

### Bony Labyrinth

Bony labyrinth consists of the following:
- Cochlea
- Vestibule
- Semicircular canals.

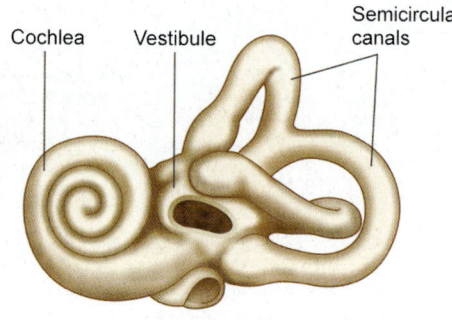

Cochlea    Vestibule    Semicircular canals

Bony labyrinth

#### Cochlea

Resembles shell of snail. The conical axis is known as modiolus around which cochlea makes two and half turns.

Spiral ridge of bone called spiral lamina projects from the modiolus and partially divides cochlea into scala vestibuli and scala tympani. Scala vestibuli and scala tympani communicate with each other at the apex by a small opening called helicotrema.

#### Vestibule

Vestibule is the central part of bony labyrinth and contains saccule and utricle. Openings in vestibule:
- Lateral wall opens at fenestra vestibuli, which is closed by foot plate of stapes
- The semicircular canals open in the vestibuli posteriorly by five openings. Medial wall: On the inner side of medial wall there is spherical recess for saccule and elliptical recess for utricle
- Medial to the medial wall is internal acoustic meatus.

#### Semicircular Canals

Semicircular canals are posterosuperior to vestibule and are at right angles to each other. Each canal has a dilated end known as ampulla. There are three semicircular canals namely superior and lateral and posterior.

Anterior canal of one side is in the same plane as the posterior canal of other side, i.e. parallel to each other, while lateral semicircular canals of both sides are in the same horizontal plane.

## Membranous Labyrinth

Membranous labyrinth consists of:

1. *Cochlear duct:*
   a. It is a continuous closed cavity, which contains receptors for sound (organ of Corti).

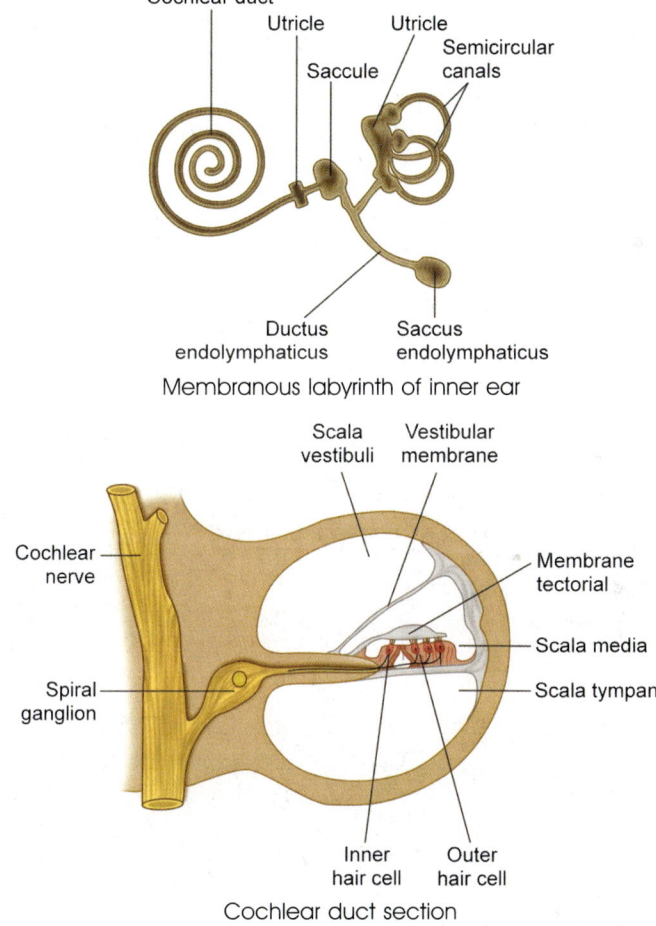

Membranous labyrinth of inner ear

Cochlear duct section

   b. Cochlear duct lies between basilar membrane and vestibular membrane. The basilar membrane has the organ of Corti, which consists of hair cells and supporting cells: Cochlear duct is connected to saccule by narrow ductus reuniens.

2. *Saccule and utricle:*
   a. Saccule lies in the anteroinferior part of vestibule.
   b. Utricle lies in the posterosuperior part of vestibule.
   c. Medial wall of saccule and utricle contains sensory organ (hair cell) known as macula.

3. *Semicircular duct:*
   a. The three ducts lie within the bony canals.
   b. Medial wall of the ampulla contains the sense organ and crista.

## Blood Supply

Labyrinthine artery a branch of basilar artery and a small twig from stylomastoid branch of posterior auricular artery supplies the labyrinth. Labyrinthine vein drains into superior petrosal or transverse sinus.

## Applied Anatomy

1. Caloric test is a test of the vestibular function based on the principle of stimulating the labyrinth by using warm and cold water.
2. Ménière's disease is characterised by periodic attacks of vertigo, tinnitus and sensorineural deafness. It is due to distension of endolymphatic sac; either due to excessive production of endolymph or inadequate drainage.
3. Labyrinthitis is viral infection of inner ear.

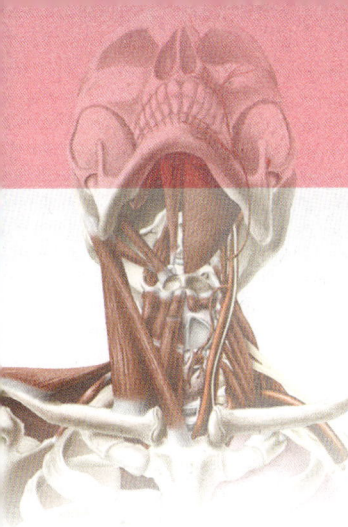

# Key Diagrams with MCQ Tips

## Q. Scalp

**Ans.**

- Skin is thick and hairy
- Wounds of scalp bleed profusely because the torn vessels are prevented from retraction and scalp has rich blood supply
- Loose areolar tissue is the 'danger area of scalp' because infection from scalp can go to cranial venous sinus
- Surgically skin, connective tissue, aponeurotic layer act as a single unit and can be peeled away from loose areolar tissues.

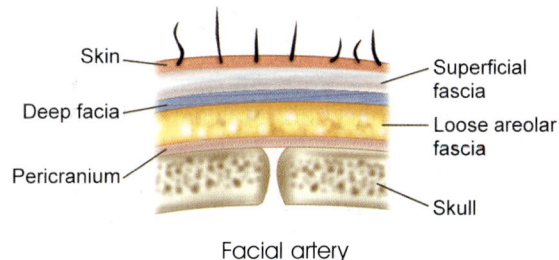

Facial artery

## Q. Sensory innervation of face

**Ans.**

- Trigeminal nerve and cervical plexus innervate the face
- Trigeminal nerve also supplies nasal cavity, paranasal sinuses, eyeball, mouth cavity, supratentorial part of dura mater, lesion in any of the above may cause referred headache
- Angle of the jaw is supplied by great auricular nerve.

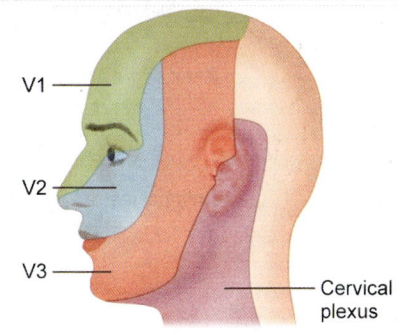

## Q. Facial artery

**Ans.**

- Branch of external carotid artery given off in carotid triangle just above the tip of greater cornu of hyoid bone

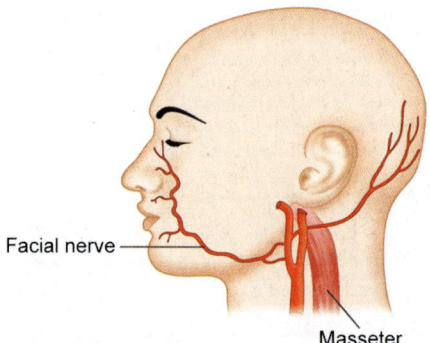

Facial nerve

Masseter

- Tortuous artery (other, e.g. uterine artery, splenic artery).

**Ans.**
- Supraorbital and supratrochlear vein join to form angular vein
- Posterior division of retromandibular vein joins posterior auricular vein to form external jugular vein
- Deep facial vein and superior ophthalmic vein are deep connections of facial vein to cavernous sinus.

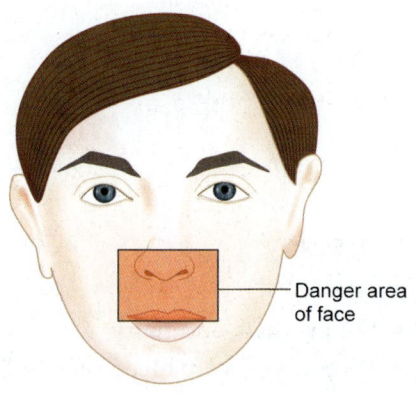

Danger area of face

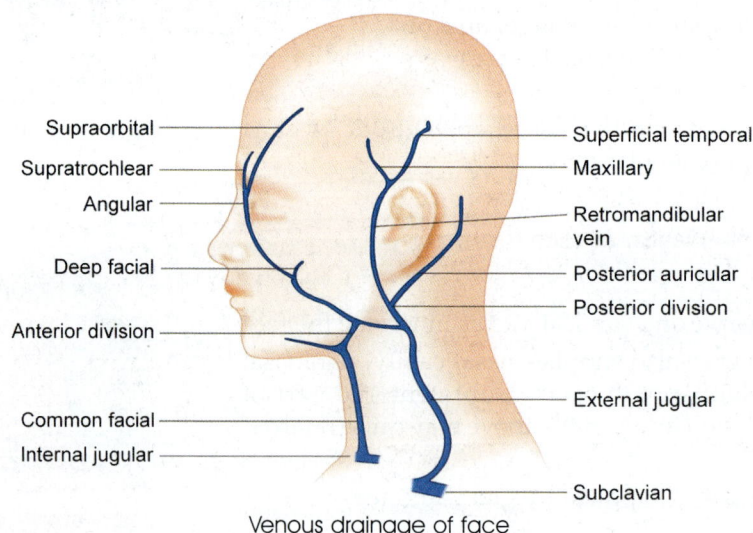

Supraorbital — — Superficial temporal
Supratrochlear — — Maxillary
Angular — — Retromandibular vein
Deep facial — — Posterior auricular
— Posterior division
Anterior division —
Common facial — — External jugular
Internal jugular —
— Subclavian

Venous drainage of face

### Q. Triangles of the neck

**Ans.**
- Sternocleidomastoid is the key muscle of the neck

- Carotid sheath lies deep to sternocleidomastoid.

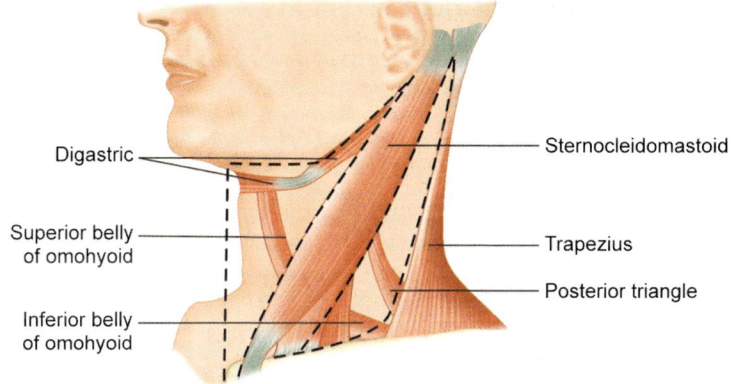

Digastric

Superior belly of omohyoid

Inferior belly of omohyoid

Sternocleidomastoid

Trapezius

Posterior triangle

### Q. Carotid sheath

**Ans.**
- Contains carotid arteries, internal jugular vein, vagus nerve
- Ansa cervicalis lies in the front
- Sympathetic chain lies behind.

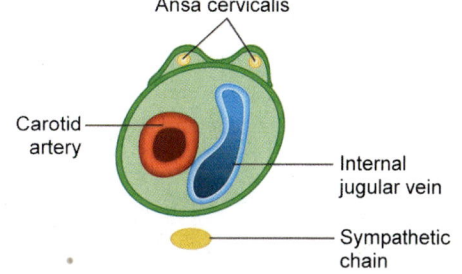

Ansa cervicalis

Carotid artery

Internal jugular vein

Sympathetic chain

### Q. Posterior triangle

**Ans.**
- Roof formed by investing layer of deep cervical fascia
- Spinal accessory nerve lies on levator scapulae muscle
- Floor is covered by prevertebral layer of deep cervical fascia
- Subclavian vein and phrenic nerve lie in front of scalenus anterior
- Subclavian artery and brachial plexus lie behind scalenus anterior.

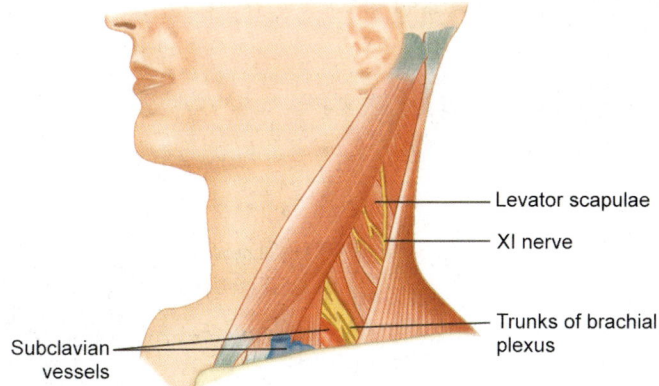

Levator scapulae

XI nerve

Subclavian vessels

Trunks of brachial plexus

### Q. Suboccipital triangle

**Ans.**
- Skin is very thick

- Greater occipital nerve is the thickest cutaneous nerves in the body
- Vertebral artery branch of first part of subclavian artery
- Third part of vertebral artery lies in suboccipital triangle.

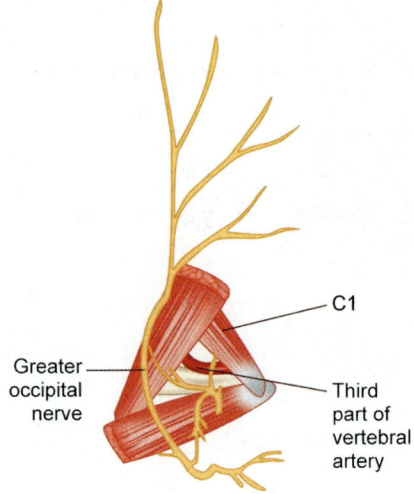

## Q. Cavernous sinus

**Ans.**
- Lateral wall related to III, IV, V1, V2 cranial nerves
- V3 is away from lateral wall.

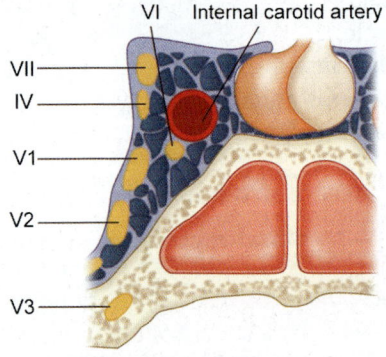

## Q. Superior orbital fissure

**Ans.**
- Common tendinous ring divides it
- Nasociliary nerve lies in between upper and lower division of III nerve.

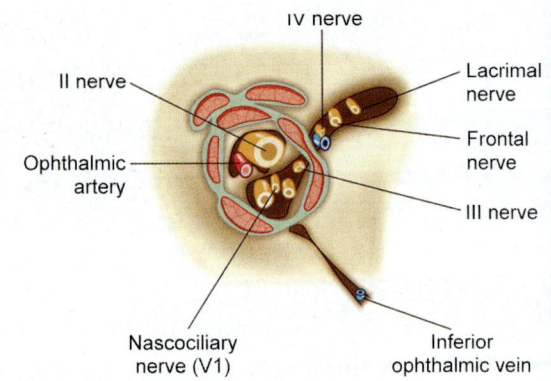

### Q. Extraocular muscles

**Ans.**
- Superior oblique supplied by trochlear nerve (SO$_4$)
- Lateral rectus supplied by abducent nerve (LR6)
- Upper division of III nerve supplies superior rectus, levator palpebrae superioris
- Lower division supplies inferior oblique, inferior rectus, medial rectus.

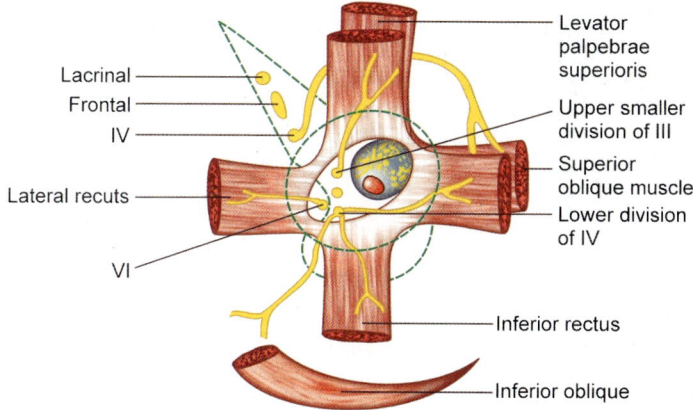

### Q. Midline structures of the neck

**Ans.**
- Internal laryngeal nerve and superior laryngeal vessels pierce thyrohyoid membrane
- Oblique line on thyroid cartilage has:
  - Sternothyroid
  - Thyrohyoid
  - Inferior constrictor.
- Cricothyroid only intrinsic muscle of larynx on external surface of larynx
- Thyroid gland lies against C5, C6, C7 and T1 vertebra
- Thyroid isthmus lies against second to third tracheal rings.

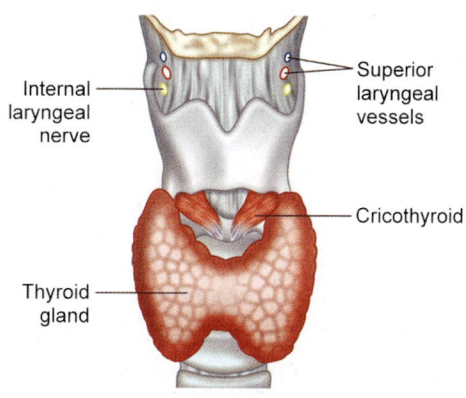

Midline structures of the neck

## Q. Carotid triangle

**Ans.**
- Common carotid artery bifurcates at upper border of thyroid cartilage
- Terminal branches of external carotid artery and posterior auricular artery are not in the carotid triangle.

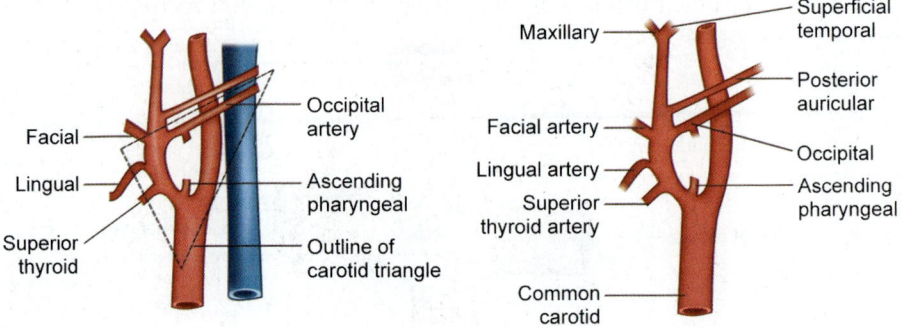

## Q. External carotid artery

**Ans.**
- Has eight branches
- First anterior branch—superior thyroid, given off just below greater cornu of hyoid bone
- Lingual artery—given off at the level of greater cornu of hyoid bone
- Facial artery—given off just above greater cornu of hyoid bone
- Posterior auricular artery—given off just above the posterior belly of digastric
- Occipital artery—given off just below the posterior belly of digastric.

| *Mnemonic* | *Branches* |
|---|---|
| "Sister | Superior thyroid |
| Lucy's | Lingual |
| Powdered | Ascending pharyngeal |
| Face | Facial |
| Often | Occipital |
| Attracts | Posterior auricular |
| Medical | Maxillary |
| Student" | Superficial temporal |

## Q. Parotid gland

**Ans.**
- Facial nerve surgically divides parotid gland into superficial and deep parts
- Facial nerve enters the gland through its posteromedial surface
- External carotid artery and retromandibular vein lie in the substance of parotid gland
- Secretomotor fibres of the gland relay in otic ganglion
- Postganglionic fibres pass through auriculotemporal nerve.

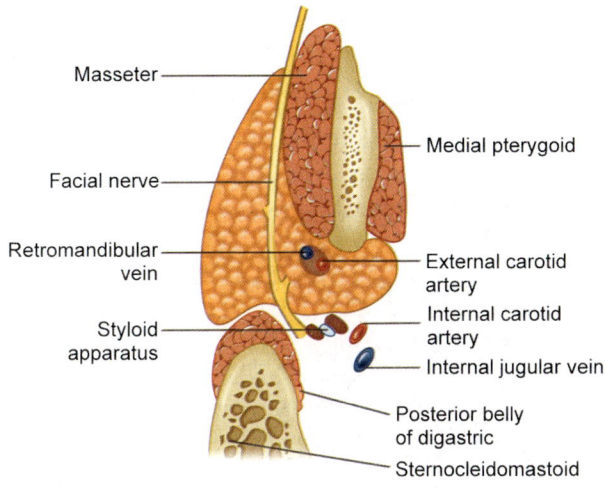

Masseter

Medial pterygoid

Facial nerve

Retromandibular vein

External carotid artery

Internal carotid artery

Styloid apparatus

Internal jugular vein

Posterior belly of digastric

Sternocleidomastoid

## Q. Muscles of mastication

**Ans.**
- Masseter, temporalis, lateral pterygoid, medial pterygoid
- Develop from first branchial arch
- The nerve of the first arch is mandibular nerve
- Lateral pterygoid is the only muscle, which opens the mouth. Other muscles close the mouth.

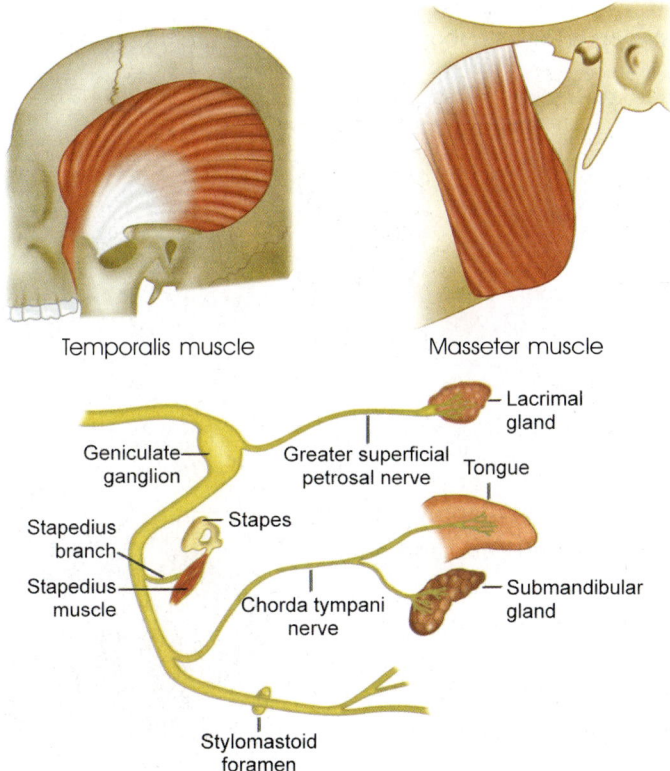

Temporalis muscle

Masseter muscle

Geniculate ganglion

Greater superficial petrosal nerve

Lacrimal gland

Tongue

Stapedius branch

Stapes

Stapedius muscle

Chorda tympani nerve

Submandibular gland

Stylomastoid foramen

### Q. Lateral pterygoid muscle

**Ans.**

Divides maxillary artery into three parts:

1. Upper border related to deep temporal and masseteric vessels and nerves
2. Buccal nerve lies between upper and lower head
3. Lingual nerve and inferior alveolar nerve and vessels are related to inferior border.

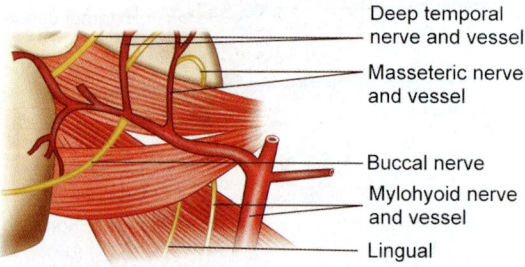

### Q. Sphenomandibular ligament

**Ans.**

- Remnant of Meckel's cartilage
- Auriculotemporal nerve lies lateral
- Chorda tympani nerve lies medial
- Pierced by mylohyoid nerve and vessels
- Auriculotemporal nerve forms a loop around middle meningeal artery.

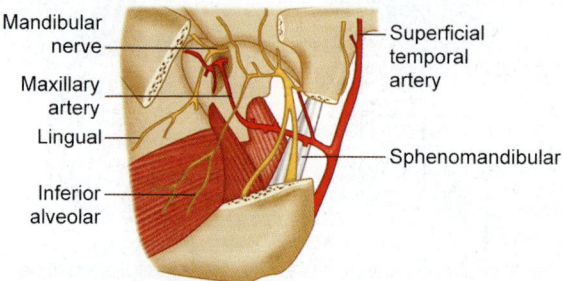

### Q. Submandibular region

**Ans.**

- Mylohyoid muscle is the oral diaphragm
- Lingual nerve winds around submandibular duct
- Lingual nerve is superficial to hyoglossus muscle
- Lingual artery is deep to hyoglossus muscle
- Facial artery forms a loop posterosuperior to submandibular gland

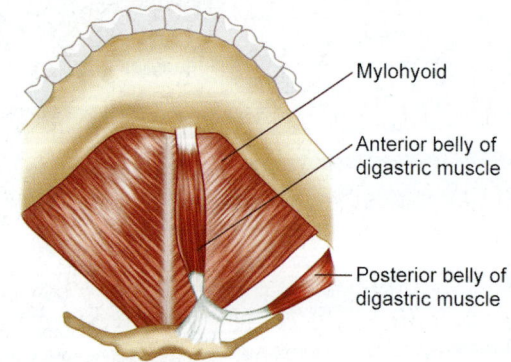

- Facial artery is deep to the gland and facial vein is superficial
- Stylomandibular ligament is present between parotid gland and submandibular gland.

## Q. Thyroid gland

**Ans.**
- Carotid sheath lies posterolateral to the gland
- Recurrent laryngeal nerve lies in the tracheoesophageal groove.

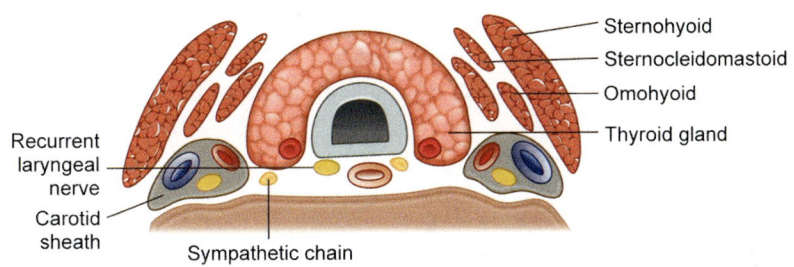

## Q. Cervical lymph nodes

**Ans.**
- Approximately 800 in whole body, approximately 300 in the neck
- Divided into superficial and deep
- Deep nodes lie along internal jugular vein.

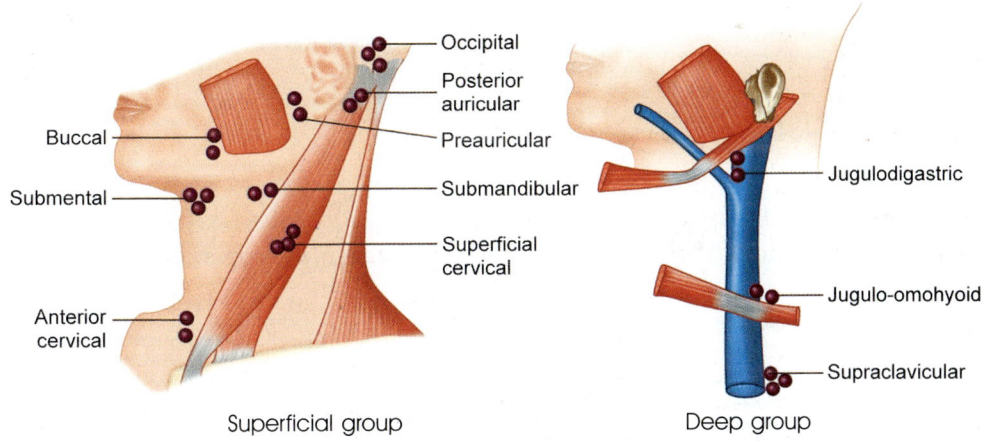

## Q. Styloid apparatus

**Ans.**
- Styloid process, stylohyoid ligament and muscle develop from second branchial arch
- Stylopharyngeus develops from third branchial arch and closely related to IX cranial nerve

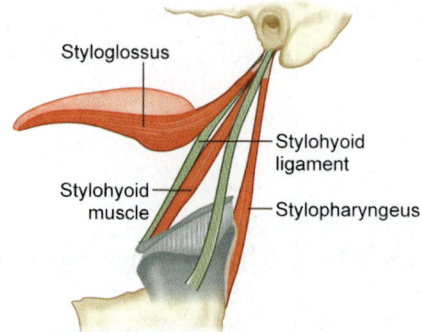

- Styloglossus develops from occipital myotomes
- Stylomandibular ligament is a part of deep cervical fascia of the neck.

## Q. Tonsillar bed

**Ans.**
- Superior constrictor muscle forms the floor
- Palatine vein is responsible for bleeding during tonsillectomy
- Internal carotid artery lies approximately 1 inch deep to tonsil.

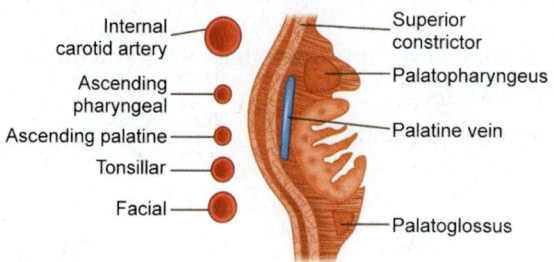

## Q. Lateral wall of nose

**Ans.**
- Sphenoid sinus opens in sphenoethmoidal recess
- Frontal, anterior ethmoidal, maxillary, middle ethmoidal sinuses open in middle meatus

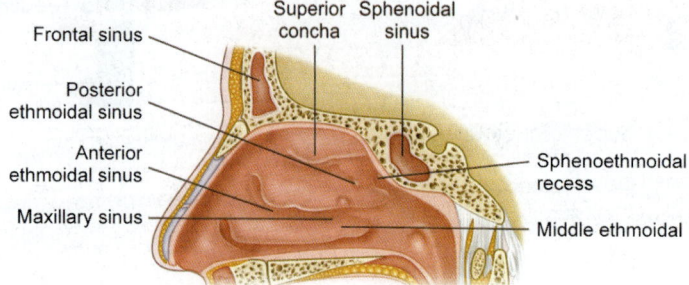

- Nasolacrimal duct opens in inferior meatus
- Posterior ethmoidal sinus opens in superior meatus.

## Q. Kiesselbach's area or Little's area

**Ans.**
- Lies on anteroinferior part of septum
- Anastomosis is between superior labial, anterior ethmoidal, sphenopalatine and greater palatine
- Sphenopalatine is the artery of epistaxis.

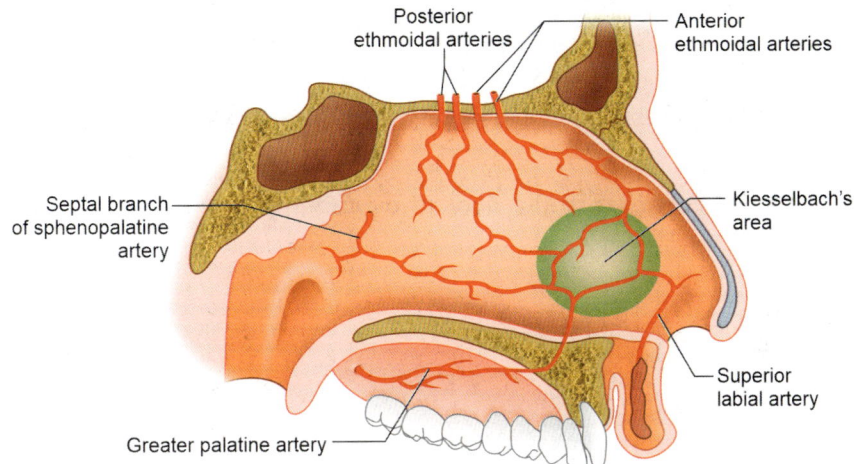

## Q. Middle ear relations

**Ans.**
- Roof—tegmen tympani
- Floor—jugular bulb, carotid canal
- Anterior wall—canal for tensor tympani, opening of auditory tube, carotid canal
- Posterior wall—aditus to antrum, fossa incudis, pyramid, posterior canaliculus for chorda tympani nerve

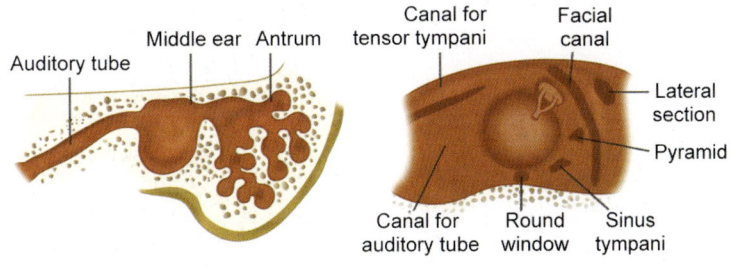

- Lateral wall—tympanic membrane, scutum
- Medial wall—promontory, fenestra vestibuli, facial canal, fenestra cochleae, sinus tympani, lateral semicircular canal.

**Q. Internal acoustic meatus**

Ans.

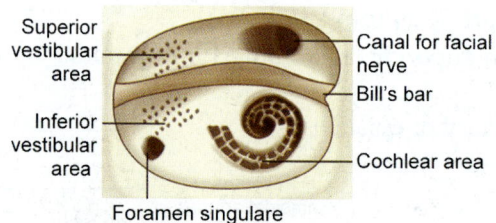

Superior vestibular area — Canal for facial nerve — Bill's bar — Inferior vestibular area — Cochlear area — Foramen singulare

**Q. Tympanic branch of glossopharyngeal nerve is known as Jacobson's nerve**

**Q. Internal laryngeal nerve lies in the floor of pyriform fossa.**

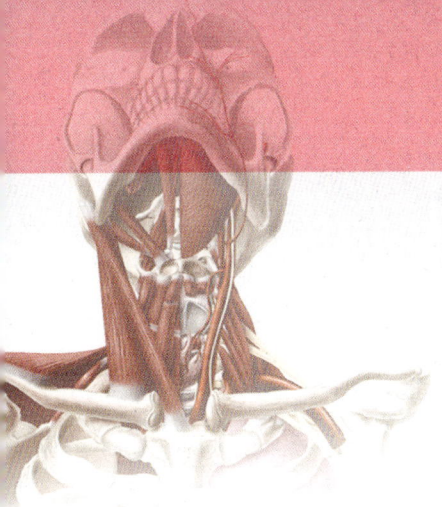

# MCQs 37

1. **'Danger layer' of scalp is ....................**

   a. Skin

   b. Superficial fascia

   c. Loose areolar tissue

   d. Pericranium

   **Answer: c**

2. **Angle of the jaw is supplied by ....................**

   a. Greater occipital nerve

   b. Great auricular nerve

   c. Lesser occipital nerve

   d. Auriculotemporal nerve

   **Answer: b**

3. **Facial artery is given off just above the level of ....................**

   a. Thyroid cartilage

   b. Hyoid bone

   c. Greater cornu of hyoid bone

   d. Lesser cornu of hyoid bone

   **Answer: c**

4. **Deep connection of facial vein is through ....................**

   a. Posterior auricular vein

   b. Superior ophthalmic vein

   c. Inferior ophthalmic vein

   d. Common facial vein

   **Answer: b**

5. **Key muscle in the neck is ....................**

   a. Sternocleidomastoid

   b. Trapezius

   c. Mylohyoid

   d. Omohyoid

   **Answer: a**

6. **Oral diaphragm is** ....................

a. Omohyoid        c. Digastric
b. Hyoglossus       d. Mylohyoid

**Answer: d**

7. **Structure posterior to carotid sheath is** ....................

a. Vagus nerve       c. Ansa cervicalis
b. Sympathetic chain       d. Internal jugular vein

**Answer: b**

8. **Floor of the posterior triangle is covered by** ....................

a. Investing layer of deep fascia       c. Prevertebral layer of deep fascia
b. Pretracheal layer of deep fascia       d. None

**Answer: c**

9. **Roof of posterior triangle of the neck is covered by** ....................

a. Prevertebral layer       c. Investing layer
b. Pretracheal layer       d. All of the above

**Answer: c**

10. **Thickest cutaneous nerve in the body is** ....................

a. Ulnar nerve       c. Peroneal nerve
b. Saphenous nerve       d. Greater occipital nerve

**Answer: d**

11. **Common carotid artery bifurcates at the level of** ....................

a. Cricoid cartilage       c. Upper border of thyroid cartilage
b. Lower border of thyroid cartilage       d. Hyoid bone

**Answer: c**

12. **Phrenic nerve is anterior to the following muscle** ....................

a. Scalenus anterior       c. Scalenus medius
b. Scalenus posterior       d. Levator scapulae

**Answer: a**

13. **Following nerves form the lateral relation of cavernous sinus except** ....................

a. III       c. V
b. IV       d. VI

**Answer: d**

14. **Nasociliary nerve lies between the divisions of following cranial nerve in superior orbital fissure** ....................

a. IV       c. III
b. VI       d. V

**Answer: c**

15. **Superioroblique muscle is supplied by .......................**

    a. IV
    b. V
    c. III
    d. VI

    **Answer: a**

16. **Lateral rectus is supplied by ......................**

    a. IV
    b. V
    c. III
    d. VI

    **Answer: d**

17. **Following structures pierce the thyrohyoid membrane ......................**

    a. External laryngeal nerve and superior laryngeal vessels
    b. Internal laryngeal nerve and superior laryngeal vessels
    c. Internal laryngeal nerve and inferior laryngeal vessels
    d. External laryngeal nerve and inferior laryngeal vessels

    **Answer: b**

18. **All the intrinsic muscles of larynx are supplied by ...................... except cricothyroid.**

    a. External laryngeal nerve
    b. Recurrent laryngeal nerve
    c. Hypoglossal nerve
    d. Glossopharyngeal nerve

    **Answer: b**

19. **Cricothyroid muscle is supplied by ......................**

    a. External laryngeal nerve
    b. Recurrent laryngeal nerve
    c. Hypoglossal nerve
    d. Glossopharyngeal nerve

    **Answer: a**

20. **Thyroid isthmus lies against ......................**

    a. 2nd, 3rd tracheal rings
    b. 1st, 2nd tracheal rings
    c. 3rd and 4th tracheal rings
    d. 1st, 2nd and 3rd tracheal rings

    **Answer: a**

21. **First branch of the external carotid artery is ......................**

    a. Superior thyroid
    b. Lingual
    c. Facial
    d. Occipital

    **Answer: a**

22. **Superior thyroid artery, a branch of external carotid artery is given off at the following level ......................**

    a. Just below greater cornu of hyoid bone
    b. At the level of greater cornu of hyoid bone
    c. Just above the level of greater cornu of hyoid bone
    d. Not related to hyoid bone

    **Answer: a**

23. **Facial artery, a branch of external carotid artery is given off at the following level** ....................

    a. Just above greater cornu of hyoid bone
    b. At the level of hyoid bone
    c. At the level of upper border of thyroid cartilage
    d. Just below greater cornu of hyoid bone

    **Answer: a**

24. **Lingual artery, a branch of ECA is given of at** ....................

    a. Just above greater cornu of hyoid bone
    b. Just below greater cornu of hyoid bone
    c. At the level of greater cornu of hyoid bone
    d. At the level of upper border of hyoid cartilage

    **Answer: c**

25. **Which nerve divides the parotid gland surgically into superficial and deep parts?**

    a. V                              c. Vll
    b. Vl                             d. Vlll

26. **Facial nerve enters the parotid gland through following surface of parotid gland** ....................

    a. Anteromedial                  c. Anterolateral
    b. Posteromedial                 d. Posterolateral

    **Answer: b**

27. **Secretomotor pathway of parotid gland relays in the following ganglion** ....................

    a. Submandibular ganglion        c. Gasserian ganglion
    b. Trigeminal ganglion           d. Otic ganglion

    **Answer: d**

28. **All are the muscles of the mastication except** ....................

    a. Lateral pterygoid             c. Mylohyoid
    b. Temporalis                    d. Medial pterygoid

    **Answer: c**

29. **Otic ganglion is located in** ....................

    a. Pterygopalatine fossa         c. Infratemporal fossa
    b. Temporal fossa                d. Trigeminal impression

    **Answer: c**

30. **All the muscles of mastication develop from** .................... **branchial arch.**

    a. I                             c. III
    b. II                            d. IV

    **Answer: a**

**31. Nerve of first branchial arch is** ......................

    a. Maxillary                   c. Ophthalmic

    b. Mandibular              d. Glossopharyngeal

**Answer: b**

**32. The muscle, which opens the mouth is** ......................

    a. Medial pterygoid           c. Masseter

    b. Lateral pterygoid          d. Temporalis

**Answer: b**

**33. The nerve in between the upper and lower head of lateral pterygoid muscle is** ......................

    a. Lingual nerve               c. Masseteric nerve

    b. Inferior alveolar nerve     d. Buccal nerve

**Answer: d**

**34. Following nerves are related to the lower border of lateral pterygoid muscle** ......................

    a. Masseteric nerve and lingual nerve

    b. Temporal nerve and inferior alveolar

    c. Lingual and inferior alveolar

    d. Masseteric and temporal nerve

**Answer: c**

**35. Sphenomandibular ligament is a remnant of** ......................

    a. Reichert's cartilage        c. Thyroid cartilage

    b. Meckel's cartilage         d. None

**Answer: b**

**36. Auriculotemporal nerve forms a loop around** ......................

    a. Maxillary artery             c. Lingual artery

    b. Tympanic artery            d. Middle meningeal artery

**Answer: d**

**37. The nerve winding the submandibular duct is** ......................

    a. Mylohyoid                 c. Lingual

    b. Buccal                    d. Facial

**Answer: c**

**38. Lingual artery is** ...................... **to hyoglossus muscle.**

    a. Superficial                 c. Medial

    b. Deep                      d. Lateral

**Answer: b**

39. The facial artery forms a loop around the ..................... aspect of submandibular gland.

    a. Inferior                              c. Anterosuperior
    b. Superior                              d. Posterosuperior

**Answer: d**

40. Carotid sheath is ..................... to thyroid gland.

    a. Lateral                               c. Posterior
    b. Medial                                d. Anterior

**Answer: a**

41. Recurrent laryngeal nerve lies in .....................

    a. Thyroid notch                         c. Tracheoesophageal groove
    b. Oblique line of thyroid cartilage     d. Vocal fold

**Answer: c**

42. All the muscles are attached on the oblique line of thyroid cartilage except .....................

    a. Sternothyroid                         c. Inferior constrictor
    b. Thyrohyoid                            d. Omohyoid

**Answer: d**

43. There are approximately ..................... number of lymph nodes in the neck.

    a. 10                                    c. 800
    b. 100                                   d. 300

**Answer: d**

44. Styloid process develops from ..................... branchial arch.

    a. I                                     c. III
    b. II                                    d. IV

**Answer: b**

45. Stylopharyngeus muscle develops from ..................... branchial arch.

    a. I                                     c. III
    b. II                                    d. IV

**Answer: c**

46. Nerve of III branchial arch is .....................

    a. X                                     c. XI
    b. IX                                    d. XII

**Answer: b**

47. Styloglossus muscle develops from .....................

    a. Occipital myotomes                    c. III branchial arch
    b. II branchial arch                     d. None

**Answer: a**

**48. Stylomandibular ligament is a part of ....................**

a. Meckel's cartilage
b. Superficial cervical fascia
c. Deep cervical fascia
d. Styloglossus muscle

**Answer: c**

**49. Muscle forming the floor of tonsillar bed is ....................**

a. Inferior constrictor
b. Superior constrictor
c. Palatoglossus
d. Palatopharyngeus

**Answer: b**

**50. Internal carotid artery is .................... inch deep to tonsil.**

a. 1/2
b. 4
c. 1
d. 0.5

**Answer: c**

**51. All the sinuses open in the middle meatus except ....................**

a. Frontal
b. Maxillary
c. Sphenoid
d. Ethmoidal

**Answer: c**

**52. Following is known as artery of epistaxis ....................**

a. Greater palatine
b. Superior labial
c. Anterior ethmoidal
d. Sphenopalatine

**Answer: d**

**53. Jacobson's nerve is ....................**

a. Auricular branch of vagus
b. Auricular branch of IX nerve
c. Tympanic branch of vagus
d. Tympanic branch of IX nerve

**Answer: d**

**54. The nerve, which lies in the floor of pyriform fossa is ....................**

a. External laryngeal nerve
b. Internal laryngeal nerve
c. Recurrent laryngeal nerve
d. Superior laryngeal nerve

**Answer: b**

**55. Auricular branch of vagus nerve is also known as ....................**

a. Arnold
b. Jacobson's
c. Gasserian
d. Meckel's

**Answer: a**

**56. Reid's baseline is an imaginary horizontal line joining infraorbital margin to ....................**

a. Upper margin of external acoustic meatus (EAM)
b. Lower margin of EAM
c. Centre of EAM
d. Condyloid process of mandible

**Answer: c**

**57. Frankfurt plane is obtained by joining infraorbital margin to** .....................
   a. Upper margin of EAM
   c. Centre of EAM
   b. Lower margin of EAM
   d. Condyloid process of mandible

   **Answer: a**

**58. Cranium is** .....................
   a. Skull with mandible
   c. Skull
   b. Skull without mandible
   d. None of the above

   **Answer: b**

**59. Bregma is** .....................
   a. Junction of coronal and sagittal
   b. Junction of coronal and lambdoid
   c. Junction of parietomastoid and lambdoid suture
   d. Junction of sagittal suture to parietomastoid suture

   **Answer: a**

**60. The fossa posterior to maxillary antrum is** .....................
   a. Temporal fossa
   c. Pterygoid fossa
   b. Infratemporal fossa
   d. Pterygopalatine fossa

   **Answer: d**

**61. What is attached to the auricular tubercle?**
   a. Fibrous capsule
   c. Lateral ligament of jaw
   b. Anterior ligament of jaw
   d. Medial ligament of jaw

   **Answer: c**

**62. Macewen's triangle has following boundaries except** .....................
   a. Supramastoid crest
   b. Anterosuperior margin of meatus
   c. Posterosuperior margin of meatus
   d. Tangent to posterior margin of meatus

   **Answer: b**

**63. All are the parts of temporal bone except** .....................
   a. Mastoid
   c. Petrous
   b. Pterygoid
   d. Tympanic

   **Answer: b**

**64. Mastoid process ossifies by the end of** .....................
   a. 1st year
   c. 3rd year
   b. 2nd year
   d. 4th year

   **Answer: b**

65. **Entomion is anterior part of** .....................

    a. Parietomastoid suture          c. Lambdoid

    b. Sagittal suture                d. Metopic suture

**Answer: a**

66. **The roof of infratemporal fossa has following foramina** .....................

    a. Foramen ovale and foramen rotundum

    b. Foramen ovale and foramen spinosum

    c. Foramen spinosum and foramen rotundum

    d. Foramen ovale and foramen lacerum

**Answer: b**

67. **Following nerve traverses the foramen rotundum** .....................

    a. Mandibular                c. Ophthalmic

    b. Maxillary                 d. Masseteric

**Answer: b**

68. **The structures passing through foramen ovale are all except** .....................

    a. Mandibular nerve         c. Maxillary nerve

    b. Lesser petrosal nerve      d. Emissary vein

**Answer: c**

69. **Middle meningeal artery passes through following foramen** .....................

    a. Spinosum               c. Ovale

    b. Rotundum             d. Lacerum

**Answer: a**

70. **Tympanic canaliculus transmits** ..................... **nerve.**

    a. X                     c. IX

    b. XI                   d. XII

**Answer: c**

71. **A 45-year-old male met with road traffic accident (RTA), where he sustained head injury. The wound on the scalp was bleeding profusely.**

    **The anatomical basis for bleeding wound is** .....................

    a. Patient had thrombocytopenia

    b. Patient had coagulation disorder

    c. Blood vessels fail to retract into fibrous trabeculae of superficial fascia

    d. Blood vessels lack tunica media

**Answer: c**

72. **A 65-year-old female diabetic patient developed a boil on the vestibule of nose. She gave history of fever and chills. Further investigations suggested that she developed cavernous sinus thrombosis.**

Anatomical basis of cavernous sinus thrombosis in 'danger area of face' is due to connection to cavernous sinus through ....................

a. Superior ophthalmic vein          c. Facial vein
b. Inferior ophthalmic vein          d. Maxillary vein

**Answer: a**

73. While operating, a house surgeon is asked to retract sternocleidomastoid muscle. What structure lies below it, which house surgeon has to beware of ....................

a. Carotid sheath                    c. External jugular vein
b. Thyroid gland                     d. Subclavian artery

**Answer: a**

74. Mother of a 3-year-old child complains of bleeding through the nose. On questioning the mother, history of the child putting fingers in the nose (nose picking) is elicited. The area traumatised is ....................

a. Posterosuperior part of nasal septum   c. Lateral nasal wall
b. Anteroinferior part of nasal septum     d. Vestibule of nose

**Answer: b**

75. Mother of 7-year-old child complains of severe pain in the left ear of the child since 1 day. Mother said that she could see a boil in the ear. Anatomical basis for severe pain is ....................

a. Richly innervated                 c. Both a and b
b. Tightly bound to perichondrium    d. None

**Answer: c**

76. 25-year-old female complains of pain in left ear for 1 month on and off. On taking full history, she also complains of toothache. What is the anatomical link?

a. Facial nerve                      c. Auriculotemporal nerve
b. IX nerve                          d. X nerve

**Answer: c**

77. While removing wax in 80-year-old male, he developed cough. This is due to stimulation of nerve.

a. Arnold's nerve                    c. IX nerve
b. Jacobson's nerve                  d. Nervus spinosus

**Answer: a**

78. An intern during his ENT posting, when saw normal tympanic membrane (TM) through otoscope.

i. The color of TM he appreciated was ....................

a. Pink                              c. White
b. Gray                              d. Pearl gray

**Answer: d**

ii. 'Cone of light' on TM, he appreciated was due to .....................

a. Color of TM
b. Light of otoscope

c. Angulation of TM to horizontal
d. None

**Answer: c**

79. After thyroid surgery, the patient lost her voice due to injury of ..................... nerve.

a. External laryngeal nerve
b. Internal laryngeal nerve

c. Recurrent laryngeal nerve
d. Hypoglossal

**Answer: c**

80. While operating on ear, the surgeon is close to oval window. What nerve lies in close relation to tympanic cavity?

a. VI
b. VII

c. VII
d. IX

**Answer: b**

81. During tonsillectomy, there is an uncontrollable bleeding.

i. The surgeon needs to tie (ligate) ..................... artery.

a. Internal carotid
b. External carotid

c. Pharyngeal
d. Lingual

**Answer: b**

ii. The level at which surgeon needs to take an incision to tie external carotid artery (ECA) ..................... is

a. Upper border of thyroid cartilage
b. Lower border of thyroid cartilage

c. At the level of cricoid cartilage
d. At the level of jugular notch

**Answer: a**

82. Bleeding from nose is profuse due to .....................

a. Lack of tunica media in blood vessels
b. Rich vascularity
c. Lack of retraction
d. All of the above

**Answer: b**

83. While operating on ear, the surgeon decides to do mastoidectomy (removal of antral cells). The surface landmark for the surgeon to do mastoidectomy is .....................

a. Spine of Henle
b. Macewen's triangle

c. Mastoid process
d. Supramastoid crest

**Answer: b**

84. The distance between the tympanic membrane and promontory is .....................

a. 1 mm
b. 2 mm

c. 3 mm
d. 4 mm

**Answer: b**

**85. While removing tonsils (tonsillectomy), there was severe bleeding. This is due to ....................**

a. Facial artery
b. Tonsillar artery
c. Pharyngeal vein
d. Palatine vein

**Answer: d**

**86. Promontory in middle ear is due to ....................**

a. Facial canal
b. Basal turn of cochlea
c. Tympanic plexus
d. Ossicles

**Answer: b**

**87. All the germ layers contribute to the formation of .................... structure.**

a. Stapes
b. External auditory canal
c. Tympanic membrane
d. Incus

**Answer: c**

**88. At birth, following structure is of adult size ....................**

a. Maxillary sinus
b. Ear
c. Frontal sinus
d. Eustachian tube

**Answer: b**

**89. Mother of 1-year-old child complains of small opening in front of both ears. It is likely to be ....................**

a. External auditory meatus
b. Sebaceous cyst
c. Preauricular sinus
d. All of above

**Answer: c**

**90. Inner ear is lodged in .................... bone.**

a. Pterygoid
b. Petrous
c. Mastoid
d. Tympanic

**Answer: b**

**91. A young male while playing on the ground had sustained blunt injury on head, half an hour back but continues to play. While playing he complains of headache and suddenly falls on the ground with loss of consciousness and hemiparesis.**

**i. The ball would have hit .................... region of temporal bone.**

a. Obelion
b. Pterion
c. Asterion
d. Glabella

**Answer: b**

**ii. The vessel that would have ruptured ....................**

a. Middle meningeal artery
b. Emissary vein
c. Middle meningeal vein
d. Supraorbital vein

**Answer: a**

### 92. Label the structures A, B, C, D in the following diagram.

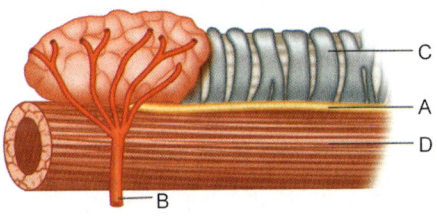

**Answer:**
- A. Recurrent laryngeal nerve
- B. Inferior thyroid artery
- C. Trachea
- D. Esophagus

### 93. Identify the marked structure in the diagram of lymphatic drainage of breast.

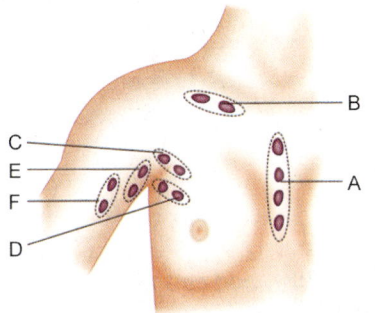

**Answer:**
- A. Internal mammary
- B. Apical
- C. Central
- D. Posterior axillary
- E. Anterior axillary
- F. Lateral

### 94. Label the midline structures of the neck.

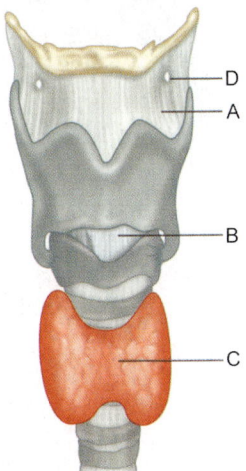

**Answer:**

    A. Thyrohyoid membrane
    B. Cricothyroid muscle
    C. Thyroid gland
    D. Superior laryngeal vessels, internal laryngeal nerve

**95. Identify the muscles dividing the triangles of the neck.**

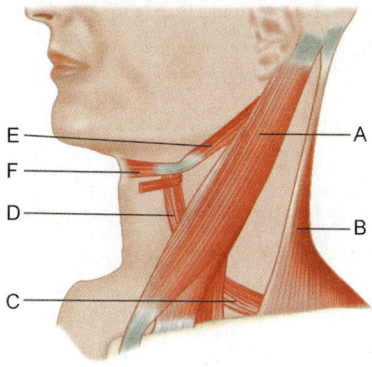

**Answer:**

    A. Sternocleidomastoid
    B. Trapezius
    C. Inferior belly of omohyoid
    D. Superior belly of omohyoid
    E. Posterior belly of digastric
    F. Anterior belly of digastric

**96. Label the structures in the diagram.**

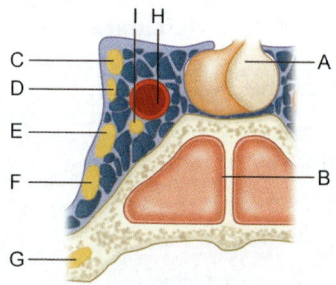

**Answer:**

    A. Pituitary gland          F. V2
    B. Sphenoid sinus         G. V3
    C. III                    H. Internal carotid artery
    D. IV                    I. VI
    E. V1

97. Label the structures in the diagram.

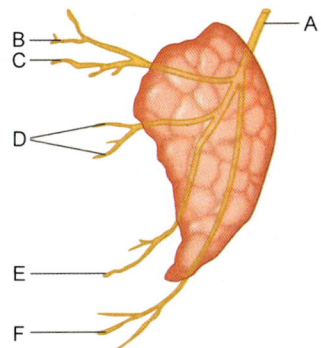

**Answer:**

A. Facial nerve

B. Temporal

C. Zygomatic

D. Buccal

E. Mandibular

F. Cervical

Facial nerve surgically divides the gland into superficial and deep parts.

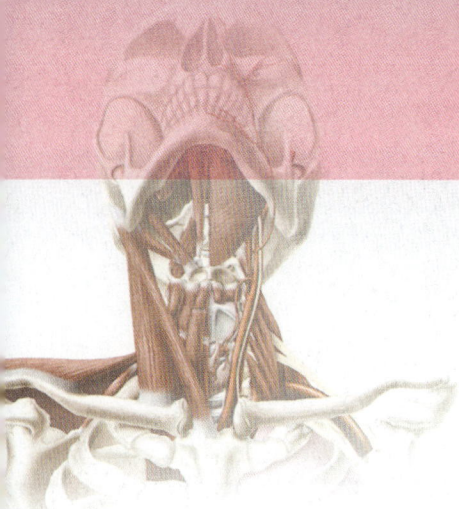

# Dissection

## 1. SCALP

### a. Incisions to be Taken

- Place a block under the head

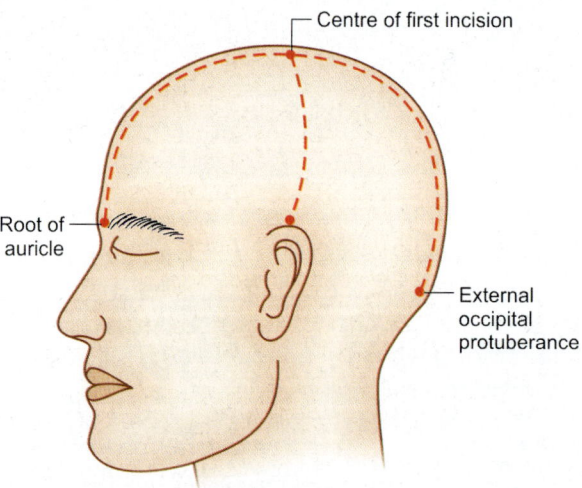

Centre of first incision

Root of auricle

External occipital protuberance

Incisions to be taken on the scalp

### b. Structures to be Identified

- Appreciate the frontal belly of occipitofrontalis muscle and then search for the supra-trochlear nerve a fingers breadth from midline.
- Supraorbital nerve lies more laterally a finger breath again.
- You will see the temporal fascia on the side of scalp, if you scrape out the fascia you can see the superficial temporal vessels and auriculotemporal nerve.

- Quite below and behind the auricle trace the great auricular and lesser occipital nerves and look for the posterior auricular vessels and nerve behind the root of auricle.

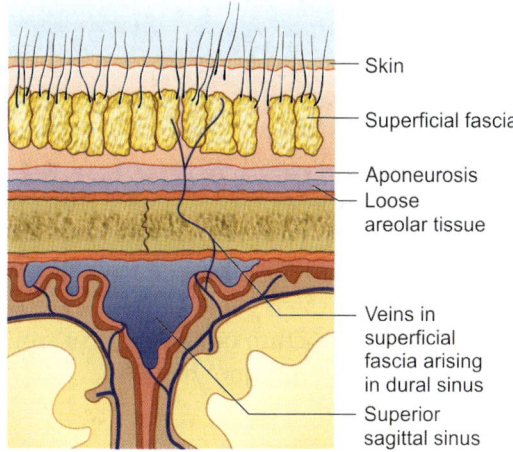

Layers of scalp

- Turn the cadaver prone and near the external occipital protuberance find the third occipital nerve.
- Take a sharp cut on the deep superficial fascia over the superior nuchal line locate occipital vessels and the greater occipital nerve and trace towards vertex.
- Look for the occipital belly of occipitofrontalis muscle.

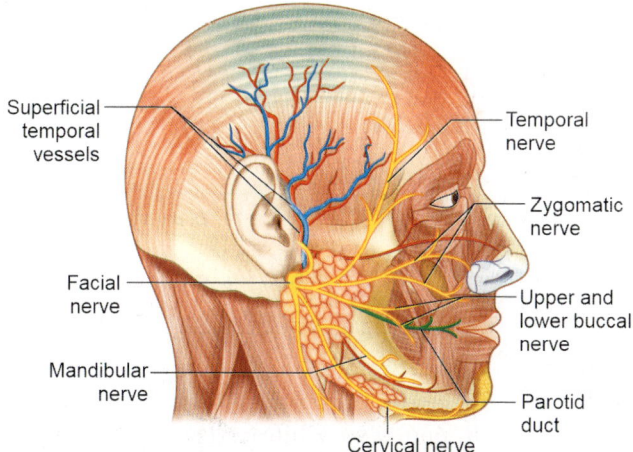

Superficial dissection of face-side view

- Make a small incision on the aponeurosis near the vertex and insert a probe, you will enter the loose areolar tissue, appreciate the extent of this space by moving the probe in all directions. You will not find any space beneath the aponeurosis near the temporal and nuchal line since, it is adherent to the periosteum below.

### c. Vivisection

- The first three layers (skin, aponeurosis, connective tissue) can be considered as a single entity and the surgeon can turn down as a single flap.

- In cases of fracture scalp, blood may get accumulated at a different site than the fracture due to the mobility of aponeurosis. The blood collection may extend all along except at the lines of firm attachment of aponeurosis to the periosteum at the nuchal line and temporal line.

### d. Viva Questions

- The danger area of scalp is the loose connective tissue since, the emissary veins opening in this layer communicate with the cranial dural sinus
- Wounds of the scalp bleed profusely due to the rich blood supply and the fibrous nature of superficial fascia which prevent the blood vessels from retracting
- Black eye can occur due to direct blow out fracture of orbit, or subcutaneous extravasation of blood into the eyelids.

Flame-shaped hemorrhage occurs in fracture orbital plate of frontal bone, the apex lies at the margin of cornea and the posterior limit cannot be seen.

## 2. FACE

### a. Incision to be Taken

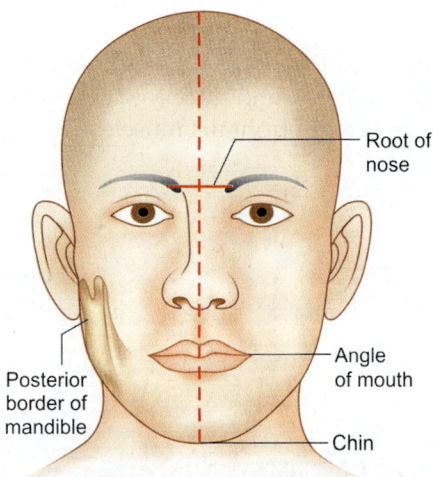

Incisions to be taken on face

### b. Structures to be Identified

- The facial muscles are subcutaneous so while reflecting the skin you may lose their attachments and also be careful not to cut the nerves
- Pull the eyelid laterally and identify the medial palpebral ligament. On the lateral part of upper eyelid you will find the palpebral branch of lacrimal nerve
- Identify the facial muscles one by one—orbicularis oculi, zygomaticus major, zygomaticus minor, orbicularis oris, along the lower border of mandible the broad thin sheet of muscle platysma (buccinators lies in a deeper plane)
- The superficial branches of facial nerve, i.e. temporal, zygomatic, buccal, mandibular and cervical
- The superficial lobe of parotid gland.

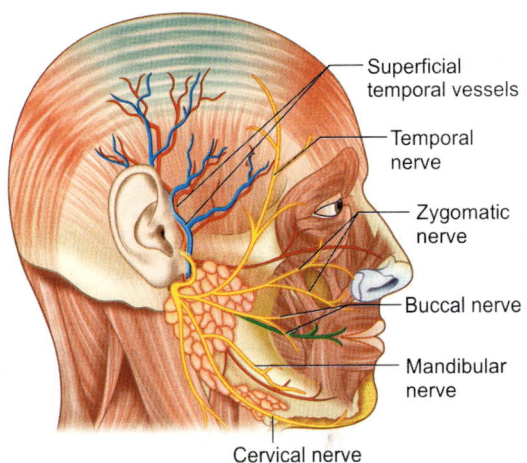

Superficial temporal vessels

Temporal nerve

Zygomatic nerve

Buccal nerve

Mandibular nerve

Cervical nerve

Superficial dissection of face-side view

## c. Vivisection

While incising the skin for any purpose the surgeon needs to remember that the facial muscles are subcutaneous and there are superficial branches of facial nerve.

## d. Viva Questions

- Facial muscles develop from second branchial arch, hence are supplied by facial nerve (motor nerve)
- Procerus, corrugator supercilli bring about frowning expression
- Risorius helps in smiling
- Laughing muscle is zygomaticus major
- Facial muscles are muscles of facial expression, and are subcutaneous. Other subcutaneous muscles are—palmaris brevis in hand, dartos muscle in scrotum.

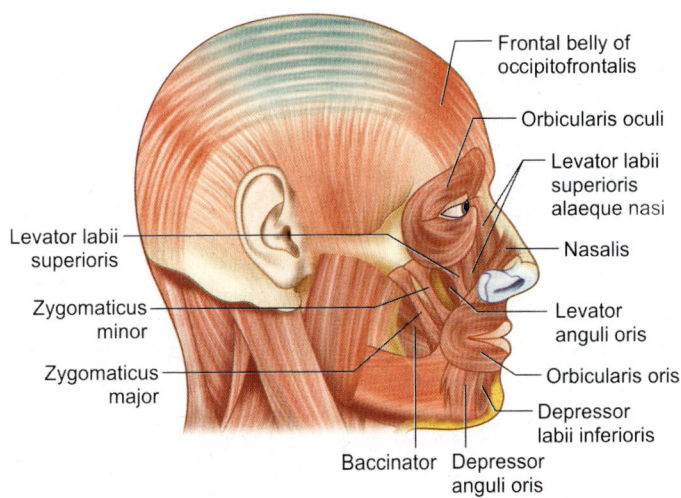

Frontal belly of occipitofrontalis

Orbicularis oculi

Levator labii superioris alaeque nasi

Nasalis

Levator labii superioris

Levator anguli oris

Zygomaticus minor

Orbicularis oris

Zygomaticus major

Depressor labii inferioris

Baccinator   Depressor anguli oris

Superficial dissection showing facial muscles

# 3. POSTERIOR TRIANGLE ON SIDE OF NECK

## a. Incisions to be Taken

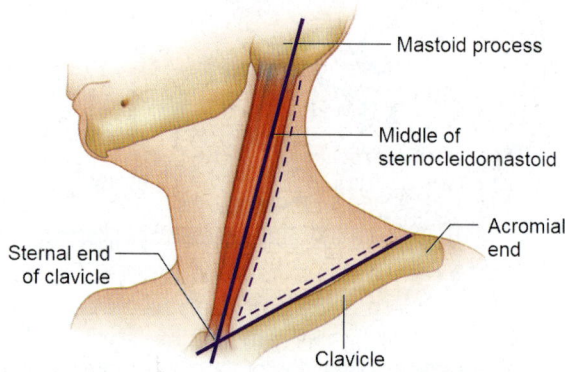

Incisions to be taken on side of the neck

## b. Structures to be Identified

- While reflecting the skin be careful not to damage the supraclavicular nerves which lie deep to platysma in the lower part of the triangle and the accessory nerve in the upper part of the triangle. Beware of the great auricular nerve, transverse cervical nerve, and external jugular vein.

- Turn platysma upwards and forwards from the clavicle in a plane above the platysma and supra-clavicular nerves.

- Trace the external jugular vein in the neck.

- Locate three cutaneous nerves approximately at the middle of the posterior border of sternocleidomastoid:
  a. Lesser occipital nerve
  b. Great auricular nerve
  c. Transverse nerve of neck

- Now incise the investing fascia along the clavicle and

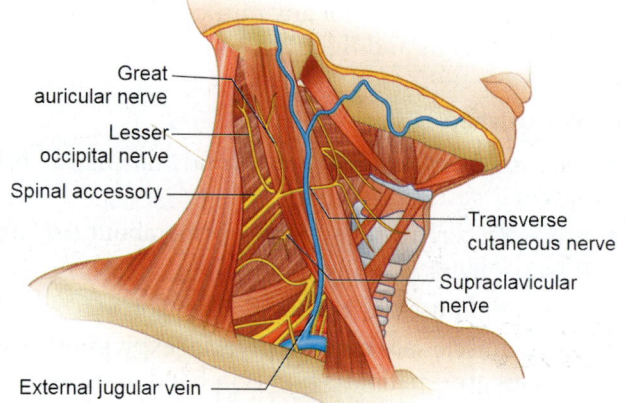

Superficial dissection of the posterior triangle of the neck

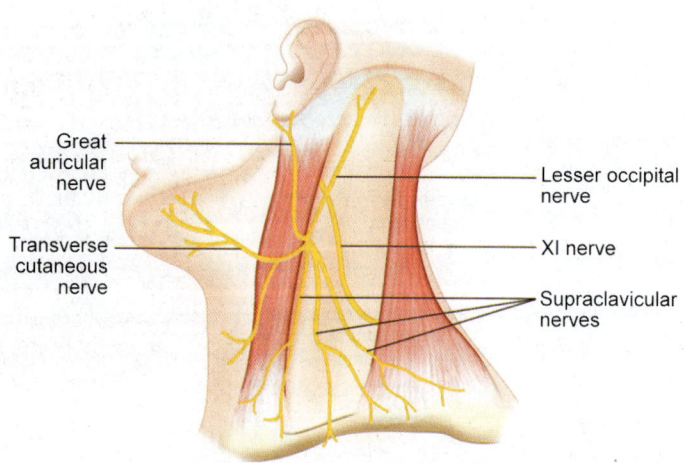

Nerves in posterior triangle

posterior border of sternocleidomastoid, reflect it to find the external jugular, transverse cervical and suprascapular veins in the lower part of the neck.

- Try to find the nerve to subclavius adjacent to the external jugular vein.
- Suprascapular artery lies deep to clavicle.
- Remove the fat from the posterior triangle starting from the apex, this exposes the deep structures of the triangle, muscle in the apex is splenius capitis.
- The first nerve from above is the accessory nerve along the posterior border of sternocleidomastoid, along with this is the third and fourth cervical nerves. The accessory nerve gives branches to the muscle on which it lies, i.e. levator scapulae.
- Clear off the fascia from the inferior belly of omohyoid and you can see the thick brachial plexus branches and transverse cervical artery at the upper border of inferior belly of omohyoid.
- Identify the dorsal scapular nerve lying on the scalenus medius muscle.
- Incise the clavicular attachment of sternocleidomastoid this will expose the scalenus anterior muscle.

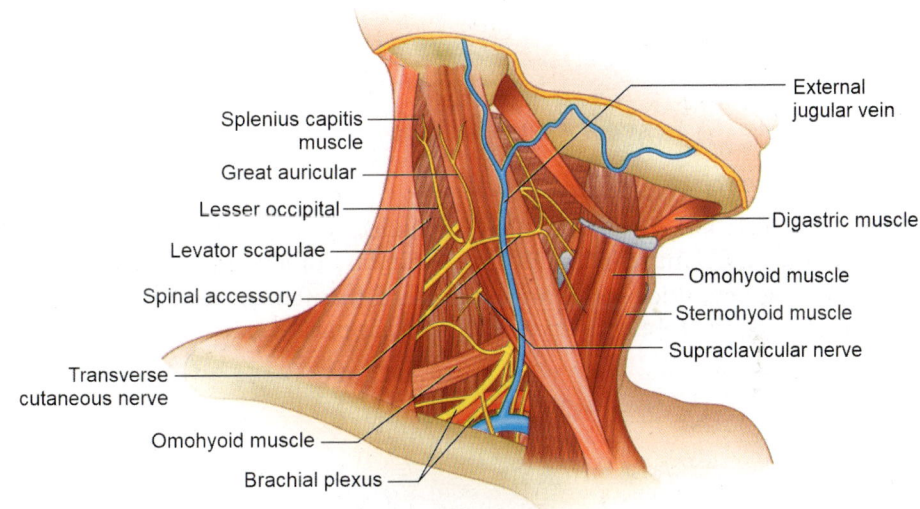

Superficial neck dissection

## c. Vivisection

Neck dissections are commonly performed in patients with cancer neck, the surgeon has to be well-versed with the anatomy of the posterior triangle, to minimise the postoperative complications.

## d. Viva Questions

- Student should be able to identify the superficial nerves in the posterior triangle. At the posterior border, mid of sternocleidomastoid where the three cutaneous nerves arise, i.e.
  a. Lesser occipital nerve
  b. Great auricular nerve
  c. Transverse nerve of neck

This point is known as Erb's point.
- The nerve on the levator scapulae is spinal accessory.

## 4. BACK OF NECK

### a. Incision to be Taken

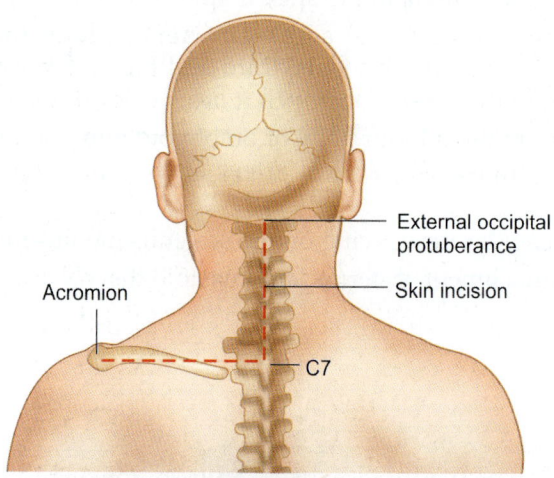

Incisions to be taken on nape of the neck

### b. Structures to be Identified

- The skin is very thick and considerable effort needed to reflect it. Appreciate the occipital belly of occipitofrontalis muscle, identify the occipital branch of posterior auricular nerve.
- Connective tissue is very thick in this area, thus it is difficult to locate the cutaneous branches however one can see the roots of nerves in the upper part of trapezius muscle.

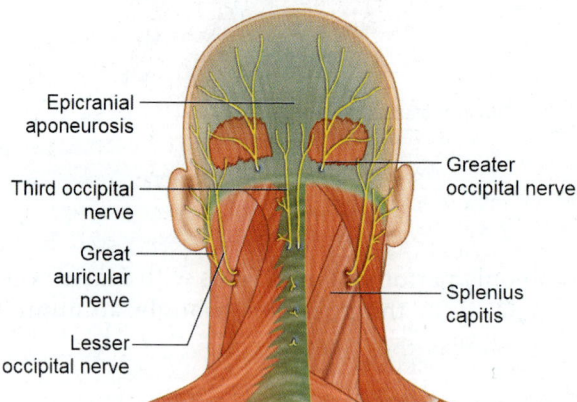

Nape of the neck-superficial dissection

- You can easily locate the occipital artery and the greater occipital nerve, which lies 2–3 cm lateral to external occipital protuberance.
- Just below the greater occipital nerve, in the superficial plane in the upper part of trapezius is third occipital nerve.

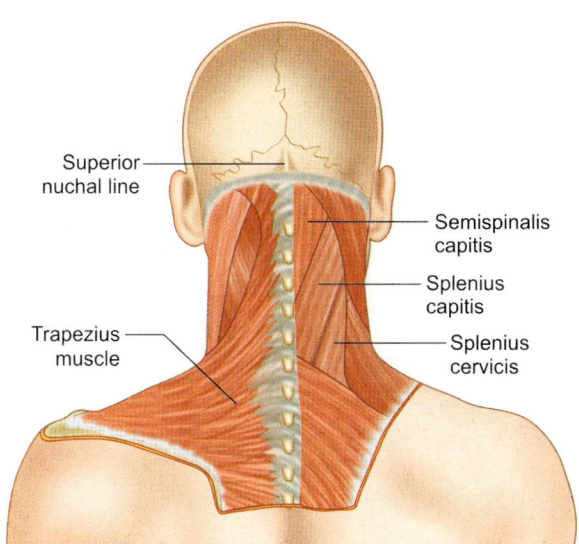

Nape of the neck-I layer

- Remove the deep fascia over the trapezius. Reflect the trapezius by incising vertically 1 cm lateral to midline on the muscle and another incision on superior nuchal line, also reflect the sternocleidomastoid which is more laterally.
- A prominent nerve can be appreciated on the deep surface of trapezius, this is the accessory nerve, other nerves along with it are third and fourth cervical nerves, and superficial branch of transverse cervical artery.

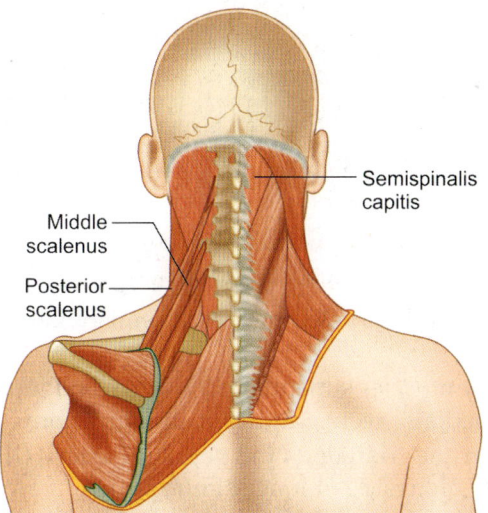

Nape of the neck-deeper plane

- After reflecting the trapezius you will see a conspicuous diagonally running muscle splenius capitis, and below it with the same direction fibres levator scapulae.
- Divide the nuchal attachment of splenius capitis and reflect downwards you will appreciate a straight muscle, running vertically the semispinalis capitis medially and laterally the longissimus capitis.

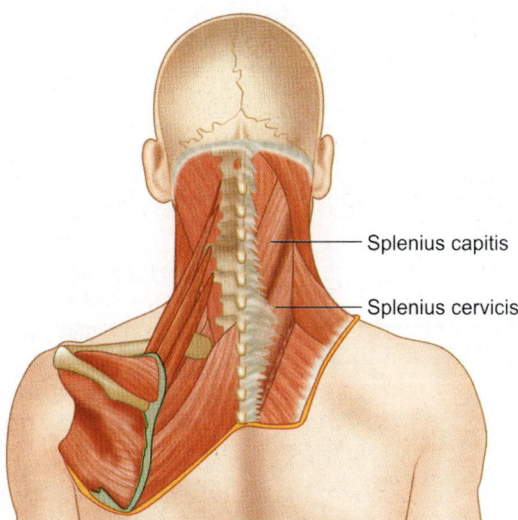

Nape of the neck-deepest layer of muscles

- Reflect the semispinalis capitis and longissimus capitis by dividing the muscles, this exposes the suboccipital triangle.

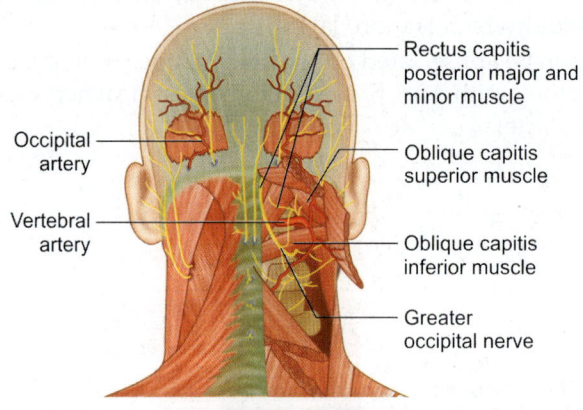

Suboccipital triangle

- Dorsal ramus of first cervical nerve going to the semispinalis can be traced into the suboccipital triangle.
- Appreciate the boundary muscles superolaterally is the obliquus superior, inferiorly minor obliquus inferior and medially rectus capitis posterior major.
- The prominent artery in the triangle is the vertebral artery (III part), while the occipital artery lies most laterally alongside of longissimus capitis.
- Trace the greater occipital nerve starting from the lower border of obliquus inferior, ascends superiorly and pierces the semispinalis capitis and finally pierces the trapezius 2–3 cm lateral to external occipital protuberance to become superficial.

## c. Vivisection

Neurosurgeons can get an access to the posterior cranial fossa by clearing the suboccipital muscles. Surgeon needs to beware of the neurovascular relations in this region.

## d. Viva Questions

- Suboccipital triangle is commonly kept as a specimen for discussion. Students should know the boundaries and contents
  - Boundaries—muscle superolaterally is the obliquus superior, inferiorly obliquus inferior and medially rectus capitis posterior major and minor
  - Third part of vertebral artery lies within the triangle.
- Greater occipital nerve is the thickest cutaneous muscle in the body. It winds the inferior border of obliquus inferior, pierce the semispinalis capitis and trapezius before becoming cutaneous. You should be able to locate the nerve, 2–3 cm lateral to external occipital protuberance.
- Trapezius is known as the shawl muscle.
- Occipital artery is a branch of external carotid artery.
- Vertebral artery is the branch of first part of subclavian artery, ascends behind the common carotid artery:

  I part—is from origin till it enters foramen transversarium. II—lies within the foramen transversarium, III—in suboccipital triangle, and IV—when it enters the cranial cavity through foramen magnum and ends by joining the other side vertebral artery at lower pons to form the basilar artery.

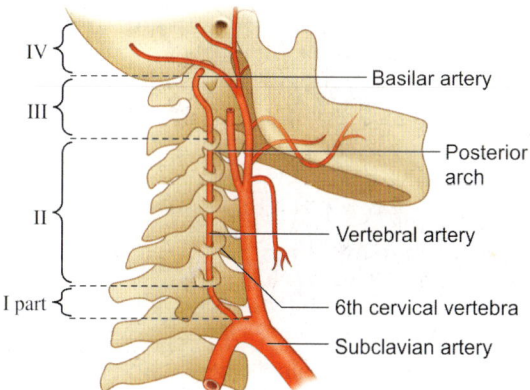

## 5. SUPERFICIAL DISSECTION IN FRONT OF NECK

## a. Incision Markings

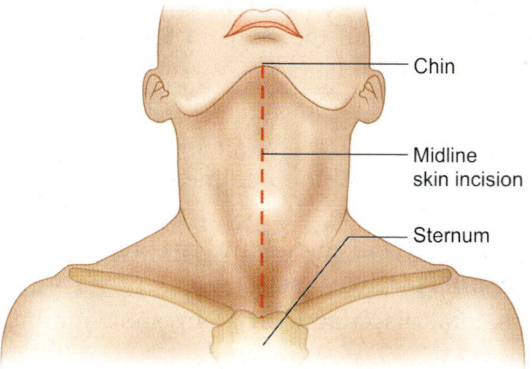

Midline skin incision to be taken on the neck

## b. Structures to be Identified

- Reflect the platysma upwards, while doing so identify the superficial branches of transverse cervical nerve, and identify the cervical branch of facial nerve
- In the midline you will see a vein variable in size this is the anterior jugular vein
- Incise the deep fascia just above the sternum horizontally and extend it few centimetres along the anterior border of sternocleidomastoid to enter the suprasternal space of Burns.
- Remove the fat and fascia from the sternocleidomastoid and the infrahyoid region this exposes the strap muscles of the neck, separate the muscles by finger dissection, identify from above downwards hyoid bone, thyroid cartilage, isthmus of thyroid gland. In the suprahyoid region, the muscle forming the floor of mouth is the mylohyoid, anterior belly of digastric can be seen, superficial lobe of submandibular gland is seen on dividing the fascia over it, facial artery along the inferior border of mandible.

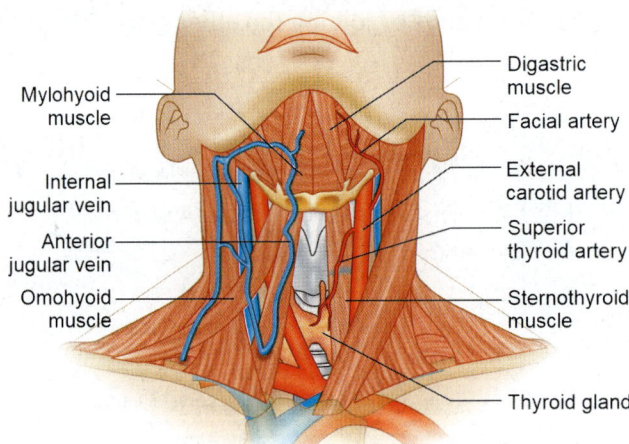

Front of neck-superficial dissection

## c. Vivisection

While doing tracheostomy, a life-saving procedure the surgeon needs to be well-versed with the midline structures, layer by layer he needs to separate, the strap muscles to reach the trachea. One needs to be vigilant about the veins in the region and the isthmus of thyroid while doing tracheostomy.

## d. Viva Questions

- Student should be able to identify all the midline structures—thyroid gland, thyrohyoid membrane, thyroid cartilage
- Structures piercing the thyrohyoid membrane is commonly asked—they are superior laryngeal vessels and internal laryngeal nerve
- Mylohyoid muscle is the oral diaphragm, dividing submandibular gland into superficial and deep parts.

# 6. ANTERIOR TRIANGLE OF THE NECK

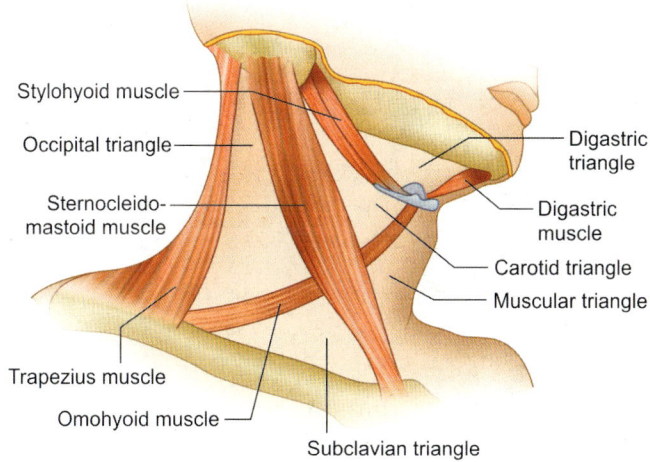

Triangles of the neck

## a. Structures to be Identified

- Pull the superficial part of submandibular gland laterally, this exposes the tendon of digastric muscle.
- Along the lower border of mandible try to locate the submental branch of facial artery, a nerve along it is the mylohyoid nerve.
- Posterior belly of digastric is closely followed by the stylohyoid muscle, follow these two muscles to the angle of mandible.
- Take the submandibular gland backwards to expose the posterior border of mylohyoid muscle and appreciate the gland hooking around the muscle.

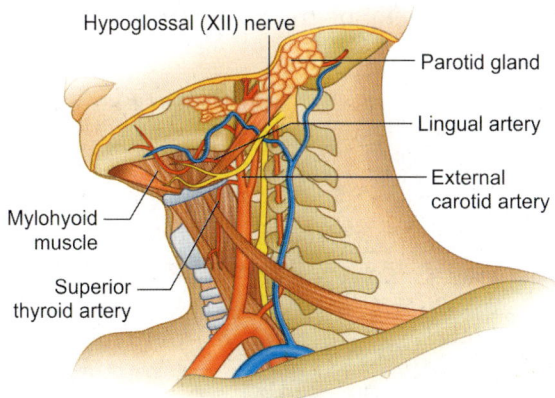

Deep dissection of submandibular region

- Dissect the facial artery which lies posterosuperior to the gland and anteriorly find the submandibular duct (Wharton's duct).

- Identify a thick nerve just superior to the greater cornu of hyoid bone, this is the hypoglossal nerve lying on the hyoglossus muscle, at a higher level above, on the hyoglossus muscle is the lingual nerve, lingual artery lies deep to hyoglossus.

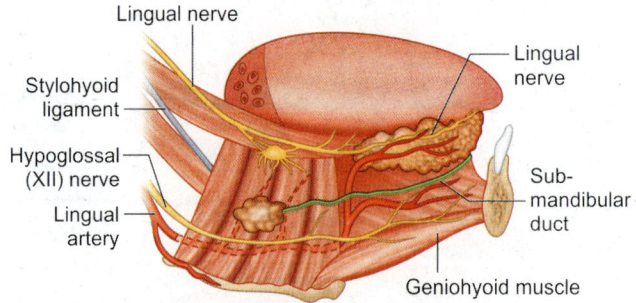

Deepest plane of the submandibular region showing relations of hyoglossus muscle

- Cut the anterior belly of digastric, sacrifice the mylohyoid nerve, study the attachments of mylohyoid muscle.
- Follow the lingual nerve posteriorly, it lies very close to the last molar tooth, it enters the mouth below the superior constrictor.
- In the upper part of hyoglossus the styloglossus muscle merges, below it, is the stylopharyngeus, glossopharyngeal nerve lies close to stylopharyngeus muscle.
- Try to identify the stylohyoid ligament to the styloid process, it lies just above stylopharyngeus.
- Divide the hyoglossus from the hyoid bone this will expose the lingual artery, genioglossus, middle constrictor, and stylohyoid ligament.
- Identify the boundaries of carotid triangle, and the branches of external carotid artery in this region
  - Superior thyroid artery, runs anteroinferiorly deep to omohyoid
  - Ascending pharyngeal artery arises from lowest part of external carotid
  - Lingual artery arises behind the tip of greater horn of hyoid bone

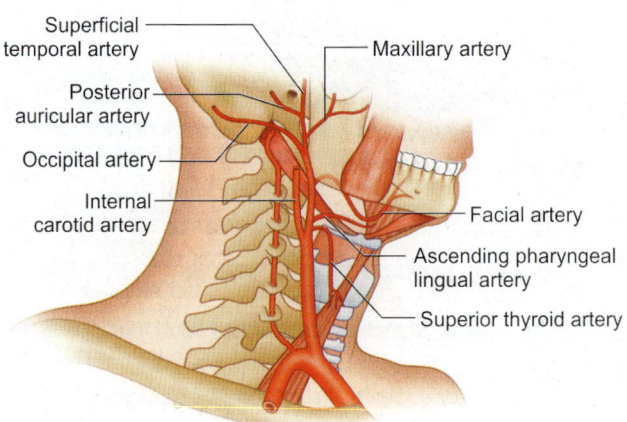

External carotid artery with its branches

- Facial artery arises above the lingual

- Occipital artery runs posterosuperiorly along the lower border of posterior belly of digastric muscle.
- To study the carotid sheath which encloses the internal jugular vein, vagus nerve, and carotid arteries, remove the fascial sheath around it.

## b. Vivisection

While doing submandibular gland resection, one needs to know all the crucial structures in vicinity, i.e. lingual artery, lingual nerve, hypoglossal nerve.

## c. Viva Questions

- Relations of hyoglossus muscle are often asked—lingual artery is deep to it while lingual nerve is superficial to it
- Mylohyoid muscle is the oral diaphragm
- Identify the posterior belly of digastric and the stylohyoid muscle with it. The occipital artery lies along the inferior border of digastric muscle.
- Carotid structures are the internal jugular vein, carotid artery and vagus nerve. Ansa cervicalis lies anterior to the sheath while the sympathetic chain lies posterior to it
- Common carotid artery divides at the upper border of thyroid cartilage.

## 7. PAROTID DISSECTION

### a. Incisions to be Taken

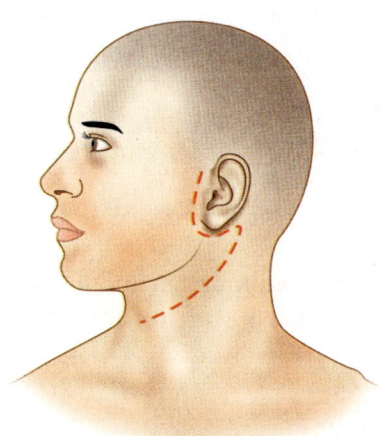

Incision to be taken to expose parotid region

### b. Structures to be Identified

- Reflect the skin carefully without damaging the underlying structures. Divide the fascia on parotid gland in front of auricle from zygomatic arch to angle of mandible.
- Dissect out the fascia around the gland anteriorly, in a horizontal fashion anticipating the presence of the terminal branches of facial nerve. It is difficult to trace the branches amongst the fascia.

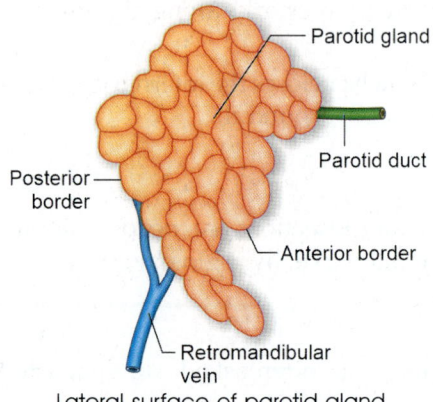

Lateral surface of parotid gland

- Trace the parotid duct to a muscle which is buccinator.
- Remove the parotid gland in piecemeal and expose the structures piercing the gland, i.e. retromandibular vein, external carotid artery, and the facial nerve.

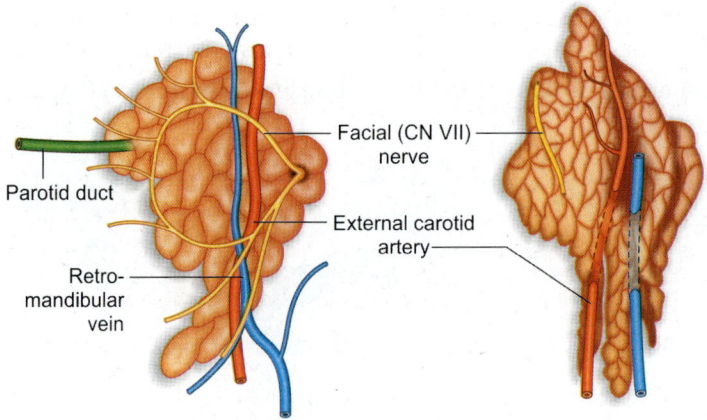

Structures piercing the parotid gland    Parotid duct

- Follow the facial nerve to stylomastoid foramen and locate the posterior auricular branch, and a branch to posterior belly of digastric on the deep surface of gland. Try to locate even the posterior auricular artery.

### c. Vivisection

Parotid surgeries are commonly performed, surgeon has to thoroughly know the anatomy of the parotid region. The facial nerve injury will lead to postoperative facial palsy, external carotid artery and retromandibular vein are major vessels traversing the parotid gland.

### d. Viva Questions

- Facial enters the parotid gland through the posteromedial surface of gland.
- The anterior border of gland is related to the terminal branches of facial nerve, i.e. temporal, zygomatic, buccal, mandibular and cervical, and the parotid duct.
- Parotid duct is also known as Stensen's duct, it opens in the vestibule of mouth against the upper second molar.

- Frey's syndrome is a clinical condition wherein a patient develops sweating while eating. This is due to the aberrant regeneration of auriculotemporal nerve with the superior cervical branch, i.e. a parasympathetic communication with the sympathetic. This syndrome occurs following direct trauma to parotid gland.
- Secretomotor pathway of parotid gland is commonly asked: Inferior salivary nucleus, tympanic branch of glossopharyngeal nerve—tympanic plexus- lesser petrosal nerve—OTIC ganglion, auriculotemporal nerve and the parotid gland.

## 8. THYROID GLAND

### a. Study of the Gland

- Identify the strap muscles, pull laterally, the sternocleidomastoid and superior belly of omohyoid, cut the strap muscles and reflect them upwards.
- Appreciate the inferior thyroid vein and then remove the fat in vicinity.
- Appreciate the location of thyroid gland, it lies against the 2nd to 4th tracheal rings, enclosed in the pretracheal fascia. Between the two lobes is the isthmus of the gland. Remove the fascia on the gland and by blunt dissection lift the lower pole of the gland to expose the lateral surface of trachea and esophagus, trace recurrent laryngeal nerve.

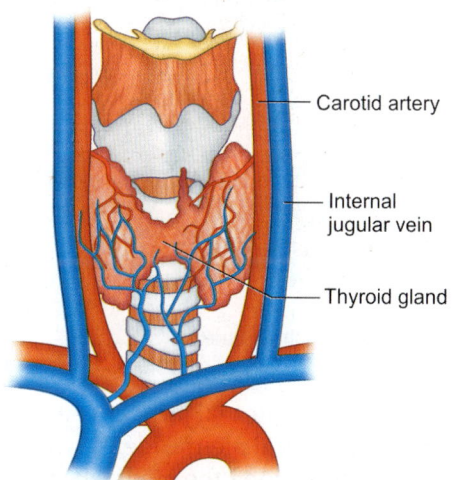

Thyroid gland *in situ*—front view

- Carotid artery
- Internal jugular vein
- Thyroid gland

- Pull the upper part of the lobe laterally and try to locate the external branch of superior laryngeal nerve reaching the cricothyroid muscle.
- Divide the isthmus, try to locate the anastomotic vessel between the superior and inferior thyroid artery, on medial part of posterior surface of the gland. Locate the yellowish-brown parathyroid gland.
- The carotid sheath lies posterolateral to the gland.
- Completely expose the trachea and esophagus and study the structures in their vicinity.

### b. Vivisection

Thyroid surgeries are the most commonly performed surgeries, while operating the surgeon has to be vigilant about the carotid sheath posterolaterally and the recurrent laryngeal nerve in the tracheoesophageal groove.

### c. Viva Questions

- Relations of thyroid gland are commonly discussed—on the viva table the crucial relations which the student should know are that the carotid sheath lies posterolaterally and the tracheoesophageal groove lodges the recurrent laryngeal nerve.
- Inferior thyroid artery is closely related to the recurrent laryngeal nerve while the superior thyroid artery is related to the external laryngeal nerve.

## 9. ROOT OF THE NECK

### a. Structures to be Identified

- Incise the carotid sheath, clear off the lymph nodes and fat from the neck. Separate the internal jugular vein and the carotid artery. Displace the artery laterally to look for the sympathetic chain.
- Dissect out the vagus nerve and vertebral artery which lie posteriorly.

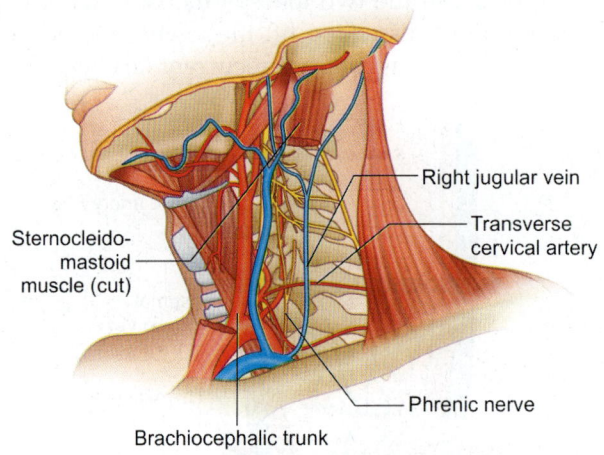

Sternocleido-
mastoid
muscle (cut)

Right jugular vein

Transverse
cervical artery

Phrenic nerve

Brachiocephalic trunk

Root of neck structures

- Identify the phrenic nerve posterior to internal jugular vein, if you turn the vein medially it exposes the subclavian artery, and cervical pleura, identify the branches of subclavian artery, you can locate the costocervical trunk along the medial border of scalenus anterior muscle. The prominent nerve in front of the scalenus anterior muscle is the phrenic nerve.

## 8. EVISCERATION OF BRAIN

### a. Incisions on the Skull

### b. Steps to Remove the Calvaria

- Mark with a chalk piece a circular incision starting 1 cm above the orbital margin all around on the side of cranium and similarly 1 cm above the external occipital protuberance.

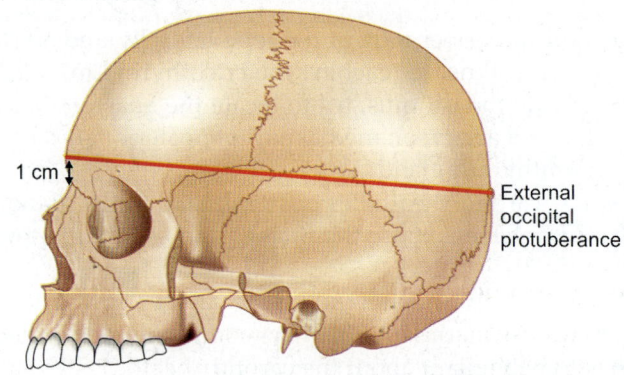

1 cm

External
occipital
protuberance

Markings on calvaria for brain evisceration

- Then with a saw, cut along the marking, do not be too hard otherwise you may cut the marrow cavity. Stop cutting with the saw, when you see the sawdust red, and the outer table has been divided.
- Remember temporal bone is thin no marrow cavity laterally, be gentle while using a saw in this region.
- Now insert a blunt chisel in the saw cut and separate the outer table of skull by sharp, definite strokes with a hammer.
- Endocranium and endosteal dura are firmly adherent to the interior of the skull, so to remove the calvaria insert the chisel through the cut and the lift the calvaria.

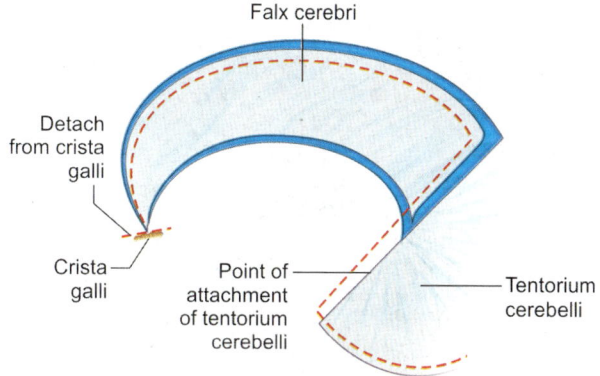

Falx cerebri and tentorium cerebelli

- After lifting the calvaria make a paramedian sagittal incision on the endocranium this will open the superior sagittal sinus.

## c. Steps to Remove the Brain Intact

- Divide the anterior attachment of falx cerebri from crista galli and then pull the falx cerebri posteriorly
- Place a wooden block under the shoulder this will create a gap between the head and table
- Now with hands gently lift the frontal lobes from the anterior cranial fossa this exposes the olfactory bulbs, which can be gently lifted from the cribriform plates of ethmoid
- Thick conspicuous optic nerves will be visible now, cut them close to the optic foramen and proceed tilting the brain backwards, now you can see the internal carotid arteries and the pituitary stalk
- While leaning the brain backwards do not allow it to be supported on the cut edge of skull otherwise the soft brain tissue may get damaged
- Behind the pituitary stalk identify the dorsum sellae, and posterior clinoid process
- Identify the oculomotor nerve
- Lateral to the oculomotor nerve is the free edge of tentorium cerebelli. Dissect the free margin of tentorium cerebella and try to locate the trochlear nerve.
- Turn the head to one side and separate the posterior lobes of cerebral hemisphere from the tentorium cerebelli with the hands, repeat the same for the other side
- Incise the tentorium along the attachment on the superior border of petrous temporal bone. While incising remain superficial to avoid damage to the cerebellum

- Pull the brain backwards so the brainstem will stand prominently and draw it away from the anterior wall of posterior cranial fossa
- Cut the cranial nerves one by one under vision
- Push the brainstem more posteriorly and cut the vertebral arteries
- Put a knife within the foramen magnum and cut the medulla this is like cutting the stalk of brain and you can deliver out the cerebrum

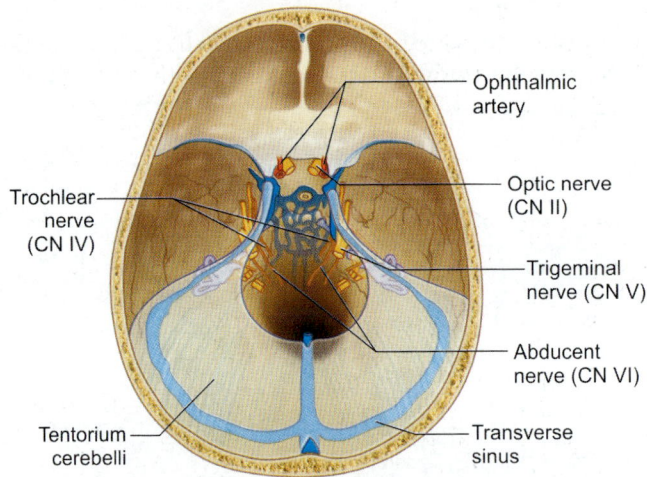

Cranial fossae as seen after brain delivery

- Incise the falx cerebri at along the left side at its junction with the tentorium, carry this incision forwards along the free edge of falx cerebri, also continue the incision laterally from the internal occipital protuberance to base of petrous temporal bone.

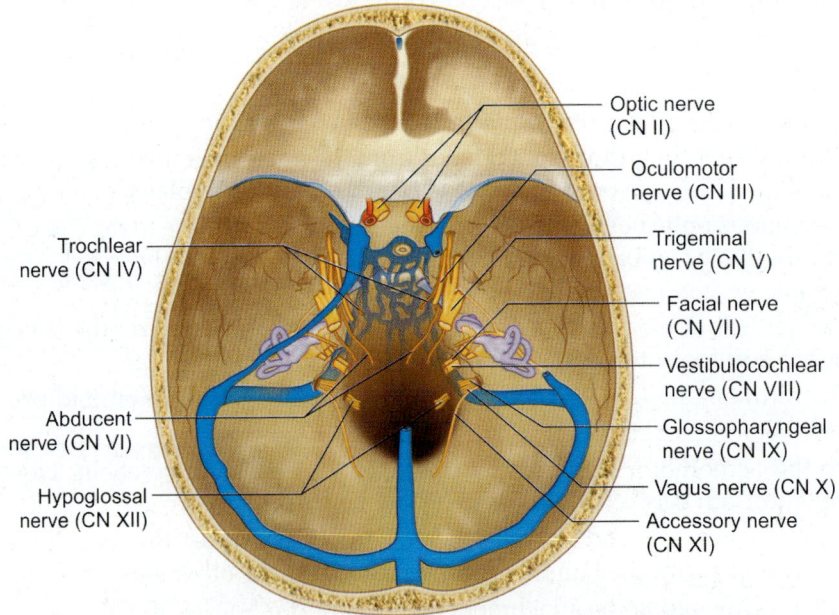

Cranial fossae showing the cut ends of all the cranial nerves

## d. Viva Questions

- Student should be able to identify all the cranial nerves (study the above diagram carefully) (there are twelve pairs of cranial nerves)

  I olfactory, II Optic, III oculomotor, IV trochlear, V trigeminal, VI abducent, VII facial, VIII auditory, IX glossopharyngeal, X Vagus, XI spinal accessory, XII hypoglossal
- Identify the various folds of dura mater namely falx cerebri, tentorium cerebelli and diaphragma sella
- Identify the petrous temporal bone, and the impression for the trigeminal ganglion in the middle cranial fossa
- Student should be able to identify the pituitary stalk piercing the diaphragma sella
- On the either side of the pituitary stalk is the cavernous sinus, lateral to cavernous sinus are the III, IV, V1 and V2 nerves
- Maxillary nerve traverses the foramen rotundum, and the mandibular nerve traverses the foramen ovale.

## 9. ORBIT DISSECTION

### a. Steps to be Taken

- Strip the periosteum from the floor of anterior cranial fossa except over the cribriform plate of ethmoid
- Engage a chisel on the roof of orbit and gently tap on it, this will break the roof into pieces, remove them this will expose the orbital contents
- Remove the remains of the lesser wing of sphenoid, but leave the margin of optic canal intact this exposes the superior orbital fissure
- Divide the periosteum of orbital roof horizontally close to the anterior margin of orbit, and then anteroposteriorly along the middle line of orbit.

### b. Structures to be Identified

- Trochlear nerve lies just below the periosteum, be careful while incising the periosteum otherwise it will get damaged.

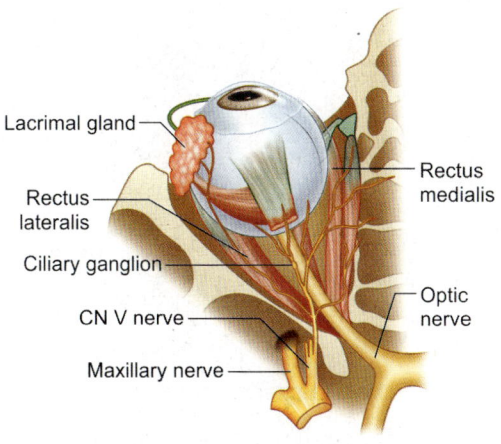

Dissected orbit—superficial plane

- Trace the trochlear nerve forwards and medial to the superior oblique muscle.

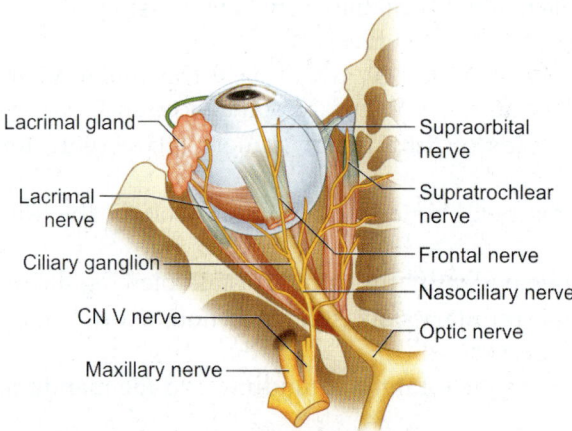

Lacrimal gland
Lacrimal nerve
Ciliary ganglion
CN V nerve
Maxillary nerve
Supraorbital nerve
Supratrochlear nerve
Frontal nerve
Nasociliary nerve
Optic nerve

Dissected orbit—deeper plane

- The frontal nerve lies on the levator palpabrae superioris in the middle of the orbit.
- Follow the tendon of superior oblique muscle at the superomedial angle of orbit.
- Follow the nerve forwards and identify its divisions into supraorbital and supratrochlear. Each nerve is accompanied by a vessel. Supratrochlear nerve runs towards the medial angle of orbit.
- Below the levator palpabrae superioris lies the superior rectus, and a branch of oculomotor nerve.
- Lacrimal nerve and artery lie along the superolateral part of the orbit.
- Locate the nasociliary nerve, ciliary ganglion, lacrimal nerve.
- Cut the levator muscle, this exposes the superior rectus, and evert the muscles.
- Inject saline in the eyeball and inflate it, pick-up the loose areolar tissue take a small cut on it and insert a probe between the fascial sheath and eyeball.

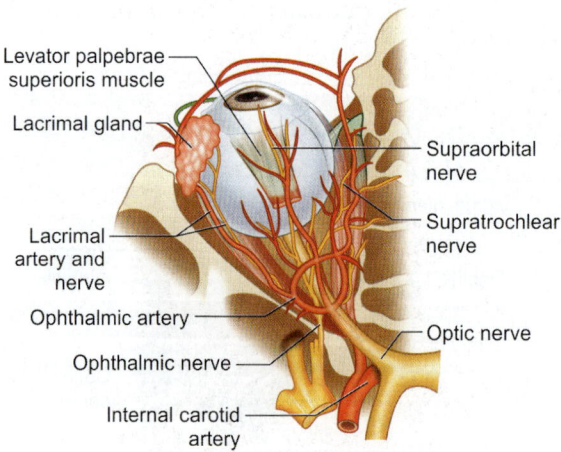

Levator palpebrae superioris muscle
Lacrimal gland
Lacrimal artery and nerve
Ophthalmic artery
Ophthalmic nerve
Internal carotid artery
Supraorbital nerve
Supratrochlear nerve
Optic nerve

Ophthalmic artery and its branches

- Remove the fat around the ciliary ganglion and expose the abducent nerve along the lateral rectus muscle.

- Study the extraocular muscles and its attachments. Cut the optic nerve close to the canal and evert it forwards to study the lateral rectus. Make an incision on the inferior fornix of conjunctiva and palpebral fascia, separate the eyeball by blunt dissection this exposes the inferior rectus muscle.

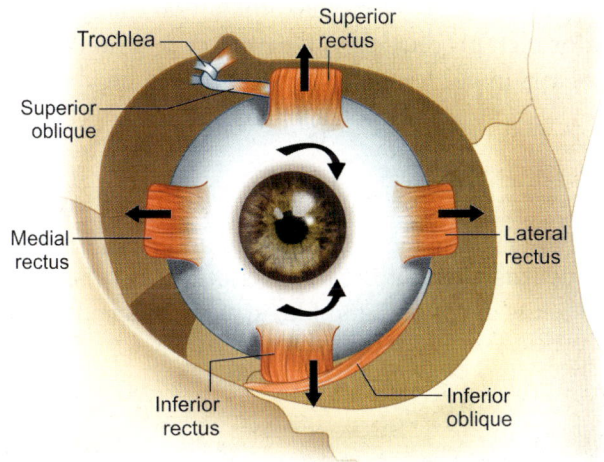

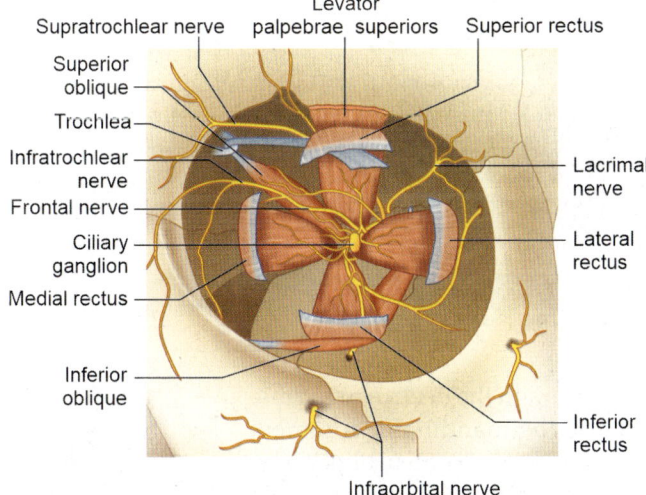

Orbit from front showing extraocular muscles

## c. Viva Questions

- Student should be able to identify each and every structure in the orbit very commonly asked in the exams
  - Frontal nerve lies on the levator palpabrae superioris muscle, and divides into supra-orbital and supratrochlear nerve
  - The first nerve encountered is the trochlear nerve, which supplies the superior oblique muscle
  - Just below the levator palpabrae superioris is the superior rectus
  - Lacrimal nerve and artery at the superolateral part of the orbit

- SO4, LR6, and other extraocular muscles supplied by the oculomotor nerve
- Student should be able to locate the ciliary ganglion, which lies within the fat between the optic nerve and the lateral rectus muscle.
- Actions of the extraocular muscles will be asked:
  - Medial and lateral recti bring about medial and lateral rotation around vertical axis
  - Superior and inferior recti produce elevation and depression around transverse axis
  - Superior oblique assists in depression and inferior oblique in elevation.

## 10. INFRATEMPORAL FOSSA

### a. Bony Incisions

- Cut the zygomatic arch by making incisions anterior and posterior to masseter and turn the cut part of bone downwards after cutting the masseteric vessels.
- Strip the masseter up to the angle of mandible, leave it attached to angle of mandible.

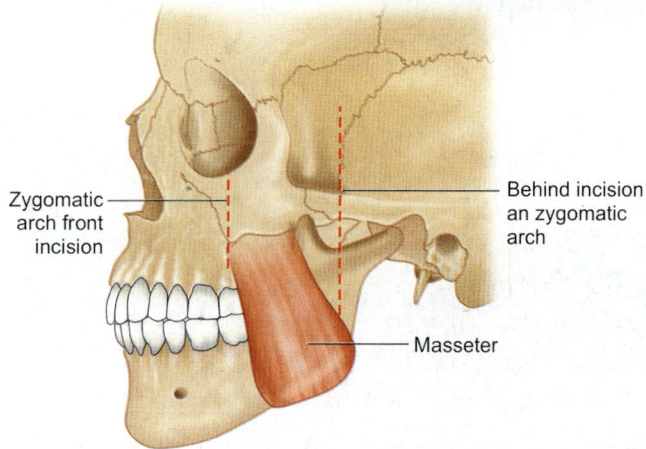

Bony cuts to be taken to expose the infratemporal fossa

- Make a horizontal cut through the neck of mandible and another just above the mandibular foramen. Mandibular foramen has to be located blindly by gliding a probe along the ramus of the mandible and subjacent soft parts. Remove the cut bone this will expose the underlying vessels and muscles in the infratemporal fossa after clearing the fat in that area.

### b. Structures to be Identified

- Identify the maxillary artery, the muscle it crosses is the lateral pterygoid muscle.
- Lateral pterygoid muscle has an upper head and lower head, by blunt dissection divide the two heads, avoid injuring the buccal nerve.

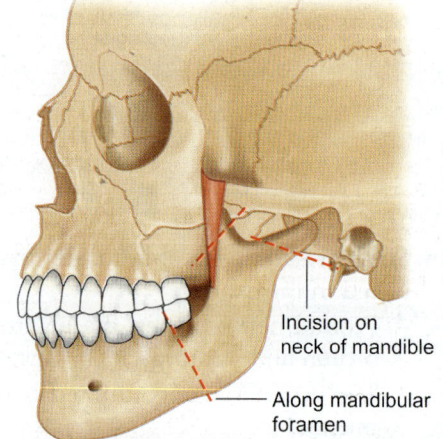

Bony cuts to be taken to expose the infra-temporal fossa

- Remove the upper head by cutting its attachment from the infratemporal fossa and the temporomandibular joint, scrape the lower head from lateral pterygoid plate laterally.
- Disarticulate the head of mandible from the articular disc and remove it with the lower head of lateral pterygoid. Be careful about the auriculotemporal nerve around the temporomandibular joint.
- Trace the middle meningeal artery to foramen spinosum and the roots of auriculotemporal nerve which loop around the artery, muscle medially is tensor palati.

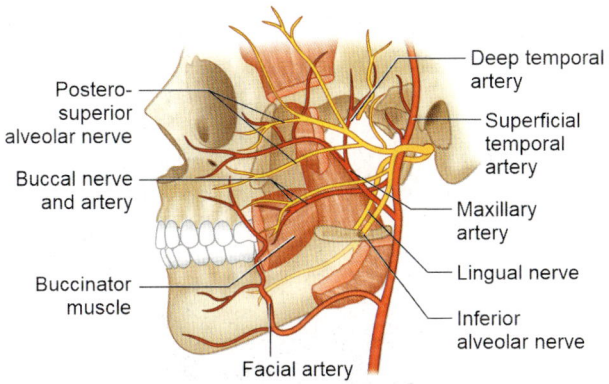

Structures in infratemporal fossa

- Trace the branches of mandibular nerve, and make an attempt to trace the otic ganglion.

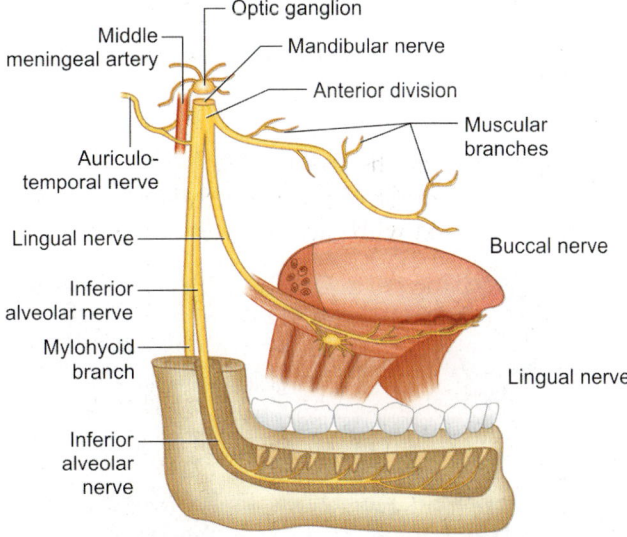

Mandibular nerve and its branches

## c. Viva Questions

- Lateral pterygoid muscle is commonly asked—student should be able to identify the muscle and know its relevant relations:
  - Maxillary artery is divided into three parts by this muscle
  - Only muscle of mastication, which opens the mouth

- Buccal nerve lies between the upper and lower head of the muscle
- Inferior alveolar nerve and lingual nerve are related to the lower border of the muscle
- Otic ganglion is located in the infratemporal fossa
- Middle meningeal artery traverses the foramen spinosum
- Auriculotemporal nerve forms a loop around the middle meningeal artery.

## 11. SAGITTAL SECTION OF NOSE, MOUTH, PHARYNX AND LARYNX

- Study the section carefully and identify the structures, turbinates and auditory tube opening is commonly asked

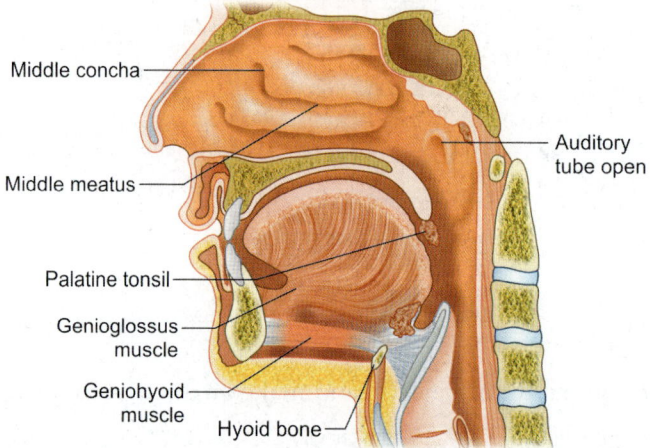

Sagittal section of head and neck, showing, oropharynx, nasopharynx, laryngopharynx

## 12. LARYNX MODEL

- Student should study the larynx with help of model:
  - Larynx is nothing but conglomeration of cartilages, thyroid, cricoid, epiglottis, arytenoids, corniculate, cuneiform connected with each other with membranes and ligaments.

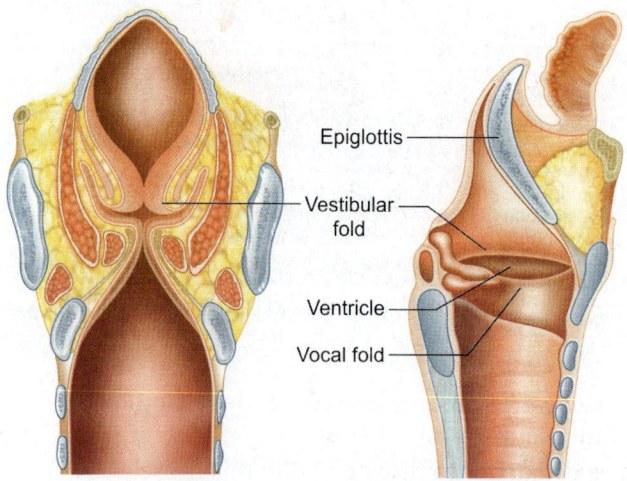

Laryngeal framework of cartilages

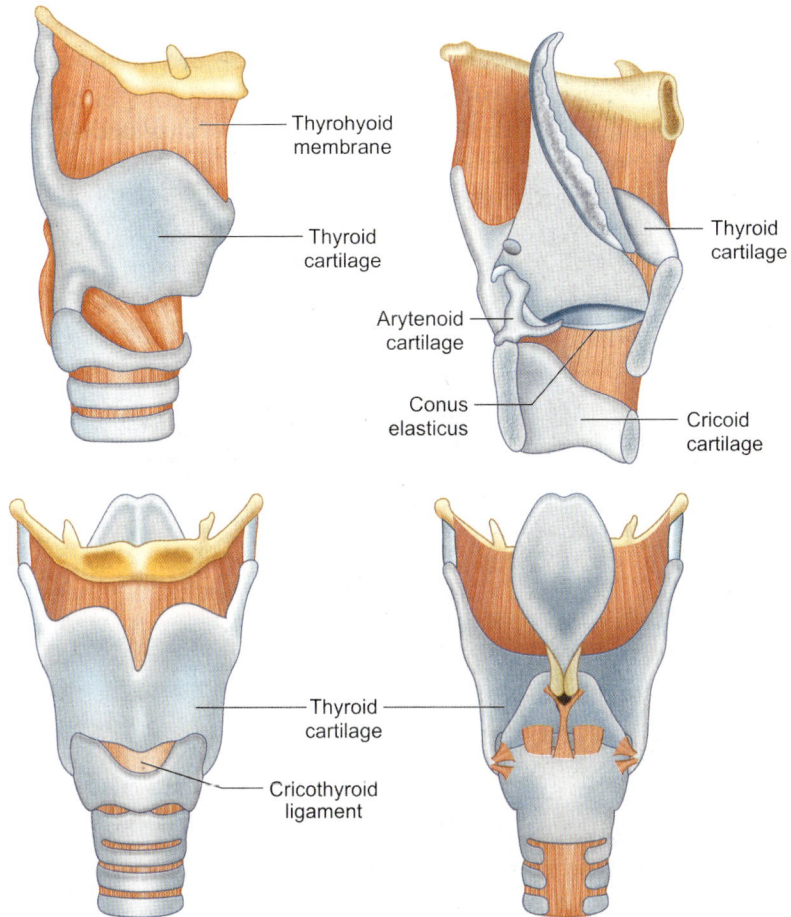

Front view and side view

- Normally a string is attached to the arytenoid cartilage in the model, to demonstrate the action of muscles on larynx one needs to pull the string, posterior cricoarytenoid muscle abducts the vocal cords.
- Study the interior of larynx, all features may not be presented in the model.

  Laryngectomy specimen can be procured from surgical department and you can appreciate the interior features of larynx very clearly.

## b. Vivisection

- Cancer larynx is very common in India due to habits like tobacco chewing and smoking. Surgically, it is divided into supraglottis, glottis, and subglottis.
  - Supraglottis includes—epiglottis, aryepiglottic folds, vestibular folds, ventricles, arytenoids cartilage
  - Glottis is vocal cords
  - Subglottis extends from vocal cords to inferior border of cricoid cartilage.
- Hypopharynx means—pyriform fossae, postcricoid region, posterior pharyngeal wall.

### c. Viva Questions

- All intrinsic muscles of the larynx are supplied by the recurrent laryngeal nerve except cricothyroid which is supplied by external laryngeal nerve
- Posterior cricoarytenoid is known as the safety muscle of the larynx as it abducts the vocal cords maintaining the patency of the airway
- Cricothyroid is the tensor of vocal cord.

## 13. SAGITTAL SECTION OF NOSE AND PALATE SHOWING THE LATERAL WALL OF NOSE

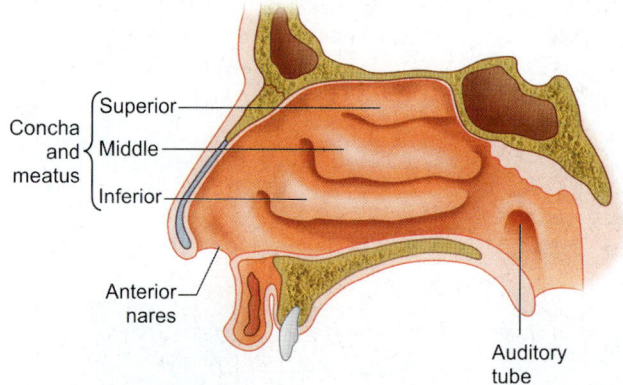

Sagittal section of nose and palate showing the lateral wall of nose

### a. Viva Questions

- Identify the turbinates—superior, middle and inferior
- Identify the nasopharyngeal opening.

### b. Vivisection

The openings in the meati can be widened for proper drainage of sinuses, with help of endoscopes. FESS—functional endoscopic sinus surgery.

## 14. SAGITTAL SECTION OF NOSE AND PALATE IN WHICH THE TURBINATES ARE SACRIFICED

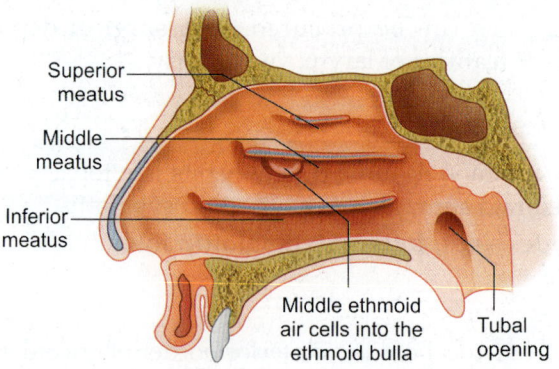

Sagittal section of nose and pharynx in which turbinates are sacrificed

## a. Viva Questions

Superior meatus has openings of posterior ethmoidal sinus, middle meatus has openings of maxillary, frontal, anterior and middle ethmoidal sinuses, inferior meatus has an opening of nasolacrimal duct.

## 15. NASAL SEPTUM

Study the components of nasal septum

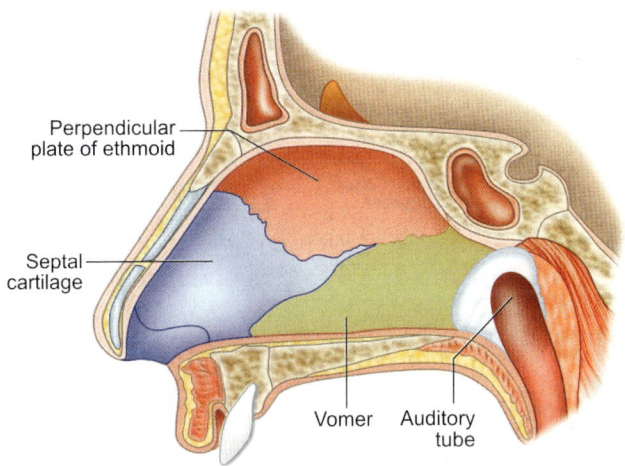

Sagittal section through nasal septum

## a. Vivisection

Septoplasty is a surgery to correct the deviation of septum, wherein the surgeon has to carefully elevate the mucoperiosteum from the underlying cartilage and bony septum later to get an access to the septum to correct the deviation.

## b. Viva Questions

- Nasal septum is mainly made-up of bones—perpendicular plate of ethmoid, vomer, cartilage forming the septum is septal cartilage
- Little's area is an area on the anteroinferior part of septum, where following arteries anastomose—anterior ethmoidal, superior labial, sphenopalatine, greater palatine
- Sphenopalatine artery is the artery of epistaxis.

## 16. MIDDLE EAR RELATIONS MODEL

## a. Viva Questions

- Students should first identify the lateral and medial side of the model to study the relations:
  - Lateral wall is formed by the tympanic membrane.
  - Medial wall features are promontory, oval window covered by foot plate of stapes, round window covered by secondary tympanic membrane, lateral semicircular canal and facial nerve produce bulges one below another posteriorly near the aditus, sinus tympani, is a depression between the two windows.

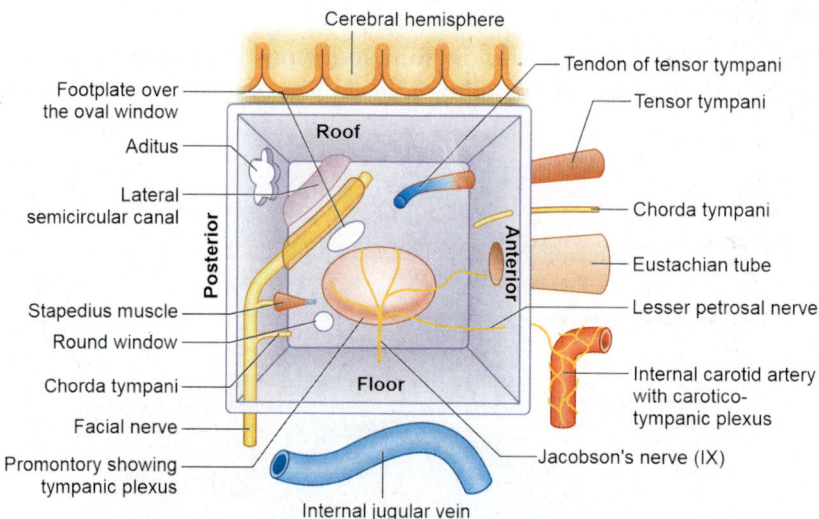

Ear model showing middle ear relations

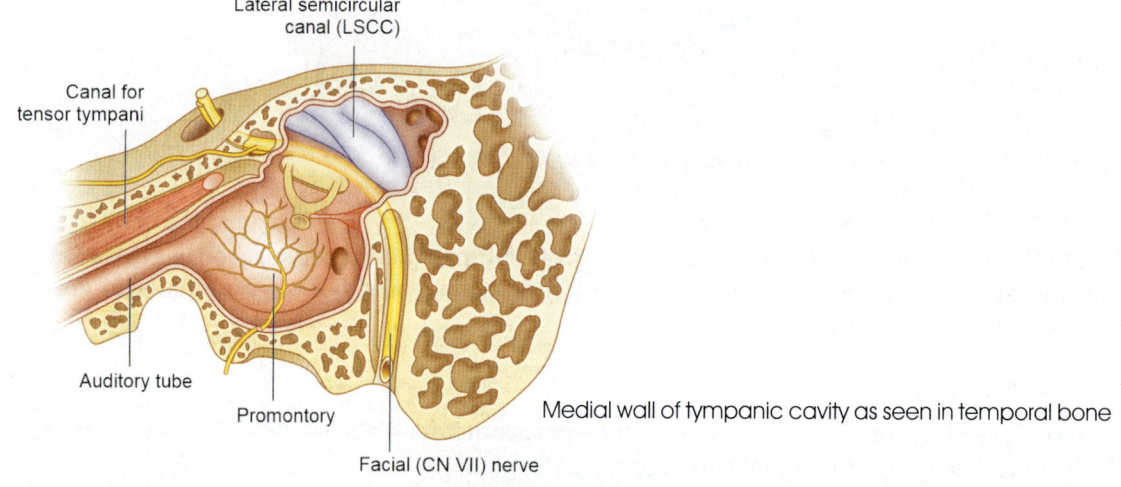

Medial wall of tympanic cavity as seen in temporal bone

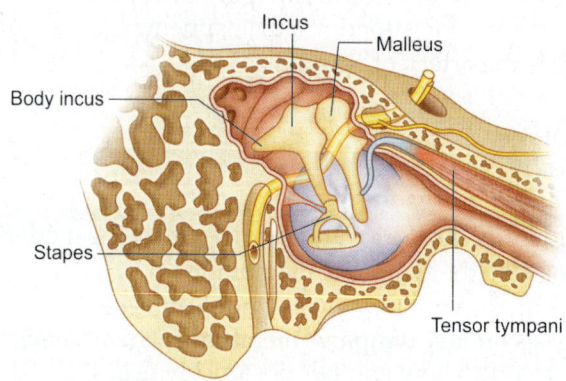

Middle ear cavity with ossicles *in situ*, tensor tympani canal

- Posterior wall shows—aditus which leads from epitympanic recess to mastoid antrum, below close to the medial wall is a small conical projection known as pyramid, it has stapedius tendon, lateral to pyramid is the opening through which the chorda tympani nerve enters.

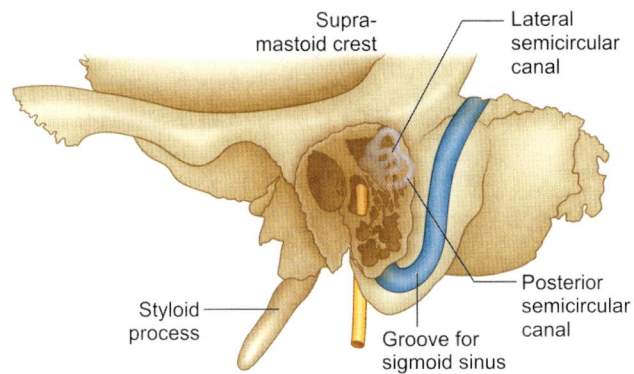

Mastoid antrum dissection

- Roof is the thin plate of bone tegmen tympani, which separates the middle ear cavity from the middle cranial fossa.
- Floor is formed by the thin bony lamina separates the middle ear cavity from the jugular vein (superior bulb).
- Promontory is a medial bulge on the medial wall of middle ear cavity produced due to the basal turn of cochlea.
- Anterior wall has superiorly an opening for semicanal for tensor tympani, opening for auditory tube, inferiorly, there is a lamina of bone separating it from carotid canal.
- Drill the mastoid bone to appreciate the antrum, and mastoid air cells.

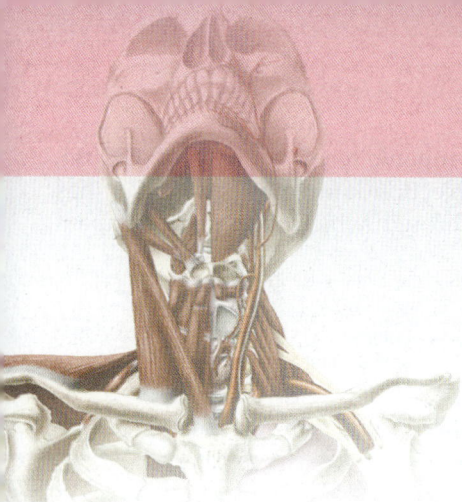

# Osteology 39

## SKULL

- Skeleton of head is skull, i.e. calvaria + facial skeleton + mandible
- Skull without mandible is cranium
- Calvaria is skull cap
- Inner surface of calvaria is cranial vault.

### Top View of Skull or Norma Verticalis

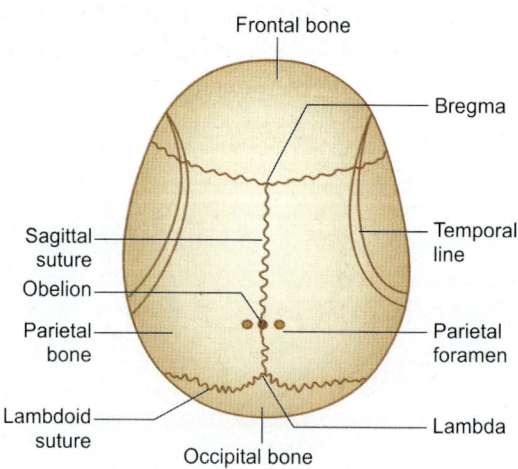

Top view of skull—external features

*Features*

- Point of junction of coronal suture with the sagittal suture is bregma
- Point of junction of lambdoid suture with the sagittal suture is lambda
- Parietal tuber is the area of maximum convexity on parietal bone

- Point in between the parietal foramen on the sagittal suture is named as obelion
- Temporal lines can also be seen.

### Foramen

Parietal foramen transmits the emissary vein from superior sagittal sinus.

### Front View of the Skull or Norma Frontalis

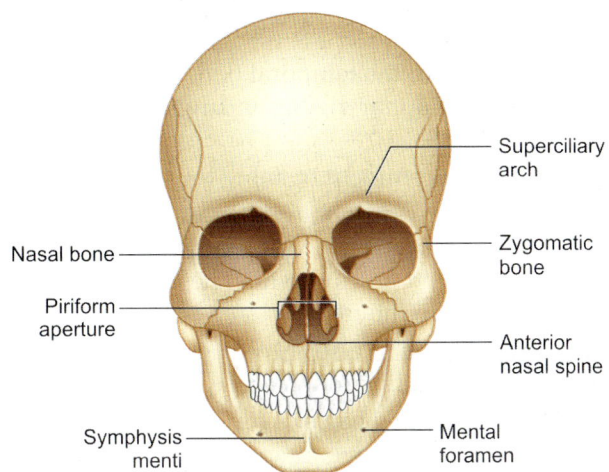

Front view of the skull—external features

### Features

- Just above the medial half of the orbit is an bony elevation, superciliary arch
- Median elevation between the 2 superciliary arches is glabella
- Framework of nose is the nasal bone and pyriform-shaped nasal aperture
- Mid of nasal aperture is a projection, anterior nasal spine
- Nasion is root of nose, rhinion is lower point of internasal suture.

### Foramen

- Supraorbital foramen—supraorbital nerve and vessels
- Infraorbital foramen—infraorbital nerve
- Mental foramen—mental nerve.

### Side View of the Skull or Norma Lateralis

### Features

- Two temporal lines can be appreciated, superior one giving attachment to epicranial aponeurosis and temporal fascia, while the inferior temporal line which continues forwards as the supramastoid crest marks the upper limit of the origin of temporalis muscle.

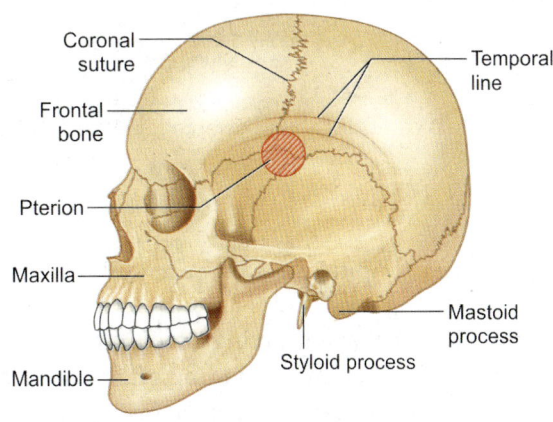

Side view of the skull—external features

- Pterion is the junctional suture between frontal, parietal, sphenoidal and temporal bone. Middle meningeal vein, anterior division of middle meningeal artery and stem of lateral sulcus lies beneath pterion (Sylvian point).
- Zygomatic arch is formed by the union of temporal process of zygomatic bone and zygomatic process of temporal bone.
- Temporal fossa is the gap deep to zygomatic arch for passage of temporal vessels.
- Quadrangular area below the temporal fossa is the infratemporal fossa which lodges the otic ganglion.
- Styloid process is a projection from the temporal bone giving attachment to three muscles- stylohyoid, styloglossus and stylopharyngeus and two ligaments—stylohyoid and stylo-mandibular.
- External acoustic meatus is the prominent opening on side of the skull.
- Suprameatal triangle or Macewan's triangle is an area bounded by supramastoid crest, posterosuperior margin of meatus and a tangent drawn from posterior margin of meatus. It forms the lateral wall of mastoid antrum which lies approximately 1.5 cm deep to it in adults and only 1 mm deep to it in infants.
- Mastoid process is another projection also seen from side of skull, which is also a part of temporal bone. It ossifies by the end of 2nd year.
- Pterygomaxillary fissure is a V-shaped gap seen on the deeper plane of the side of the skull, it communicates with the pterygopalatine fossa.
- Thin plate of bone forming a frill around the external acoustic meatus is the tympanic plate of temporal bone.

## View of the Skull from Behind or Norma Occipitalis

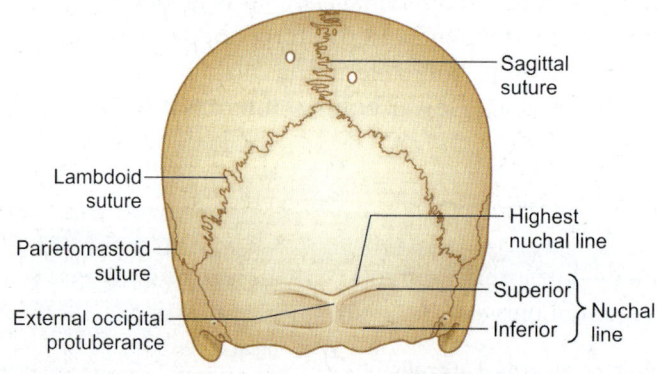

Skull from behind—external features

*Features*

- External occipital protuberance with the highest point on it, inion, giving attachment at the base to trapezius and ligamentum nuchae
- Superior nuchal line giving attachment to trapezius, sternocleidomastoid and splenius capitis
- Highest nuchal line providing attachment to epicranial aponeurosis and occipitalis muscle
- Diagonally opposite to glabella is a point, occipital point, a little above inion
- Asterion is a junctional point between lambdoid and parietomastoid suture.

## Foramen

Mastoid foramen transmits emissary vein connecting sigmoid sinus to posterior auricular vein and meningeal branch of occipital artery.

## View of the Skull from Below or Norma Basalis

For study purpose it can be divided into anterior 1/3rd, middle 1/3rd and posterior 1/3rd.

### *Anterior 1/3rd*

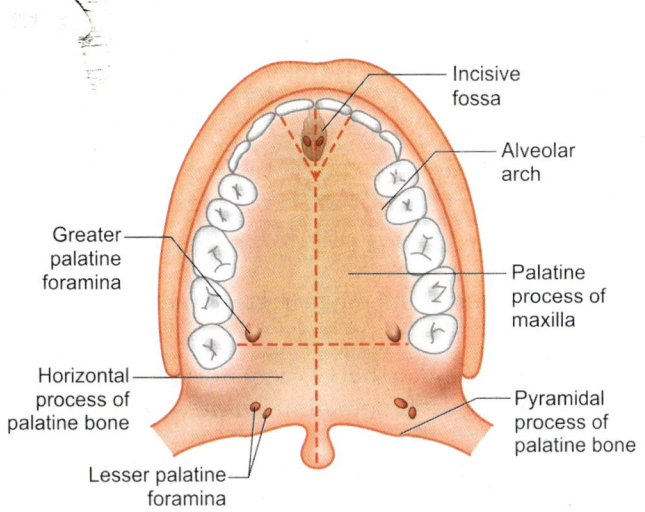

Anterior 1/3rd of base of skull—external features

## Features

- Alveolar arch, hard palate with small processes projecting posterolaterally, pyramidal process of palatine bone perforated by lesser palatine foramen
- Incisive fossa a deep fossa in the median plane of anterior most end of hard palate
- In the centre, along the posterior border of hard palate is the posterior nasal spine, giving attachment to musculus uvulae while posterior border gives attachment to palatine aponeurosis
- Just in front of posterior border is an elevation, palatine crest providing attachment to tendon of tensor palate muscle.

## Foramina

- Incisive foramen transmits greater palatine vessels from palate to nose and nasopalatine nerve from nose to palate
- Greater palatine foramen transmits greater palatine vessels and anterior palatine nerve
- Lesser palatine foramen transmits the middle and posterior palatine nerve.

### *Middle 1/3rd*

## Features

- Vomer, a thin plate of bone forming the posterior most part of nasal septum
- Pterygoid process at the junction of greater wing of sphenoid and body of sphenoid, it has lateral and medial pterygoid plates. The lateral pterygoid plate gives attachment to lateral and medial pterygoid muscles to its respective surfaces

- Basiocciput has a pharyngeal tubercle in its mid, proving attachment to superior pharyngeal constrictor
- Pterygoid hamulus, grooved anteriorly by tendon of tensor veli palatini
- Sulcus tubae, a linear depression which holds the cartilaginous portion of auditory tube
- Spine of sphenoid, mandibular fossa and articular tubercle are the other important features.

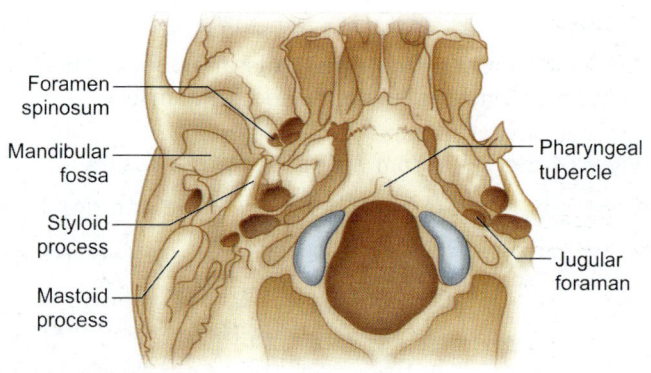

Middle 1/3rd base of skull—external features

*Foramen*

- Foramen spinosum transmits middle meningeal artery and meningeal branch of mandibular nerve
- Foramen ovale (MALE)—mandibular nerve, accessory meningeal artery, lesser petrosal nerve, emissary vein connecting cavernous sinus to pterygoid plexus of veins and anterior trunk of middle meningeal vein
- Foramen lacerum—meningeal branch of ascending pharyngeal artery and an emissary vein from cavernous sinus
- Carotid canal transmitting internal carotid artery with its venous and sympathetic plexus.

*Posterior 1/3rd*

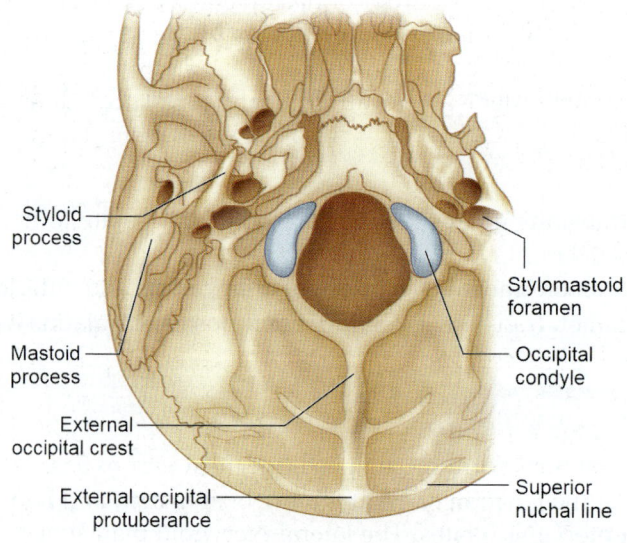

Posterior 1/3rd base of skull—external features

*Features*
- Occipital condyles, roughened medial surface gives attachment to alar ligament
- External occipital crest gives attachment to ligamentum nuchae
- Glossopharyngeal notch lodging the inferior ganglion of IX nerve.

*Foramen*
- Foramen magnum transmitting lower part of medulla, tonsils of cerebellum, meninges, spinal accessory nerve, vertebral artery with its sympathetic plexus, anterior and posterior spinal arteries, apical ligament of dens and membrane tectoria. Margins provide attachment to anterior and posterior atlanto-occipital membrane.
- Jugular foramen provides passage for IX, X, XI cranial nerves, ascending pharyngeal and occipital arteries, internal jugular vein and inferior petrosal sinus
- Mastoid canaliculus—auricular branch of vagus
- Stylomastoid foramen—VII nerve and stylomastoid branch of posterior auricular artery
- Cochlear canaliculus at the apex of glossopharyngeal notch transmits aqueduct of cochlea
- Mastoid process forms lateral wall of mastoid notch which provides attachment to posterior belly of digastric and is grooved medially by occipital artery.

## Cranial Vault

*Features*

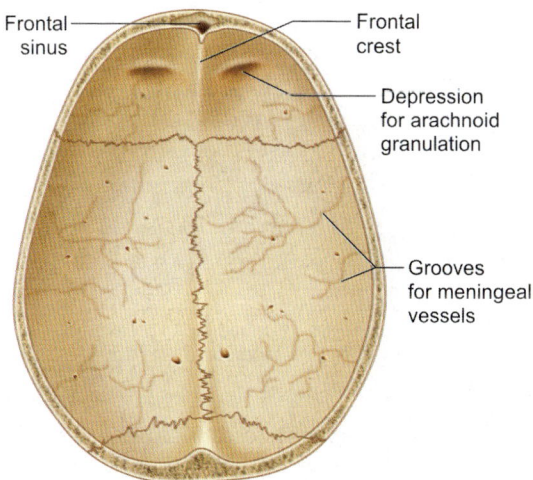

Cranial vault—endocranium

- Cranial bones are made-up of inner and outer table made-up of compact bone in between these tables is sandwiched the spongy bone, diploe filled with red bone marrow
- Internal surface of cranial vault has several markings produced by meningeal vessels, arachnoid granulations and venous sinuses
- Frontal crest in the anterior part of the vault in the midline provides attachment to the falx cerebri.

## Internal Surface of Base of Skull

This area is divided into anterior cranial fossa, middle cranial fossa and posterior cranial fossa.

## Anterior Cranial Fossa

### Features

- Cribriform plate is perforated by several foramina, for passage of olfactory nerves
- Crista galli, a projection on the cribriform plate provides attachment to falx cerebri
- Posterior part of this fossa is the lesser wing of sphenoid, whose posterior border fits into the stem of lateral sulcus of brain
- Anterior clinoid process provides attachment to the free margin of tentorium cerebella
- Orbital plate shows undulations on its surface produced by the frontal lobe orbital surface

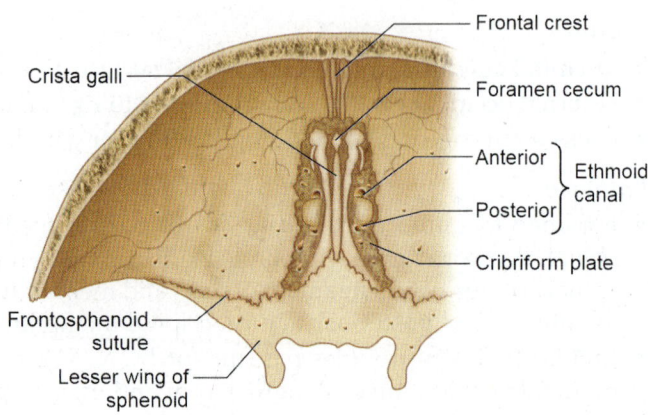

Anterior cranial fossa features

### Foramen

- Anterior ethmoidal canal—anterior ethmoidal vessels and nerve
- Posterior ethmoidal canal—posterior ethmoidal vessels and nerves.

## Middle Cranial Fossa

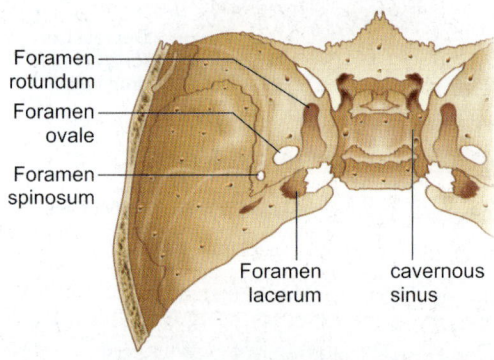

Middle cranial fossa features

### Features

- Sella turcica is a very deep fossa on the upper surface of sphenoid bone, it lodges the pituitary gland
- Cavernous sinus lies on each side of pituitary fossa
- Thick pyramidal bone marks the posterior limit of the middle cranial fossa, this is the petrous temporal bone
- Apex of the petrous temporal bone anteriorly, has a shallow depression for lodging the trigeminal ganglion (student should be able to locate it)
- Arcuate eminence lies on the middle of the anterior surface of petrous temporal bone and this eminence is produced by the superior (= anterior) semicircular canal
- Tegmen tympani is the thin plate of bone forming the roof of middle ear.

*Foramen*
- Foramen rotundum—maxillary nerve
- Foramen ovale—mandibular nerve, accessory meningeal artery, lesser petrosal nerve, emissary vein
- Foramen spinosum—middle meningeal artery, meningeal branch of mandibular nerve
- Superior orbital fissure—structures passing through this can be well-studied in the following diagram

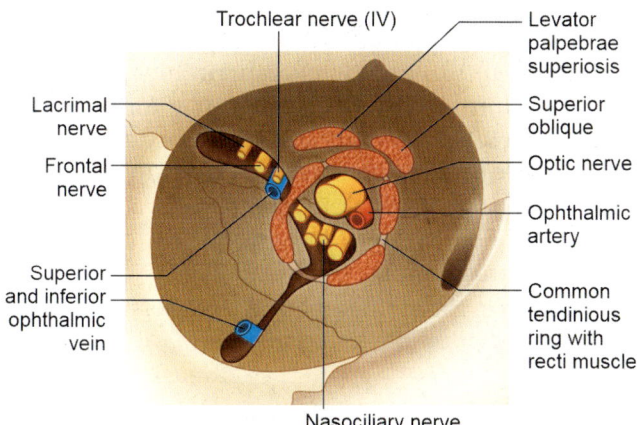

Superior orbital fissure with its contents

- Optic canal lies in between the roots of lesser wing of sphenoid and transmit optic nerve and ophthalmic artery
- Foramen lacerum—meningeal branch of ascending pharyngeal artery, emissary vein. In fetal life it is covered by cartilage.

*Posterior Cranial Fossa*

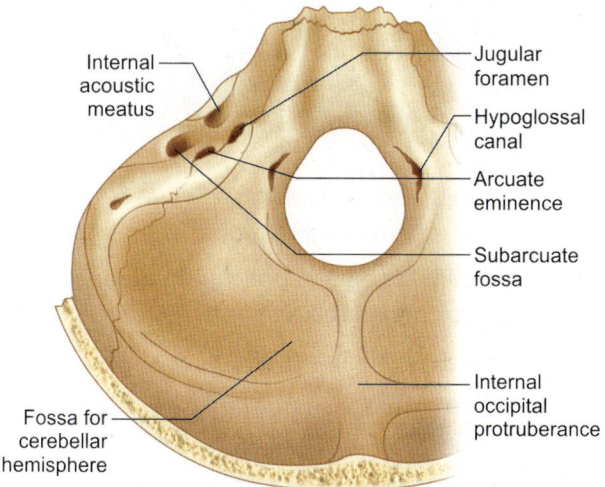

Posterior cranial fossa features

*Features*
- Clivus is the sloping bone in front of foramen magnum, related to basilar plexus of veins and supports the pons and medulla
- Internal occipital crest provides attachment to the falx cerebelli
- Internal occipital protuberance related to confluence of sinuses
- Internal acoustic meatus transmits VII, VIII and labyrinthine vessels
- Arcuate eminence is lateral to the meatus
- Subarcuate fossa lodges the flocculus of cerebellum.

*Foramen*
- Internal acoustic meatus—VII, VIII nerves and labyrinthine vessels.
- Foramen magnum transmitting lower part of medulla, tonsils of cerebellum, meninges, spinal accessory nerve, vertebral artery with its sympathetic plexus, anterior and posterior spinal arteries, apical ligament of dens and membrane tectoria (margins provide attachment to anterior and posterior atlanto-occipital membrane).
- Jugular foramen—IX, X, XI nerves, ascending pharyngeal and occipital arteries, internal jugular vein and inferior petrosal sinus.
- Hypoglossal canal—XII nerve, ascending pharyngeal artery, emissary vein.

## Orbit

*Features*
- Roof—orbital plate of frontal bone
- Lateral wall—greater wing of sphenoid posteriorly and frontal process of zygomatic bone anteriorly

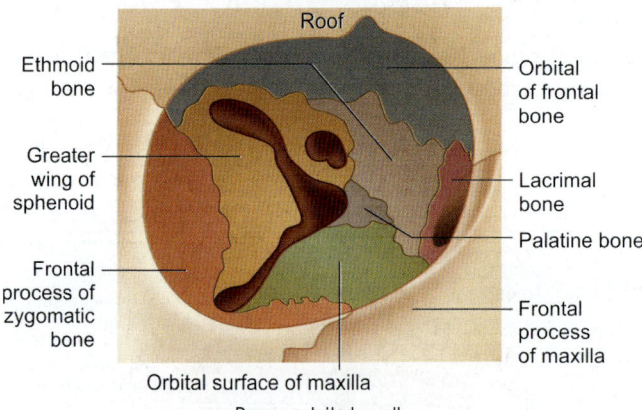

Roof

Ethmoid bone

Greater wing of sphenoid

Frontal process of zygomatic bone

Orbital of frontal bone

Lacrimal bone

Palatine bone

Frontal process of maxilla

Orbital surface of maxilla

Bony orbital walls

- Floor—orbital surface of maxilla, zygomatic bone and palatine bone
- Medial wall—frontal process of maxilla, lacrimal bone, orbital plate of ethmoid, body of sphenoid.

## Fetal Skull

*Features*
- Skull is proportionately large
- Facial skeleton is very small

- Base of skull is short
- Skull bones have no diploe
- Frontal and parietal tuber are prominent
- Glabella, superciliary arch, mastoid process not developed
- Frontal bone and mandible are in 2 halves
- Internal ear, tympanic cavity, of adult size
- Membranous gaps at the parietal bone angles
- Paranasal sinuses rudimentary
- Stylomastoid foramen is exposed.

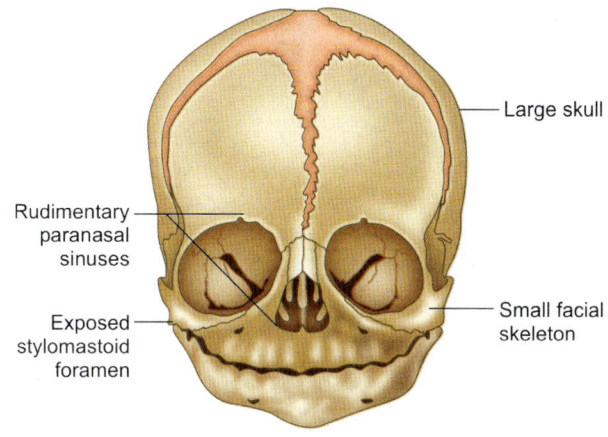

Large skull

Rudimentary paranasal sinuses

Exposed stylomastoid foramen

Small facial skeleton

Fetal skull

## SOLITARY SKULL BONES

### Occipital Bone

Occipital bone external features

*Features*

- Markedly internally concave
- Foramen magnum is the distinct feature
- Expanded flat part postero-superior to this foramen is squamous part
- Stout quadrilateral part anterior to the foramen is basilar part
- On each side of the foramen is the basioccipital part

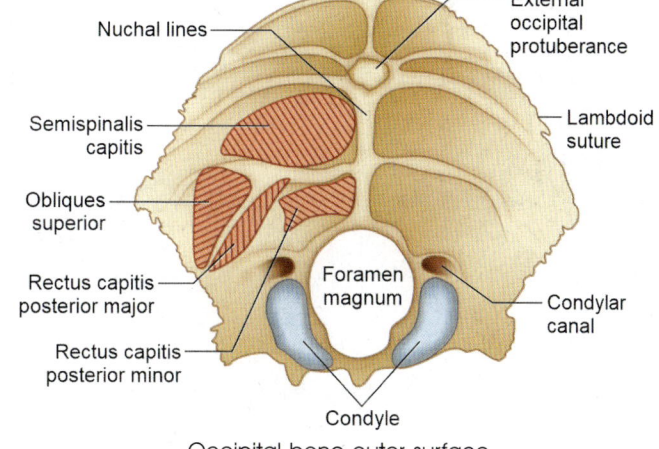

Nuchal lines

External occipital protuberance

Semispinalis capitis

Lambdoid suture

Obliques superior

Rectus capitis posterior major

Foramen magnum

Condylar canal

Rectus capitis posterior minor

Condyle

Occipital bone-outer surface

- External occipital protuberance and nuchal lines are the prominent feature on the exterior
- Internal occipital protuberance is internally present
- Base has two oblong condyles
- Condylar canal and foramen magnum are the foramen in the bone

- Two primary centres for squama during 8th week of IUL, rest is cartilaginous framework, additional centre may appear in posterior rim of foramen magnum during 16th week, Kerckring's centre.

## Sphenoid Bone

### Features

- Optic canal lies in between the roots of lesser wing of sphenoid
- Superior orbital fissure lies between the greater and lesser wings of sphenoid
- Hypophyseal fossa
- Foramen rotundum, foramen ovale and optic canal.

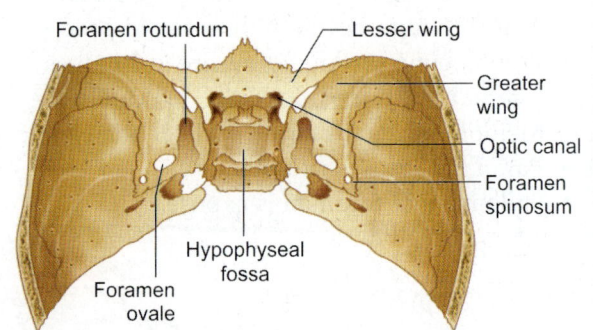

Sphenoid bone—external features

## Temporal Bone

### Side Determination

- External surface has features like external acoustic meatus, mandibular fossa, styloid process, zygomatic arch, mastoid process
- Mastoid process is behind
- Zygomatic process is in the front
- Internal surface has undulations for the temporal lobe
- Internal acoustic meatus is seen.

### Parts

- Mastoid
- Styloid
- Petrous
- Tympanic
- Squamous.

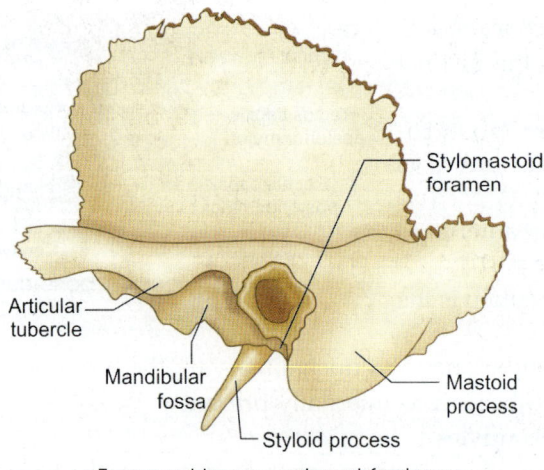

Temporal bone—external features

## Parietal Bone

### Side Determination

- Superior border is smooth
- Serrated anterior border is longer in length compared to posterior border
- Inferior border is undulated
- Internal surface has grooves for the middle meningeal vessels.

## Frontal Bone

Identify the bone

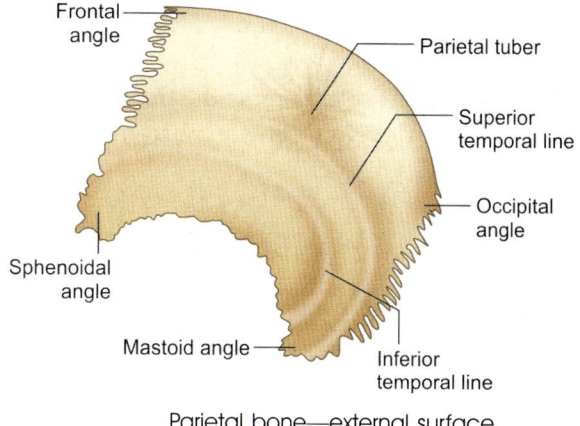

Parietal bone—external surface

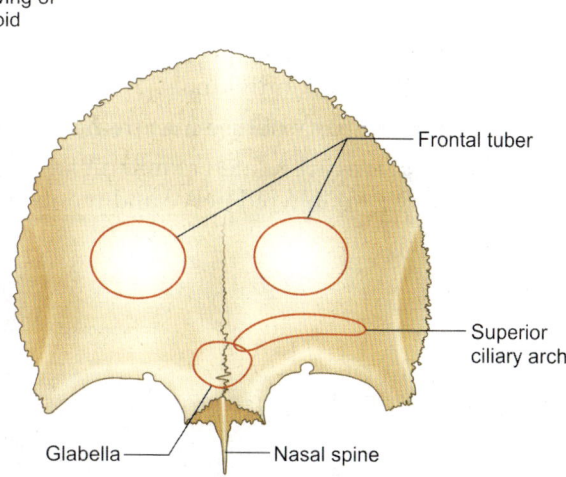

Frontal bone—internal surface

## Maxilla

Appreciate the features of maxilla bone.

Frontal bone—external surface

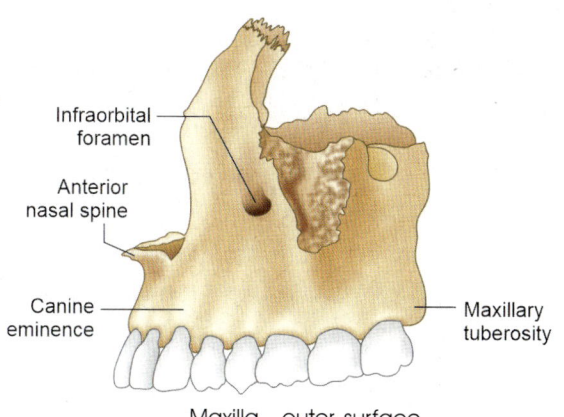

Maxilla—outer surface

## *Mandible*

### Features

- Masseteric vessels traverse the mandibular fossa
- Mandible develops in the fibro-membranous tissue and lower part of membranous cartilage

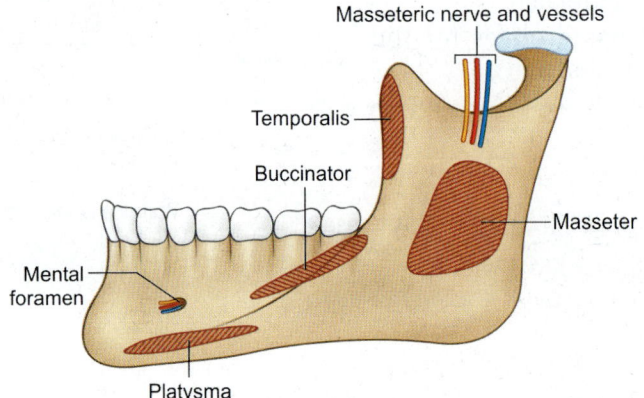

Mandible—outer surface (features and attachments)

- Mental foramen is near the lower border in childhood, midway in adults and near the upper border in old individuals
- Angle of mandible is obtuse in extremes of age (140) little less obtuse in adult (110)
- Following nerves are related to mandible—auriculotemporal nerve, inferior alveolar nerve, lingual nerve, mylohyoid nerve and mental nerve.

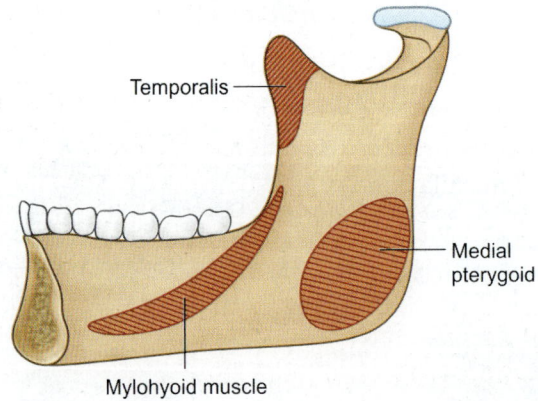

Mandible—inner surface (features and attachments)

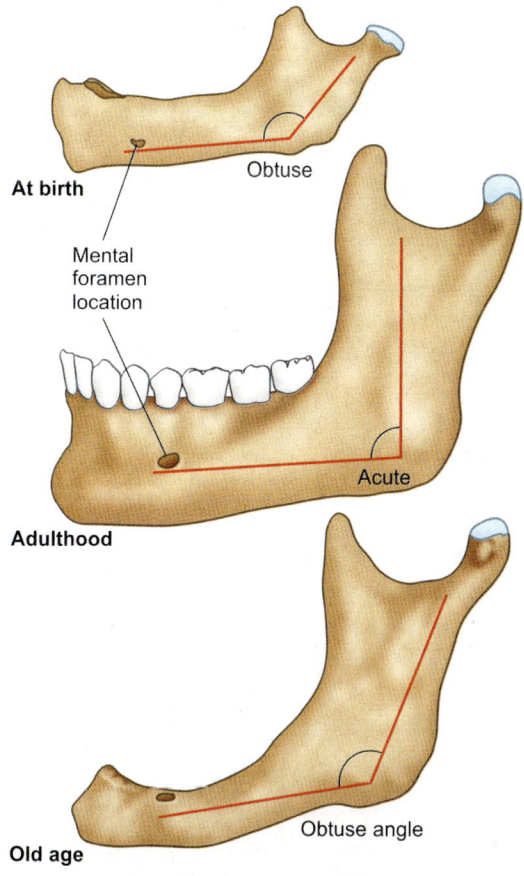

**Age changes in mandible**

## Typical Cervical Vertebra

*Identification Points*

- Body of this vertebra is relatively small compared to other vertebrae. Looks ring like prima facie
- Most typical feature of cervical vertebra is the presence of foramen transversarium, i.e. a foramen in the transverse process
- Vertebral foramen is large and triangular
- Spinous process is short and bifid
- Pedicles diverge sharply.

*First Cervical Vertebra or Atlas*

### Identification points

- Has no body (this site is taken by the dens of 2nd cervical vertebra)

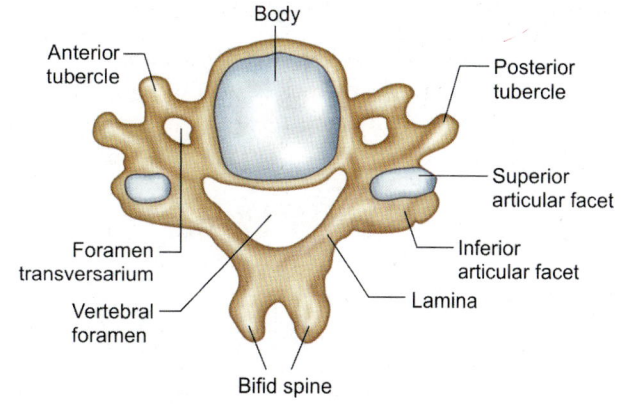

Typical cervical vertebra

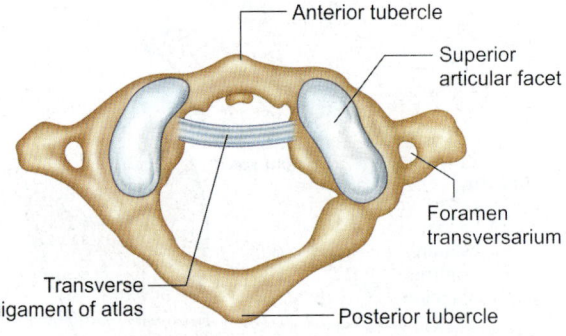

First cervical vertebra or atlas

- Has no spine
- Thin anterior and posterior arch
- Has lateral masses.

### Second Cervical Vertebra or Axis

***Identification points:*** Can be distinctly identified by a projection, dens

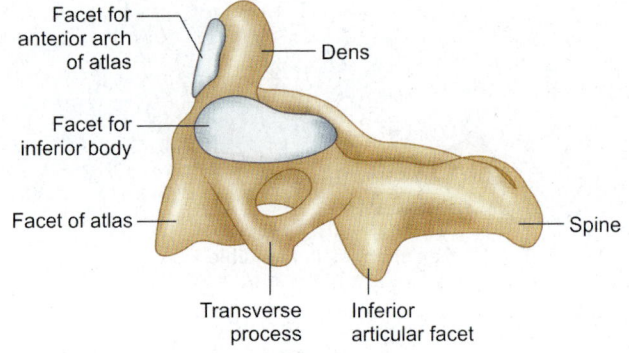

Second cervical vertebra or axis

### Seventh Cervical Vertebra or Vertebra Prominens

***Identification points:*** It has a very prominent spine, easily palpable on the lower part on the nape of the neck.

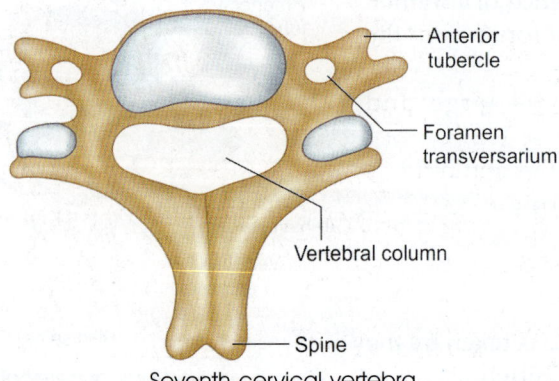

Seventh cervical vertebra

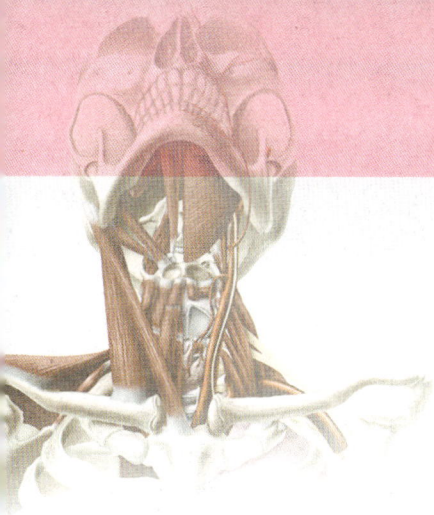

# Surface Anatomy

## 1. FACIAL ARTERY

### Position to be Taken

Ask the subject to clench the teeth.

### Points to be Marked

- Palpate the contracted masseter, and mark a point along the inferior border of mandible just in front of contracted masseter
- Second point 1.25 cm lateral to the angle of mouth
- Third point at the medial angle of eye.

It is a tortuous artery, join the points in a serpentine manner (same markings for the facial vein, but a straight line, not tortuous)

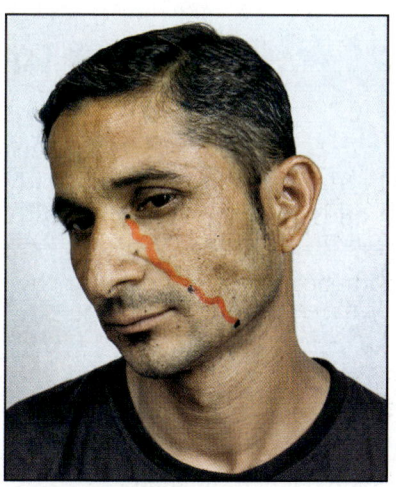

Markings for facial artery

## 2. COMMON CAROTID ARTERY

### Position of the Subject

Ask the subject to sit on a chair.

### Points to be Marked

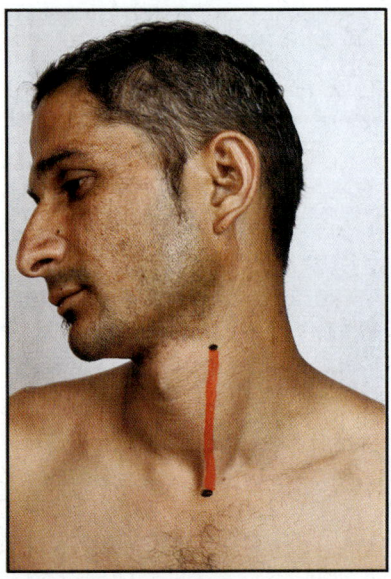

Common carotid artery marking

- Mark one point at the sternoclavicular joint
- Another point along the anterior border of sternocleidomastoid at the level of upper border of thyroid cartilage.

## 3. EXTERNAL CAROTID ARTERY

### Position of the Subject

Let the subject sit on the chair.

### Points to be Marked

- A point along the anterior border of sternocleidomastoid where the common carotid ends at the level of thyroid cartilage
- Another point at the posterior border of the neck of the mandible.

## 4. PAROTID GLAND

### Position of the Patient

Subject can be sitting on chair ask to clench the teeth.

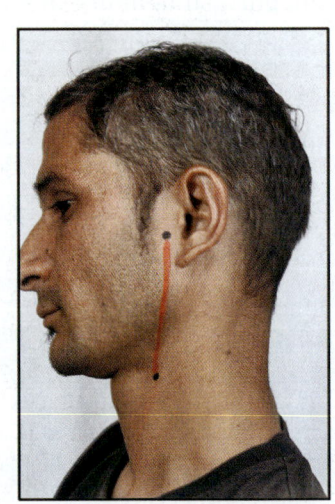

Marking for external carotid artery

## Points to be Marked

- Upper border of head of mandible
- Centre of masseter
- Posteroinferior to the angle of mandible
- Upper part of the anterior border of sternocleidomastoid

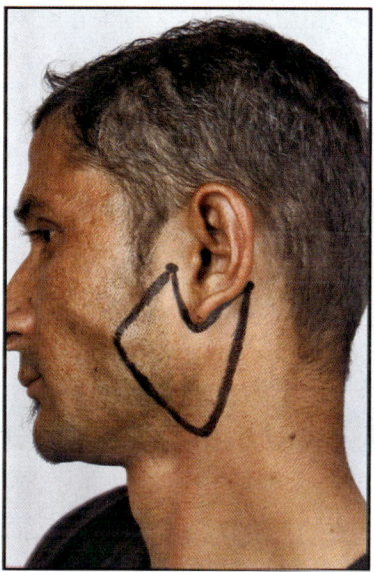

Marking for parotid gland

## 5. PAROTID DUCT (STENSON'S DUCT)

### Position of the Subject

Patient can be sitting in the chair.

### Points to be Marked

- Lower limit of tragus
- A mid between ala of nose and red margin of upper lip.
  Draw a thick line joining these points, middle third of this
line represents the parotid duct.

## 6. THYROID GLAND

### Position of the Subject

Ask the subject to lie supine with neck extended (place a
sandbag below the neck).

### Points to be Marked

- Isthmus is marked as 2 lines 1.5 cm apart 2 finger breath
  from jugular notch mark 1 line and another line 1.5 cm
  above it

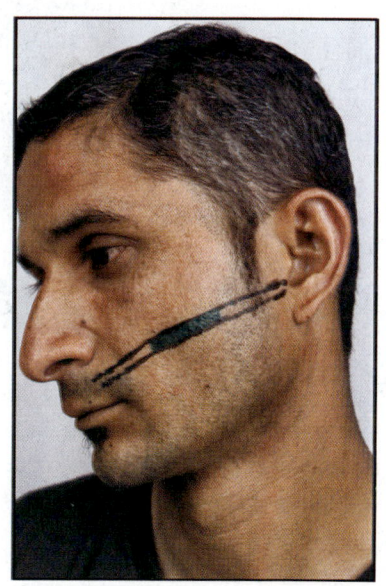

Markings for parotid duct

- Lobe extends up to middle of thyroid cartilage, above and below just above clavicle and laterally it overlaps the sternocleidomastoid.

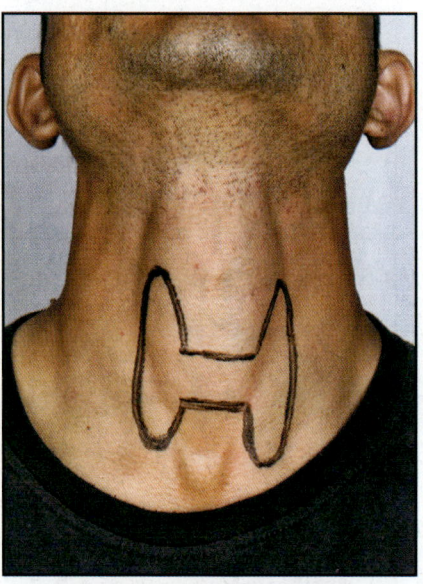

Thyroid gland marking

## 7. SUBMANDIBULAR GLAND

### Points to be Marked

Student can mark an oval area over posterior part of base of mandible.

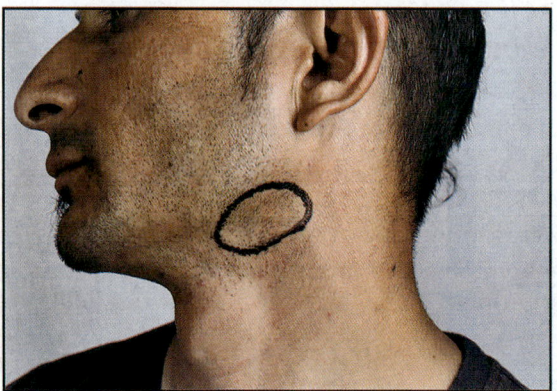

Marking for submandibular gland

## 8. MAXILLARY SINUS

### Points to be Marked

- Infraorbital margin
- Alveolus of maxilla
- Lateral wall of nose
- Apex is at the zygomatic process of maxilla.

## FRONTAL SINUS

### Points to be Marked

- Nasion
- 2.5 cm above the nasion medial 1/3 rd of supraorbital margin.

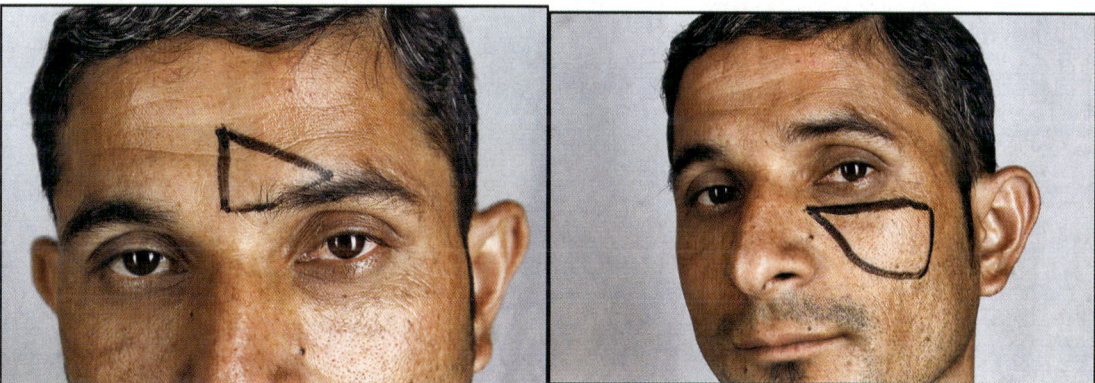

Markings for maxillary sinus and frontal sinus

Give the shape of respective sinuses by joining the points as shown in the photos.

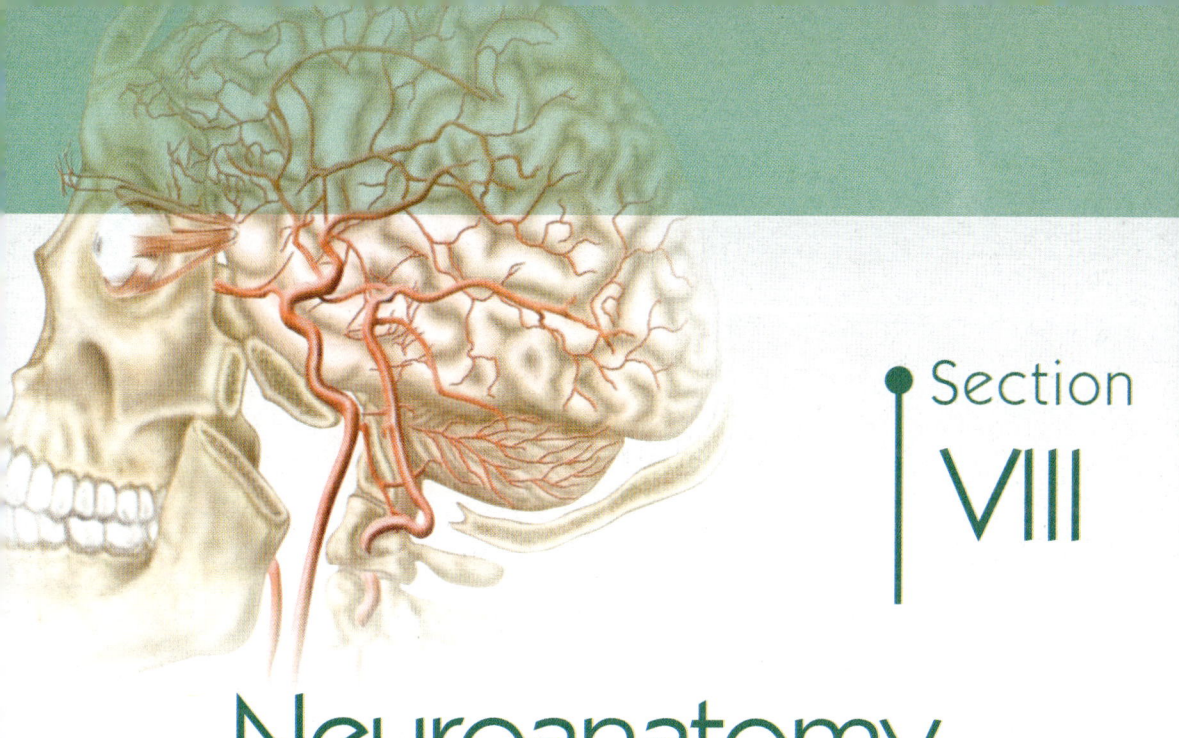

# Neuroanatomy

# Key Questions

### Q. How is the nervous system classified?

**Ans.** The nervous system is classified as follows:
- Central nervous system (CNS)
- Peripheral nervous system (PNS).

### Q. What are the parts of central nervous system?

**Ans.** The parts of CNS are brain (encephalon) and spinal cord (medulla spinalis).

### Q. What is included in peripheral nervous system?

**Ans.** Peripheral nervous system includes following structures:
- 12 pairs of cranial nerves
- 31 pairs of spinal nerves.

### Q. Is autonomic nervous system a part of CNS or PNS?

**Ans.** Autonomic nervous system by and large is considered as a separate functional unit. Since it is connected anatomically to CNS and PNS, it is included under both classifications.

### Q. What are the subdivisions of brain?

**Ans.** The subdivisions of brain are:
- Cerebral hemispheres
- Brainstem
- Cerebellum.

## Q. What are the parts of brainstem?

**Ans.** Following are the parts of brainstem:
- Mesencephalon (midbrain)
- Metencephalon (pons)
- Myelencephalon (medulla).

## Q. What is included in hindbrain?

**Ans.** Metencephalon (pons) and myelencephalon (medulla) together form hindbrain.

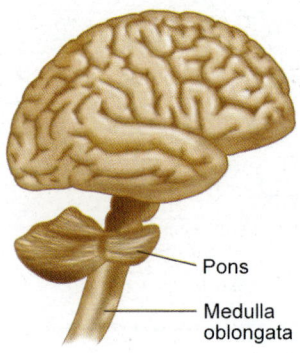

Parts of brainstem

## Q. What are the coverings of brain and spinal cord?

**Ans.** Three membranes surround the brain and spinal cord for protection, and support of these delicate structures. The membranes are as follows:
- Outer dura mater (pachymeninx)
- Middle arachnoid mater
- Inner pia mater.

## Q. What are leptomeninges?

**Ans.** The pia mater and arachnoid mater together are known as leptomeninges.

## Q. What are the layers of dura mater in the cranium?

**Ans.** The cranium dura has outer periosteal layer and inner meningeal layer. The meningeal layer gives rise to several folds (falx cerebri, tentorium cerebelli, falx cerebelli, diaphragma sellae), which divides the cranial cavity into compartments.

## Q. Which main artery supplies blood to dura mater?

**Ans.** The middle meningeal artery, a branch of maxillary artery mainly supplies blood to dura mater. Middle meningeal artery enters the skull through foramen spinosum.

## Q. Depict the covering of CNS.

**Ans.** Anesthetic drugs when injected in epidural space produce epidural anesthesia.

## Q. Discuss the normal cerebrospinal fluid (CSF) composition.

**Ans.** Following are the properties of normal CSF:
- Clear, colorless fluid

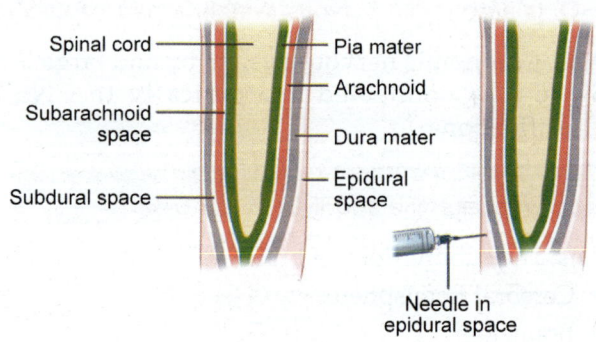

Coverings of CNS

- By and large considered as ultrafiltrate of blood plasma
- Contains small quantities of protein and glucose
- Higher quantities of $Na^+$, Cl and $Mg^{2+}$
- Lower quantities of $K^+$, $Ca^{2+}$
- No cellular component.

### Q. How is the CSF produced and what is its quantity?

**Ans.** About 70% of CSF is secreted by choroid plexus present in lateral ventricles, third and fourth ventricles. 30% of CSF is water produced due to metabolic reactions like oxidation of glucose.
- Total quantity of CSF is approximately 140 mL
- CSF production: 0.35 mL/min, 400–500 mL/24 hours.

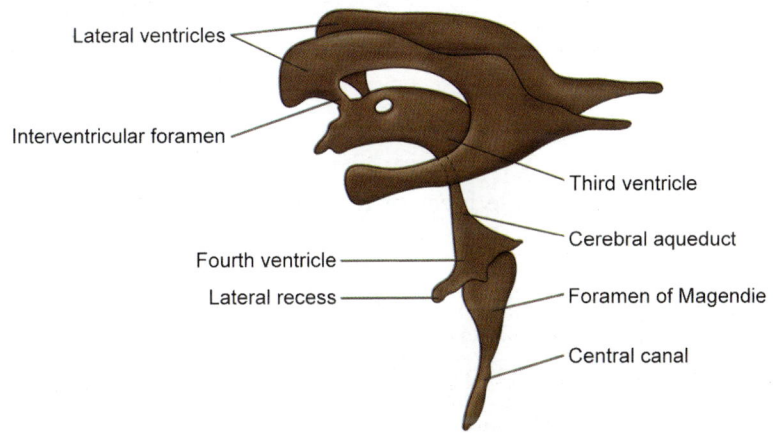

Ventricles of brain and choroid plexus

### Q. What are the functions of CSF?

**Ans.** Following are the functions of the CSF:
- It protects and cushions the CNS from trauma
- By virtue of buoyancy in case of any sudden movement of brain, the CSF reduces the damage to brain
  - Buoyancy: The brain weighs only 50 g when immersed in CSF. The gross weight of brain is around 1,500 g.
- It clears waste products of metabolism, anesthetic drugs that diffuse in the brain
- It clears the particulate matter from venous blood via arachnoid villi
- Coordinates endocrine function
  - Releasing hormones are directly secreted in CSF.
- Influences function of neurons and glial cells by altering the ionic composition.

### Q. What do you understand by lumbar puncture?

**Ans.** It is also known as spinal tap. A needle is inserted into spinal canal to collect CSF for analysis in lumbar region.

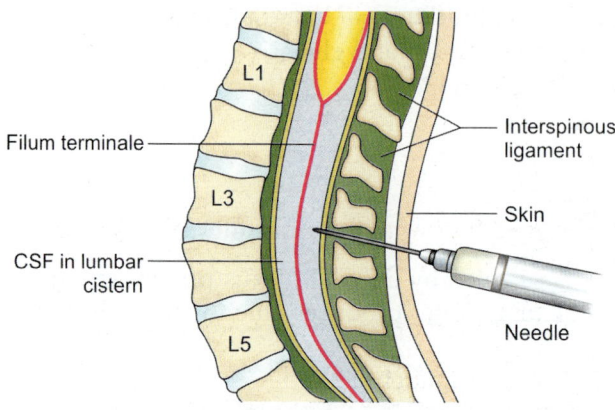

Lumbar puncture—needle in the spinal canal

While doing procedure one should keep in mind that spinal cord ends at lower border of L1 in adults.

### Q. What is choroid plexus?

**Ans.** Choroid plexus consist of single layer of folded cuboidal epithelium with a mesh of capillaries within it.

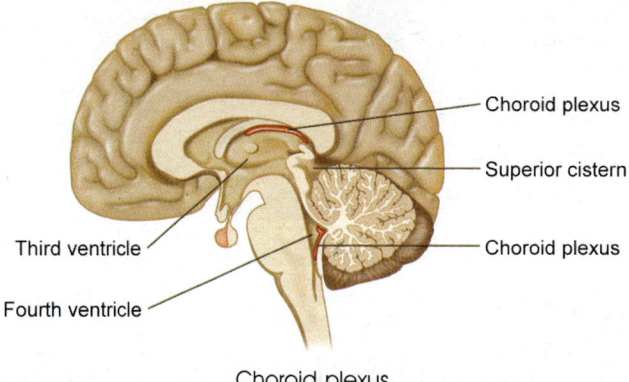

Choroid plexus

### Q. What is the extent of spinal cord?

**Ans.** The spinal cord extends from foramen magnum to the lower border of first lumbar vertebra (medulla continues as spinal cord).

### Q. What are the peculiarities of the structure of spinal cord?

**Ans.** Following are the peculiarities of the structure of the spinal cord:
- There are two enlargements cervical and lumbar
- Cervical enlargement consists of four cervical nerve roots and one thoracic nerve root forming brachial plexus

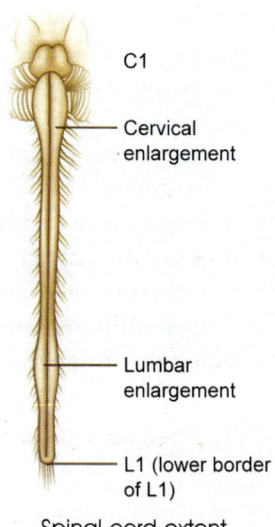

Spinal cord extent

- Lumbar enlargement consists of four lumbar nerve roots and two sacral nerve roots giving rise to lumbar plexus and sacral plexus respectively
- Distal to lumbar enlargement the spinal cord becomes conical and is known as conus medullaris
- Pia mater condenses into singular filament distal to conus known as filum terminale
- Spinal cord consists of 31 segments namely 8 cervical, 12 thoracic, 5 lumbar, 5 sacral and 1 coccygeal.
- In cut section spinal cord can be distinctly divided into H-shaped gray matter (cell bodies) and surrounding white matter (myelinated fibers).

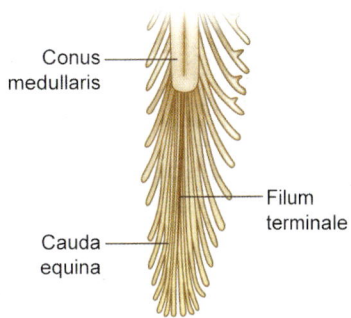

Terminal segment of spinal cord

**Q. Depict the transverse section of spinal cord (important cell groups and fiber tract to be shown).**

**Ans.**

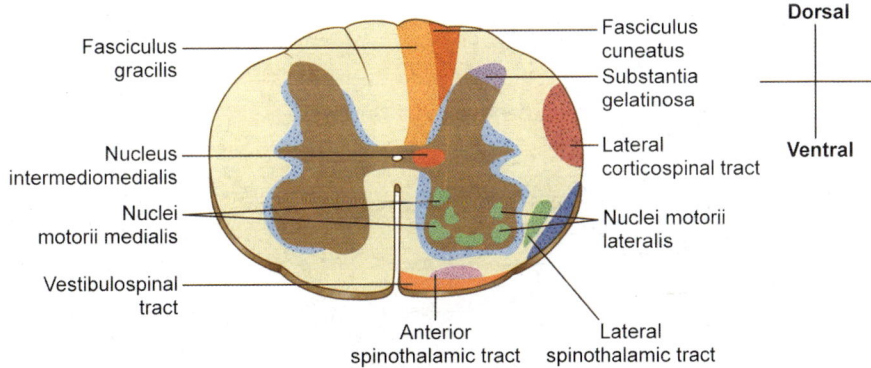

**Q. How are the cells of the gray matter of spinal cord classified?**

**Ans.** There are two types of cells:

1. *Root cells:* These are present in anterior and lateral horns of spinal cord and gives rise to axons, which leave through ventral root.
2. *Column cells:* These are neurons whose peripheral processes are within CNS.

**Q. At what level does the conus medullaris lie at birth?**

**Ans.** The conus medullaris is at the level of L3 vertebra at birth.

**Q. What are the components of reflex arc?**

**Ans.** Following are the components of reflex arc:

- Receptor
- Sensory root
- Dorsal root ganglion

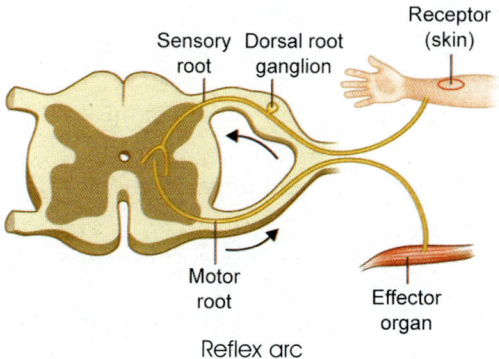

Reflex arc

• Motor root
• Effector organ.

### Q. Draw a neat labeled diagram of a neuron.

**Ans.**

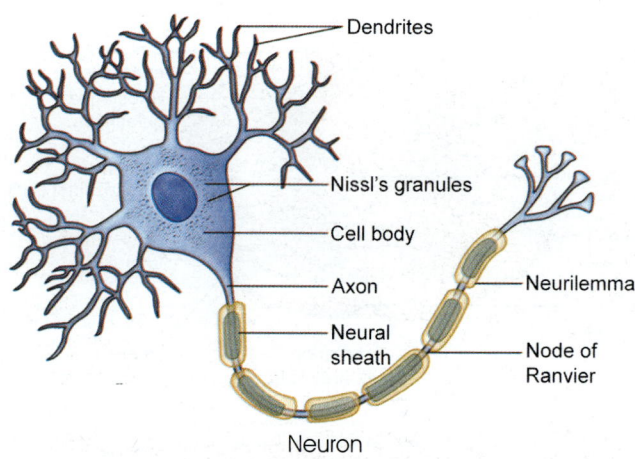

Neuron

### Q. What do you understand by nuclei and ganglia?

**Ans.** • Collection of cell bodies of neuron within CNS is known as nuclei
• Collection of cell bodies of neuron within PNS is known as ganglia.

### Q. What are the major cell types of nervous system?

**Ans.** There are mainly two cell types of nervous system:
1. *Excitable cells:* Neurons
2. *Non-excitable cells:* Neuroglia, ependyma, Schwann cells.

### Q. How do you classify neuroglial cells?

**Ans.** Neuroglial cells are broadly classified into:
• *Macroglia:* Astrocytes, oligodendrocytes
• *Microglia:* Phagocytes.

# Key Short Notes

---

### Q. White matter of cerebrum.

**Ans.** The core of cerebral hemisphere consists of thick myelinated fibers interconnecting subcortical nuclei, this forms the white matter of cerebrum.

The fibers of white matter can be subdivided into three types:
1. Projection fibers
2. Association fibers
3. Commissural fibers.

### Projection Fibers

The fibers transmit impulses to and fro from cerebral cortex, and form fan-like bundle of fibers known as corona radiata.

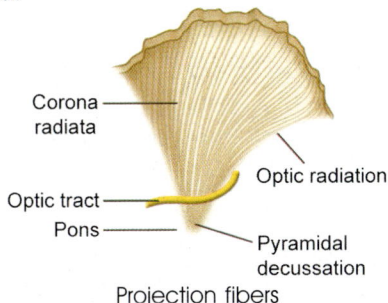

Projection fibers

### Association Fibers

The fibers interconnect different cortical areas within the same cerebral hemisphere, e.g. uncinate fasciculus.

### Commissural Fibers

The fibers interconnect similar cortical areas between the two cerebral hemispheres, e.g. corpus callosum.

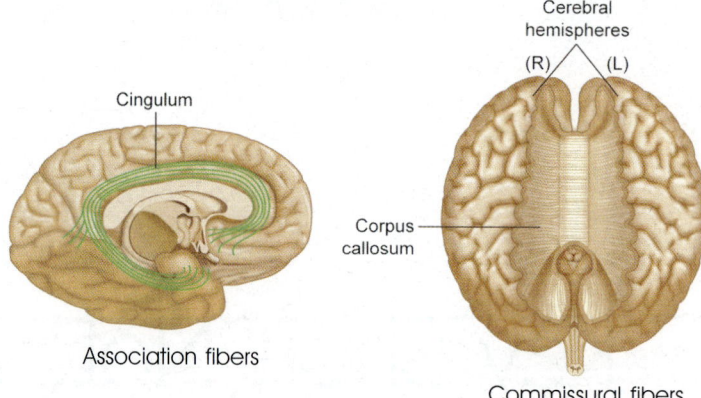

Cingulum

Cerebral hemispheres
(R)  (L)

Corpus callosum

Association fibers

Commissural fibers

## Q. Superolateral surface and medial surface of cerebral hemisphere (diagram only).

**Ans.**

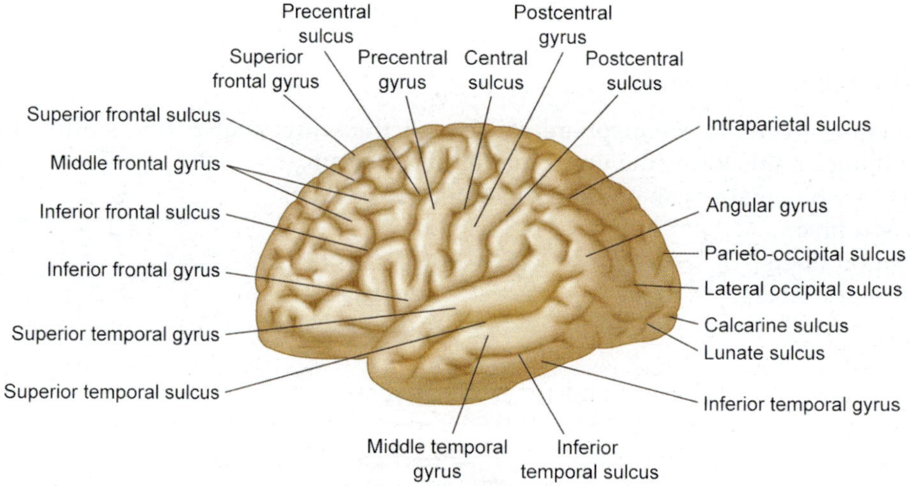

Precentral sulcus
Postcentral gyrus
Superior frontal gyrus
Precentral gyrus
Central sulcus
Postcentral sulcus
Superior frontal sulcus
Intraparietal sulcus
Middle frontal gyrus
Inferior frontal sulcus
Angular gyrus
Inferior frontal gyrus
Parieto-occipital sulcus
Lateral occipital sulcus
Superior temporal gyrus
Calcarine sulcus
Lunate sulcus
Superior temporal sulcus
Inferior temporal gyrus
Middle temporal gyrus
Inferior temporal sulcus

Superolateral surface of cerebral hemisphere

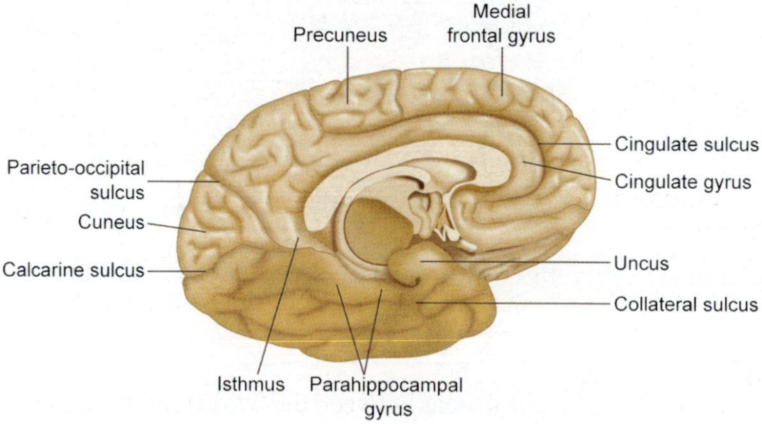

Medial frontal gyrus
Precuneus
Parieto-occipital sulcus
Cingulate sulcus
Cingulate gyrus
Cuneus
Calcarine sulcus
Uncus
Collateral sulcus
Isthmus
Parahippocampal gyrus

Medial surface of cerebral hemisphere

### Q. Limbic system.

**Ans.** It is an additional neural network of brain concerned with memory, learning ability, emotional and motivational activity. *Composition:* Limbic Brain + Hippocampus

a. *Limbic brain comprises of:*
  - Amygdaloid nuclear complex
  - Hypothalamic nuclei (especially connected with mammillary body)
  - Septal nuclei
  - Nucleus accumbens
  - Cingulate cortex
  - Prefrontal cortex habenula
  - Anterior thalamic nuclei
  - Parts of basal ganglia
  - Limbic midbrain areas

b. *Hippocampal formation:*
  It comprises of:
  - Dentate gyrus
  - Hippocampus proper
  - Subicular complex
  - Entorhinal cortex.

## Connections

It is connected to forebrain, midbrain, lower brainstem, limbic spinal system via following connections:
- Fornix
- Stria terminalis
- Ventral amygdalo-fugal pathway
- Mammillothalamic tract.

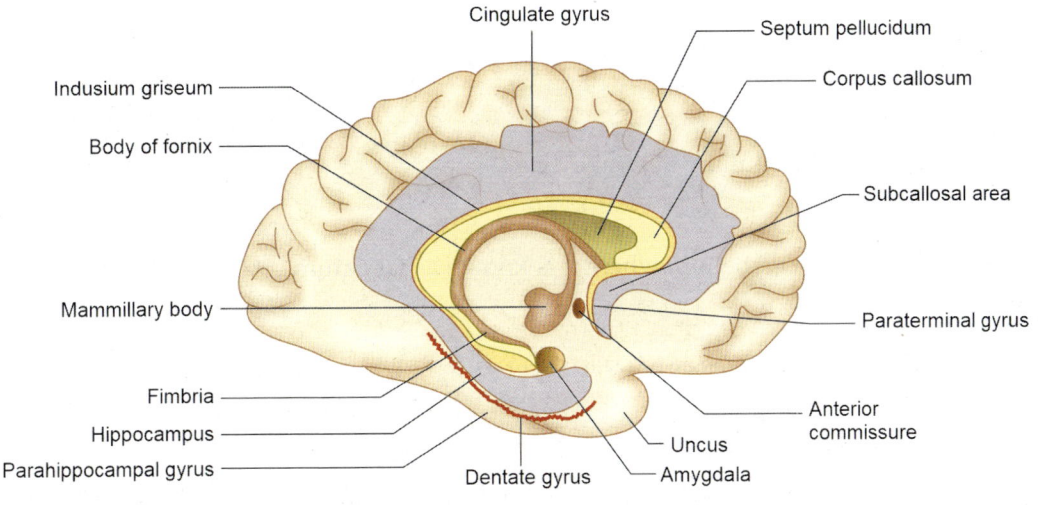

Limbic system with its connections

## Q. Components of basal ganglia.

**Ans.** Basal ganglia are subcortical nuclei derived principally from telencephalon. The components of basal ganglia are:

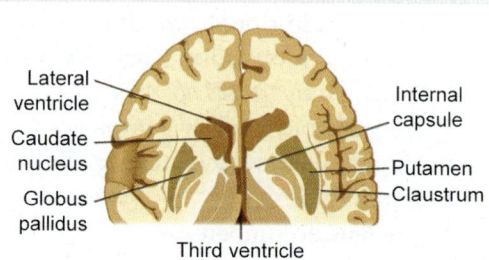

Coronal section of the cerebral hemisphere

- Caudate nucleus
- Putamen
- Globus pallidus
- Amygdaloid nuclear complex:
  - Caudate nucleus, putamen and globus pallidus are known as corpus striatum
  - Putamen and globus pallidus together are known as lentiform nucleus.

## Applied Anatomy

Movement disorders are associated with the diseases of basal ganglia. Two types of abnormalities are identified:

1. Involuntary movements known as dyskinesia
2. Changes in the muscle tone.

(*Dyskinesia types:* Tremor, athetosis, chorea, ballism).

## Q. Fourth ventricle.

**Ans.** Fourth ventricle is a rhomboid-shaped cavity overlying the pons and medulla and hence it can be subdivided into pontine part and medullary part.

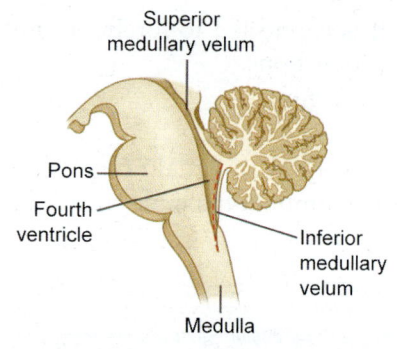

Fourth ventricle location

## Extent

- *Above:* Cerebral aqueduct of midbrain
- *Below:* Central canal of upper cervical spinal cord.

## Roof

Superior and inferior medullary veli (like a tent).

## Apex

Apex extends into the cerebellum where it is known as fastigium.

## Recess

*Lateral recess:* Lies over the surface of inferior cerebellar peduncle and opens into the cerebello-medullary cistern.

## Communications

Communicates with the subarachnoid space through foramen of Luschka and foramen of Magendie.

## Floor

### Features

- Vertically in the center, divided by median sulcus and paramedially divided by sulcus limitans
- Horizontally, it is divided by stria medullaris
- Paramedian area has a bulge known as median eminence
- Caudal area of fourth ventricle is known as calamus scriptorius
- The apex of the ventricle is known as obex.

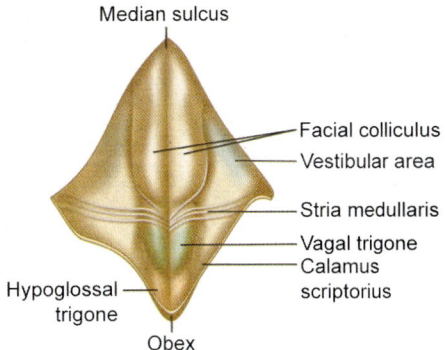

Floor of fourth ventricle

## Specific Area

- Just above the stria medullaris paramedially is facial colliculus and vagal trigone is just below it
- Hypoglossal trigone lies paramedially toward the caudal part of fourth ventricle
- Just above the stria medullaris laterally is vestibular area beneath, which is vestibular nuclei
- Just above the obex is a paired circumventricular organ known as area postrema.

**Q. Draw a diagram of cut section of medulla passing through the floor of fourth ventricle.**

**Ans.**

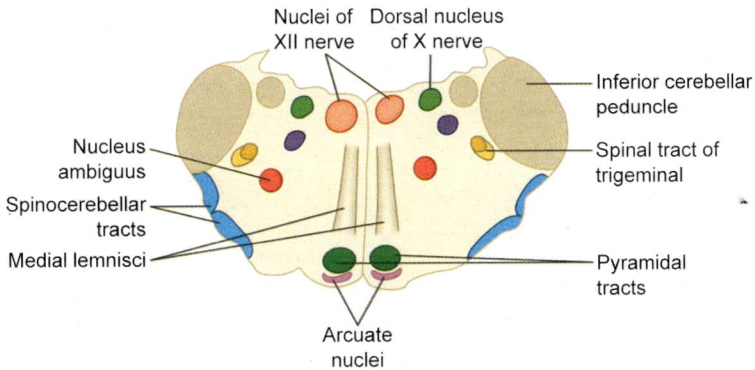

**Q. Features of midbrain.**

**Ans.** Midbrain is smallest and least differentiated portion of brainstem. The features of midbrain are as follows:

- *Tectum comprises of superior and inferior colliculus:*
  - Superior colliculus is part of visual pathway
  - Inferior colliculus is part of auditory pathway.
- *Tegmentum:* It is ventral to cerebral aqueduct
- Crura cerebri

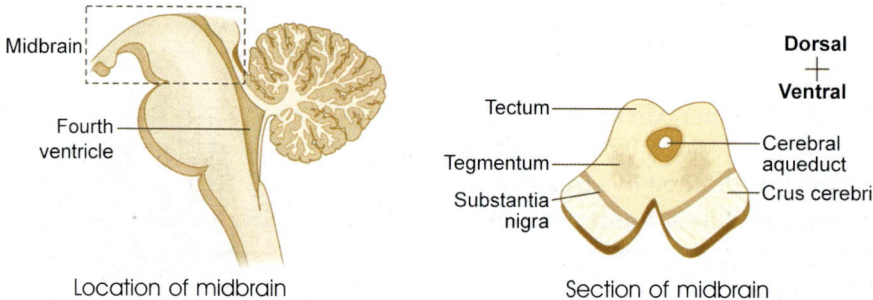

Location of midbrain                    Section of midbrain

- *Substantia nigra:* It is a pigmented area between tegmentum and crura cerebri: The cells of substantia nigra produce dopamine.
- Superior colliculus and an area just above it, is known as pretectum
- Two cranial nerves are related to midbrain namely oculomotor and trochlear
- Superior cerebellar peduncle decussates in caudal midbrain and surrounds a discrete nuclear mass known as red nucleus.

**Q. Draw a neat labeled diagram showing fissures and lobules of cerebellum.**

**Ans.**

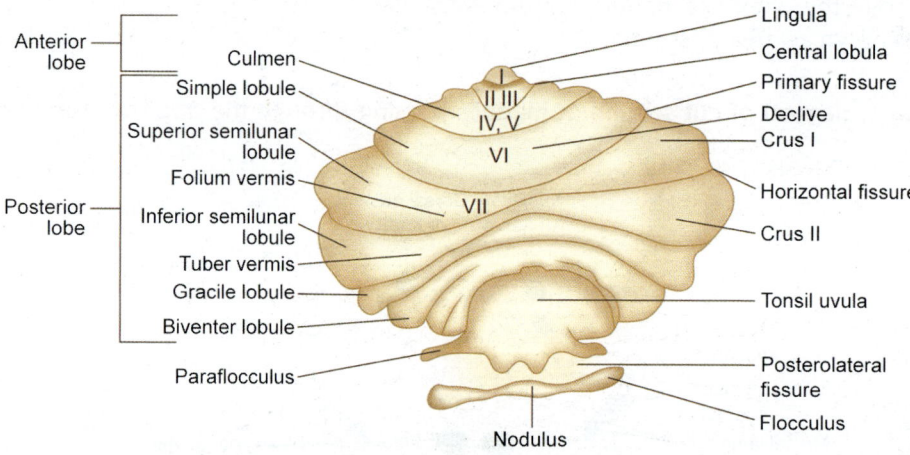

Cerebellum showing lobes and fissures

- Cerebellum—two main parts:
  a. Cerebellar hemispheres
  b. Vermis
- Two main fissures—primary fissure, paramedian fissure.
- Primary fissure divides the hemisphere into anterior lobe and posterior lobe; while paramedian fissure lies between vermis and hemispheres.
- Cerebellar hemispheres and vermis are further divided into lobes, lobules and folia (leaflets) by various sulci and gyri.
  (*Mnemonic:* Lal Chand could die for tereylene pants unnecessarily)
  L—lingula, C—central lobule, C—culmen, D—declive, F—folium, T—tuber, P—pyramis, U—uvula, F—flocculus

## Q. Components of diencephalon.

The most proximal segment of brainstem is known as diencephalon. It is a paired structure on each side of third ventricle (area between cerebral hemisphere). It can be subdivided into four parts namely:

a. Epithalamus

b. Thalamus

c. Hypothalamus

d. Subthalamic region.

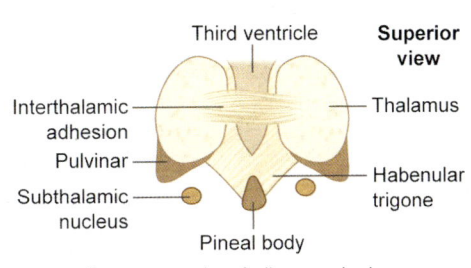

Components of diencephalon

| Epithalamus | Thalamus | Hypothalamus | Subthalamic region |
|---|---|---|---|
| Pineal body | Pulvinar (expanded posterior part) | Optic chiasm | Subthalamic nucleus |
| Habenular nuclei | Medial and lateral geniculate bodies (meta-thalamus) | Infundibulum | Zona incerta |
| Striae medullares | Anterior, lateral, medial and ventral nuclear groups | Tuber cinereum | |
| Tenia thalami | | Mammillary bodies | |

## Q. Depict cut section of medulla at motor (pyramidal) decussation and sensory (medial lemniscus) decussation.

**Ans.**

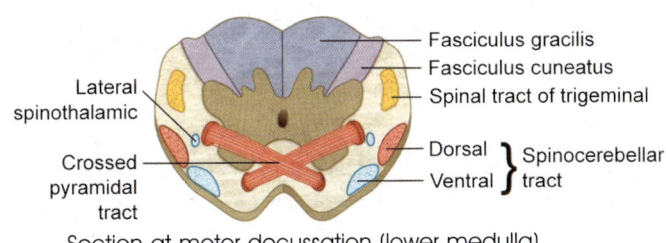

Section at motor decussation (lower medulla)

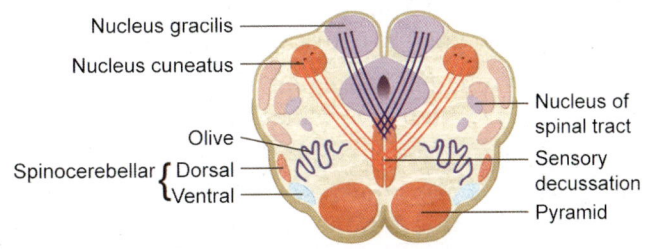

Section at sensory decussation (upper medulla)

## Q. Depict cut section of lower and upper pons.

**Ans.**

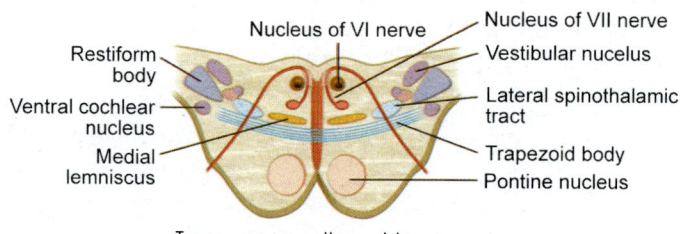

Transverse section at lower pons

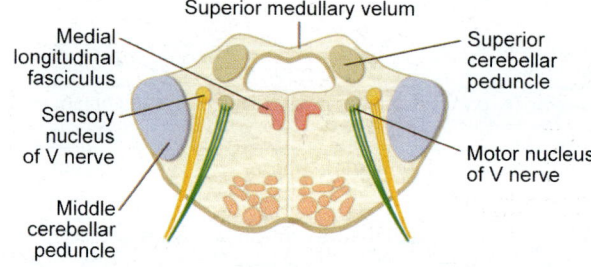

Transverse section at upper pons

## Q. Laminar pattern of spinal cord.

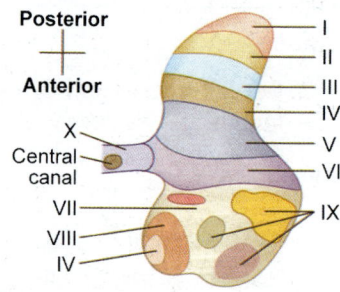

Laminar pattern of spinal cord

**Ans.** The cells in the gray matter of spinal cord are arranged in the form of layers (like a marble print); this constitutes the laminar pattern of spinal cord.

The layers (laminae) are given in roman numbers. It includes:

*Lamina I:* Caps the posterior horn, has posteromarginal nucleus, receives axons from lamina II. Cells in the lamina respond to pain and temperature stimuli, and contribute fibers to contralateral spinothalamic tract.

*Lamina II:* Corresponds to substantia gelatinosa, found at all spinal levels, send axons to dorsolateral fasciculus, transmits pain impulses also has opiate receptors.

*Lamina III:* Axons of the neurons in this lamina divide number of times to form thick plexus in laminae III and IV; most cells in this laminae are interneurons.

*Lamina IV:* Contains cells, which respond to light touch.

*Lamina V:* Divided into medial and lateral parts (except in thoracic region). Lateral part in cervical region gives rise to reticular process.

*Lamina VI:* Present in the region of cord enlargements, divided into medial and lateral parts, group I muscle afferent terminate in medial zone and descending spinal tracts are present in lateral zone.

*Lamina VII:* It is also known as zona intermedia, dorsal nucleus of Clarke forms an important cell group in this lamina, gives rise to uncrossed posterior spinocerebellar tract, intermediolateral nucleus gives rise to preganglionic sympathetic fibers.

*Lamina VIII:* Most of the descending tracts of spinal cord terminate in the cells of this lamina.

*Lamina IX:* Consist of many discrete groups of somatic motor neurons and involved in maintaining muscle tone.

*Lamina X:* It is a gray matter around the central canal.

### Q. Corpus callosum.

**Ans.** The most prominent structure on the medial surface of cerebral hemisphere is corpus callosum. It comprises of bunch of myelinated fibers, which interconnect specific areas of cerebral hemisphere.

*Following are the parts of corpus callosum:*
- Rostrum
- Genu
- Body
- Splenium.

*Subdivisions of fibers of corpus callosum:*
- Fibers connecting frontal lobes are known as anterior forceps (forceps minor)
- Fibers connecting occipital lobes are known as posterior forceps (forceps major)
- Fibers in splenium lying between lateral wall of posterior horn of lateral ventricle and optic radiation are known as tapetum.

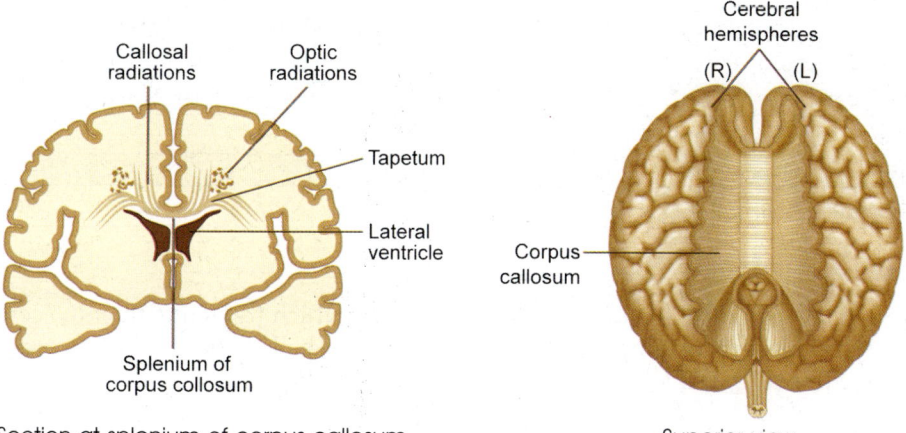

Section at splenium of corpus callosum          Superior view

### Relations of Corpus Callosum
- *Above:* Longitudinal fissure
- *Below:* Lateral ventricle.
  Callosal sulcus separates the corpus striatum from cingulate gyrus.

### Function

Corpus callosum helps in transferring information learned by one cerebral hemisphere to another, e.g. some experiences in the past memory of certain events.

However, surgical transection of corpus callosum does not show any obvious neurological deficit in experimental animals.

### Q. Cerebellar peduncles.

**Ans.** The cerebellum is connected to the brainstem by cerebellar peduncles.

There are three cerebellar peduncles:
1. Superior cerebellar peduncle
2. Middle cerebellar peduncle
3. Inferior cerebellar peduncle.

The fibers reaching the cerebellum (afferent system) enter via inferior and middle cerebellar peduncle by and large.

The fibers leaving the cerebellum (efferent system) enter the superior cerebellar peduncle by and large.

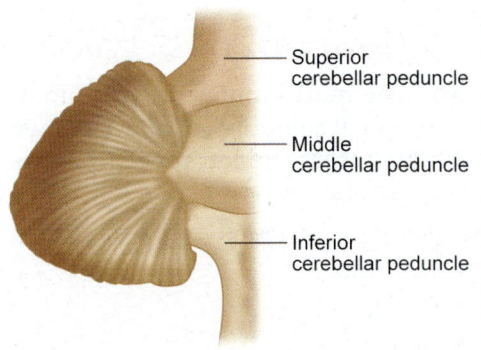

Cerebellar peduncle

### Inferior Cerebellar Peduncle

Inferior cerebellar peduncle can be subdivided into two portions:
1. Lateral restiform body
2. Medial juxta-restiform body.

| Afferent fibers | Efferent fibers |
|---|---|
| Posterior spinocerebellar tract | Cerebelloolivary fibers |
| Cuneocerebellar tract | Cerebellovestibular fibers |
| Olivocerebellar tract | Cerebelloreticular fibers |
| Parolivocerebellar tract | |
| Reticulocerebellar tract | |
| Vestibulocerebellar tract | |

### Middle Cerebellar Peduncle

Middle cerebellar peduncle is the most-thick peduncle, which transmits fibers to cerebellum, i.e. pontocerebellar fibers originating from pontine precerebellar nuclei. Pontine precerebellar nuclei receive fibers from ipsilateral cerebral cortex.

### Superior Cerebellar Peduncle

Superior cerebellar peduncle comprises of efferent bundle of fibers arising from deep nuclei of cerebellum mostly dentate nucleus. The efferent fibers end in inferior olivary nuclei, reticular formation, red nucleus and thalamus.

Accordingly the fibers are classified as detailed below.

| Efferent fibers | Afferent fibers |
|---|---|
| Cerebello-olivary | Anterior spinocerebellar |
| Cerebelloreticular | Tectocerebellar |
| Cerebellorubral | Dentatothalamic |

## Q. Visual pathway (diagram only).

**Ans.**

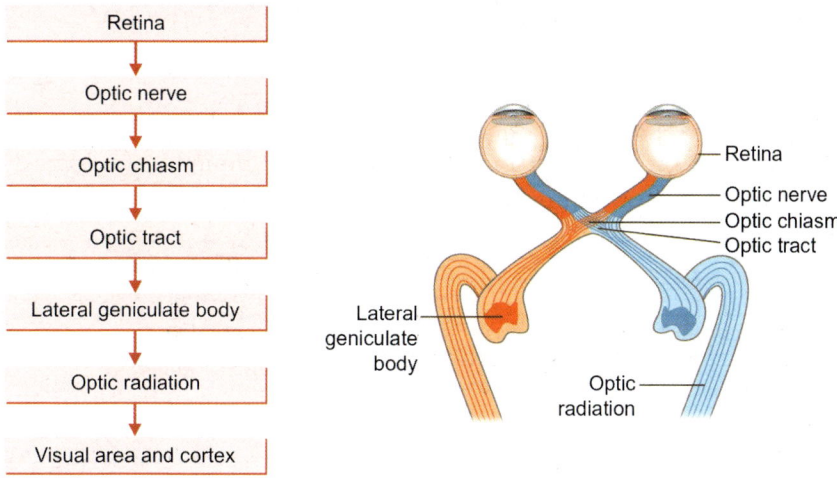

Retina → Optic nerve → Optic chiasm → Optic tract → Lateral geniculate body → Optic radiation → Visual area and cortex

## Q. Auditory pathway.

**Ans.** Auditory receptors (hair cells of organ of corti in cochlea).

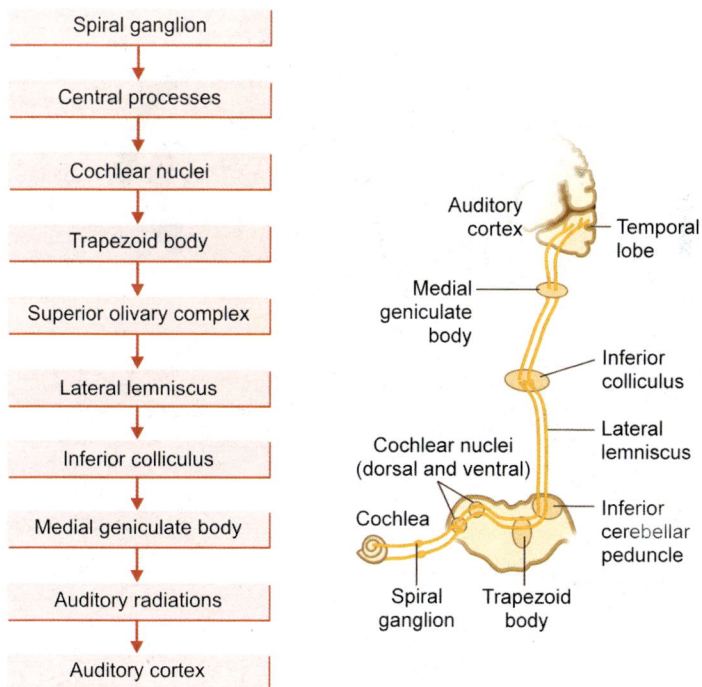

Spiral ganglion → Central processes → Cochlear nuclei → Trapezoid body → Superior olivary complex → Lateral lemniscus → Inferior colliculus → Medial geniculate body → Auditory radiations → Auditory cortex

## Q. General features of tracts of the spinal cord.

- Tracts or fasciculi are bundles of nerve fibers having same origin, course and termination (functionally and anatomically having a single link)

- Funiculus is a distinct area in the spinal cord having different tracts
- By and large, long tracts are located peripherally in the white matter and small tracts are close to the gray matter.

## Classification

Tracts are classified into:

- Ascending tracts that carry sensory impulses towards the brain by and large
- Descending tracts that carry motor impulses away from the brain.

| Ascending tracts | Descending tracts |
|---|---|
| Posterior white column in spinal cord | Corticospinal (lateral and anterior) |
| Medial lemniscus in brainstem | Rubrospinal |
| Spinotectal | Reticulospinal |
| Lateral spinothalamic | Lateral spinothalamic |
| Posterior spinocerebellar autonomic pathways | |
| Anterior spinocerebellar | |

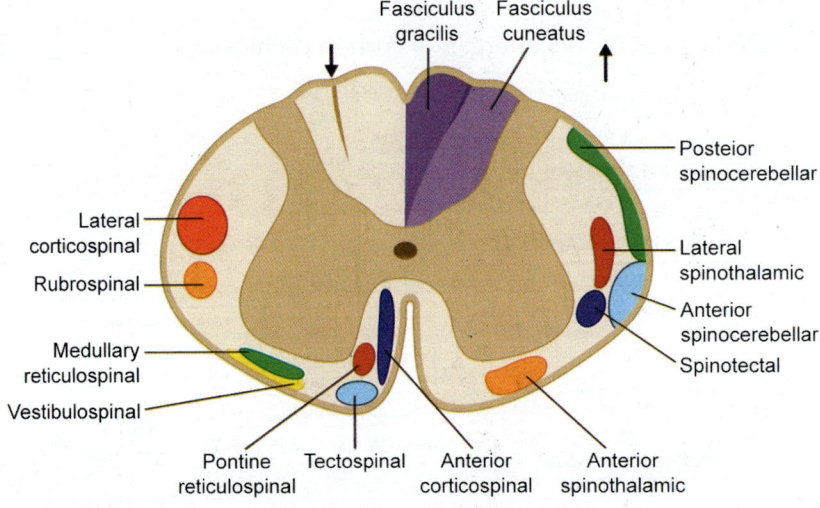

Ascending and descending tracts

## ASCENDING TRACTS

### Q. Posterior white column.

**Ans.**

**Functions**

Concerned with touch, pressure sensation and proprioception (joint position).

*Origin*

Dorsal root ganglion (first order neuron) and uncrossed ascending branches of spinal ganglion cells.

## Course

1. Fibers ascend in posterior funiculus medially and dorsally (in thoracic and cervical region, a septum appears within the posterior funiculus dividing it into fasciculus gracilis and fasciculus cuneatus).
2. The fibers synapse at nuclei gracilis and cuneatus (second order neuron).
3. Second order fibers arise from above neurons, which curve anteriorly and medially as internal arcuate fibers.
4. The fibers after crossing the midline, form a bundle known as medial lemniscus. This crossing over occurs at lower medulla.
5. The fibers of medial lemniscus ascend in the brainstem to synapse with ventral posterolateral nucleus of thalamus (third order neuron).

## Termination

Ventral posterolateral nucleus of thalamus (third order neuron).

## Clinical Importance

Lesions of the posterior column abolish sense of proprioception, touch and pressure.

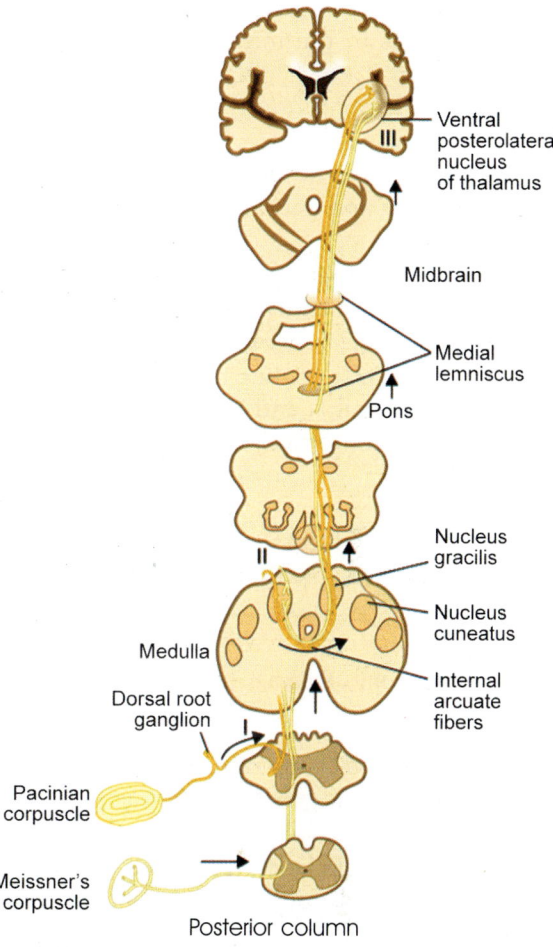

## Q. Anterior spinothalamic tract.

**Ans.**

## Function

Conveys light touch sensation (like produced by wisp of cotton).

## Origin

Cells within the gray matter of spinal cord and the tract arise from laminae I, IV and V contra-laterally.

## Course

- The fibers of the tract ascend in the anterior aspect of the white matter of the spinal cord to reach the medulla
- In the medulla, the thickness of the tract reduces since collateral fibers are given to the nuclei in reticular formation
- The tract is closely associated with medial lemniscus in pons and midbrain

- The tract is subdivided into medial and lateral components in the midbrain depending upon its termination.

## Termination

1. Medial component terminates into periaqueductal gray matter and the intralaminar thalamic nuclei bilaterally.
2. Lateral component terminates into caudal parts of ventral posterolateral thalamic nuclei.
3. Spinotectal tract is in close association with anterior spinothalamic tract, but terminates in contralateral superior colliculus and periaqueductal gray matter. This tract is concerned with nociceptive sensation.

## Clinical Importance

Lesion of this tract does not cause significant changes since the major sensations are carried by posterior column.

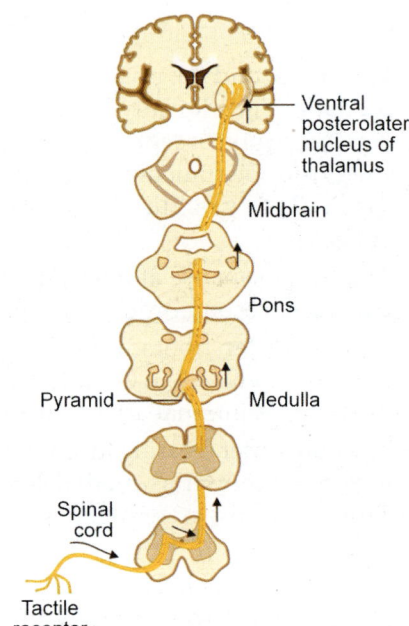

Anterior spinothalamic tract

## Q. Lateral spinothalamic tract.

**Ans. Function**

Conveys pain and temperature sensation.

## Origin

Cells in laminae I, IV and V gives rise to fibers that cross the spinal cord anteriorly and ascend in contralateral lateral funiculus as lateral spinothalamic tract.

## Course

- The tract ascends upwards just medial to anterior spinocerebellar tract in spinal cord
- The fibers concerned with temperature sensation are posterior to the fibers concerned with pain
- In the brainstem, collateral fibers are given to the reticular formation
- It terminates in thalamus.

## Termination

Ventral posterolateral nucleus of thalamus.

## Clinical Importance

Lesion on one side of the lateral spinothalamic tract causes loss of pain and temperature on the opposite side of the body.

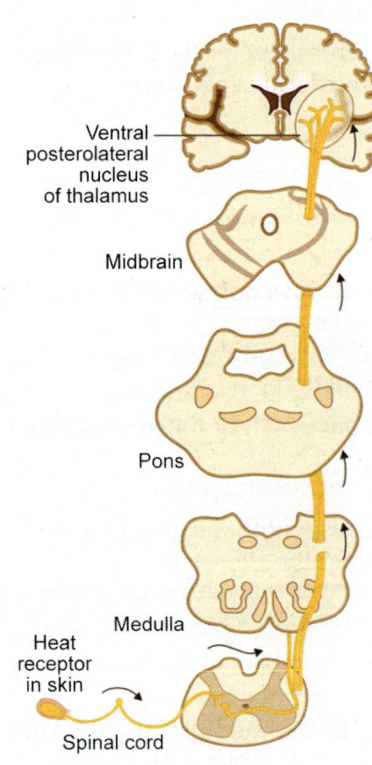

Lateral spinothalamic tract

## Q. Posterior spinocerebellar tract.

**Ans.**

### Functions

Posterior spinocerebellar tract is involved in fine coordination of posture and movement of individual limb muscles.

### Origin

Arises from dorsal nucleus of Clarke (lamina VII).

### Course

- Ascends in the posterolateral part of lateral funiculus
- In the medulla, the fibers enter the inferior cerebellar peduncle and end in the vermis of cerebellum.

### Termination

Vermis of cerebellum.

## Q. Anterior spinocerebellar tract.

**Ans.**

### Functions

Concerned with coordination of movement and maintenance of posture of lower limb.

### Origin

Arise from cells of laminae V, VI and VII.

### Course

1. Dorsal root ganglion is first order neuron where the sensory fiber synapse with the gray cell neuron, i.e. second order neuron.
2. The fibers from second order neuron cross the midline of spinal cord to ascend upwards anteriorly.
3. In the brainstem, at the level of upper pons, the fibers course on the dorsal surface of superior cerebellar peduncle. The tract terminates contralaterally in the anterior cerebellar vermis (lobules I–IV).

Spinocerebellar tracts

### Clinical Importance

Lesions of spinocerebellar tract do not cause any significant loss of sensation since the impulses enter the cerebellum and not the cerebrum, which is a conscious brain.

## DESCENDING SPINAL TRACTS

### Q. Corticospinal tract.

**Ans.**

**Function**

Concerned with voluntary skilled movements.

*Origin*

Arises from the cells in the cerebral cortex lamina V (motor area 4, premotor area 6 mainly).

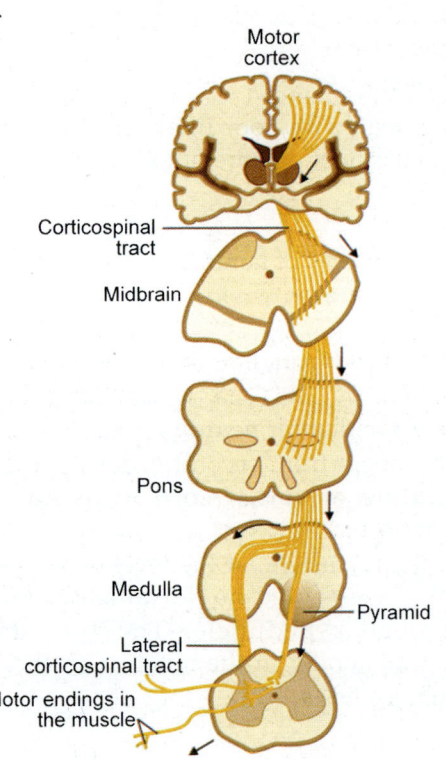

Origin of corticospinal tract

*Course*

1. The fibers arising from the cerebral cortex converge in corona radiata and descend downwards to enter the posterior limb of internal capsule and form crus cerebri at midbrain level.
2. In the medulla, the fibers form massive pyramids.
3. At the junction of medulla and spinal cord, the tract divides into three separate parts:
   a. 90% of the fibers cross the midline to form lateral corticospinal tract.
   b. 8% forms uncrossed anterior corticospinal tract.
   c. 2% forms uncrossed lateral corticospinal tract.

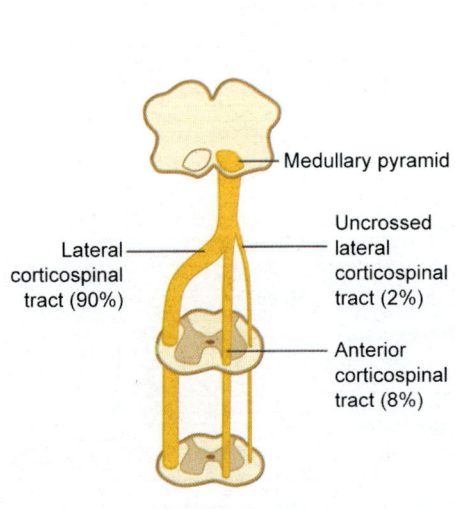

Corticospinal tract

4. The lateral corticospinal tract as it descends along the spinal cord gives fibers to gray matter of laminae IV, V, VI and VII of spinal cord.

## Termination

Terminates in the gray matter of laminae IV, V, VI and VII of spinal cord.

## Clinical Importance

Lesions involving this tract lead to:
- Loss of muscle tone
- Hyperactive deep tendon reflexes
- Loss of superficial abdominal and cremasteric reflex
- Extensor toe response (Babinski sign).

### Q. Vestibulospinal tract.

**Ans.**

### Function

Vestibulospinal tract exerts an excitatory influence on spinal reflex and muscle tone.

### Origin

Arises mainly from lateral vestibular nucleus present in the floor of fourth ventricle (the vestibular nuclei receive afferent impulses from vestibular nerve and the cerebellum).

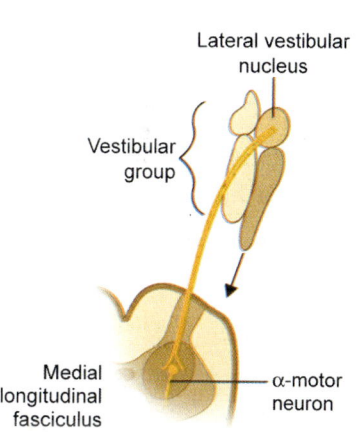

Origin of vestibulospinal tract

### Course

- It descends in the anterior part of lateral funiculus of spinal cord
- It ends in the laminae IX (VII and VIII), by synapsing with the alpha motor neurons.

### Termination

Vestibulospinal tract ends in the laminae IX (VII and VIII), by synapsing with alpha motor neurons.

### Q. Medial longitudinal fasciculus.

**Ans.**

1. Medial longitudinal fasciculus is present in the posterior part of anterior funiculus.
2. It connects the different nuclei in the brainstem.
3. Fibers from superior vestibular nuclei ascend to ipsilateral trochlear nucleus and oculomotor nucleus and also few fibers to contralateral oculomotor nucleus.

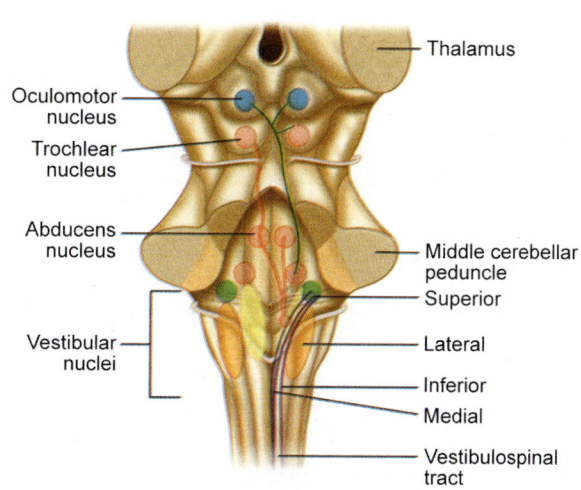

Medial longitudinal fasciculus

4. Fibers arising from medial vestibular nuclei ascend to contralateral abducens nucleus and trochlear and oculomotor nucleus, and few fibers to ipsilateral abducens nucleus.
5. This interconnection between vestibular, abducens, trochlear and oculomotor nucleus forms a composite ascending medial longitudinal fasciculus.
6. The descending medial longitudinal fasciculus begins from the medial vestibular nuclei, and terminate in the laminae VIII and VII of spinal cord.

### Clinical Significance

Medial longitudinal fasciculus plays important role in conjugate eye movements. Stimulation of a nerve in the semicircular duct (vestibular component) produces deviations in both eyes by virtue of extraocular muscle action.

### Q. Cranial nerves.

**Ans.** There are 12 pairs of cranial nerves, namely:

| | |
|---|---|
| I—Olfactory nerve | VII—Facial nerve |
| II—Optic nerve | VIII—Vestibulocochlear nerve |
| III—Oculomotor nerve | IX—Glossopharyngeal nerve |
| IV—Trochlear nerve | X—Vagus nerve |
| V—Trigeminal nerve | XI—Spinal accessory nerve |
| VI—Abducens nerve | XII—Hypoglossal nerve. |

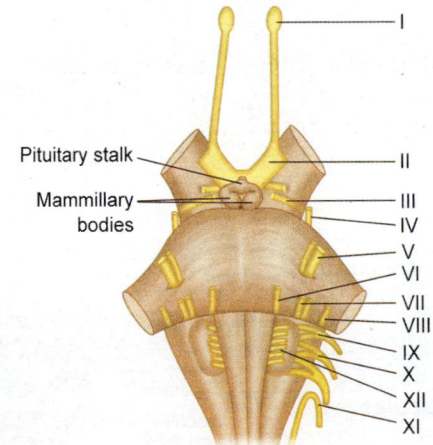

Ventral view of brainstem showing cranial nerves

### General Features

**General understanding regarding the functions of the cranial nerves (= functional components)**
- Each nerve may have a specific or general function and afferent (sensory) or efferent (motor) fibers
- A nerve supplying specific group of muscle, e.g. facial muscles, which are derived from branchial arch, will have a branchial efferent (special efferent) component
- A nerve supplying a gland will produce secretion by contraction of myoepithelial cell, which is considered to have general efferent component

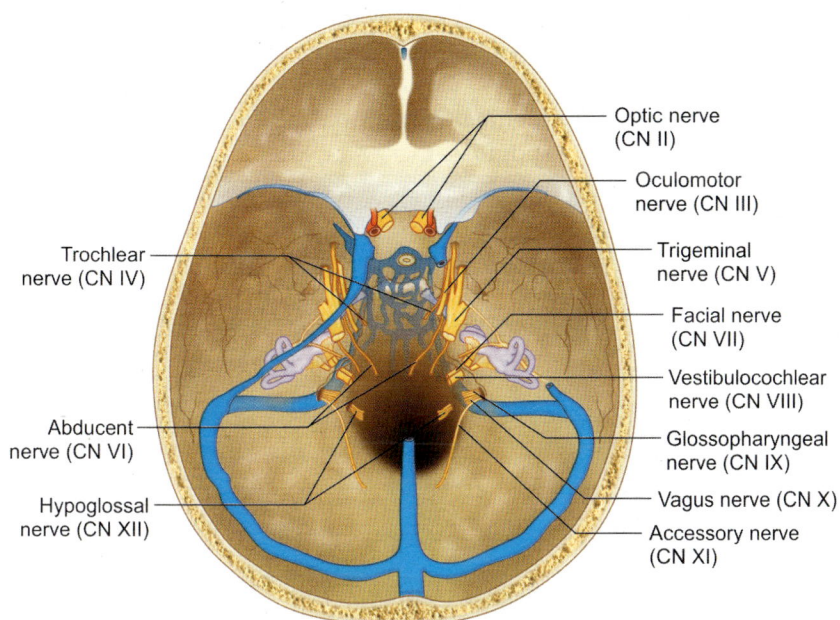

Cranial nerves as seen in the floor of cranial cavity

- Glands are considered as general viscera, and tongue and branchial muscles are considered as special viscera
- Skin, eye, pinna, nose are organs on the exterior and fibers starting from them are considered as somatic afferent
- Fibers going to the muscles or glands are known as efferent fibers
- Regarding the specific positions of cranial nerve nuclei, one should understand the phenomenon of neurobiotaxis.

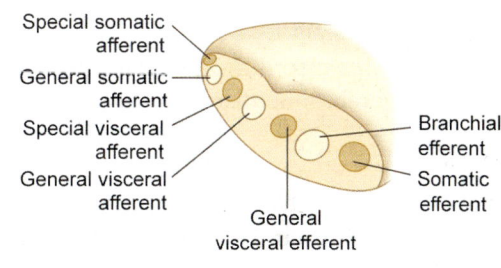

Cranial nerve fibers

### Q. Neurobiotaxis.

**Ans.** • The dorsolateral lamina of spinal cord has specific locations of the nuclei within, in the developmental stage.
- Most of the nuclei retain their primitive positions, but some move out. This displacement of the nuclei is due to differential growth patterns and by appearance and growth of neighboring fiber tracts and by active migration. This migration of nuclei in the direction of stimuli is known as neurobiotaxis like chemotaxis. Facial nerve nucleus and nucleus ambiguus assume different adult position by virtue of neurobiotaxis.

### General understanding regarding the course of cranial nerves.

- *Function of the nerve itself will act as a guide to its course. For example: Olfactory nerve, is a nerve which carries sensation of smell from nose to the brain and thus follow the same course. Nerves end by branching out. Each nerve has a root of origin, a pathway to traverse and ends by branching. There could be crucial relations as they reach their destination.*

**(Remember; there are 12 pairs of cranial nerves, not 12 cranial nerves)**

*Mnemonic:* **o**ops! **O**n **o**ccasion of **2** **t**rue **a**nnual-exams, **f**unny, **v**ery **g**ood, **v**ery **a**ttractive, **h**appened

- **Optic, ophthalmic, oculomotor, trochlear, trigeminal, abducent, facial, vestibulocochlear, glosso-pharyngeal, accessory, hypoglossal.**

## CRANIAL NERVES (Functional Components, Course, and its Distribution)

### Olfactory Nerve (I)

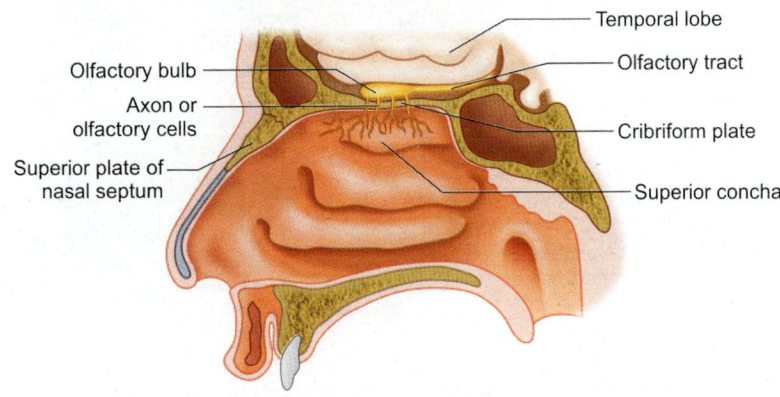

- *Function:* Smell
- *Component:* It carries smell (special sense) from exterior, so functionally the fibers are named special somatic afferent.
- *Origin:* Olfactory cells are on the mucosa of the superior nasal concha and upper part of nasal septum.

Olfactory nerve (schematic diagram)

- *Course:* Axons of the olfactory cells pass through the cribriform plate of the ethmoid bone to reach the olfactory bulb in anterior cranial fossa.
- *Termination:* From the olfactory bulb the olfactory tract begins to reach the medial surface of the cerebral hemisphere (temporal lobe).

### Optic Nerve (II)

- *Function:* Vision
- *Component:* It conveys the sight (special sense) of objects in the external environment to brain. So functionally the fibers are named special somatic afferent.
- *Origin:* Axons of ganglion cells of retina.
- *Course:* Axons converge at the optic disc.
  (optic disc itself is a blind spot has no rods and cones.)
  - Orbital course—extends from where the optic nerve pierces the sclera to optic foramen in the skull.
  - The nerve leaves the orbit through the optic foramen where nerve from both sides unite to form optic chiasma.
  - At this juncture it is important to know the crucial relations of optic chiasma. It is related above to third ventricle, below to pituitary gland and on either side to internal carotid artery.

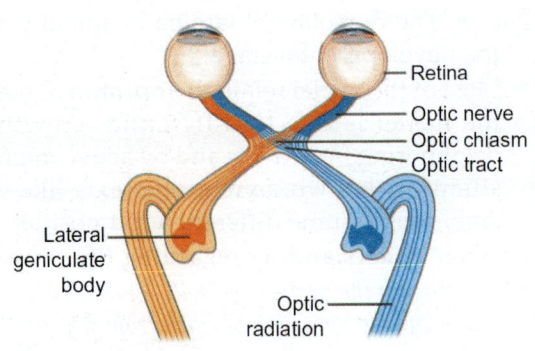

Optic pathway

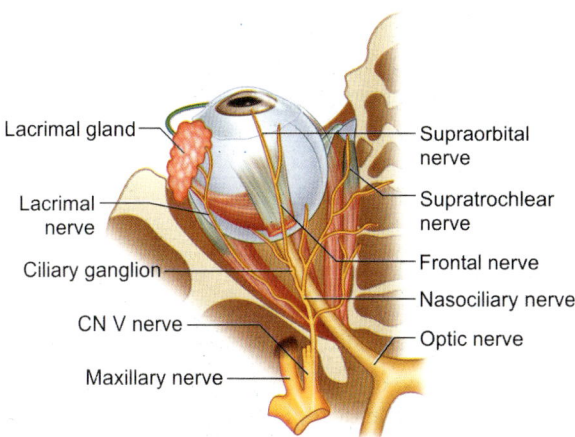

Dissected orbit

## Oculomotor Nerve (III)

- *Function:* Bring about movements in extraocular muscles (special muscles)
- *Component:* Eye is on exterior aspect, so considered somatic; and fiber is going to the muscle. So, the component of the nerve is considered as somatic efferent.

- *Function:* Constriction of pupil
- *Component:* It is due to contraction of pupillary muscles and hence the functional component is considered as general visceral efferent.
- *Origin:* Nucleus in the midbrain

*Course*: Nerve emerges from the midbrain between posterior cerebral and superior cerebellar arteries and lies lateral to posterior communicating artery.

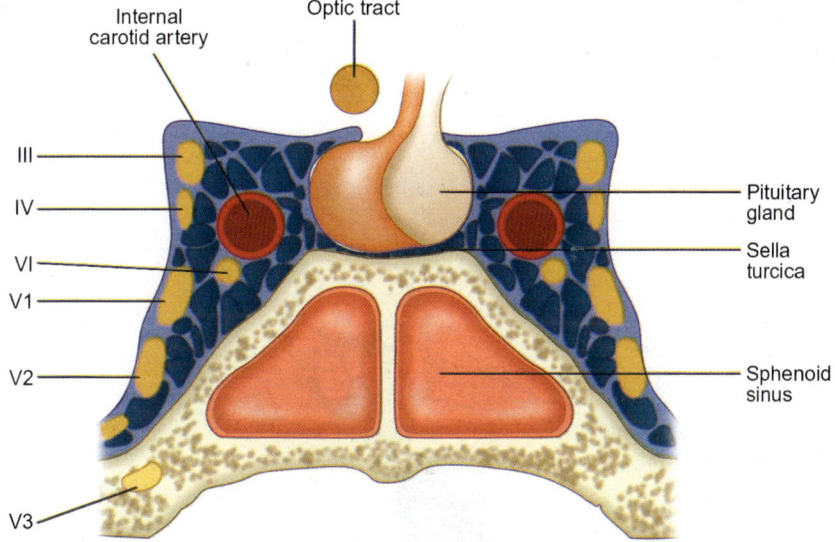

Cavernous sinus relations

Ahead, it lies on the lateral wall of cavernous sinus and enters orbit through superior orbital fissure.

- The nerve also carries parasympathetic fibres which synapse in ciliary ganglion and supply the constrictors of the pupil and ciliary muscle.
- The nerve also relays sympathetic fibres from the carotid plexus and enter the orbit through ophthalmic artery.

*Branches:* Supplies most of extraocular muscles.

### Trochlear Nerve (IV)

- *Function:* Bring about movements in extraocular muscles (special muscles)
- *Component:* Eye is on exterior aspect, so considered somatic; and fiber is going to the muscle. So, the component of the nerve is considered as somatic efferent.
- *Origin:* Nucleus lies in the midbrain.
  (it is the only nerve which lies on the dorsal aspect of brainstem).
- *Course:* The nerve fibres crosses the midline, ascends up to reach the orbit through superior orbital fissure to end by supplying superior oblique muscle.

### Trigeminal Nerve (V)

- *Functions:* As follows:
  - Movement of jaw is brought about by pterygoid muscles (branchial muscles); so, the component is named branchial efferent
  - Carry touch, pain, temperature general sensations from face (exterior) and hence the component considered is general somatic afferent.
- *Origin:* Arises from the pons, from two roots sensory and motor.
- *Course:* The two roots traverse forwards in the posterior cranial fossa to reach the trigeminal depression on the anterior aspect of pterous temporal bone.
  - Anterior part of the ganglion gives off three major divisions—ophthalmic, maxillary and mandibular.

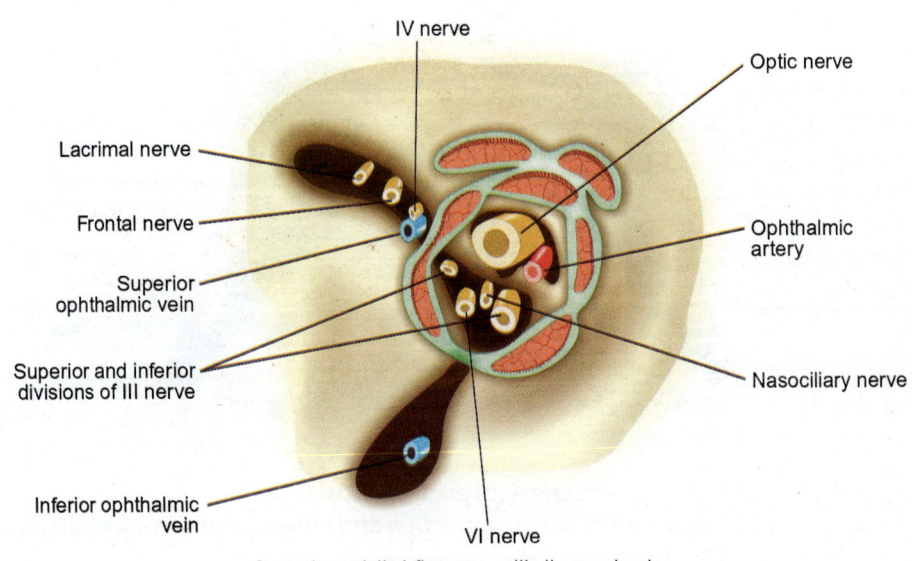

Superior orbital fissure—with its contents

- Ophthalmic nerve reaches the orbit by traversing lateral wall of cavernous sinus and superior orbital fissure. It supplies the cornea, conjunctiva, upper eyelid, forehead, nose and anterior part of the scalp.
- Maxillary nerve exits from middle cranial fossa through foramen rotundum, enters the pterygopalatine fossa, hence the orbit through infraorbital fissure. Lies on the floor of orbit to emerge through the infraorbital foramen. It supplies skin of cheek, nose, upper lip and mucosal surface of uvula, hard palate, nasopharynx and inferior part of nasopharynx.

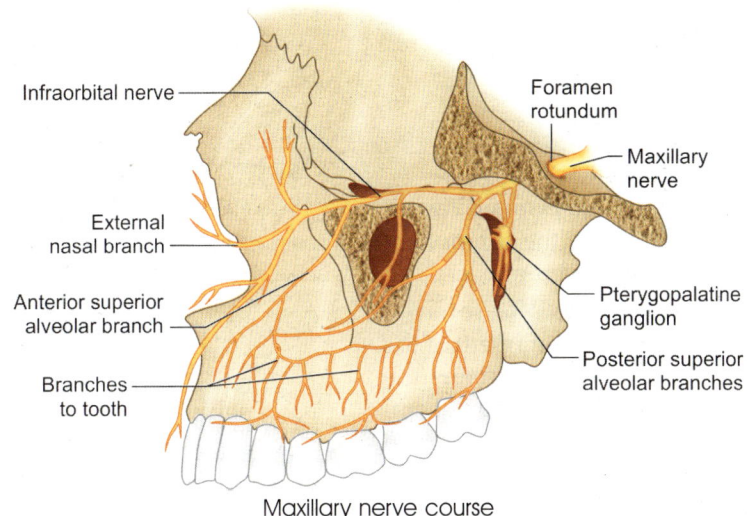

Infraorbital nerve

Foramen rotundum

Maxillary nerve

External nasal branch

Anterior superior alveolar branch

Pterygopalatine ganglion

Posterior superior alveolar branches

Branches to tooth

Maxillary nerve course

- Mandibular nerve leaves the cranial cavity through foramen ovale (mandibular nerve further details discussed in long question section).
- Ganglia associated with trigeminal nerve—ciliary, pterygopalatine, otic and submandibular.

## Abducent Nerve (VI)

- *Function:* Bring about movements in extraocular muscles (special muscles)
- *Component:* Eye is on exterior aspect, so considered somatic; and fiber is going to the muscle. So, the component of the nerve is considered as somatic efferent.
- *Origin:* Emerges from the brainstem at the junction of pons and pyramid of medulla.
- *Course:* It runs upwards, forwards and laterally in the subarachnoid space initially lateral and then inferolateral to internal carotid artery. It ends by entering the orbit through superior orbital fissure and supplying the lateral rectus muscle.

### OCULOMOTOR, TROCHLEAR, ABDUCENT NERVES

Points common about these nerves are:
- They all supply muscles of eyeball
- They traverse on either lateral or medial wall of cavernous sinus
- They all enter the orbit through superior orbital fissure
- Since all these nerves have to reach orbit, they traverse upwards and forwards.

## Facial Nerve (VII)

- *Functions:* As follows:
  - – Supply fibers to facial muscles (branchial), so the component is named branchial efferent
  - – Carry special taste sensation from tongue (viscera), so the component is named special visceral afferent
  - – Supply fibers to salivary glands (viscera) like submandibular and produce secretion (general saliva), so the component is named general visceral efferent (for the details of facial nerve refer the long question section).

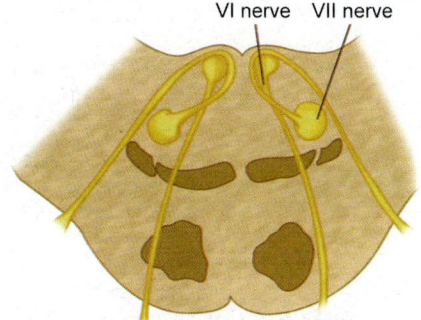

Brainstem showing origin of VII and VIII nerves

## Vestibular Cochlear Nerve (VIII)

- *Function:* Hearing (special sense)
- *Component:* Ear is on the exterior and carries special hearing sense, hence the component is named special somatic afferent.
- *Course:* It runs laterally in the internal acoustic meatus. Cochlear component of the nerve is sensory for hearing, contains the central process of bipolar neuron, peripheral process of which end on hair cells of organ of Corti.

  Vestibular nerve senses balance during head movements, the peripheral processes end on the hair cells of semicircular canals, utricle and saccule.

**FACIAL AND VESTIBULOCOCHLEAR NERVE**

*Common points:* Both the nerves emerge from lower pons and run laterally and little forwards to enter the internal acoustic meatus. The anterior inferior cerebellar artery lies in close proximity to both the nerves.

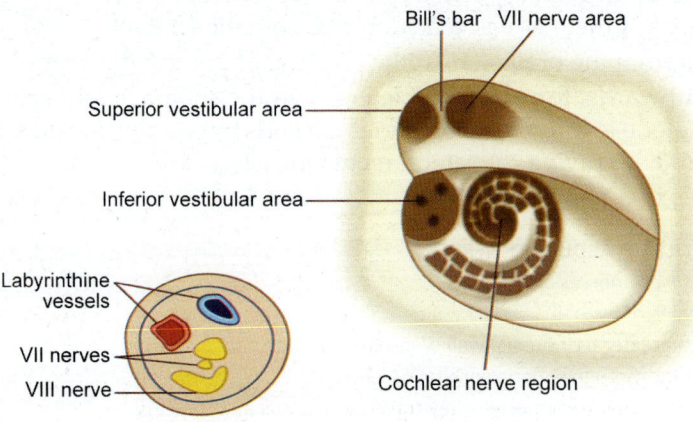

Internal acoustic meatus—with its structures

### Glossopharyngeal Nerve (IX)

- *Functions:* As follows:
  - Brings about movement in special (branchial) muscles of larynx, hence the component is named branchial efferent.
  - Supplies fibers to parotid (viscera) gland and produces secretion of saliva (general fluid) and hence the component is named general visceral efferent.
  - Carries special taste sensation from posterior one-third of tongue (viscera) and hence the component is named special visceral afferent.
- *Course:* It exits through the jugular foramen in its own dural sheath, between sigmoid and inferior petrosal sinus. At this juncture it has 2 ganglia superior and inferior and runs downwards between internal jugular vein and internal carotid artery, follows the stylopharyngeus muscle to end by supplying the pharynx, in between superior and middle constrictors. It runs forwards into the tongue, deep to hyoglossus. Terminates by giving sensory fibers to posterior third of tongue, epiglottis, soft palate.
- *Branches:* Tympanic nerve, twig to stylopharyngeus and pharyngeal branches.

### Vagus Nerve (X) and Cranial Part of XI Nerve

- *Functions:* As follows:
  - Brings about movements in special (branchial) muscles of palate, pharynx and larynx, hence the component is named branchial efferent
  - Produces general secretions in the bronchi and gut, hence the component is named general visceral efferent
  - Carries general sensations from abdominal viscera, so the component is named general visceral afferent
  - Carries special taste sensation from epiglottis (viscera) and hence the component is named special visceral afferent.

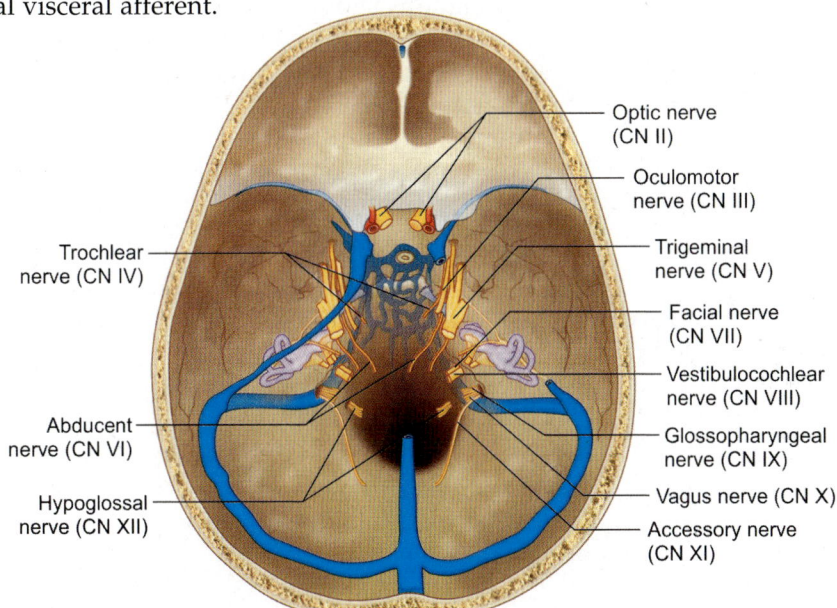

Cranial fossae after removing brain

- *Course and distribution of vagus nerve; (longest cranial nerve):* As it leaves the jugular foramen it possesses 2 sensory ganglia at this juncture like glossopharyngeal nerve, and runs downwards in carotid sheath to lie posteromedial to IJV, and posterolateral to ICA. At the root of neck, it crosses the anterior surface of subclavian artery. As the nerve descends it lies posterior to brachiocephalic vessels on right side and arch of aorta on left side enters abdomen through oesophageal opening.
- *Branches:* Meningeal, auricular, pharyngeal, superior laryngeal, cardiac, recurrent laryngeal.

## Spinal Part of Spinal Accessory (XI)

- *Function:* Supplies fibers to special (branchial) muscles, i.e. sternocleidomastoid and trapezius, and hence the component is named branchial efferent—course of accessory nerve
- *Origin:* Cranial root arise from side of medulla along with vagus and spinal root arise from the first 5 cervical segments of spinal medulla. These spinal rootlets ascend through foramen magnum to join cranial roots in the skull.
- *Course:* The nerve leaves the jugular foramen in the same dural sheath as the vagus. As it leaves the foramen the cranial part enters the laryngeal branches of vagus while the spinal part turns posteroinferiorly in close relation to IJV, and crosses the tip of 6th cervical vertebra and the upper part of carotid triangle.

  It lies deep to sternocleidomastoid and goes under the trapezius posteriorly and gives branches to the same muscles.

### GLOSSOPHARYNGEAL, VAGUS and ACCESSORY NERVES
Common points: All arise from the side of medulla and enter the jugular foramen to exit.

## Hypoglossal Nerve (XII)

- *Function:* Brings about movements of tongue by supplying fibers to tongue muscles. Tongue is considered on exterior aspect, so the component is named somatic efferent.
- *Course:* As the nerve emerges from the medulla it enters the hypoglossal canal in two separate dural sheaths. For a short distance it adheres to the vagus nerve and then runs forwards and upwards and lies deep to posterior belly of digastric muscle. At this juncture it lies anterior to root of occipital artery and enters submandibular triangle lateral to external carotid artery.

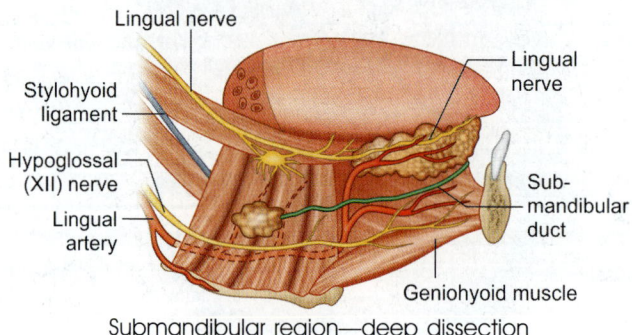

Submandibular region—deep dissection

- *Branches:* Meningeal, superior root of ansa cervicalis, nerves to thyrohyoid and geniohyoid and all intrinsic and extrinsic muscles of the tongue except palatoglossus.

## Q. Autonomic nervous system.

**Ans.**

- Autonomic nervous system comprises of sympathetic and parasympathetic components, which are under the control of centers in the brainstem, hypothalamus and cerebral cortex
- Each component has efferent and afferent fibers
- All efferent fibers synapse on its way with a ganglion
- All afferent fibers have their cell bodies in cranial and dorsal spinal nerve
- Preganglionic fibers are medullated
- Postganglionic fibers are nonmedullated
- Afferent sensory fibers from blood vessels viscera traverse via both pre- and post-ganglionic fibers.

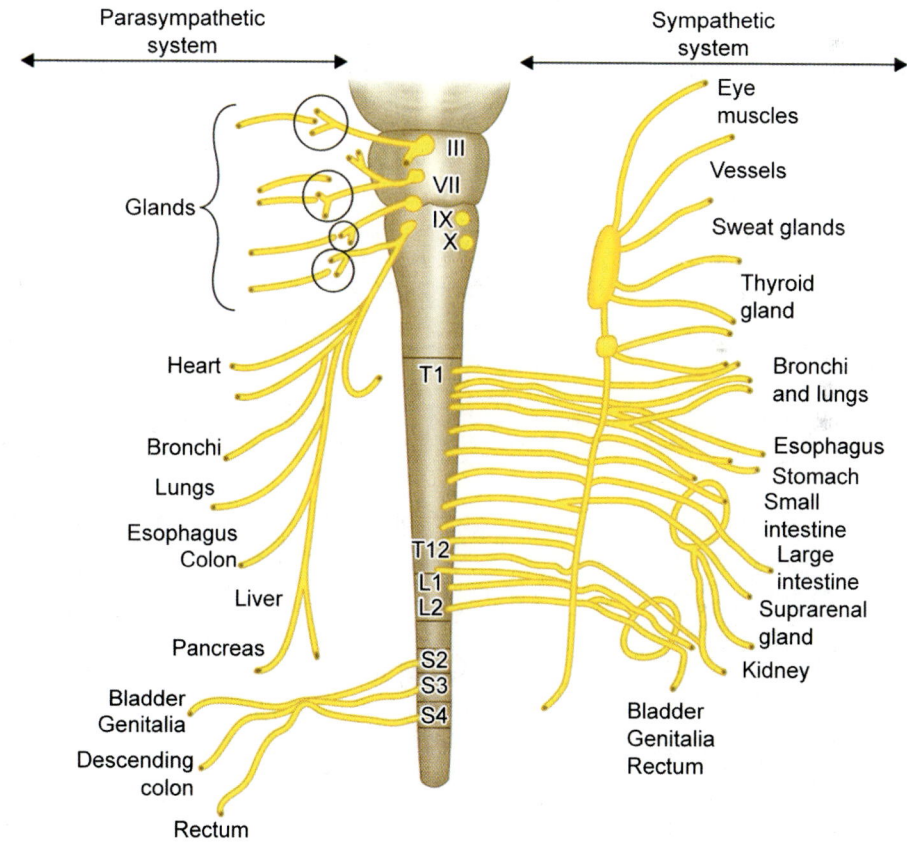

Autonomic nervous system

| Features | Sympathetic system | Parasympathetic system |
|---|---|---|
| Preganglionic fibers arise from | Axons of lateral column of gray matter | III, VII, IX, X cranial nerve nuclei Gray matter of S2, S3, S4 |
| Origin | Thoracolumbar outflow | Craniosacral outflow |
| Preganglionic fibers length | Short | Long |
| Postganglionic synapse | Many | Few |
| Effect | Widespread | Limited |
| Ganglia | Away from the structure to be innervated | Close to the structure to be innervated |
| Neurotransmitters: <br> in preganglionic <br> in postganglionic | Acetylcholine <br> Noradrenaline (except sweat glands, it is acetylcholine) | Acetylcholine <br> Acetylcholine |
| Spinal cord segments giving origin | All thoracic, L1, L2 | III, VII, IX, X cranial nerve nuclei and S2, S3, S4 |
| Distribution of fibers | Vasoconstrictors <br> To arterioles, sweat glands, skin | Mainly visceral |

# Key Long Questions

**Q. Describe internal capsule in detail (parts, ascending and descending fibers, blood supply, applied anatomy).**

**Ans.** Internal capsule is a bundle of fibers stacked between the basal nuclei components. It has both ascending and descending fibers interconnecting the cortex to brainstem, spinal cord. Since it is a closely packed area, damage to even a small region will cause involvement of many fibers leading to extensive signs and symptoms.

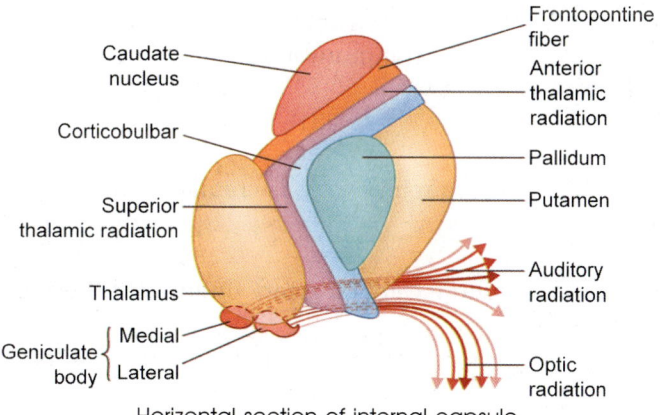

Horizontal section of internal capsule

## Parts

In horizontal section, it can be subdivided into following parts:
- Anterior limb
- Genu
- Posterior limb
- Retrolentiform part
- Sublentiform part.

*Composition of Each Part*

1. ***Anterior limb:*** It lies between caudate nucleus and lentiform nucleus. It contains anterior thalamic radiation and frontopontine fibers.
2. ***Genu:*** The anterior and the posterior limb meet at an angle known as genu. It contains corticobulbar and corticoreticular fibers.
3. ***Posterior limb:*** It lies between lentiform nucleus and thalamus. It contains superior thalamic radiation, corticopontine fibers, corticofugal fibers and corticospinal fibers.
4. ***Retrolentiform part:*** It is a part behind the lentiform nucleus. It contains posterior thalamic radiation including optic radiation and other fibers included are parietopontine and occipito-pontine fibers.
5. ***Sublentiform part:*** It is a part below the lentiform nucleus. It contains inferior thalamic peduncle auditory radiation and other fibers included are parietopontine and temporo-pontine.

## Blood Supply

*Arterial Supply*

The chief source of arterial blood is lenticulostriate branches of middle cerebral artery.

Following is the blood supply of various parts of internal capsule:

- *Anterior limb:* It is supplied by central branches of middle cerebral artery and anterior cerebral artery
- *Genu:* It is supplied by central branches of middle cerebral artery
- *Posterior limb:* It is partly supplied by central branches of middle cerebral artery, posterior communicating artery and anterior choroidal artery.

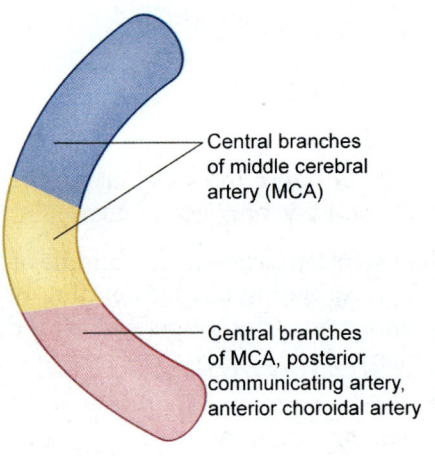

Arterial supply of internal capsule

## Venous Drainage

Striate branches of cerebral veins drain into various cranial venous sinuses.

## Applied Anatomy

Thrombosis or hemorrhage of middle cerebral artery or anterior choroidal artery lead to the lesions of internal capsule, i.e.:

- Vascular injury in the posterior limb of internal capsule results in the contralateral hemianesthesia
- Lesion in the genu leads to contralateral hemiplegia
- Vascular lesion in the retro- or sub-lentiform part causes hemianesthesia, hemianopsia and hemihypoacusis.

**Q. Discuss ventricles of brain in detail with its clinical significance.**

**Ans.** Cavities within the forebrain, midbrain and hindbrain form ventricular system of the brain. These cavities communicate with each other and then the subarachnoid space and permit circulation of cerebrospinal fluid (CSF).

The choroid plexus within the ventricular system, produces the CSF. Following are the divisions of ventricles:

- *Lateral ventricle:* Cavity in cerebral hemisphere
- *Third ventricle:* Cavity in diencephalon
- *Cerebral aqueduct:* It is a passage connecting third ventricle to fourth ventricle
- *Fourth ventricle:* Cavity within the medulla.

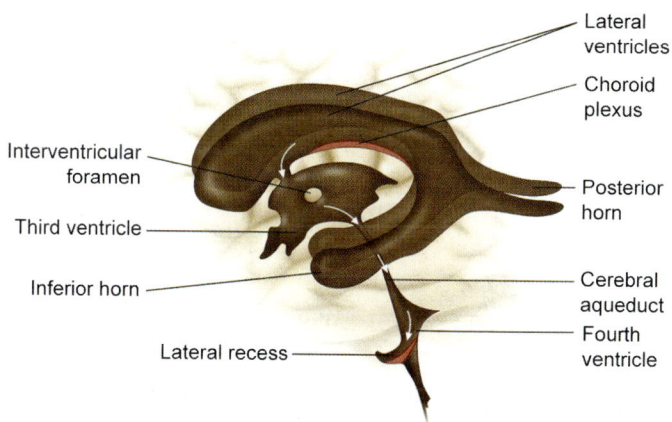

Ventricles of brain (arrow shows flow of CSF)

## Communications

- The lateral ventricles communicate with third ventricle through interventricular foramen (foramen of Monro)
- The third ventricle communicates with fourth ventricle through the cerebral aqueduct
- The fourth ventricle communicates with subarachnoid space through foramen of Magendie and foramen of Luschka.

## Lateral Ventricle: Cavity in Cerebral Hemisphere

*Lateral ventricle has following parts:* A central part and three horns—anterior, posterior and inferior.

### Central Part

Central part is related to corpus callosum. It extends from interventricular foramen to splenium of corpus callosum.

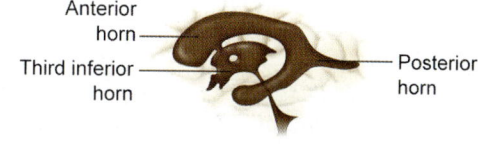

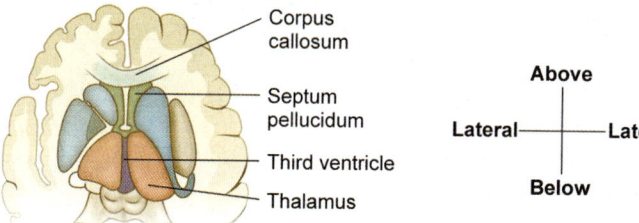

Relations of lateral ventricle body

*Relations*
- *Above:* Corpus callosum
- *Below:* Caudate nucleus and thalamus
- *Medially:* Septum pellucidum.

### Anterior Horn

The part lies in front of interventricular foramen and extends into frontal lobe.

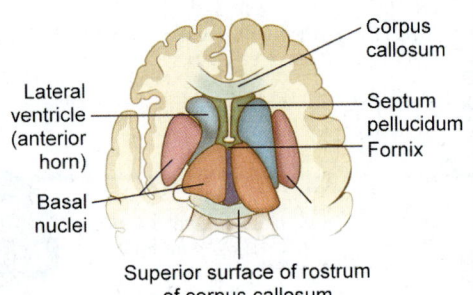

*Relations*
- *In front:* Genu and rostrum of corpus callosum
- *Above:* Body of corpus callosum
- *Below:* Caudate nucleus and superior surface of rostrum of corpus callosum.

### Posterior Horn

The part lies behind the splenium of corpus callosum and extends into occipital lobe.

*Relations*
- *Above and laterally:* Tapetum and optic radiation
- *Below and medially:* Forceps major (fibers of corpus callosum).

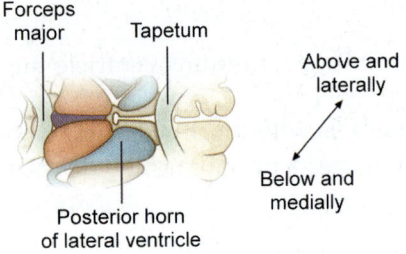

### Inferior Horn

Inferior horn is the largest horn of lateral ventricle extending into the temporal lobe.

*Relations*
- *Above and laterally:* Tapetum and caudate nucleus
- *Below and medially:* Collateral sulcus and hippocampus.

### Third Ventricle

Cavity of diencephalon has extensions namely suprapineal, pineal, infundibular and optic. The cavity lies between thalami on either side.

*Relations*
- *In front:* Lamina terminalis
- *Behind:* Pineal body, posterior commissure, cerebral aqueduct
- *Above:* Choroid plexus
- *Below:* Optic chiasma, tuber cinereum, pituitary stalk, mammillary bodies, posterior perforated substance and tegmentum of midbrain
- *On either side:* Thalamus.

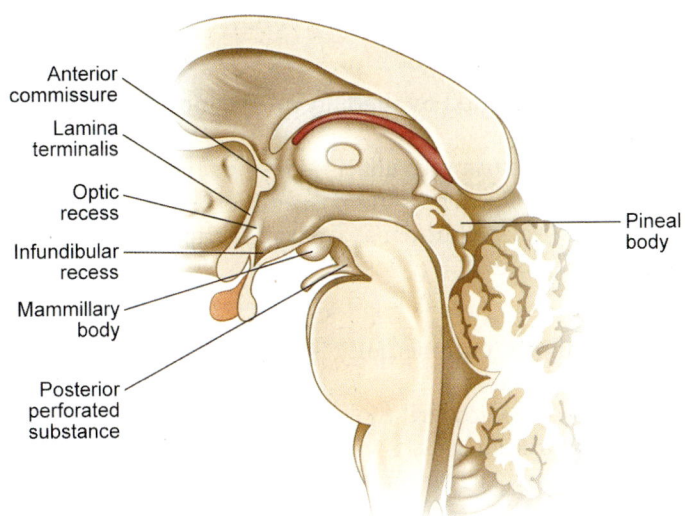

Boundaries of III ventricle

## Fourth Ventricle: Cavity within the Medulla

Fourth ventricle is a rhomboid-shaped cavity overlying the pons and medulla and hence it can be subdivided into pontine part and medullary part.

### Extent

- *Above:* Cerebral aqueduct of midbrain
- *Below:* Central canal of upper cervical spinal cord.

### Roof

Superior and inferior medullary vela (like a tent).

### Apex

Apex extends into the cerebellum, where it is known as fastigium.

### Recess

Lateral recess: It lies over the surface of inferior cerebellar peduncle and opens into the cerebello-medullary cistern.

### Communications

Communicates with subarachnoid space through foramen of Luschka and foramen of Magendie.

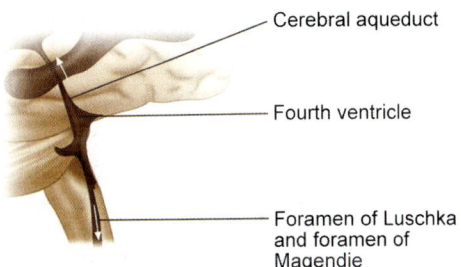

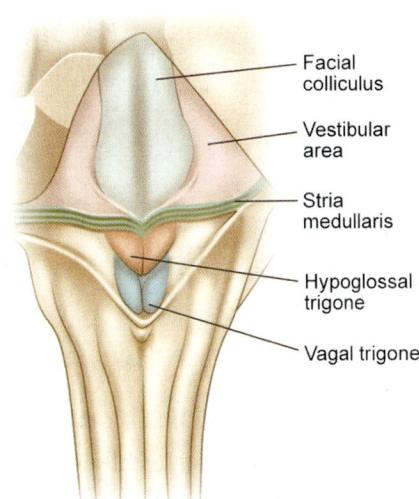

Floor of fourth ventricle

## Floor

### Features

- Vertically in the center, it is divided by median sulcus and paramedially divided by sulcus limitans
- Horizontally, it is divided by stria medullaris
- Paramedian area has a bulge known as median eminence
- Caudal area of fourth ventricle is known as calamus scriptorius
- The apex of the ventricle is known as obex.

### Specific area

- Just above the stria medullaris, paramedially is facial colliculus and hypoglossal trigone is just below it
- Vagal trigone lies paramedially toward the caudal part of fourth ventricle
- Just above the stria medullaris, laterally is vestibular area beneath, which is vestibular nuclei
- Just above the obex is a paired circumventricular organ known as area postrema.

### Clinical Importance

In case of blockage of communicating passages of ventricular system or excessive production of CSF, due to brain tumors will lead to dilatation of ventricles giving rise to hydrocephalus.

### Q. Discuss the blood supply of brain and spinal cord.

**Ans.** Brain is the most active system of the body with an average blood supply of 50 mL/100 g of brain tissue per minute. Compromise of the blood supply to the brain even for 5 minutes can cause neurological deficit. Thus, the blood supply of brain and spinal cord assumes great clinical significance.

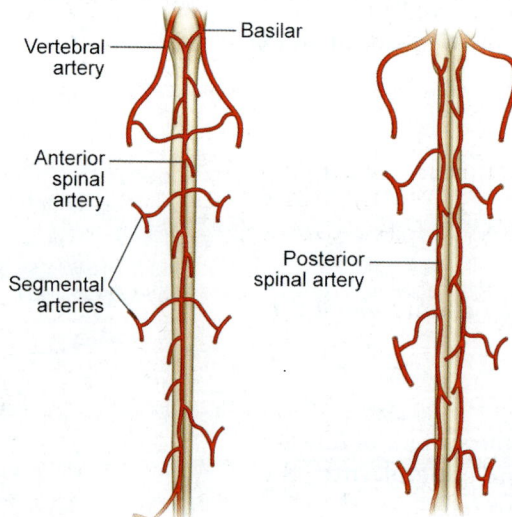

### Arterial Supply of Spinal Cord

The spinal cord receives blood from following sources:
- Branches of vertebral arteries
- Branches of segmental arteries.

### Branches of Vertebral Arteries

*Posterior spinal artery:* These are paired arteries on posterior surface of spinal cord and form plexiform channels or may be so small in size, hardly visible.

*Anterior spinal artery:* Paired anterior spinal arteries soon unite after its origin from vertebral arteries and form a single midline vessel, which lies on the anterior median fissure of the spinal cord. They anastomose with radicular arteries.

### Branches of Segmental Arteries

*Radicular arteries:* These arteries traverse the intervertebral foramina and divide into anterior and posterior radicular arteries. A prominent anterior radicular artery in lumbar region is known as artery of Adamkiewicz.

Spinal arteries and radicular arteries through their small branches, i.e. sulcal branches, form a rich network of arteries all-around the spinal cord.

## Venous Drainage of Spinal Cord

The venous blood of the spinal cord is drained mainly by two venous trunks namely:

- Anterior longitudinal venous trunk, which consist of anteromedian and anterolateral spinal veins
- Posterior longitudinal venous trunk, which consist of posteromedial vein and paired posterolateral vein.

### Communications of Venous Channels

The internal vertebral venous plexus lies between dura mater and vertebral periosteum. At the level of intervertebral space, the plexus is connected to thoracic, abdominal and intercostal veins and also with the external vertebral venous plexus. The blood can flow in both directions since there are no valves. When there is rise in intra-abdominal pressure or block in jugular veins the blood may flow in the internal vertebral venous system. This communication within the venous channels may cause spread of tumor.

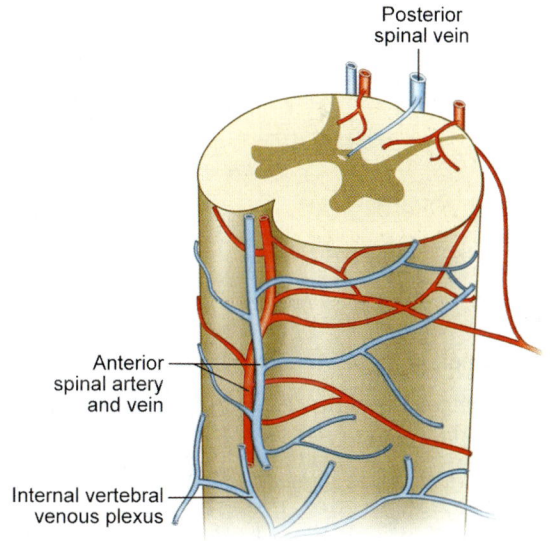

Blood supply of spinal cord

## Arterial Supply of the Brain

The brain is supplied by the branches of internal carotid artery and vertebral artery. Following are the branches of internal carotid artery.

### Internal Carotid Artery

- Anterior cerebral
- Middle cerebral
- Ophthalmic

- Posterior communicating
- Anterior choroidal.

## Vertebral Artery

Vertebral artery arises from the first part of subclavian artery and runs along the anterolateral surface of medulla, and unites to form basilar artery at the lower border of pons.

Intracranial branches of vertebral and basilar artery supply the brainstem, cerebellum, posterior parts of diencephalon and occipital, and temporal lobes of the brain. Labyrinthine, a branch of basilar artery, supplies the inner ear.

An anastomotic arterial circle is formed by branches of internal carotid artery and basilar artery. This arterial circle is known as circle of Willis.

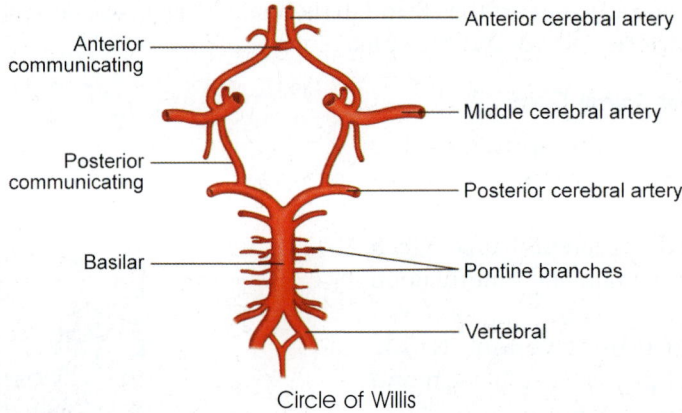

Circle of Willis

## Regional Arterial Supply

1. Cortical branches of anterior, middle and posterior cerebral arteries supply the cerebral hemisphere.
2. The anterior choroidal artery supplies the choroidal plexus, hippocampal formation, portions of globus pallidus, posterior limb of internal capsule and retrolenticular portion of internal capsule. Small branches also supply portions of basal ganglia and ventrolateral part of thalamus.
3. The posterior choroidal artery supplies the choroid plexus in lateral ventricle mainly.

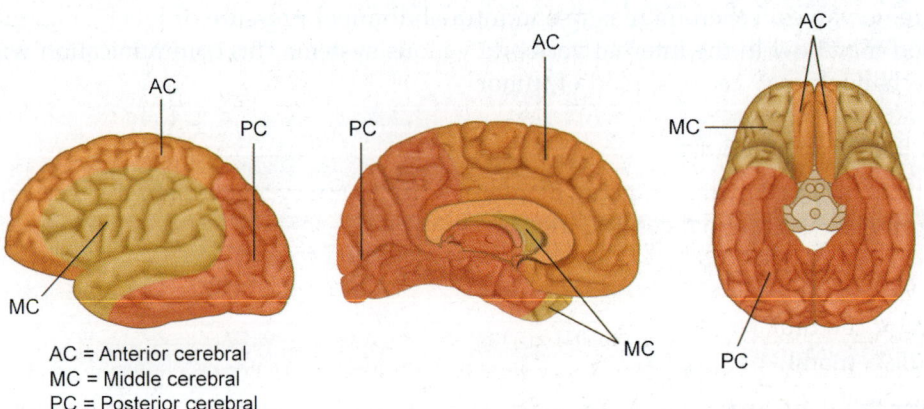

AC = Anterior cerebral
MC = Middle cerebral
PC = Posterior cerebral

4. The corpus striatum, internal capsule (anterior and posterior limb) receives arterial blood mainly from lateral striate branches of middle cerebral artery.
5. Thalamus receives blood mainly from posterior cerebral artery.
6. Pons and medulla receive arterial blood from spinal arteries, cerebellar arteries, and branches of vertebral and basilar arteries.
7. The cerebellum is supplied by superior, anterior and posterior inferior cerebellar arteries.

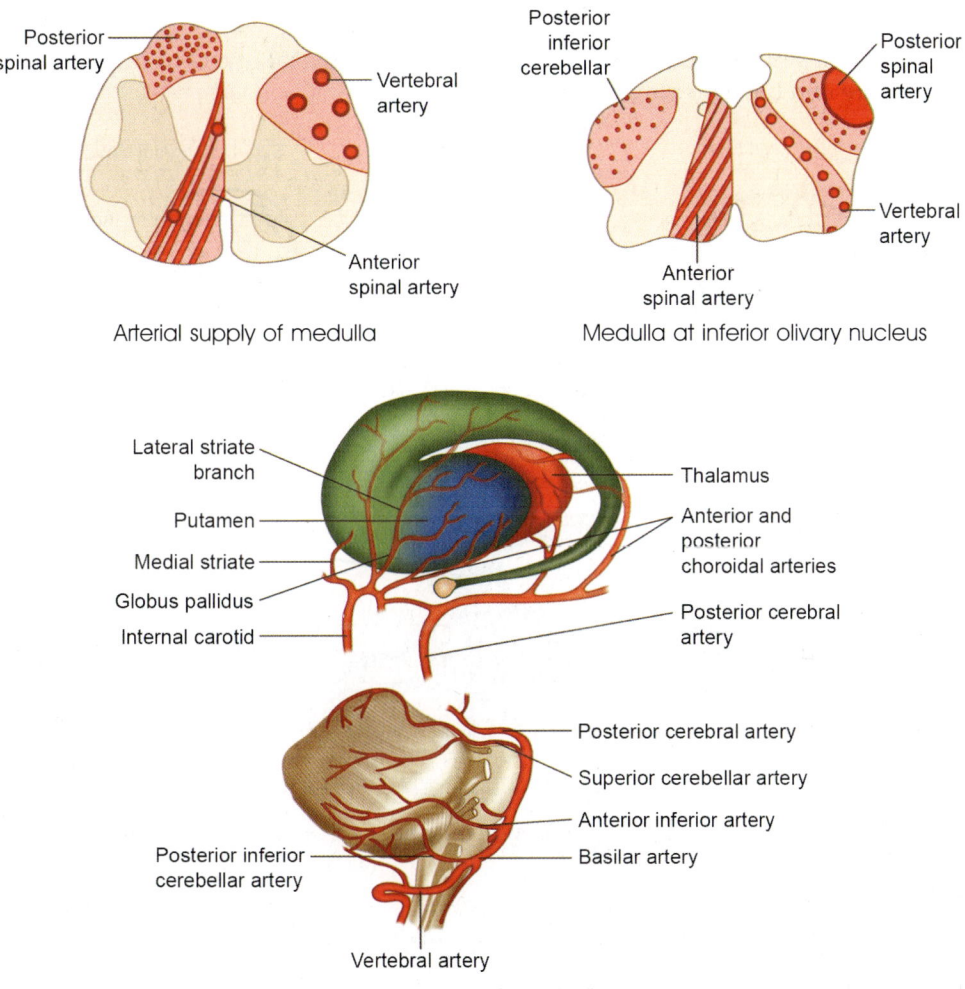

Arterial supply of medulla

Medulla at inferior olivary nucleus

Arterial supply of cerebellum

## Venous Drainage

The venous blood of brain is mainly drained by cerebral veins and dural venous sinuses.

### Cerebral Vein

- The cerebral veins can be classified into superficial and deep groups
- Superficial cerebral veins drain the cortex and the subcortical white matter and ends in various cranial sinuses.

*Tributaries*

| Superficial cerebral vein | Deep cerebral vein |
|---|---|
| Superior cerebral | Internal cerebral |
| Inferior cerebral | Basal (Rosenthal) |
| Superficial middle cerebral | Great cerebral (Galen) |

## Dural Venous Sinuses

The dural venous sinuses lie between periosteal and meningeal layers of dura, and are very tough in nature and have no valves.

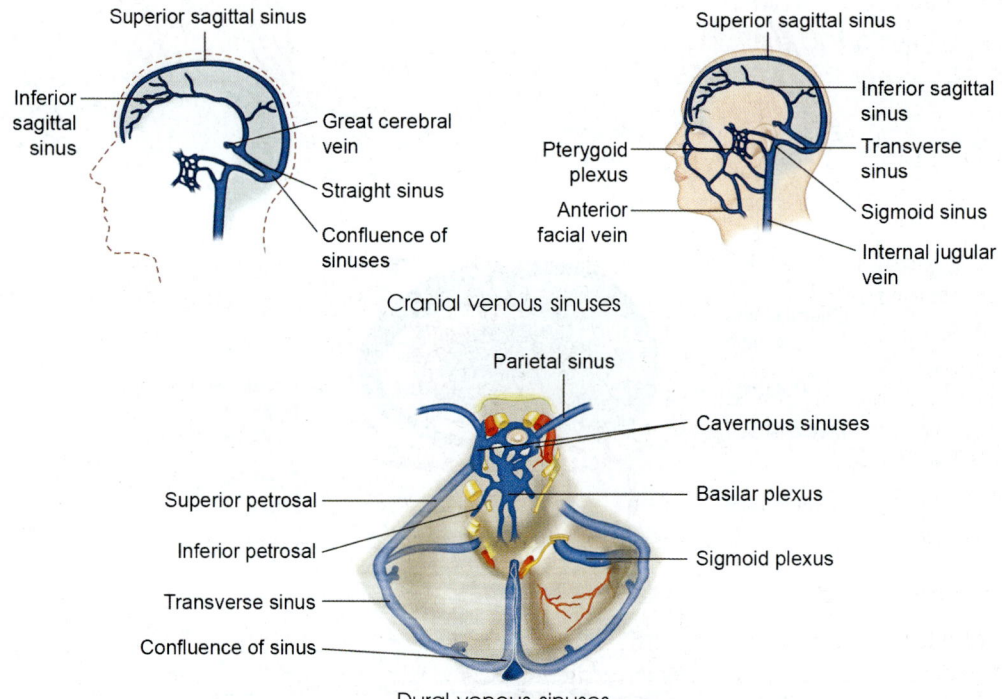

Cranial venous sinuses

Dural venous sinuses

*Following are the dural sinuses:*
- Superior and inferior sagittal sinus
- Transverse sinus
- Cavernous sinus
- Sigmoid sinus.

## Clinical Importance

- Sudden occlusion of posterior inferior cerebellar artery gives rise to lateral medullary syndrome. In this syndrome, there is loss of pain and temperature on the same side of the face and opposite side of the body, dysphagia and Horner's syndrome
- Thrombosis of lenticulostriate branch of middle cerebral artery gives rise to hemiplegia
- Sudden rupture of pontine artery can be fatal.

**Q. Discuss thalamus under following headings: Location, gross features, relations, connections and applied anatomy.**

**Ans.** Thalamus is a large mass of gray matter, which constitutes one of the subdivisions of diencephalon and is a sensory relay station for the ascending tracts.

## Location

Thalamus lies on either side of third ventricle and is disposed obliquely with the axis running backward and laterally.

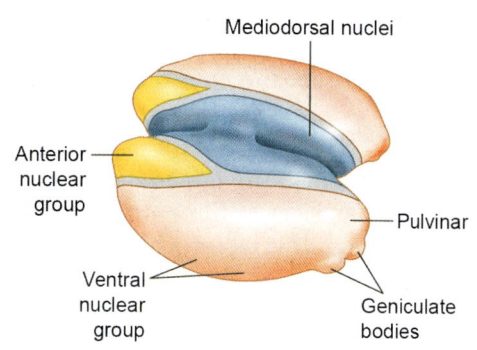

## Gross Features

- *Shape:* Oval (like an egg)
- *Surfaces:* Medial, superior, lateral and inferior
- *Ends:* Anterior end, posterior end.

Anterior two-thirds of medial surface is covered by ependyma and form lateral wall of third ventricle above hypothalamic sulcus.

Posterior end of thalamus is wide and is known as pulvinar and overhangs the midbrain. The superior surface tapers anteriorly in a rounded tubercle just posterior to interventricular foramen.

Posterior part of inferior surface of thalamus has two swellings namely medial and lateral geniculate bodies (metathalamus).

## Important Relations

- *Medially:* Third ventricle, habenular triangle
- *Laterally:* Stria terminalis, internal capsule.

## Subdivisions

Major thalamic nuclei can be classified into specific relay nuclei and association nuclei. Specific relay nuclei receive definite ascending pathways and project to definite cerebral areas. Association nuclei of thalamus project to associated areas of cerebrum. Following are the nuclear groups of thalamus and their main connections.

*Anterior Nuclear Group*

- Anteroventral (AV)
- Accessory nuclei
- Anterodorsal (AD)
- Anteromedial (AM).

Receives fibers from mammillothalamic tract, fornix projects fibers to cingulate gyrus via anterior limb of internal capsule.

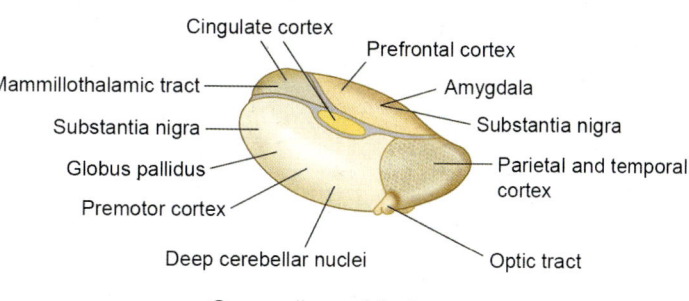

Connections of thalamus

## Mediodorsal Nuclear Group

Mediodorsal nuclear group portion is subdivided into three parts namely:
1. Magnocellular portion
2. Parvocellular portion
3. Paralaminar portion.

    Receives fibers from amygdaloid complex, temporal neocortex, frontal cortex. Projects fibers to frontal cortex and coordinates somatic and visceral activities.

## Lateral Nuclear Group

Lateral nuclear group lies on the dorsomedial surface of the thalamus caudal to anterior nuclear group. It consists of three nuclear masses—lateral dorsal nucleus, lateral posterior nucleus and pulvinar. It is reciprocally connected to temporal cortex.

## Ventral Nuclear Group

Ventral nuclear group is subdivided into three nuclei namely:
1. Ventral anterior
2. Ventral lateral
3. Ventral posterior.

    The ventral posterior is further subdivided into ventral posterolateral and ventral posteromedial nuclei. It receives impulses from substantia nigra, globus pallidus, contralateral deep cerebellar nuclei, medial lemniscus and spinothalamic tract; project fibers to premotor cortex and sensory cortex.

    There are other less distinct nuclei groups like midline nuclei and intralaminar nuclei group. Thalamic reticular nucleus is a neuronal shell, which surrounds lateral, superior and anteroinferior aspect of dorsal thalamus.

## Applied Anatomy

Neurosurgically, thalamotomy may control rigidity and tremors in diseases of corpus striatum.

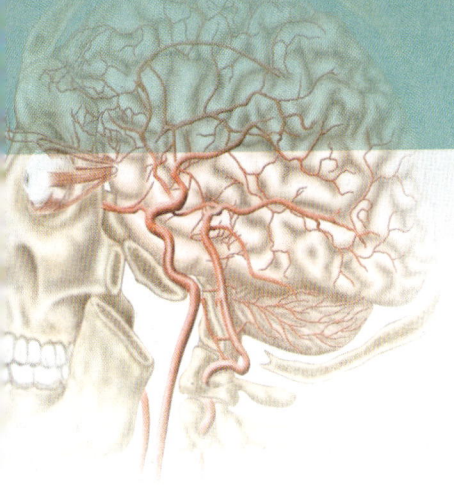

# MCQs

## 44

**1. Weight of the adult brain is approximately** ....................

    a. 1,500 g

    b. 500 g

    c. 1,500 mg

    d. 500 mg

**Answer: a**

**2. Following constitute hindbrain** ....................

    a. Diencephalon + Metencephalon

    b. Mesencephalon + Metencephalon

    c. Metencephalon + Myelencephalon

    d. Diencephalon + Myelencephalon

**Answer: c**

**3. Leptomeninges means** ....................

    a. Dura + Pia

    b. Pia + Arachnoid

    c. Dura + Arachnoid

    d. Dura + Pia + Arachnoid

**Answer: b**

**4. Dura chiefly receives blood from** .................... **artery.**

    a. Middle meningeal

    b. Ophthalmic

    c. Ethmoidal

    d. All of the above

**Answer: a**

**5. What is the approximate quantity of CSF?**

    a. 1 L

    b. 500 mL

    c. 150 mL

    d. 5 mL

**Answer: c**

**6.** Match the following spinal cord segments:

| Column A | Column B |
|----------|----------|
| 1. Cervical | a. 12 |
| 2. Thoracic | b. 1 |
| 3. Lumbar | c. 5 |
| 4. Coccygeal | d. 8 |

**Answer: 1-d, 2-a, 3-c, 4-b**

**7.** The spinal cord ends at ..................... level in adults.
- a. L1
- b. L2
- c. L3
- d. L4

**Answer: a**

**8.** The spinal cord ends at ..................... level at birth.
- a. L1
- b. L2
- c. L3
- d. L4

**Answer: c**

**9.** Lentiform nucleus is a combination of following nuclei ....................
- a. Caudate nucleus + Putamen
- b. Putamen + Globus pallidus
- c. Caudate nucleus + Globus pallidus
- d. Caudate nucleus + Putamen + Globus pallidus

**Answer: b**

**10.** The least differentiated segment of brainstem is ....................
- a. Pons
- b. Medulla
- c. Midbrain
- d. All of the above

**Answer: c**

**11.** Following cranial nerves are related to midbrain:
- a. I, II
- b. III, IV
- c. IV, V
- d. V, VI

**Answer: b**

**12.** Following are the areas noted in the floor of fourth ventricle except ....................
- a. Facial colliculus
- b. Vestibular area
- c. Hypoglossal trigone
- d. Oculomotor area

**Answer: d**

**13.** Which lamina surrounds the central canal?
- a. Lamina I
- b. Lamina IV
- c. Lamina X
- d. Lamina VIII

**Answer: c**

14. The lamina, which forms many discrete groups in the anterior horn of the gray matter of spinal cord is ....................

   a. Lamina IX
   b. Lamina VII
   c. Lamina III
   d. Lamina V

**Answer: a**

15. Zona intermedia is following ....................

   a. Lamina I
   b. Lamina VII
   c. Lamina IX
   d. Lamina VIII

**Answer: b**

16. The tract, which carries crude touch and pressure is ....................

   a. Posterior white column
   b. Anterior spinothalamic tract
   c. Lateral spinothalamic tract
   d. Posterior spinocerebellar tract

**Answer: a**

17. The tract, which carries light touch sensation is ....................

   a. Posterior white column
   b. Anterior spinothalamic tract
   c. Lateral spinothalamic tract
   d. Posterior spinocerebellar tract

**Answer: b**

18. The tract, which conveys pain and temperature is ....................

   a. Posterior white column
   b. Anterior spinothalamic tract
   c. Lateral spinothalamic tract
   d. Posterior spinocerebellar tract

**Answer: c**

19. The sensory relay station in the brain is ....................

   a. Epithalamus
   b. Hypothalamus
   c. Metathalamus
   d. Thalamus

**Answer: d**

20. Following are the ascending crossed tracts except ....................

   a. Lateral spinothalamic
   b. Medial lemniscus
   c. Anterior spinocerebellar
   d. Posterior spinocerebellar

**Answer: d**

21. Following are the uncrossed descending fibers except ....................

   a. Lateral corticospinal
   b. Anterior corticospinal
   c. Uncrossed lateral corticospinal
   d. Vestibulospinal

**Answer: a**

22. Medial longitudinal fasciculus connects following nucleus except ....................

   a. Oculomotor
   b. Trochlear
   c. Abducens
   d. Facial

**Answer: d**

23. **Carotid siphon is referred to ..................... parts of internal carotid artery.**

    a. Cervical + Cerebral portion         c. Intracavernous + Cerebral portion

    b. Intrapetrosal + Intracavernous      d. Intrapetrosal + Cervical

            **Answer: c**

24. **The lateral medullary syndrome is produced by ....................**

    a. Anteroinferior cerebellar artery     c. Middle cerebral artery

    b. Posteroinferior cerebellar artery    d. Basilar artery

            **Answer: b**

25. **Pulvinar is a portion of ....................**

    a. Hypothalamus             c. Thalamus

    b. Epithalamus              d. Internal capsule

            **Answer: c**

26. **Fornix is an efferent system of ....................**

    a. Hypothalamus             c. Thalamus

    b. Epithalamus              d. Hippocampus

            **Answer: d**

27. **Following is a part of metathalamus ....................**

    a. Habenular trigone         c. Medial geniculate body

    b. Pineal body              d. Thalamus

            **Answer: c**

28. **Restiform body is ....................**

    a. Superior cerebellar peduncle     c. Middle cerebellar peduncle

    b. Inferior cerebellar peduncle     d. All of the above

            **Answer: b**

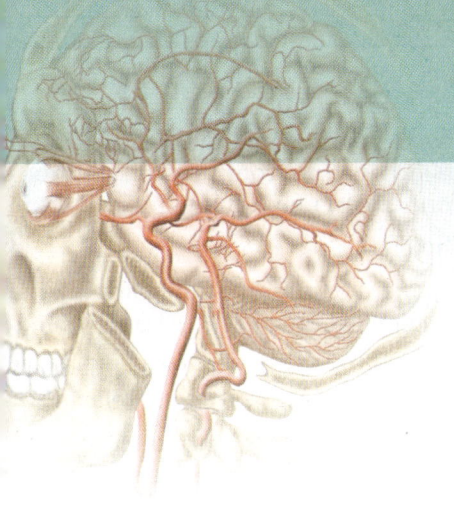

# Glossary

## 45

**Fornix:** It is a main efferent system of hippocampus, which includes projection and commissural fibers. The fibers are axons of cells in subicular cortex and pyramidal cells of hippocampus. The fibers from fornix end in mammillary body and from the mammillary body, the fibers go to anterior nuclei of thalamus.

**Hypothalamus:** It is a part of diencephalon, which lies ventral to hypothalamic sulcus and extends from optic chiasm to mammillary bodies. It is divided into medial and lateral nuclear groups by fornix. It grossly comprises of infundibulum, tuber cinereum and mammillary bodies. Functionally related to visceral, endocrine, metabolic activities and temperature regulation, sleep and emotional behavior.

**Habenular nuclei:** Part of epithalamus, which consist of medial and lateral nuclei, receive fibers from stria medullaris and gives rise to fasciculus retroflexus; it is a site of convergence of limbic pathway, which conveys impulses to midbrain.

**Limbus of the cerebrum:** The hippocampus, dentate gyrus, indusium griseum, septum pellucidum and fornix form the limbus of the cerebrum. It forms a part of rhinencephalon (literally means smell brain).

**Olivary complex:** It has two subdivisions namely, superior and inferior:

1. *Superior olivary complex:* It comprises of several nuclei, located in lateral position in reticular formation, medial to it is trapezoid body. It is involved in auditory sound source localization and are main relay stations of cochlear nuclei.
2. *Inferior olivary complex:* It is the most striking feature in medulla comprising of three parts—principal nuclei, medial accessory nuclei and dorsal accessory nuclei. These nuclei have short dendrites, and the axons of the cells cross the median raphe to enter the inferior cerebellar peduncle. These fibers end as climbing fibers in cerebellar cortex, which cause excitatory action upon Purkinje cells.

**Pre-cerebellar nuclei:** The nuclei in the brainstem, which project to cerebellum are collectively known as pre-cerebellar nuclei.

*Pyramid:* On the anterior surface of medulla, there are two pyramids separated by anterior median fissure. The pyramids are bundles of nerve fibers originating from precentral gyrus and descend downward through crura and the pons to form the pyramid in medulla.

*Restiform body:* It is equivalent to inferior cerebellar peduncle.

*Red nucleus:* It is an ovoid mass, dorsomedial to substantia nigra of midbrain, appear pink in fresh specimens due to ferric pigment in the neurons. Its function in human beings is uncertain.

*Reticular formation:* It lies dorsal and lateral to red nucleus, and fibers of superior cerebellar peduncle traverse this nucleus and referred as locomotor center (walking movements elicited).

*Stria terminalis:* It is a well-defined amygdaloid nuclear complex. Fibers of stria terminalis arch along medial border of caudate nucleus to end in nuclei of stria terminalis. Amygdaloid complex stimulation causes fear confusion and amnesia.

*Stria medullaris of diencephalon:* It is a bundle of fibers arising from septal nuclei, lateral preoptic region and anterior thalamic nuclei.

*Septal area:* The subcallosal region and paraterminal gyrus constitute septal area. Beneath this area lie septal nuclei. The septal nuclei receive afferent from hippocampus via fornix and efferent fibers project via stria medullaris to medial habenular nucleus, medial forebrain bundle to lateral hypothalamus and fornix to hippocampus.

*Syndrome of Benedict:* Ipsilateral III nerve paresis and contralateral involuntary motor movements like tremor, ataxia is known as syndrome of Benedict. It occurs in the lesions of midbrain tegmentum.

*Stria medullaris of fourth ventricle:* Arcuate nucleus is an inferior extension of pontine nuclei; fibers arising from arcuate nucleus pass posteriorly through midline of medulla and run across the floor of fourth ventricle forming the striae medullares of fourth ventricle.

*Trapezoid body:* Mostly regarded as auditory relay station, but the axons of trapezoid body may enter medial longitudinal fasciculus connecting V, VII, III, IV, VI nuclei. Thus, coordinating stapedial reflex, action of tensor tympanic and extraocular muscle.

*Tectum of midbrain:* It is the roof of midbrain (dorsal to cerebral aqueduct) bearing two dorsal swellings namely, superior colliculus and inferior colliculus, detailed as follows:
1. *Superior colliculi:* It is a laminated structure having alternate gray and white matter. Superficial layers receive fibers from retina and visual cortex, and are involved in detection of movements in visual field. The deep layers receive fibers from auditory system, motor cortex, reticular formation. Efferent fibers of deep layers are concerned with head and eye movements.
2. *Inferior colliculi:* It is an ovoid cellular mass in caudal tectum concerned with transmitting signals from lateral lemniscus to medial geniculate body involved in auditory pathway.

*Weber's syndrome:* Lesions affecting III nerve and corticospinal fibers in midbrain cause ipsilateral III nerve paralysis and contralateral hemiplegia. This is known as Weber's syndrome (superior alternating hemiplegia).

Wallenberg's syndrome or lateral medullary syndrome; occurs due to thrombosis of posterior inferior cerebellar artery in the brainstem, with clinical features of sudden onset vertigo, dysphagia, vomiting, ataxia, ipsilateral anesthesia of face and nasal twang.

# Neuroanatomy Specimens

## 46

## FLOOR OF THE CRANIAL CAVITY

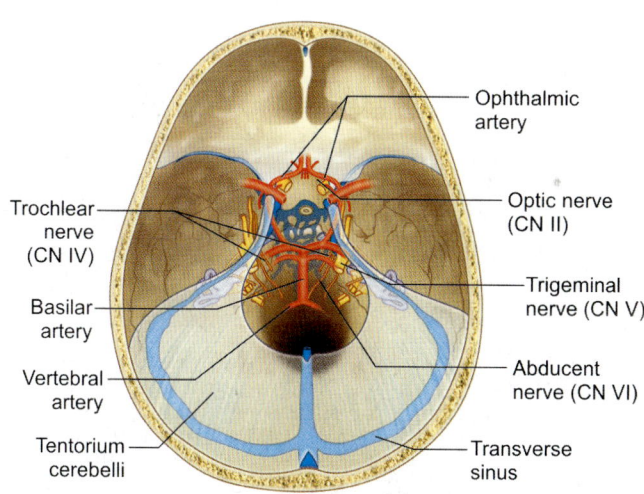

Floor of cranial cavity

### Viva Questions

Student should be able to identify the structures in the floor of the cavity as shown in above figure

| | |
|---|---|
| I—Olfactory | VII—Facial |
| II—Optic | VIII—Vestibulocochlear (auditory) |
| III—Oculomotor | IX—Glossopharyngeal |
| IV—Trochlear | X—Vagus |
| V—Trigeminal | XI—Spinal accessory |
| VI—Abducent | XII—Hypoglossal |

*Mnemonic:* oops! On occasion of 2 true annual-exams, funny, very good, very attractive, happened

## CEREBRAL HEMISPHERES

### a. Superolateral Surface

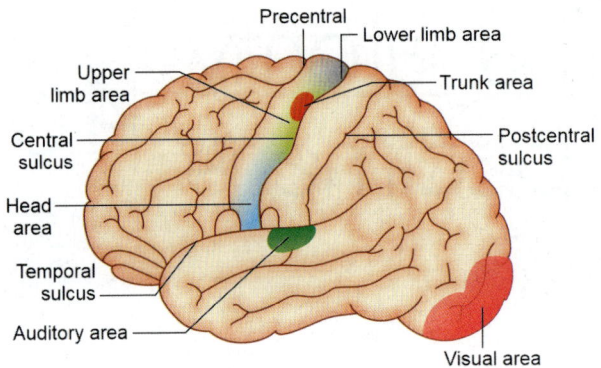

Superolateral surface of brain

### b. Viva Questions

- Students should be able to identify the sulci and gyri on the cerebrum; first try to locate the central sulci, and then identify other sulci and gyri.
- Cerebrum is supplied by the anterior, middle and posterior cerebral artery.
- Precentral gyrus is the motor cortex, while the postcentral gyrus is the sensory gyrus, visual area is the gyrus around the calcarine sulcus, while the auditory area is around the temporal sulcus.

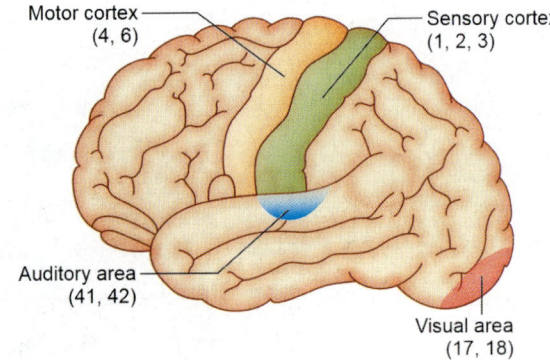

Functional cortical areas on superolateral surface of cerebrum

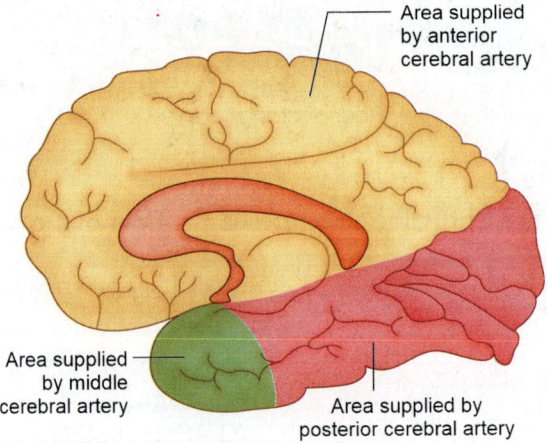

Vascular territories of cerebral arteries

## INFERIOR SURFACE OF BRAIN

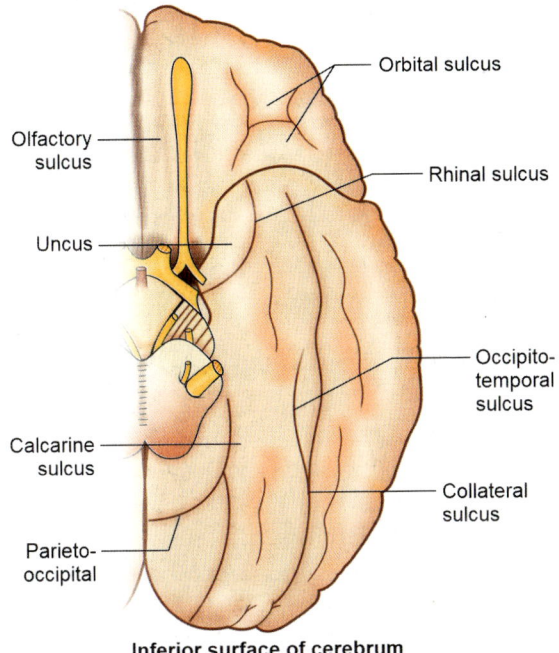

**Inferior surface of cerebrum**

### Viva Questions

- Identify the sulci and gyri on this surface (study above the diagram)
- Identify the mammillary body, pituitary stalk.

## MEDIAL SURFACE OF CEREBRUM

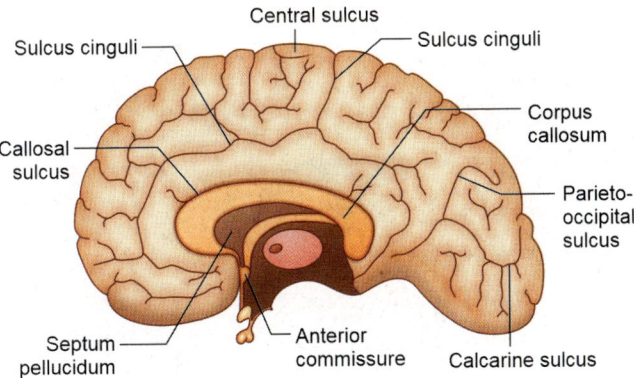

Medial surface of cerebrum features

## Viva Questions

- Corpus callosum is the largest commissural fiber, parts are rostrum, genu, body, splenium

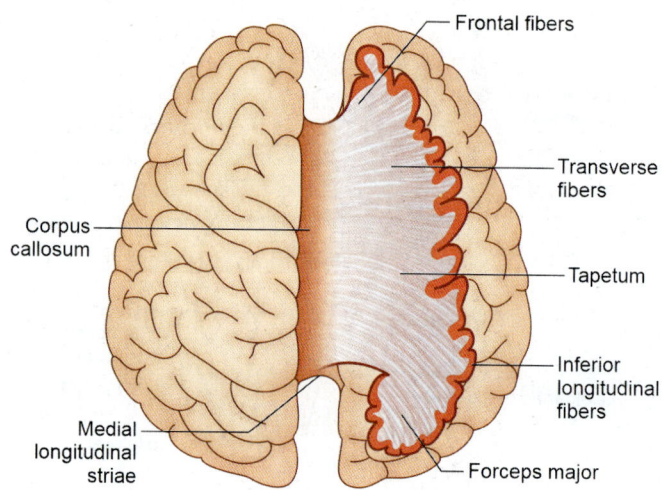

Corpus callosum as seen from above

- White matter of cerebrum is classified into:
  - Association fibers—connect various regions of cerebral cortex within one hemisphere
  - Commissural fibers—connect a region of one hemisphere to the other on the other hemisphere, after crossing the midline
  - Projection fibers—connect the cerebral cortex to the other parts of central nervous system.
- Cingulum is the largest association fiber, while corpus callosum is the largest commissural fiber.

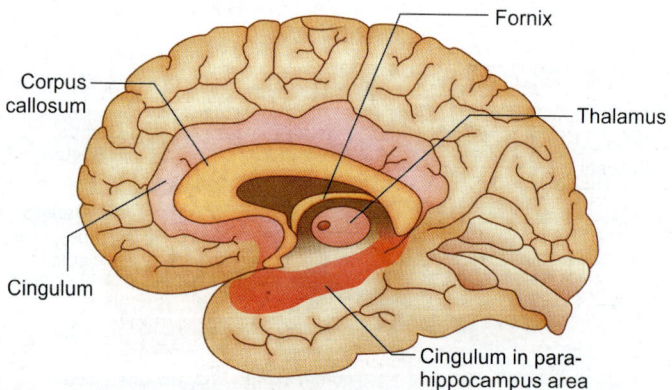

Medial aspect of cerebral hemisphere

## MEDIAN SECTION THROUGH THIRD AND FOURTH VENTRICLE

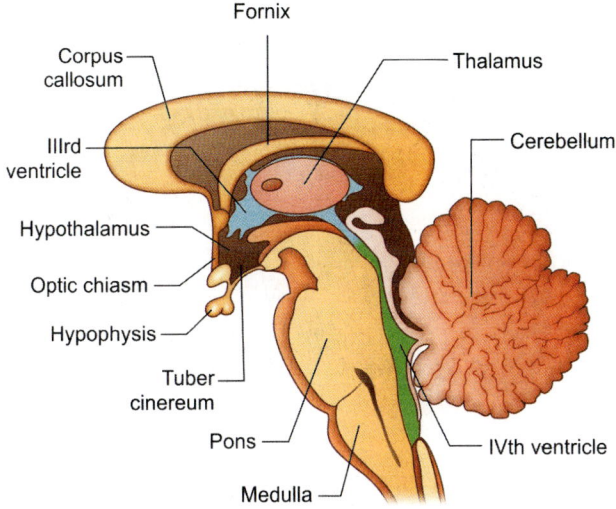

Median section through III and IV ventricle

### Viva Questions

Study the specimen carefully, student should be able to identify and name the structures as shown in the above figure.

## HORIZONTAL SECTION AT THE LEVEL OF INTERVENTRICULAR FORAMEN

### Viva Questions

- Internal capsule lies between the putamen globus pallidus, and caudate nucleus
- Claustrum is a thin layer of gray matter lying outside the external capsule and the insula
- Student should be able to identify external capsule and optic radiation
- Corpus striatum consists of caudate nucleus and lentiform nucleus

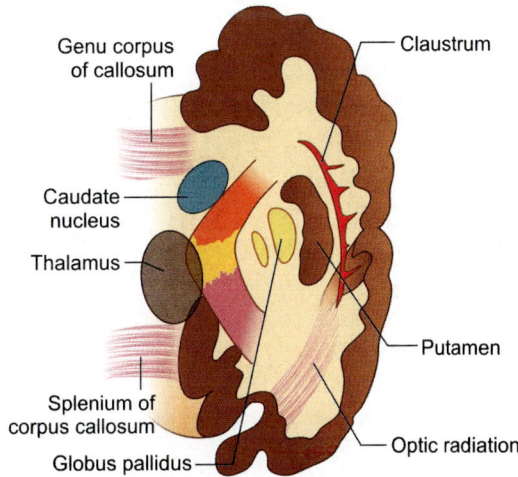

Horizontal section of cerebrum at the level of interventricular foramen

## CORONAL SECTION OF BRAIN

Study the specimen carefully

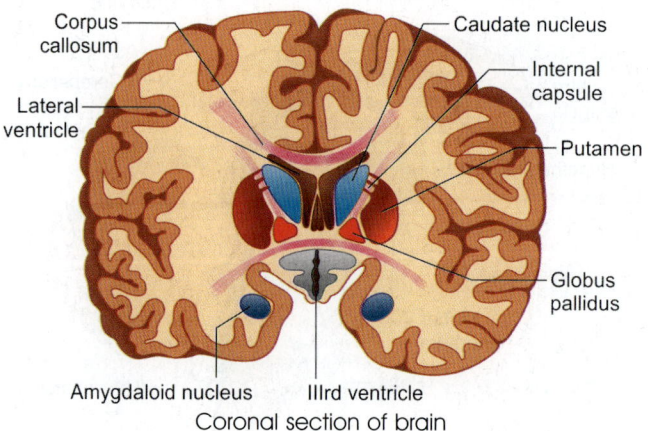

Coronal section of brain

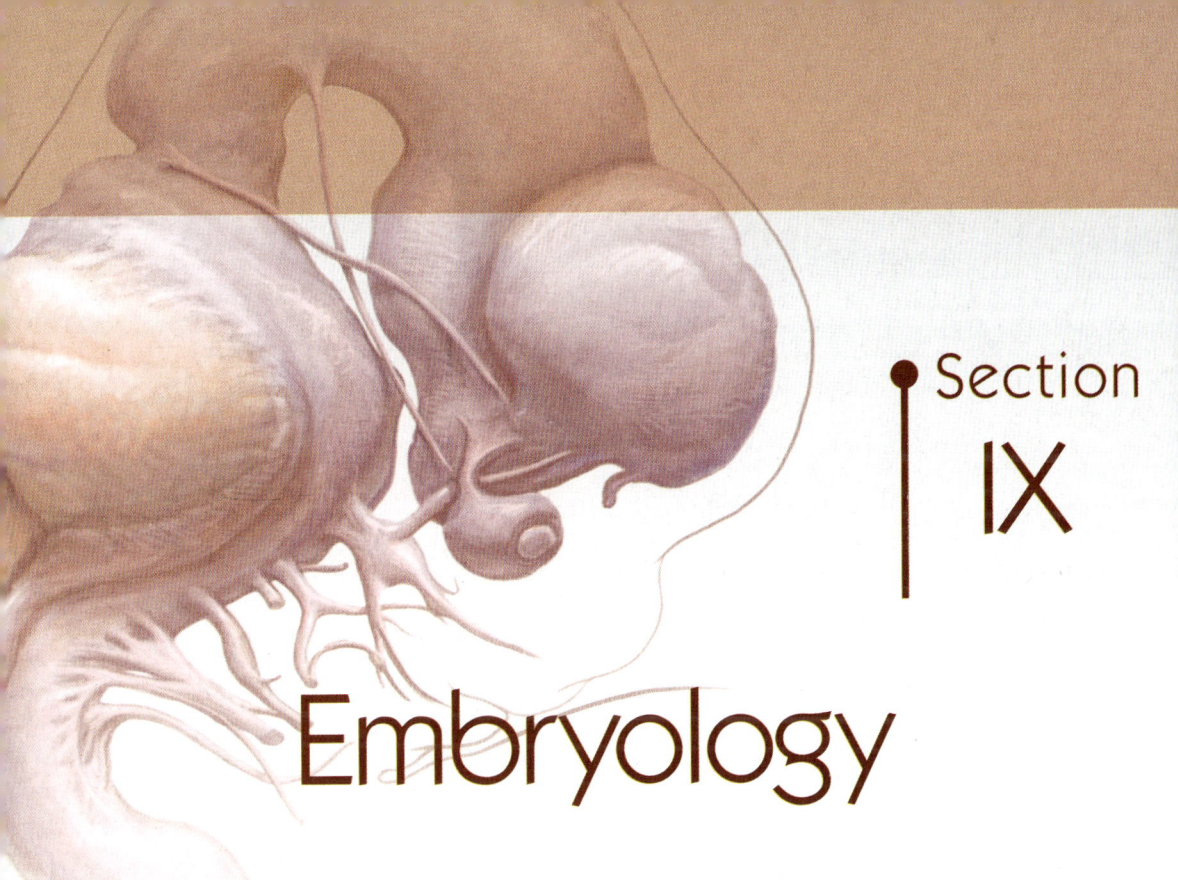

Section

IX

Embryology

# General Embryology Key Questions

### Chapter 47

### Q. What do you understand by embryology?

**Ans.** Embryology can also be described as developmental anatomy. Embryology is the study of the formation and development of the embryo from the time of its inception till birth.

### Q. What is an embryo?

**Ans.** From the time of inception to first 2 months (8 weeks) is known as an embryo.

### Q. What is a fetus?

**Ans.** From 3rd month onwards till birth is known as fetus.

### Q. What are gametes?

**Ans.** The sex organs, i.e. testes and ovaries produce highly specialized cells known as gametes. Male gamete is spermatozoa and female gamete is ova.

### Q. What is fertilization?

**Ans.** Fusion of male and female gamete is known as fertilization.

### Q. Where does fertilization take place?

**Ans.** Fertilization occurs in the ampulla of uterine tube.

### Q. Why does fertilization take place in ampulla?

**Ans.** Fertilization takes place in ampulla for following reasons:
- Ampulla is the widest portion of uterine tube
- Close to ovary and is easy to pick up ova.

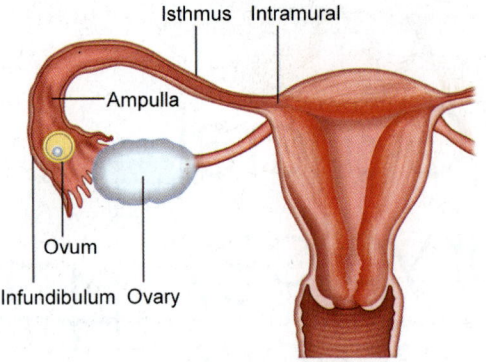

Parts of fallopian tube

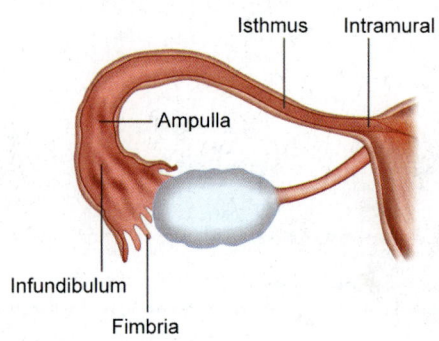

Fallopian tube showing ampulla

## Q. Draw a neat labeled diagram of DNA.

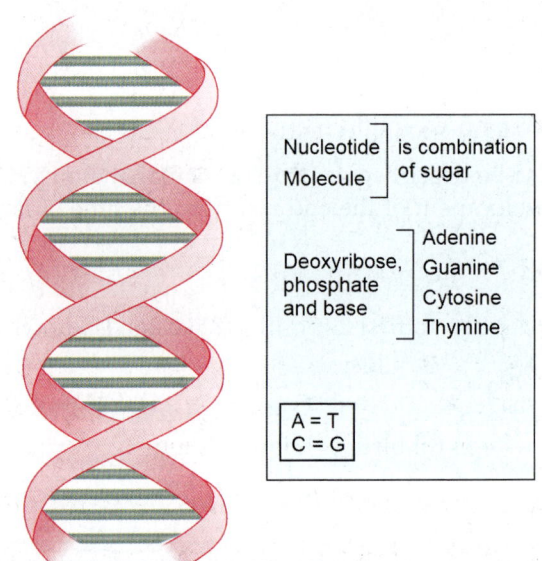

Double helical structure. Diagram of DNA

## Q. What is a chromosome?

**Ans.** In the nucleus of the cell, DNA molecule is packed in a thread like structure called chromosome. Each chromosome has DNA and supporting molecules histones.

## Q. How many chromosomes are therein each human cell?

**Ans.** The number of chromosomes in each human cell is 46. This is a diploid number.

## Q. How many chromosomes are therein the gametes?

**Ans.** The gametes, i.e. spermatozoa and ova have 23 number of chromosomes. It is a haploid number.

**Q. How are the chromosomes classified in each cell?**

**Ans.** The 46 chromosomes in each cell can be divided into 44 autosomes and two sex chromosomes.

**Q. Draw a neat labeled diagram of typical chromosome.**

**Ans.**

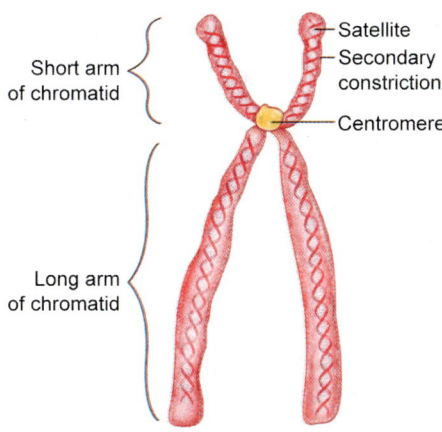

**Q. What are sex chromosomes?**

**Ans.** Sex chromosomes are of two types: X and Y.

**Q. How are the chromosomes classified in man and woman?**

**Ans.** In man, there are 44 autosomes and one X and one Y chromosome. In woman, there are 44 autosomes and two X chromosomes.

**Q. How are the chromosomes classified?**

**Ans.** Chromosomes are classified depending upon their length, position of centromere and presence of satellite bodies, i.e. depending upon the morphology.

**Q. What is Denver classification?**

**Ans.** In this system of classification, all the chromosomes are assigned groups from A to G, in order of decreasing length, i.e. depending on size of chromosome:

Group A—1, 2, 3 chromosomes.
Group B—4, 6 chromosomes.
Group C—6, 7, 8, 9, 10, 11, 12, X chromosomes.
Group D—13, 14, 15 chromosomes.
Group E—16, 17, 18 chromosomes.
Group F—19, 20 chromosomes.
Group G—1, 22, Y chromosomes.

**Q. Classify X chromosome.**

**Ans.** X chromosome is a member of group C, it is a submetacentric chromosome.

**Q. Classify Y chromosome.**

**Ans.** Y chromosome is a member of group G and is an acrocentric chromosome.

**Q.  How do you classify chromosomes depending upon the position of centromere?**

**Ans.** 1. Telocentric—centromere is at one end.

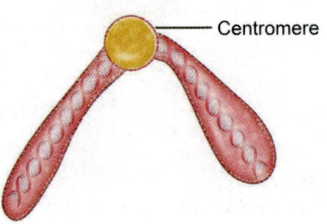

2. Acrocentric—centromere is near one end.

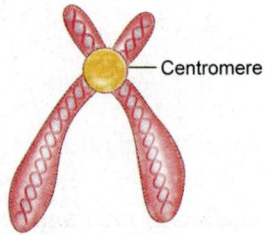

3. Submetacentric—centromere is submedian.

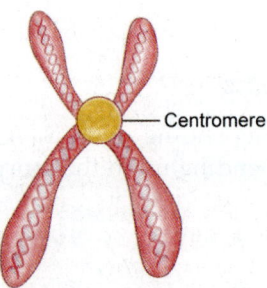

4. Metacentric—centromere is in the center.

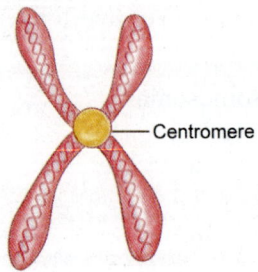

## Q. What is a barr body?

**Ans.** It is an inactive chromosome in female somatic cell. This is rendered inactive by a process called Lyonisation.

## Q. What is Lyon hypothesis?

**Ans.** Lyon hypothesis states, in cells with multiple X chromosomes, all but one is inactivated during development.

## Q. What are mendelian disorders?

**Ans.** Single gene disorders are mendelian disorders. They can be depicted in chart form known as Pedigree chart.

## Q. What are the different inheritance patterns?

**Ans.** Autosomal dominant, autosomal recessive, X-linked recessive and X-linked dominant.

## Q. How are genetic diseases classified?

**Ans.** Chromosomal abnormalities, mendelian disorders and complex diseases.

## Q. Describe in few characteristics of autosomal dominant trait.

**Ans.**
- Dominant mutation manifests even in heterozygous trait
- Male and female offsprings equally affected, 50% chance of transmission, delayed age of onset
- Vertical transmission

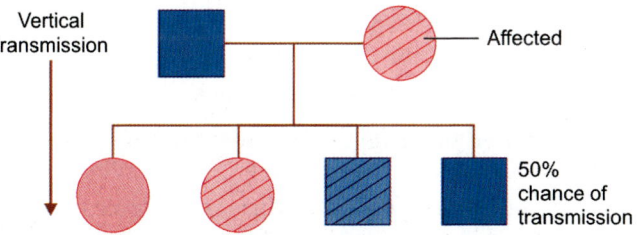

Autosomal dominant trait-pedigree chart

- For example, neurofibromatosis, tuberous sclerosis, achondroplasia.

## Q. Describe few features of autosomal recessive state.

**Ans.**
- These are clinically apparent only in homozygous state
- Parents are normal, siblings are affected
- Consanguinity contributory for this type of inheritance
- Horizontal transmission

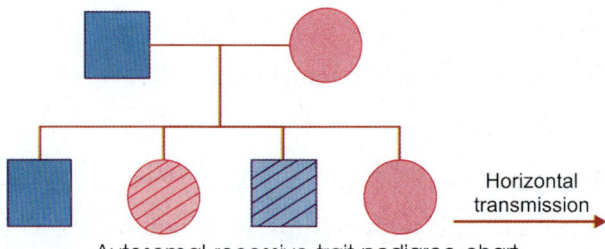

Autosomal recessive trait-pedigree chart

- For example, deafness, Wilson's disease.

### Q. Define peculiarities of X dominant mutant gene.

**Ans.** Either 46XY or 46XX, affected male will transmit the trait to all daughters.

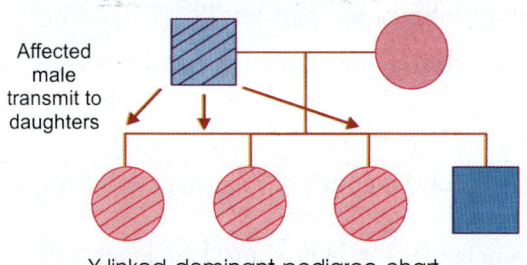

Affected male transmit to daughters

X-linked dominant pedigree chart

### Q. Describe features of X-linked recessive trait.

**Ans.**
- Males are affected
- Transmits abnormal gene only to daughters.

### Q. What do you understand by mosaic, chimera?

**Ans.**
- Presence of two different genotypes in an individual which developed from a single fertilized egg—Mosaic pattern.
- Two different cell types developed from two different zygotes is known as chimera (two different phenotypes) (genotype is genetic make-up; phenotype pertains to the external features of the individual).

### Q. What is phylogeny, ontogeny?

**Ans.** Phylogeny refers to evolutionary history of species; while ontogeny is development of organism from egg stage to mature form.

### Q. What is the significance of chromosomes?

**Ans.** Chromosomes are made up of predominantly nucleic acid called deoxyribonucleic acid (DNA). It carries the information necessary for the formation of numerous tissues and organs of the body, and for their orderly assembly and function. This information is imprinted on genes, i.e. structural units of chromosomes.

### Q. In what ways the cells divide?

**Ans.** There are two types of cell divisions:
1. Mitosis
2. Meiosis.

### Q. What is the main difference between mitosis and meiosis?

**Ans.** In mitosis, daughter cells have identical number of chromosomes and genetic information as that of the mother. In meiosis, the number of chromosomes in daughter cells is reduced to half that of mother cell and genetic information is not identical.

### Q. What is interphase?

**Ans.** The period between the two successive divisions is interphase.

### Q. What are the stages of mitosis?

**Ans.** Following are the stages of mitosis:
1. Prophase
2. Metaphase
3. Anaphase
4. Telophase.

### Q. What happens in interphase?

**Ans.** During specific period of interphase, the DNA content of chromosome is duplicated.

### Q. What important events occur during prophase?

**Ans.** Chromosomes become more prominent and the two centrioles move to opposite poles in early prophase. In late prophase, a significant number of microtubules develop giving rise to spindle formation.

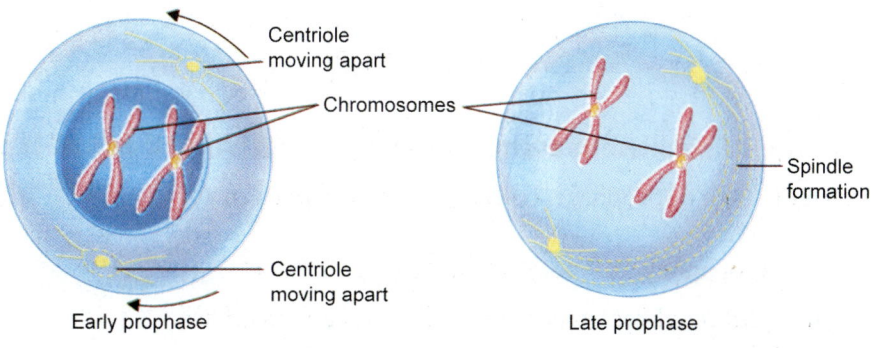

**Q. What happens in metaphase?**

**Ans.** Chromosomes occupy a central position in between the centrioles and get attached to the microtubule of the spindle.

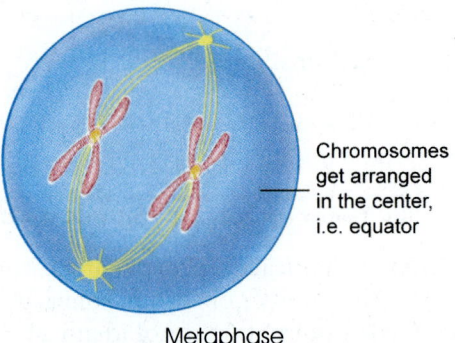

Chromosomes get arranged in the center, i.e. equator

Metaphase

**Q. What events occur in anaphase?**

**Ans.** The centromere of each chromosome splits longitudinally to give rise to independent chromosomes.

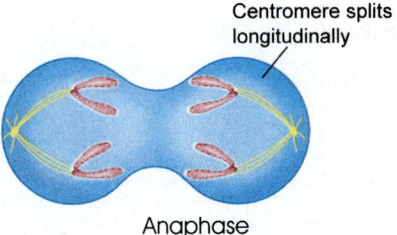

Centromere splits longitudinally

Anaphase

**Q. How is the telophase marked by?**

**Ans.** During telophase, nuclear membrane appears and two daughter cells are formed, cytoplasm also divides.

**Q. What are the stages of prophase in first meiotic division?**

**Ans.** Following are the stages of prophase in first meiotic division:
1. Leptotene
2. Zygotene
3. Pachytene
4. Diplotene.

**Q. In what stage of prophase 'crossing over' takes place?**

**Ans.** In pachytene stage of prophase, crossing overtakes place.

**Q. How does the anaphase of meiosis differ from mitosis?**

**Ans.** There is no splitting of centromere in meiosis during anaphase.

## Q. How does the interphase of meiosis differ from mitosis?

**Ans.** There is no duplication of DNA during the interphase of meiosis.

## Q. Differentiate meiosis from mitosis.

**Ans.**

| Stages | Mitosis | Meiosis |
|---|---|---|
| Interphase | Duplication of DNA | No duplication of DNA |
| Prophase | Single stage | Four stages |
| Prophase I | No crossing over | Crossing over takes place |
| Anaphase | Centrioles split | No splitting of centrioles |
| Metaphase | Spindle formation | No spindle formation |
| Anaphase | One chromosome moves to pole | One pair moves to pole |

## Q. To what does second meiotic division resemble?

**Ans.** Second meiotic division resembles mitosis.

## Q. Enumerate spermatogenesis.

**Ans.**

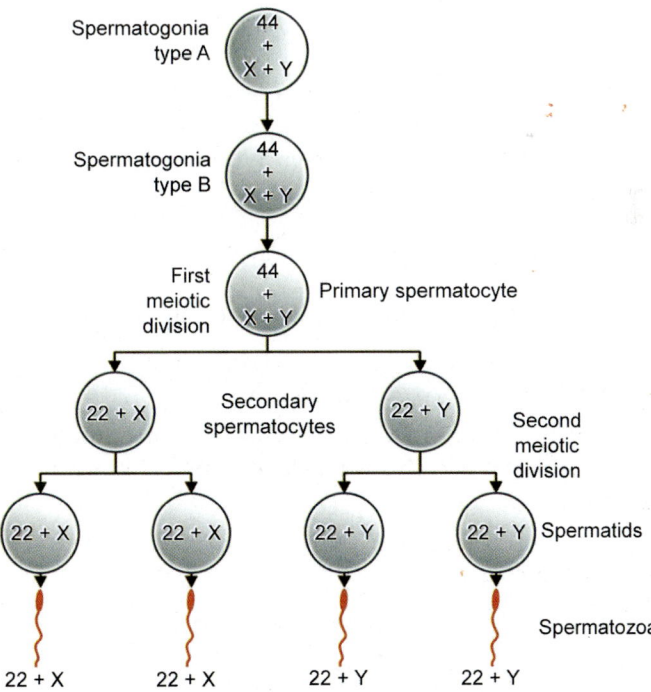

## Q. What is spermiogenesis?

**Ans.** The process of transformation of spermatid to spermatozoa is known as spermiogenesis.

# Q. Enumerate stages in oogenesis.

**Ans.**

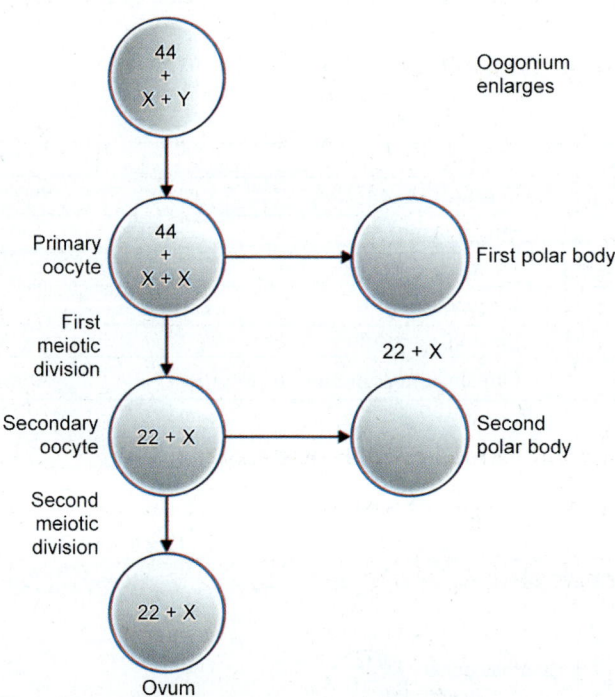

# Q. How is the sex of offspring decided?

**Ans.** Sex of the offspring is determined by which type of sperm unites with ovum. Sperm could be either 22X or 22Y, while ovum is only 22X.

# Q. What are the parts of spermatozoa?

**Ans.** A spermatozoa has a head, neck, middle piece and tail.

# Q. What is capacitation?

**Ans.** Spermatozoa acquire the ability to fertilize ovum only after they have been in the female genital tract. This final stage of maturation is called capacitation.

# Q. What is spermiogenesis?

**Ans.** The process by which a spermatid becomes spermatozoa is called spermiogenesis.

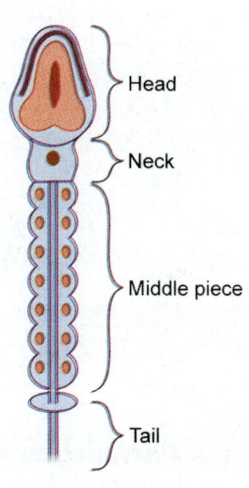

Spermatozoa pouts

## Q. How are the parts of spermatozoa derived?

**Ans.**

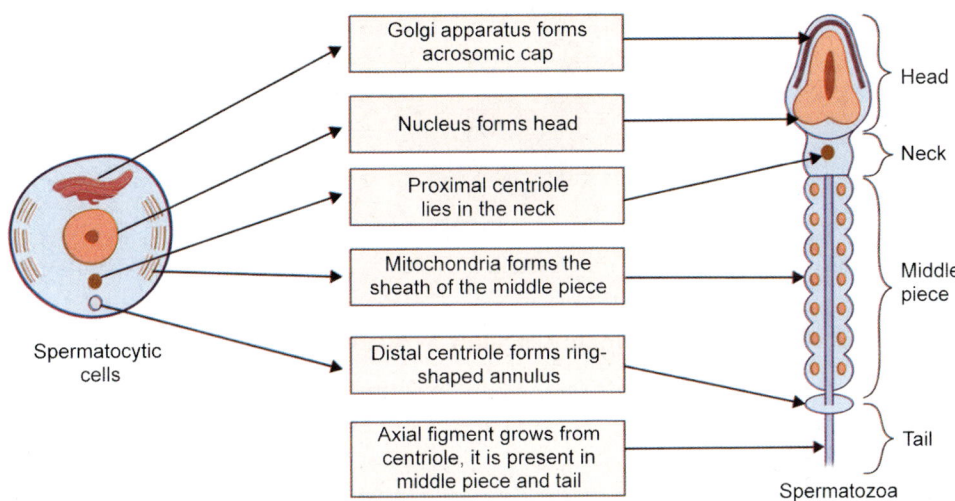

Spermatocytic cells

| Golgi apparatus forms acrosomic cap |
| Nucleus forms head |
| Proximal centriole lies in the neck |
| Mitochondria forms the sheath of the middle piece |
| Distal centriole forms ring-shaped annulus |
| Axial figment grows from centriole, it is present in middle piece and tail |

Head
Neck
Middle piece
Tail

Spermatozoa

## Q. How is the Graafian follicle formed?

**Ans.** Oogonia are surrounded by stromal cells, which form Graafian follicle. Following are the stages in the formation of graafian follicle:

1. Some stromal cells become flattened and surround an oocyte. These flattened cells ultimately form ovarian follicle and therefore called follicular cells.
2. Flat cells become columnar and a homogenous layer appears between oocyte and follicular cells. This is known as zona pellucida.
3. Follicular cells proliferate to form several layers, which constitute membrana granulosa.

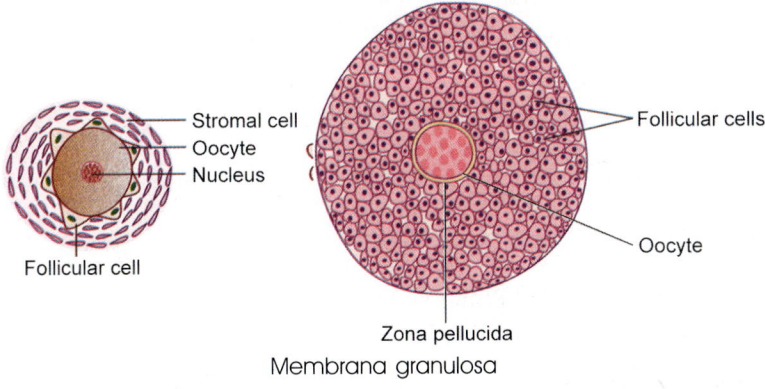

Stromal cell
Oocyte
Nucleus

Follicular cell

Follicular cells

Oocyte

Zona pellucida
Membrana granulosa

4. A cavity appears within membrana granulosa, which gradually increase in size. Oocyte lies eccentrically surrounded by granulosa cells, i.e. cumulus oophorus. The cells which attach it to the wall are discus proligerus.
5. Stromal cells surrounding the membrana granulosa become condensed to form theca interna, while the surrounding fibrous tissue forms theca externa.

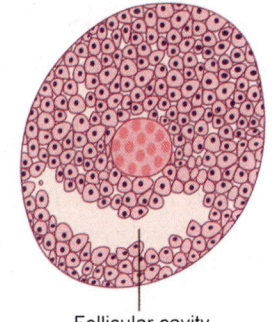

Follicular cavity

Formation of graafian follicle

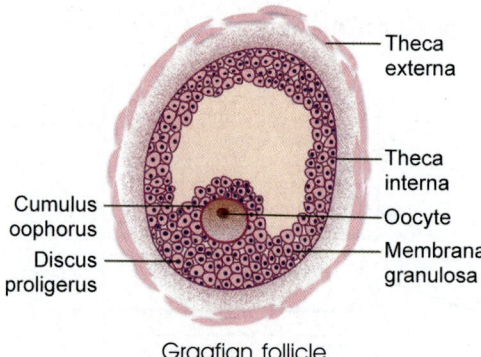

Graafian follicle

## Q. What is the stage of ovum, when it is shed from the ovary?

**Ans.** Ovum is in the secondary oocyte stage, which is undergoing division to shed off second polar body.

## Q. Depict the structure of ovum at the time of ovulation.

**Ans.**

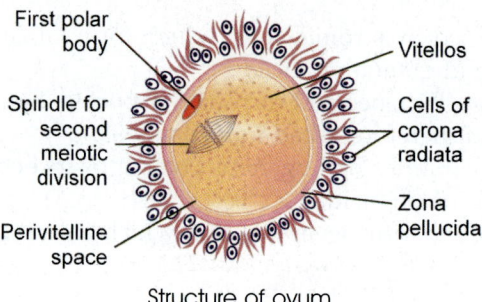

Structure of ovum

## Q. How long does the ovum take to reach the uterus?

**Ans.** Ovum takes 3–4 days to reach the uterus.

## Q. What is corpus luteum?

**Ans.** Ovarian follicle after ovulation is corpus luteum.

## Q. What is the fate of corpus luteum?

**Ans.** Fate of corpus luteum depends upon whether the ovum is fertilized or not. If the ovum is not fertilized, the corpus luteum persists for 14 days. It is known as corpus luteum of menstruation. At the end of 14 days it degenerates and forms a fibrous mass known as corpus albicans.

If ovum is fertilized and pregnancy results, corpus luteum persists for 3–4 months and is known as corpus luteum of pregnancy.

## Q. What is the importance of corpus luteum?

**Ans.** Corpus luteum secretes hormone progesterone, which maintains pregnancy.

## Q. What is non-disjunction?

**Ans.** During the first meiotic division, the two chromosomes of the pair instead of separating at anaphase may both go to the same pole. This is known as non-disjunction.

## Q. What is the chromosomal abnormality in Down syndrome?

**Ans.** Trisomy of chromosome 21 results in Down syndrome.

## Q. What are the features of Down syndrome?

**Ans.** Child has a broad face, obliquely placed palpebral fissures, epicanthus, furrowed lower lip and broad hands with single palmar crease. By and large are mentally retarded and have heart defects.

## Q. What are the features associated with extra X or Y chromosome?

**Ans.** The presence of extra X or Y chromosome can give rise to syndromes associated with abnormal genital development, mental retardation and abnormal growth.

## Q. Who are superfemales?

**Ans.** These are patients with XXX chromosomes.

## Q. What are the features of Turner syndrome?

**Ans.** When both chromosomes of a pair go to one gamete, the other gamete resulting from the division has only 22 chromosomes and at fertilization zygote has 45 chromosomes. This is monosomy. In this syndrome, the subject is always female. There is agenesis of ovary associated with mental retardation, skeletal abnormalities and webbed neck.

## Q. What are isochromosomes?

**Ans.** During cell division, centriole splits transversely to give rise to isochromosomes.

## Q. What are the phases of menstrual cycle?

**Ans.** Menstrual cycle is divided into following phases:

1. Postmenstrual
2. Proliferative
3. Secretory
4. Menstrual

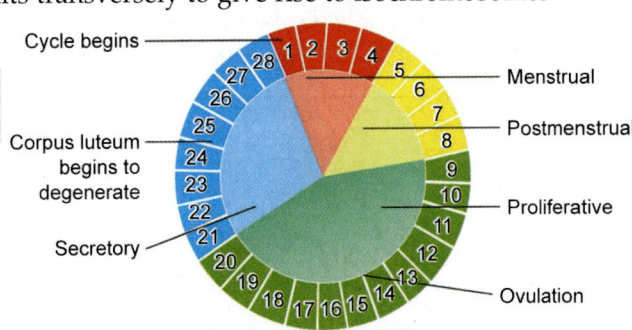

Phases of menstrual cycle

*It is also divided in other ways:*
1. Follicular phase.
2. Luteal phase.

**Q. Which hormone influences the luteal phase?**

**Ans.** Progesterone hormone influences the luteal phase.

**Q. Which hormone influences the follicular phase?**

**Ans.** Estrogen hormone influences the follicular phase.

**Q. Depict the changes in the epithelium of uterine glands during a menstrual cycle.**

**Ans.**

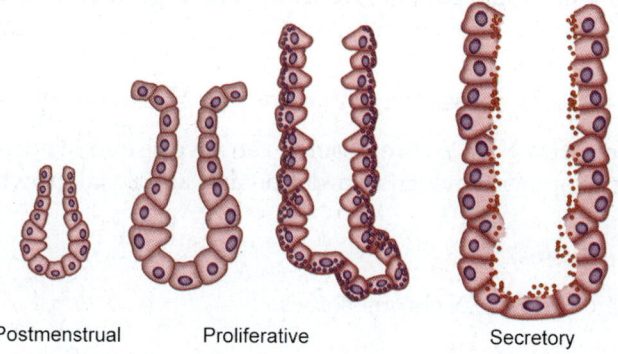

| Postmenstrual | Proliferative | Secretory |

**Q. What layers of endometrium are shed off during menstruation?**

**Ans.** Stratum compactum and stratum spongiosum are shed off during menstruation.

**Q. When does ovulation occur? How does one detect ovulation?**

**Ans.** In a 28 days cycle, ovulation takes place at about middle of the cycle. The period between ovulation and next menstrual cycle is fixed, i.e. 14 days.

At about middle of the cycle, there is a sudden fall in temperature followed by a rise in temperature. This rise in temperature is a crude indicator of ovulation.

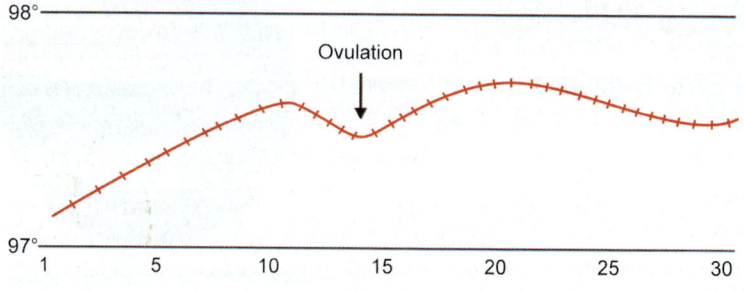

### Q. What is rhythm method of family planning?

**Ans.** After ovulation, ovum remains viable for maximum 2 days. Spermatozoa introduced into vagina die within 4 days. Therefore, fertilization occurs only if intercourse takes place during a period between 4 days before ovulation to 2 days after ovulation. The remaining days have been regarded as safe period. This forms the basis of rhythm method of family planning.

### Q. What hormones influence the ovulation and menstruation?

**Ans.** Follicular stimulating hormone (FSH)—stimulates formation of follicle. Luteinizing hormone (LH)—converts follicle into corpus luteum.

Secretions of both the above mentioned hormones are under the influence of gonadotropin-releasing hormone. Secretion of LH is also under the influence of estrogens.

### Q. What are oral contraceptive pills?

**Ans.** Oral contraceptive pills are hormonal pills, which contain progestin as nor-ethisterone acetate (1 µg) and estrogen as estradiol (50 µg).

### Q. Describe the formation of blastocyst.

**Ans.**

1. After fertilization, the two-cell stage undergoes further divisions to give rise to 16-cell stage known as morula.

2. A section of morula shows inner cell mass covered by outer layer of cells known as trophoblast.

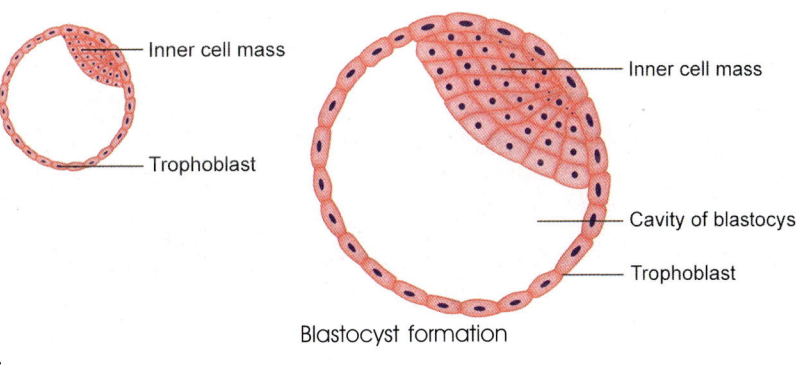

Blastocyst formation

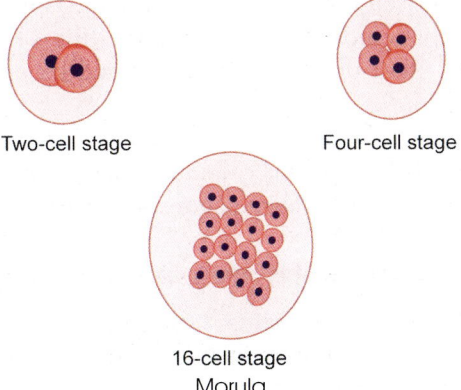

Two-cell stage

Four-cell stage

16-cell stage
Morula

3. Fluid appears between trophoblast and inner cell mass. As the fluid accumulates, the cells of the trophoblast become flattened.
4. The inner cell mass gets attached to the inner side of the trophoblast. This is known as the blastocyst.

### Q. What is the function of the zona pellucida?

Ans. Trophoblast has the property of being able to stick to uterine epithelium and eat up other cells. They can invade and burrow into tissues. Zona pellucida prevents abnormal implantation of blastocyst.

### Q. Discuss the formation of primary yolk sac.

**Ans.**
1. Few cells of the inner cell mass of blastocyst get converted into flattened cells that lie against the free surface. This forms the endoderm.

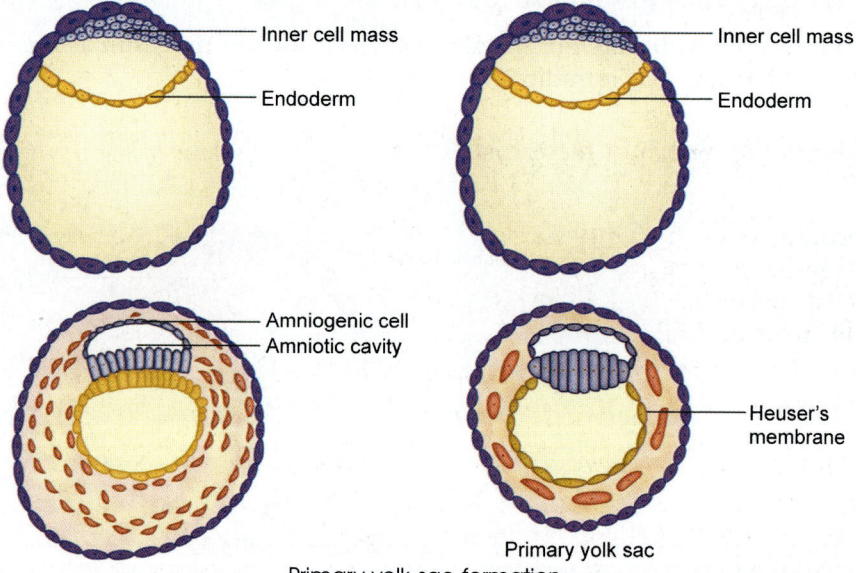

Primary yolk sac formation

2. Remaining cells of the inner cell mass become columnar. These form the ectoderm.
3. A space appears between the ectoderm and trophoblast this is known as the amniotic cavity, filled with amniotic fluid. Roof of this cavity is formed by amniogenic cells and floor is formed by ectoderm.
4. Flattened cells arising from the endoderm spread and line the inside of the blastocystic cavity. This lining of the flattened cells is called Heuser's membrane.
5. A cavity lined from all sides by endoderm is known as primary yolk sac.

### Q. Describe the formation of extraembryonic mesoderm and extraembryonic celom.

**Ans.** The trophoblastic cells lining the primary yolk sac gives rise to the extraembryonic mesoderm. These cells come to lie between the endoderm and trophoblast below, and amniogenic cells and trophoblast above.

Small cavities appear in the extraembryonic mesoderm, which coalesce to form a large cavity, i.e. extraembryonic celom.

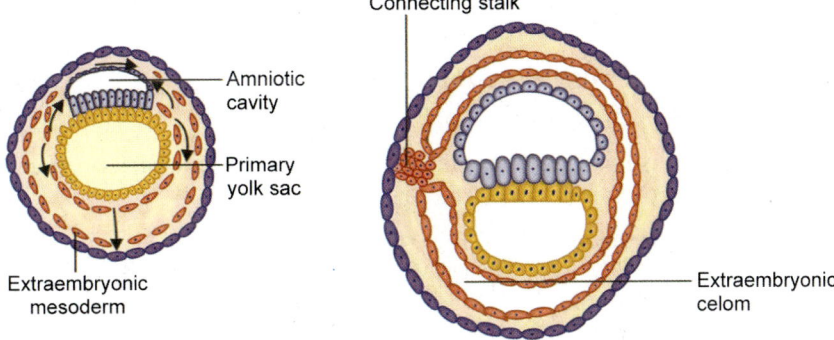

Secondary yolk sac formation

Because of the appearance of the celom, the extraembryonic mesoderm is split into two layers. The part lining the outside of the amniotic cavity is parietal extraembryonic mesoderm. The part lining the yolk sac is visceral extraembryonic mesoderm. The extraembryonic celom does not extend beyond the amniotic cavity and this region of unsplit extraembryonic mesoderm forms connecting stalk. The yolk sac becomes smaller and now known as secondary yolk sac.

## Q. How is the chorion formed?

Ans. The chorion is formed by the combination of parietal extraembryonic mesoderm and overlying trophoblast.

## Q. What is amnion?

Ans. The amnion is constituted by amniogenic cells forming the wall of amniotic cavity.

## Q. How does one decide about the head end or tail end of the embryo?

Ans. When the embryo is made of bilaminar disk, made up of ectoderm and endoderm one cannot make out, which is the head end or tail end.

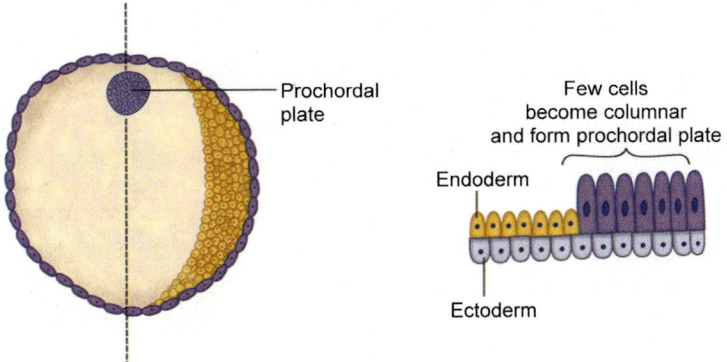

Axis of embryonic disk formation of prochordal plate

Soon a circular area develops near the margin of the embryonic disk, the cubical cells of endoderm become columnar. This area is known as prochordal plate. It determines the central axis of the embryo.

### Q. What is primitive streak? What is its importance?

**Ans.**

1. Some of the ectodermal cells toward the tail end of the embryonic disk proliferate (increase in number). This elevation is known as the primitive streak.

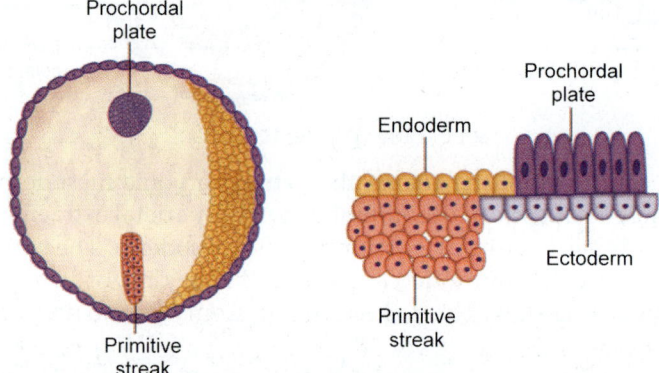

2. The cells of the primitive streak proliferate and grow in between the ectoderm and endoderm. These cells form the intraembryonic mesoderm.
3. With the formation of the primitive streak, the third germinal layer is formed. This marks the process of gastrulation.

### Q. What is gastrulation?

**Ans.** The process of formation of primitive streak and of intraembryonic mesoderm is referred to as gastrulation.

### Q. What is Sacrococcygeal teratoma?

**Ans.** Remnants of primitive streaks persist in sacrococcygeal region. These clusters of pleuri-potent cells proliferate and form sacrococcygeal teratoma.

### Q. In which two areas the intraembryonic mesoderm does not split?

**Ans.** The intraembryonic mesoderm does not spread in the region of prochordal plate, which forms the buccopharyngeal membrane.

It also does not spread in an area caudal to primitive streak. This region forms the cloacal membrane.

Here, arrows depict the spread of intraembryonic mesoderm.

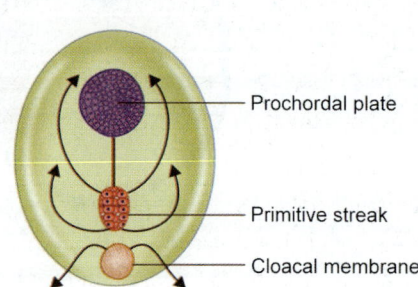

## Q. Which is the critical period of development?

**Ans.** Critical period of development is considered for 3–8 weeks since this period is characterized by organogenesis and any environmental insult in the form of drugs, radiation, infections, etc. can lead to development of congenital anomalies.

## Q. After how many days of fertilization morula is formed?

**Ans.** Embryo becomes morula 3 days after fertilization.

## Q. When does the blastocyst form?

**Ans.** On day 4, the blastocyst is formed.

## Q. When does intraembryonic mesoderm develops?

**Ans.** Intraembryonic mesoderm develops by day 16.

## Q. Describe the formation of notochord and its importance.

**Ans.** The cranial end of primitive streak becomes thickened. This thickened part is called primitive knot or Hensen's node. Cells in the primitive knot proliferate grow cranially in midline between ectoderm and endoderm reaching up to the caudal margin of prochordal plate. These cells form a solid rod called notochord.

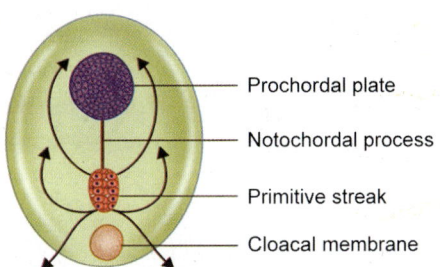

- Prochordal plate
- Notochordal process
- Primitive streak
- Cloacal membrane

Formation of notochord

Notochord remains in the center position later to be occupied by the vertebral column. Most of the notochord disappears, but parts of it remain in the region of each intervertebral disk as nucleus pulposus.

## Q. At which sites in an embryo the ectoderm and the endoderm are in close contact? Or at which sites the intraembryonic mesoderm does not reach?

**Ans.** The intraembryonic mesoderm does not develop in the following regions:
1. Prochordal plate.
2. Cloacal membrane.
3. In the midline caudal to prochordal plate.

**Q. How is the intraembryonic mesoderm divided?**

**Ans.** The intraembryonic is subdivided into:

1. Para-axial mesoderm.
2. Lateral plate mesoderm.
3. Intermediate mesoderm.

**Q. What is the fate of intraembryonic mesoderm?**

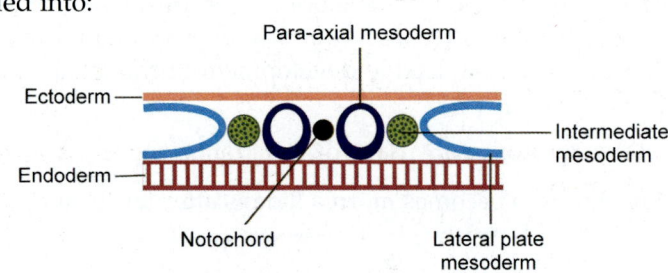

Intraembryonic mesoderm

**Ans.**

1. Para-axial mesoderm gives rise to somites.
2. Intermediate mesoderm gives rise to nephrogenic cord.
3. A cavity develops in the lateral plate mesoderm, which gives rise to pericardial, pleural and peritoneal cavities.

**Q. What is septum transversum?**

**Ans.** With the appearance of the cavity in lateral plate mesoderm it gets split into parietal intraembryonic mesoderm and visceral intraembryonic mesoderm.

However, it does not get split cranial to cardiogenic area. This unsplit area forms the septum transversum.

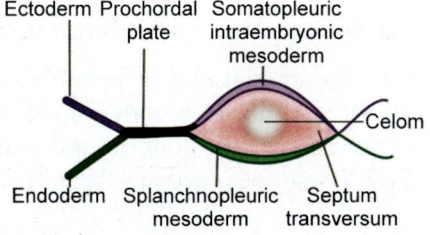

Septum transversum

**Q. Draw neat labeled diagrams to depict folds of embryonic disk and formation of primitive gut.**

**Ans.**

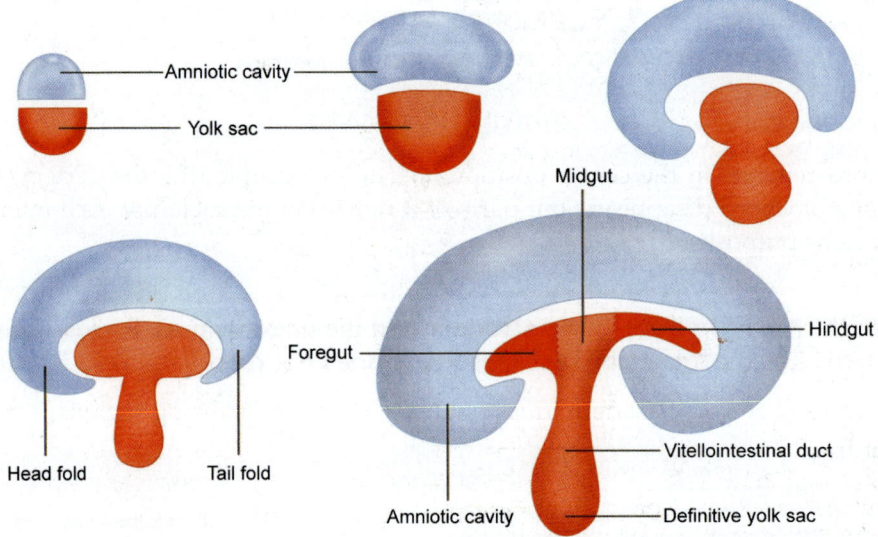

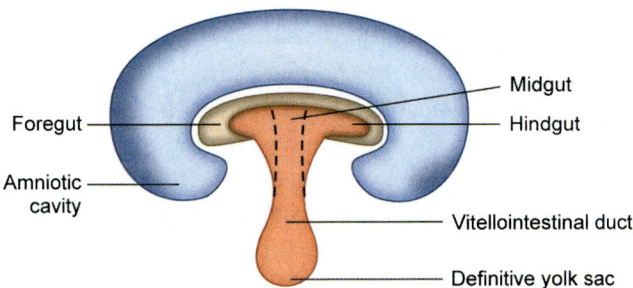

Q. Draw neat labeled diagrams to show embryonic disk before and after formation of head and tail end.

Ans.

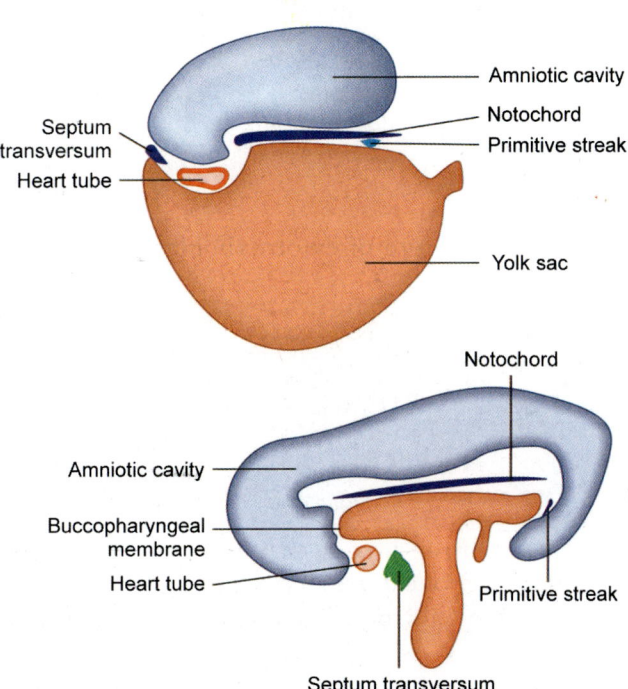

Q. When does the implantation of blastocyst occur?

**Ans.** Implantation begins after 6 days of fertilization. Blastocyst goes deeper and deeper into uterine mucosa till it lies within the thickness of the endometrium. This is called interstitial implantation.

Q. What is decidual reaction?

**Ans.** After implantation, the uterine endometrium is known as decidua. The stromal cells of the endometrium enlarge, become vacuolated, store glycogen and lipids. This change in stromal cells is called decidual reaction.

### Q. What are the parts of decidua?

**Ans.**
1. The portion of decidua, where placenta is to be formed is called decidua basalis.
2. The part of the decidua that separates the embryo from the uterine lumen is called decidua capsularis.
3. The part lining the rest of the uterine cavity is decidua parietalis.

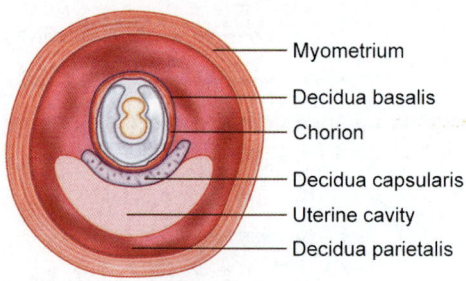

Myometrium

Decidua basalis

Chorion

Decidua capsularis

Uterine cavity

Decidua parietalis

Parts of decidua

### Q. What are the different types of villi?

**Ans.** *There are three types of villi:*
1. Primary villi consist of central core of cytotrophoblast covered by layer of syncytio-trophoblast.

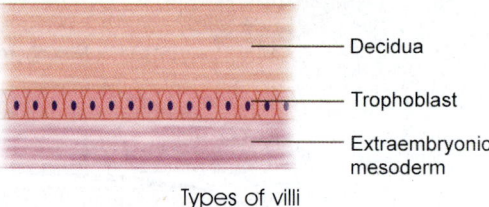

Decidua

Trophoblast

Extraembryonic
mesoderm

Types of villi

2. Secondary villi consist of three layers—outer syncytiotrophoblast, intermediate cytotrophoblast and inner layer of extraembryonic mesoderm.
3. Tertiary villi are like secondary villi, but also have blood capillaries in the mesoderm.

### Q. What is placental barrier?

**Ans.** *The structure, which constitutes placental barrier:*
1. Endothelium of fetal blood vessels and its basement membrane.
2. Surrounding mesoderm.
3. Cytotrophoblast and its basement membrane.
4. Syncytiotrophoblast.

### Q. What are the functions of placenta?

**Ans.**
1. Placenta helps in transport of oxygen, water, electrolytes and nutrition from maternal blood to fetal blood.

2. It provides excretion of carbon dioxide, urea and other waste products produced by fetus.
3. Maternal antibodies reach fetus through the blood and give immunity to fetus.
4. It prevents bacteria and other harmful substances reaching the fetus.
5. Progesterone secreted by the placenta is essential for the maintenance of pregnancy.
6. Estrogen produced by placenta reach maternal blood and promotes uterine growth and development of mammary gland.
7. Human chorionic gonadotropin and somatomammotropin are other hormones secreted by placenta.

### Q. What are upper and lower uterine segments?

**Ans.** Uterus can be divided into two parts. An upper part, consisting of the fundus and the greater part of the body.

The lower part of the body and cervix forms the lower uterine segment respectively.

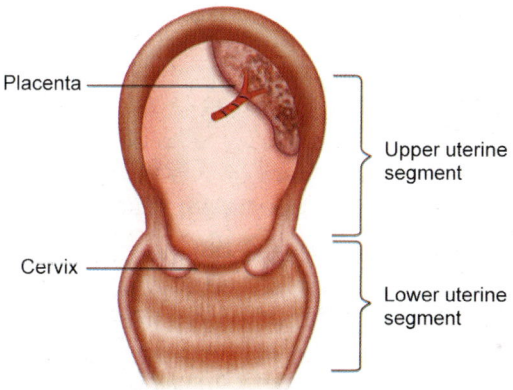

Upper and lower uterine segments

### Q. What is the normal site of implantation of placenta?

**Ans.** The placenta is normally attached to the upper uterine segment only.

### Q. What is placenta previa? What are its various degrees?

**Ans.** The attachment of placenta may partially or completely extend into lower uterine segment. This condition is known as placenta previa.

*Various degrees of placenta previa are as follows:*

*First degree:* The attachment of placenta extends into the lower uterine segment, but does not reach internal os.

*Second degree:* The margin of the placenta reaches the internal os, but does not cover it.

*Third degree:* The edge of the placenta covers the internal os, but when the os dilates during childbirth, the placenta no longer occludes it.

*Fourth degree:* The placenta completely covers the internal os even after it is dilated.

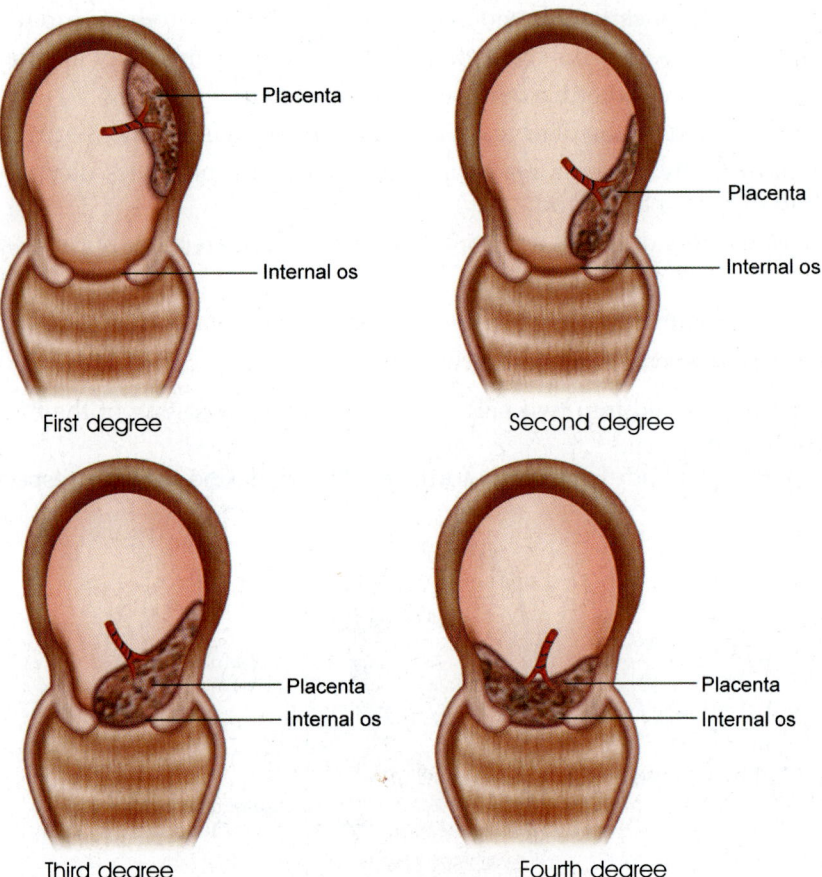

First degree           Second degree

Third degree           Fourth degree

Types of placenta previa

### Q. What are the sites of ectopic pregnancy?

**Ans.** When the fertilized ovum gets implanted at any site outside the uterus, is called ectopic pregnancy. Following are the sites of ectopic pregnancy:

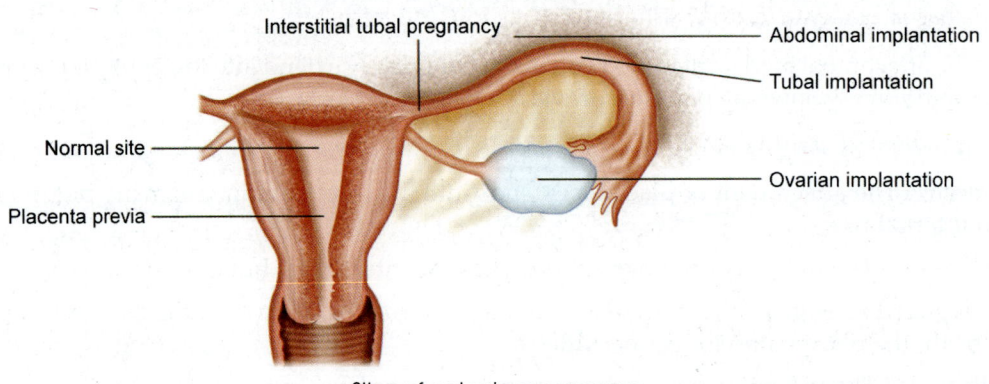

Sites of ectopic pregnancy

1. Tubal pregnancy—the blastocyst gets implanted in the uterine tube. Such a pregnancy cannot go onto full term, may result into rupture of the tube. After the rupture, the blastocyst may acquire a secondary implantation in the abdominal cavity giving rise to abdominal pregnancy.
2. Interstitial tubal implantation—the blastocyst gets implanted in the intramural part of the uterine tube.
3. Implantation in the ovary—fertilization and implantation may occur in the ovary.

### Q. What are the common tools of prenatal diagnosis?

**Ans.** Following are commonly used tools for prenatal diagnosis:
- **Amniocentesis** (aspirating amniotic fluid for analysis), alpha-feto protein level estimations, done in 16–19 weeks, helps in detection of neural tube defects, etc.
- Chorion villous biopsy (done early, 9 to 11 weeks, for chromosomal analysis, to detect defects like Down's syndrome, etc.).

### Q. What do you understand by trimester, viability?

**Ans.** A period of 3 months during pregnancy is called **trimester**. First 3 months is referred as first trimester, next 3 months as second trimester and last 3 months as third trimester
   **Viability** is the ability to continue to exist or develop into living being.

### Q. What is surrogacy?

**Ans.** A woman who bears child on behalf of other woman (her own fertilized egg) or even implanting in the uterus, fertilized egg of another woman is surrogacy.

### Q. Describe features of placenta.

**Ans.**
- The formation begins at the start of 4th week, i.e. end of 1st trimester
- 15–25 cm, in diameter, 3 cm thick, 500–600 gm
- Has 2 parts—fetal portion and maternal portion.

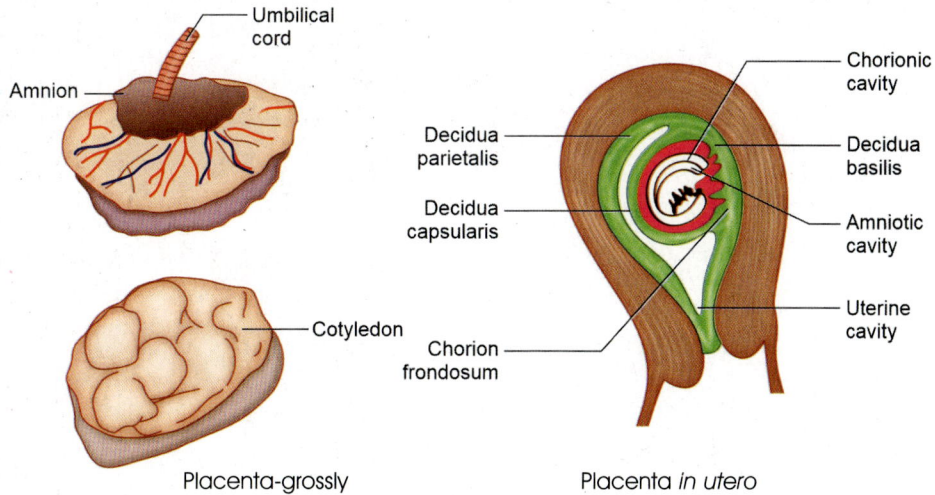

Placenta-grossly

Placenta *in utero*

## Q. How can one estimate fetal age?

**Ans.** Fetal age estimation is of medicolegal importance. Following ways will give an approximate estimate of fetal age:

- **Hess's rule**—formula states, square of number of months of gestation gives the length of fetus in centimeters up to 5th month, e.g. 2 months (4 cm); after 5 months the formula is number of months × 5 = length of fetus, e.g. 6 months fetus, 6 × 5 = 30 cm
- Biparietal diameter of skull, femur length, abdominal circumference are other parameters of fetal age estimation
- Ossification center appears just before birth in lower end of femur.

## Q. What does abortion mean?

**Ans.** Termination of pregnancy by surgical or medical methods, or spontaneous expulsion of products of conception anytime before 20 weeks of gestation is known as abortion.

## Q. Depict structure of umbilical cord.

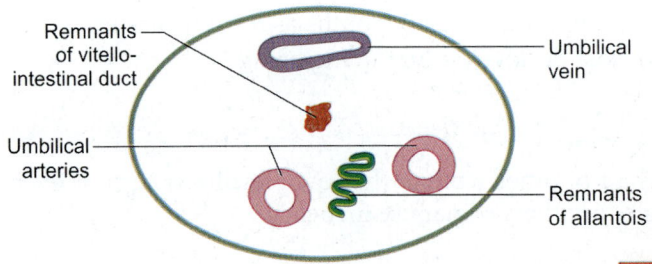

Umbilical cord section

## Q. Draw neat labeled diagrams of anomalies of placenta.

**Ans.** Variations in the attachment of umbilical cord to placenta are shown in figures below.

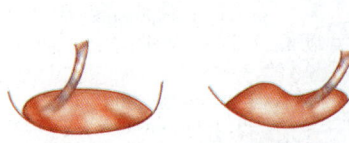

Placental anomalies

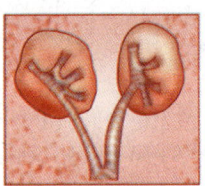

Bidiscoidal

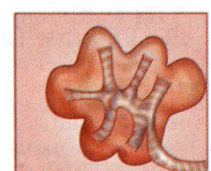

Multilobed

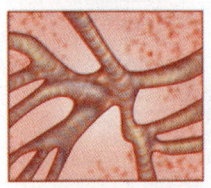

Diffuse

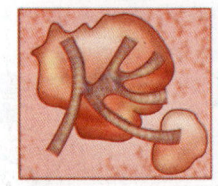

Placenta succenturiata

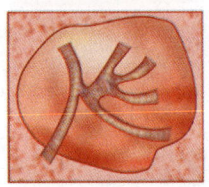

Fenestrated placenta

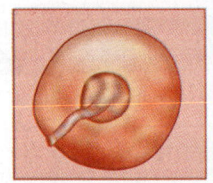

Circumvallate placenta

**Q. Depict a diagram showing normal disposition of embryo in uterine cavity.**

**Ans.**

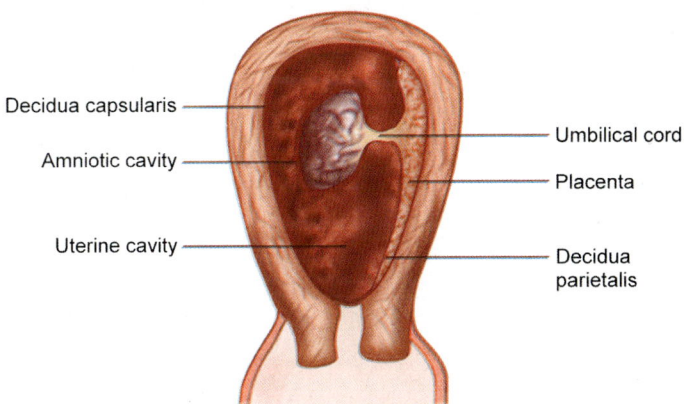

**Q. What do you understand by the term membranes?**

**Ans.** At the time of childbirth, the fused amnion and chorion along with the greatly thinned decidua capsularis constitutes membranes.

**Q. Discuss the fate of somites.**

**Ans.** Para-axial mesoderm becomes segmented to form a number of somites that lie on either side of developing neural tube. The somite is divisible into three parts namely:
- Dermatome
- Myotome
- Sclerotome.

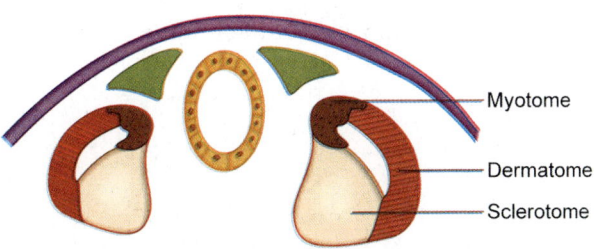

Fate of somites

1. *Fate of dermatome:* The cells of dermatome also migrate and come to lie beneath the ectoderm and give rise to dermis of skin and subcutaneous tissue.
2. *Fate of myotome:* It gives rise to striated muscle.
3. *Fate of sclerotome:* It gives rise to vertebral column and ribs.

**Q. What is mesenchyme? What are the derivatives of mesenchyme?**

**Ans.** Cells of mesoderm, which gives rise to loose connective tissue are known as mesenchymal cells. Following are the derivatives of mesenchyme (as shown in the figure).

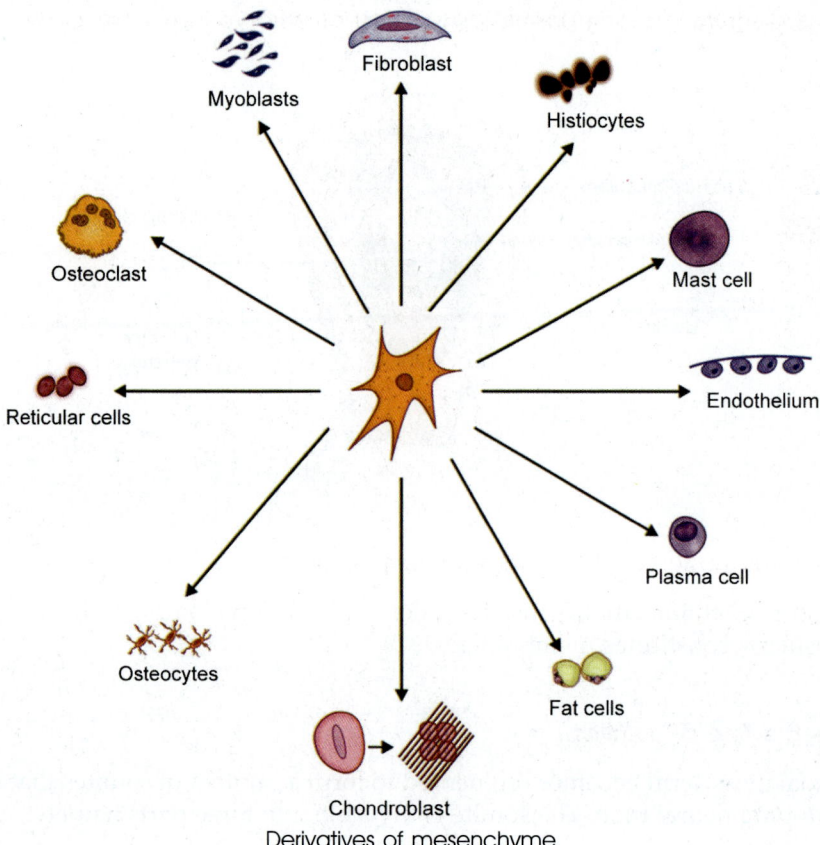

Derivatives of mesenchyme

## Q. What is the fate of occipital myotomes?

**Ans.** Occipital myotomes give rise to muscles of the tongue.

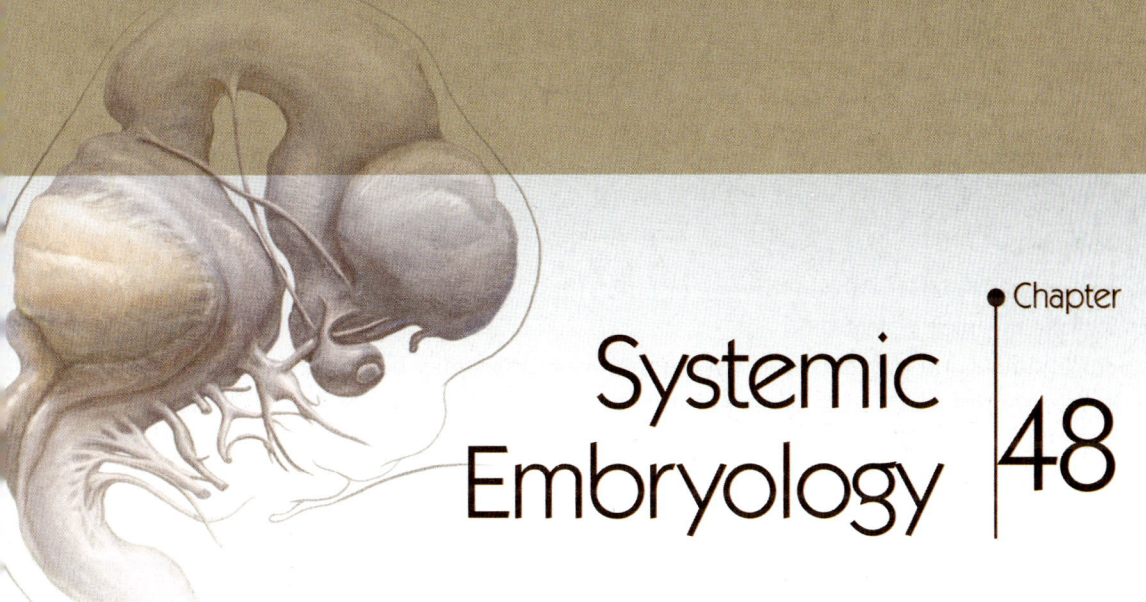

# Systemic Embryology

### Q. What components take part in the formation of skin?

**Ans.** Skin is derived from three diverse components:
1. Epidermis is derived from surface ectoderm.
2. Melanoblasts of the epidermis are derived from the neural crest.
3. Dermis is formed by condensation and differentiation of mesenchymc underlying the surface ectoderm. This mesenchyme is a derivative of dermatome of somites.

### Q. What are skin appendages? How do they develop?

**Ans.** Following are the skin appendages:
1. Nails.
2. Hair.
3. Sebaceous glands.
4. Sweat glands.
   All the above structures develop from the ectoderm.

### Q. Discuss the development of mammary gland. Add a note on its anomalies.

**Ans.** The ectoderm becomes thickened along a line from axilla to inguinal region. This is known as milk line or mammary ridge or line.

In the region, where the mammary gland is to form, a thickened mass of epidermal cells is seen projecting into the dermis. From this thickened mass, 16–20 solid outgrowths arise. Eventually these thickened outgrowths get canalized. The secretory elements are formed by the proliferation of the terminal parts of the outgrowths. The proximal part forms the lactiferous duct.

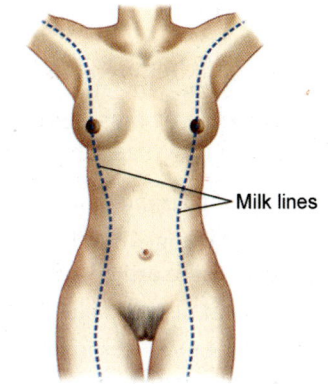

Milk lines

Development of mammary gland

The ducts open into a pit. However due to growth of underlying mesoderm, the pit is pushed outside and forms the nipple.

## Anomalies

1. Amastia—gland is absent on one or both sides.
2. Athelia—nipple is absent.
3. Polythelia and polymastia—supernumerary nipples may be present along the milk line.
4. Accessory breasts may be found outside the milk line, like in the neck, cheeks, femoral triangle and vulva.
5. Inverted/crater nipple—failure of development of nipple.
6. Gland may be abnormally small (micromastia) or abnormally large (macromastia).

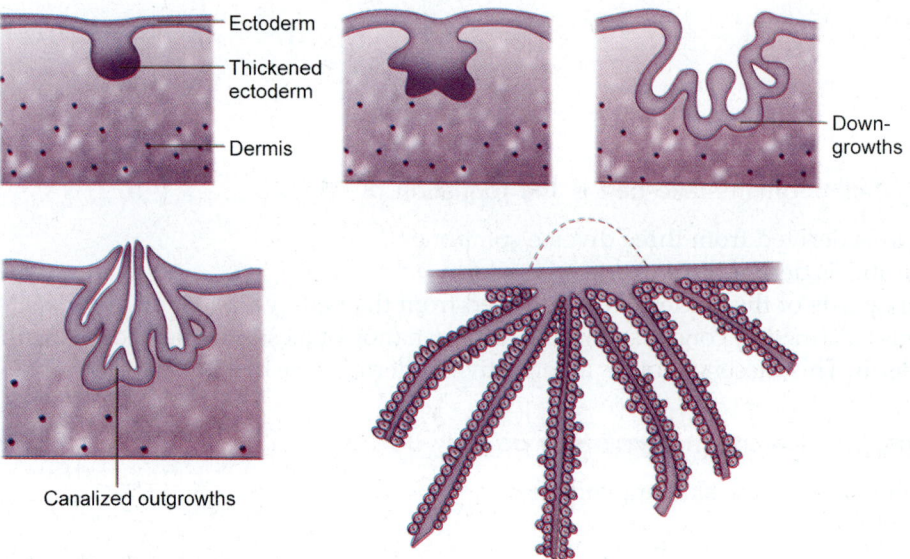

Canalized outgrowths

## Q. What are pharyngeal arches?

**Ans.** A series of mesodermal thickenings appear in the cranial most portion of the foregut. These are known as the pharyngeal arches or branchial arches.

*Structure of pharyngeal arch is as follows:*

1. Each pharyngeal arch has an endodermal lining, which dips outward to form endodermal pouch (there are six pharyngeal arches, arch five disappears).
2. Ectoderm also dips at the same place to form ectodermal cleft.
3. In between the ectoderm and endoderm is the mesoderm. The mesoderm gives rise to the following structures:
   a. Cartilage
   b. Nerve
   c. Striated muscle
   d. Arterial arch.

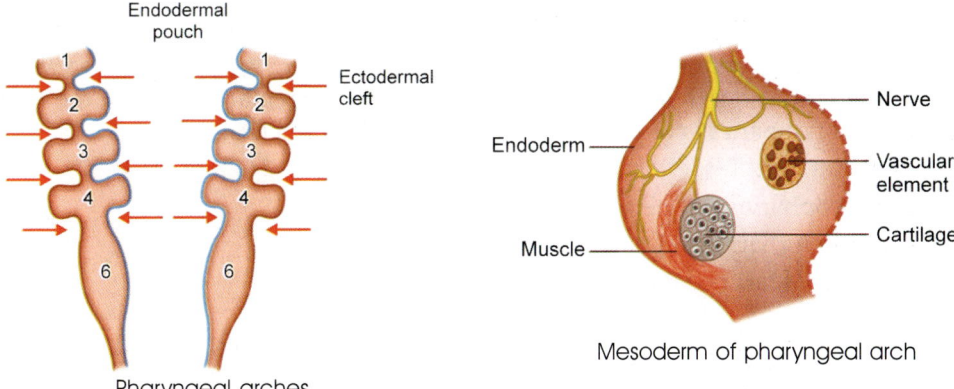

Pharyngeal arches

Mesoderm of pharyngeal arch

### Q. What do you understand by pre- and post-trematic nerve?

**Ans.** In some lower animals, each arch has two nerves. A nerve of the arch itself, which runs along the cranial side of the arch. This is the post-trematic nerve of the arch.

Each arch also receives a branch from the nerve of the succeeding arch. This runs along the caudal border of the arch. This is known as the pretrematic nerve of the arch.

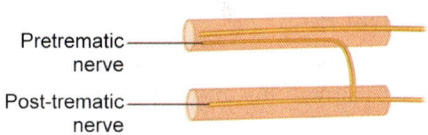

### Q. Discuss the derivatives of the skeletal elements of all pharyngeal arches.

**Ans.**

#### First Arch

1. Cartilage of first arch is known as Meckel's cartilage.
2. Incus and malleus are derived from its dorsal end.
3. Ventral part of the cartilage is surrounded by developing mandible and is absorbed.
4. The part of perichondrium from middle ear to mandible forms the anterior ligament of malleus and sphenomandibular ligament.

#### Second Arch

Cartilage of second arch gives rise to: (5S)
1. Stapes.
2. Styloid process.
3. Stylohyoid ligament.
4. Smaller cornu of hyoid bone.
5. Superior part of the body of hyoid bone.

#### Third Arch

Cartilage of third arch gives rise to:
1. Greater cornu of hyoid bone.
2. Lower part of the body of hyoid bone.

#### Fourth and Sixth Arches

Cartilages of larynx develop from these arches.

## Q. What are the nerves of each pharyngeal arch?

**Ans.**

*First arch*—mandibular nerve (mandibular nerve is the post-trematic nerve of the first arch, while the chorda tympani nerve is the pre-trematic nerve of the first arch).

*Second arch*—facial nerve.

*Third arch*—glossopharyngeal nerve.

*Fourth arch*—superior laryngeal nerve.

*Sixth arch*—recurrent laryngeal nerve.

## Q. What are the muscles developing from each arch?

**Ans.**

### First Arch

Tensor tympani, tensor palati, medial and lateral pterygoids, masseter, temporalis, mylohyoid and anterior belly of digastric.

### Second Arch

Stapedius, stylohyoid, posterior belly of digastric, muscles of the face, auricular muscles, occipitofrontalis and platysma.

### Third Arch

Stylopharyngeus.

### Fourth and Sixth Arches

Muscles of pharynx, soft palate and larynx.

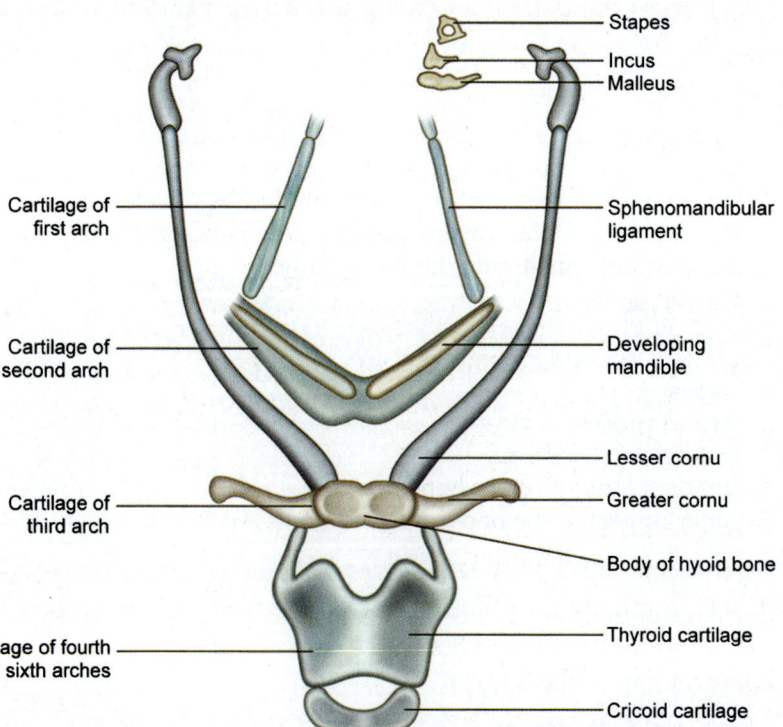

Derivatives of the skeletal elements of pharyngeal arches

**Q. How does the pinna and external auditory meatus develop?**

**Ans.**

1. The dorsal part of the first cleft develops into the epithelial lining of external auditory meatus.
2. The pinna is formed from the series of swellings that arise around the first and the second arch, where they adjoin the first cleft.
3. Swellings around the mandibular arch form the tragus, while rest of the auricle develops from the hyoid arch.

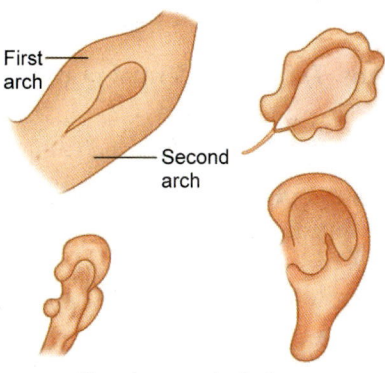

Development of pinna

**Q. What is cervical sinus?**

**Ans.** The second arch grows much faster than the succeeding arches and overhangs them. The space between the overhanging second arch and third, fourth and sixth arches is called the cervical sinus.

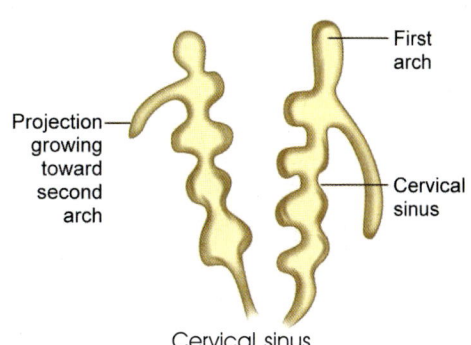

Cervical sinus

**Q. What is the embryological basis of branchial cyst and branchial sinus?**

**Ans.** Normally, the cavity of cervical sinus gets obliterated. Sometimes part of the cavity may persist and gives rise to swellings that lie in the neck along the anterior border of sterno- cleidomastoid, these are branchial cysts. If such a cyst opens on the surface, it becomes branchial sinus.

**Q. What is the fate of first pharyngeal pouch?**

**Ans.**

1. Ventral part of first pharyngeal pouch gets obliterated due to formation of tongue.
2. Dorsal part of first pouch and a part of second pouch form a diverticulum toward developing ear. This diverticulum is called tubotympanic recess.

**Q. What is the fate of the tubotympanic recess?**

**Ans.**

1. Proximal part of tubotympanic recess gives rise to auditory tube.
2. Distal part of tubotympanic recess gives rise to middle ear cavity.

**Q. Discuss the fate of second pharyngeal pouch.**

**Ans.**

1. Epithelium of the ventral part of this pouch contributes to the formation of tonsil.
2. Dorsal part takes part in the formation of the tubotympanic recess.

**Q. Third endodermal pouch gives rise to which structures?**

**Ans.** Third endodermal pouch gives rise to inferior parathyroid glands and thymus.

**Q. What is the fate of fourth endodermal pouch?**

**Ans.** Fourth endodermal pouch gives rise to superior parathyroid glands and may contribute to thyroid gland.

**Q. What is the fate of ultimobranchial body?**

**Ans.** Ultimobranchial body gives rise to para-follicular cells of thyroid gland.

**Q. Draw a diagram to show the fate of pharyngeal pouches.**

**Ans.**

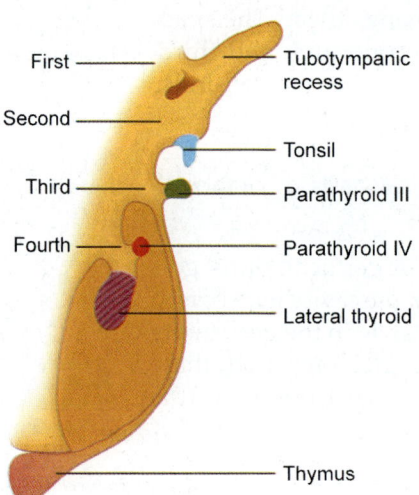

**Q. Discuss the development of parathyroid glands.**

**Ans.**

1. Endoderm of third pharyngeal pouch gives rise to inferior parathyroid gland (parathyroid IV).
2. Endoderm of fourth pharyngeal pouch gives rise to superior parathyroid gland (parathyroid III).

Third pouch also gives rise to thymus; this organ is closely related to parathyroid III. When the thymus descends towards the thorax parathyroid III is carried caudally along with it.

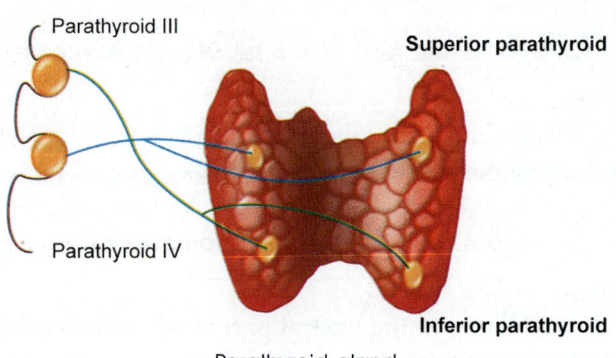

Parathyroid gland

## Q. Discuss the development of thyroid gland.

**Ans.** Thyroid gland development begins immediately behind tuberculum impar. The epithelium of the floor of the pharynx shows a thickening in the midline. This is the site of foramen cecum.

This region soon gets depressed to form a diverticulum called thyroglossal duct.

The diverticulum grows down in the midline into the neck. Its tip soon bifurcates. Proliferation of the cells of this bifid end gives rise to the two lobes of the thyroid gland.

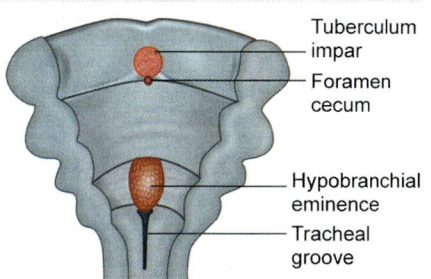

Thyroid gland

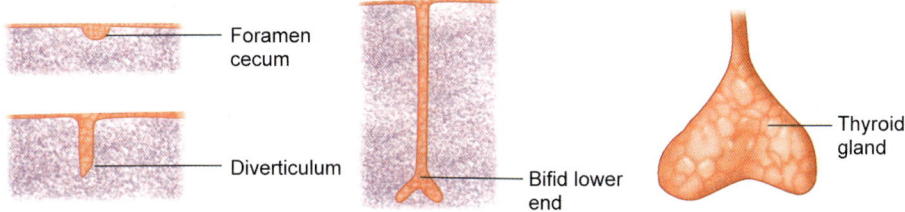

Development of thyroid gland

## Q. Discuss the anomalies of thyroid gland.

**Ans.** Anomalies of thyroid gland can be classified under following headings.

### Anomalies of the Shape

1. The pyramidal lobe may arise from isthmus or from one of the lobes.
2. The isthmus may be absent.
3. One of the lobes may be small.

### Anomalies of the Position

1. Lingual thyroid—the thyroid tissue may be under the mucosa of the tongue.
2. Suprahyoid thyroid—the gland may lie in the midline of the neck.
3. Infrahyoid thyroid.
4. Intrathoracic.

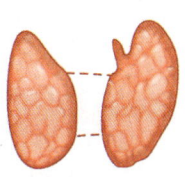

A. No isthmus

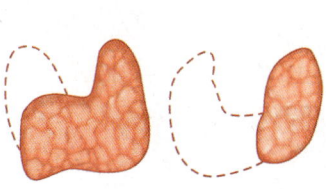

B. Partially developed lobes

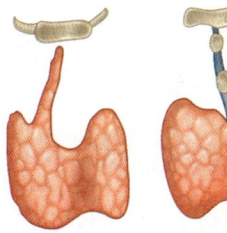

C. Anomalies of thyroid gland

*Ectopic Thyroid Tissue*

Small masses of thyroid tissue have been observed in the larynx, trachea, esophagus, pons, pleura, pericardium and ovaries.

Remnants of thyroglossal duct may be in the form of thyroglossal cysts or thyroglossal fistula.

**Q. Trace the path of thyroglossal duct (diagram only).**

**Ans.**

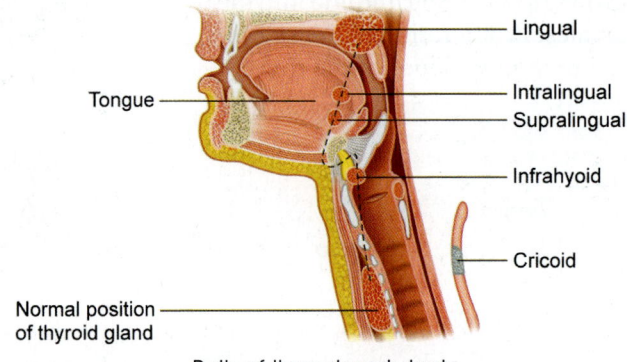

Path of thyroglossal duct

**Q. What embryological structures take part in the formation of face?**

**Ans.** The face is derived from following embryological structures:
1. Frontonasal process.
2. First pharyngeal or mandibular arch.

**Q. Development of limbs.**

**Ans.** Limb buds develop from the somatic layer of lateral plate mesoderm. Upper limb (UL) buds develop in mid of 4th week of fetal life, while lower limb (LL) bud develop 1 to 2 days later.

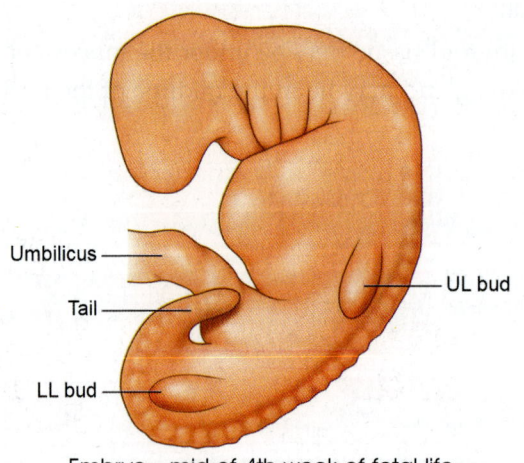

Embryo—mid of 4th week of fetal life

## Q. What is frontonasal process?

**Ans.** Mesoderm over the developing forebrain proliferates and forms a downward projection that overlaps the upper part of the stomodeum. This forms the frontonasal process.

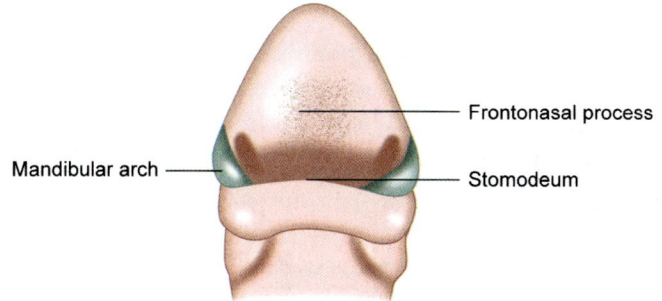

Development of face

## Q. What are nasal placodes?

**Ans.** The ectoderm over the frontonasal process shows bilateral localized thickenings. These are called nasal placodes. The nasal placodes soon sink to form nasal pits. The edges of nasal pits are raised above the surface, the medial raised edge is called medial nasal process and lateral edge is called lateral nasal process.

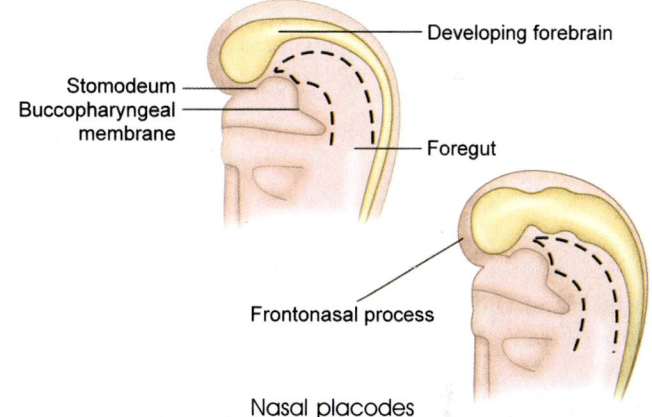

Nasal placodes

## Q. Describe the formation of lower lip.

**Ans.** Mandibular process of the two sides grows toward each other and fuses in the midline to form the lower lip. The mouth develops from the stomodeum.

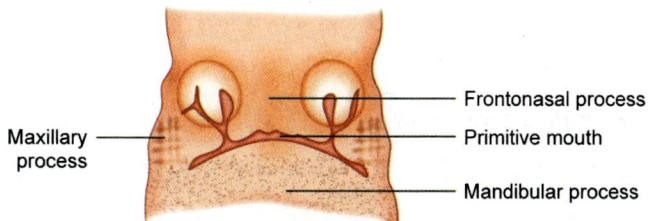

## Q. Discuss the formation of upper lip.

**Ans.** Each maxillary process grows medially and fuses with the lateral nasal process, and then the medial nasal process. The two nasal processes also fuse with each other. All the above mentioned structures contribute to the formation of upper lip.

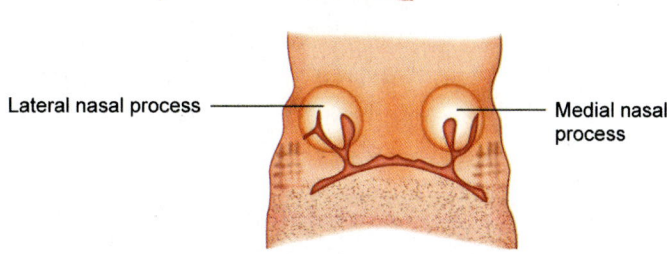

Formation of lower lip

**Q. What structures form the philtrum?**

**Ans.** Frontonasal process forms the philtrum.

**Q. What is the origin of the muscles of the face?**

**Ans.** Muscles of the face are derived from second branchial arch and are therefore supplied by the facial nerve.

**Q. Depict derivatives of the face in the form of a diagram.**

**Ans.**

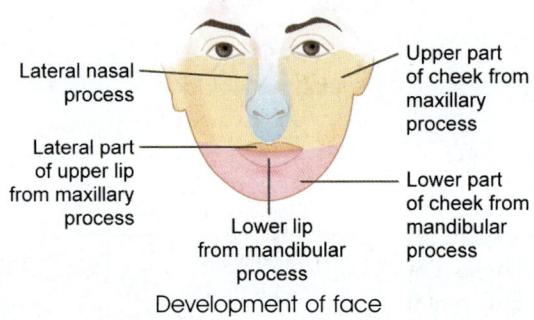

Development of face

**Q. Discuss the embryological basis of harelip, i.e. cleft lip.**

**Ans.** Non-fusion of the maxillary process with medial nasal process gives rise to the defects of upper lip.

**Q. What are the embryological basis of oblique facial cleft?**

**Ans.** Non-fusion of the maxillary process with lateral nasal process gives rise to oblique facial cleft.

**Q. Underdevelopment of first arch leads to which anomaly?**

**Ans.** Underdevelopment of first arch leads to mandibulofacial dysostosis.

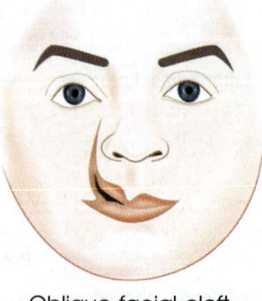

Oblique facial cleft

**Q. Discuss the development of nose, i.e. nares, nasal septum, lateral nasal wall.**

**Ans.**

1. Nasal cavities are formed as extension of nasal pits.

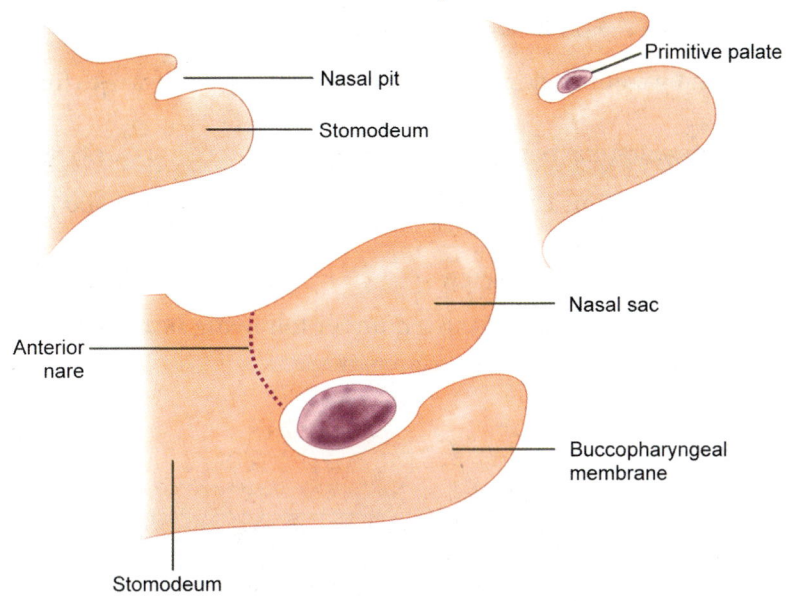

Development of nose

2. Nasal pits deepen to form nasal sac, which expands dorsally and caudally. Anterior opening of nasal sac forms the anterior nares, which opens on the face. Dorsal opening into the stomodeum forms the posterior nares.
3. The nasal sacs are separated from each other by frontonasal process. With the enlargement of nasal sacs the frontonasal process diminishes in size to form the nasal septum.
4. Lateral wall of the nose is derived from lateral nasal process.

**Q. How do the paranasal sinuses develop?**

**Ans.** The paranasal sinuses appear as a diverticuli from nasal cavities. The diverticuli grow within the facial bones after which they are named. Maxillary and sphenoidal sinuses begin to develop before birth and are rudimentary at birth. Frontal and ethmoidal sinuses begin to develop after birth (i.e. they are absent at birth).

**Q. Discuss the embryological basis of palatal development.**

**Ans.** Three components contribute to the development of palate:

1. Primitive palate, which develops from the frontonasal process.
2. Palatal process, which is an outgrowth of maxillary process.

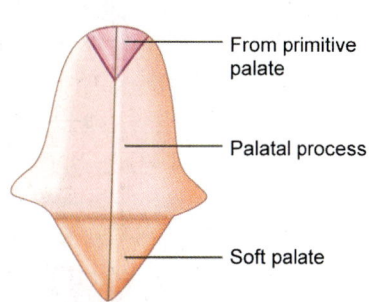

Development of palate

3. Medial edge of palatal process fuse with lower edge of nasal septum.

Mesoderm in the palate undergoes intramembranous ossification to form the hard palate. This ossification fails to extend backwards; this unossified part forms the soft palate.

**Q. Why are cleft palates associated with cleft lips?**

**Ans.** Both upper lip and palate develop from fusion of maxillary process with frontonasal process.

**Q. What is the embryological basis of cleft palate?**

**Ans.** Defective fusion of various components of palate, i.e. premaxilla and palatal process.

**Q. Discuss the development of tongue.**

**Ans.** Development of tongue can be discussed under following headings:

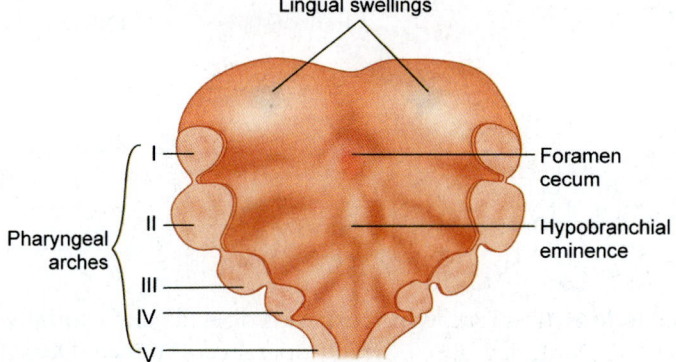

1. Development of anterior two-thirds of tongue develops from:
   a. Lingual swellings.
   b. Tuberculum impar.
   c. Cranial part of hypobranchial eminence.
2. Development of posterior one-third of tongue. The third pharyngeal arch grows over the second and thus contributes to the development of posterior one-third of tongue.

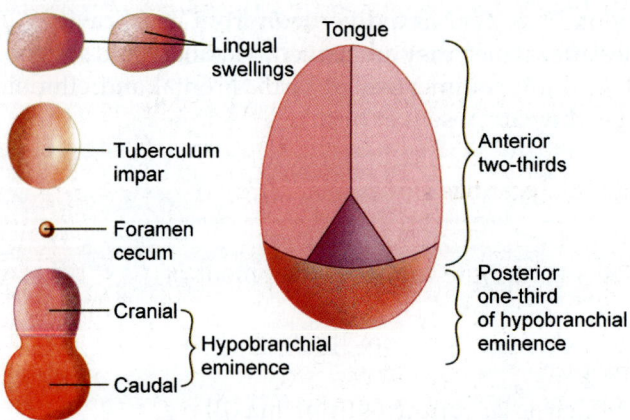

Embryological basis of tongue innervation

**Q. Discuss the embryological basis of tongue innervations.**

**Ans.**

1. Anterior two-thirds of tongue are supplied by lingual branch of mandibular nerve, which is the post-trematic nerve of first arch and by the chorda tympani, which is the pretrematic nerve of this arch.

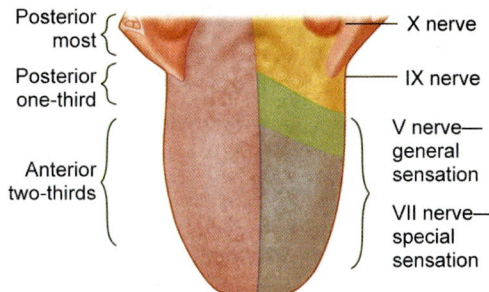

2. Posterior one-third of tongue is supplied by glossopharyngeal nerve, i.e. nerve of third arch.
3. Posterior most part is supplied by superior laryngeal nerve (branch of vagus), which is the nerve of fourth arch.

**Q. Discuss the origin of muscles of tongue.**

**Ans.** Musculature of tongue is derived from occipital myotomes. Occipital myotomes are supplied by hypoglossal nerve, thus the muscles of the tongue have the same innervation.

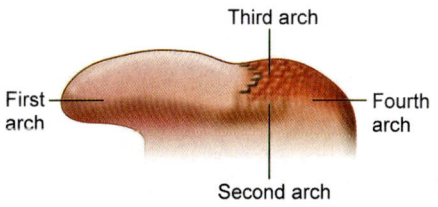

**Q. In relation to which pouch palatine tonsils develop?**

**Ans.** Palatine tonsils develop in relation to second pharyngeal pouch.

**Q. Draw a diagram showing parts of the primitive gut.**

**Ans.**

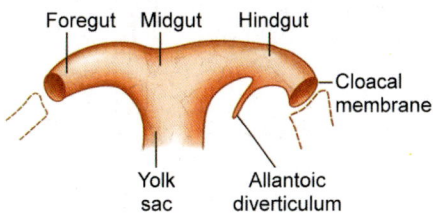

**Q. What are the arteries of primitive gut?**

**Ans.**

1. The artery of abdominal part of foregut is celiac artery.
2. The artery of midgut is superior mesenteric artery.
3. The artery of hindgut is inferior mesenteric artery.

## Q. Discuss rotation of midgut loop.

**Ans.** Rotation of midgut loop can be studied in three stages (refer page 828).

### Begins

1. Between 5th and 10th weeks within the umbilical cord.
2. Development of liver, forces the portion of midgut proximal to superior mesenteric artery, downwards and to the right.
3. Thus, the postarterial segment goes upwards and to the left.
4. Viewed from ventral side, the loop undergoes anticlockwise rotation by 90°, so that it lies in horizontal plane.
5. The prearterial segment now undergoes great increase in length to form coils of jejunum and herniate.

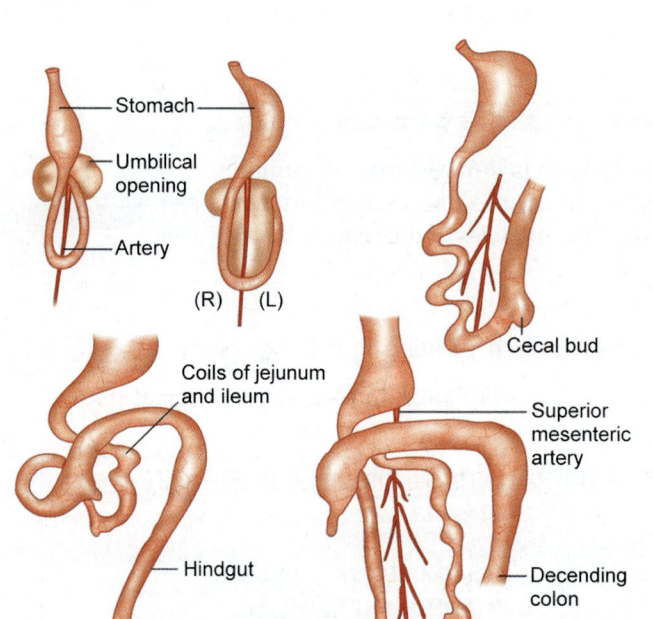

Rotation of midgut

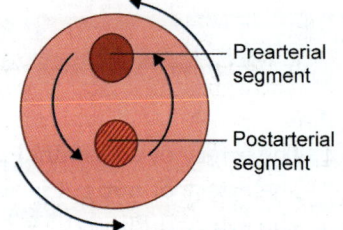

6. The coils of jejunum and ileum now return to abdominal cavity. As they do so the midgut loop undergoes a further anticlockwise rotation. As a result, the coils of jejunum and ileum pass behind the superior mesenteric artery (11th week).
7. Finally, the postarterial segment returns to the abdominal cavity. As it returns, it goes in anticlockwise direction (rotation of the gut takes place in anticlockwise direction).

## Q. What are the derivatives of foregut?

**Ans.** Following are the derivatives of foregut:
1. Part of the floor of mouth including the tongue.
2. Pharynx.
3. Various derivatives of the pharyngeal pouches and the thyroid.
4. Esophagus.
5. Stomach.
6. Duodenum.
7. Liver and extrahepatic biliary system.
8. Pancreas.
9. Respiratory system.

## Q. What are the subdivisions of cloaca?

**Ans.** With the formation of urorectal septum, cloaca divides into primitive urogenital sinus and rectum (dorsally).

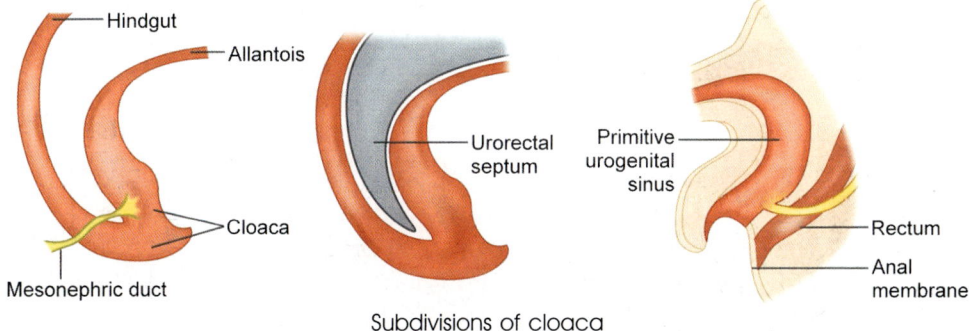

Subdivisions of cloaca

## Q. Draw a diagram showing derivatives of primitive gut.

**Ans.**
1. Duodenum below entry of bile duct, jejunum and most of ileum from prearterial segment of midgut.
2. Terminal ileum, cecum, ascending colon, right two-thirds of transverse colon from postarterial segment of midgut.

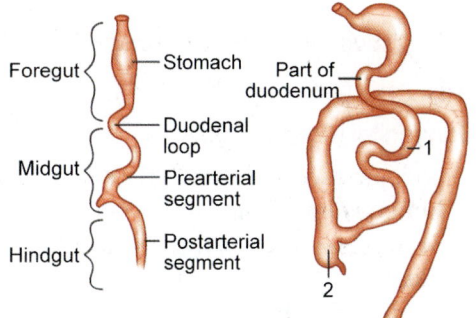

## Q. What are the derivatives of midgut?

**Ans.** Following are the derivatives of midgut:
1. Duodenum.
2. Jejunum.
3. Ileum.
4. Cecum and appendix.
5. Ascending colon.
6. Right two-thirds of transverse colon.

## Q. What are the derivatives of hindgut?

**Ans.** Following are the derivatives of hindgut:
1. Left one-third of transverse colon.
2. Descending and pelvic colon.
3. Rectum.
4. Upper part of anal canal.
5. Parts of the urogenital system are derived from primitive urogenital sinus.

## Q. Discuss the development of cecum (diagram only).

**Ans.** Cecal bud is a diverticulum that arises from the postarterial segment of midgut loop. The cecum and appendix are formed by enlargement of this bud.

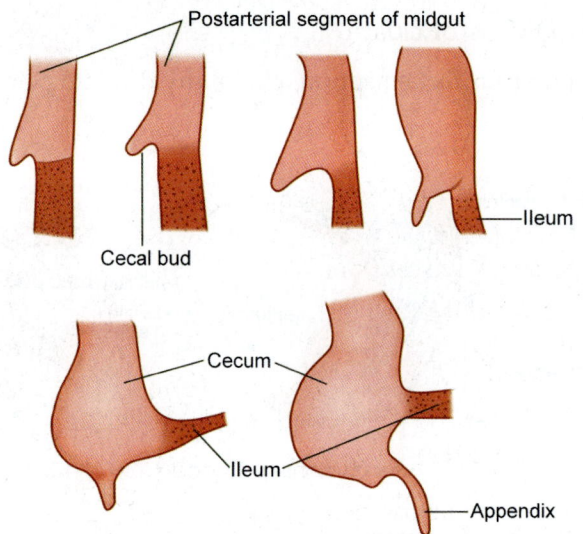

Development of cecum and appendix

## Q. Discuss the developmental anomalies of the gut.

**Ans.**

### Congenital Obstruction

1. Atresia—continuity of the lumen is interfered.
2. Stenosis—narrowing of the lumen.
3. Abnormal thickening of the muscular wall is seen at the pyloric end of the stomach.
4. External pressure by abnormal peritoneal bands.

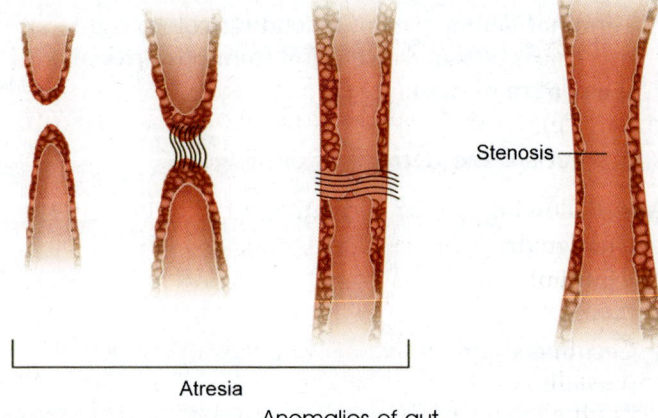

Anomalies of gut

## Abnormal Communications

Tracheoesophageal fistula.

## Duplication

Various lengths of intestine may get duplicated.

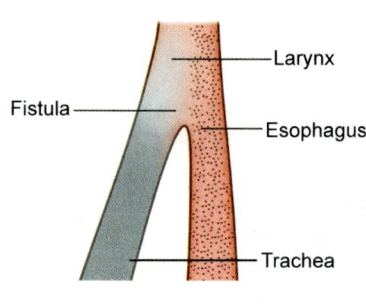

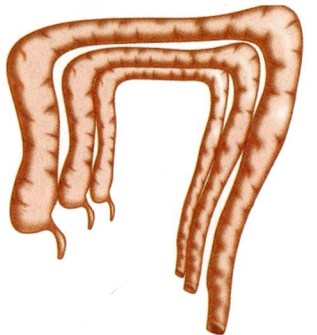

Tracheoesophageal fistula

Intestinal duplication

## Diverticuli

Persistence of vitellointestinal duct may give rise to the presence of diverticulum attached to the terminal part of ileum. This is called Meckel's diverticulum.

## Errors of Rotation

- Nonrotation of the loop
- Reversed rotation
- Nonreturn of umbilical hernia, i.e. wherein the coils of intestine remain outside the abdominal cavity. Such a condition is known as exomphalos.

## Errors of Fixation

Parts of intestine, which are normally retroperitoneal may get suspended by mesentery.

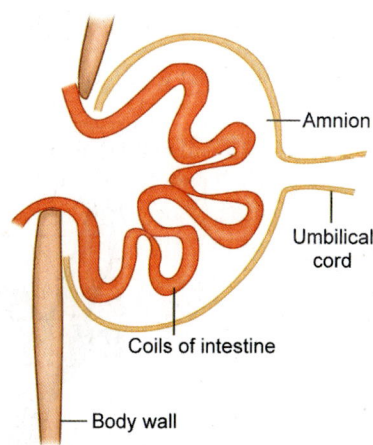

Exomphalos

## Situs Inversus

There is a lateral inversion of all the abdominal organs (e.g. liver is on the left side, heart on right side).

### Q. Discuss the development of liver.

**Ans.** Liver develops from an endodermal bud that arises from the ventral aspect of the gut at the point of junction between foregut and midgut. This bud grows into ventral mesogastrium and passes through it into the septum transversum.

This bud enlarges and soon shows a division into larger cranial part called pars hepatica and smaller caudal portion pars cystica. Pars hepatica divides into right and left parts, which forms the lobes of the liver.

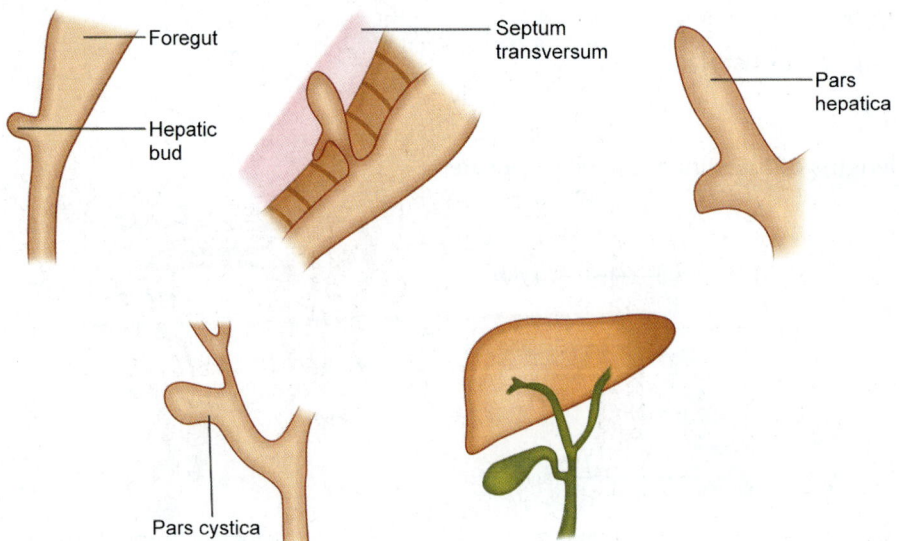

Development of liver

## Q. Which embryonic structure gives rise to gallbladder?

**Ans.** Pars cystica gives rise to gallbladder.

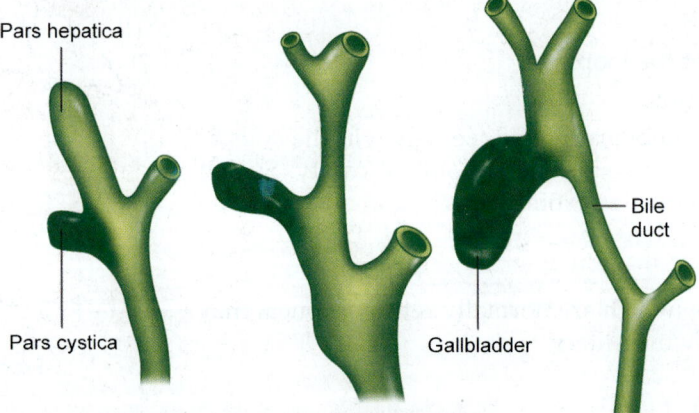

Development of gallbladder

## Q. How does the pancreas develop?

**Ans.** Pancreas develops by two buds originating from the endoderm lining of the duodenum:
- Dorsal pancreatic bud is in the dorsal mesentery
- Ventral pancreatic bud is close to the bile duct.

When the duodenum rotates to the right and becomes C-shaped, the ventral pancreatic bud moves dorsally, and comes to lie immediately below and behind the dorsal bud.

Ventral bud forms the lower part of the head and the uncinate process. Dorsal bud forms the upper part of the head, body and tail.

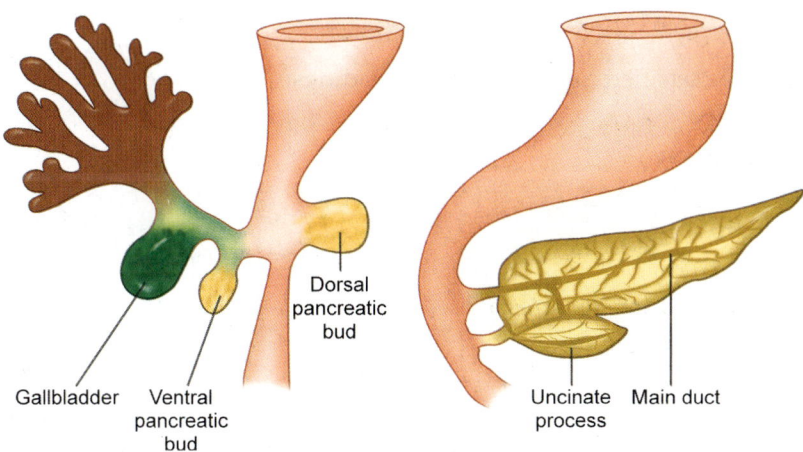

Development of pancreas

## Duct System of Pancreas

The ducts of dorsal and ventral bud anastomose with each other.

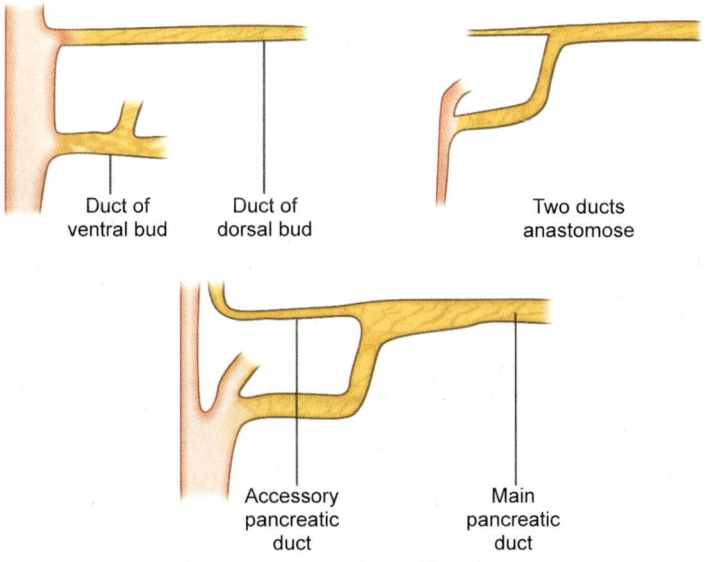

Duct system of pancreas

Part of dorsal duct proximal to anastomosis forms accessory pancreatic duct. Main pancreatic duct is a combination of ventral duct and dorsal duct distal to the anastomosis.

### Q. How does the spleen develop?

**Ans.** Spleen develops as a collection of mesenchymal cells in the dorsal mesogastrium. Some cells of the celomic epithelium also contribute in the development of spleen.

## Q. How do you classify anomalies of any system?

**Ans.** Anomalies are classified under following headings:
- Anomalies of shape
- Anomalies of position
- Duplication
- Abnormal length
- Abnormal termination
- Nondevelopment of duct, i.e. atresia
- Accessory tissue at ectopic sites.

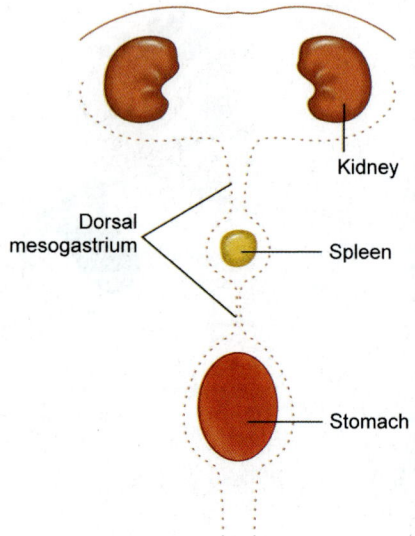

Spleen development

## Q. How does the respiratory diverticulum develop? What is its fate?

**Ans.** The diverticulum, which is destined to form respiratory system is initially spotted as midline groove, i.e. tracheoesophageal groove in the floor of developing pharynx just caudal to hypobranchial eminence.

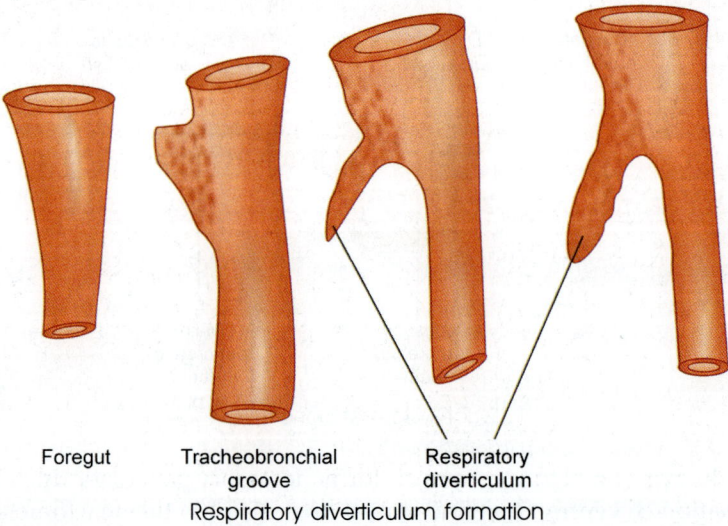

Respiratory diverticulum formation

This groove is flanked by sixth pharyngeal arches. The free caudal end of the diverticulum becomes bifid giving rise to lung bud.

Respiratory diverticulum gives rise to larynx, trachea, bronchi and lung parenchyma. The connective tissue, cartilage and muscle in relation to the organs of respiratory system are derived from splanchnopleuric mesoderm.

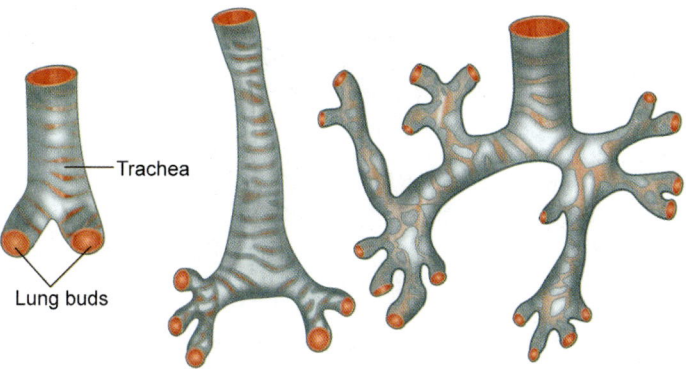

Trachea

Lung buds

## Q. Cavities of the body develop from which structure?

**Ans.** The pericardial, pleural and peritoneal cavities are derivatives of the intraembryonic celom.

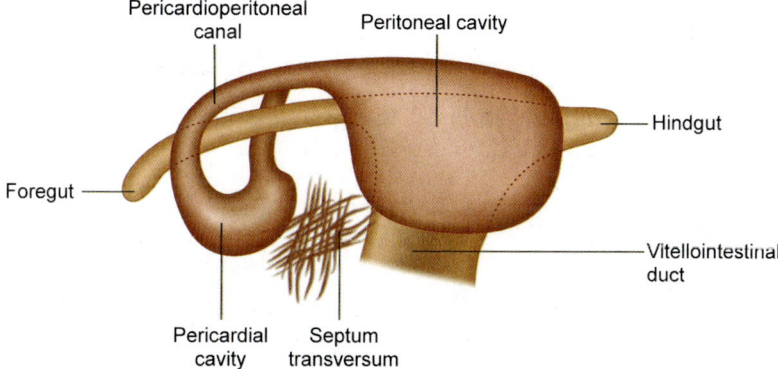

Pericardioperitoneal canal

Peritoneal cavity

Hindgut

Foregut

Vitellointestinal duct

Pericardial cavity    Septum transversum

## Q. Discuss the development of diaphragm.

**Ans.** Diaphragm develops from following components:
- Septum transversum
- Pleuroperitoneal membranes
- Ventral and dorsal mesenteries of esophagus
- Mesoderm of body wall, including mesoderm around the dorsal aorta.

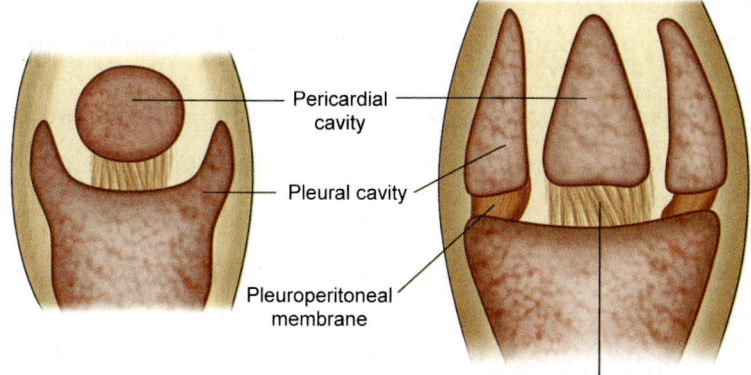

Pericardial cavity

Pleural cavity

Pleuroperitoneal membrane

Septum transversum

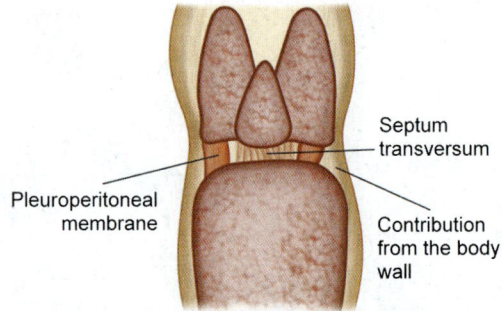

Development of diaphragm

### Q. Give the embryological basis of the innervation of diaphragm.

**Ans.** Diaphragm is supplied by C3, C4, C5 and intercostal nerve. Innervation by C3, C4 and C5 implies the migration of diaphragm to caudal direction. Intercostal nerve innervations depict the contribution of body wall.

### Q. From which embryological structure does the heart develop?

**Ans.** The heart develops from angioblastic tissue that arises from this splanchnopleuric mesoderm, i.e. from the cardiogenic area.

### Q. Depict the parts of heart tube.
**Ans.**

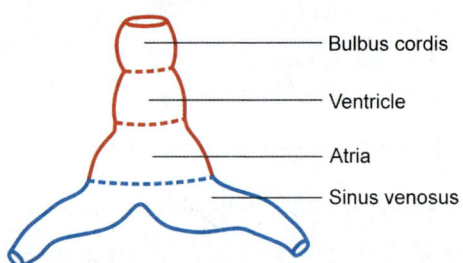

### Q. Which veins drain into sinus venosus?
**Ans.** Common cardinal vein, umbilical vein and vitelline vein drains into sinus venosus.

### Q. Which is the arterial end and venous end of the heart tube?

**Ans.** Bulbus cordis represents the arterial end of the heart tube, while sinus venosus represents the venous end of the heart tube.

### Q. Discuss the embryological basis of the openings in the right atrium.

**Ans.**
1. The body and right horn of sinus venosus are absorbed into common atrial chamber and form part of right atrium.

2. The common cardinal vein, which forms the terminal part of superior vena cava and right vitelline vein which forms the terminal part of inferior vena cava, opens into right atrium.
3. The left horn of the sinus venosus forms part of the coronary sinus, which opens into right atrium.

### Q. What are the derivatives of pericardium?

**Ans.** Visceral layer of pericardium is derived from splanchnopleuric mesoderm. The parietal layer is derived from somatopleuric mesoderm.

### Q. Depict the fate of heart tube.

**Ans.**

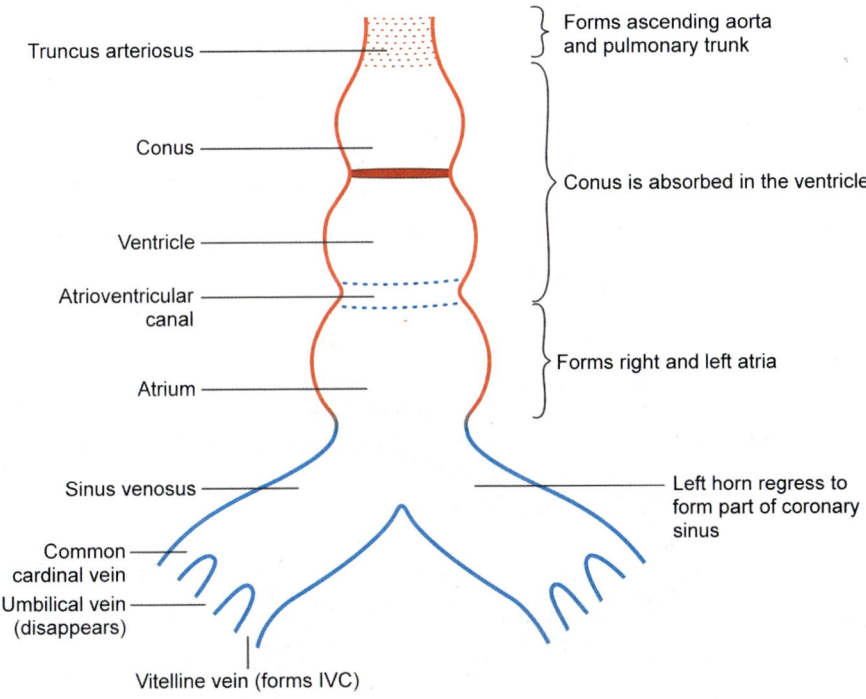

### Q. Discuss the fate of sinus venosus (diagram only).

**Ans.**

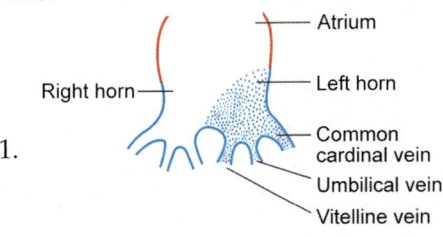

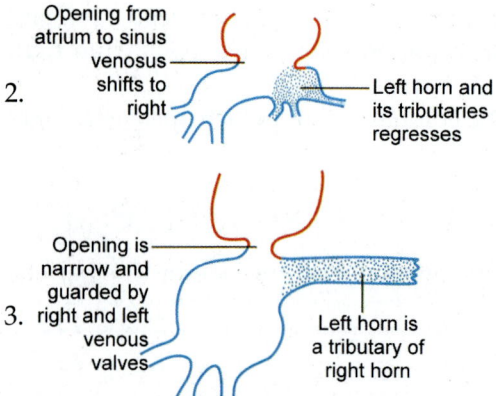

2. Opening from atrium to sinus venosus shifts to right — Left horn and its tributaries regresses

3. Opening is narrrow and guarded by right and left venous valves — Left horn is a tributary of right horn

## Q. Discuss the formation of interatrial septum.

**Ans.**

1. A septum arises from the roof of the atrial chamber, a little to the left of the opening of sinus venosus. This is septum primum.

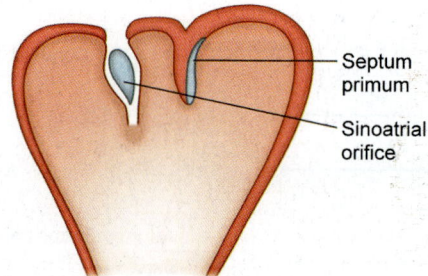

Septum primum

Sinoatrial orifice

2. The septum primum grows downwards towards atrioventricular cushions.

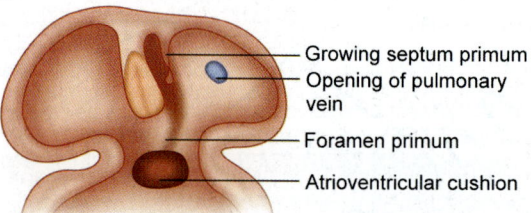

Growing septum primum
Opening of pulmonary vein
Foramen primum
Atrioventricular cushion

3. A second septum arises from the roof of atrial chamber, i.e. to the right of septum primum.

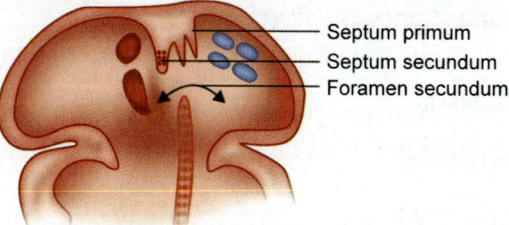

Septum primum
Septum secundum
Foramen secundum

4. As septum primum gets detached from the roof, it gives rise to foramen secundum.
5. Septum secundum grows downwards from the roof towards septum primum.

6. An oblique valvular gap remains between septum primum and secundum.

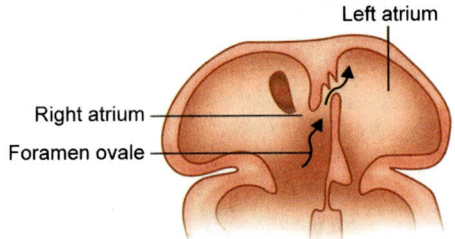

Pressure changes in the atrial chamber closes the foramen ovale.

**Q. What are the remnants of septum primum and septum secundum in adult life?**

**Ans.** Annulus ovalis represents the lower free edge of septum secundum. Fossa ovalis represents the lower free edge of septum primum.

**Q. What embryological components give rise to right atrium?**

**Ans.** The right atrium develops from:
• Right half of primitive atrium
• Sinus venosus
• Right half of atrioventricular canal.

**Q. What embryological components give rise to left atrium?**

**Ans.** The left atrium is derived from:
• Left half of primitive atrial chamber
• Left half of atrioventricular canal
• Absorbed parts of the pulmonary veins.

**Q. What are the subdivisions of bulbus cordis? What is their fate?**

**Ans.**
• Bulbus cordis is divisible into proximal part, the conus and the distal part called the truncus arteriosus
• The truncus arteriosus gets divided into two parts by means of spiral septum into ascending aorta and pulmonary trunk
• Conus merges with the cavity of primitive ventricle.

**Q. What is the remnant of first arch artery in adult life?**

**Ans.** In adult life, the first arch artery is represented by maxillary artery.

**Q. What are the components of interventricular septum?**

**Ans.** Following are the components of interventricular septum:
• Bulbar septum

- Atrioventricular cushions
- Proliferation of tissue from bulboventricular cavity.

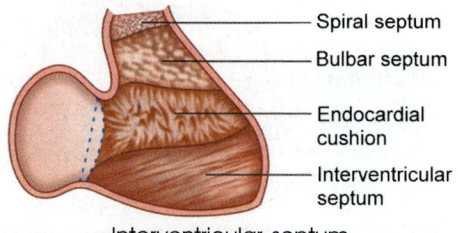

Interventricular septum

## Q. Depict the components of tetralogy of Fallot.

**Ans.**

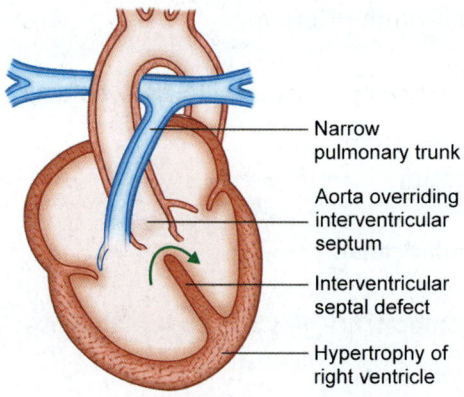

Tetralogy of Fallot components

## Q. Give the genesis of following arteries:
- Ascending aorta and pulmonary trunk
- Arch of aorta
- Descending aorta
- Subclavian artery right and left
- External carotid artery.

**Ans.**

1. Ascending aorta and pulmonary trunk are formed from truncus arteriosus.
2. Ventral part of aortic sac, left horn and left fourth arch, form arch of aorta.
3. Left dorsal aorta below the attachment of fourth arch artery with fused median vessel form descending aorta.
4. Right fourth arch artery and seventh cervical intersegmental artery form right subclavian artery. Left subclavian artery is derived from seventh intersegmental artery.
5. External carotid artery arises as a bud from third arch artery.

**Q. Discuss the relationship of recurrent laryngeal nerve on right and left side.**

**Ans.**
1. The nerve of sixth arch is caudal to sixth arch artery on both sides initially.
2. With the disappearance of part of sixth arch artery on right side the nerve moves cranially and comes into relationship with right fourth arch artery (subclavian). On left side, it retains its relationship to that part of sixth arch, which forms ductus arteriosus.
3. With the elongation of the neck and the descent of the heart these nerves are dragged downwards and therefore have to follow a recurrent course back to larynx.

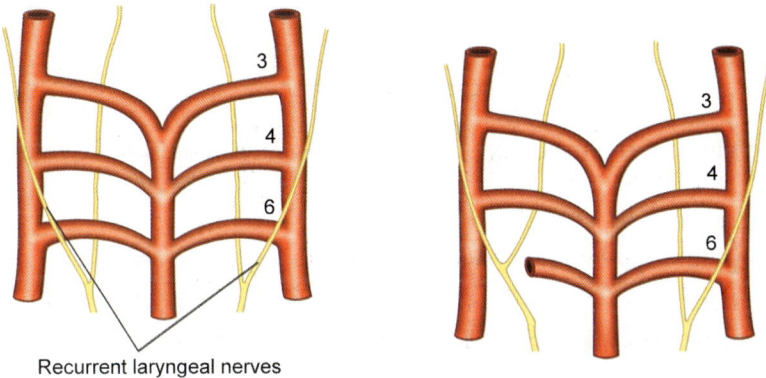

Recurrent laryngeal nerves

**Q. What is the axis artery of upper limb and lower limb?**

**Ans.** Axis artery of the upper limb is formed by the seventh intersegmental artery. Axis artery of lower limb is derived from fifth lumbar intersegmental artery.

**Q. How is portal vein formed?**

**Ans.** Portal vein develops from following embryological components:

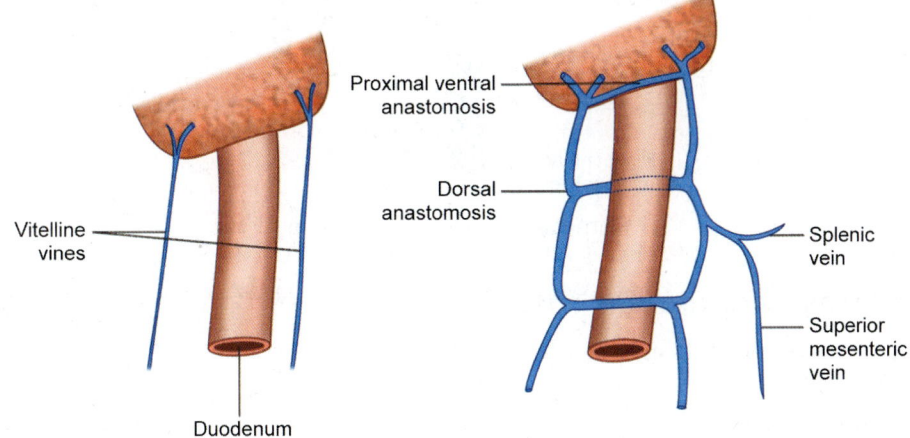

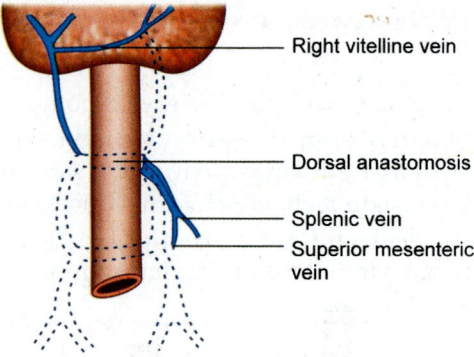

Portal vein formation

- Left vitelline vein between the entry of superior mesenteric and splenic veins and the dorsal anastomosis
- Dorsal anastomosis itself
- Right vitelline vein between the dorsal anastomosis and the cranial ventral anastomosis.

### Q. How is superior vena cava formed?

**Ans.** Superior vena cava is derived from:
- Right anterior cardinal vein caudal to the transverse anastomosis
- Right common cardinal vein.

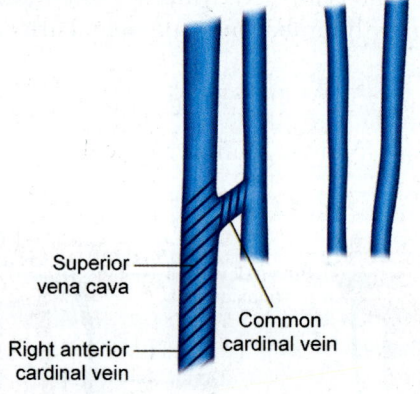

Formation of superior vena cava

### Q. What are the components of inferior vena cava?

**Ans.** Following components give rise to inferior vena cava, i.e.:
- Subcardinal veins
- Supracardinal veins
- Subcardinal hepatocardiac anastomosis
- Hepatocardiac channel
- Supracardinal subcardinal anastomosis.

**Q. Discuss the features of fetal circulation.**

**Ans.**
1. The source of oxygenated blood is placenta.
2. Oxygenated blood from placenta passes through ductus venosus to inferior vena cava.
3. Most of the oxygenated blood from right atrium passes through foramen ovale into left atrium. Rest goes from right atrium into right ventricle.
4. Most of the blood from right ventricle is directed into ductus arteriosus and thence into the aorta.

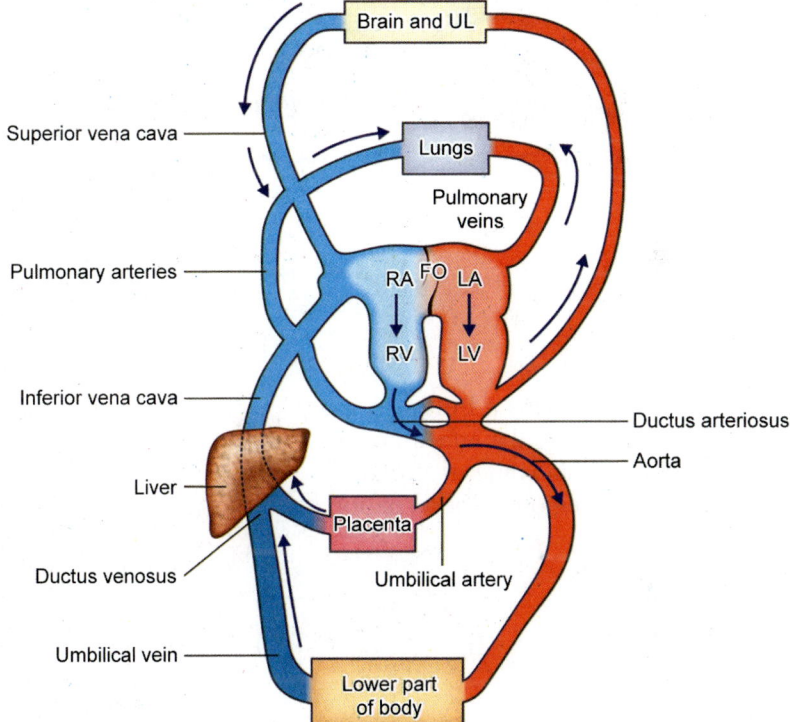

Fetal circulation (FO, foramen ovale; LA, left atrium; LV, left ventricles; RA, right atrium; RV, right ventricle; SVC, superior vena cava)

**Q. Discuss the remnants of the components of fetal circulation.**

**Ans.**
- Umbilical arteries—medial umbilical ligament
- Left umbilical vein—ligamentum teres of liver
- Ductus venosus—ligamentum venosum
- Ductus arteriosus—ligamentum arteriosum.

**Q. What are the changes in fetal circulation at birth?**

**Ans.**
1. The muscle in the wall of umbilical arteries immediately contracts after birth. This prevents loss of fetal blood into the placenta.

2. Lumen of umbilical vein and ductus venosus is also occluded, but this takes few minutes after birth.
3. Ductus arteriosus is occluded.
4. Pulmonary vessels increase in size and proportionately a much larger volume of blood reaches left atrium from lungs.

### Q. Which embryological structure plays role in the formation of urogenital system?

**Ans.** The intermediate mesoderm plays an important role in the development of urogenital system.

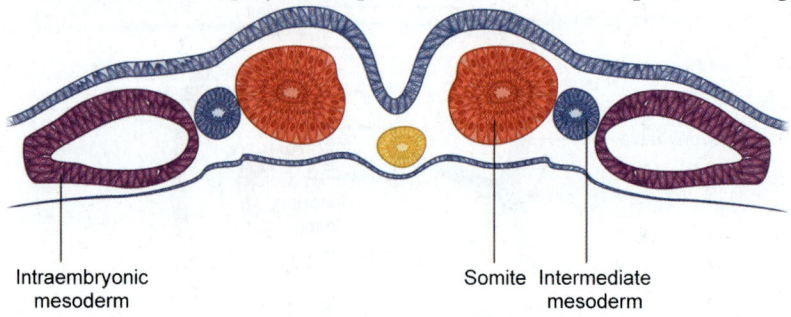

Intraembryonic mesoderm

Somite Intermediate mesoderm

### Q. What is nephrogenic cord?

**Ans.** Intermediate mesoderm forms a bulge on the posterior abdominal wall lateral to the attachment of dorsal mesentery of the gut. This is the nephrogenic cord. It extends from cervical region to sacral region.

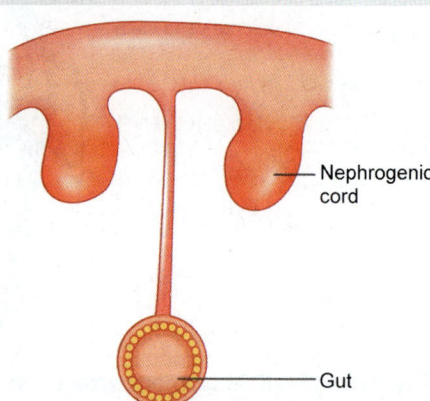

Nephrogenic cord

Gut

### Q. What components give rise to urethra?

**Ans.** Definitive urogenital sinus and caudal part of vesicourethral canal give rise to urethra.

### Q. What are the subdivisions of cloaca?

**Ans.** Cloaca is subdivided into:
- Primitive urogenital sinus
- Rectum.

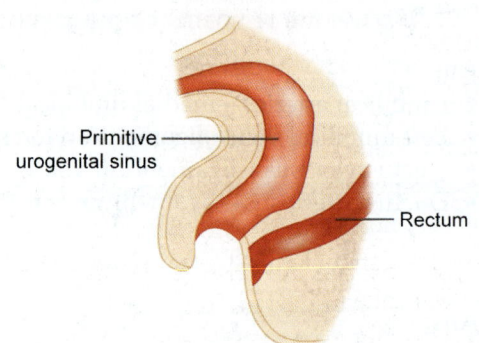

Primitive urogenital sinus

Rectum

Primitive urogenital sinus

**Q. Depict the subdivisions of urogenital sinus.**

**Ans.**

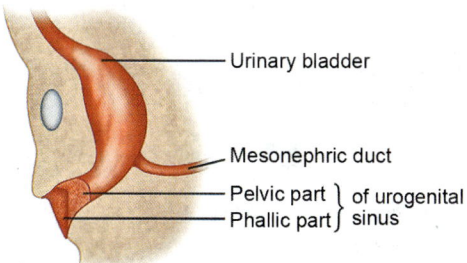

**Q. What are the two distinct sources of kidney?**

**Ans.**
- The excretory tubules are derived from the lowest part of nephrogenic cord of cells of which form the metanephric blastema
- The collecting part of the kidney is derived from a diverticulum called ureteric bud.

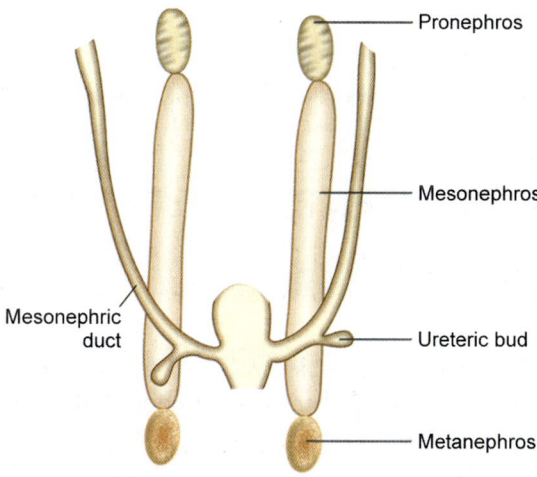

**Q. How do you classify anomalies of kidney?**

**Ans.** Following anomalies may be encountered:
- Agenesis
- Duplication
- Horseshoe kidney
- Pancake kidney
- Lobulated kidney.

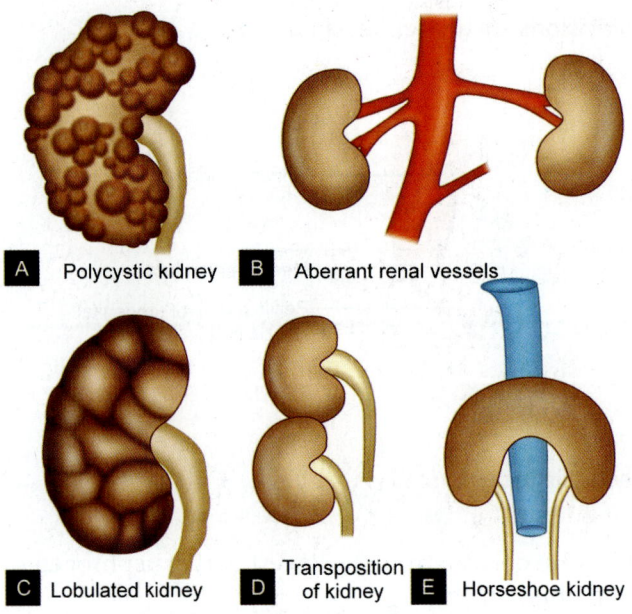

A   Polycystic kidney     B   Aberrant renal vessels

C   Lobulated kidney     D   Transposition of kidney     E   Horseshoe kidney

Anomalies of kidney

### Q. How does the ureter develop?

**Ans.** Ureter is derived from the part of ureteric bud that lies between the pelvis of the kidney and the vesicourethral canal.

### Q. Discuss the development of urinary bladder.

**Ans.**
- The epithelium of urinary bladder develops from the cranial part of vesicourethral canal
- Epithelium of trigone of the bladder is derived from the absorbed mesonephric duct
- Muscular and serous walls are derived from splanchnopleuric mesoderm.

### Q. What is the fate of paramesonephric ducts in females?

**Ans.** In the females, paramesonephric duct gives origin to uterine tubes, uterus and part of vagina.

### Q. What is the fate of paramesonephric ducts in males?

**Ans.**
- Paramesonephric duct remains rudimentary in males
- Cranial end of each duct persists as a small rounded body attached to the testis—appendix of testis
- Uterovaginal canal remnant is prostatic utricle.

**Ans.**

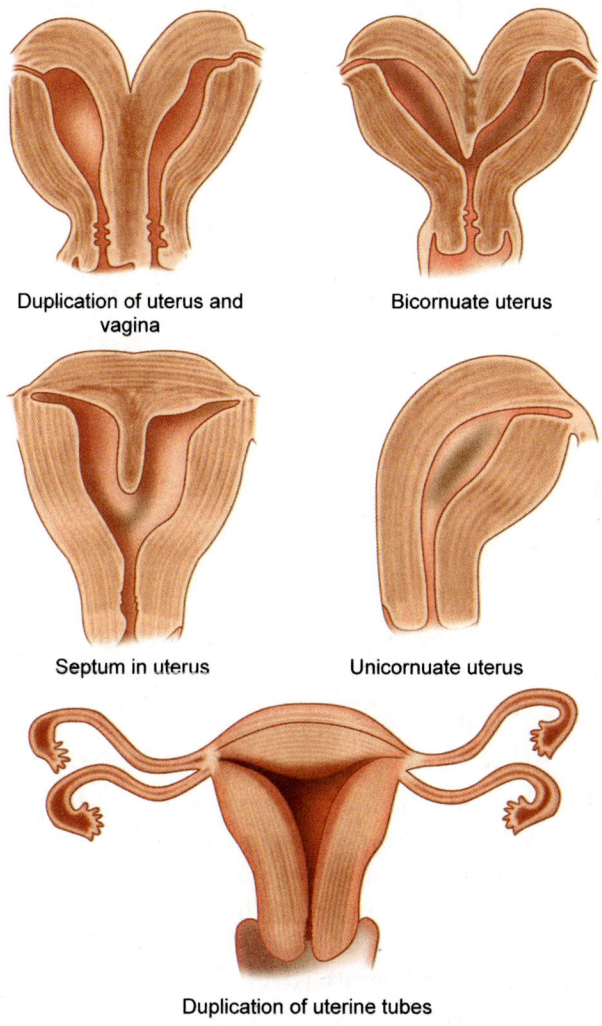

Duplication of uterus and vagina

Bicornuate uterus

Septum in uterus

Unicornuate uterus

Duplication of uterine tubes

Anomalies of uterus

**Q. What is the male homologue of uterus?**

**Ans.** Prostatic utricle is the male homologue of uterus.

**Q. Discuss the development of external genitalia.**

**Ans.** *In females:*
- Genital tubercle forms clitoris
- Genital swellings form labia majora
- Primitive urethral folds form labia minora.

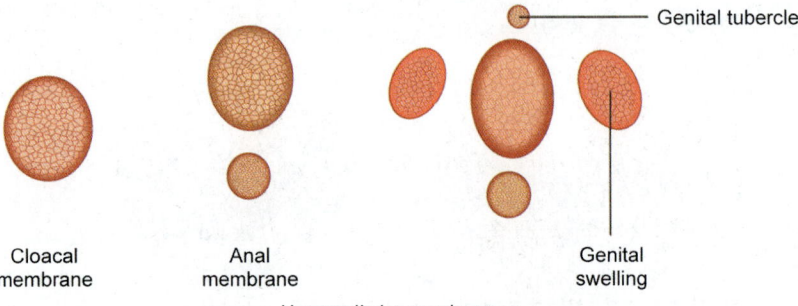

Cloacal membrane

Anal membrane

Urogenital membrane

Genital swelling

Genital tubercle

*In males:*
- Genital tubercle forms penis
- Genital swellings form scrotal sac
- Urethral folds form penile urethra.

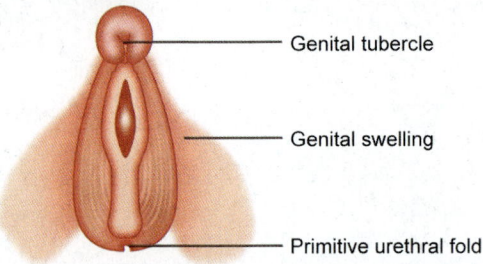

Genital tubercle

Genital swelling

Primitive urethral fold

## Q. Discuss the descent of testis.

**Ans.**
- The testis develops in relation to the lumbar region of the posterior abdominal wall
- During fetal life, they gradually descend to the scrotum
- They reach the iliac fossa during the third month
- They lie at the site of deep inguinal ring up to 7th month of intrauterine life (IUL)
- They pass through the inguinal canal during the 7th month (IUL)
- They reach the scrotum during 8th month (IUL).

*Factors affecting descent of testis:*
- Differential growth of the body wall
- Formation of inguinal bursa
- Shortening of gubernaculums
- Processus vaginalis is a diverticulum of peritoneal cavity, which grows towards scrotum
- The descent of testis is greatly influenced by hormones
- Appendix of epididymis represents the remnant of mesonephric duct
- Appendix of testis is the remnant of paramesonephric duct.

## Q. Discuss the formation of neural tube.

**Ans.**
1. Whole of the nervous system is derived from ectoderm.

2. The part of ectoderm overlying the notochord on the dorsal aspect of embryonic disk becomes thickened to form neural tube.
3. The neural plate becomes depressed so that neural groove is formed.
4. The neural groove grows deeper and the edges come close to each other and fuse thus converting neural groove into neural tube.

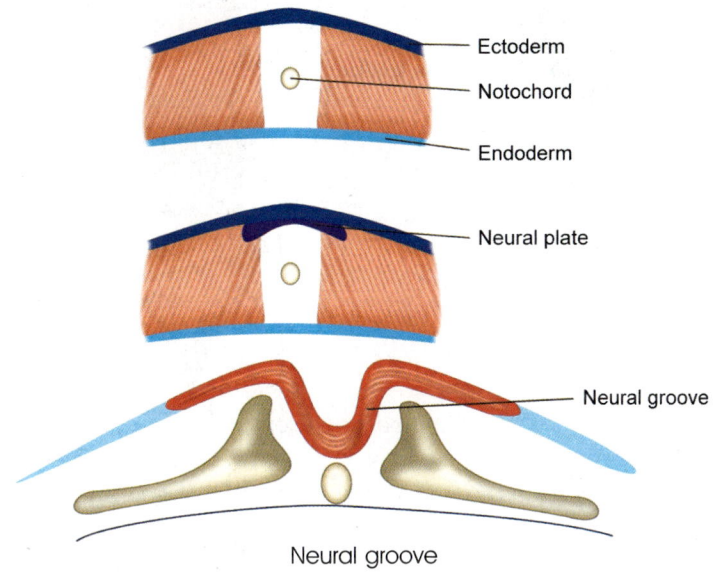

Neural groove

**Q. What are the subdivisions of neural tube?**

**Ans.** Neural tube is broadly divided into three parts:
1. Prosencephalon.
2. Mesencephalon.
3. Rhombencephalon.

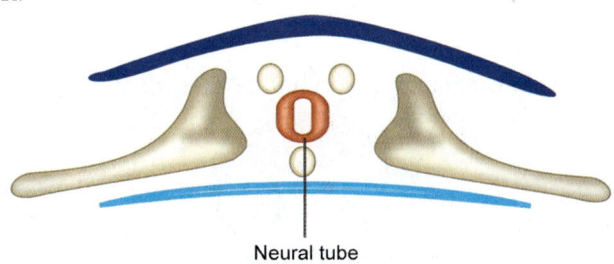

Neural tube

**Q. What is the fate of neural tube in adult?**

**Ans.**
- Telencephalon—cerebral cortex, corpus striatum
- Diencephalon—thalamus, hypothalamus, optic stalk, pars nervosa of hypophysis
- Mesencephalon—midbrain
- Metencephalon—pons, cerebellum
- Myelencephalon—medulla oblongata.

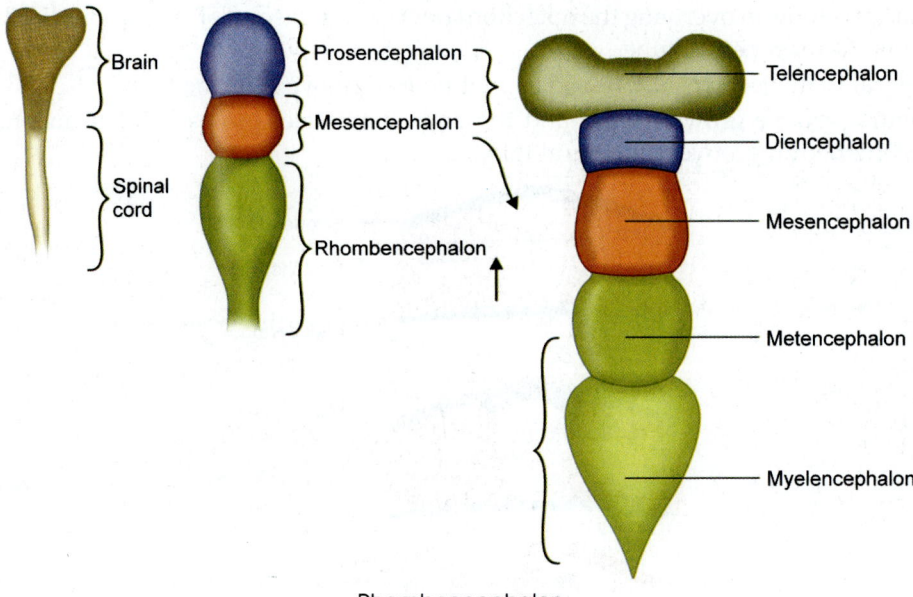

Rhombencephalon

**Q. How does the neural tube fold?**

**Ans.** Neural tube folds by the development of several flexures such as:

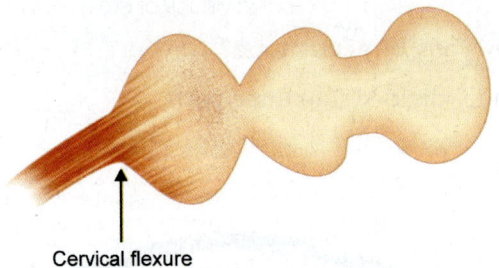

Cervical flexure

1. Cervical flexure between rhombencephalon and spinal cord.

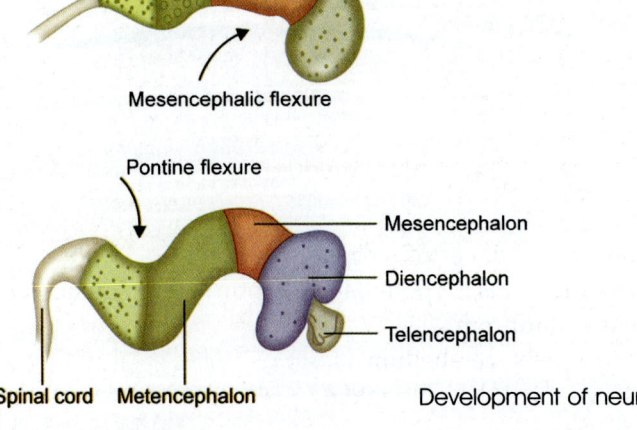

Development of neural tube fold

2. Mesencephalic flexure in the region of midbrain.
3. Pontine flexure at the middle of rhombencephalon dividing into metencephalon and myelencephalon.

## Q. What are the cavities of subdivisions of brain?

**Ans.** The cavities of subdivisions of brain are explained in the table given below.

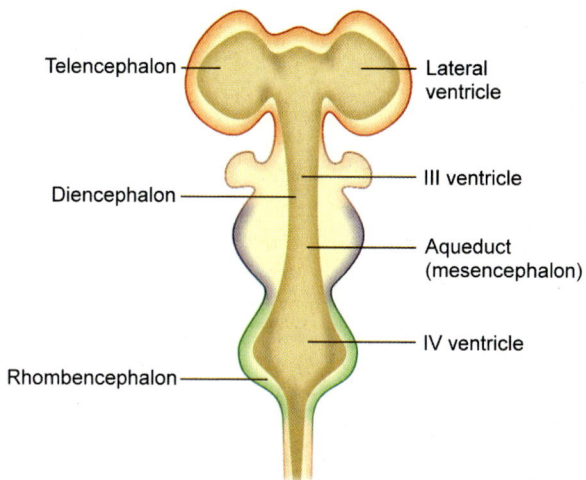

Cavities of subdivisions of brain

| Subdivision of brain | Cavity |
| --- | --- |
| Telencephalon | Lateral ventricle |
| Diencephalon | Third ventricle |
| Mesencephalon | Aqueduct |
| Rhombencephalon | Fourth ventricle |

## Q. What are neural crest cells?

**Ans.** At the time when the neural plate is being formed, some cells at the junction between the neural plate and rest of the ectoderm becomes specialized to form the primordium of neural crest.

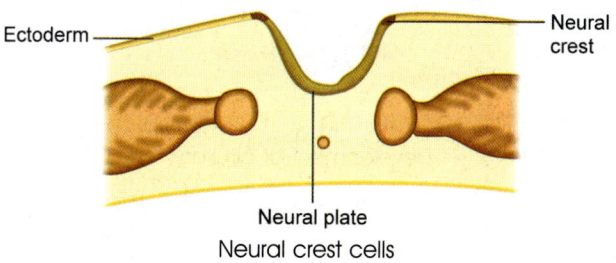

Neural crest cells

## Q. What are the derivatives of neural crest cells?

**Ans.** Following are the derivatives of neural crest cells:
- Neurons of the spinal posterior nerve root ganglia
- Neurons of the sensory ganglia of V, VII, VIII, IX and X cranial nerves
- Neurons of sympathetic ganglia
- Schwann cells
- Some cells of adrenal medulla
- Chromaffin cells, pigment cells
- Pia- and arachnoid-mater
- Mesenchyme of dental papillae.

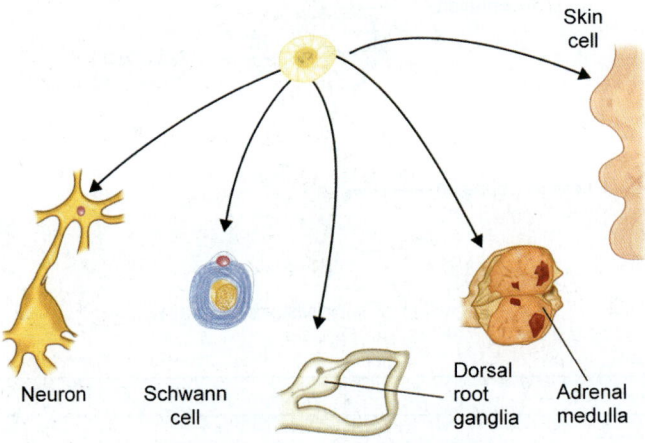

Neural crest cell derivatives

## Q. How does pituitary gland develop?

**Ans.**
1. The anterior and the intermediate part of the organ develops from ectodermal diverticulum that grows upwards from the roof of stomodeum, i.e. Rathke's pouch.

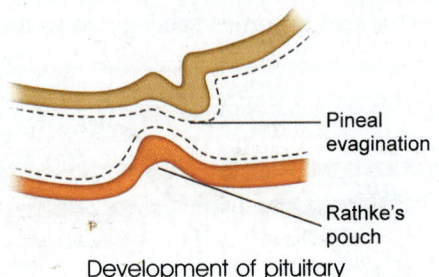

Development of pituitary

2. Posterior lobe is formed as downgrowth of infundibulum from the floor of third ventricle.

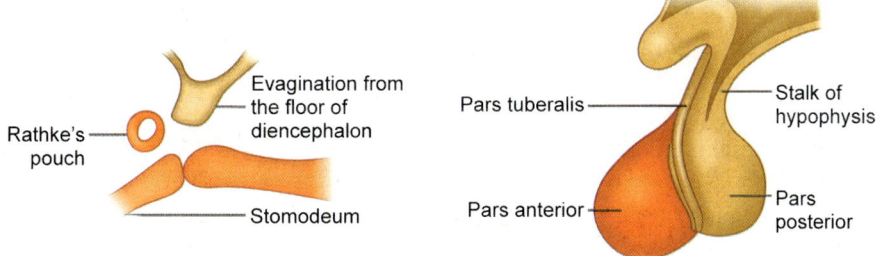

### Q. Depict the layers of neural tube.

**Ans.**

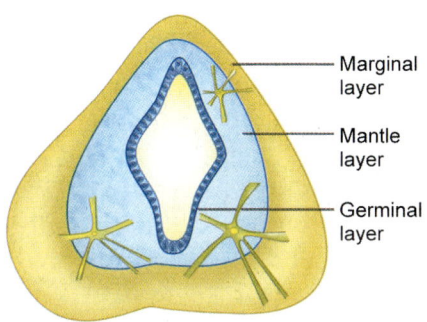

Layers of neural tube

### Q. What embryological components give rise to eyeball?

**Ans.** The various components are derived from following primordia:
- Outgrowth from prosencephalon called optic vesicle
- Specialized area of surface ectoderm gives rise to lens
- Mesoderm covering optic vesicle.

### Q. Depict the formation of optic vesicle.

**Ans.**

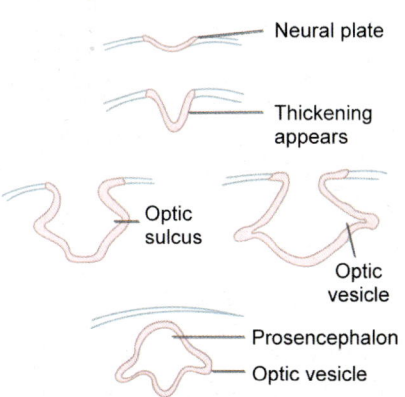

**Q. How does the lens vesicle form?**

**Ans.**

- Optic vesicle grows laterally and comes to lie into relation with surface ectoderm
- An area of this surface ectoderm overlying optic vesicle becomes thickened to form lens placode.

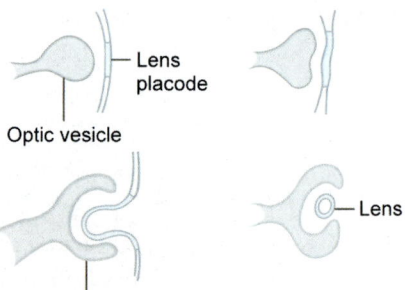

**Q. How does otic vesicle develop? What is its fate?**

**Ans.**

- Part of surface ectoderm overlying the developing hindbrain gets thickened
- This area of thickening is called otic placode
- Otic placode soon gets depressed to form otic pit
- Otic vesicle by differential growth gives rise to membranous labyrinth.

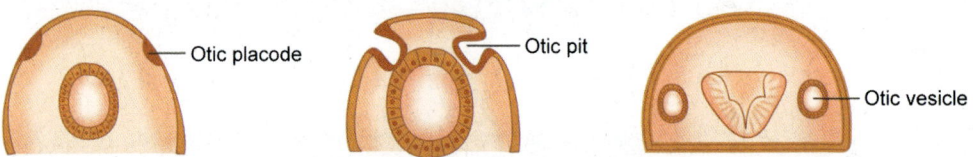

**Q. Discuss the middle ear development.**

**Ans.**

1. Epithelial lining of middle ear and of the pharyngotympanic tube is derived from tubo-tympanic recess.
2. Mastoid antrum is a dorsal extension of tympanic cavity.

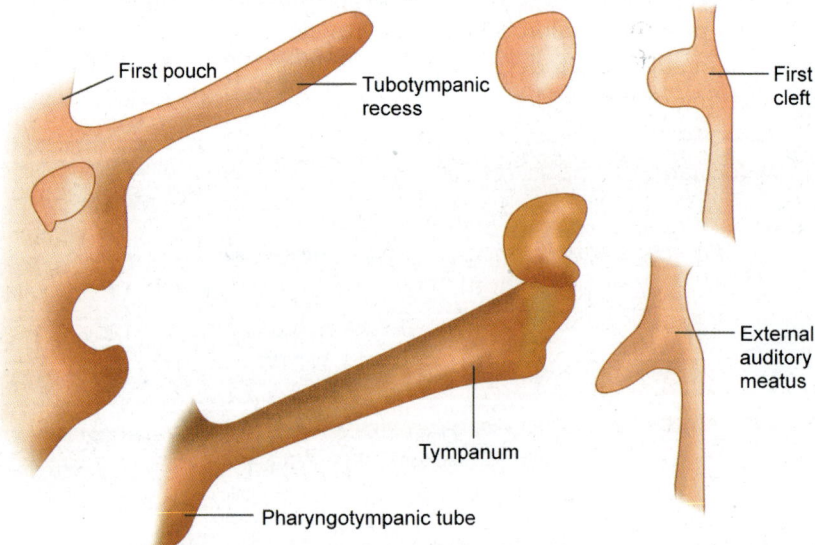

3. Tubotympanic recess is an outgrowth of first pharyngeal pouch.
4. Tympanic cavity and auditory tube develop from tubotympanic recess.

5. Malleus and incus are derived from the dorsal end of Meckel's cartilage.
6. Stapes is derived from the dorsal end of the cartilage of the second pharyngeal pouch.
7. Tensor tympani muscle is derived from the mesoderm of the first pharyngeal pouch.
8. Stapedius muscle from second pharyngeal pouch.

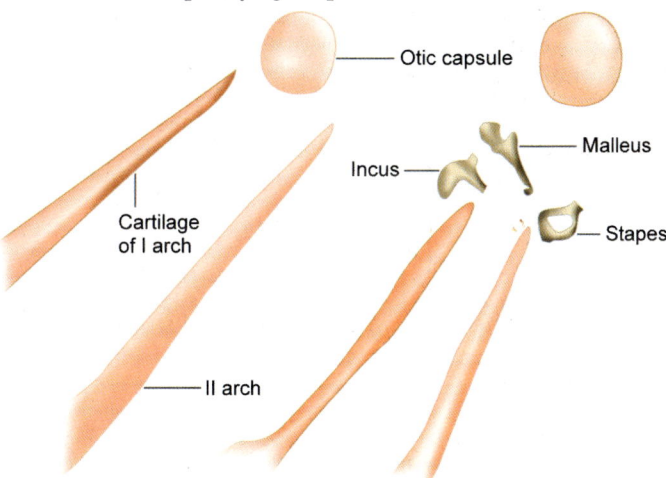

Development of middle ear

**Q. How does the external auditory canal develop?**

**Ans.** External auditory canal develops from the dorsal part of first ectodermal cleft.

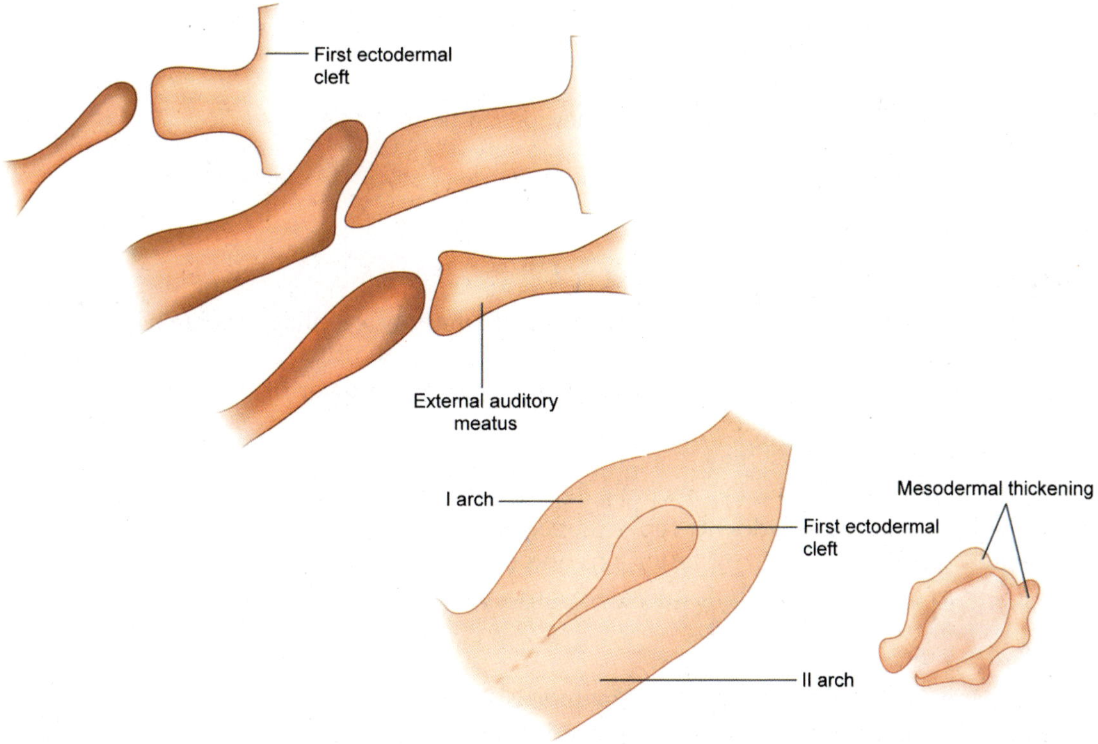

### Q. How is pinna formed?

**Ans.** Pinna is formed from a series of mesodermal thickenings that appear on the mandibular and hyoid arches around the opening of the dorsal part of the first ectodermal cleft.

Tympanic membrane is formed by the contribution of tubotympanic recess and outer epithelial layer.

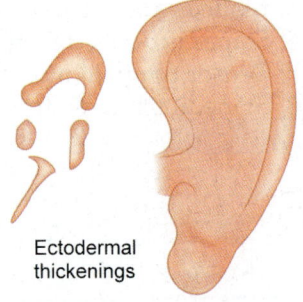

Ectodermal thickenings

Development of pinna

### Q. What are the derivatives of ectoderm?

**Ans.**

### Lining Epithelia

- Skin
- Mucous membrane of lips, cheeks, gums, floor of mouth, part of palate, nasal cavities paranasal sinuses
- Lower part of anal canal
- Terminal part of male urethra
- Outer surface of labia minora and whole of labia majora
- Anterior epithelium of cornea, conjunctiva, epithelial layers of ciliary body and iris
- Outer layer of tympanic membrane.

### *Glands*

- Exocrine glands, i.e. sweat glands, sebaceous glands, parotid, mammary glands, lacrimal glands
- Endocrine glands, i.e. hypophysis cerebri, adrenal medulla.

### *Other Derivatives*

- Hair, nails, enamel of teeth, lens of eye, nervous system.

### Q. What are the derivatives of endoderm?

**Ans.**

### Lining Epithelia

- Epithelia of mouth, part of palate, tongue, tonsil, pharynx, esophagus, stomach, small and large intestine, upper part of anal canal
- Epithelium of pharyngotympanic tube, middle ear, inner layer of tympanic membrane, mastoid antrum and air cells
- Epithelium of respiratory tract
- Epithelium of gallbladder, extrahepatic duct system, pancreatic duct
- Epithelium of urinary bladder except trigone, female urethra except its posterior wall, male urethra except its prostatic posterior part and penile urethra
- Epithelium of vagina, vestibule and inner surface of labia minora.

### Glands

- Endocrine, i.e. thyroid, parathyroid, thymus, islets of Langerhans
- Exocrine, i.e. liver, pancreas, glands of gastrointestinal tract (GIT) and greater part of prostate.

## Q. What are the derivatives of mesoderm?

**Ans.**

1. All connective tissue including loose areolar tissue, superficial and deep fascia, ligaments, tendons, aponeuroses, dermis of skin.
2. Adipose tissue, reticular tissue, cartilage and bone.
3. Dentine of teeth.
4. All the muscles—smooth, striated, cardiac.
5. Heart, blood vessels, lymphatics, blood vessels.
6. Kidneys, ureters, trigone of bladder, posterior wall of part of female and male urethra.
7. Ovary, uterus, uterine tube.
8. Testis, epididymis, vas deferens, seminal vesicle, ejaculatory ducts.
9. Lining mesothelium of pleura, pericardia, peritoneal cavities.
10. Lining epithelium of bursae and joints.

## Q. What are Neural tube defects?

**Ans.** Common neural tube defects are:

- If neural tube does not close in the cranial region—brain development does not occur, this is termed anencephaly.
- If neural tube fails to close anywhere below cervical region it leads to an entity termed spina bifida.

## Q. Which vitamin prevents neural tube defects?

**Ans.** Folic acid administration prevents neural tube defects.

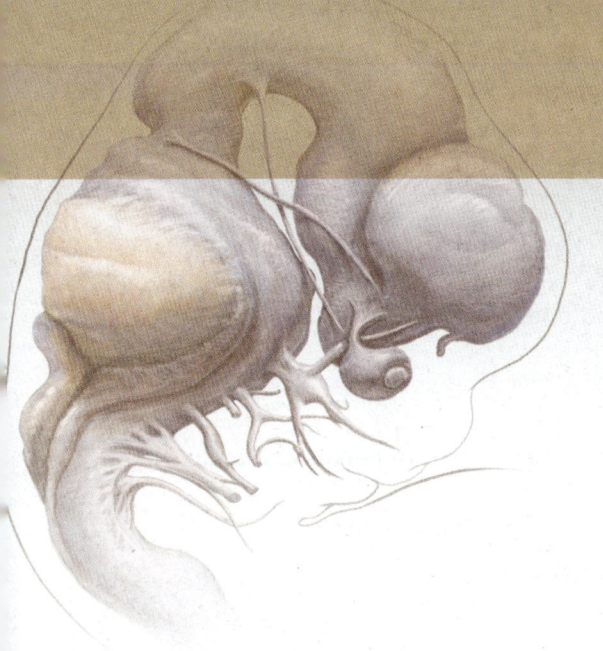

1. Embryo is from the time of inception till first .................... weeks.

   a. 4                              c. 6

   b. 8                              d. 2

   **Answer: b**

2. From .................... month till birth is called fetus.

   a. 1st                            c. 3rd

   b. 2nd                            d. 4th

   **Answer: c**

3. Fertilization occurs in .................... part of the fallopian tube.

   a. Intramural

   b. Isthmus

   c. Ampulla

   d. Infundibulum

   **Answer: c**

4. X chromosome is a member of .................... group (Denver classification).

   a. A                              c. C

   b. B                              d. D

   **Answer: c**

5. Y chromosome is a member of .................... group.

   a. E                              c. G

   b. F                              d. E

   **Answer: c**

6. DNA content of chromosome is duplicated during ..................... phase.

   a. Prophase                         c. Metaphase
   b. Interphase                       d. Anaphase

   **Answer: b**

7. Spindle formation occurs during ..................... of cell division.

   a. Prophase                         c. Anaphase
   b. Metaphase                        d. Telophase

   **Answer: a**

8. 'Crossing over' takes place during what stage of prophase?

   a. Leptotene                        c. Pachytene
   b. Zygotene                         d. Diplotene

   **Answer: c**

9. At the time of ovulation, the stage of ovary is .....................

   a. Primary oocyte                   c. Oogonium
   b. Secondary oocyte                 d. None of the above

   **Answer: b**

10. How many days it takes for the ovum to reach the uterus?

    a. 1–2 days                        c. 3–4 days
    b. 2–3 days                        d. Within 24 hours

    **Answer: c**

11. If the ovum is not fertilized, the corpus luteum persists for ..................... days.

    a. 10                              c. 14
    b. 12                              d. 16

    **Answer: c**

12. Corpus luteum secretes ..................... hormone.

    a. Estrogen                        c. Progesterone
    b. Luteinizing hormone             d. Follicle-stimulating hormone

    **Answer: c**

13. Superfemales have ..................... number of chromosomes.

    a. XX                              c. XO
    b. XXY                             d. XXX

    **Answer: d**

14. In isochromosomes, the centriole splits .....................

    a. Longitudinally                  c. Obliquely
    b. Transversely                    d. Diagonally

    **Answer: b**

15. **Hormone influencing luteal phase is** ....................

    a. Estrogen                        c. LH
    b. Progesterone                    d. FSH

                                                    **Answer: b**

16. **Hormone influencing follicular phase is** ....................

    a. Estrogen                        c. LH
    b. Progesterone                    d. FSH

                                                    **Answer: a**

17. **Ovum remains viable for** .................... **days.**

    a. 1                               c. 3
    b. 2                               d. 4

                                                    **Answer: b**

18. **Spermatozoa introduced into vagina die within** .................... **days.**

    a. 2                               c. 4
    b. 3                               d. 5

                                                    **Answer: c**

19. **Chorion is formed by the union of** ....................

    a. Visceral extraembryonic mesoderm with trophoblast
    b. Parietal extraembryonic mesoderm and trophoblast
    c. Parietal extraembryonic mesoderm with amnion
    d. Visceral with parietal extraembryonic mesoderm

                                                    **Answer: b**

20. **Morula is** .................... **cell stage.**

    a. 10                              c. 14
    b. 12                              d. 16

                                                    **Answer: d**

21. .................... **decides the axis of embryonic disk.**

    a. Primitive streak                c. Prochordal plate
    b. Chorion                         d. Amnion

                                                    **Answer: c**

22. **Prochordal plate is the modification of** .................... **cells of embryonic disk.**

    a. Ectoderm                        c. Endoderm
    b. Mesoderm                        d. None

                                                    **Answer: c**

**23. Primitive streak is the proliferation of .................... cells toward tail end of disk.**

a. Ectoderm                               c. Endoderm

b. Mesoderm                               d. All

**Answer: a**

**24. What gives rise to intraembryonic mesoderm?**

a. Prochordal plate                       c. Trophoblast

b. Primitive streak                       d. Extraembryonic mesoderm

**Answer: b**

**25. Gastrulation is the formation of ....................**

a. Prochordal plate and primitive streak

b. Prochordal plate and extraembryonic mesoderm

c. Primitive streak and intraembryonic mesoderm

d. Primitive streak and extraembryonic mesoderm

**Answer: c**

**26. Morula formation occurs after .................... days of embryo formation.**

a. 1                                      c. 3

b. 2                                      d. 4

**Answer: c**

**27. Blastocyst formation occurs in .................... days after embryo formation.**

a. 2                                      c. 5

b. 4                                      d. 6

**Answer: b**

**28. Intraembryonic mesoderm develops by the day ....................**

a. 8                                      c. 14

b. 10                                     d. 16

**Answer: d**

**29. Hensen's node is the thickened part of ....................**

a. Cranial end of primitive streak        c. Cranial end of prochordal plate

b. Caudal end of primitive streak         d. Caudal end of prochordal plate

**Answer: a**

**30. Para-axial mesoderm gives rise to ....................**

a. Nervous system                         c. Somites

b. Body cavities                          d. Vertebral column

**Answer: c**

31. **Pleural, pericardial and peritoneal cavities develop from** .....................
    a. Para-axial mesoderm
    b. Lateral plate mesoderm
    c. Intermediate mesoderm
    d. Extraembryonic celom

    **Answer: b**

32. **Intermediate mesoderm gives rise to** .....................
    a. Cardiogenic area
    b. Peritoneal cavities
    c. Nephrogenic area
    d. Genitalia

    **Answer: c**

33. **Normally, placenta is implanted in** .....................
    a. Upper uterine segment
    b. Lower uterine segment
    c. Both (a and b)
    d. Partially in upper segment

    **Answer: a**

34. **Muscles of tongue develop from** .....................
    a. Mesoderm of 1st branchial arch
    b. Occipital myotomes
    c. Sclerotome
    d. Dermatome

    **Answer: b**

35. **Meckel's cartilage is the cartilage of** ..................... **pharyngeal arch.**
    a. 1st
    b. 2nd
    c. 3rd
    d. 4th

    **Answer: a**

36. **Which of the following pharyngeal arch disappears during embryological development?**
    a. 2nd
    b. 3rd
    c. 4th
    d. 5th

    **Answer: d**

37. **Stapes develops from** ..................... **pharyngeal arch.**
    a. 1st
    b. 2nd
    c. 3rd
    d. 4th

    **Answer: b**

38. **Hyoid bone develops from** ..................... **pharyngeal arch.**
    a. 1st
    b. 2nd
    c. 3rd
    d. 4th

    **Answer: c**

39. **Cartilages of larynx develop from** ..................... **pharyngeal arches.**
    a. 1st and 2nd
    b. 2nd and 3rd
    c. 3rd and 4th
    d. 4th and 6th

    **Answer: d**

40. **Pretrematic nerve of 1st pharyngeal arch is** ....................

   a. Chorda tympani             c. XI
   b. Mandibular                 d. X

41. **Post-trematic nerve of 1st arch is** ....................

   a. Chorda tympani             c. Facial
   b. Mandibular                 d. Glossopharyngeal

42. **Third pharyngeal arch nerve is** ....................

   a. V                          c. X
   b. VII                        d. IX

43. **Muscles of mastication develop from** .................... **pharyngeal arch.**

   a. 1st                        c. 3rd
   b. 2nd                        d. 4th

44. **Anterior belly of digastric develops from** .................... **pharyngeal arch.**

   a. 1st                        c. 3rd
   b. 2nd                        d. 4th

45. **Posterior belly of digastric develops from** .................... **pharyngeal arch.**

   a. 1st                        c. 3rd
   b. 2nd                        d. 4th

46. **Auditory tube develops from** ....................

   a. Proximal part of tubotympanic recess
   b. Distal part of tubotympanic recess
   c. Second pharyngeal pouch
   d. Ventral part of first pharyngeal pouch

47. **Tubotympanic recess is formed by contribution of following two structures** ....................

   a. Ventral and dorsal part of 1st pouch
   b. Dorsal part of 1st pouch and 2nd pouch
   c. Dorsal and ventral part of 2nd pouch
   d. Tympanic cavity

48. **Third endodermal pouch gives rise to** .....................

    a. Superior parathyroid           c. Inferior parathyroid

    b. Thyroid                         d. Thymus

**Answer: c**

49. **Fourth endodermal pouch gives rise to** .....................

    a. Superior parathyroid           c. Inferior parathyroid

    b. Thyroid                         d. Thymus

**Answer: a**

50. **Ultimobranchial body gives rise to** .....................

    a. Follicular cells of thyroid       c. Stromal cells of thyroid

    b. Parafollicular cells of thyroid    d. Myoepithelial cells of thyroid

**Answer: b**

51. **Face develops from** .....................

    a. Frontonasal process and 1st arch    c. Frontonasal process only

    b. 1st and 2nd arch               d. 1st pharyngeal arch only

**Answer: a**

52. **Lower lip develops from** .....................

    a. Maxillary process            c. Nasal process

    b. Mandibular process          d. All of the above

**Answer: b**

53. **All contributes to the formation of upper lip except** .....................

    a. Maxillary process            c. Medial nasal process

    b. Lateral nasal process        d. Mandibular process

**Answer: d**

54. **Philtrum develops from** .....................

    a. Mandibular process          c. Frontonasal process

    b. Medial nasal process        d. Lateral nasal process

**Answer: c**

55. **Muscles of the face develop from** ..................... **branchial arch.**

    a. 1st                            c. 3rd

    b. 2nd                          d. 4th

**Answer: b**

56. **Harelip is due to non-fusion of** .....................

    a. Maxillary process with medial nasal process

    b. Mandibular process with medial nasal process

c. Maxillary process with lateral nasal process

d. Medial and lateral nasal process

57. **Oblique facial cleft is due to non-fusion of .....................**

a. Mandibular process with lateral nasal process

b. Maxillary process with the medial nasal process

c. Maxillary process with lateral nasal process

d. Mandibular process with medial nasal process

Answer: c

58. **Lateral wall of nose is derived from ....................**

a. Frontonasal process          c. Lateral nasal process

b. Medial nasal process         d. Maxillary process

Answer: c

59. **The paranasal sinus absent at birth is ....................**

a. Frontal                      c. Sphenoid

b. Maxillary                    d. All

Answer: a

60. **The paranasal sinus absent at birth is ....................**

a. Ethmoid                      c. Sphenoid

b. Maxillary                    d. All

Answer: a

61. **Sinuses rudimentary at birth are ....................**

a. Frontal and sphenoidal       c. Maxillary and sphenoidal

b. Frontal and ethmoidal        d. Maxillary and ethmoidal

Answer: c

62. **Palatine tonsils develop in relation to .................... pharyngeal pouch.**

a. 1st                          c. 3rd

b. 2nd                          d. 4th

Answer: b

63. **Artery of foregut is ....................**

a. Celiac                       c. Gastric

b. Superior mesenteric          d. Duodenal

Answer: a

64. **Artery of midgut is ....................**

a. Inferior mesenteric          c. Superior mesenteric

b. Celiac                       d. Duodenal

Answer: c

65. Artery of hindgut is .....................

    a. Inferior mesenteric
    b. Celiac
    c. Superior mesenteric
    d. Duodenal

    **Answer: a**

66. Rotation of midgut loop occurs between .....................

    a. 3rd and 8th week
    b. 5th and 10th week
    c. 4th and 6th week
    d. 2nd and 6th week

    **Answer: b**

67. Spleen develops in .....................

    a. Dorsal mesogastrium
    b. Ventral mesogastrium
    c. Midgut
    d. Foregut

    **Answer: a**

68. Arterial end of the heart tube is .....................

    a. Bulbus cordis
    b. Sinus venosus
    c. Ventricle
    d. Atria

    **Answer: a**

69. Annulus ovalis is the remnant of .....................

    a. Septum primum
    b. Septum secundum
    c. Foramen ovalis
    d. Foramen primum

    **Answer: b**

70. First arch artery remnant in adult life is .....................

    a. Facial artery
    b. Superior thyroid artery
    c. Maxillary artery
    d. Superficial temporal artery

    **Answer: c**

71. External carotid artery is a bud from ..................... arch artery.

    a. 1st
    b. 2nd
    c. 3rd
    d. 4th

    **Answer: c**

72. Axis artery of upper limb is .....................

    a. 1st intersegmental
    b. 4th intersegmental
    c. 7th intersegmental
    d. None

    **Answer: c**

73. Axis artery of lower limb is .....................

    a. 1st lumbar intersegmental
    b. 2nd lumbar intersegmental
    c. 4th lumbar intersegmental
    d. 5th lumbar intersegmental

    **Answer: d**

74. Ligamentum teres is the remnant of ....................
    a. Umbilical artery
    b. Right umbilical vein
    c. Left umbilical vein
    d. Ductus venosus

    **Answer: c**

75. A 2 months pregnant woman happens to get exposed to radiation; there is a risk of development of anomalies to the baby due to ....................
    a. Radiation is dangerous
    b. Exposure to radiation falls in period of organogenesis
    c. Genetic predisposition
    d. All the above

    **Answer: b**

# Embryology Models

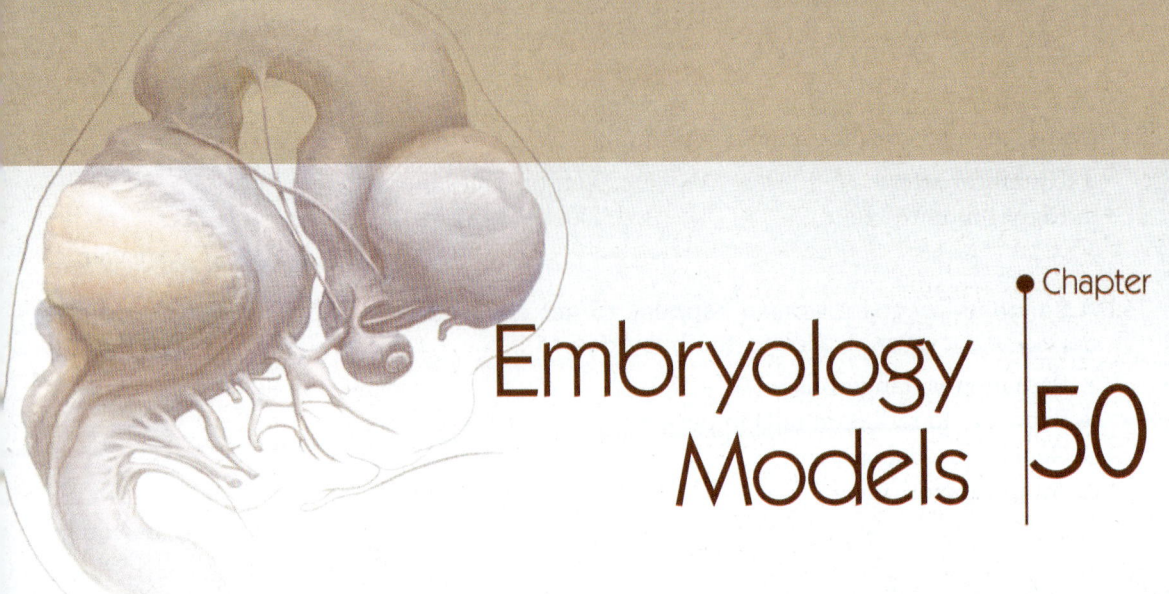

## 50

Following section will first have unlabeled model as kept in exam for practice purpose; and then labeled model, and related viva questions on each model.

## SPERMATOGENESIS

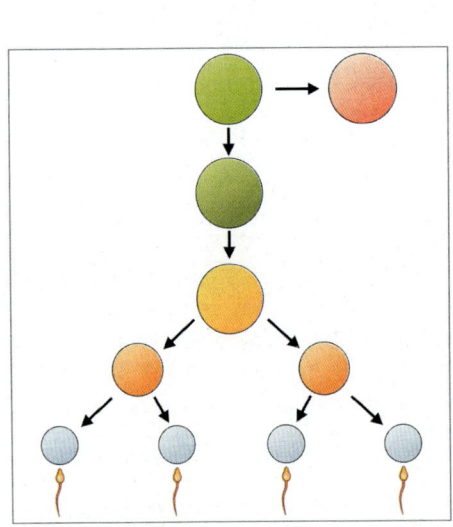

Spermatogenesis model unlabeled

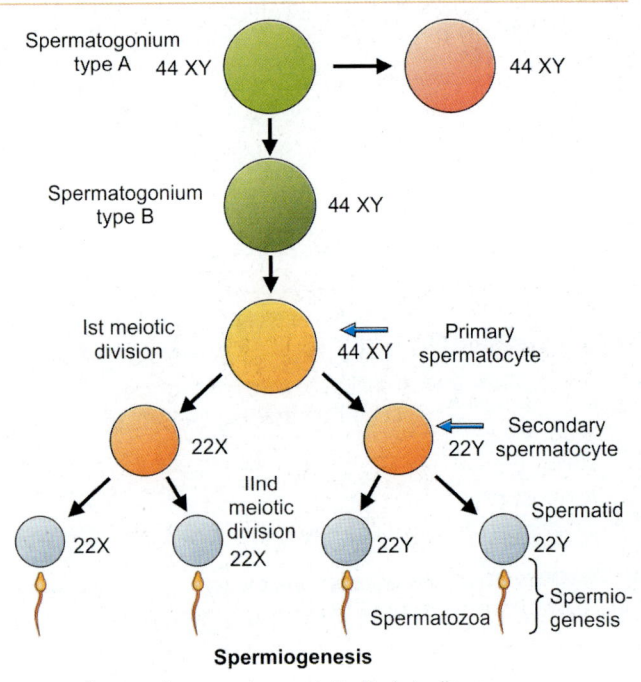

Spermatogenesis model with labelings

## Viva Questions

- **Type A**—spermatogonia are the germ cells giving rise to similar cells by dividing mitotically
- **Type B**—take origin from type A, and are bit large in size, give rise to primary spermatocyte
- **Primary spermatocyte**—undergo first meiotic division to form secondary spermatocyte
- **Secondary spermatocyte** is either 22X or 22Y, haploid number chromosome. It divides mitotically to give rise to spermatids
- **Spermatid** undergoes metamorphosis to form spermatozoa
- The transformation of spermatids to spermatozoa is known as spermiogenesis
- Spermatozoa arise from primordial germ cells.

## OOGENESIS

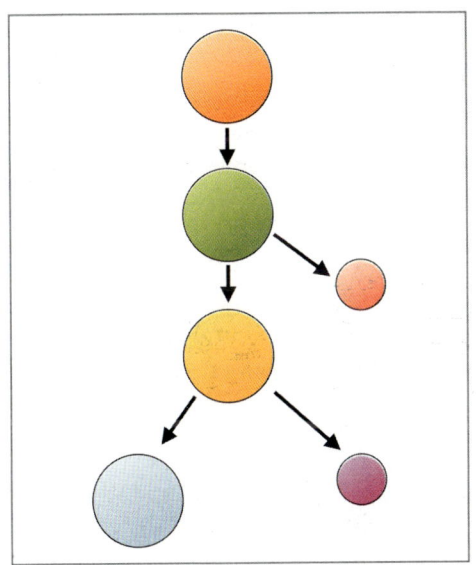

Oogenesis model unlabeled

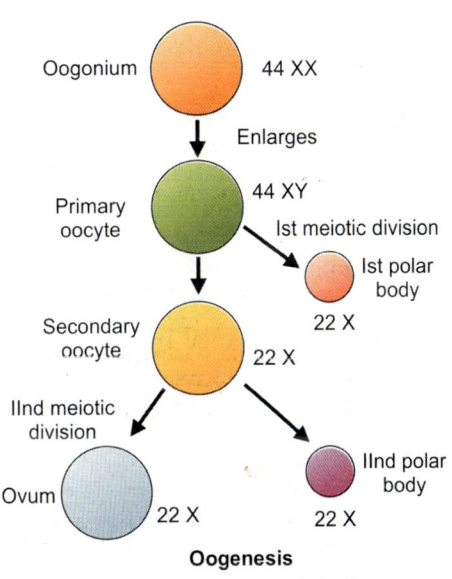

Oogenesis model with labelings

## Viva Questions

- Germ cells for oogenesis are **oogonia**
- Oogonia enlarges to form primary oocyte
- **Primary oocyte** undergoes first meiotic division to give rise to one secondary oocyte and polar body
- **Secondary oocyte** undergoes second meiotic division (=mitosis) to form ovum and second polar body
- Ova arise from primordial germ cells.

## SEX DETERMINATION

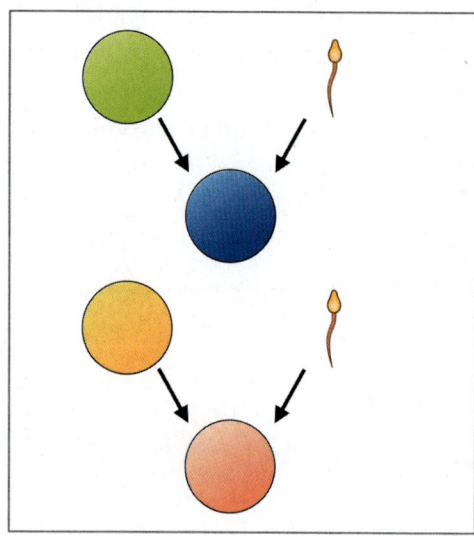

Sex-determination model unlabeled

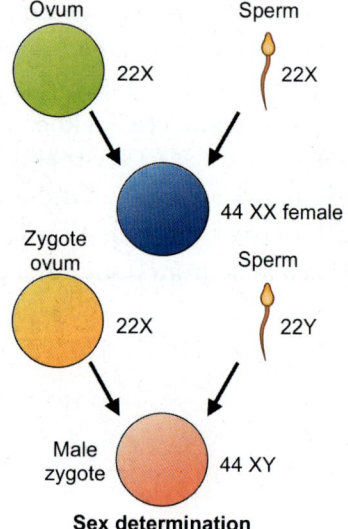

**Sex determination**

Sex determination model labeled

### Viva Questions

- All ova contain 22X, chromosomes
- Spermatozoa are of two types—22X, and 22Y chromosomes
- Sex of child is determined by what type of spermatozoa (X or Y) unites with ova (all X)
- If spermatozoa Y unites ova then male zygote is formed, while when spermatozoa X unites ova a female zygote is formed.

## MATURE SPERMATOZOA

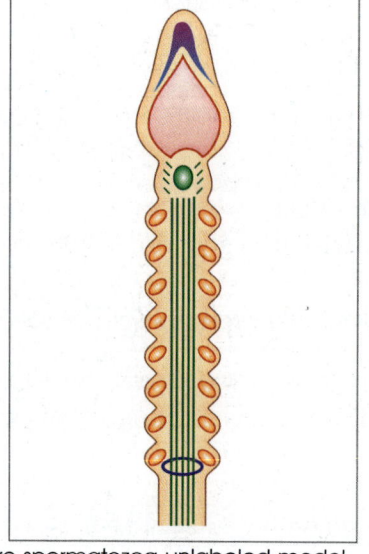

Mature spermatozoa unlabeled model

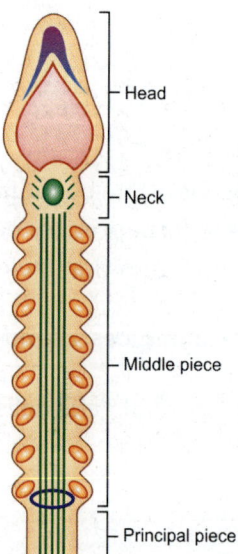

Mature spermatozoa labeled model

## Viva Questions

- Golgi apparatus of spermatid forms acrosomic cap
- Nucleus of spermatid forms head
- Mitochondria of spermatid form sheath of middle piece
- Proximal centriole of spermatid lies in the neck of spermatozoa
- Distal centriole forms the annulus of spermatozoa
- Centrioles have very crucial role in formation of sperm flagellum which gives motility to sperm thus helps in fertilization
- Spermatozoa acquires the capacity to fertilize the ovum only in the female genital tract, this final stage of maturation of spermatozoa is known as **capacitation** it lasts for 7 hours (appx).

## KARYOTYPE OF TRISOMY 21

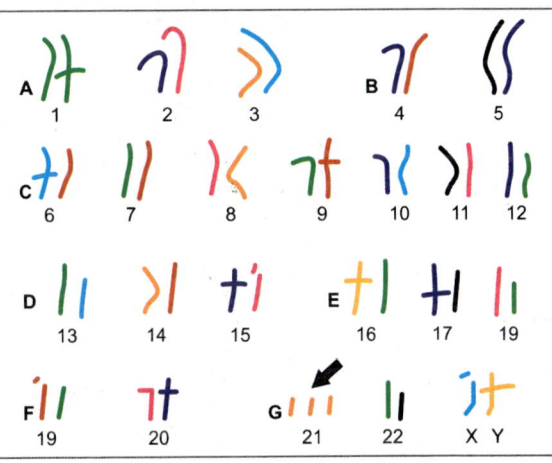

Down syndrome unlabeled model

Down syndrome labeled model

## Viva Question

- Down syndrome—Trisomy 21, characterised by flat, broad face, slanting palpebral fissures, epicanthus and furrowed lower lip.
- These children are mentally retarded, have simian crease, i.e. single palmar crease, often have congenital heart diseases.

## OVARIAN FOLLICLE FORMATION

## Viva Questions

- Some stromal cells get flattened and surround the oocyte, these are the follicular cells
- Follicular cells become columnar, and a well-defined membrane appears between the oocyte and stromal cells this is the **zona pellucida**
- Follicular cells proliferate vigorously to form multilayered, **membrana granulosa**, or granulosa cells
- Cavity appears within the membrana granulosa, known as follicular cavity
- Towards the final stage of development the cavity grows in size, oocyte comes to lie at a corner as shown in above diagram.

(study the diagram, and the labelings of mature Graffian follicle as shown in the figure)

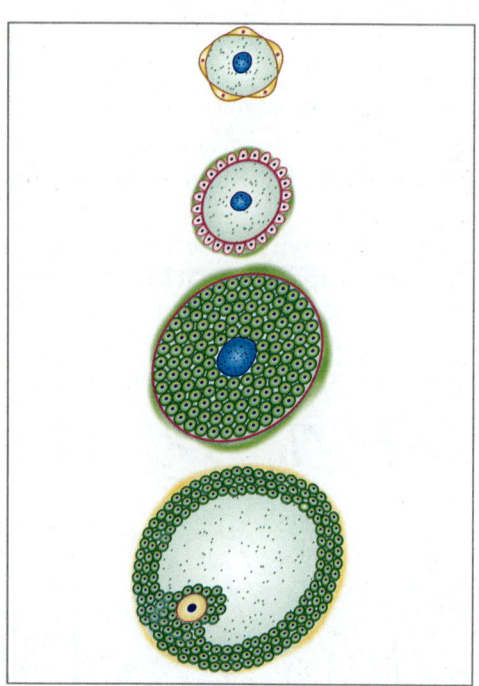

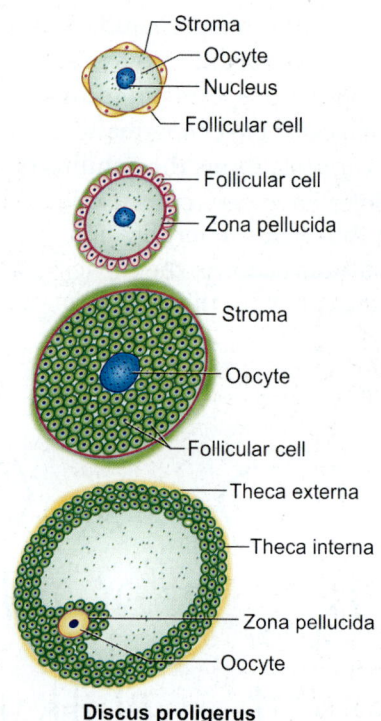

**Discus proligerus**

Ovarian follicle model unlabeled       Ovarian follicle model labeled

## UTERINE GLANDS AT VARIOUS STAGES OF MENSTRUAL CYCLE

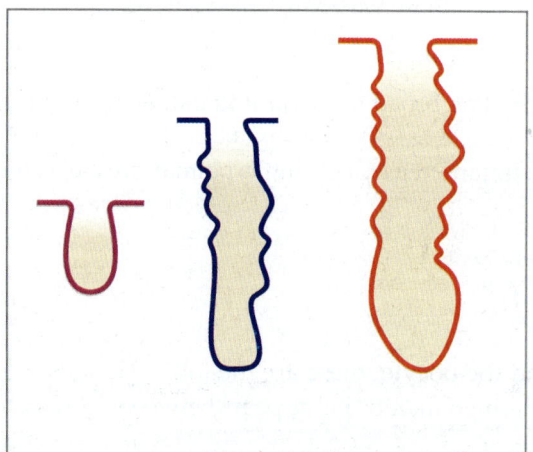

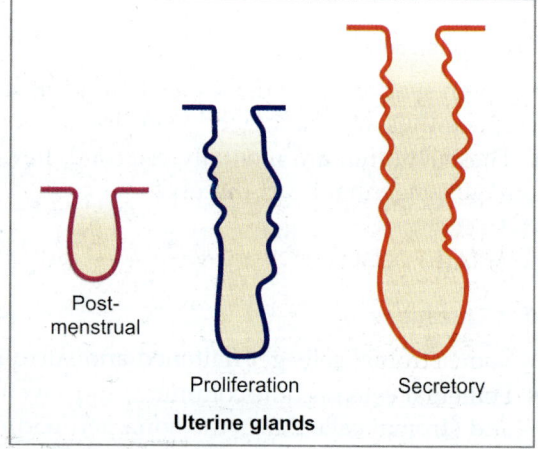

Post-menstrual

Proliferation          Secretory

**Uterine glands**

Unlabeled model          Labeled model

Uterine glands at various stages of menstruation

### Viva Question

Uterine glands grow in shape, size, get convoluted, saw-toothed during menstrual cycle.

## STAGES OF MENSTRUAL CYCLE

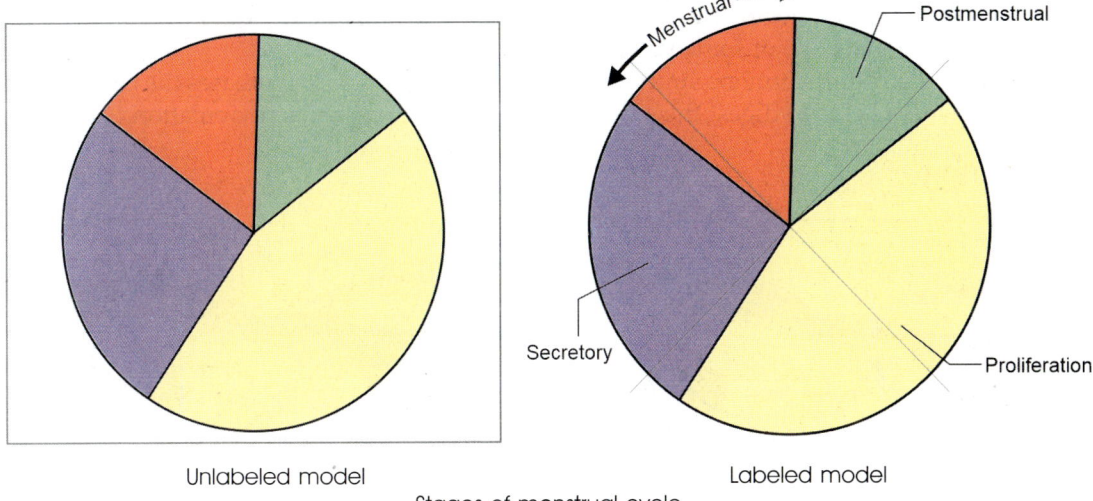

Unlabeled model        Labeled model

Stages of menstrual cycle

### Viva Questions

- Menstrual cycle is divided into—postmenstrual, proliferative, secretory, menstrual
- Cycle begins from the day of menstruation
- Ovulation takes place in mid of cycle, period between ovulation and next menstrual bleeding is constant it is 14 days
- Ova remain viable for 2 days, while sperm which have been deposited in the vaginal tract remain viable for 4 days. Fertilisation can occur 4 days prior to ovulation, to 2 days after ovulation. Remaining days chances of pregnancy are less. This is the **rhythm method of contraception**.

## INDICATORS OF OVULATION

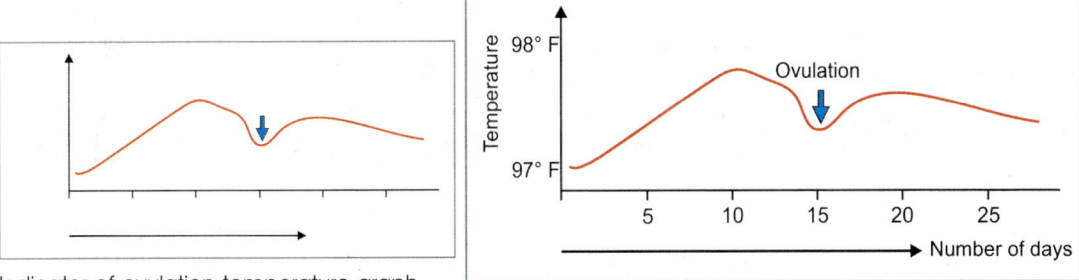

Indicator of ovulation temperature graph unlabeled model

Indicator of ovulation temperature graph labeled mode

### Viva Questions

- At the time of ovulation, a slight abdominal discomfort and pain in lower abdomen occurs almost during middle of menstrual cycle. This is known as middle pain, or **Mittelmertz syndrome** and is an indicator of ovulation. The oocyte is in second meiotic stage at the time of ovulation.

- If basal body temperature is monitored during menstrual cycle, there is initially fall and then rise in temperature (as shown in the graph) at the time of ovulation.
- In cases of infertility, doctor has to define whether it is an ovulatory or anovulatory cycle, these indicators may be of some value.
- There is a luteinising hormone spurt just prior to ovulation which increases the collagenase activity; which helps to digest the surrounding collagen and helps in ovulation.

## FERTILISATION

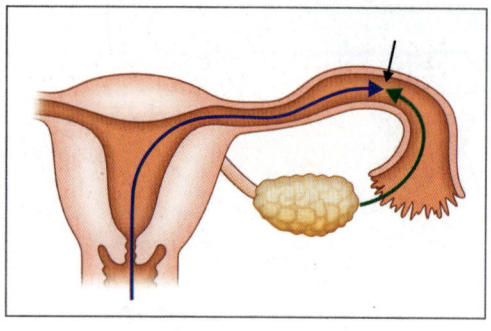

Site of fertilization unlabeled model

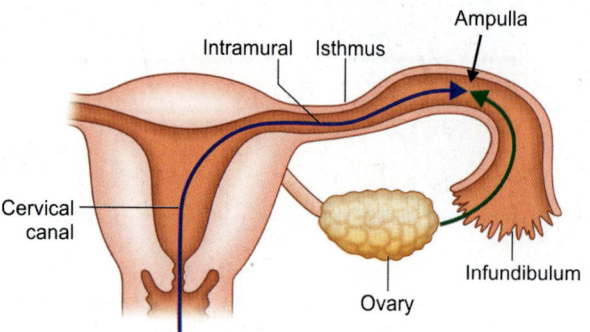

Site of fertilization labeled model

### Viva Questions

- Fusion of male and female gamete occurs in the ampulla of Fallopian tube, since it is the widest part of Fallopian tube.
- The spermatozoa, to fertilise the ovum has to penetrate corona radiata, zona pellucida and oocyte cell membrane. As the spermatozoa fertilises the oocyte, it completes the second meiotic division. Now further the zona pellucida is refractory to penetration by the spermatozoa.

## MORULA FORMATION

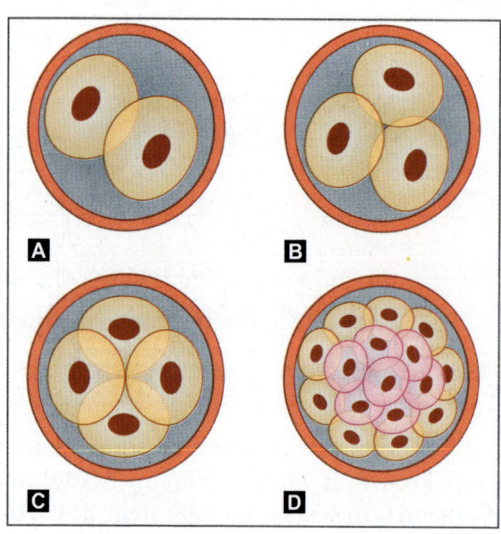

Morula formation unlabeled model

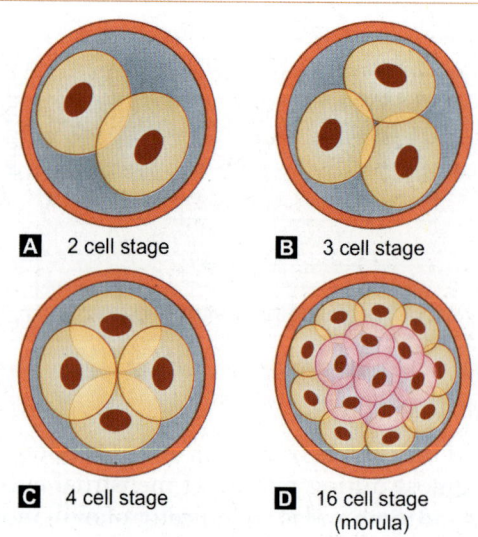

Morula formation labeled model

## Viva Questions

- 2-celled staged after fertilization undergoes repeated division, becomes 3-celled, 4-celled, and then sixteen cell stage, which is known as the morula stage. It is surrounded by zona pellucida
- Zona pellucida prevents the implantation of blastocyst at abnormal site of tube
- In section of morula, one can appreciate inner cell mass and neatly arranged outer layer of cells.

## BLASTOCYST FORMATION

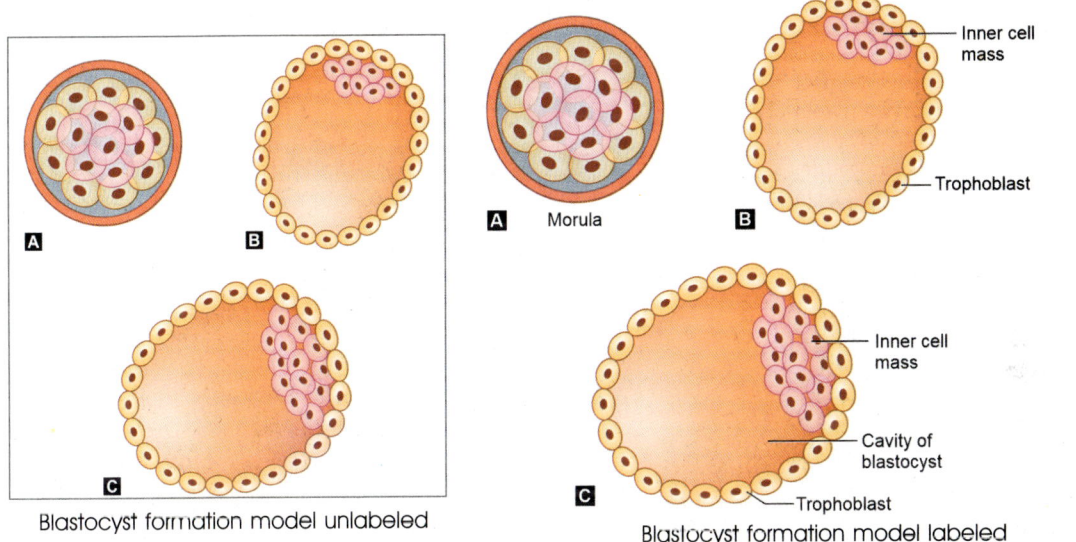

Blastocyst formation model unlabeled

Blastocyst formation model labeled

## Viva Questions

- Morula gets differentiated into inner cell mass and outer layer forming the trophoblast
- Fluid accumulates in the morula between the inner cell mass and the outer cell layer and now, the solid morula becomes cystic. Now, it is known as the blastocyst.

## BILAMINAR STAGE

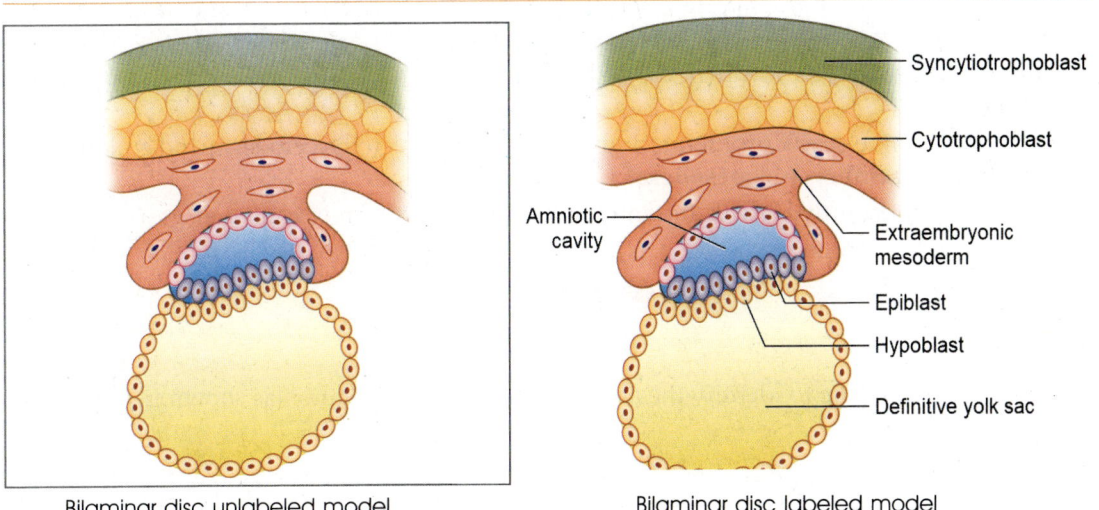

Bilaminar disc unlabeled model

Bilaminar disc labeled model

## Viva Questions

- Model shows a 2 weeks stage of blastocyst. The cells of inner cell mass differentiate into endoderm (Hypoblast) and ectoderm (Epiblast).
- **Second week is known as week of twos**, because trophoblast differentiates into cytotrophoblast and syncytiotrophoblast, endoderm and ectoderm two germ layers, extra-embryonic mesoderm splits into two layers somatopleuric and splanchnopleuric layers, and there are two cavities amniotic and yolk sac cavities.

## EMBRYONIC DISC

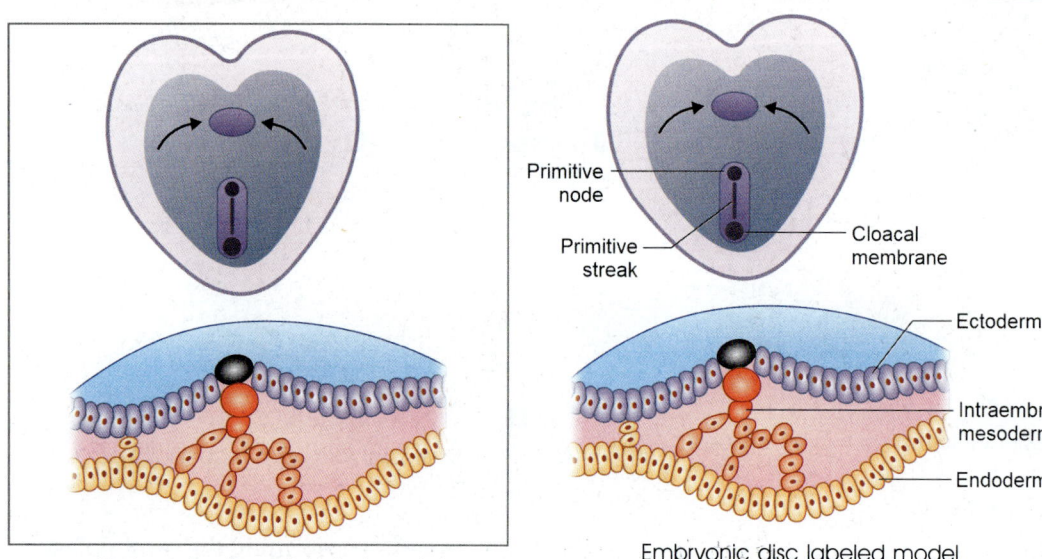

Embryonic disc unlabeled model

Embryonic disc labeled model

## Viva Questions

- Appearance of **prochordal plate** wherein, cubical cells of endoderm become columnar. This defines the embryonic axis, i.e. head end and tail end
- Few ectodermal cells towards the tail end begin to proliferate to form the **primitive streak**
- Cells of primitive streak proliferate and come to lie between the ectoderm and endoderm to form the **intraembryonic mesoderm**
- Formation of primitive streak and intraembryonic mesoderm is known as **gastrulation.**

## ECTOPIC SITES OF BLASTOCYST IMPLANTATION

## Viva Question

Student should be able to identify the abnormal sites of implantation as shown in the labeled model.

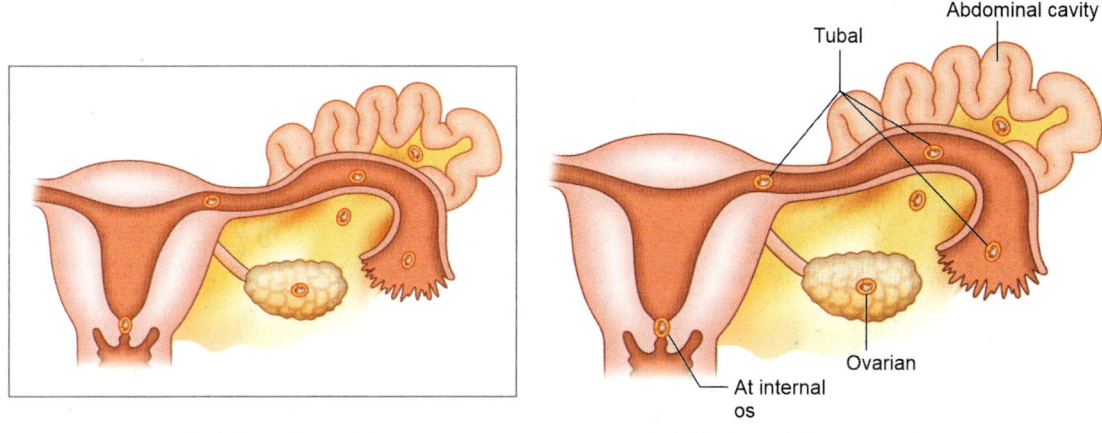

Ectopic sites of blastocyst implantation

Unlabeled model    Labeled model

## DEVELOPMENT OF VILLI

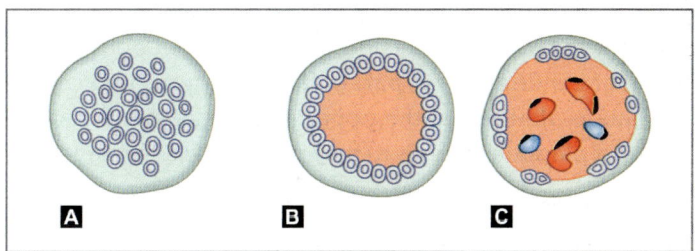

Development of villi unlabeled model

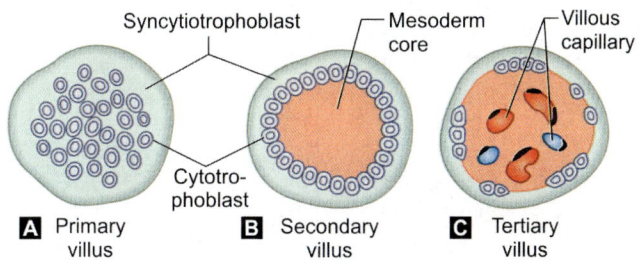

Development of villi labeled model

### Viva Questions

- During the third week, the trophoblast shows villi formation. Primary villi have a central core of cytotrophoblast covered by syncytiotrophoblast
- Secondary villi comprise of central core of mesoderm surrounded by cytotrophoblast and syncytiotrophoblast
- Blood vessels develop within the mesodermal core giving rise to the formation of tertiary villi, which are also surrounded by cytotrophoblast and syncytiotrophoblast.

## UTERINE SEGMENTS

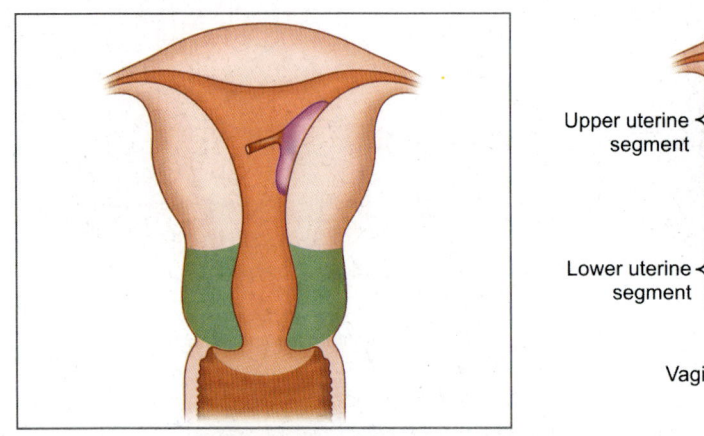
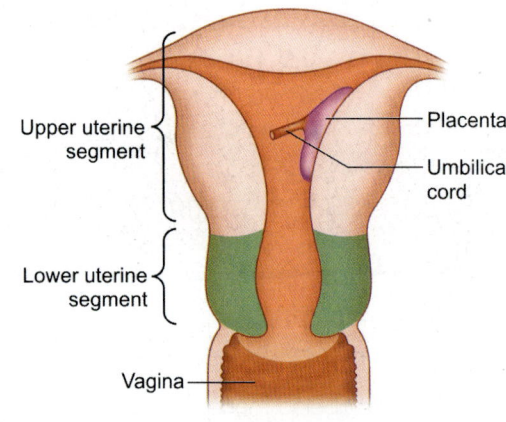

Unlabeled model        Labeled model

Upper and lower uterine segments

### Viva Questions

- Upper uterine segment includes fundus and greater parts of body of uterus
- Lower uterine segment includes lower part of body of uterus and cervix
- Normally, the placenta is attached to the upper uterine segment
- When the attachment of placenta extends to the lower uterine segment it is known as placenta previa.

## TYPES OF PLACENTA PREVIA

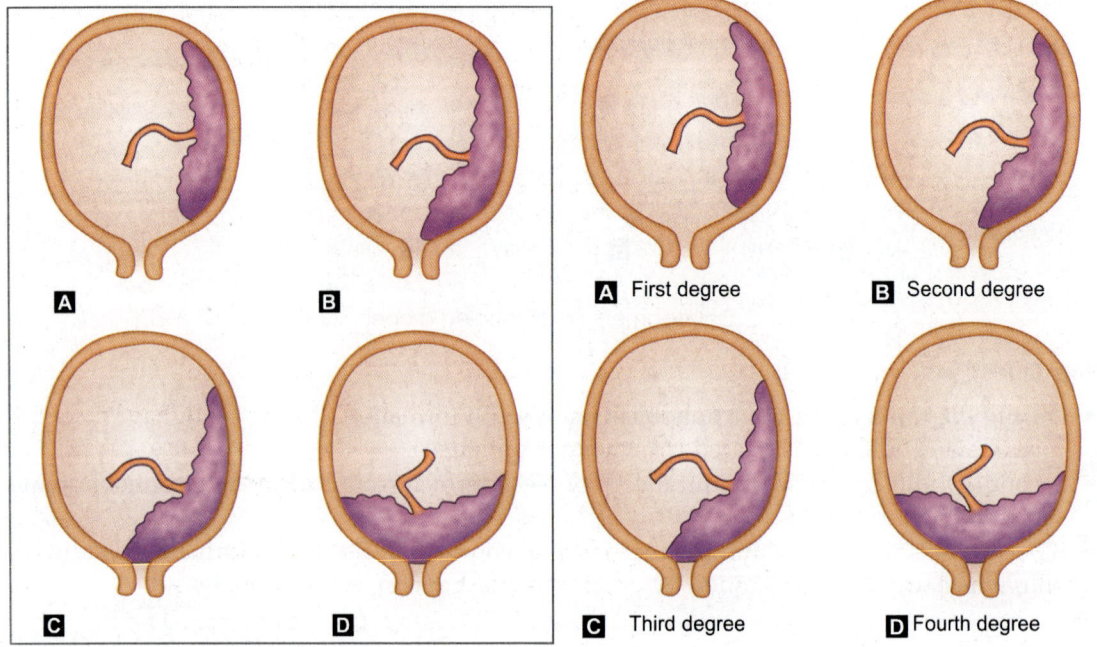

Unlabeled model        Labeled model

Types of placenta previa

## Viva Questions

- Attachment of placenta extends to lower uterine segment, but does not reach the internal os—this is first degree placenta previa
- When the placenta reaches the internal os but does not cover it—this is second degree placenta previa
- Placenta covers the os when it is closed, but when it dilates it does not close it. This is third degree
- When the placenta completely covers the os even after dilatation. This is fourth degree placenta previa.

## PLACENTAL ANOMALIES

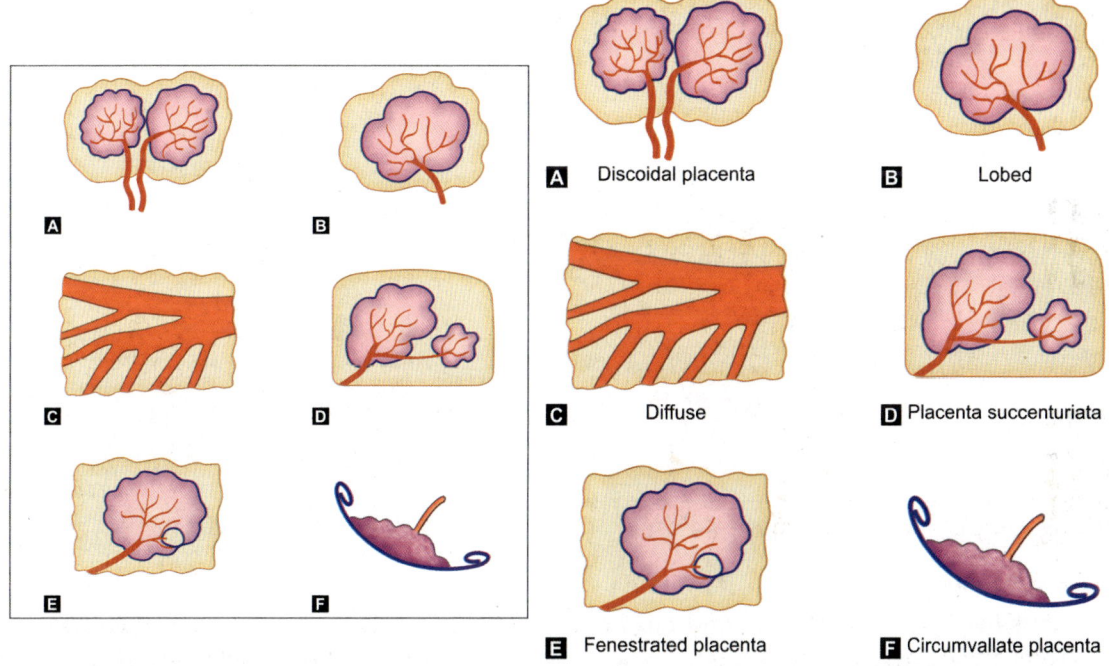

Anomalies of placenta unlabeled model

A  Discoidal placenta  B  Lobed

C  Diffuse  D  Placenta succenturiata

E  Fenestrated placenta  F  Circumvallate placenta

Anomalies of placenta labeled model

## VARIATIONS IN THE ATTACHMENT OF UMBILICAL CORD

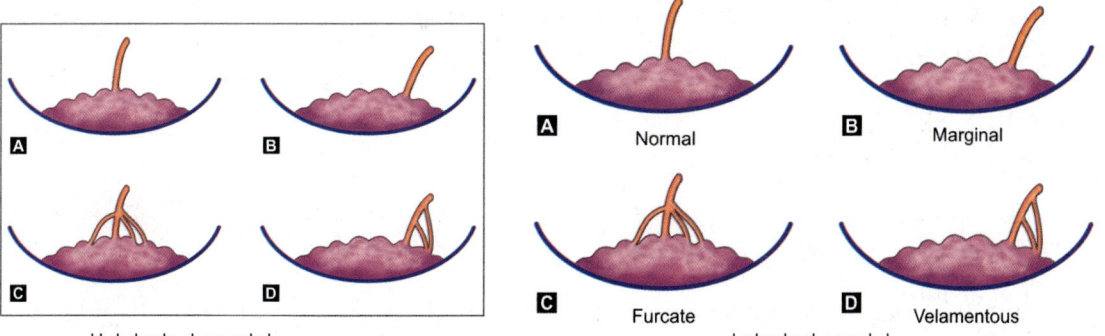

Unlabeled model

A  Normal  B  Marginal

C  Furcate  D  Velamentous

Labeled model

Variations in attachment of umbilical cord

## FOLDING OF EMBRYO

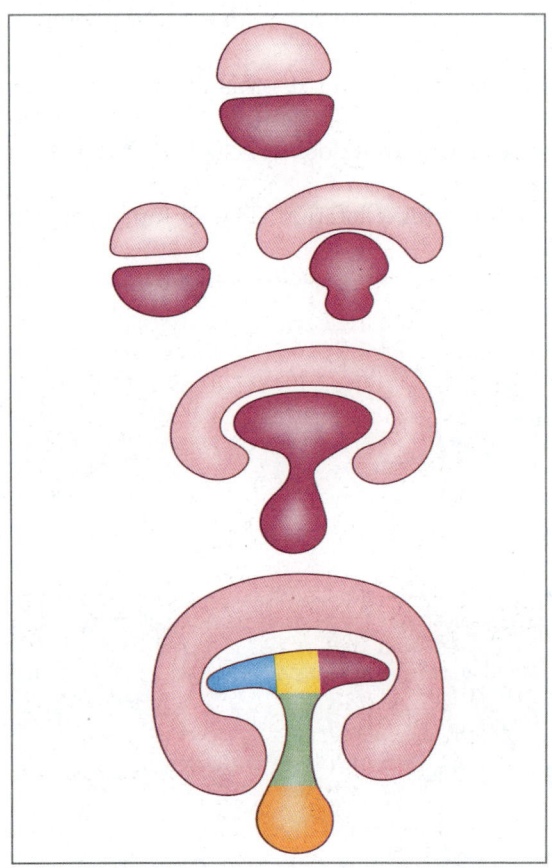

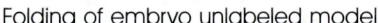

Folding of embryo unlabeled model

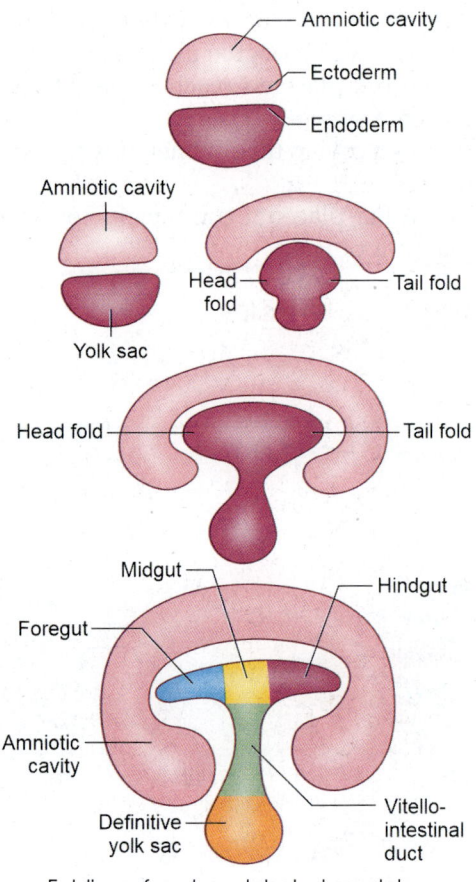

Folding of embryo labeled model

### Viva Questions

- After the formation of head and tail folds the yolk sac gets enclosed within the embryo. Thus, the embryo assumes tubular shape forming the so-called **primitive gut.**
- The primitive gut freely communicates with the yolk sac to begin with. Part of the gut proximal to this communication is foregut, part distal to this communication is hindgut and the part in between is midgut.
- The narrow communicating channel between the yolk sac and the primitive gut is the vitello-intestinal duct.

## ALLANTOIC DIVERTICULUM

### Viva Questions

- Before the formation of the tail fold, a small endodermal diverticulum arises from the caudal end of yolk sac. This diverticulum grows into the mesoderm of yolk sac. This is the allantoic diverticulum.
- Allantois forms the primitive urogenital sinus which gives rise to urinary bladder and urethra.

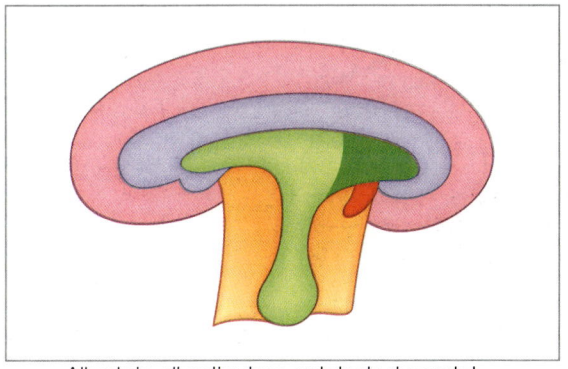

Allantoic diverticulum unlabeled model

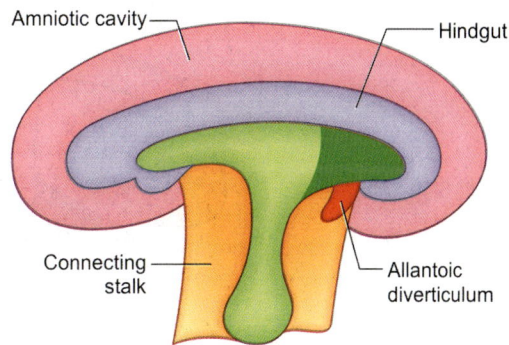

Amniotic cavity · Hindgut

Connecting stalk · Allantoic diverticulum

Allantoic diverticulum labeled model

## INTRAEMBRYONIC MESODERM

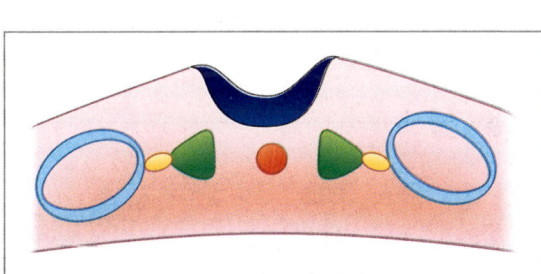

Unlabeled model

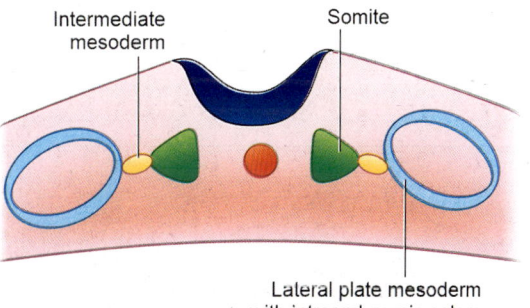

Intermediate mesoderm · Somite

Lateral plate mesoderm with intraembryonic celom

Labeled model

Subdivisions of intraembryonic mesoderm

### Viva Questions

- Paraaxial mesoderm gets segmented to form somites.
- Intraembryonic celom develops within the lateral plate mesoderm.
- Intermediate mesoderm gives rise to urogenital system.

## FATE OF SOMITES

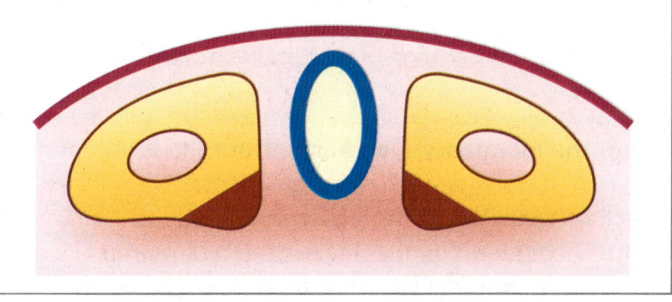

Subdivisions of somites unlabeled model

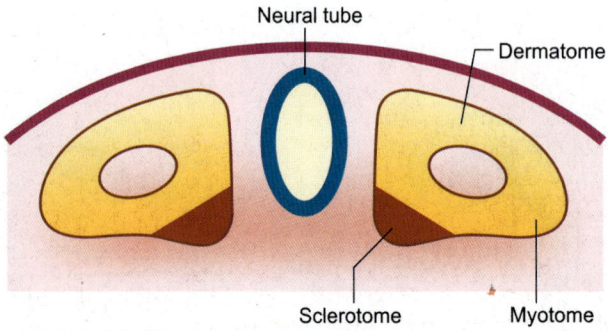

Subdivisions of somites labeled model

## Viva Questions

- The somites subdivide into three portions—sclerotome, dermatome and myotome.
- Sclerotome surround the neural tube and further develop into vertebral column and ribs.
- Dermatome gives rise to dermis of the skin and subcutaneous tissue.
- Myotome gives rise to striated muscles of the body.

## DEVELOPMENT OF MAMMARY GLAND

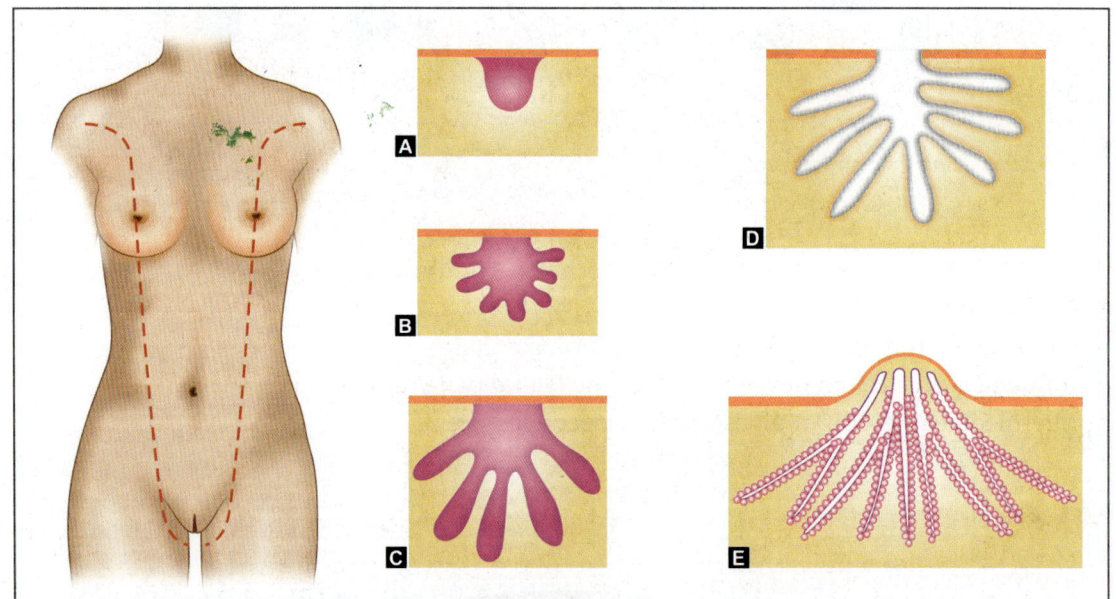

Development of mammary gland—unlabeled model

## Viva Questions

- Secretory elements of the mammary gland arise from the terminal parts of the epidermal outgrowths.
- Proximal part of each outgrowths forms lactiferous duct.
- Several anomalies are encountered in the development of mammary gland like—absence of gland (amastia), absent nipple (athelia), supernumerary nipples may be present along the milk line (polythelia, polymastia), accessory breast, inverted nipple, micro- or macro-mastia.

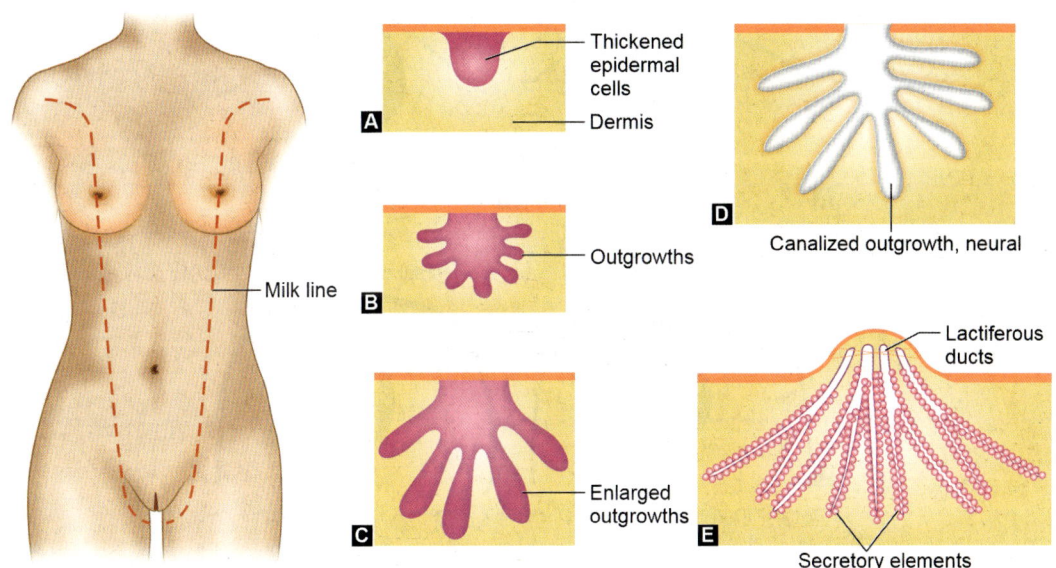

Development of mammary gland—labeled model

## FORMATION AND MIGRATION OF NEURAL CREST CELLS

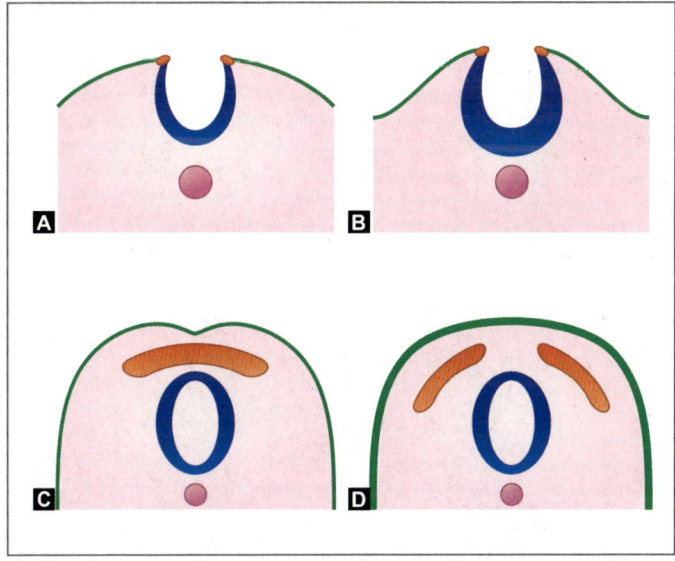

Formation and migration of neural crest cells unlabeled model

### Viva Question

Neural crest derivatives are—connective tissue, bones of the face and skull, cranial nerve ganglia, C cells of thyroid gland, cono-truncal septum of the heart, odontoblasts, dermis in face and neck, spinal ganglia, sympathetic chain and preaortic ganglia, parasympathetic ganglia of gastrointestinal tract, adrenal medulla, Schwann cells, glial cells, arachnoid and pia mater, melanocytes.

Neural crest

Neural groove

**A**

Notochord

**B**

Neural crest

Dorsal root ganglion

**C**

**D**

Formation and migration of neural crest cells labeled model

## FORMATION OF PHARYNGEAL ARCHES

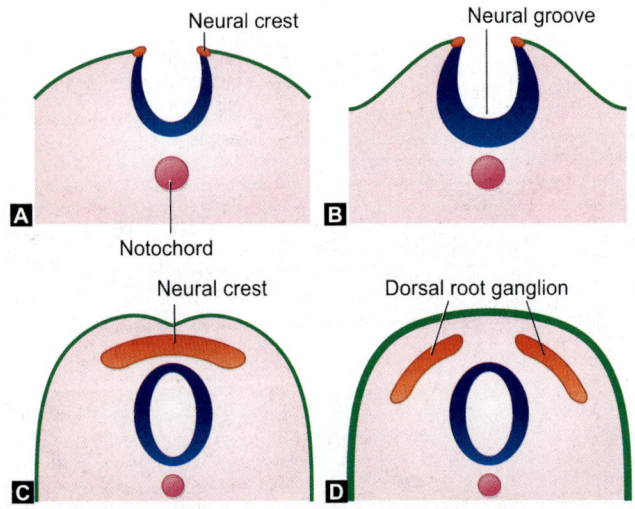

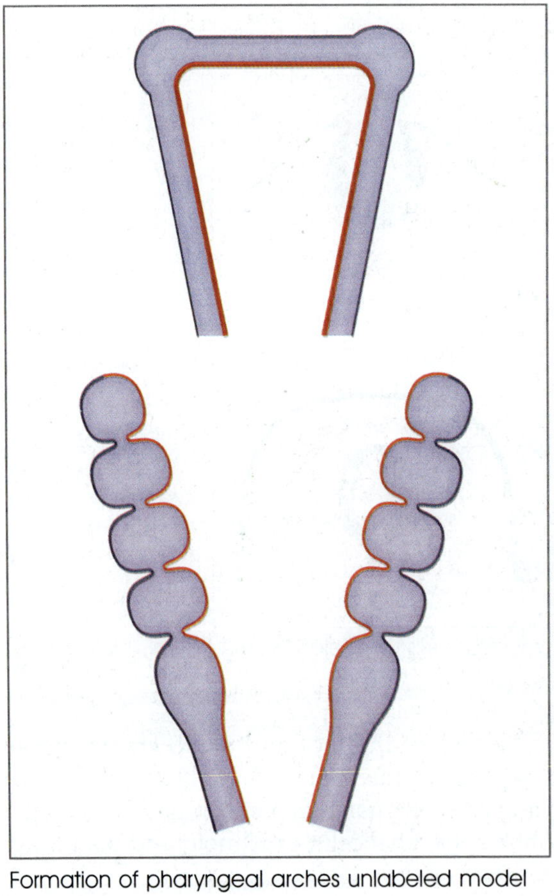

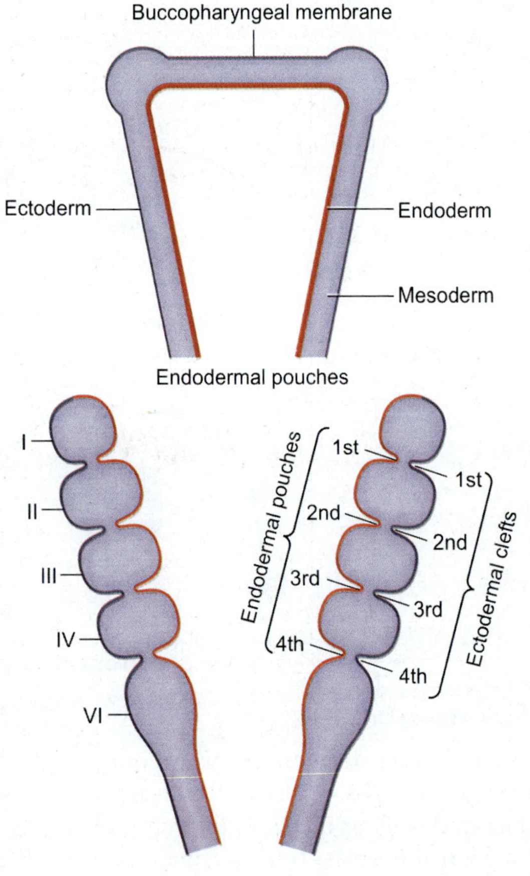

Buccopharyngeal membrane

Ectoderm

Endoderm

Mesoderm

Endodermal pouches

I

II

III

IV

VI

Endodermal pouches

1st

2nd

3rd

4th

1st

2nd

3rd

4th

Ectodermal clefts

Formation of pharyngeal arches unlabeled model

Formation of pharyngeal arches labeled model

## Viva Questions

- There are 5 pharyngeal arches. First arch also known as **mandibular arch**, and second arch known as hyoid arch, fifth arch disappears. Each arch has ectodermal cleft and endodermal pouch and intervening mesoderm.

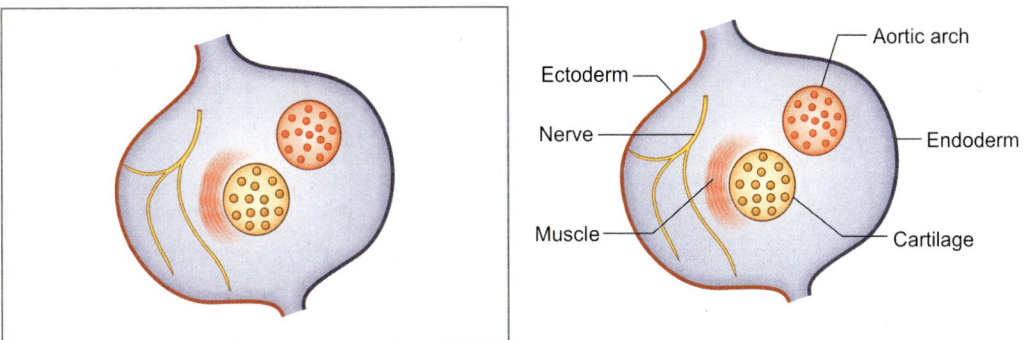

Pharyngeal arch elements (diagram)

- Mesodermal elements comprise of cartilage, nerve, artery. Each arch has its own cartilage, muscle and nerve supply.
- Nerve of arch is known as post-trematic, it lies along the cranial border of arch. Each arch also receives a branch from the succeeding arch, it lies caudally this is pretrematic nerve. First arch post-trematic nerve is mandibular nerve while the chorda tympani nerve is the pretrematic nerve.
- Nerve of first arch is mandibular, second is facial, third is glossopharyngeal, fourth arch is superior laryngeal and sixth arch is recurrent laryngeal

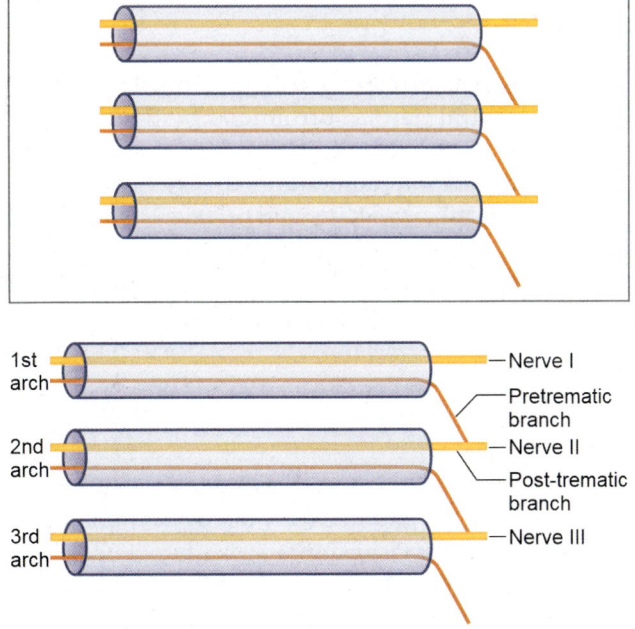

Nerve pattern in pharyngeal arches (diagram)

# FATE OF CARTILAGES OF PHARYNGEAL ARCHES

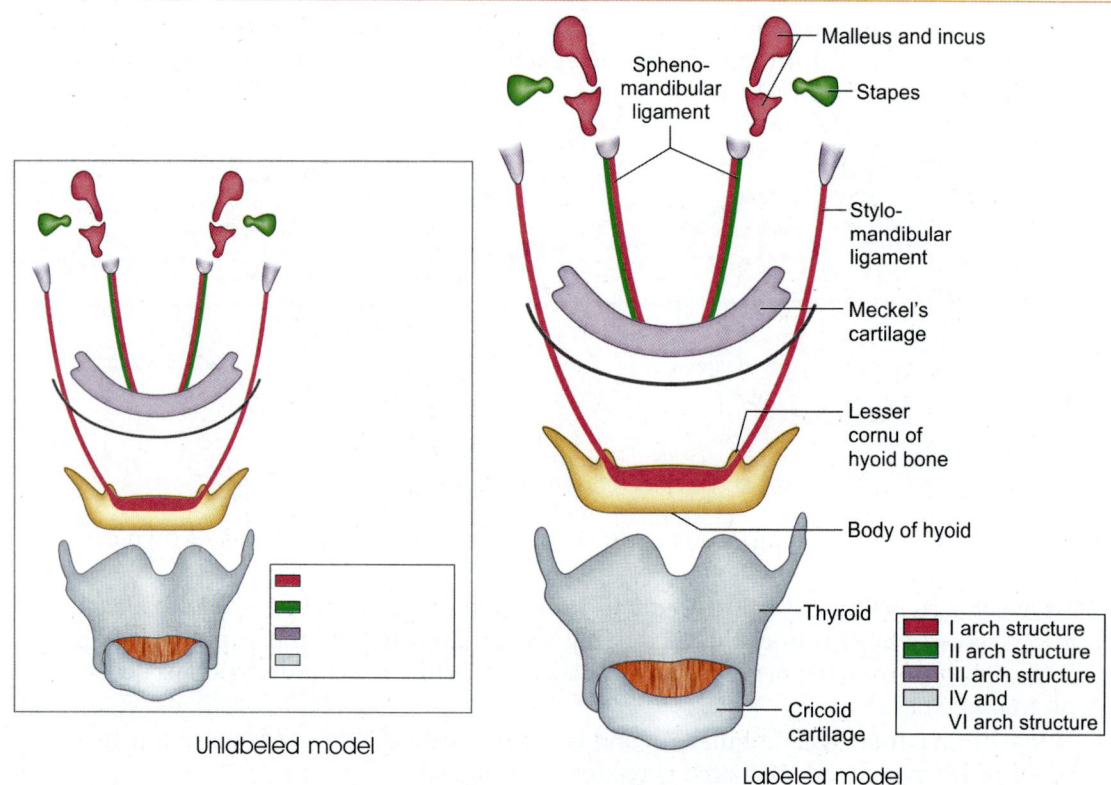

Unlabeled model

Malleus and incus

Spheno-
mandibular
ligament

Stapes

Stylo-
mandibular
ligament

Meckel's
cartilage

Lesser
cornu of
hyoid bone

Body of hyoid

Thyroid

Cricoid
cartilage

Labeled model

| | I arch structure |
| | II arch structure |
| | III arch structure |
| | IV and VI arch structure |

Fate of cartilages of pharyngeal arches

## Viva Questions

- Cartilage of first arch is known as Meckel's cartilage. Dorsal end of Meckel's cartilage gives rise to malleus and incus, ventral part is surrounded by the developing mandible. Part of cartilage between the ear and mandible remains in the form of sheath which gives rise to anterior ligament of malleus and sphenomandibular ligament.
- Second arch cartilage gives rise to—stapes, styloid process, stylohyoid ligament, lesser cornu of hyoid bone, superior part of body of hyoid bone.
- Third arch gives rise to greater cornu and lower part of hyoid bone.
- Fourth and fifth cartilages give rise to laryngeal cartilages.

## CERVICAL SINUS

## Viva Questions

- Growth rate of second pharyngeal arch is very rapid, as a result of which it overhangs the third, fourth and fifth arches. This gap between the overhanging part of second arch and the other arches is known as the cervical sinus.
- Normally, the cervical sinus gets obliterated, occasionally it may persist in the form of nodular swellings along the anterior border of sternocleidomastoid. These swellings are known as branchial cysts; if it has a communication with the skin it is termed branchial sinus.

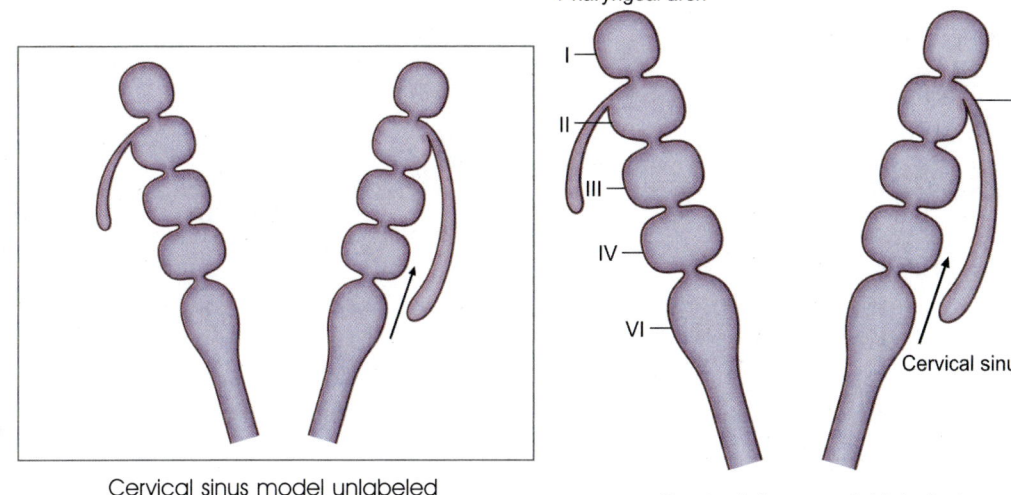

Pharyngeal arch

I
II
III
IV
VI

Cervical sinus model unlabeled

Projection of II arch

Cervical sinus

Cervical sinus model labeled

## FATE OF PHARYNGEAL POUCHES

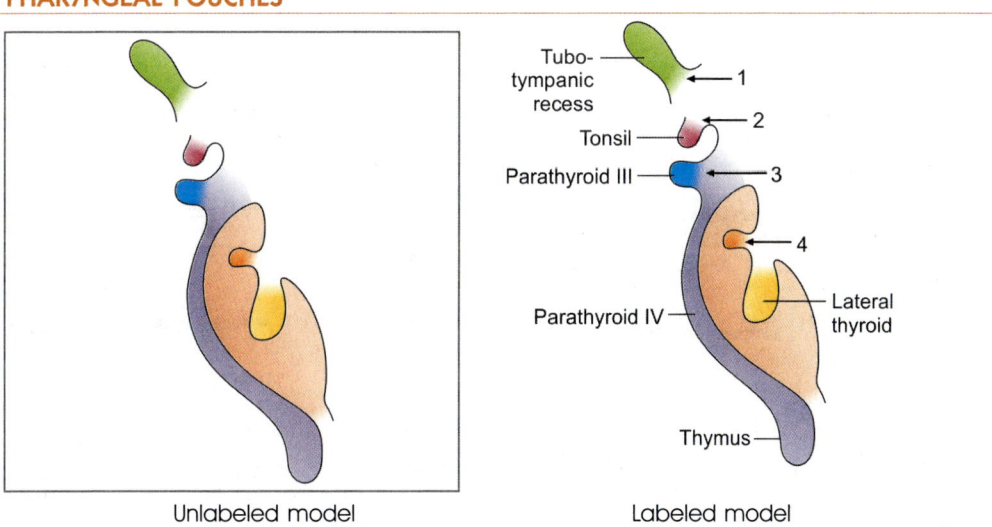

Unlabeled model

Tubo-
tympanic
recess — 1
— 2
Tonsil — 
Parathyroid III — 3
— 4
Parathyroid IV — 
Lateral thyroid
Thymus — 

Labeled model

## Viva Questions

- Dorsal part of first and second pouch form the tubotympanic recess. Proximal part of tubotympanic recess gives rise to auditory tube while the distal part gives rise to middle ear cavity.
- Ventral part of second pouch takes part in formation of tonsil
- Third pouch gives rise to inferior parathyroid gland and thymus
- Fourth pouch gives rise to superior parathyroid gland
- Fifth pouch also known as ultimobranchial arch gives rise to parafollicular cells of the thyroid gland.

## FATE OF THIRD AND FOURTH POUCH

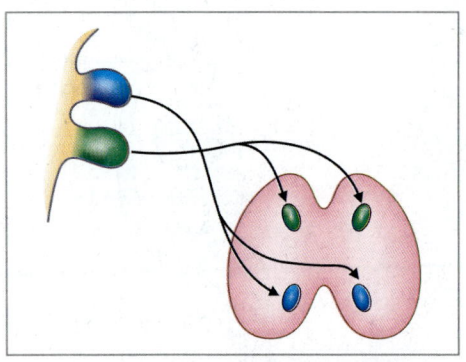

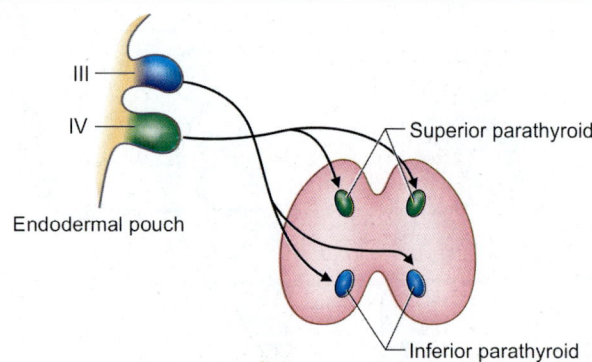

Fate of 3rd and 4th pouch, unlabeled model

Fate of 3rd and 4th pouch, labeled model

### Viva Questions

- Fourth endodermal pouch gives rise to superior parathyroid gland
- Third endodermal pouch gives rise to inferior parathyroid gland and thymus.

## DEVELOPMENT OF THYROID GLAND

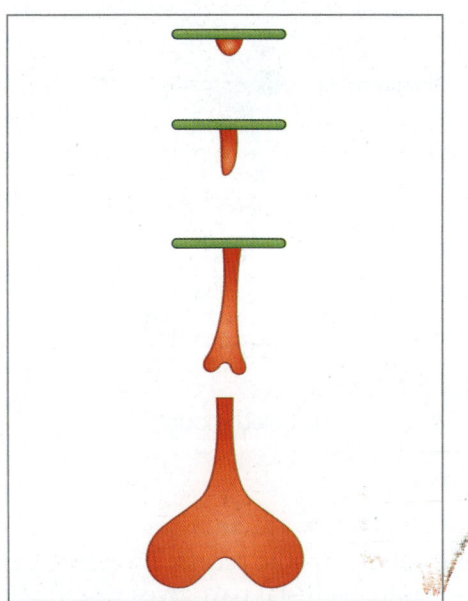

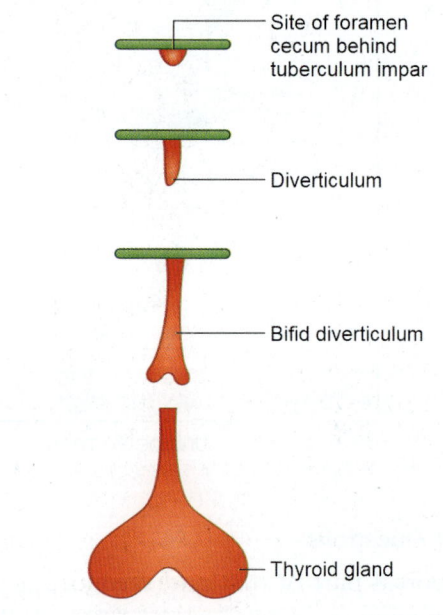

Development of thyroid gland unlabeled model

Development of thyroid gland labeled model

### Viva questions

- A midline swelling appears within the floor of mandibular arch, this is known as tuberculum impar. Just behind this swelling a thickening appears which soon depresses within itself, the depressed site known as foramen cecum.

- The diverticulum grows downwards in the neck, which soon bifurcates. This gives rise to the lobes of thyroid gland.
- When this developing lobe comes in contact with the ultimobranchial arch the para-follicular cells are formed.

## ECTOPIC SITES OF THYROID GLAND

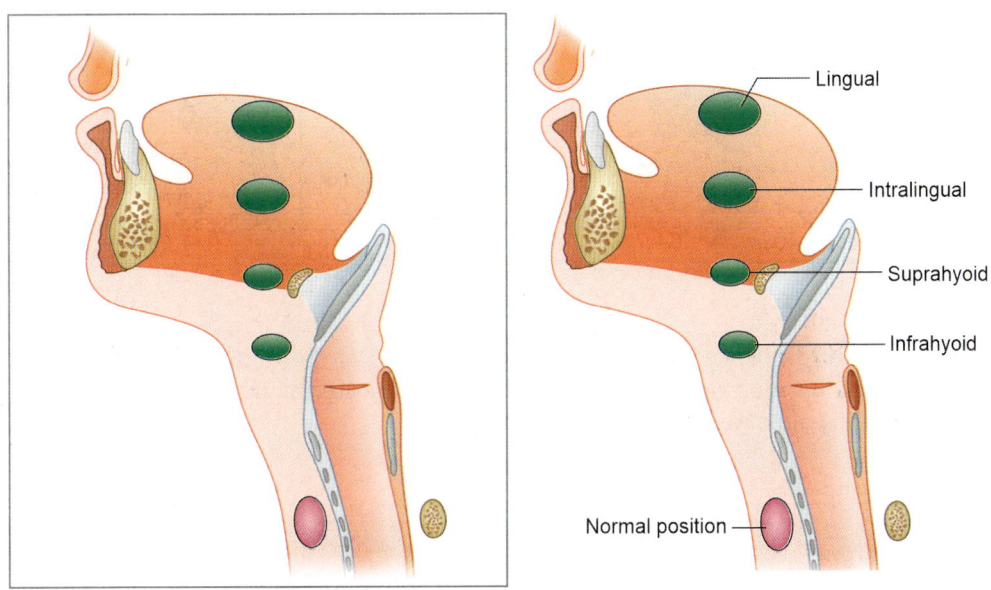

Lingual

Intralingual

Suprahyoid

Infrahyoid

Normal position

Unlabeled model                    Labeled model
Model of ectopic sites of thyroid gland

### Viva Questions

- The model depicts the path of thyroglossal duct follows. The thyroid gland may be encountered anywhere in the path, e.g. on the surface of tongue, within the tongue, above the hyoid bone, below the hyoid bone.
- Thyroglossal cyst may occur anywhere along the path. If the cyst communicates with the skin it is known as thyroglossal fistula.
- While operating on the thyroglossal cyst or fistula. All the remnants of the tract need to be excised.

## DEVELOPMENT OF TONGUE

### Viva Questions

- Medial most parts of mandibular arch proliferate to form lingual swellings, there is also another swelling in between the lingual swelling, this is the tuberculum impar.
- Against the medial end of the 2nd, 3rd, and 4th arch another swelling appears, this is known as hypobranchial eminence.
- Anterior two-thirds of the tongue is formed from tuberculum impar and lingual swellings, while the posterior one-third is formed from cranial part of hypobranchial eminence.

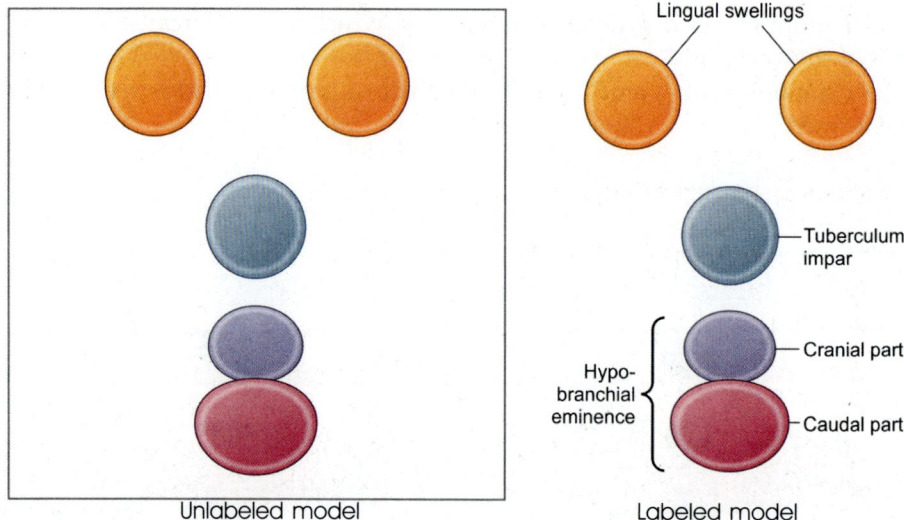

Development of tongue

- Anterior two-thirds nerve supply is lingual and chorda tympani nerve, while posterior 1/3rd supplied by glossopharyngeal nerve and the posterior most part of the tongue is supplied by the vagus nerve.

## DEVELOPMENT OF FACE

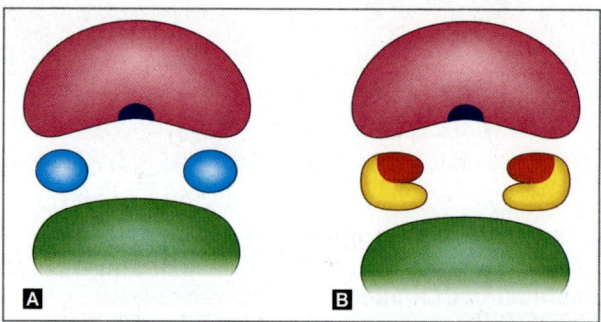

Development of face unlabeled model

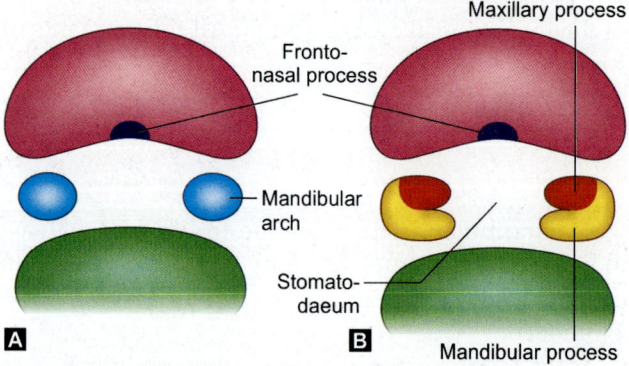

Development of face labeled model

## Viva Questions

- Face develops from frontonasal process and mandibular arch which forms the lateral wall of stomatodaeum.
- Mandibular arch gives off dorsal bud maxillary process and rest cranial part is the mandibular process.

## DEVELOPMENT OF LIPS

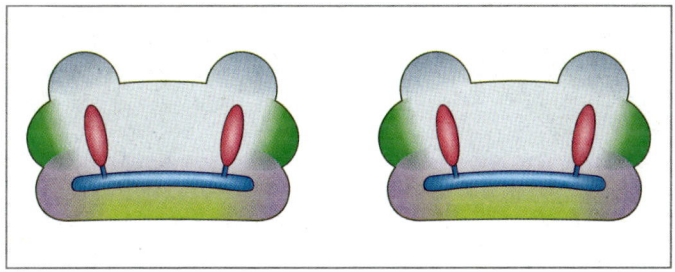

Development of lips unlabeled model

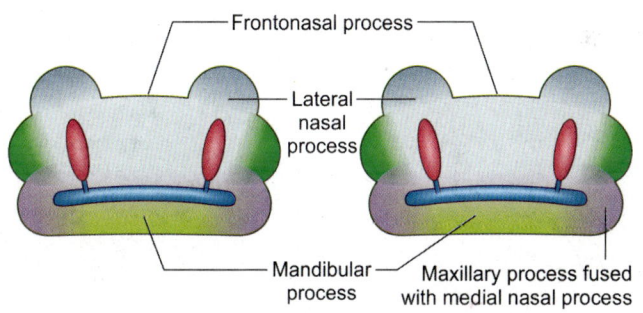

Development of lips labeled model

## Viva Questions

- Lower lip formed by the fusion of mandibular processes, while the upper lip is formed by fusion of maxillary process and frontonasal process.
- Deeper part of frontonasal process forms the septum, muscles of face develop from mesoderm of second branchial arch.
- Non-fusion of maxillary process with lateral nasal process gives rise to oblique facial cleft.
- Failure of fusion of maxillary process with the medial nasal process leads to defects in upper lip.

## DEVELOPMENT OF PALATE

## Viva Questions

- Primitive palate is formed from the frontonasal process and the remaining palate from the palatal process which is a part of maxillary process.
- The two palatal processes fuse with each other in midline.
- Mesoderm in the palate undergoes intramembranous ossification giving rise to hard palate. The ossification does not extend posteriorly thus forming the soft palate.

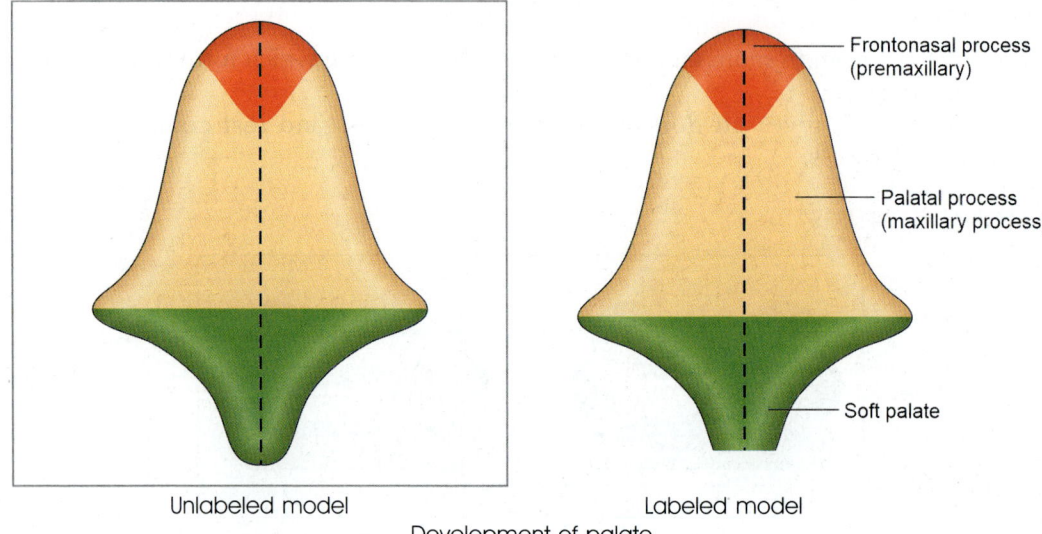

Unlabeled model    Labeled model

Frontonasal process
(premaxillary)

Palatal process
(maxillary process)

Soft palate

Development of palate

## PARTS OF PRIMITIVE GUT

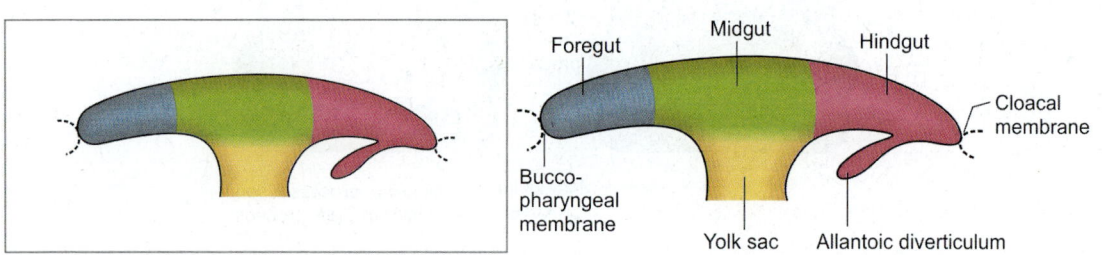

Parts of primitive gut unlabeled model

Parts of primitive gut labeled model

Foregut    Midgut    Hindgut

Bucco-
pharyngeal
membrane

Yolk sac    Allantoic diverticulum

Cloacal
membrane

### Viva Questions

- After the formation of head and tail fold the yolk sac gets well within the embryo forming the primitive gut. This is in communication with the yolk sac.
- Gut proximal to communication is foregut, while distal to it is hindgut and the intermediate part is the midgut.
- Artery of foregut is celiac, that of midgut is superior mesenteric while hindgut is inferior mesenteric.

## MIDGUT LOOP FORMATION

### Viva Questions

- The primitive gut enlarges and at the same time the communication with the yolk sac narrows thus it assumes a shape of loop forming the midgut loop.
- Superior mesenteric artery forms the axis of the midgut for the rotation of the gut.

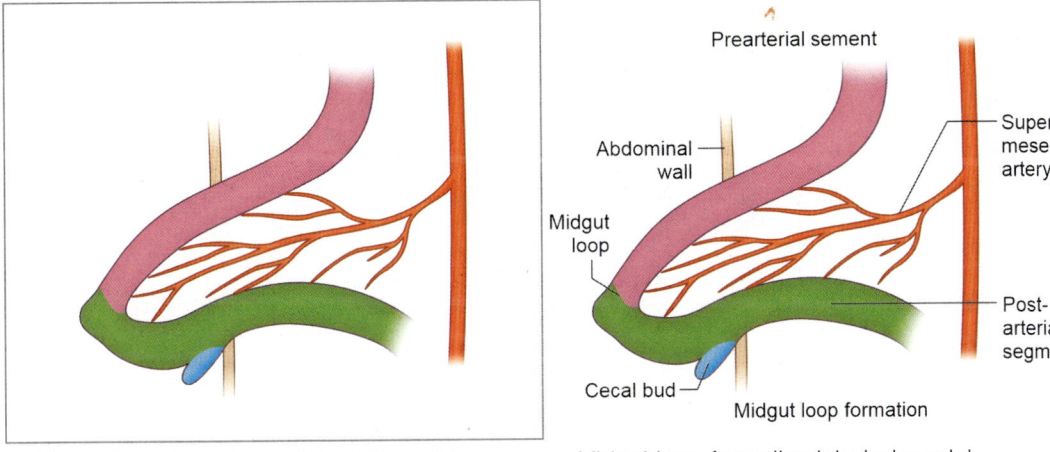

Midgut loop formation unlabeled model          Midgut loop formation labeled model

## CLOACAL SUBDIVISIONS

### Viva Questions

- Student should be able to identify the urorectal septum, ventral division of cloaca is primitive urogenital sinus and the dorsal part is primitive rectum.
- Primitive urogenital sinus forms the urogenital system while the primitive rectum forms the rectum and anal canal.

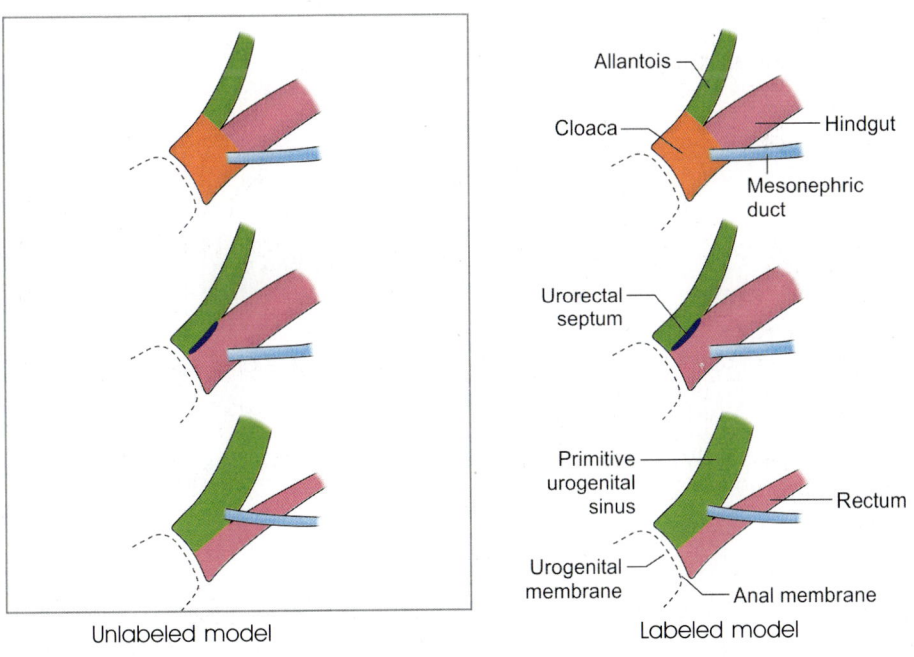

Subdivisions of cloaca

## DEVELOPMENT OF CECUM AND APPENDIX

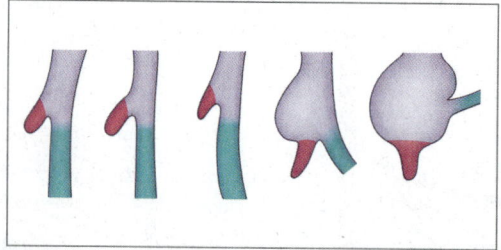

Development of cecum and appendix unlabeled model

### Viva Question

Cecal bud is an outgrowth from the postarterial segment of midgut loop.

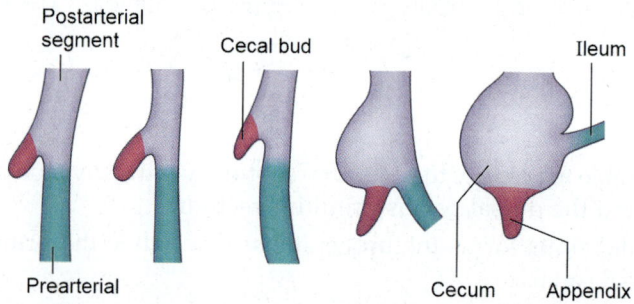

Development of cecum and appendix labeled model

## DEVELOPMENT OF ANAL CANAL

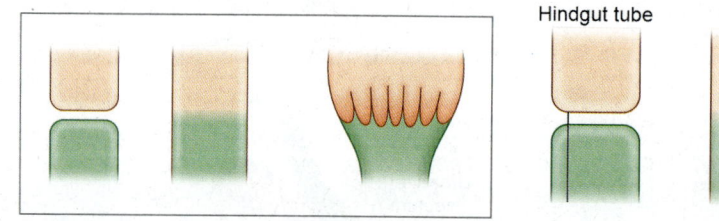

Development of anal canal unlabeled model

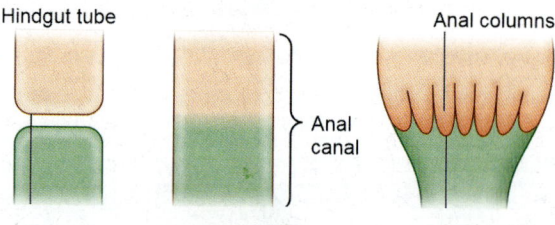

Development of anal canal labeled model

### Viva Question

Anal canal develops partly from ectoderm and endoderm, the line of junction between the two is pectinate line.

## ROTATION OF GUT

### Viva Questions

*I Stage of Rotation*

Rotation of gut occurs around 5th to 10th weeks of intrauterine life and largely influenced by the growth of liver. The pressure of growing liver forces rotation of gut in such a way that the prearterial segment lies down and to the right, while postarterial segment lies upwards and to the left. In this stage midgut loop rotates 90° anticlockwise.

### II Stage of Rotation

Occurs between 10 to 11 weeks, during this period the midgut loop increases in size, post-arterial segment increases in thickness, and umbilical hernia starts returning to the abdominal cavity in a specific order proximal part of prearterial segment returns first.

Midgut rotates around the superior mesenteric artery 270°.

### III Stage of Rotation

Occurs around, 11 weeks of gestation and after birth during this stage most of the gut gets fixed to the posterior abdominal wall.

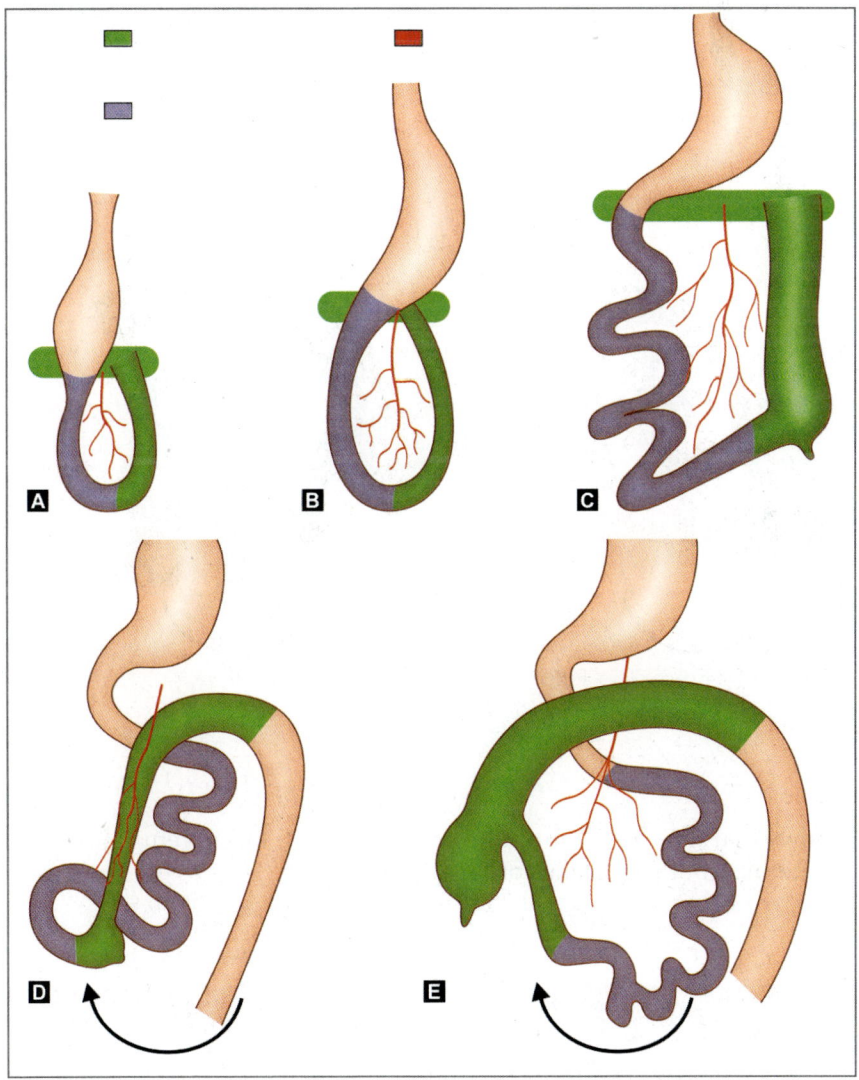

Rotation of gut unlabeled model

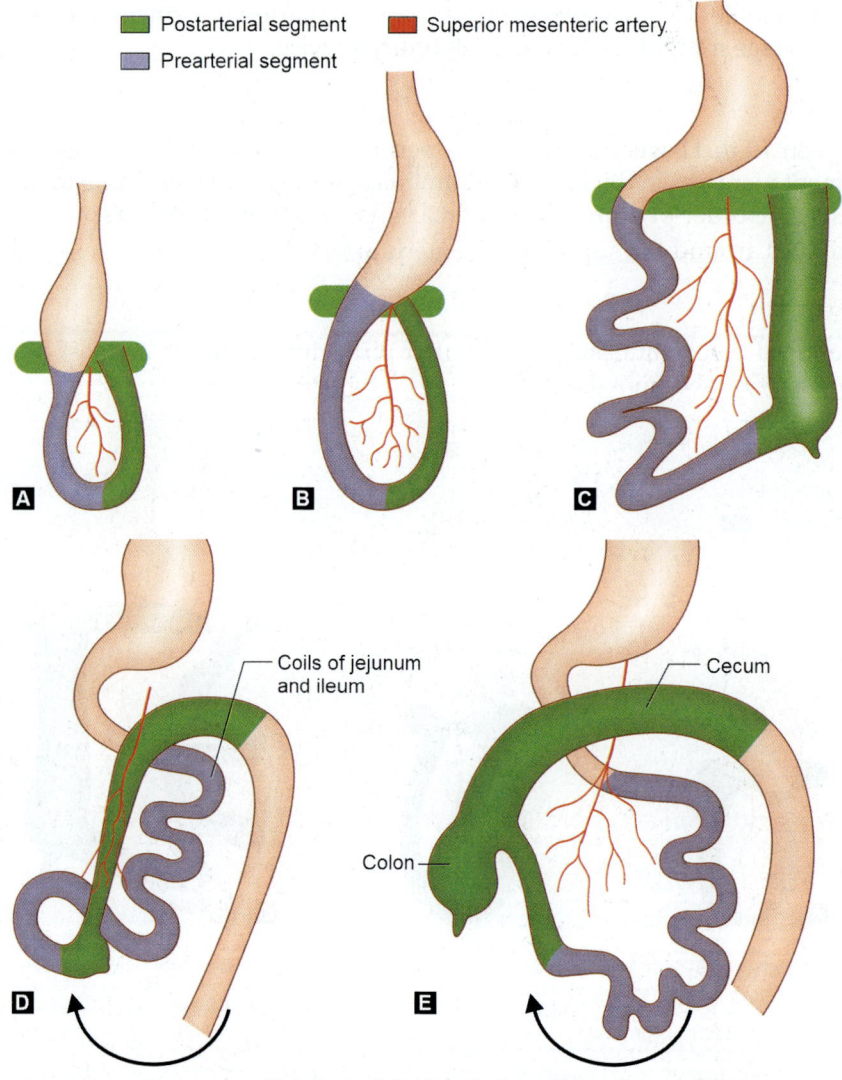

Postarterial segment
Prearterial segment
Superior mesenteric artery

A

B

C

D — Coils of jejunum and ileum

E — Cecum

Colon

Rotation of gut labeled model

## EXOMPHALOS

### Viva Question

The model shows that the coils of intestine of midgut loop fail to return into the abdominal cavity. This is nothing but persistence of umbilical hernia.

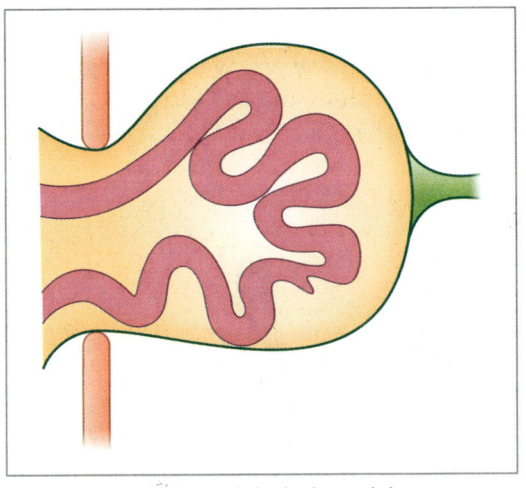

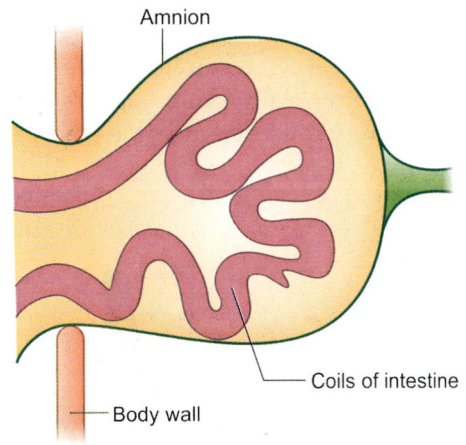

Exomphalos unlabeled model

Exomphalos labeled model

## LOWER RESPIRATORY TRACT DEVELOPMENT

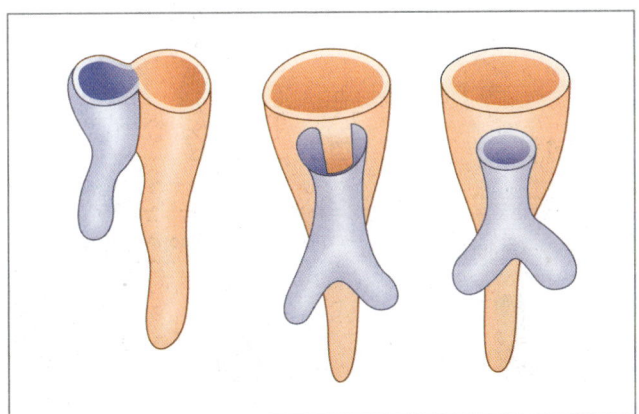

Development of respiratory system unlabeled model

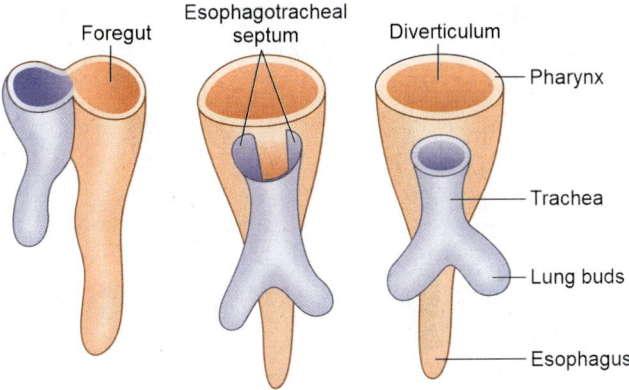

Development of respiratory system labeled model

## Viva Questions

- Around 4 weeks, respiratory diverticulum appears on the ventral wall of foregut. Later a esophagotracheal septum appears between the diverticulum and the foregut.
- Respiratory diverticulum gives rise to trachea and lung buds.

### ESOPHAGEAL ATRESIA AND TRACHEOESOPHAGEAL FISTULA

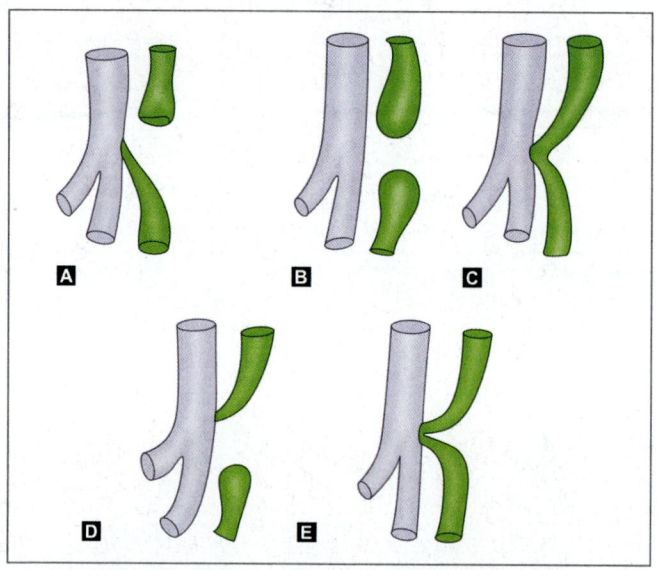

Various types of tracheoesophageal fistula unlabeled model

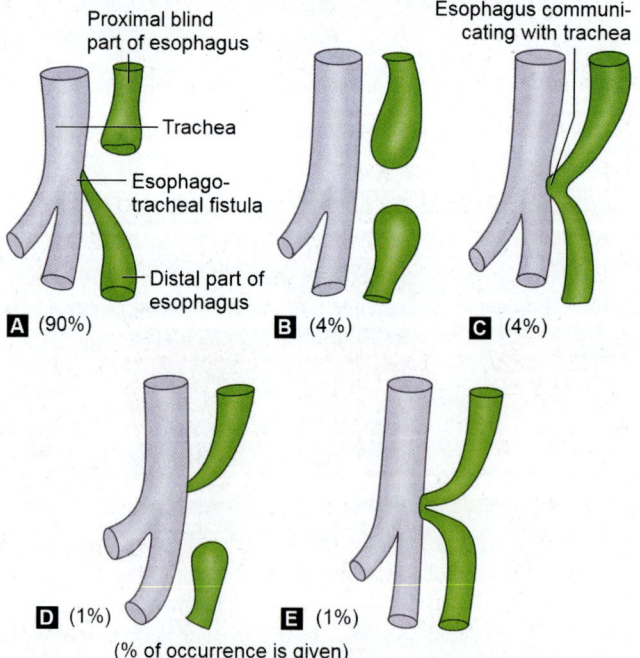

(% of occurrence is given)

Various types of tracheoesophageal fistula labeled model

## Viva Questions

- These abnormalities occur either due to posterior deviation of esophagotracheal septum or dorsal wall of foregut getting inclined anteriorly.
- Most common form of esophageal atresia, is where the proximal part of esophagus is a blind sac.
- Atresia of esophagus leads to excessive collection of amniotic fluid. This is known as polyhydramnios.

## DEVELOPMENT OF PANCREAS

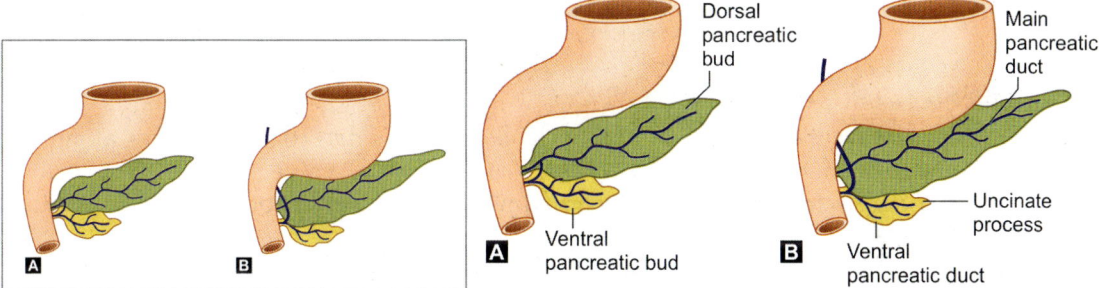

Development of pancreas unlabeled model

Development of pancreas labeled model

## Viva Questions

- Pancreas develops from two pancreatic buds, dorsal bud and ventral bud during sixth week of development.
- After the rotation of duodenum to the right, the ventral bud comes to lie below and behind the dorsal bud.
- Ventral bud forms the lower part of the head of pancreas and the uncinate process remaining gland develops from the dorsal bud
- Main pancreatic duct is formed by the distal part of the dorsal pancreatic duct and whole of the ventral pancreatic duct.

## REMNANTS OF VITELLINE DUCT

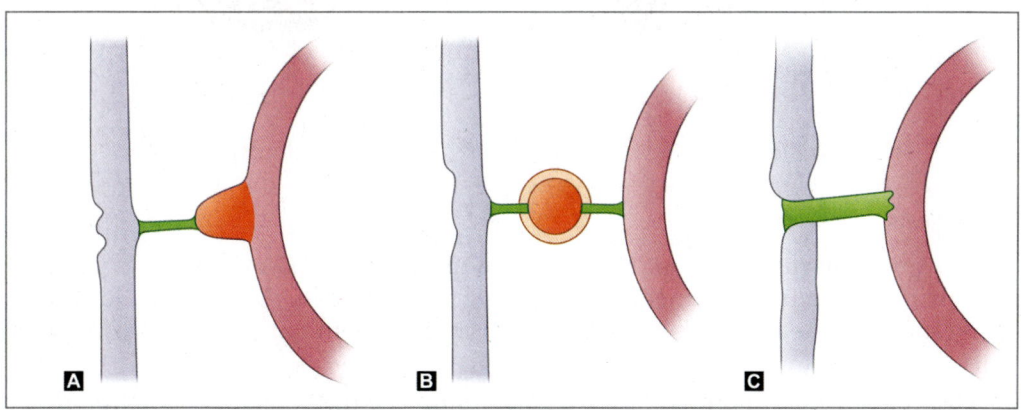

Remnants of vitellointestinal duct unlabeled model

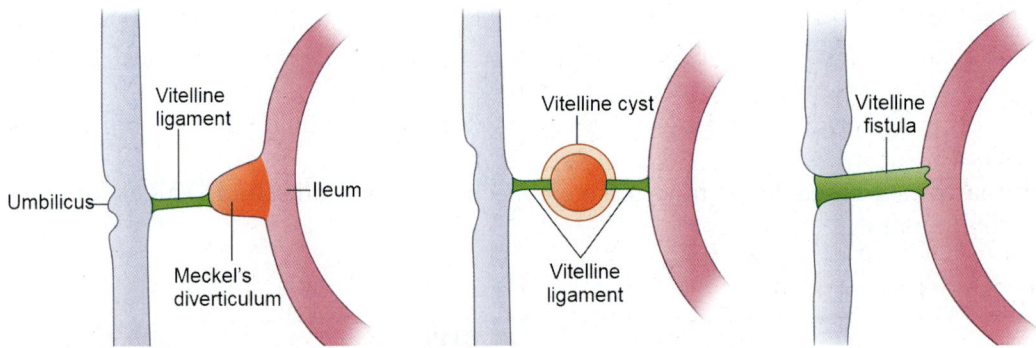

Remnants of vitellointestinal duct labeled model

## Viva Questions

- 2–4% of population the vitelline duct persists as Meckel's diverticulum, it lies along the antimesenteric border, around 40 to 60 cm from ileocecal valve, if gastric mucosa or pancreatic tissue is found in the diverticulum it will cause symptoms like ulceration, bleeding.
- Vitelline duct may remain in the form of fibrous cord, or cyst.

## DIAPHRAGMATIC HERNIA

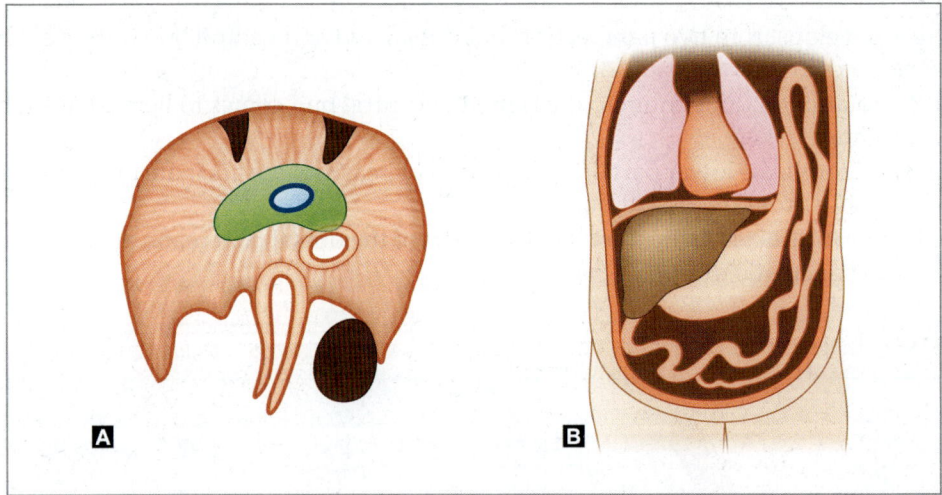

Unlabeled models. (A) Development of diaphragm; (B) Diaphragmatic hernia

## Viva Questions

- Diaphragmatic hernia is one of the most common congenital malformation caused by the failure of pleuroperitoneal membranes to fuse with the pericardioperitoneal membrane. This defect leads to the herniation of abdominal viscera into the pleural cavity.
- Diaphragm develops from septum transversum (central tendon), pleuroperitoneal membranes, dorsal body wall (muscular component), mesentry of esophagus.

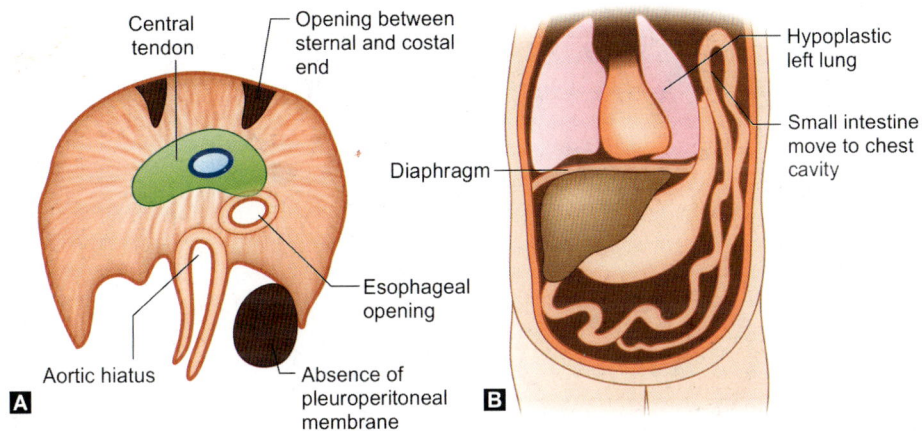

Labeled models. (A) Development of diaphragm; (B) Diaphragmatic hernia

## HEART TUBE

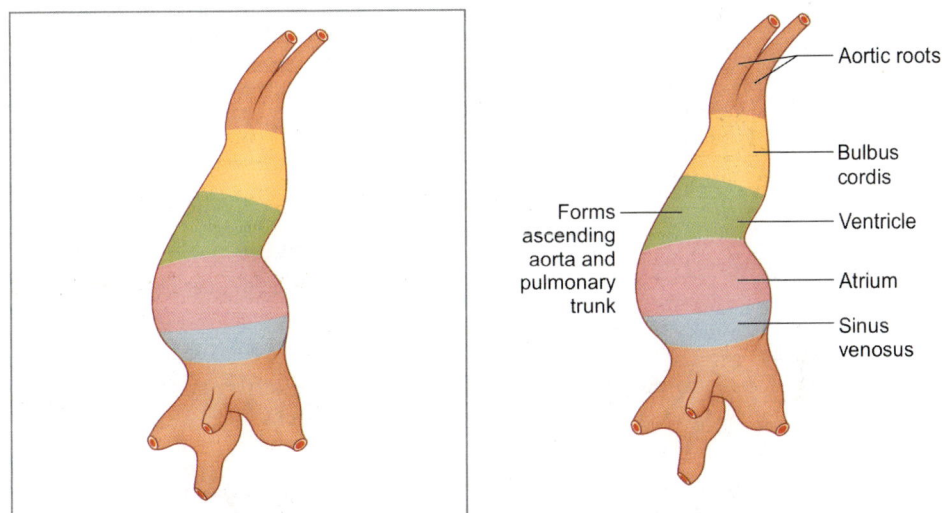

Parts of heart tube unlabeled model          Parts of heart tube labeled model

### Viva Question

Student should be able to identify the parts of heart tube and tell the derivatives as shown in the figure.

## FORMATION OF INTERATRIAL SEPTUM

### Viva Questions

- A septum appears from the roof of the atrial wall a little left to the sinus venosus, this is septum primum. It grows downwards leaving a gap above the endocardial cushion known as foramen primum.
- Septum primum fuses below with the endocardial cushion and gets freed from above leaving a gap foramen secundum.

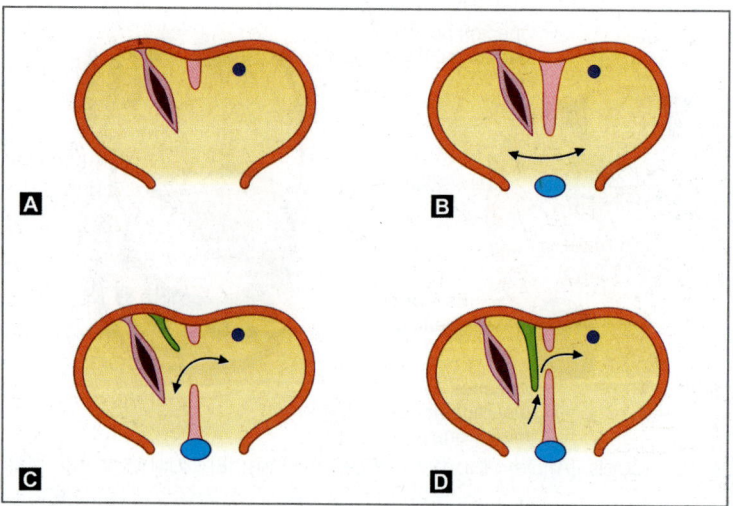

Formation of interatrial septum unlabeled model

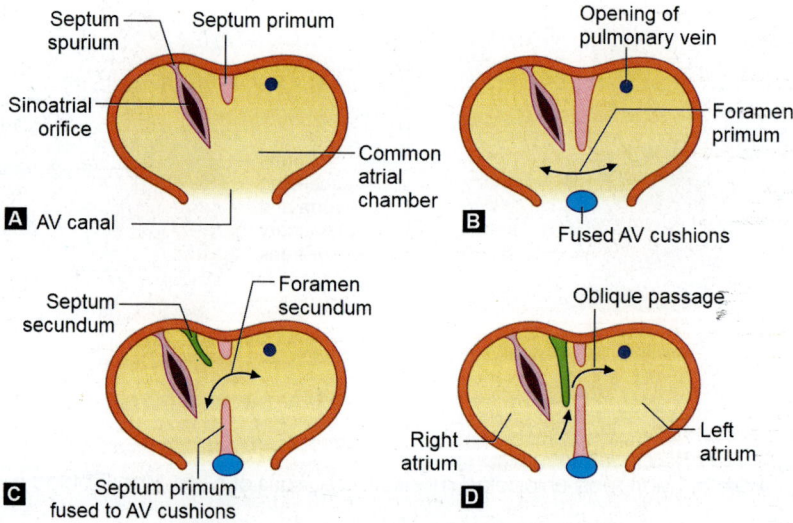

Formation of interatrial septum labeled model

- Another septum appears between the septum primum and septum spurium of sinus venosus known as septum secundum.
- Septum secundum grows downwards and overlaps the foramen secundum leaving an oblique valvular gap known as foramen ovale.
- Within the features of atrium in adults, fossa ovalis is a remnant of septum primum while annulus ovalis is the lower edge of septum secundum.

## DEVELOPMENT OF INTERVENTRICULAR SEPTUM

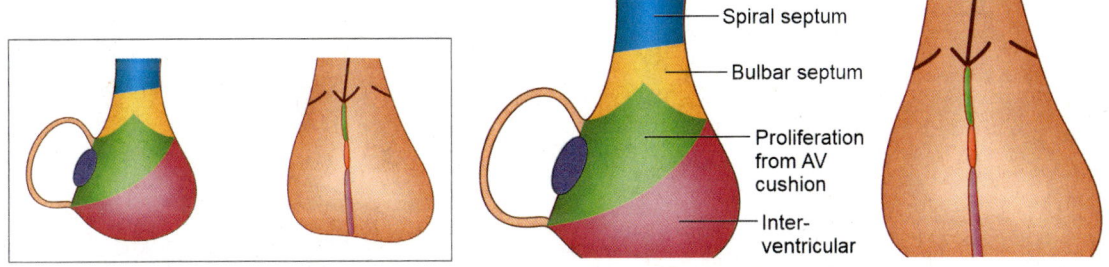

Unlabeled model    Labeled model

Development of interventricular septum

### Viva Question

During the fifth week, medial walls of gradually expanding ventricles and the endocardial cushions form the interventricular septum.

## FALLOT'S TETRALOGY

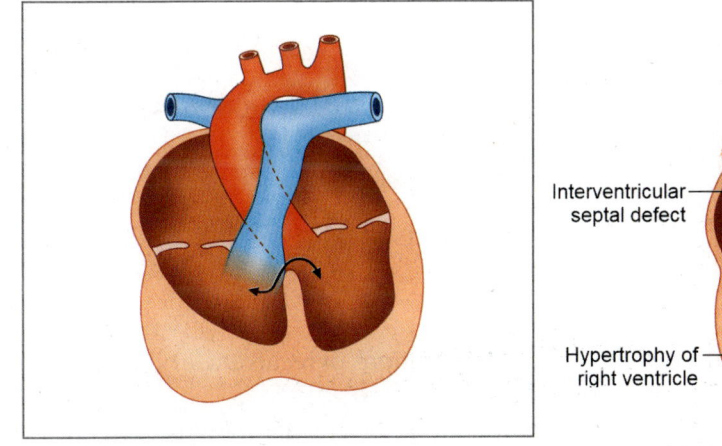

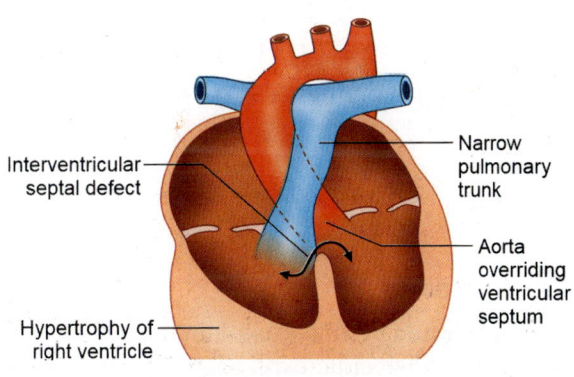

Tetralogy of Fallot unlabeled model    Tetralogy of Fallot labeled model

### Viva Question

Student should be able to identify the model and tell the components of tetralogy of Fallot.

## POSITION OF RECURRENT LARYNGEAL NERVE

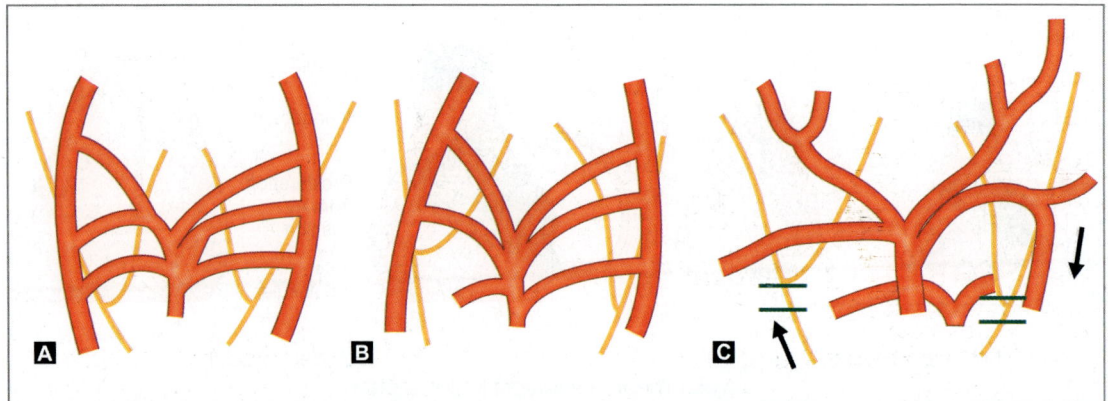

Relationship of recurrent laryngeal nerves (right and left) to aortic arches unlabeled model

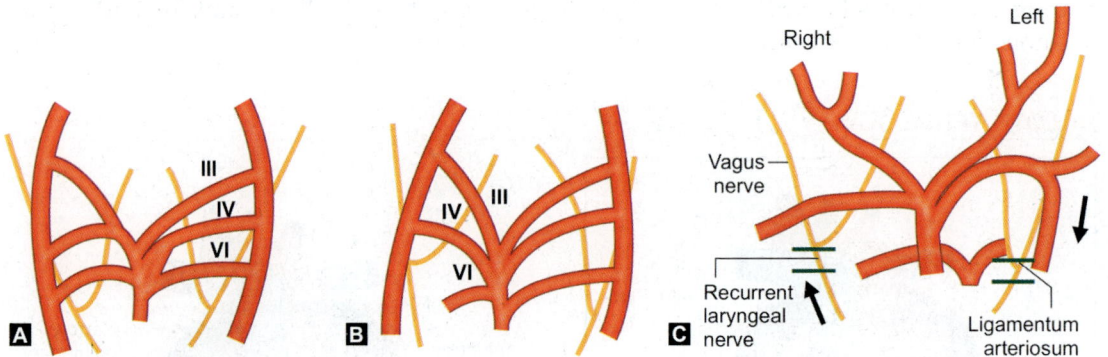

Relationship of recurrent nerves (right and left) to aortic arches labeled model

### Viva Questions

Student should be able to explain the discrepancy in the positions of recurrent laryngeal nerve on right and left side (explanation given below).

- Recurrent laryngeal nerve is first, caudal to sixth arch on both sides. However, with the disappearance of sixth arch artery on the right side the nerve on right side moves cranially to lie against fourth arch, i.e. subclavian artery, (fifth arch disappears), while on the left side the nerve retains the position with the sixth arch.

- As the embryo develops there is elongation of the neck and descent of heart, the nerves have to return back to their destination larynx and hence follow a recurrent course.

## DEVELOPMENT OF PORTAL VEIN

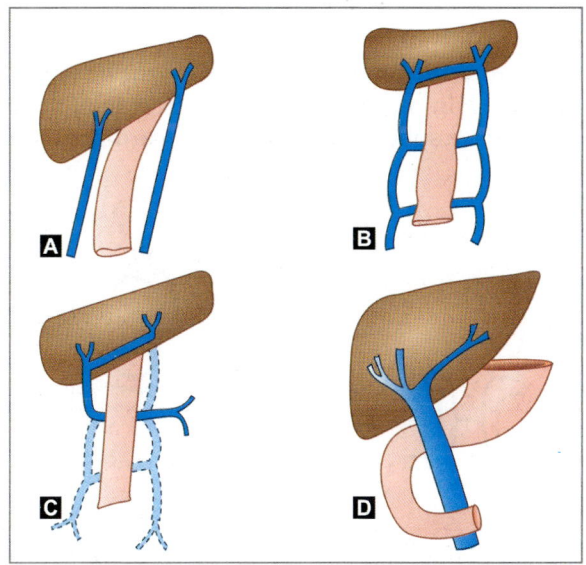

Development of portal vein unlabeled model

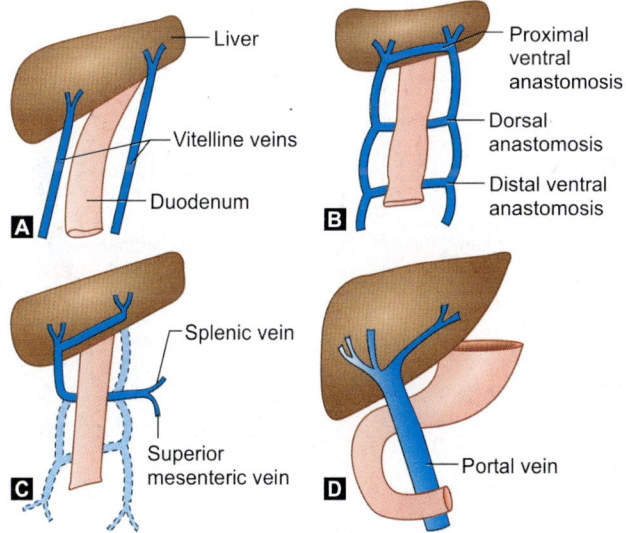

Development of portal vein labeled model

### Viva Question

The vitelline vein lies on either side of duodenum and get connected to each other by transverse communicating channels, 2 ventral and in between 1 dorsal. Portal vein develops from the parts of vitelline vein and the dorsal anastomosis.

## DEVELOPMENT OF INFERIOR VENA CAVA

### Viva Question

Inferior vena cava develops from the lowest part of the right posterior cardinal vein, lower part of the right supracardinal vein, right supra- and subcardinal anastomosis, chip of subcardinal vein, anastomosis between subcardinal and hepatocardiac veins, and the right hepatocardiac channel.

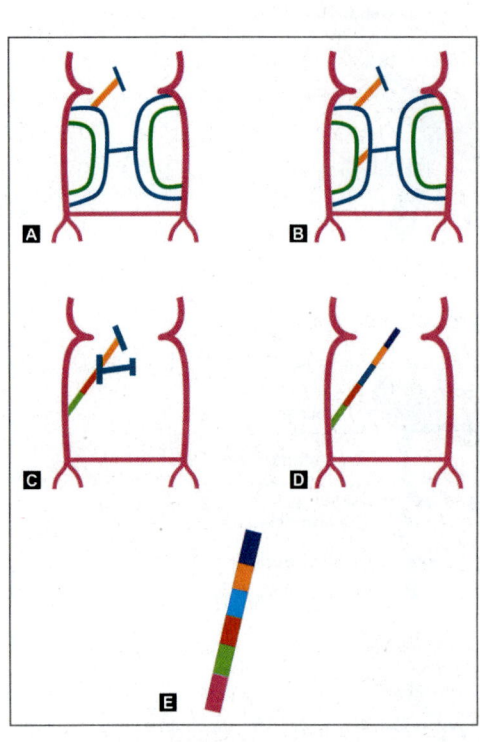

Unlabeled model

Development of inferior vena cava

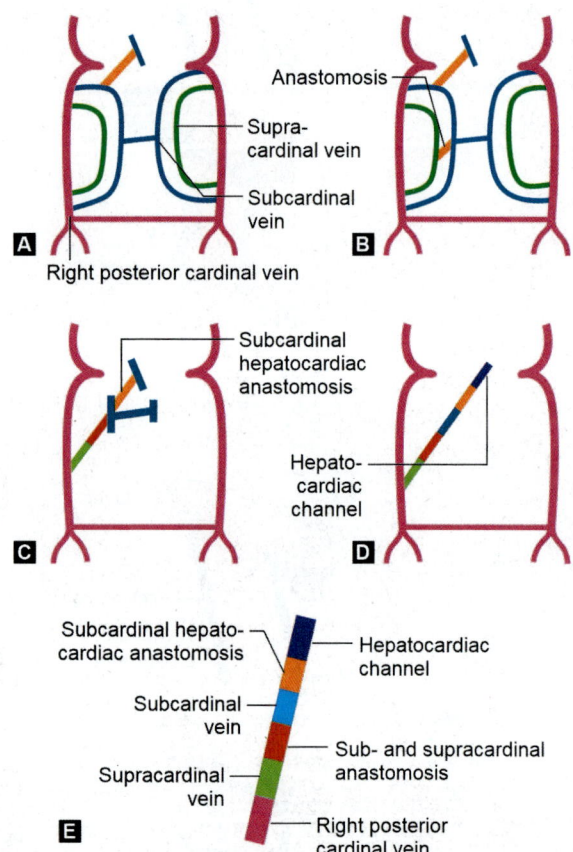

Development of inferior vena cava labeled model

## FETAL CIRCULATION

### Viva Questions

Student should be able to quote the differences between the adult and fetal circulation (given below)

|  | *Fetal* | *Adult* |
|---|---|---|
| Saturation site | Placenta | Lungs |
| Bypass channels | Ductus venosus | None |
|  | Ductus arteriosus | None |

*Contd...*

| Oxygenated blood channel | Umbilical vein | Pulmonary vein |
|---|---|---|
| Communications within the chambers (between right and left channel) | Foramen ovale | Right and left no inter-communication |
| Nonfunctional organs | Lungs | None |
| Saturation | Falls step by step | Maintained all throughout |
| Pathway | Placenta | Vena cavae |
| | Umbilical veins | Right atrium |
| | Ductus venosus | Right ventricle |
| | Inferior vena cava | Pulmonary artery |
| | Right atrium | Lungs |
| | Left atrium | Pulmonary veins |
| | Left ventricle | Left atrium |
| | Ascending aorta | Left ventricle |
| | Arch and descending | Ascending, arch, descending |
| | Umbilical arteries | Vena cavae |
| | Placenta | Right atrium |

- At the time of birth foramen ovale, ductus venosus, ductus arteriosus, umbilical arteries and veins close. Closure of these channels is by and large initiated either by pressure changes or release of bradykinin like substances.
- Left umbilical vein is left behind in the form of ligamentum teres.

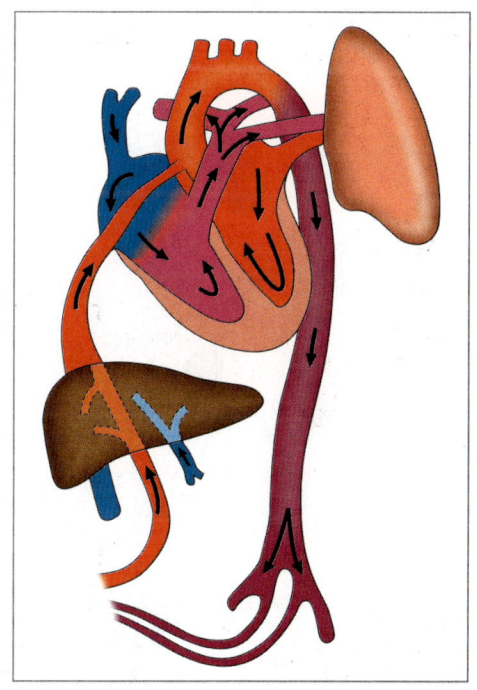

Fetal circulation unlabeled model

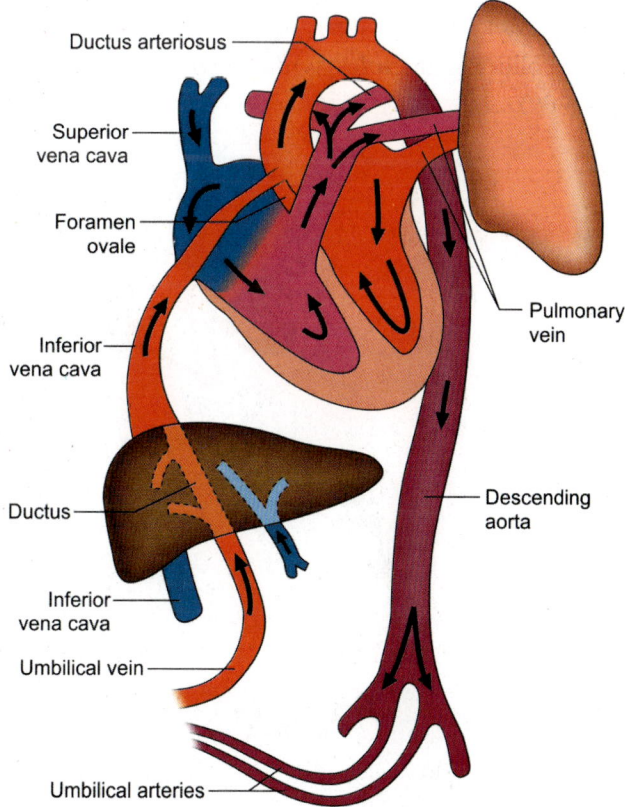

Fetal circulation labeled model

## HINDGUT AND CLOACA

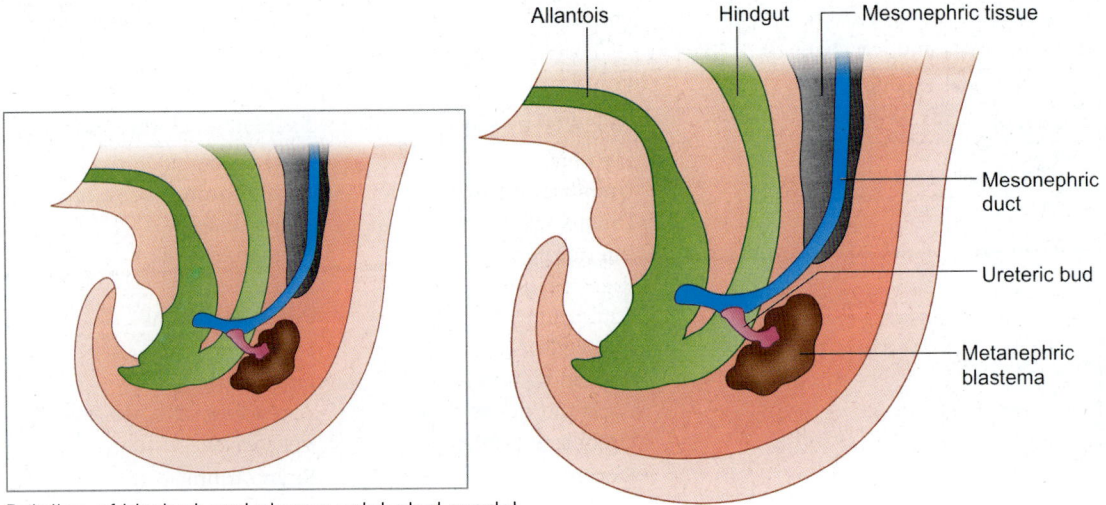

Relation of hindgut and cloaca unlabeled model

Relation of hindgut and cloaca labeled model

### Viva Questions

- Urinary as well as genital system develop from the intermediate mesoderm
- Ureteric bud forms the collecting system of kidney namely ureter, renal pelvis, calyces and the collecting ductules, while the metanephric blastema forms the excretory components of kidney.

## ANOMALIES OF URINARY SYSTEM

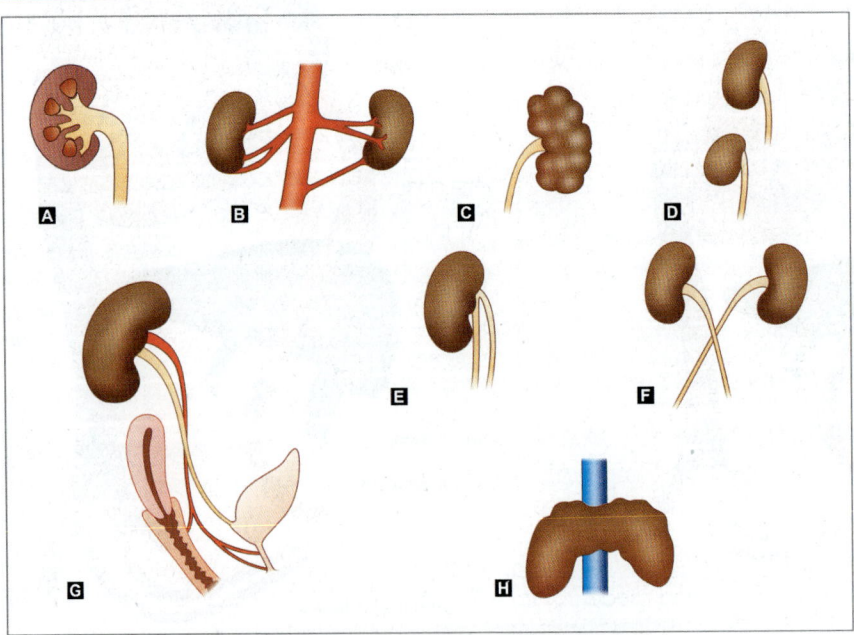

Anomalies of urinary system unlabeled model

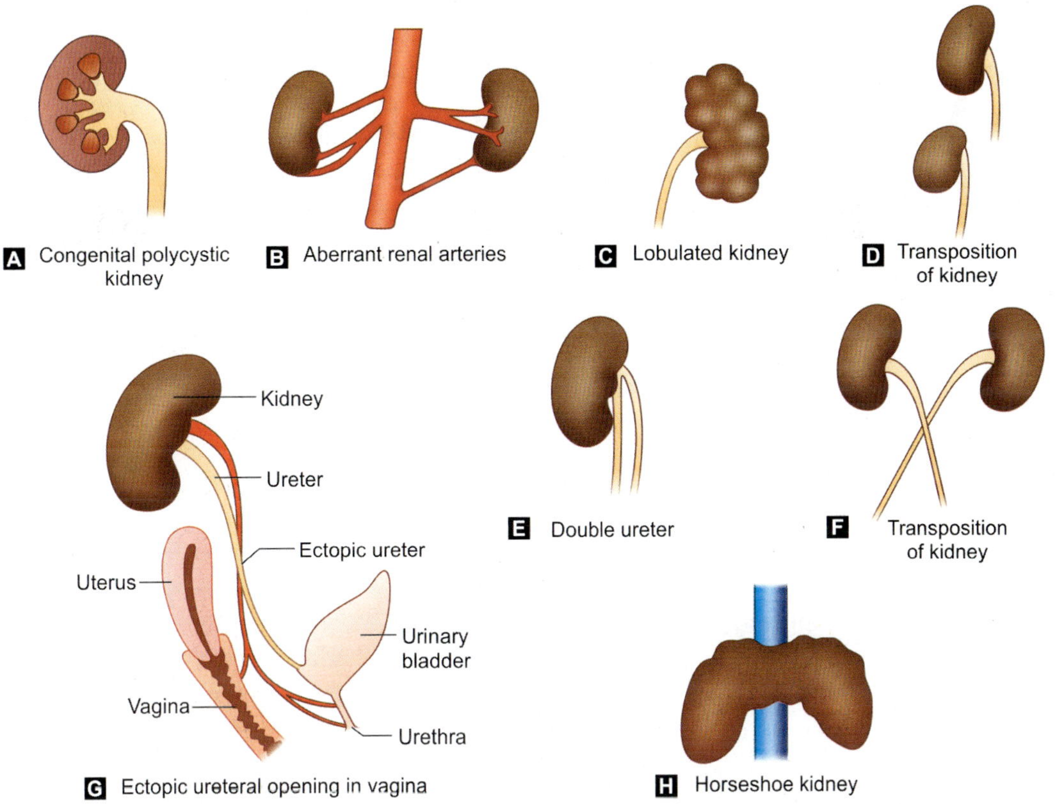

A  Congenital polycystic kidney

B  Aberrant renal arteries

C  Lobulated kidney

D  Transposition of kidney

Kidney

Ureter

Ectopic ureter

Uterus

Urinary bladder

Vagina

Urethra

E  Double ureter

F  Transposition of kidney

G  Ectopic ureteral opening in vagina

H  Horseshoe kidney

Anomalies of urinary system labeled model

## Viva Question

Student should be able to identify the anomalies as labeled in the diagram

## URINARY BLADDER ANOMALIES

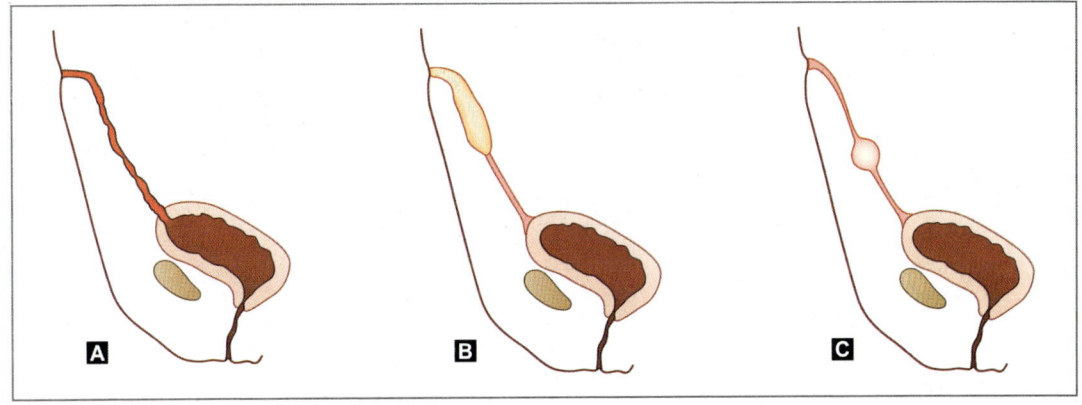

A

B

C

Model showing urinary bladder anomalies unlabeled

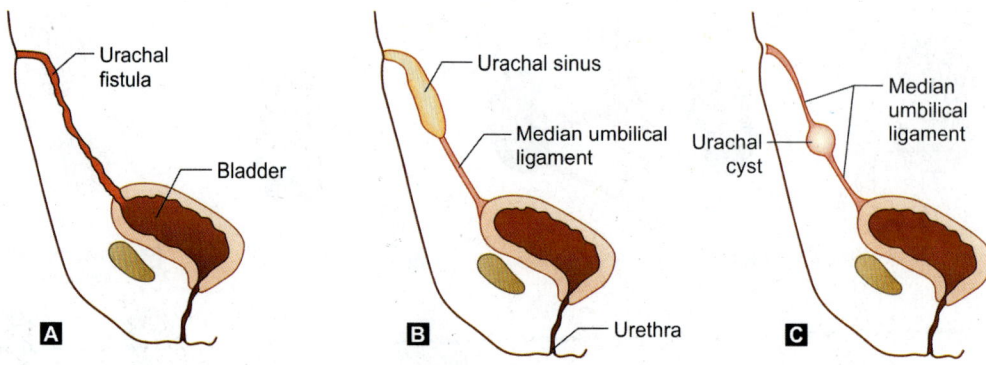

Model showing urinary bladder anomalies labeled

## Viva Question

Patent allantois lumen may cause urine to drain from the umbilicus, this is the urachal fistula, small remnant of allantois may persist as urachal cyst, sometimes only patent in the upper part in the form of urachal sinus.

## DEVELOPMENT OF UTERUS AND VAGINA

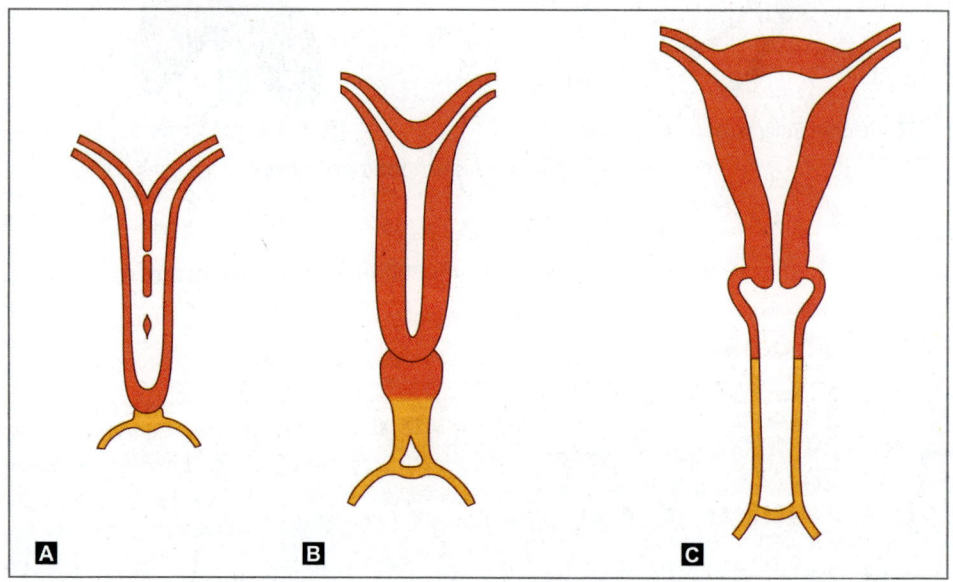

Development of uterus and vagina unlabeled model

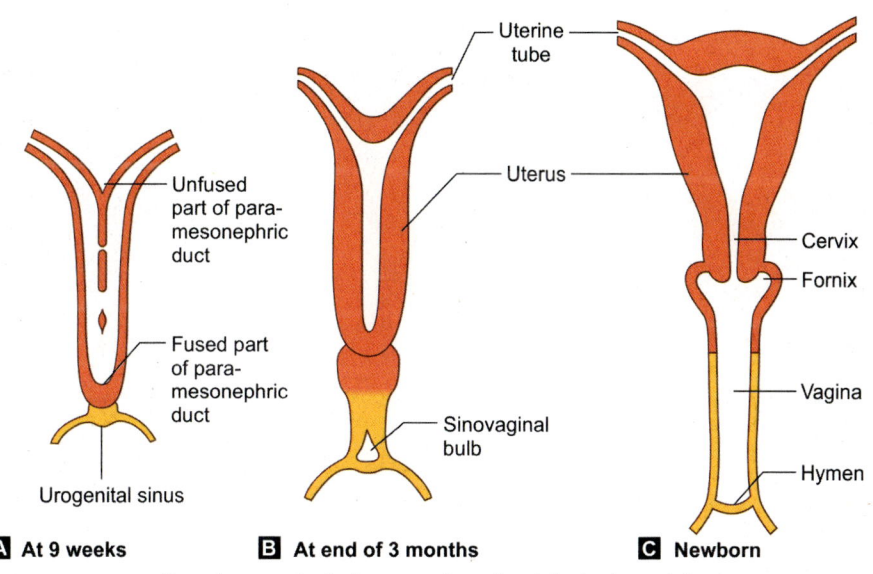

A **At 9 weeks**    B **At end of 3 months**    C **Newborn**

Development of uterus and vagina labeled model

## Viva Questions

- Paramesonephric ducts give rise to the uterus (fused part), and uterine tubes (unfused part) partly vagina
- Endodermal cells of urogenital sinus proliferate to form sinovaginal bulbs. This forms vagina.

*Also remember:* Testis develops close to mesonephros; and duct system of testis develops from mesonephric duct.

## ANOMALIES OF UTERUS AND VAGINA

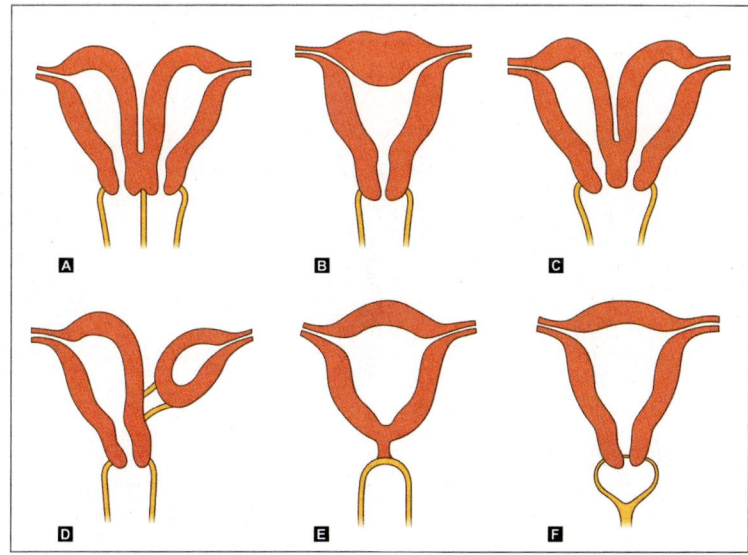

Anomalies of uterus and vagina unlabeled model

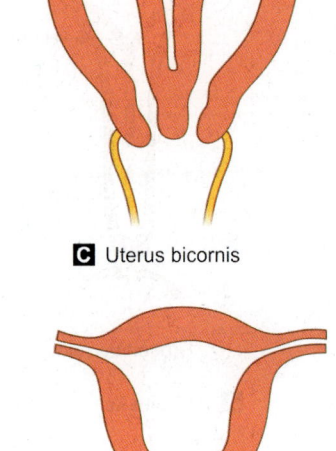

**A** Uterus didelphys with double vagina

**B** Uterus arcuatus

Indentation

**C** Uterus bicornis

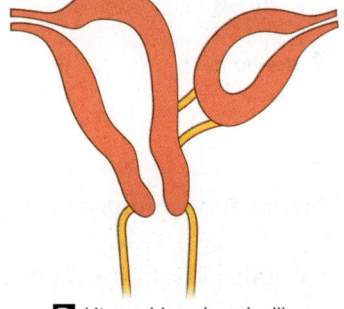

**D** Uterus bicornis unicollis with rudementary horn

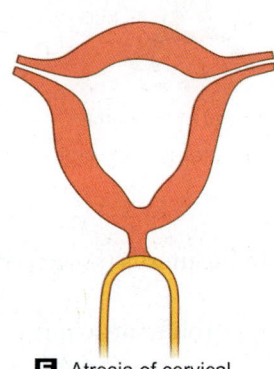

**E** Atresia of cervical

**F** Partial atresia of vagina

Open part of vagina

Anomalies of uterus and vagina labeled model

## Viva Question

Student should be able to name the anomalies (shown in the figure).

## EXTERNAL GENITALIA OF FEMALES

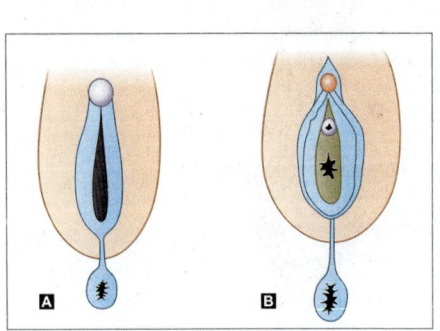

Model of externl genitalia of females unlabeled

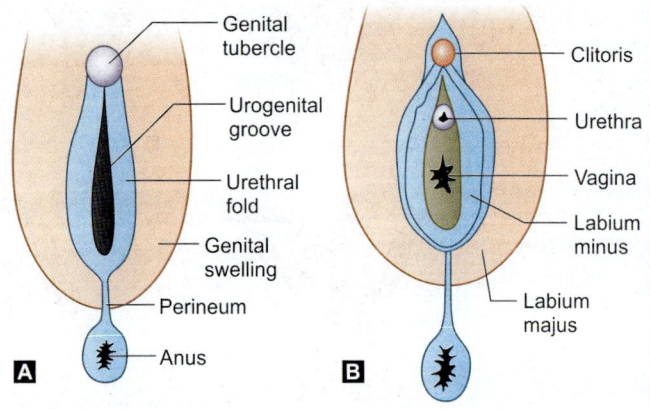

Genital tubercle

Urogenital groove

Urethral fold

Genital swelling

Perineum

Anus

Clitoris

Urethra

Vagina

Labium minus

Labium majus

Model of external genitalia of females labeled

## Viva Question

Genital tubercle gives rise to clitoris, urethral folds form the labia minora, genital swellings form the labia majora, urogenital groove forms the vestibule.

## BRANCHIAL FISTULAS

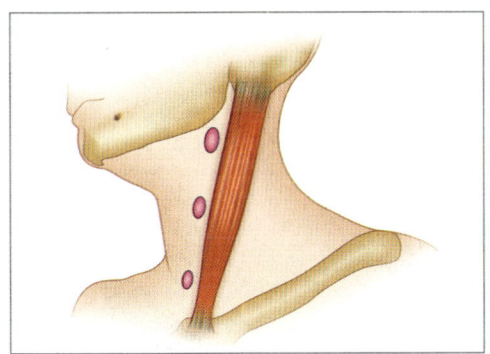

Model of branchial fistulas unlabeled

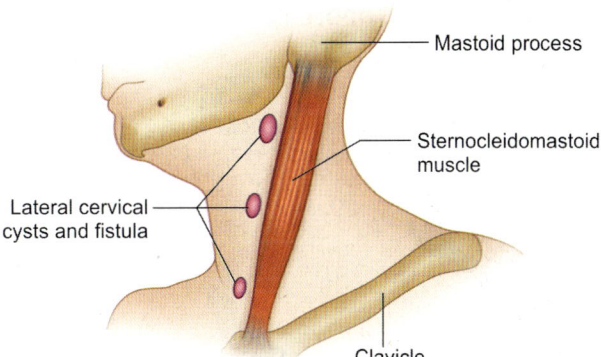

Model of branchial fistulas labeled

## Viva Questions

- Model shows branchial fistulas normally detected on the patient just below angle of mandible but can lie anywhere in front of sternocleidomastoid. They develop when the second pharyngeal arch does not over grow the third and fourth arches, thus the remnants of 2nd, 3rd, and 4th clefts come to lie on surface.
- Branchial fistulas facilitate the drainage of cervical cyst.

## FORMATION OF OTIC VESICLE

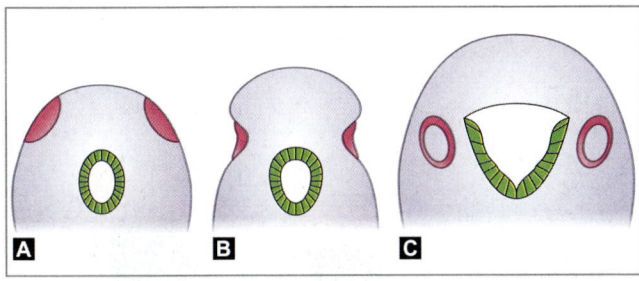

Formation of otic vesicle unlabeled model

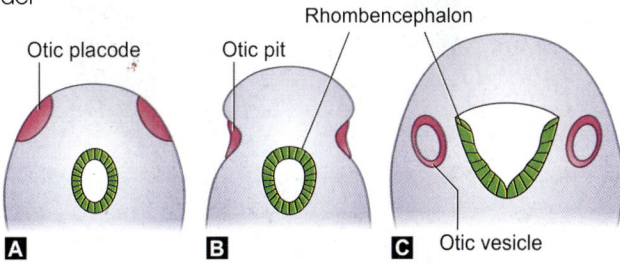

Formation of otic vesicle labeled model

## Viva Question

Otic placode is a specialized area, on surface ectoderm; over the developing hindbrain, this depresses on itself and now called otic pit, slowly the pit separates from the ectoderm to form otic vesicle. This vesicle undergoes differential growth to give rise to membranous labyrinth.

## DEVELOPMENT OF MIDDLE EAR AND AUDITORY TUBE

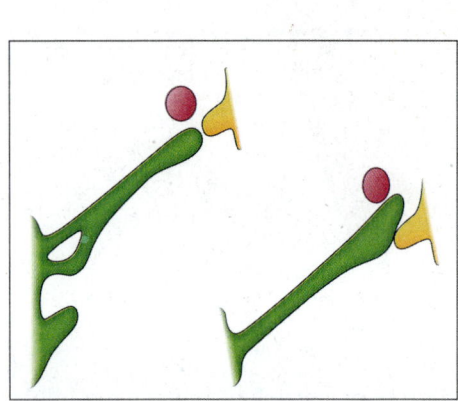

Development of middle ear and auditory tube unlabeled model

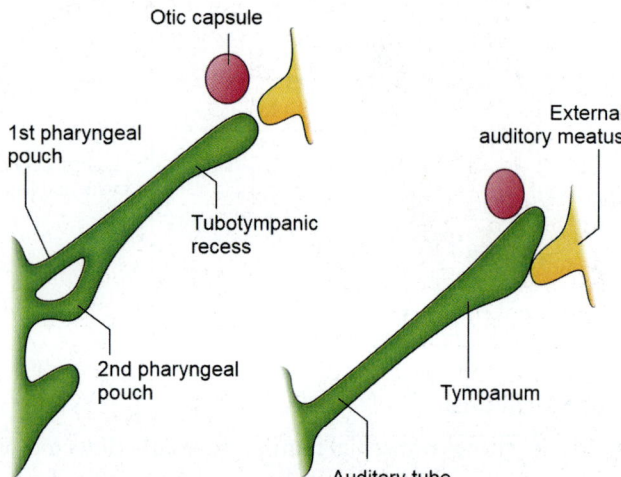

Development of middle ear and auditory tube labeled model

## Viva Questions

• Middle ear and auditory tube develop from the tubotympanic recess.
• Tubotympanic recess develops from the dorsal part of first pharyngeal pouch and a small part of the second pharyngeal pouch.

## DEVELOPMENT OF PINNA

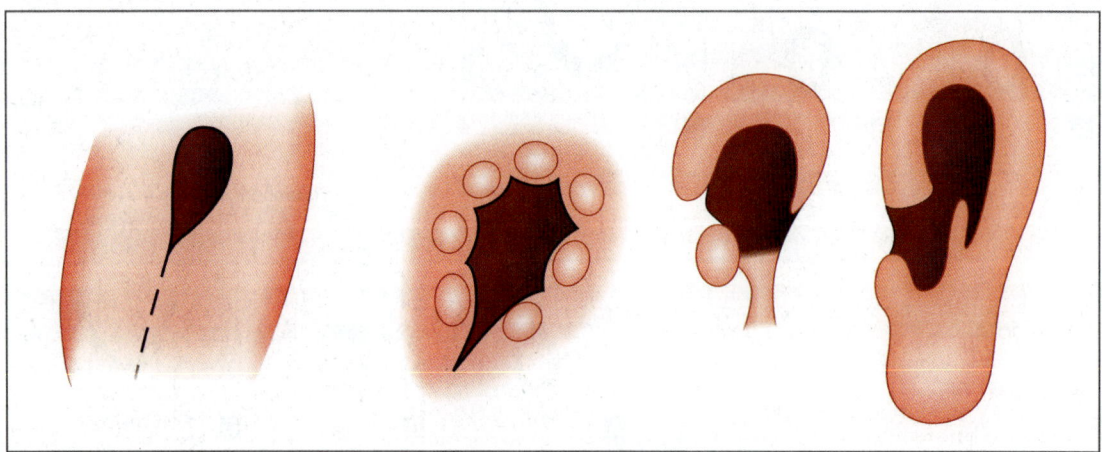

Development of pinna unlabeled model

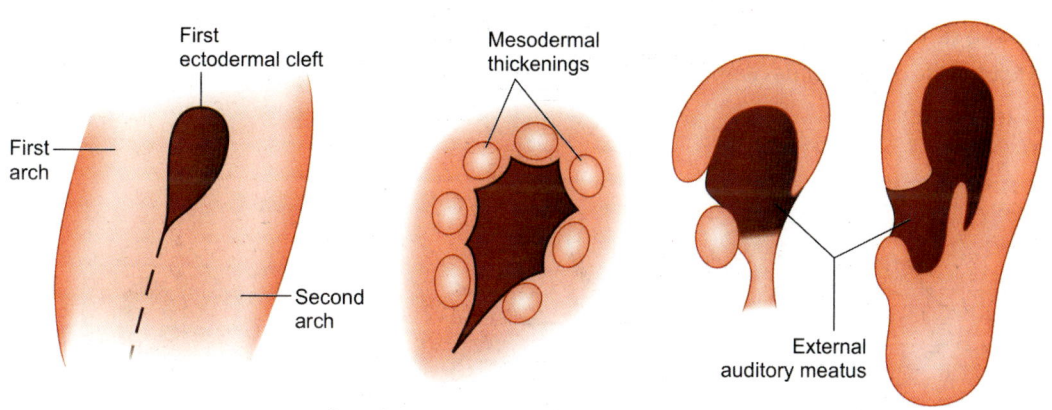

First arch

First ectodermal cleft

Second arch

Mesodermal thickenings

External auditory meatus

Development of pinna labeled model

## Viva Questions

- Mesodermal thickenings appear on the mandibular and hyoid arch around the opening of the external auditory meatus (= First ectodermal cleft).
- Tragus is formed from mandibular arch while rest of auricle from hyoid arch.

## DEVELOPMENT OF OPTIC VESICLE

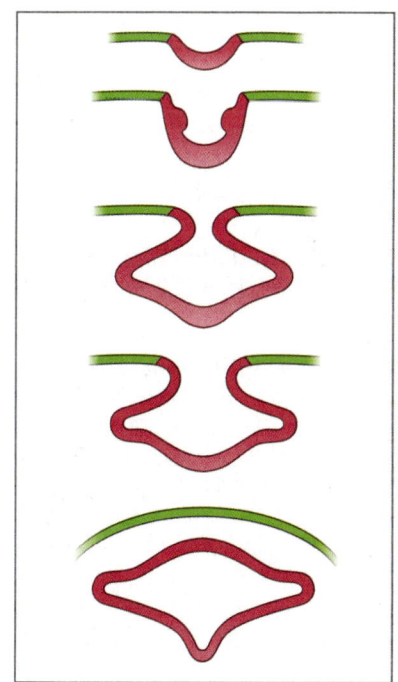

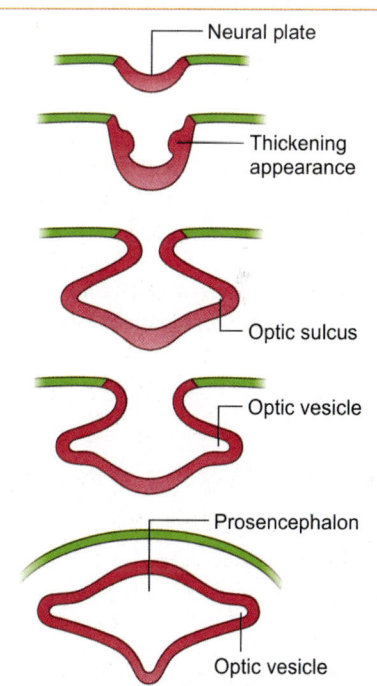

Neural plate

Thickening appearance

Optic sulcus

Optic vesicle

Prosencephalon

Optic vesicle

Development of optic vesicle unlabeled model

Development of optic vesicle labeled model

## Viva Questions

- A region on the neural plate which will further develop into prosencephalon, gets thickened, and depresses to form optic sulcus.

- As the development progresses, neural plate transforms into prosencephalic vesicle.
- Meanwhile optic sulcus deepens, prosencephalon over the sulcus bulges to form optic vesicle.

## DEVELOPMENT OF LENS VESICLE

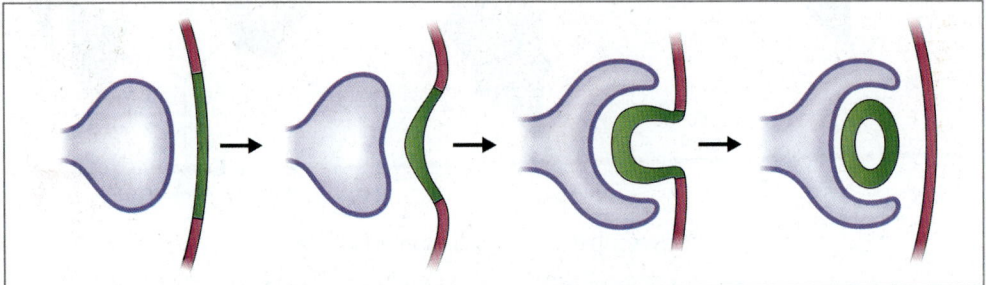

Development of lens vesicle unlabeled model

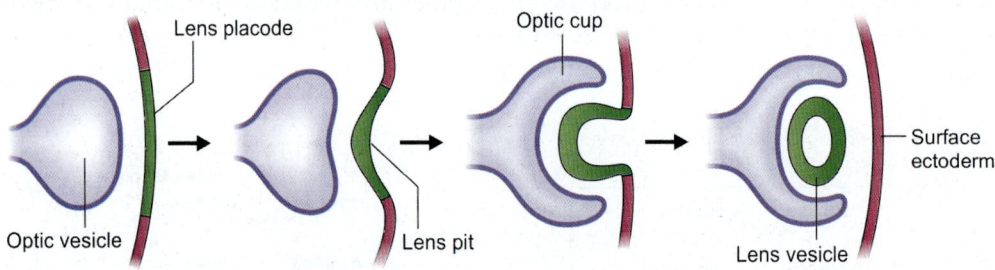

Development of lens vesicle labeled model

### Viva Questions

- Optic vesicle grows laterally to come to lie close to a specialized area on surface ectoderm, lens placode. This area sinks on itself to form lens vesicle; eventually it gets detached from surface ectoderm.
- As the lens vesicle develops optic vesicle gets converted into optic cup.

### Different Parts of Eyeball and its Source of Development

- Retina—layers of optic cup
- Lens—Lens vesicle
- Vitreous—partly from optic cup, mesoderm, lens vesicle partly
- Muscles of iris:
    - Sphincter pupillae and dilator pupillae—ectodermal origin
    - Ciliary muscle—mesodermal origin
- Sclera, cornea—mesoderm around optic cup
- Choroid—Vascular layer of mesoderm around optic cup
- Eyelids—Reduplication of surface ectoderm
- Lacrimal sac, nasolacrimal duct—nasolacrimal furrow.

## COLOBOMA IRIS

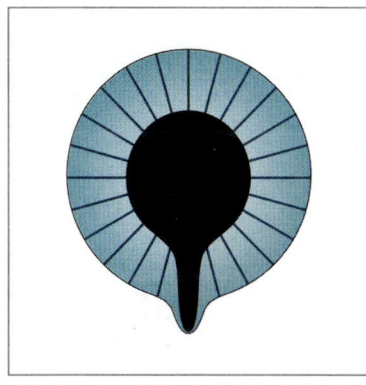

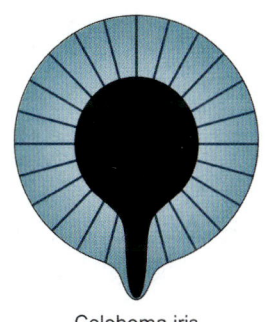

Coloboma iris

Model of coloboma iris unlabeled    Model of coloboma iris labeled

## Viva Question

Failure of choroidal fissure to disappear leads to coloboma iris.

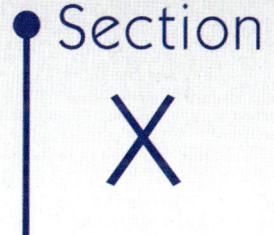

Section

X

Histology

# Histology Slides

## 51

## Q. Cell structure

**Ans.** Cell is bounded by cell membrane (plasma membrane):

- Within the cell membrane is protoplasm
- Protoplasm consists of central nucleus and surrounding cytoplasm
- Nucleus is covered by nuclear membrane
- Many structures are present within the cytoplasm, which are referred as organelle.

| Organelles | Functions |
|---|---|
| Endoplasmic reticulum (ER) (smooth, rough) | Rough ER-protein synthesis; smooth ER-metabolic processes, e.g. carbohydrate metabolism |
| Ribosomes (free in cytoplasm) | Protein synthesis |
| Mitochondria | ATP, GTP are produced, exhibit important part in Krebs cycle |
| Golgi complex | Protein-carbohydrate complexes are formed |
| Phagosomes | Engulf bacteria by phagocytosis |
| Pinocytic vesicle | Fluid taken in by pinocytosis |
| Exocytic vesicle | Cell products expelled out by exocytosis |
| Storage vesicle | Stores lipid, carbohydrate |
| Lysosomes | Contain enzymes, which destroy unwanted material in the cell |
| Microtubule | Provide stability to cell, facilitate transport within the cell, form mitotic spindle in dividing cell |
| Centriole | Crucial role in formation of cilia, flagella, mitotic spindles |

- **Tissue**—collection of cells which have similar structure and function, e.g. bone
- **Organ**—collection of tissue with same function form organ, e.g. liver, lungs
- **System**—organs performing same function form the system, e.g. respiratory system—nose, trachea, bronchi, lungs.

855

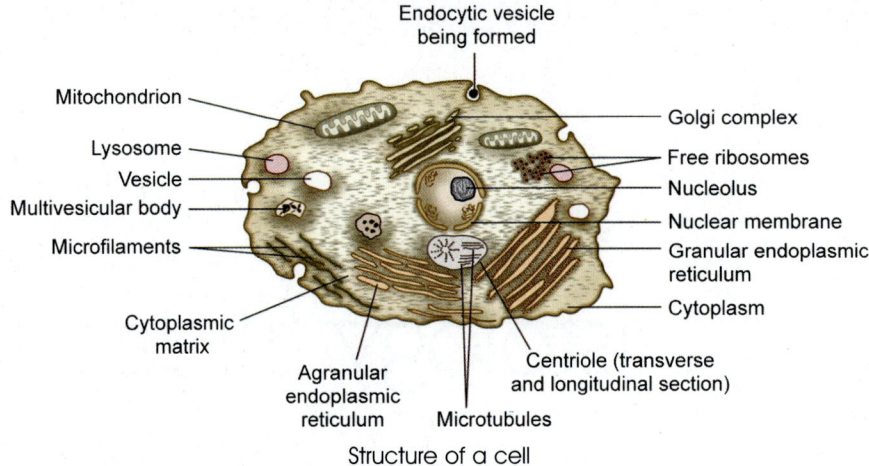

Structure of a cell

## Q. Simple squamous epithelium

**Ans.**
- Single layer of flattened cells
- Very thin cell membrane; hence the nuclei bulge on the surface
- Lines the alveoli of lungs, free surface of serous pericardium, pleura peritoneum
- Lines the interior of heart (endocardium), blood vessels and lymphatics (endothelium).

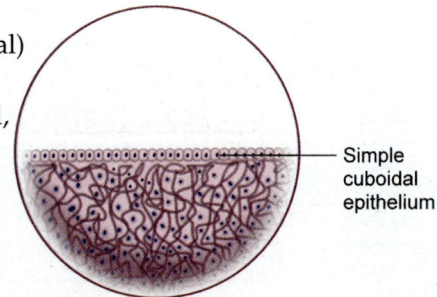

## Q. Simple cuboidal epithelium

**Ans.**
- Single layer of cube-like cells (length and breadth equal)
- By and large, lines the glands
- Typical cuboidal epithelium is seen in thyroid gland, surface of ovary
- Cuboidal epithelium with brush border is seen in proximal convoluted tubule of kidney.

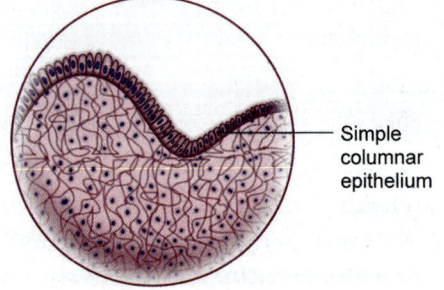

## Q. Simple columnar epithelium

**Ans.**
- Single layer of tall cells (height > width)
- Nuclei oval vertically lie near the base of the cell
- At certain sites, columnar epithelium has cilia and is known as ciliated columnar epithelium, e.g. respiratory tract, uterus, uterine tube
- In some other sites, the surface is covered by microvilli and is known as striated or brush border, e.g. small intestine, gallbladder.

## Q. Pseudostratified columnar epithelium

**Ans.**

- Gives a false appearance of multiple layers of cells
- The nuclei are arranged at different levels and hence gets a multilayered appearance
- At certain sites, may have cilia and is known as ciliated pseudostratified columnar epithelium, e.g. trachea and bronchi
- Pseudostratified columnar epithelium present in auditory tube partly, ductus deferens, parts of male urethra.

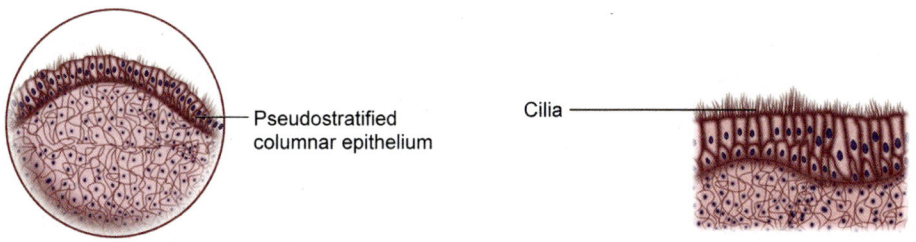

Pseudostratified columnar epithelium

Cilia

## Q. Transitional epithelium

**Ans.**

- Multilayered (4–6 layers thick)
- Basal layer is columnar or cuboidal, middle layer is pear-shaped, upper layer is large umbrella-shaped cells
- Found in urinary system.

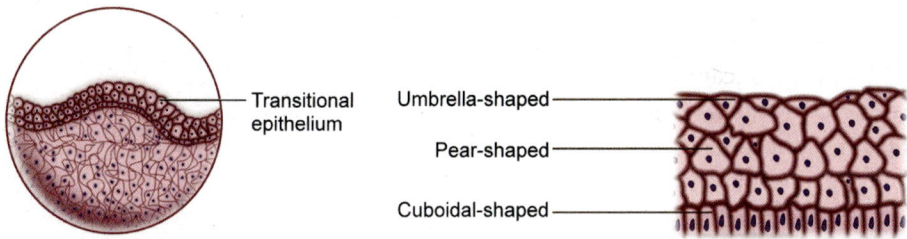

Transitional epithelium

Umbrella-shaped

Pear-shaped

Cuboidal-shaped

## Q. Stratified squamous epithelium

**Ans.**

- Multilayered epithelium
- Basal layer is columnar, middle layer polyhedral, while superficial layer is made-up of flat cells
- Nuclei are oval in basal layer, round in middle layer, transversely elongated in superficial layer, e.g. epidermis of skin
- Following layers are identified in the epidermis of skin:
  - Basal layer, stratum spinosum, stratum granulosum, stratum lucidum, stratum corneum.

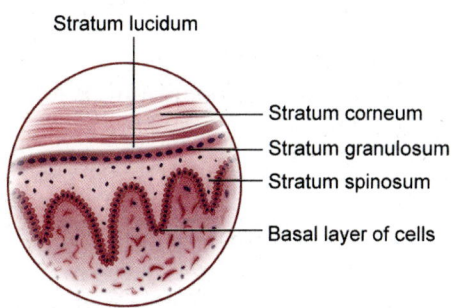

Stratum lucidum

Stratum corneum

Stratum granulosum

Stratum spinosum

Basal layer of cells

| Mnemonic | Layers |
|----------|--------|
| "Bombay | Basal |
| Shall | Spinosum |
| Give | Granulosum |
| Lot of | Lucidum |
| Coins" | Corneum |

- Thick skin has prominent stratum corneum
- Stratum lucidum is present only in thick skin
- Majority of the body is covered by thin hairy skin
- Thick hairless skin is present on the palms of the hand and sole of the feet.

## Q. Loose areolar tissue

**Ans.**
- Bundle of collagen fibers are seen and have a wavy course
- Dark branching elastic fibers visible
- Connective tissue cells are mostly fibroblasts
- Elastic fibers need special stains for visualization, e.g. omentum.

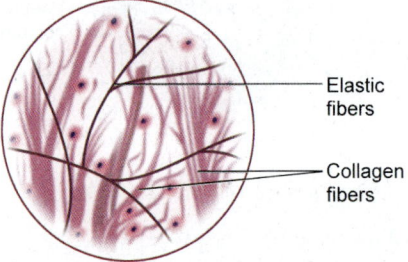

Loose areolar tissue

## Q. Adipose tissue

**Ans.**
- Made-up of fat cells
- The cells appear vacant, since the fat gets dissolved during the preparation of section
- Cytoplasm reduced to thin rim and nucleus lies at a periphery, e.g. omentum.

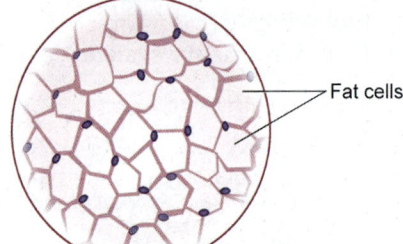

Adipose tissue

## Q. Hyaline cartilage

**Ans.**
- On the surface of cartilage, the cells are flat and in continuation with the overlying connective tissue forming perichondrium
- Within the perichondrium, is a homogenous matrix (glass like)
- The matrix is packed with collagen fibers
- The groups of cartilage cells that are present within the matrix known as chondrocytes
- Groups of cells formed due to mitosis are known as cell nests, e.g. articular cartilage, costal cartilage, laryngeal cartilage, trachea and bronchial cartilage.

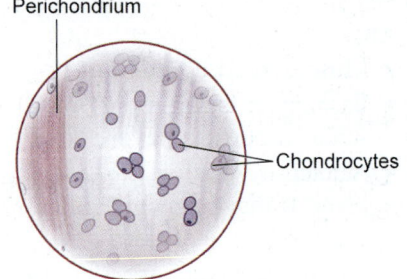

Hyaline cartilage

## Q. Elastic cartilage

**Ans.**
- Special stain needed
- Dense elastic fibers seen in the slide
- Between the dense fibers are the cartilage cells
- Perichondrium is visible at upper end, e.g. pinna, lateral part of external acoustic meatus, medial part of auditory tube, epiglottis.

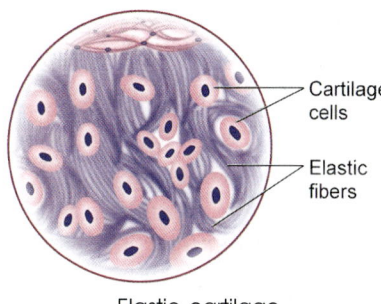

Elastic cartilage

## Q. Fibrocartilage

**Ans.**
- Section contains typical cartilage cell groups surrounded by capsule
- Dense collagen bundles are present within the matrix
- Has no perichondrium, e.g.:
  - Secondary cartilaginous joints, pubic symphysis, intervertebral disk, manubriosternal joints
  - Synovial joints of membrane bones like clavicle, mandible is covered by fibrocartilage.

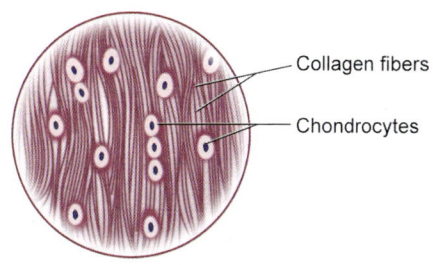

Fibrocartilage

## Q. Compact bone

**Ans.**
- Made-up of haversian system, i.e. ring like osteons
- In the center has a canal known as haversian canal
- Around the canal are layers of lamellae of bone
- Within the lamellae are small spaces, lacunae filled with osteocytes
- Canaliculi radiate from lacunae.

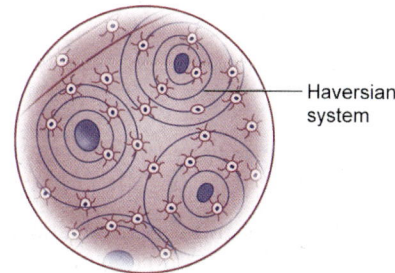

Compact bone

## Q. Cancellous bone

**Ans.**
- Incomplete bony trabeculae are seen
- Within the trabeculae are osteocytes
- The spaces within the trabeculae are filled by bone marrow in which fat cells are present
- Blood-forming elements are present within the bone forming space.

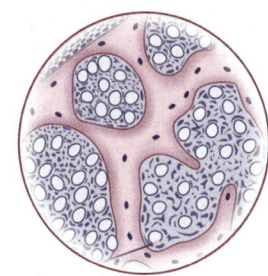

Cancellous bone

## Q. Skeletal muscle (LS)

**Ans.**
- Vertical bundle of the muscle fibers is identified

- Cross striations are visible on the muscle fibers
- Peripherally located nuclei.

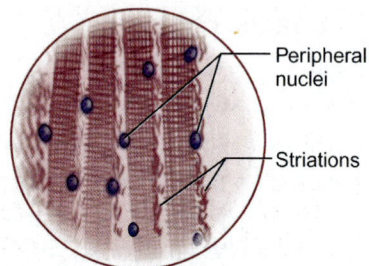

Skeletal muscle

## Q. Smooth muscle (LS)

**Ans.**
- Spindle-shaped cells with broad central part and tapering ends
- Nucleus is oblong along the axis of the cell
- No striations visible, e.g. walls of stomach, intestine.

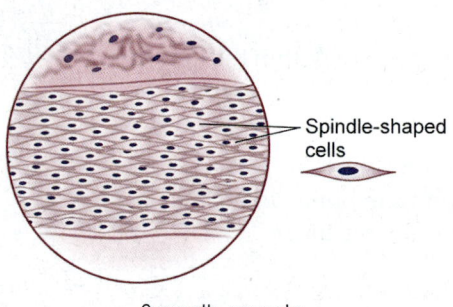

Smooth muscle

## Q. Cardiac muscle (LS)

**Ans.**
- Bundles of muscle fibers show faint striations
- Nuclei of the cells of muscle fibers are centrally located
- The muscle fibers branch and anastomose with each other
- Presence of intercalated disk is characteristic of cardiac muscle.

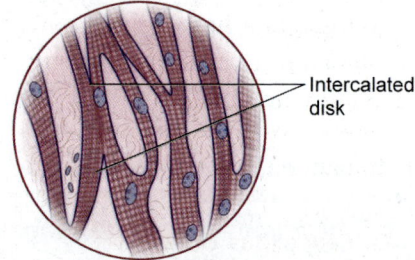

Cardiac muscle

## Q. Peripheral nerve (TS)

**Ans.**
- The nerve tissue fixation needs special stain, osmic acid
- The myelin sheaths are stained black
- Group of nerve fibers appear as collection of empty black rings
- The bundle of nerve fibers is covered by connective tissue known as perineurium.

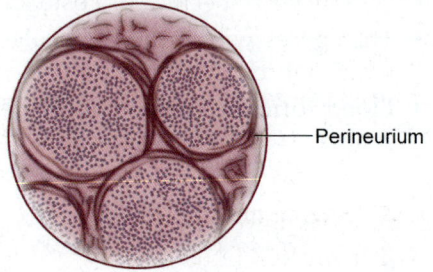

Peripheral nerve

## Q. Sensory ganglion

**Ans.**

- Groups of neurons can be identified
- Each neuron has vesicular nucleus with prominent nucleoli
- Neuron is surrounded by satellite cells
- Collection of nerve fibers can be identified between groups of neurons.

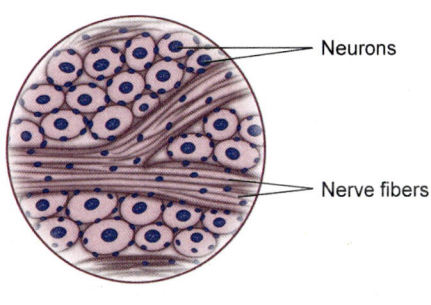

Sensory ganglion

## Q. Elastic artery

**Ans.**

- Tunica media is very thick
- It is made-up of fenestrated concentric elastic membranes
- In between the membranes there is connective tissue and few smooth muscle cells
- Internal elastic lamina is not distinct
- Tunica adventitia is thin, e.g. aorta, large arteries supplying head, neck and limbs.

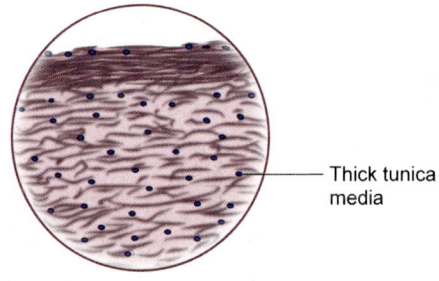

Elastic artery

## Q. Muscular artery

**Ans.**

- The internal elastic membrane is very distinct
- Clear separation of tunica media and tunica intima can be appreciated
- Tunica media is made-up of smooth muscle cells
- Tunica adventitia is made-up of collagen and elastic fibers, e.g. all other arteries in the body except aorta, the large arteries supplying head, neck and limbs.

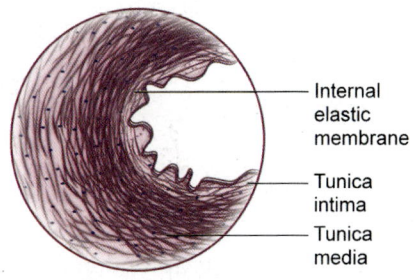

Muscular artery

## Q. Vein

**Ans.**

- Vein has a collapsed wall and a large lumen within
- Tunica intima, media and adventitia cannot be separately identified and merge with each other
- Tunica adventitia is very thick
- Tunica media is thin and contain few muscle fibers.

Vein

## Q. Lymph node

**Ans.**

- Demarcated into outer cortex and inner medulla
- The cortex is made-up of lymphatic follicles

- Each follicle has a pale staining germinal center and peripheral, closely packed lymphocytes
- Lymphocytes are present within the follicles
- Medulla consists of blood vessels and collection of lymphocytes in the form of cords.

## Q. Spleen

**Ans.**
- Parenchyma of spleen is divisible into red pulp and white pulp
- Red pulp comprises of numerous sinusoids and few lymphocytes
- White pulp is a dense collection of lymphocytes in the form of cords
- Capsule can be identified
- Incomplete septae or trabeculae can be identified within the parenchyma.

Lymph node

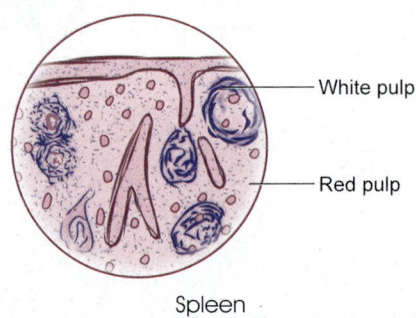

Spleen

## Q. Thymus

**Ans.**
- Distinct lobules can be identified
- Each lobule has an outer cortex and inner medulla
- Cortex is made-up of densely packed lymphocytes
- Medulla has few lymphocytes and pink rounded masses of cells known as corpuscles of Hassall
- In between the lobules, connective tissue can be identified.

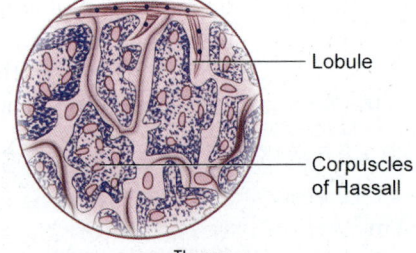

Thymus

## Q. Palatine tonsil

**Ans.**
- It is the only lymphatic tissue covered by stratified squamous epithelium
- Epithelium dips at certain places and these sites are known as crypts
- Beneath the epithelium, there are lymphatic follicles, which have densely packed lymphocyte in the periphery and diffuse lymphocytes in the center.

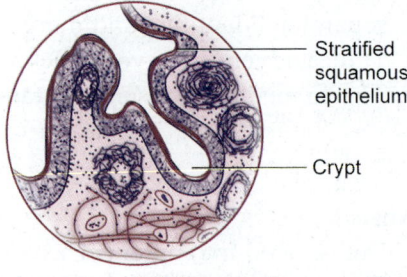

Palatine tonsil

## Q. Skin—Thin skin

**Ans.**

- Comprises of epidermis and dermis
- Hair follicle with arrector pili muscle visible
- Sebaceous gland present near the hair follicle
- The parts of sweat gland can be appreciated.
- For example: Eyelid skin.

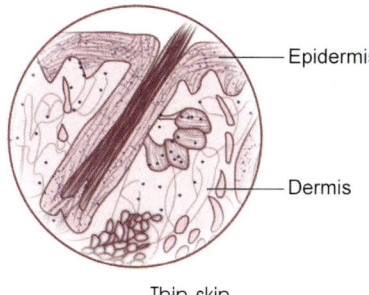

Thin skin

## Q. Skin—Thick skin

**Ans.**

- Comprises of epidermis and dermis
- Keratin layer thickest, i.e. thick stratum corneum
- Does not have hair, sebaceous or sweat glands.
- Dermis is thin
- For example: Sole of foot.

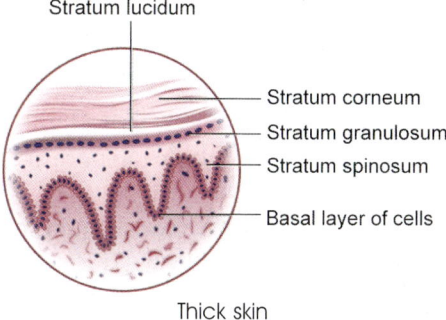

Thick skin

## Q. Tongue

**Ans.**

- Section of tongue shows group of skeletal muscle fibers in various directions
- Collection of serous and mucous glands are present in between the muscle fibers
- Surface is covered by stratified squamous epithelium
- Papillae are seen on the dorsum, each papilla has connective tissue covered by stratified squamous epithelium.

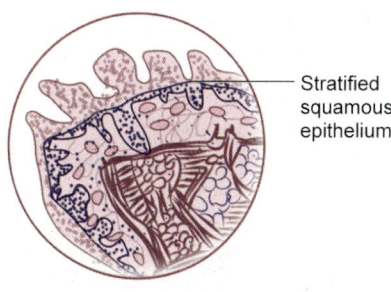

Tongue

## Q. Circumvallate papilla

**Ans.**

- It is the largest papilla of the tongue
- Top of the papilla is broad and covered by stratified squamous epithelium
- It has a lateral wall that forms deep groove
- The lateral wall has taste buds
- Core of the papilla shows serous glands and muscle fibers.

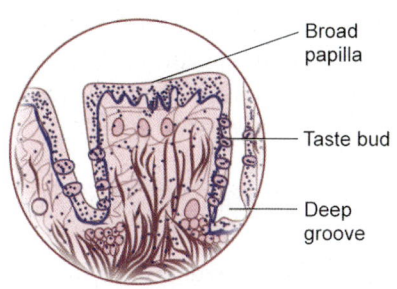

Circumvallate papilla

### Q. Serous salivary gland

**Ans.** (Darkly stained section)
- Compound tubuloalveolar gland
- Section shows lobules separated by inter lobular connective tissue
- Each lobule shows collection of serous acini mainly and few mucous acini
- Connective tissue has blood vessels, adipose tissue, e.g. parotid salivary gland.

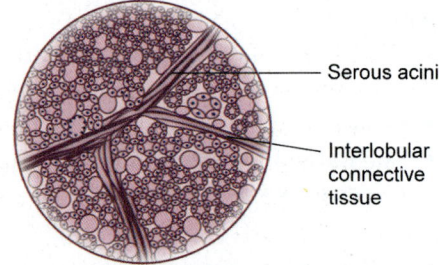

Serous salivary gland

### Q. Mixed salivary gland

**Ans.**
- Compound tubuloalveolar gland
- Section shows lobules separated by interlobular connective tissue
- Each lobule shows almost equal collection of serous acini and mucous acini
- Connective tissue has blood vessels, adipose tissue, e.g. submandibular salivary gland.

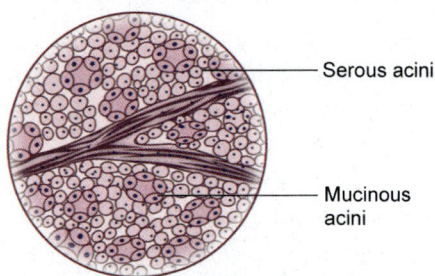

Mixed salivary gland

### Q. Mucous salivary gland

**Ans.** (Lightly stained section)
- Compound tubuloalveolar gland
- Section shows lobules separated by interlobular connective tissue
- Each lobule shows collection of only mucous acini; occasionally a serous demilune may be seen
- Connective tissue has blood vessels, adipose tissue, e.g. sublingual salivary gland.

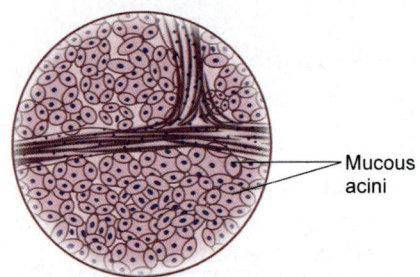

Mucous salivary gland

### Q. Esophagus

**Ans.**
- Lining of nonkeratinized stratified squamous epithelium seen
- Beneath the epithelium is lamina propria, a connective tissue layer
- Cut muscle fibers are seen below the lamina propria
- Thick submucosal layer comprising of mucous glands, lymphoid tissue, plasma cells, macrophages
- Muscular layer consists of inner circular and outer longitudinal muscles.

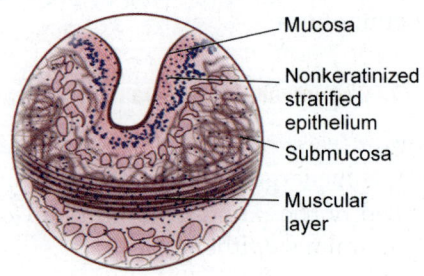

Esophagus

## Q. Cardiac end of stomach

**Ans.**

- The mucosa is thin in this area and gastric pits are shallow
- Junction of stratified squamous epithelium of esophagus and columnar epithelium of stomach is seen
- Cardiac glands are simple tubular or compound tubuloalveolar packed within the mucosa
- Other layers seen are muscularis mucosa, submucosa, circular muscle layer and longitudinal muscle layer.

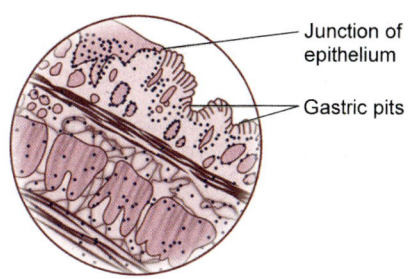

Junction of epithelium

Gastric pits

Cardiac end of stomach

## Q. Body of the stomach

**Ans.**

- Mucosal lining is of the columnar epithelium
- Relatively deep gastric pit
- Numerous gastric glands are visible in the mucosa, viz. chief cells (peptic cells), parietal cells (oxyntic cells)
- Near the neck of the gastric glands are mucous neck cells, while at the base are endocrine cells and some undifferentiated cells
- Other layers seen are muscularis mucosa, submucosa, circular muscle layer and longitudinal muscle layer.

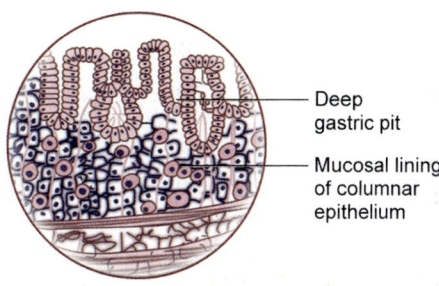

Deep gastric pit

Mucosal lining of columnar epithelium

Body of the stomach

## Q. Pyloric end of stomach

**Ans.**

- Gastric pits are deep and occupy two-thirds of the mucosa
- Pyloric glands are seen in the deeper part of mucosa
- Other layers seen are muscularis mucosa, submucosa, circular muscle layer and longitudinal muscle layer.

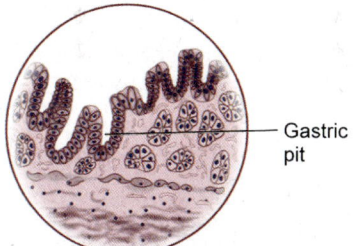

Gastric pit

Pyloric end of stomach

## Q. Jejunum

**Ans.**

- Mucosa shows numerous finger-like projections known as villi
- Each villus is covered by columnar epithelium and has a central connective tissue; few goblet cells are seen
- Deep crypts reaching muscularis mucosal layer are seen
- Single lymph nodule is present in the mucosa
- Other layers seen are the muscularis mucosa, submucosa, circular muscle layer and longitudinal muscle layer.

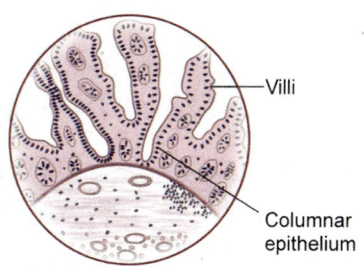

Villi

Columnar epithelium

Jejunum

## Q. Duodenum

**Ans.**

- Mucosa shows numerous finger-like projections known as villi
- Each villus is covered by columnar epithelium and has a central connective tissue; few goblet cells are seen
- Intestinal crypts lie above muscularis mucosa
- Glands of Brunner lie below the muscularis mucosa
- Glands of Brunner pack the submucosa and is distinguishing feature of duodenum.

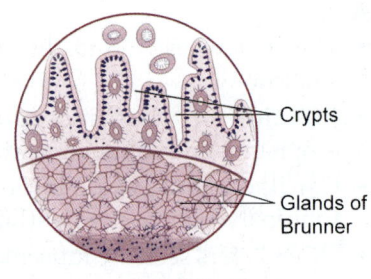

Duodenum

## Q. Ileum

**Ans.**

- Presence of lymphatic follicles (Peyer's patch) is the distinguishing feature
- The lamina propria is filled with lymphocytes
- Villi are rudimentary or absent just above the follicle
- The muscularis mucosae are not well-developed
- Other layers seen are submucosa, circular muscle layer and longitudinal muscle layer.

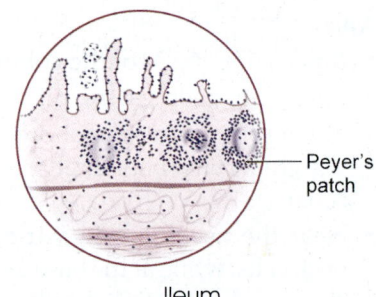

Ileum

## Q. Large intestine

**Ans.**

- Mucosal surface and the crypts are lined by columnar cells amongst which are numerous goblet cells
- Villi are absent
- Paneth cells absent
- Lymphatic nodule is seen in lamina propria
- Longitudinal muscle coat is in the form of three bands called *Taenia coli*
- Other layers seen are muscularis mucosa, submucosa and circular muscle layer.

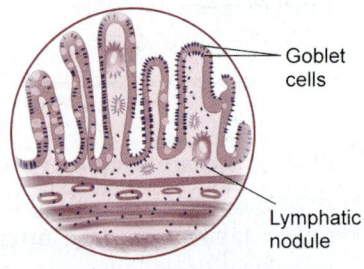

Large intestine

## Q. Vermiform appendix

**Ans.**

- Mucosa is poorly developed
- Lamina propria filled with lymphocytes and numerous lymphatic nodules
- Other layers seen are muscularis mucosa, submucosa, circular muscle layer and longitudinal muscle layer.

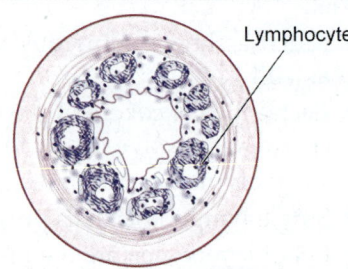

Vermiform appendix

## Q. Liver

**Ans.**

- Section is made-up of hexagonal hepatic lobules
- Each lobule has a central vein from which radial sinusoids are visible
- Lobules are separated by connective tissue
- Within connective tissue is portal triad, which comprises of branch of portal vein, hepatic artery and interlobular bile duct.

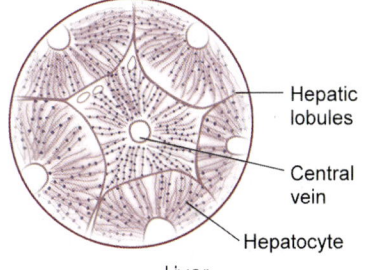

Liver

## Q. Gallbladder

**Ans.**

- The mucosa is lined by tall columnar epithelium
- Goblet cells are absent
- Muscularis mucosa is absent
- Mucosa is highly folded
- Muscle coat is poorly developed and has connective tissue within lined by mesothelium.

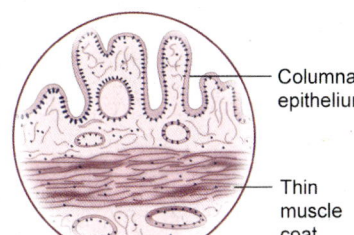

Gallbladder

## Q. Trachea

**Ans.**

- The mucous membrane is lined by pseudostratified ciliated columnar epithelium
- Hyaline cartilage structure seen in the section
- Connective tissue contains serous and mucous glands.

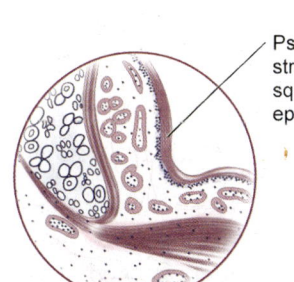

Trachea

## Q. Lung

**Ans.**

- Section is filled up by thin-walled spaces known as alveoli
- Alveoli filled up with air
- Cut section of bronchi can be seen in the slide
- Wall of the alveoli is lined by simple squamous epithelium
- Smooth muscle, cartilage and glands are seen in the wall of the bronchus
- Lining of mesothelium can be appreciated in the section.

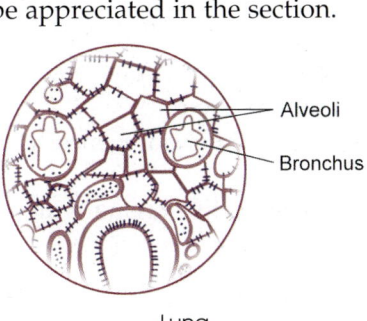

Lung

## Q. Kidney

**Ans.**

- Covered by a capsule
- Substance of a kidney can be divided into outer cortex and inner medulla
- Cortex is made-up of renal corpuscles and cut section of tubules around it
- Cut sections of collecting ducts running vertically can be seen in medulla
- Few collecting duct sections may extend into the cortex known as medullary ray
- Cut sections of blood vessels can be seen in the cortex.

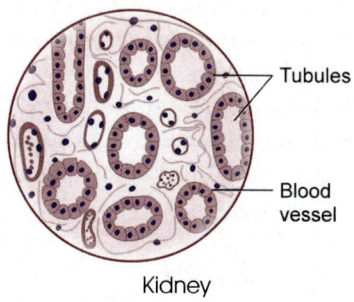

Tubules

Blood vessel

Kidney

## Q. Ureter

**Ans.**

- Slide shows star-shaped lumen
- Mucous membrane is lined by transitional epithelium
- Muscle coat comprises of inner longitudinal layer and outer circular layer
- Muscle layer is covered by connective tissue layer in which fat cells and blood vessels are seen.

Transitional epithelium

Star-shaped lumen

Ureter

## Q. Urinary bladder

**Ans.**

- Mucous membrane is lined by transitional epithelium
- Subepithelial connective tissue layer is present
- Very thick muscular layer is present
- No clear demarcation can be appreciated between longitudinal and circular muscle
- By and large, circular muscle fibers are seen in between outer and inner longitudinal layer.

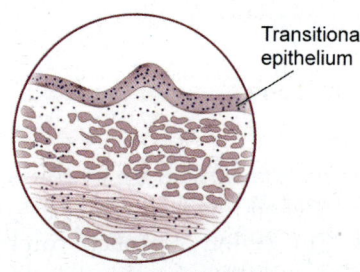

Transitional epithelium

Urinary bladder

## Q. Testis

**Ans.**

- Outer fibrous layer, tunica albuginea can be appreciated
- Cut section of seminiferous tubules are seen
- Several layers of cells (different stages of spermatogenesis) can be appreciated within the tubules
- In between the tubules, there is connective tissue with blood vessels and groups of interstitial cells.

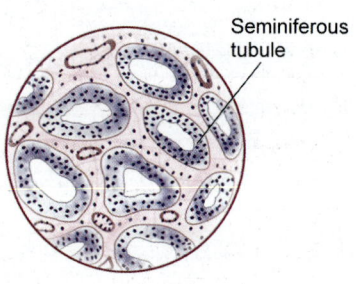

Seminiferous tubule

Testis

## Q. Epididymis

**Ans.**
- Slide shows cut sections of convoluted duct
- Duct is lined by pseudostratified columnar epithelium
- Spermatozoa groups can be identified within the lumen of the duct
- Smooth muscle can be identified in the wall of the duct.

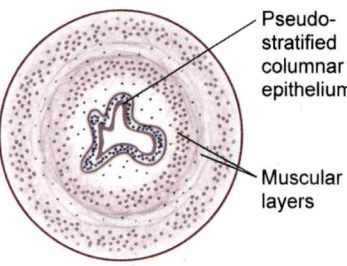

Pseudo-stratified columnar epithelium

Epididymis

## Q. Ductus deferens

**Ans.**
- Mucous membrane lined by pseudostratified columnar epithelium
- Below the mucosa is lamina propria
- Thick muscle coat comprises of inner longitudinal, middle circular and outer longitudinal.

Pseudo-stratified columnar epithelium

Muscular layers

Ductus deferens

## Q. Seminal vesicle

**Ans.**
- The mucosal lining of cut tubule is folded several times and branch and form a network
- Lining epithelium is simple columnar or pseudo-stratified
- Smooth muscle layer is very thin
- Tube is covered by thick connective tissue layer.

Markedly folded muscle

Smooth muscle

Seminal vesicle

## Q. Prostate

**Ans.**
- Section shows collection of glandular tissue interspersed between thick fibromuscular tissue
- Glands are irregular in shape and lined by columnar epithelium
- Lumen may show amyloid bodies
- Fibromuscular tissue is very thick and is the peculiarity of prostate
- Cut section of urethra lined by transitional epithelium can be appreciated in low power.

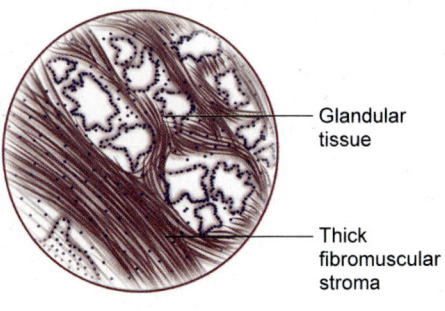

Glandular tissue

Thick fibromuscular stroma

Prostate

## Q. Penis (low magnification)

**Ans.**

- Outer covering of skin can be seen
- Three masses of erectile tissue can be appreciated
- Masses adjacent to each other are corpora cavernosa
- Center of each corpus cavernosum shows cut section of artery
- Mass in front of corpora cavernosa is corpus spongiosum
- Corpus spongiosum is traversed by urethra
- Erectile masses are covered by thick fibrous sheath
- Urethra is lined by pseudostratified columnar epithelium
- Diverticula are seen within the urethral opening
- Outside the erectile masses, cut section of dorsal arteries can be seen within the connective tissue layer.

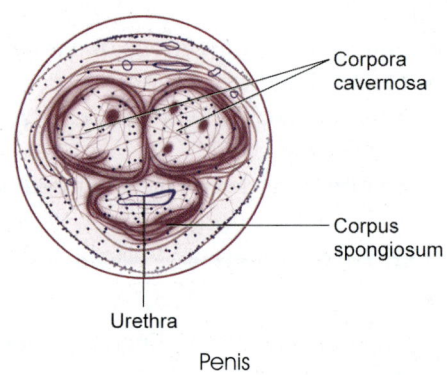

Penis

## Q. Ovary

**Ans.**

- Surface covered by cuboidal germinal epithelium
- Below the epithelium is connective tissue layer known as tunica albuginea
- Substance of ovary divisible into outer cortex and inner medulla
- Cortex comprises of follicles, which contain developing ovum surrounded by follicular cells
- Cells surrounding the ovum form corona radiata
- Different stages of follicles can be appreciated
- Pink body corpus luteum can be seen in some slides
- The medulla comprises of connective tissue with blood vessels within.

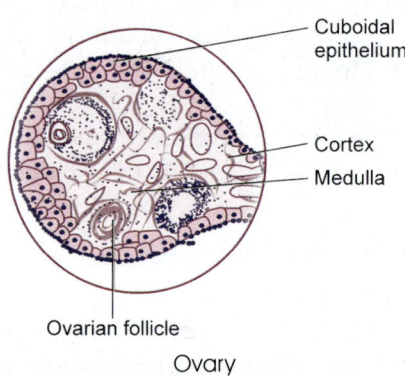

Ovary

## Q. Uterine tube

**Ans.**

- Mucous membrane shows intricate branching pattern, which fills up the lumen of the tube
- Muscular wall of the tube is made-up of outer longitudinal and inner circular layer
- Mucosa is lined by ciliated columnar epithelium.

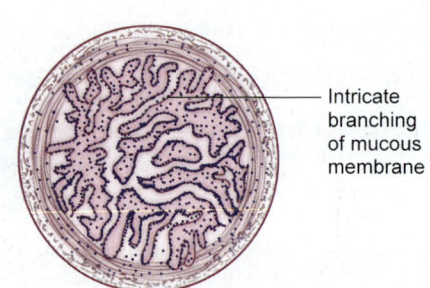

Uterine tube

## Q. Uterus in proliferative stage

**Ans.**
- Uterine wall comprises of mucous membrane known as endometrium and a thick muscle layer known as myometrium
- Columnar epithelium lines the endometrium and is thin
- Under the epithelium is the stroma of connective tissue
- Numerous cut sections of tubular glands, which are straight, can be seen in the stroma
- Smooth muscle fibers running in different directions with cut sections of blood vessels can be seen.

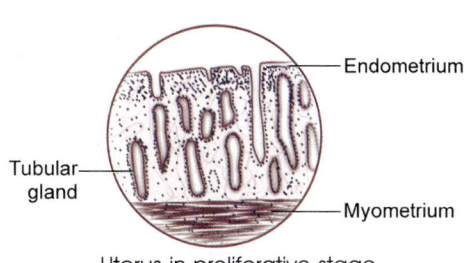

Uterus in proliferative stage

## Q. Uterus in secretory phase

**Ans.**
- Uterine wall comprises of mucous membrane known as endometrium and a thick muscle layer known as myometrium
- Columnar epithelium lines the endometrium and is thick
- Under the epithelium is the stroma of connective tissue
- Tubular glands become elongated, dilated and tortuous
- Stroma is divisible into superficial stratum compactum, middle stratum spongiosum and stratum basale
- The smooth muscle fibers running in different directions with cut sections of blood vessels can be seen
- Blood vessels are prominently visible.

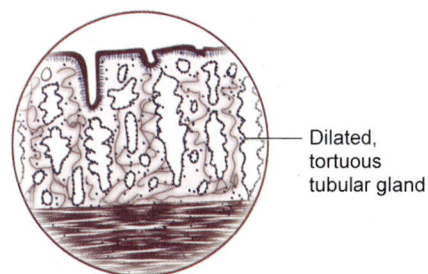

Uterus in secretory phase

## Q. Vagina

**Ans.**
- Mucosa lined by nonkeratinized stratified squamous epithelium
- There are no glands in the mucosa
- Subepithelial connective tissue layer shows cut sections of blood vessels and lymphatic follicles
- Thin layer of circular muscle fibers running in different directions can be appreciated.

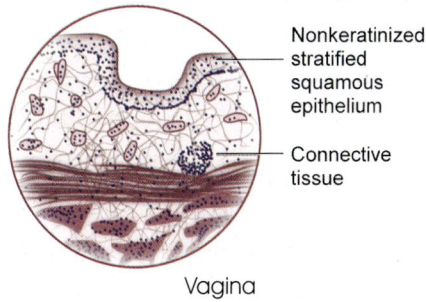

Vagina

## Q. Mammary gland

**Ans.**
- Comprises of lobules of glandular tissue with intervening connective tissue and fat
- Cut sections of glands are lined by cuboidal epithelium and have large lumen
- Within the connective tissue cut section of duct can be appreciated lined by two layers of cuboidal or squamous epithelium.

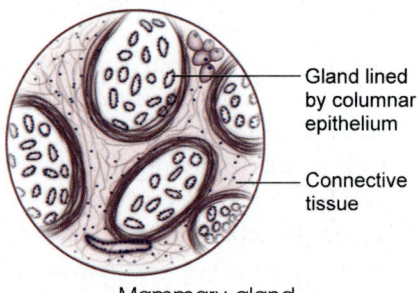

Gland lined by columnar epithelium

Connective tissue

Mammary gland

## Q. Pituitary gland

**Ans.**
- Section shows pars anterior, pars intermedia and pars posterior
- Pars anterior comprises of groups of cells, and chromophobe
- Cells of acidophils are pink
- Cells of basophils are blue
- Nuclei are closely packed and cytoplasm not distinct in chromophobe cells
- Pars intermedia comprises colloid filled vesicle, blood vessels and few cells
- Pars posterior is collection of nerve fibers and neuroglial cells.

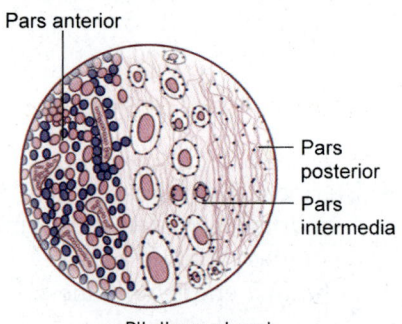

Pars anterior

Pars posterior

Pars intermedia

Pituitary gland

## Q. Thyroid gland

**Ans.**
- Numerous follicles are seen in the section lined by cuboidal epithelium
- Follicles contain homogenous pink colloid within
- In between the follicles is connective tissue
- Parafollicular cells can be seen adjacent to the follicles and in the connective tissue.

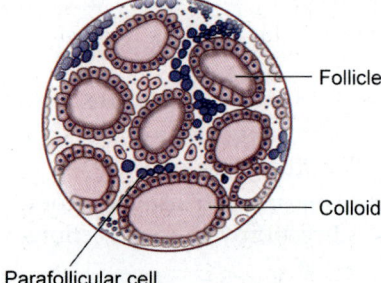

Follicle

Colloid

Parafollicular cell

Thyroid gland

## Q. Parathyroid gland

**Ans.**
- Comprise of clusters of cells with different stains
- Most of the cells are blue staining and are known as chief cells
- Scattered within the chief cells are large pink staining cells known as oxyphil cells
- Cut sections of blood vessels can be appreciated in the slide.

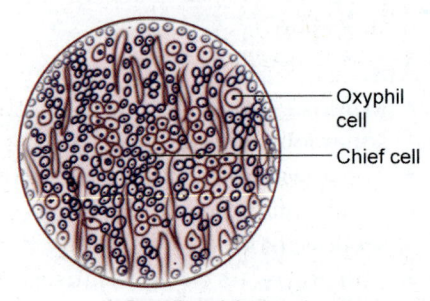

Oxyphil cell

Chief cell

Parathyroid gland

## Q. Suprarenal gland

**Ans.**

- Gland is covered by capsule, it can be seen in the form of connective tissue layer
- Substance of the gland is divided into outer cortex and inner medulla
- Cortex is made of zona glomerulosa, zona fasciculata and zona reticularis
- Zona glomerulosa is made-up of horseshoe-shaped clusters of cells
- Zona fasciculata is made-up of vertical columns of cells with interspersed sinusoids
- Zona reticularis is made-up of network of cords of cells
- Medulla is made-up of groups of cells, sympathetic neurons and sinusoids between the cells.

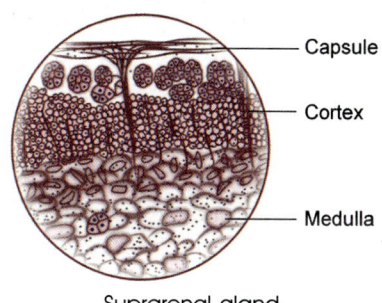

Suprarenal gland

## Q. Cornea

**Ans.**

- Glance at the slide will show several layers
- Outermost layer is nonkeratinized stratified squamous epithelium
- Next layer is anterior limiting membrane appreciated as a thin homogenous pink layer
- A very thick collagen fiber layer known as substantia propria embedded in ground substance is the peculiar feature
- Below the propria is posterior limiting lamina
- Innermost layer is a single layer of cuboidal cells.

Cornea

## Q. Wall of eyeball

**Ans.** Following layers of eyeball can be appreciated:

- Sclera in the form of collagen fibers
- Choroid made-up of blood vessels and pigment cells
- Pigment cell layer of retina
- Rods and cones layer
- Outer nuclear layer
- Outer plexiform layer
- Inner nuclear layer
- Inner plexiform layer
- Ganglion cell layer
- Layer of optic nerve fibers.

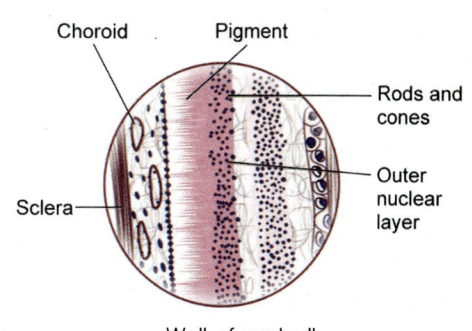

Wall of eyeball

## Q. Cochlea

**Ans.**
- Bony tissue can be appreciated outside the cochlea
- Cochlea is in the form of spiral canal seen as six cut section
- Modiolus contains a canal through which cochlear nerve fibers pass
- Group of spiral ganglion neurons can be appreciated near the canal section
- Three parts can be identified in the cochlea namely scala vestibuli, scala tympani and cochlear duct
- Vestibular membrane lies between scala vestibuli and cochlear duct
- On the basilar membrane is organ of Corti.

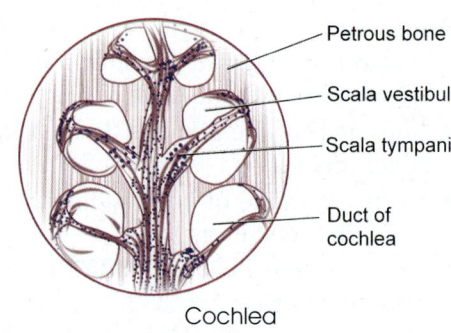

Cochlea

## Q. Spinal cord (special stain)

**Ans.**
- H-shaped lightly stained gray matter (groups of cell bodies) can be appreciated
- Around the gray matter is densely stained myelinated fibers, which forms the white matter of spinal cord
- Central canal can be seen within the gray matter
- Vertically long and thin posterior median septum can be seen
- Wide and short anterior median sulcus can be appreciated.

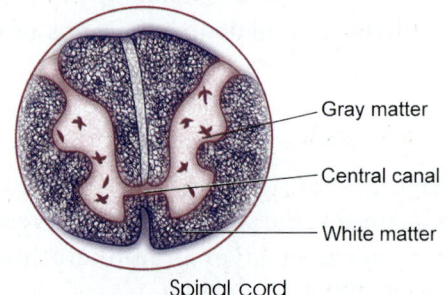

Spinal cord

## Q. Cerebellum

**Ans.**
- Section depicts leaf-like folia
- Each folia has central blue-stained fibers of white matter
- Outer cortex comprises of molecular layer, Purkinje cells and granule cell layer
- Covered by pia mater.

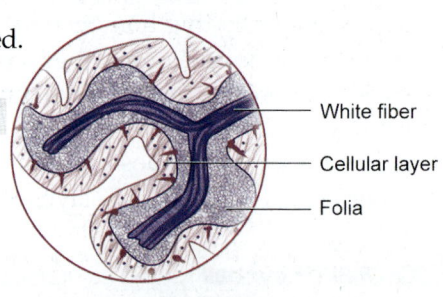

Cerebellum

## Q. Cerebral cortex

**Ans.** Following are the layers of cells and nerve fibers, which form the cerebral cortex:
- Molecular layer
- External granular
- Pyramidal cell layer
- Internal granular layer
- Ganglionic layer
- Multiform layer.

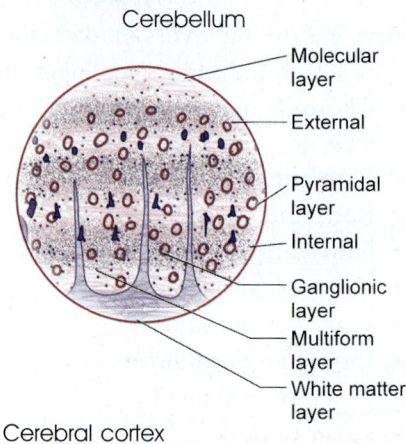

Cerebral cortex

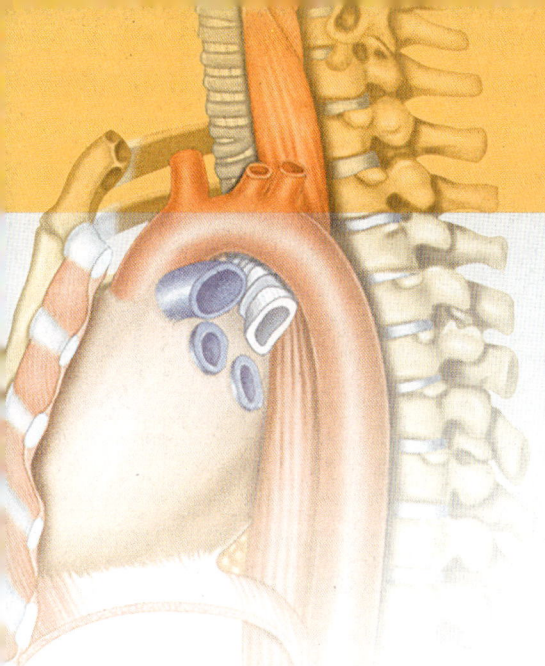

# Great Vessels of the Body

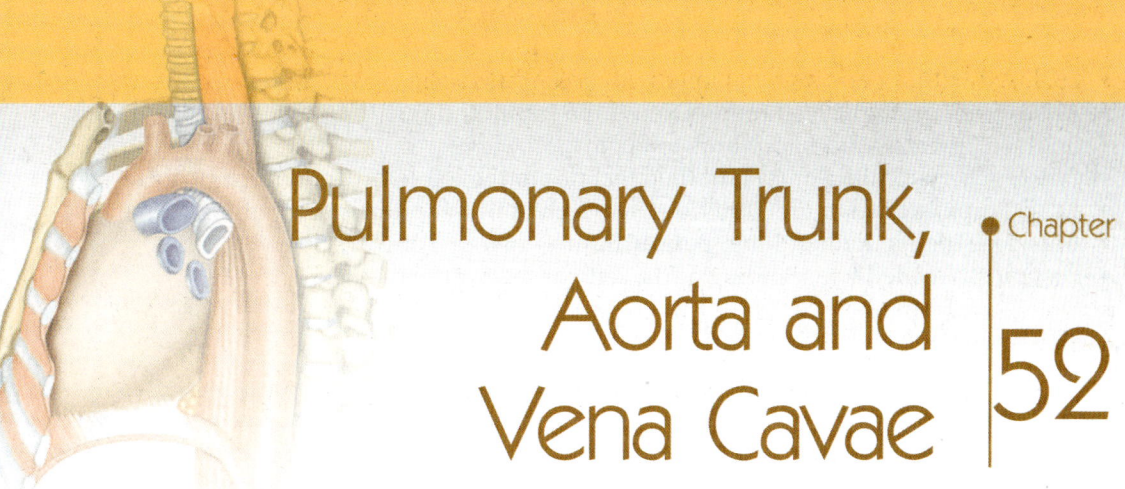

# Pulmonary Trunk, Aorta and Vena Cavae

The great vessels of the body are:
1. Pulmonary trunk
2. Aorta
3. Superior vena cava
4. Inferior vena cava

## PULMONARY TRUNK

Carries deoxygenated blood from right ventricle to lungs.

*Features and crucial relations:*
• It is short and thick, like trunk of a tree

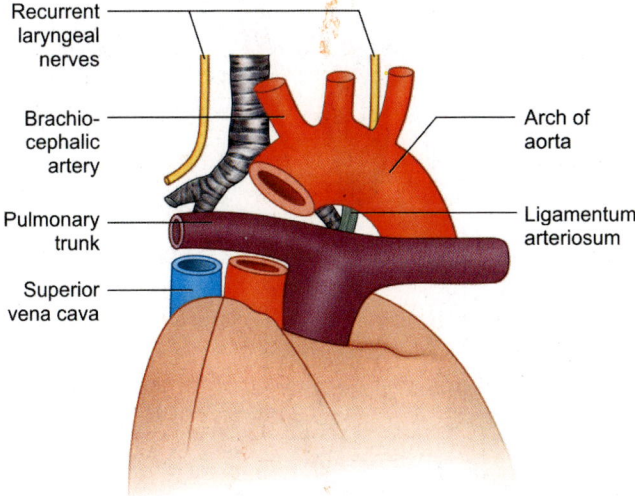

Pulmonary trunk front view

- Enclosed within pericardium along with ascending aorta
- Arises from pulmonary annulus around the infundibulum
- Courses upwards and backwards to begin
- Crosses the ascending aorta and then inclines to the left to lie under arch of aorta
- At T5 (appx. sternal angle) it divides into right and left pulmonary trunk
- Anteriorly lie pleura, left lung, pericardium
- Posteriorly related to ascending aorta, left coronary artery.

## AORTA

It is a major vessel distributing oxygenated blood to all parts of the body.

### Parts

1. Depending upon location
   a. Thoracic
   b. Abdominal
2. Depending on direction and shape of vessel:
   a. Ascending
   b. Arch
   c. Descending
   Ascending and arch of aorta lie in thorax while most of descending part lies in the abdomen.

### Course

Remember the vessel starts from left ventricle; has to end on left side and more posteriorly, so most of the time it is on left side of body except has little inclination to the right before it forms the arch.

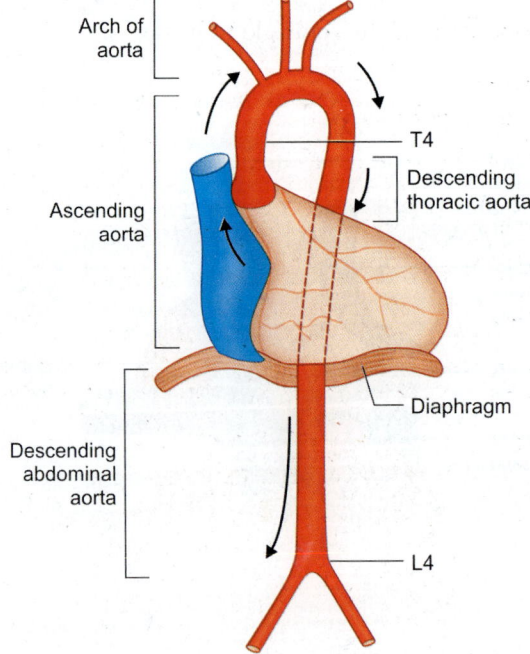

Course of aorta and its parts

**Ascending aorta** arises from base of left ventricle runs obliquely upwards to the right and then turns left to continue as **arch of aorta**, at the level of sternal angle. The arch of aorta begins and ends at the sternal angle. Arch continues as **descending thoracic aorta** at the level of lower border of T4 and ends at T12; further the abdominal descending aorta part begins at T12 and ends at L4.

## Crucial Relations

Remember aorta begins in middle mediastinum proceeds to superior mediastinum and then descends to abdomen through posterior mediastinum. Structures in all these mediastinum will form strategic relations of the vessel.

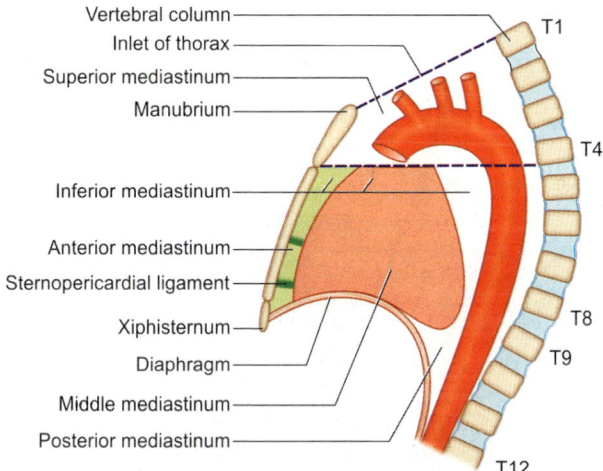

Aorta traversing all the mediastinum

- **Ascending aorta relations**
  - *Anteriorly:* Infundibulum of pulmonary trunk right appendage, pericardium, pleura
  - *Posteriorly:* Left atrium, right pulmonary artery, right principal bronchus
  - *To the right:* SVC
  - *To the left:* Left atrium, pulmonary trunk.

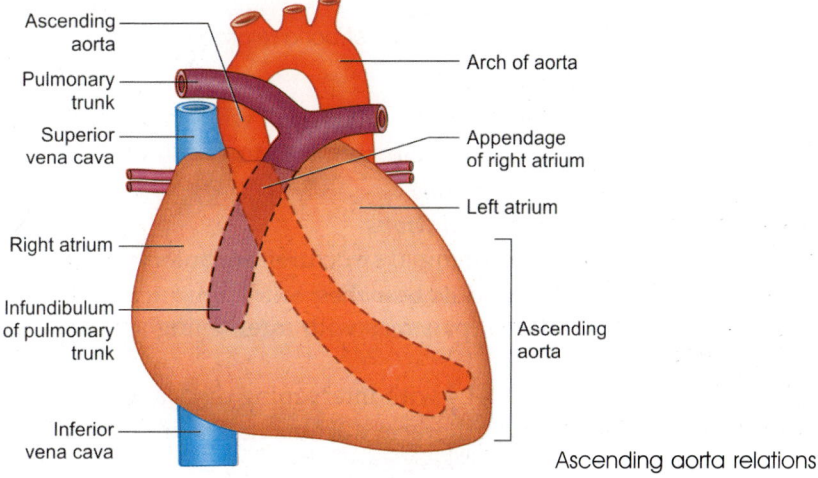

Ascending aorta relations

- *Arch of aorta relations*
  - *Anteriorly:* Left phrenic nerve, left vagus, cardiac branches of vagus and sympathetic trunk, left mediastinal pleura, left superior intercostal vein
  - *Posteriorly:* Trachea, deep cardiac plexus, esophagus, thoracic duct, vertebra
  - *Superiorly:* Its own branches, i.e. brachiocephalic trunk, left common carotid and left subclavian
  - *Inferiorly:* Pulmonary trunk bifurcation, left principal bronchus ligamentum arteriosum, superficial cardiac plexus left recurrent laryngeal nerve as it winds the arch.

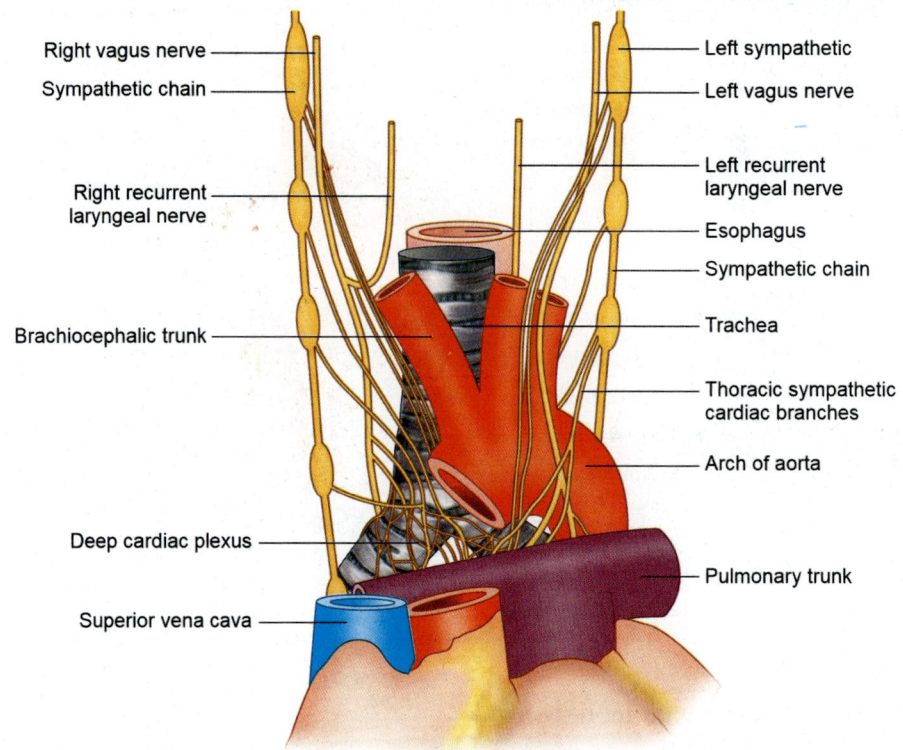

Arch of aorta relations

- *Descending thoracic aorta relations*
  - *Anteriorly:* Left pulmonary hilum, left atrium with its pericardium
  - *Posteriorly:* Vertebra, azygous vein, thoracic duct
  - *Inferiorly:* Right pleura and lungs.
- *Descending abdominal aorta relations*
  It is most posterior, so all abdominal structures are anterior to it:
  - *Anteriorly:* Celiac trunk and its branches, autonomic nerve plexus, lymphatics, superior mesenteric artery, body of pancreas with intervening splenic vein, lesser sac, stomach, 3rd part of duodenum
  - *Posteriorly:* T12, L1, L2, L3, L4 with intervening discs and anterior longitudinal ligament
  - *To the right:* Cistern chyli, thoracic duct, azygos vein, right crus of diaphragm (upper part), inferior vena cava in lower part

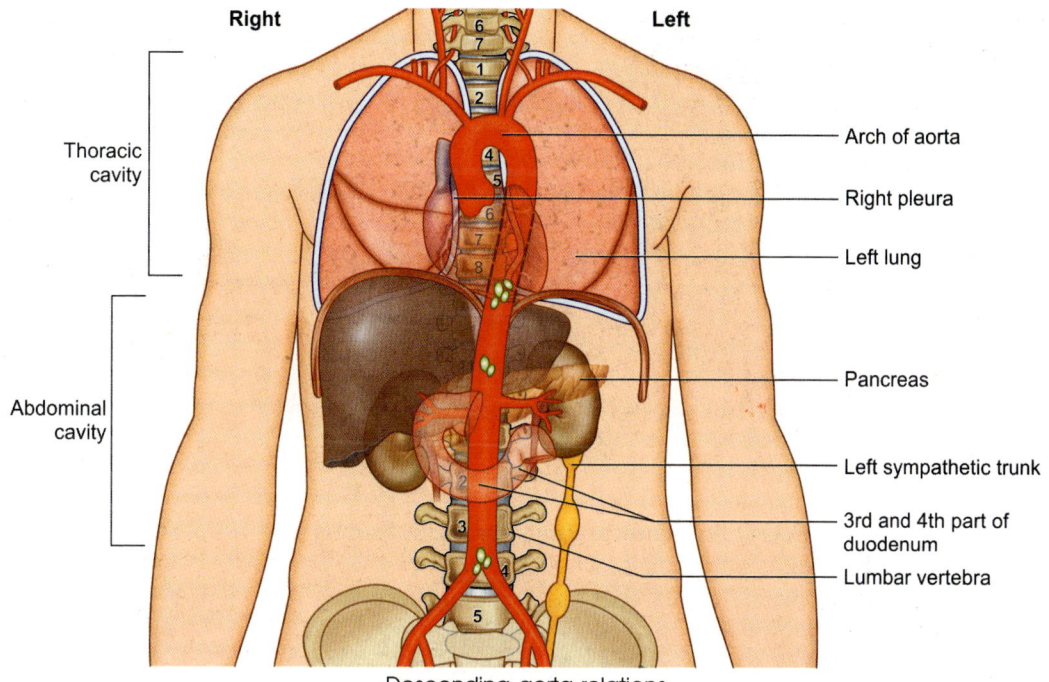

Descending aorta relations

– *To the left:* Left crus of diaphragm, left celiac ganglion, (upper part), 4th part of duodenum, left sympathetic trunk, inferior mesenteric vein.

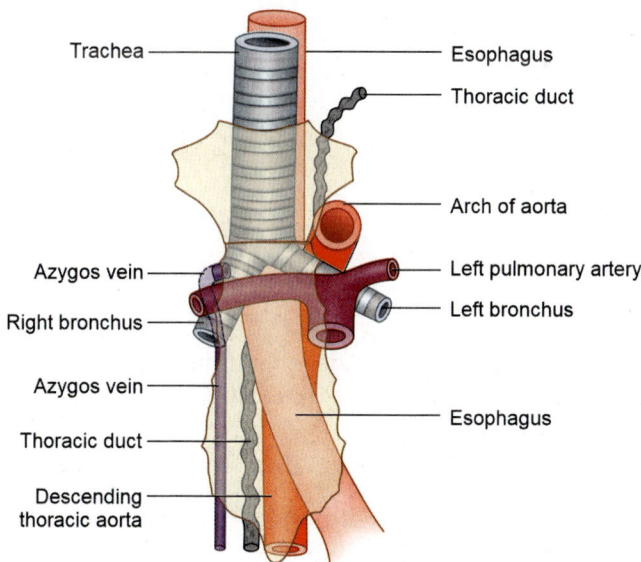

Relations of descending aorta

## Branches of Aorta

- *Ascending aorta:* Coronary arteries
- *Arch of aorta:* Brachiocephalic, left common carotid, left subclavian.

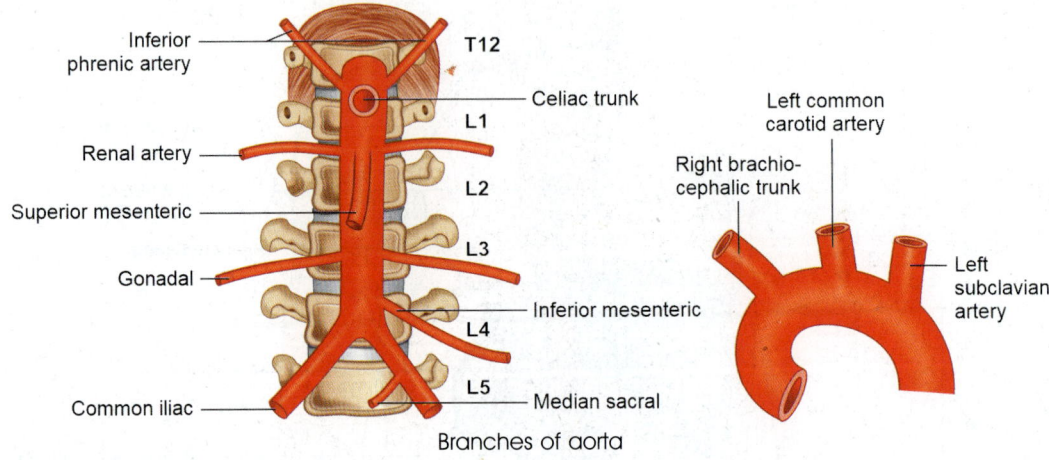

Branches of aorta

- *Descending aorta:*
  - Thoracic part—visceral branches to lungs, bronchi, esophagus and parietal branches to thoracic body wall
  - Abdominal part.

### Anterior Group of Branches

- Celiac trunk
- Superior mesenteric
- Inferior mesenteric.

### Lateral Group of Branches

- Suprarenal
- Renal
- Gonadal.

### Dorsal Group of Branches

- Inferior phrenic artery
- Lumbar artery
- Median sacral artery.

*Applied anatomy:* Aortic aneurysm is due to degeneration of tunica media of the aorta leading to intimal weakening of vessel wall and thus dissection of aorta. The common predisposing factors are aging and hypertension.

## SUPERIOR VENA CAVA (SVC)

This vessel collects deoxygenated blood from tissues above diaphragm to the right atrium
- *Formation:* Right and left brachiocephalic veins unite to form SVC
- *Site:* Behind lower border of first right costal cartilage
- *Crucial relations*
  - *Anteriorly:* 2nd, 3rd costal cartilages and intercostal spaces. Internal thoracic vessels, right lung and pleura

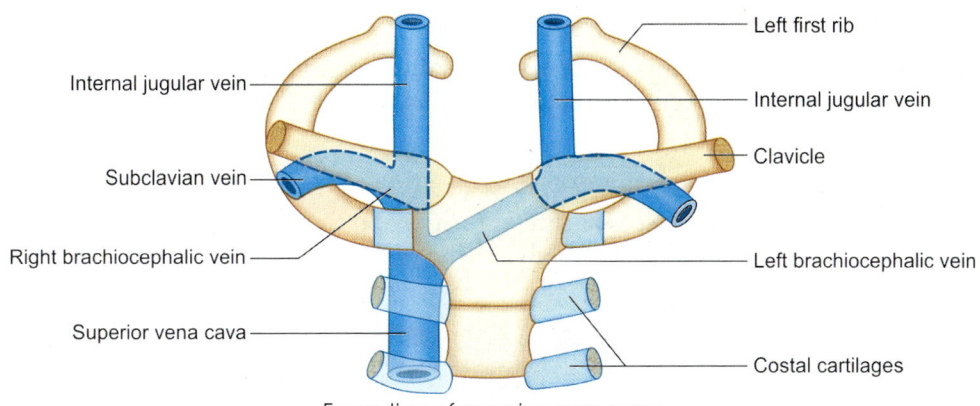

Formation of superior vena cava

- Posteromedial—trachea, right vagus
- Posterolateral—right lung, and pleura
- Posterior—right pulmonary hilum
- Right lateral—right phrenic nerve, pleura
- Left lateral—ascending aorta, brachiocephalic trunk.

- **Tributaries**
  - Azygos veins
  - Small veins from mediastinum and pericardium

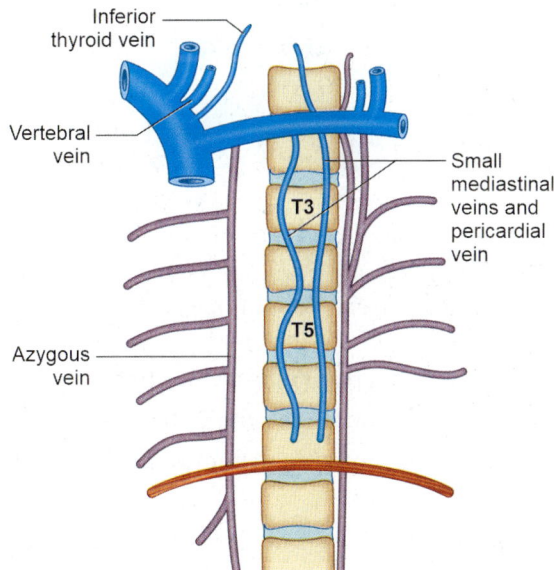

Tributaries of superior vena cava

*Applied anatomy:* SVC obstruction can be due to lung cancer wherein the venous drainage of head and neck is compromised; leading to headache, facial and venous congestion and development of collaterals on the chest wall in patients.

## INFERIOR VENA CAVA (IVC)

This vessel collects deoxygenated blood from infradiaphragmatic tissues to the right atrium. Most of it is in the abdomen; while some portion is in thorax:

- *Formation:* Union of right and left common iliac veins
- *Site:* Front of L5 (1 cm right of midline)
- *Course:* After its formation it ascends upwards (more on right) and enters thorax by passing through the central tendon of diaphragm at level of T8

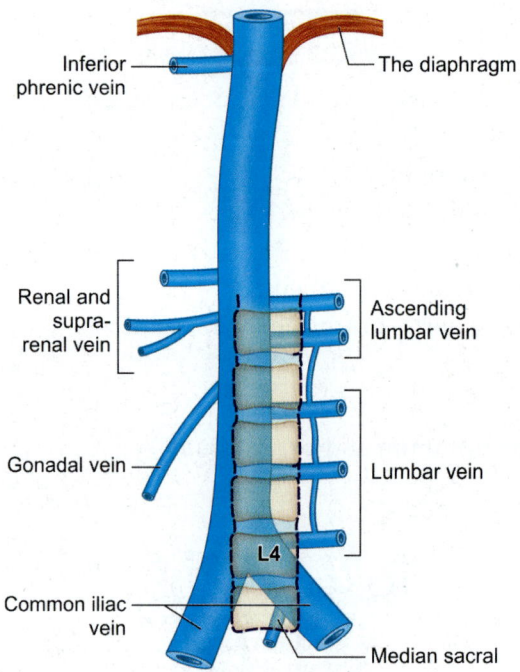

Inferior vena cava formation

- *Crucial relations:* Abdominal part
  - *Anteriorly:* Right common iliac artery, root of mesentery, right gonadal artery 3rd part of duodenum.
  - *Anteriorly and above:* Head of pancreas, 1st part of duodenum
  - *Posteriorly:* Vertebral column, sympathetic chain, lumbar arteries, right psoas major
  - *Posteriorly and above:* Right renal, suprarenal, inferior phrenic arteries, right celiac ganglion
  - *To the left:* Aorta
  - *To the right:* Right ureter, right kidney, 2nd part of duodenum.

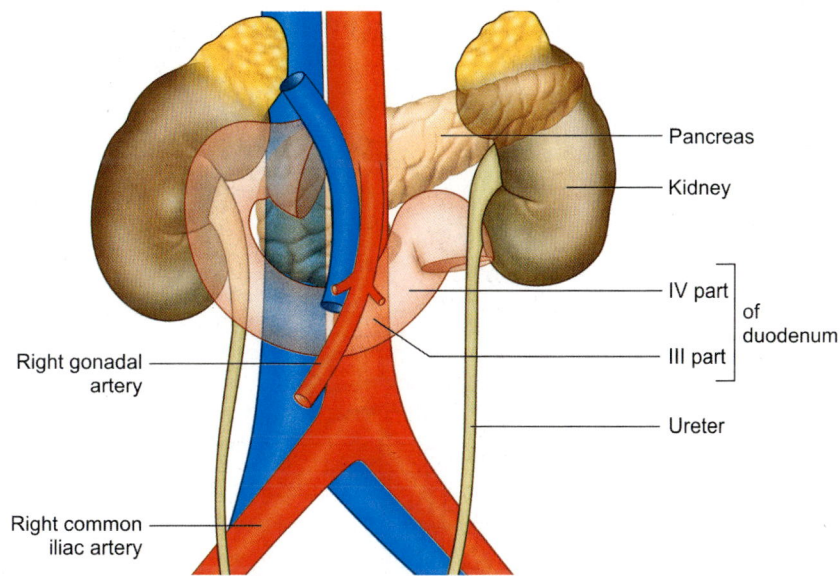

Abdominal part of inferior vena cava—relations

- *Crucial relations of thoracic part:* Lies in the pericardium, extrapericardial part is related to right lung and pleura and right phrenic nerve

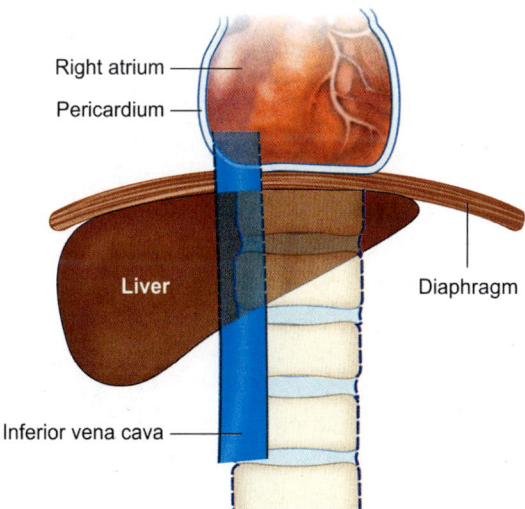

Thoracic part of inferior vena cava—relations

- *Tributaries*
  - Lumbar veins
  - Ascending lumbar veins
  - Gonadal veins
  - Renal, suprarenal veins
  - Inferior phrenic veins.
- *Applied anatomy:* In event of obstruction of IVC, due to thrombosis, or external compression; azygos veins, hemiazygos veins and vertebral venous plexus, superficial body wall veins

form the alternate venous drainage system. An extensive collateral circulation becomes functional between SVC and IVC.

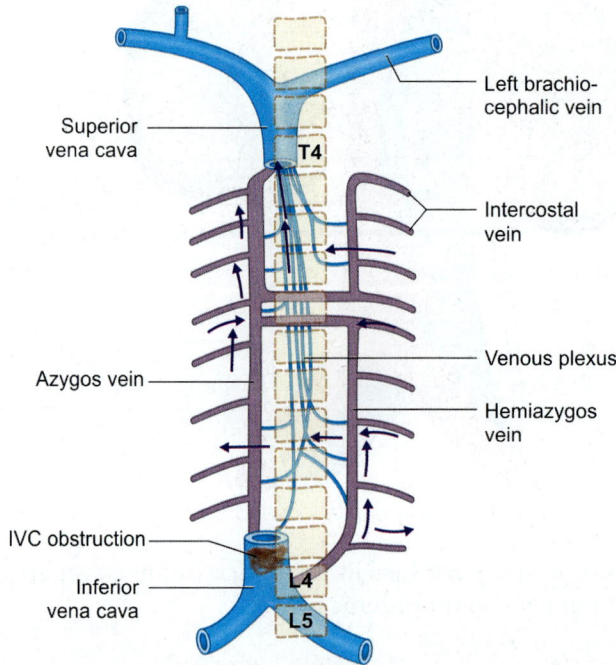

Inferior vena caval obstruction and opened up collaterals

# Radiological Anatomy

# Basics of Radiological Anatomy

Student needs to know few points of radiological anatomy before going to clinical studies ahead in the medical career. Only those points are given below. Several images provided below for study purpose.

- When a film is given to you during the viva, the student should read the film as given below:
- For example: **Chest radiograph**

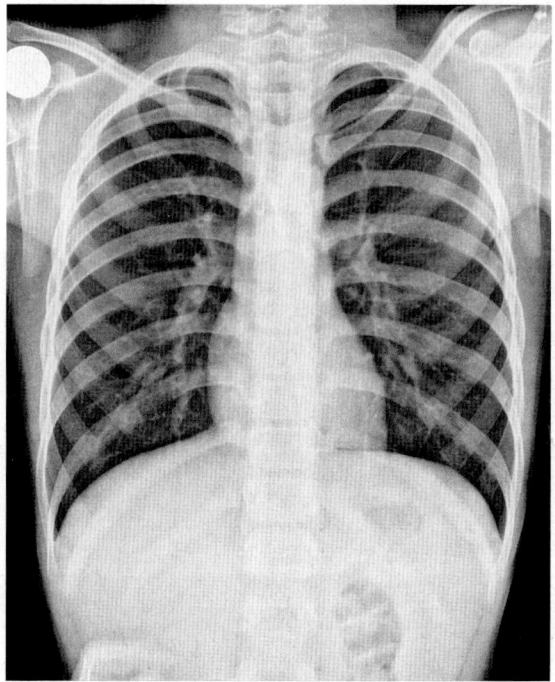

Chest X-ray image PA view

- Please remember when a film is given in your hand that film is the radiograph, so say this is a plain radiograph of chest. (no dye has been used to enhance the anatomical structure, so it is called plain radiography, if any such dye is used it is known as contrast radiography).
- Hazy shadow is of the soft tissue, (bone is the hard tissue, while rest is the soft tissue).
- Radiolucent is the dark black shadow, produced due to air in the body.
- Radiopaque tissue appears as plane homogenous white shadow, density of this shadow varies, e.g. bone has very dense uniform appearance while soft tissue is also plane white but little less dense.
- Identify the soft tissue and the bony shadow on the radiograph.
- Chest radiography is always a posteroanterior view = PA view while most of the other views in the body are anteroposterior view = AP view.

## RADIOGRAPHS OF LIMBS

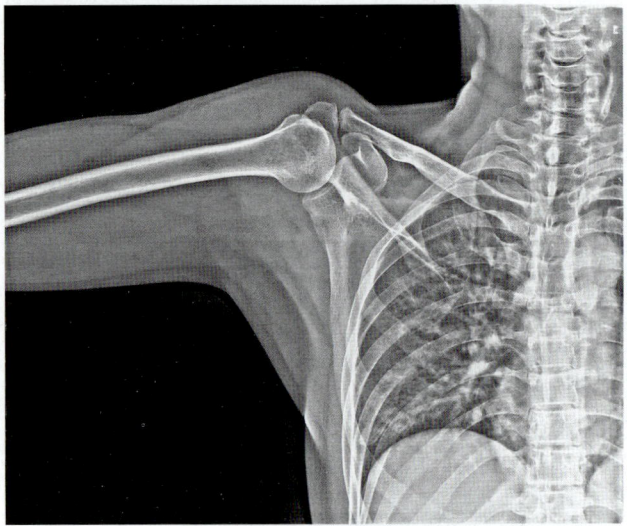

X-ray films of upper limb

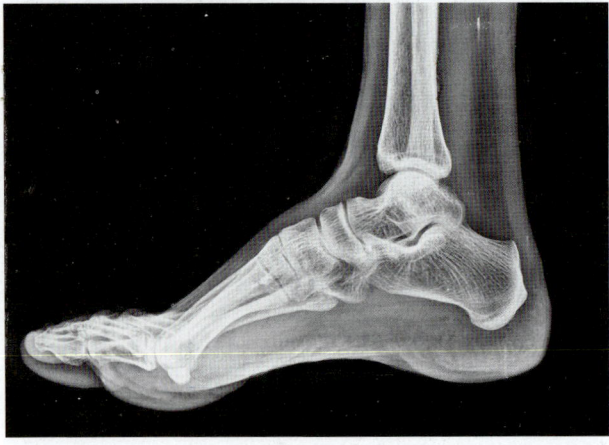

X-ray films of lower limb

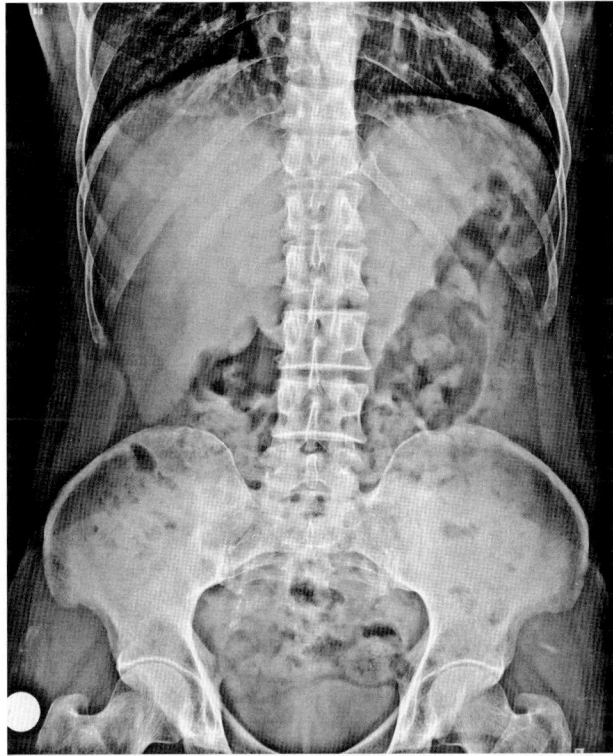

Plain X-ray abdomen (appreciate the gas shadow)

- Student should be able to identify the soft tissue shadow and bony shadow on the film.
- Identify the bones and the joints, visible on the film.
- Discontinuity in the bony margins is known as fracture. Be careful while seeing the film there could be a very thin fracture line, hair line fracture or an obvious break on the long bone.
- **Contrast radiography.**
- To visualise hollow viscera one needs to enhance the organ by injecting a dye this is contrast radiography done for gastrointestinal tract, (Barium swallow), or to visualise uterus and the fallopian tube (hysterography).
- **Computed tomography** (CT scan) provides transverse sectional anatomy information. Body is scanned into slices 3–6 mm size and the cross-sectional anatomy can be studied.
- **Magnetic resonance imaging**.
- This technique has rapidly evolved over the years and most preferred, best suited to study the soft tissue of the body, e.g. MRI brain, MRI of menisci of knee joint.

# Literal Meanings of Anatomical Words

| TERM | DESCRIPTION |
|------|-------------|
| **A** | |
| Acetabulum | Vinegar cup, Latin word, 'Acetum'—vinegar |
| Acoustic | Greek word, 'Akouein'—to hear |
| Adenoid | Greek word, 'Glandular' |
| Adenoids | Enlarged adenoid glands |
| Affinitas | Latin word, Affinity |
| Amnion | Greek word, 'Amnion'—lamb |
| Amygdaloid | Latin word, 'Almond' |
| Amyloid | Latin word, 'Amylum'—starch |
| Anatomy | Greek word, 'Ana'—up or through, 'Tomy'—cutting |
| Antrum | Latin word, cavity or a chamber |
| Aqueduct | Latin word, 'Aquaeductus', 'Aqua'—water, 'Ductus'—a leading pipe |
| Arachnoid | Greek word, 'Arachne'—like a spider |
| Arcuate | Latin word, 'Arcuatus'—curved like a bow |
| Argentaffin | Latin word, 'Argentum'—silver |
| Arytenoid | Shaped like a jug or pitcher |
| Auditory | Latin word, 'Auditories'—to hear |
| **B** | |
| Bregma | Latin word—top of head |
| Brevis | Latin word—short |
| Bulla | Latin word—bubble/seal |
| Bursa | Latin word—purse/pouch |

## C

| | |
|---|---|
| Calamus | Latin word—cane, Greek word, 'Kalamos'—reed |
| Calcaneus | Latin word, 'Calx'—limestone; heel bone looked like a lump of chalk |
| Capitate | Latin word, 'Caput'—head |
| Carpus | Greek word, 'Karpos'—wrist |
| Caudate | Latin word—having a tail/tail-like appendage |
| Cavernous | Spongy |
| Cerebellum | Latin word—diminutive of cerebrum; 'Cartesian maze' (plural—cerebella) |
| Cerebrum | Latin word, 'Cerebrate'—to use the mind to think; Rome—understanding a fiery |
| Cervix | Neck |
| Chiasm | Decussation/crossing over |
| Chorea | Latin word—ceaseless occurrence of rapid, jerky movements |
| Cinereum | Latin word—ashes, ash colored |
| Cingulate | Latin word, 'Cingulum'—a belt worn by roman soldiers to protect their groin |
| Cingulate gyrus | Girdle—like marking; band or ridge zone |
| Claustrum | Latin word—barrier (plural—claustra) |
| Clavicle | Latin word, 'Clavicula'—little key |
| Clinoid | Greek word, 'Kline'—bed; 'Oid'—resemblance |
| Clivus | Latin word—slope |
| Coccyx | Greek word, 'Kokku'—cuckoo |
| Cochlea | Latin word—snail; Greek word, 'Kokhlias'—spiral, snail shell |
| Colliculus | Latin word—a small elevation |
| Condyloid | Latin word, 'Condylus'—knuckle |
| Corniculate | Shaped like a small horn |
| Coronal | Latin word—crown |
| Coronoid | Crown like |
| Cribriform | Perforated like sieve |
| Crura | Latin word—leg/leg like |
| Cubital | Latin word, 'Cubit'—elbow, unit of length |
| Cuboid | Cube like |
| Culmen | Upper ridge of bird's bill |
| Culmus | Latin word—stalk |
| Cuneatus | Latin word—tapering/pointed like a wedge |
| Cuneiform | Latin word—shaped like wedge |

## D

| | |
|---|---|
| Deltoid | Shaped like a delta, triangular |
| Diaphragm | Latin word—midriff; Greek word—partition |
| Diencephalon | Greek word—portion of brain between the cerebrum and the mesencephalon |

| Diploë | Greek word—fold |
| Duodenum | Latin word, 'Duodenum digitorum'—12 fingers' breadth |
| Dura | Hard |

## E

| Ecto | Outside |
| Emissary | Latin word—to send out; an agent sent on a mission to represent or advance the interests of others |
| Encephalon | En—in; Greek word, 'Kephale'—head |
| Epi | Above |
| Epididymis | Greek word, 'Epi'—on; 'Didymos'—twin |
| Ethmoid | Spongy |

## F

| Falx | Latin word—sickle shaped |
| Fastigium | Latin word—summit |
| Fibula | Latin word, 'Clasp'—brooch |
| Flexion | Latin word, 'Flexus'—to bend |
| Fontanel | Old French, 'Fontanel'—fountain |
| Foramina | Latin word—opening |
| Fornix | Latin word—arch-like structure |
| Fossa | Latin word—ditch |
| Fundus | Latin word—bottom |

## G

| Gaster | Greek word—belly |
| Gastrocnemius | Latin word—calf of leg, 'Gastro'—belly |
| Glabella | Latin word, 'Glabellus'—hairless |
| Glenoid | Saucer like |
| Glial | Greek word—glue |
| Globus Pallidus | Latin word—sphere, globe; 'Pallidus'—pale |
| Gluteal | Greek word, 'Gloutos'—buttock |
| Goblet | French word—drinking cup with a thin stem |
| Griseum | Latin word, 'Griseus'—bluish or gray |

## H

| Habenula | Latin word, 'Habena'—rein |
| Hallux | Latin word, 'Hallex'—big toe |
| Hamulus | A hook |
| Hiatus | Latin word, 'Hiare'—an opening, to gape or yawn |
| Hilum | Latin word, depression/pit |
| Hippocampus | Greek word, 'Hippokampus', 'Hippos'—horse, 'Kampos'—sea monster |

| Holo | Greek word, whole, entire |
| Hyoid | Greek word, 'Hyoeides'—shaped like a letter epsilon |
| Hypo | Below |

## I

| Ileum | Greek word, 'Eileo'—to roll up, twist |
| Ilium | Latin word—groin |
| Incus | Anvil |
| Indusium | Latin word, 'Induere'—to put on, kind of tunic |
| Inguinal | Latin word, 'Inguin'—groin |
| Innominate | No name |
| Ischium | Greek word, 'Ishion'—hip joint |

## J

| Jejunum | Latin word, 'Jejunus'—fasting |
| Jugular | Latin word, 'Jugulum'—throat |
| Juvenile | Latin word, 'Juvenis'—young |

## L

| Labrum | Latin word—lip edge |
| Lamella | Latin word—diminutive of lamina |
| Lamina | Latin word—thin plate |
| Lepto | Greek word—thin |
| Limbus | Latin word, 'Limbus'—border |
| Linea aspera | Latin word, 'Spera'—rough or hard |
| Lumbricals | Earthworm |
| Lunate | Moon shaped |

## M

| Malleus | Latin word—hammer |
| Mammillary | Resembling breast or nipple |
| Mandible | Latin word, 'Mandere'—to chew |
| Masseter | Latin word—chewer |
| Mastoid | Greek word,—'Mastoeides', breast like |
| Mater | Latin word—mother (slang) |
| Maxilla | Latin word—jawbone |
| Meatus | Latin word—opening, to go |
| Mesencephalon | Greek word, 'Mesos'—middle |

## N

| Navicular | Latin word—boat |
| Nidus | Latin word—nest |

## O

| | |
|---|---|
| Obex | Latin word—barrier |
| Obturator | Latin word, 'Obturare'—to stop up or closing on opening |
| Olive | Latin word—symbol of piece |
| Ovary | Latin word—egg |
| Oxyntic | Greek word, 'Oxyno'—secreting acid, to make sour acid |

## P

| | |
|---|---|
| Parietal | Latin word—belonging to the wall |
| Patella | Latin word, 'Dish/Pan'—saucer like |
| Pectineus | Latin word, 'Pecten'—comb |
| Pellucidum | Per—through, 'Lucere'—to shine |
| Peritoneum | Greek word, 'Tonos'—stretching, 'Peri'—around |
| Peroneus | Greek word, 'Perone'—pin of a brooch or buckle |
| Petrous | Latin word, 'Petra'—stone |
| Phalanx | Greek word, 'Phalangos'—finger |
| Physis | Greek word—growth |
| Pia mater | Latin word—tender mother |
| Pilus | Latin word—hair |
| Pineal | Latin word—pine cone |
| Piriformis | Latin word—pear shaped |
| Pisiform | Latin word, 'Pisum'—pea shaped |
| Pituitary | 'Phlegm'—gland that produces mucus |
| Pons | Latin word—bridge |
| Popliteus | Latin word, 'Poples', 'Poplit'—back of the knee |
| Postrema | Latin word—for back end area |
| Profunda | Deep |
| Propria | Latin word, 'Proprius'—proper, own |
| Prostate | Greek word, 'Prostates'—one who stands before, protector, guardian |
| Psoas | Greek word, 'Psoa'—loin region, either of muscle of the loin that rotate the hip joint and flex the spine |
| Pterygoid | Like bird's wings |
| Pulvinar | Latin word—a cushion |
| Putamen | Latin word—falls off in pruning |
| Putane | To prune/to think |

## R

| | |
|---|---|
| Ramus | Branch |
| Restiform | Latin word, 'Restis'—rope, 'Forma'—form; shaped like a rope |
| Rima | A gap or cleft between two symmetrical parts |
| Rostrum | Roused platform on which person stands |

## S

| | |
|---|---|
| Sacrum | Latin word—sacred/strong bone |
| Saphenous | Greek word—easily seen |
| Sartorius | Latin word, 'Sartor'—tailor |
| Scaphoid | Greek word—shaped like a boat |
| Scapula | Greek word, 'Scaphein'—to dig |
| Sciatic | Latin word, 'Sciaticus'—derived from Greek word, 'Ischiadikos'—pertaining to/located near ischium |
| Septum | Latin word—dividing wall, partition |
| Sinus | Space |
| Soleus | Latin word, 'Solea'—sandal |
| Sphenoid | Shaped like a wedge |
| Spine | Latin word—point |
| Splenium | Band—like structure |
| Stapes | Latin word—stirrup |
| Sternum | Breast, chest |
| Striae | Latin word—thin line or band |
| Stroma | Greek word—bed |
| Subiculum | Latin word—support |
| Sural | Latin word, 'Sura'—calf of leg |

## T

| | |
|---|---|
| Tapetum | Latin word—coverlet |
| Tarsus | Latin word—tarsus, Greek word—wicker |
| Tectum | Latin word—roof |
| Tegmentum | Latin word—covering |
| Tela | Latin word—web-like tissue |
| Temporal | Not lasting forever |
| Tenia | Greek word—headband |
| Tentorium | Latin word—tent |
| Teres | Latin word—round and long |
| Testis | Latin word—witness |
| Thalamus | Greek word, 'Thalamos'—chamber |
| Thyroid | Greek word—shield like |
| Tibia | Latin word—flute, shinbone |
| Tissue | French word — to weave |
| Tonsils | Check posts |
| Trapezoid | Greek word—table shaped; Latin word—shaped like a trapezium |
| Triceps | Latin word, 'Caput'—3 heads |
| Triquetral | Latin word—3 cornered |
| Trochanter | Greek word—wheel |
| Trochlea | Latin word—system of pulleys, Greek word, 'Trokhileia'—to run |
| Tubercle | Wart—like growth |
| Tympanic | Drum |

## U

| | |
|---|---|
| Ulna | Yard, 3 feet |
| Urethra | Greek word, 'Ourein'—to urinate |
| Uterus | Latin word—womb |

## V

| | |
|---|---|
| Vagina | Latin word—sheath/scabbard |
| Vastus | Latin word—vast, huge |
| Vertebra | Latin word, 'Vertere'—to turn, joint, spinal column |
| Vomer | Latin word—plowshare, ploughshare |

## X

| | |
|---|---|
| Xiphoid | Like a sword |

## Z

| | |
|---|---|
| Zygoma | Greek word, 'Zygon'—a yoke |

# Index

**A**bdominal
  policeman 269
  regions 287, 352
  tonsil 343
Adductor canal 173
Adson's test 397
Alderman's nerve 465, 467
Anastomosis
  back of thigh 165
  definition 26
  elbow 58
  Galen's 499
  genicular 165
  palmar arches
    deep 59
    superficial 59
  porto-systemic 337
  scapular 57
  types of 26
Anatomical snuff box 72
Anatomy
  anatomical position 7
  anatomical terms 8
  anatomy act 34
  classification 7
  definition 7
  general anatomy
    bones 9
    muscles 18
      division of 23
    nerves 31
      referred pain 31
    vessels 24
Aneurysm 26
Angles
  angle of ante-flexion of uterus
    264, 324, 345
  angle of ante-version of
    uterus 264, 324, 345
  angle of femoral torsion 147
  angle of humeral torsion 43
  carrying angle 73
  renal angle 341
  sternal angle 395
    events occurring at 395
Ansa cervicalis 499

Aponeurosis 23
  external oblique 339, 340
  internal oblique 261
Arnold's nerve 465
Arteries
  aorta 878
    abdominal 880
    thoracic 879
  arteria profunda femoris 163
  artery of epistaxis 479
    Little's area/Kiesselbach's
      plexus 591
  axillary 79
  basilar 580
  carotid
    external 500, 503
    internal
      iliac 281, 346
      thoracic 402, 431
  celiac (coeliac) trunk 277, 882
  central artery of retina 504
  cerebellar
    inferior 690, 704, 712
  cerebral
    anterior 696, 701
    middle 696
    posterior 703, 714
  clinical terms related to
    vessels in the body
    aneurysm 26
    infarction 26
    lymphedema 26
    thrombosis 26
  coronary 422
  end-arteries 26
  facial 500, 581
  femoral 162
  maxillary 485, 559, 773
  mesenteric
    inferior 280, 343
    superior 278, 343
  popliteal 164, 225
  vertebral 473, 501, 617
    events occurring at C6 473
Axon types 31

**B**lood supply to brain and spinal
  cord 700
Bone marrow
  composition 11
  differences 12
  types 11
Bones
  blood supply of long bones 10
  bregma 460
  calvaria 460, 638
  carpal bones 130, 131, 132
    mnemonic 130
  centres
    primary 11
    secondary 11
  cephalic index 474
  clavicle 39, 40, 121
  coracoid process 12, 40, 68
  cranial vault (endocranium)
    638, 643
  differences between fetal and
    adult skull 474
  ethmoid 476
  femur 236
    adductor tubercle 147
    greater trochanter 236
    lesser trochanter 236
    medico-legal importance
      of lower end 147
    third trochanter 147, 196
  fibula 11, 243
    head 149
  foramina see under f
  frontal 649
    cribriform plate 470, 476
  hip
    iliac crest 143
    ischial spine 145
    ischial tuberosity 144, 145
    pre-auricular sulcus 144
  humerus 41, 125
    anatomical neck 126
    inter-tubercular sulcus 42, 126
    radial (spiral) groove 56,
      82, 116
    surgical neck 41, 116

lambda 460
mandible 650
　age changes 472
　nerves related 472
maxilla 649
　age changes 477
navicular 149, 246
norma basalis 641
norma frontalis 639
norma lateralis 639
norma occipitalis 640
norma verticalis 638
nuchal lines 647
occipital 647
parietal 460, 649
　tuber 460, 638
patella 148, 239
peculiarities 40
pelvis 145
　differences between male
　　and female pelvis 146,
　　258, 383
points
　asterion 465, 640
　entomion 465
　gonion 461
　inion 461
　jugal 463
　mental 463
　nasion 461, 639
　obellion 460, 639
　pterion 466, 640
　sylvian 466, 640
pterygoid plates lateral 468
　medial 468
radius 127
ribs 393
　cervical 397
　first 394, 430
　twelveth 430
sacrum 258, 382
scapula 123, 40
sesamoid 42, 148, 149
skull 460
sphenoid 478, 648
　spine 469, 515
sub-talar 171, 200
temporal bone
　lines 460, 639
　parts 464, 648
thoracic cage 448
　sternum 448
tibia 240

tubercles
　adductor 147
　articular 464
　pharyngeal 468, 642
tuberosities
　ischial 144, 195, 235
　maxillary 462, 649
vertebrae
　cervical
　　atlas 473, 651
　　axis 473, 651
　　seventh 473, 652
　lumbar 257
　　events occurring at L1 259
　thoracic 395, 396, 451
vertebral column 17
　curvatures 17
Broncho-pulmonary segments
　418, 434
Bursae around knee joint 178

Caecum (cecum) posterior
　relations 366
Calcaneal tendon rupture 194
Canals
　adductor 173, 215
　inguinal 288, 355
　optic 470, 648
　pudendal 292, 345
Capillaries
　definition 25
　meta-arteriole 25
　pre-capillary sphincter 25
Cardiac silhouette 405, 432
Cartilage
　elastic 12
　fibrocartilage 12
　hyaline 12
　peculiarities 12
Celiac trunk (coeliac) 277
Cerebellum
　inferior peduncle 676, 712
Cerebrum 903, 904
　association fibres 667, 716
　commissural fibres 667, 716
　medial surface 715
　superolateral surface 668, 714
Cervical rib 397
Choroid plexus 664
Claw hand 56
Club foot 232
Cochlea section 531
Common abdominal incisions 286

Comparison between carpal and
　tarsal bones 149
Cubital fossa 69, 88
Cysterna chyli 281

Danger area of
　face 504, 582
　scalp 534, 581
Deep vein thrombosis 183
Definitions
　joint 12
　organ 855
　system 855
　tissue 855
Dehiscence
　Killian's 490
Dermatomes
　lower limb 202
　perineum 294
　upper limb 91
Diaphragm
　oral 521
　pelvic 326
　thoracic 415
Diencephalon 673
Dissections
　**abdomen and pelvis**
　　anterior abdominal wall 353
　　common abdominal
　　　incisions 286
　　bladder
　　　gall bladder 310
　　　urinary bladder 313
　　　　posterior surface 315, 380
　　caecum (cecum)
　　　posterior relations 366
　　colon—features 366, 367
　　diaphragm 375, 415
　　evisceration of spleen 374
　　evisceration of stomach 360
　　　stomach bed 295, 361
　　inguinal canal 355
　　inguinal region
　　　superficial and deep 355
　　kidney 370
　　liver 371
　　　Couinaud's liver
　　　　segments 373
　　　surgical lobes 372
　　　visceral impressions on
　　　　postero-inferior surface
　　　　of liver 373
　　loin 358
　　male external genitalia 356

muscles of anterior
abdominal wall 353
omentum
greater 268
lesser 359
pelvic viscera arrangement 377
male and female pelvis
sagittal section 379, 380
penis 358
perineum 377
peritoneal cavity 358
epiploic foramen 360
lesser sac 362
posterior abdominal cavity 376
rectus sheath 354
small intestine 362
duodenum 362
ileum 364
jejunum 364
**head and neck**
back (nape) of neck 614
sub-occipital triangle 616
cranial nerves on base of
skull 626
evisceration of brain 624
face—superficial dissection 611
front of neck 617
glands
parotid 621
sub-mandibular 620
thyroid 623
infra-temporal fossa 630
larynx model 632
lateral wall of nose 634
middle ear relations 635
nasal septum 635
functional cortical areas 714
median section through
3rd and 4th ventricles 717
orbit 627
root of neck 624
sagittal section of nose,
mouth, pharynx 632
triangles of neck
anterior 619
carotid 619
sub-mandibular 620
posterior 612
sub-occipital 616
**lower limb**
back of knee 224
back of leg 226
back of thigh 222

dorsum of foot 219
front of leg 217
front of thigh 212
adductor canal 215
femoral region 214
gluteal region 220
lateral side of leg (peroneal
compartment) 228
medial side of leg 227
sole of foot 228
**neuroanatomy specimens**
cerebral hemispheres
coronal section 718
medial surface 715
superolateral surface 714
floor of cranial cavity 713
median section through 3rd
and 4th ventricles 717
principles 35
tools 34
**thorax**
anterior thoracic wall 439
important vertebral levels 439
diaphragm 375
heart 444
anatomical position 444
pericardial sinuses 447
lungs 441
fissures, lobes 442
hilum hilar structures 441
mediastinal surface 442
mediastinum 440
**upper limb**
axillary region 100
back of arm 114
back of forearm 116
back of hand 118
cubital fossa 105
front of arm 103
front of forearm 107
scapular region 113
Diverticulum Meckel's 765
DNA (diagram) 722

Ear ossicles 530
Embalming 34
Embalming fluid 34
Embryology
**anomalies (see under
malformations)**
**general embryology**
amnion 737, 747
Barr body 725

blastocyst formation 735
capacitation 730
chimera 726
chorion 737
chromosomes
classification 723
non-dysjunction 733
types 724
corpus luteum fate 732
critical period 739
decidual reaction 741
Denver's classification 723
Down's syndrome 733
embryo 721
embryonic disc 737
extra-embryonic
mesoderm 736
fertilization 721
fetal age estimation 746
fetus 721
gastrulation 738
genetic diseases
autosomal dominant 725
autosomal recessive 725,
726
classification 725
X-linked dominant and
recessive 726
Graffian follicle 731, 806
inheritance pattern 725
intra-embryonic
mesoderm 738, 739
Lyon hypothesis 725
meiosis 728, 729
mendelian disorders 725
menstrual cycle 733
rhythm method of
contraception 735
mitosis 727
morula 735, 739
mosaic 726
notochord 739
ontogeny 726
oogenesis 730
oral contraceptive pills 735
parts of decidua 742
phylogeny 726
placenta
functions 742
previa 743
placental barrier 742
primary yolk sac 736
primitive gut formation 761

primitive streak  738
septum transversum 740
sex determination 804
spermatogenesis   729
spermiogenesis 729
super females 733
trimester 745
  Turner's syndrome 733
  types of villi 742
  umbilical cord structure 746
  viability 745
**systemic embryology**
  **derivatives of**
    ectoderm 790
    endoderm 790
    foregut 763
      hindgut 764
      mesenchyme 747
    mesoderm 791
    midgut 763
    neural crest  786
  **development of**
    arteries 774
    ascending aorta 774
    atrium 773
    auditory canal 789
    axis artery of upper and
      lower limb 775
    brain 783
    caecum (cecum) 764
    cloacal sub-divisions 763
    diaphragm 769
    external ears 753
    external genitalia (males,
      females) 781, 782
    eyeball 787
    face 758
      facial muscles 758
    gall bladder 766
    inter-atrial septum 772
    inter-ventricular septum
      773, 779
    kidney 779
    limbs 756
    lips (upper and lower) 757
    liver  765
    mammary gland 749
      middle ear 788
    neural tube 782
    nose 759
    optic vesicle 787
    otic vesicle 788
    palate 759
    pancreas 766

parathyroid  754
pinna 753, 790
portal vein 775
prostate 790
spleen 767
superior vena cava 776
thyroid gland 755
tongue 760
ureter 780
urinary bladder 780
uterus 780
  urinary bladder  780
  villi 742
**embryological basis of**
  **innervation of** diaphragm
    770
  **innervation of** tongue 761
  openings in right atrium 770
**embryology models**
  allantoic diverticulum 814
  anomalies of urinary
    system 842
  anomalies of uterus and
    vagina 845
  bilaminar stage  809
  blastocyst formation 809
  branchial fistula 847
  cloacal sub-divisions 827
  coloboma iris 851
  **development of**
    anal canal 828
    caecum and appendix 828
    face 824
    lens vesicle 850
    lips 825
    mammary gland 816
    middle ear and auditory
      tube 848
    3rd and 4th pharyngeal
      pouch 822
    optic vesicle 849
    palate 825
    pinna 848
    portal vein 839
    thyroid gland 822
    villi 811
  diaphragmatic hernia 834
  ectopic sites of blastocyst
    implantation 810
  ectopic sites of thyroid
    gland 823
  embryonic disc 810
  exomphalos 830

external genitalia of
  females 846
fate of cartilages of
  pharyngeal arches 820
fate of pharyngeal
  pouches 821
fertilisation 808
fetal circulation 840
folding of embryo 814
heart tube 835
hindgut and cloaca 842
indicators of ovulation 807
intra-embryonic
  mesoderm 815
karyotype21 805
lower respiratory tract
  development 831
mature spermatozoa 804
mid-gut loop formation 826
morula formation 808
oesophageal atresia and
  tracheo-oesophageal
  fistula 832
oogenesis 730
ovarian follicle formation
  805, 806
parts of primitive gut 826
placental anomalies 746, 813
position of recurrent
  laryngeal nerve 838
remnants of vitello-
  intestinal duct 833
rotation of gut 828
sex determination 804
spermatogenesis 802
spermatozoa-mature 804
stages of menstrual cycle 807
types of placenta previa 812
uterine segments 812
variations in attachment of
  umbilical cord 813
**fate of**
  heart tube 771
    neural tube 783
    notochord 739
    para-mesonephric duct
      in females 780
      in males 780
    pharyngeal arches 751
    pharyngeal pouches 754
    respiratory diverticulum
      768

septum transversum 740, 769
  sinus venosus 770
  somites 746
**malformations (anomalies)**
  anencephaly 791
    cleft lip 758
    cleft palate 760
    Fallot's tetralogy 774
    gut 764
    kidney 780
    mammary gland 750
    neural tube defects
      anencephaly 791
      spina bifida 791
    sacro-coccygeal
      teratoma 738
    uterus and vagina 845, 846
    vitamin preventing
      neural tube defect 791
**remnants of**
  allantois 844
  descent of testis 782
  differences between fetal
    and adult circulation 840
  fetal age estimation 746
  fetal circulation 777
  first arch 773
  homologue of uterus 781
  mesonephric duct 782
  paramesonephric 782
  path of thyroglossal duct 756
  pre- and post-trematic
    nerve 751
  pre-natal diagnosis 745
  rotation of gut 762, 781
  septum primum 773
  septum secundum 773
  vitello-intestinal duct 291
Erb's paralysis 55
Erb's point in
  neck 614
  upper limb 79
Events occurring at
  C6 473
  L1 259
  the level of insertion of
    coracobrachialis 46
  sternal angle 395, 449
Eyeball (diagram) 530

Fabella 149
Falx cerebri 519

Fascia
  cervical 539
  clavipectoral 68
  deep fascia 33
  modifications 33
  superficial fascia 33
FESS 634
Fetal skull 474, 646
Fibrous skeleton of heart 404
Fissures
  inferior orbital 480, 571
  pterygopalatine 571, 640
  superior orbital 470
Fistula—definition 462
Flat foot 194
Foot drop 174
Foramina (table) 479
  epiploic 270
  of base of skull with structures
    passing through 479
Fossae
  cubital 69, 88, 105
  duodenal 273
  ischio-rectal 336
  pterygo-palatine 463, 466, 571
  pyriform 592
    boundaries 532
Frankfurt's plane 459
Frey's syndrome 499, 623

Galen's anastomosis 499
Ganglia
  basal 670
  definition 666
  gasserion (trigeminal) 469, 493
  otic 494
  pterygopalatine 495
  spinal 31
  stellate 496
  sub-mandibular (Langley's) 497
  sympathetic 31
Glands
  parathyroid 572
  parotid 548
    Frey's syndrome 499, 551
    relations 549
    secretomotor pathway 492, 551
  pituitary 575
  thyroid 564, 585
Gluteal region
  intra-muscular injections 187

Heart-blood supply 422, 444
Hilton's law 17

**Histology slides**
  adipose tissue 858
  appendix (vermiform
    appendix) 866
  artery
    elastic 861
    muscular 861
  bone
    cancellous (spongy) 859
    compact 859
  cartilage
    elastic 859
    fibro-cartilage 859
    hyaline 858
  cell structure 855
    definition of organs, tissue,
      system 855
  cerebellum 874
  cerebral cortex 874
  cochlea 874
  cornea 873
  ductus deferens 869
  epididymis 869
  epithelium
    pseudo-stratified 857
    simple cuboidal 856
    simple squamous 856
    transitional 857
  gall bladder 867
  glands
    mammary 872
    mixed salivary 864
    mucinous salivary 864
    parathyroid 872
    pituitary 872
    serous salivary 864
    suprarenal 873
  kidney 868
  large intestine 866
  liver 867
  loose areolar tissue 858
  lungs 867
  lymph node 861
  muscles
    cardiac 860
    skeletal 859
    smooth 860
  oesophagus 864
  ovary 870
  palatine tonsil 862
  penis 870
  peripheral nerve 860
  prostate 869

seminal vesicle 869
sensory ganglia 861
skin
    thick 863
    thin 863
small intestine
    duodenum 866
    ileum 866
    jejunum 865
spinal cord 874
spleen 862
stomach
    body 865
    cardiac end 865
    pyloric end 865
testis 868
thyroid 872
tongue
    circumvallate papillae 863
thymus 862
trachea 867
ureter 868
urinary bladder 868
uterine tube 870
uterus
    proliferative phase 871
    secretory phase 871
vagina 871
vas deferens 869
vein 861
vermiform appendix 866
wall of eyeball 873
Holden's line 298
Horner's syndrome 496
Hydrocele 313, 358

Infarction 26
Interior of right atrium 406, 433
Inter-muscular spaces of upper
    limb 48, 115
Internal capsule 695
Intestines
    cardinal features of large
    intestine 365, 366, 367
    differences between large and
    small intestines 291
Jacobson's nerve 469, 592
Joints
    amphiarthrosis 17
    ankle 169
    atlanto-axial 514
    atlanto-occipital 513
    biaxial 17
    cartilaginous

primary 15
    secondary 15
classification 12
complex 17
compound 17
definition 12
diarthrosis 17
elbow 84
fibrous 16
first carpo-metacarpal 13, 67
gomphosis 16
hip 183
    ligaments 184
    movements 186
    relations 185
    Trendelenburg's sign 187
joints of thorax 424
    bucket handle movement 429
    pump handle movement 428
knee 188
    ligaments 189
    menisci 190
locking and unlocking 191
    relations 190
multiaxial 17
radio-ulnar 82
shoulder 82
    abduction at shoulder joint 66
sternoclavicular 65
sub-talar 171, 200
synarthrosis 17
synovial joint-sub types 13
uniaxial 17

Kehr's sign 299
Killian's dehiscence 532
Klumpke's paralysis 56

Lacrimal apparatus 538
Larynx 566
Leptomeninges 662
Ligaments
    arcuate popliteal 189
    deltoid 176
    ilio-femoral 184
    inguinal 339
    ischiofemoral
    pubofemoral 184
    sacroiliac 259
    spheno-mandibular 515, 561
    spring 177
    stylo-mandibular 515, 561
Limbic system 669

Lines
    Cantlie's 372
    Holden's 298
    pectinate 297
    trans-pyloric 384
Liver
    bare areas and peritoneal
    reflections 271
    lobes 272
    surgical 372
Locking of knee joint 191
Lumbar puncture 663
Lymph nodes
    axillary 62
    cervical 551, 589
    deep 511
    superficial 509
    Cloquet's 198
    inguinal
    deep 168
    superficial 167
    levels 511
    structure 27
    Virchow's 512
Lymphatic drainage
    anal canal 335
    breast 63, 89
    broadly classified 27
    differences between other
    lymphatic tissue and
    Waldeyer's ring 509
    larynx 566
    rectum 283
    stomach 282
    tongue 512
Lymphedema 568

McBurney's point 298
Medial longitudinal fasciculus 683
Mediastinum 420, 440
Meta-tarsalgia 194
Middle ear relations 568
Mid-inguinal point 216
Mid-line structures of the neck 521
Mid-point of inguinal ligament 217
Muscles
    adductor hallucis 156
    anterior abdominal wall 353
    biceps brachii 46
    cardiac 18
    common extensor origin 90
    common flexor origin 90
    constrictors of pharynx 488
    coracobrachialis 46
    peculiarities 46

dartos 358
definition 18
differences between tendon
  and muscle 23
external oblique 260
extra-ocular 483, 585
facial 481
flexor digitorum profundus 89
flexor digitorum superficialis 89
gluteus maximus 153
    structures under the cover of
       gluteus maximus 154, 221
hamstrings 154
intercostal 400
internal oblique 261
interossei of hand
    dorsal 49
    palmar 48
intrinsic muscles of larynx 491
    safety muscle of larynx 491
involuntary 18
lateral pterygoid 485
    relations 486
levator ani 266
lumbricals 50
muscle layers of foot 157
muscles of mastication 557, 587
mylohyoid 521, 542, 562
palmaris brevis 90, 611
pectineus 153
pectoralis major 44
pharyngeal 573
posterior crico-arytenoid 491, 634
psoas major 150
quadriceps femoris 152
rectus sheath 262
rotator cuff 41, 47
sartorius 152
scalenus anterior 430, 450, 490
serratus anterior 44
    winging of scapula 45
shunt 22
skeletal 18
smooth 19
spurt 22
sternocleidomastoid 482
transverses abdominus 261
triceps surae 155
voluntary 18
**testing of muscles**
    biceps brachii 140
    brachio-radialis 140
    deltoid 140

gluteus maximus and
    hamstrings 252
pectoralis major 139
psoas major and hamstrings 252
serratus anterior 139
tendo achilles and flexors of
    leg 253
tibialis anterior and
extensors 253
transversus abdominus 261
triceps surae 155
voluntary 18

Neck spaces 539
Nerves
    afferent 28
    axillary 51
    common peroneal 174
    cranial 684
        general understanding
            regarding course of cranial
            nerves 685
        general understanding
            regarding function of
            cranial nerves 684
        general features 684
    efferent 28
    facial 554, 690
    femoral 160
    intercostal 401
        atypical 409
        typical 408, 409
    median 53
    musculocutaneous 51
    petrosal
        greater 495, 556
        lesser 479, 495, 556
    phrenic (right and left) 409
    radial 81
    sciatic 160
    spinal 28
        reflex arc 28
    splanchnic (greater and
    lesser) 397
    sural 199
    types 31
    ulnar 52
Nervous system
    cell types 666
    classification 661
    coverings (meninges) 662
Neurobiotaxis 685
Neuroglial cells 29, 666

Neuron
    diagram 29
    parts 29
    types of 29
Nose
    bones forming lateral wall of
        nose 475, 569
    lateral wall 569
    osteo-meatal complex 571
    septum
        blood supply 526
        formation 635
        Little's area/Kiesselbach's
            plexus 527, 591
    nerve supply 526
Nuclei
    brainstem with all cranial
        nerve nuclei (diagram) 684
    definition 29, 666
    facial nerve 554

Omentum
    greater 268
        policeman of abdomen 269
    lesser (omentum) 269, 359
Openings in diaphragm
    (apertures of diaphragm) 433
Organs
    anal canal 333
    brain
        brainstem 662
        cerebellum 672
        cerebrum 714
    diencephalon 673
    ductus deferens 317
    duodenum 303
    extra-hepatic biliary apparatus 309
    gall bladder 310
    heart
        chambers 444
        fibrous skeleton 404
        interior of right atrium 406,
            433, 445
        pericardium 404
        sinuses 405
    hypothalamus 673, 711
    kidney
        anterior relations 296, 370
        posterior relations 297, 341
    large intestine-cardinal
        features 291, 366, 367
    liver
        bare areas and peritoneal
            reflections 297

lobes 373
   postero-inferior surface
    relations 372
lungs 442, 443
oesophagus constrictions and
  their levels from upper incisor
  410
ovary 328
pancreas 307
prostate 320
rectum 330
small intestine differences
  between large and small
  intestine 291
spleen 305
stomach 300
testis 312
ureter 322
urethra (male) 319
uterine tubes 327
uterus 324
   supports of uterus 325
**Ossification**
carpal bones 133
  pisiform 132
clavicle 122
femur 239
fibula 11, 244
general understanding about
  ossification 121
hip 235
humerus 126, 127
laws of ossification 11
  exception for the rule 11
mandible 473
patella 240
radius 128
ribs 451
sacralization 257, 382
scapula 125
skull bone 647
sternum 449
tarsal bones 247
ulna 130

**P**athways
acoustic (auditory) 677
optic (visual) 677
secretomotor pathways
  lacrimal 493
  parotid 492
  sub-mandibular 492
Pectinate line

anatomical and surgical
  importance 345
Peduncles
cerebellar 676
Penis
transverse section (diagram
  only) 290
Perforators (venous)
direct 182
indirect 182
Pericardium
blood supply, nerve supply 404
cavity 444
fibrous, serous 404
sinuses 405
Perineal body 263
Perineal membrane (diagram)
  male, female 293
Peritoneal cavity 358
greater sac 270
horizontal disposition
  (diagram) through supra-colic
  compartment 269
lesser sac 270
supra-colic compartment 269
vertical disposition(diagram) 270
Per-rectal examination 293
Per-vaginal examination 294
Pharynx
hypopharynx 633
nasopharynx, oropharynx 632
Phimosis 299
Planes
trans-pyloric 259, 352
trans-tubercular 353
Plantar fasciitis 194
Plexus
brachial 77
cardiac 408
lumbar 157
on posterior wall 285
sacral 285
Pouch
Douglas 273
Morrison's 271
Prussack's 529
Principles of skin incisions 32
Process
mastoid 464, 474
plates
  medial and lateral pterygoid
  641
tympanic (tegmen tympani)
  591, 644

styloid 465
  styloid apparatus 522
zygoma 463
Pyriform fossa boundaries 532

**Q**uadriceps femoris 152
Quinsy 524

**R**adial incisions on breast 90, 100
Radiological anatomy
basic 889
computed tomography (CT) 891
contrast 891
CXR 889
MRI 891
plain X-rays 891
Recesses
pleural (costodiaphragmatic,
  costomediastinal) 402
Reflex arc 665, 666
Regions of abdomen and pelvis 352
Reid's baseline 459
Retinaculum
extensor (hand) 73
flexor (hand) 70
flexor retinaculum of lower
  limb 175

**S**clero-corneal junction 532
Segments
broncho-pulmonary 418
liver 373
uterine 743
Sensory innervation of face 537
Sheaths
carotid 583, 623
digital synovial 74
femoral 173
fibrous flexor sheath 74
Shoulder girdle 90
Sinuses
cavernous—relations 471
cranial dural venous 546, 704
definition 462
para-nasal 475, 590
pericardial 447
Skeleton axial, appendicular 9
Skin
appendages 749
structures under the skin 35
thick 863
thin 863
Spaces
aorto-pulmonary 414

intercostal 400
intermuscular 48, 115
neck 539
of Whitlow 76
pterygomaxillary 541
Sphincters
anal 267, 334
crico-pharyngeal 490, 574
Spinal cord
laminar pattern 674
termination
in adults 664
in newborn 665
transverse section 665
Stomach bed 295, 301, 361
Styloid apparatus 522
Supports of uterus 264, 325, 326
**Surface anatomy**
abdominal planes and
quadrants 384
anatomical snuff box 137
appendix 385
axillary artery 134
brachial artery 135
colon 387
common carotid 654
dorsalis pedis artery 250
duodenum 388, 389
extensor retinaculum of upper
limb 138
external carotid 654
facial artery 653
femoral artery 248
flexor retinaculum of lower
limb 251
flexor retinaculum of upper
limb 138
great saphenous vein 251
heart 454, 455
heart valves 455
inguinal canal 386
internal mammary artery 455
kidneys (from front and
behind) 387, 388
liver 386
lungs 453, 454
mid-inguinal point 216, 217
mid-point of inguinal ligament
216, 217, 248
palmar arch
deep 137
superficial 136
parotid duct 655

parotid gland 655
pleura 452, 453
popliteal artery 249
radial artery 135
sinuses
frontal 657
maxillary 656
spleen 388
sternal angle 452
stomach 385
sub-mandibular gland 656
surface projection of heart
valves 455
thyroid gland 655
tibial
anterior (photo only) 250
posterior 250
ulnar artery 136
Surgeon's graveyard 533
Sutures
bregma 460
lambdoid 460
metopic 475
tympanomastoid 465
Synapse-types 31
Syndromes
Benedickt's 712
carpal tunnel 56
Down's 733
Horner's 79
Turner's 733
Wallenberg's 712
Weber's 712
Systems
limbic 669
lymphatic 26
pulmonary 25
systemic 25
vascular 26

**T**entorium cerebelli 520
Testis
appendix 312, 782
coverings 312
descent 782
Thoracic duct 421
Thoracic inlet
boundaries 398
clinical significance 399
structures passing through 398
Tonsil
abdominal 344
palatine 523, 862

Trachea parts 411
extent 411
relations 411, 412
**Tracts of spinal cord**
anterior spinocerebellar 681
anterior spino-thalamic 679
cortico-spinal 682
lateral spino-thalamic 680
medial longitudinal fasciculus 683
posterior spino-cerebellar 681
posterior white column 678
vestibulo-spinal 683
Transverse sections (diagrams)
medulla
pyramidal decussation 673
sensory decussation 673
pons (upper and lower) 674
spinal cord 665
Trendelenberg's sign (anatomical
basis) 187
Triangles
Beahr's 478
Calot's 276
carotid 518
femoral 172, 197
Hesselbach's 276
Joll's 478
Koch's 413
Macewan's 464
neck 516
scalene 477
sub-occipital 583
Tubercles
adductor 147
articular (surgical importance) 642
pharyngeal 468, 642
Tuberosities
ischial 144, 145, 195, 235
navicular 149
radial 42, 246
tibial 149
Turbinates
inferior 475, 476
middle 475, 476
ground lamella 476
superior 475, 476
Tympanic membrane 528
myringotomy incisions 529

**U**rinary bladder
innervation 284
reflex/neurogenic bladder 317
supra-pubic cystostomy 317
Uvula 487

**V**aricocele 313
  nutcracker 358
Vascular arcades ileum 364
  jejunum 364
Veins
  azygous 417
  basalic 61
  cephalic 61
  definition 24
  external jugular vein 507
  features 24
  femoral 166

great saphenous vein 180
internal jugular 505
portal 337
porto-systemic anastomosis
  337, 338
short saphenous vein 167
Venous drainage of face 582
  danger area of face 582
Venous drainage of lower limb 180
  peripheral heart 182
Ventricles
  floor of 4th ventricle 671, 699

of brain 696
of heart 446
Vertebral levels 439
Virchow's triad 183

**W**aldeyer's ring 508
Wallenberg's syndrome 712
Weber's syndrome 712
Wrist drop 56

**X**iphoid process 448
  ossification 449

**Z**ona pellucida 731, 736

# Reader's Notes

# Reader's Notes

# Reader's Notes

# Reader's Notes